NINTH EDITION

PEDIATRIC INJECTABLE DRUGS

THE TEDDY BEAR BOOK

Stephanie J. Phelps
Emily B. Hak
Catherine M. Crill

American Society of Health–System Pharmacists®
Bethesda, Maryland

Any correspondence regarding this publication should be sent to the publisher, American Society of Health-System Pharmacists, 7272 Wisconsin Avenue, Bethesda, MD 20814, attention: Special Publishing.

Director, Special Publishing: Jack Bruggeman
Acquisitions Editor: Jack Bruggeman
Senior Editorial Project Manager: Dana Battaglia
Production Editor: Kristin Eckles
Cover and Page Design: David Wade

ISBN 978-1-58528-243-2

Dedication

According to the National Academy of Sciences' independent Institute of Medicine, roughly 1.5 million individuals are given the wrong dose of a medication every year in the U.S., and about 7,000 people die from such mistakes each year. During the 18 months ending in July 2008, about 250 cases of heparin errors were reported in children less than one year of age in the U.S. Unfortunately, some were fatal. Prevention of harm from medication errors has become a national priority and a major area of emphasis in children's hospitals. This edition is dedicated to those pharmacists who create, implement, and evaluate strategies that enhance medication safety and prevent medication errors in children of all ages.

Table of Contents

About the Editors

Stephanie J. Phelps, Pharm.D., BCPS, FCCP, F.A.Ph.A.

Dr. Phelps was born in August Georgia but spent her formative years in Niceville, Florida—a small town in the pan-handle of the state. She attended high school and junior college in the area before moving to Birmingham, Alabama to pursue a B.S.Pharm. degree from Samford University (1979). She relocated to Memphis where she obtained a Pharm.D. degree from The University of Tennessee in 1982 and subsequently completed a pediatric subspecialty residency at Le Bonheur Children's Medical Center. She is board certified as a Pharmacotherapy Specialist and is an elected fellow of both the American College of Clinical Pharmacy and the American Pharmaceutical Association. Dr. Phelps is currently a professor in the Departments of Clinical Pharmacy and Pediatrics at The University of Tennessee Health Science Center. She also serves as Associate Dean of Academic Affairs and Vice-Chair, Professional Programs in the Department of Clinical Pharmacy. She is a member of various national pharmacy organizations and has held elected offices in AACP, APhA, ASHP, ASPEN and PPAG. In addition to serving as an editor of *Pediatric Injectable Drugs*, she is also editor-in-chief of *the Journal of Pediatric Pharmacology and Therapeutics*. She has published numerous manuscripts, book chapters, and reviews that focus on pediatric pharmacotherapy.

Emily B. Hak, Pharm.D., BCPS, FCCP

Dr. Hak received her B.S.Pharm. and Pharm.D. degrees from the University of Tennessee Health Science Center in 1984 and 1985, respectively. She completed a pediatric pharmacotherapy residency at the University of Tennessee and Le Bonheur Children's Medical Center in 1986. She completed the ASHP Fellowship in Pediatric Pharmacy Practice at the same institution in 1986–1988. She currently works as a Post-Retirement Professor in the Departments of Clinical Pharmacy and Pediatrics at the University of Tennessee. Dr. Hak's research interests are in the area of nutrition focusing on pediatric nutrition support and micronutrients. In addition, she teaches an elective course in Complementary and Alternative Medicine. Her teaching and research has resulted in the publication of nearly 50 journal articles including case reports, reviews, and letters-to-the editor. She has also published book chapters in pediatric nutrition support, immunizations and immunoglobulin therapy, and complementary medicine in addition to her co-editorship of *Pediatric Injectable Drugs*.

Catherine M. Crill, Pharm.D., BCPS, BCNSP

Dr. Crill received her Pharm.D. degree from the University of Tennessee College of Pharmacy in 1996. She completed residency and fellowship training in pediatric pharmacotherapy and nutrition support at Le Bonheur Children's Medical Center and the University of Tennessee from 1996 to 1999. Dr. Crill is Associate Professor of Clinical Pharmacy and Pediatrics at the University of Tennessee Health Science Center in Memphis, Tennessee. Her practice site is Le Bonheur Children's Medical Center where she serves as Clinical Pharmacy Specialist and Director of the Parenteral Nutrition Service. Dr. Crill's research interests are in the area of neonatal and pediatric parenteral nutrition, focusing on micronutrients and patient safety. In addition to her co-editorship of *Pediatric Injectable Drugs*, she is also a co-editor of the *A.S.P.E.N. Parenteral Nutrition Handbook* and has published over 20 papers in peer reviewed journals, six book chapters, and over 30 scientific abstracts.

Preface

Those who practice in pediatrics understand that the majority of medications given to children are used off label because research to validate safety and efficacy has not been conducted in children. The reason for the lack of studies in children is multifactorial and relates to priorities in pharmaceutical industry and federal funding, the need to protect our most vulnerable from medication-associated harm, and ethical considerations such as voluntary participation and informed consent/assent, which in many cases is not possible to obtain due to the patient's young age.

In 1957, the use of thalidomide to prevent nausea and vomiting during early pregnancy resulted in babies who were born with significant birth defects; thalidomide was not tested for teratogenic effects prior to marketing. In December 1983, the intravenous vitamin E supplement, E-Ferol, was marketed. Within three months its use was associated with ascites, liver and renal failure, thrombocytopenia, and death in low birth weight infants. This tragedy was ultimately attributed to the polysorbates added as emulsifiers; a new drug application had not been submitted to the FDA prior to use. Other noteworthy "therapeutic disasters" include sulfanilamide elixir, chloramphenicol gray-syndrome, valproate hepatotoxicity in young children, aspirin and Reye's syndrome, benzyl alcohol and fatal gasping syndrome, and the list goes on.

During the late 1960s, Dr. Harry Shirkey coined the term *therapeutic orphan*. Although pharmacokinetic and pharmacodynamic research has increased our understanding of medication therapy in neonates, infants, and children, unfortunately, the use of the term *therapeutic orphan* continues to be applicable to the pediatric population.

In 1994, the NIH established Pediatric Pharmacology Research Units (PPRUs) whose mission is to support the attainment of pediatric labeling of new and currently marketed drugs. The Food and Drug Administration Modernization Act (FDAMA) of 1998 provided an incentive to study drugs in children by extending the manufacturer's patent right for six months if they conducted pediatric studies. The impact of FDAMA was noted when, from 1998 to 2000, over 90 industry-sponsored primarily pharmacokinetic and pharmacodynamics studies were conducted in children, including neonates. In addition, NIH supported, investigator initiated trials have been conducted for older, off-patent drugs to assist in validation of their use in pediatric populations where they have been used for years.

The ninth edition of *Pediatric Injectable Drugs* (The Teddy Bear Book), has been revised to include 220 parenteral medications. Information included in this text was compiled in an evidence-based manner from, in most cases, the primary literature including case reports, observational reports, and comparative trials. Limited information is available for some of the frequently used older drugs in which case recommendations may come from textbooks. Importantly, the references are provided in the back of the book according to generic drug names, thereby allowing readers to know the source of the information provided. All monographs have been updated to improve existing sections and to make them more user-friendly through their placement in the monograph and with the addition of more specific subheadings. The monographs also include four new sections in the ninth edition: Medication error potential, Contraindications and warnings, Suitable diluents, and Preparation and delivery. Finally, a new feature is the inclusion of an additional appendix that summarizes information regarding extravasation treatment for medications known to cause effects from infiltration or extravasation.

Yes, drugs are used off-label in children all the time. We do hope that this text improves medication use and delivery in children that will facilitate recovery and improve their quality of life.

Stephanie J. Phelps
Emily B. Hak
Catherine M. Crill
2010

Acknowledgments

The editors and ASHP gratefully acknowledge the following individuals for their contributions to this edition:

Drug Information Center
The University of Tennessee Health Science Center
Memphis, TN

Jennifer S. Chung, Pharm.D.*
The University of Tennessee Health Science Center
Memphis, TN

Carolyn Cummings, Pharm.D.*
The University of Tennessee Health Science Center
Memphis, TN

Daniel Gharbawy, Pharm.D.
Drug Information and Health Outcomes Resident
The University of Tennessee Health Science Center
MED Communications, Inc.
St. Jude Children's Research Hospital
Memphis, TN

Kelley R. Lee, Pharm.D., BCPS
Clinical Pharmacy Manager
Le Bonheur Children's Medical Center
Professor
Department of Clinical Pharmacy
The University of Tennessee Health Science Center
Memphis, TN

Katherine E. Marks, Pharm.D., BCPS
The University of Tennessee Health Science Center
Memphis, TN

Lacey McRae, Pharm.D.*
The University of Tennessee Health Science Center
Memphis, TN

Brian Marlow, Pharm.D.*
The University of Tennessee Health Science Center
Memphis, TN

Johanna L. Norman, BA*
Pharm.D. Candidate 2011
The University of Tennessee Health Science Center
Memphis, TN

Malinda Parman, Pharm.D.*
The University of Tennessee Health Science Center
Memphis, TN

Jasmine Sahni, Pharm.D., BCPS
Assistant Professor
Department of Clinical Pharmacy
The University of Tennessee Health Science Center
Memphis, TN

Chasity M. Shelton, Pharm.D., BCPS, BCNSP
Assistant Professor
Department of Clinical Pharmacy
The University of Tennessee Health Science Center
Memphis, TN

Mina Tadrous, Pharm.D., M.Sc.
Drug Information and Health Outcomes Resident
The University of Tennessee Health Science Center
MED Communications, Inc.
St. Jude Children's Research Hospital
Memphis, TN

Julia Underwood, Pharm.D.*
The University of Tennessee Health Science Center
Memphis, TN

Morgan Weaver, Pharm.D.*
The University of Tennessee Health Science Center
Memphis, TN

*Contributed while a student pharmacist at the University of Tennessee College of Pharmacy

Introduction

The following guidelines were developed to provide a single authoritative source of information on the parenteral administration of medications to pediatric patients. All recommendations should be individualized in accordance with the clinical situation.

This ninth edition of ASHP's *Pediatric Injectable Drugs* has been updated to improve existing sections and to make them more user-friendly through their placement in the monograph and with the addition of more specific subheadings. The monographs include four new sections: Medication error potential, Contraindications and warnings, Suitable diluents, and Preparation and delivery. The ninth edition provides the following information for updates to 220 drugs and all references that support information contained in the text.

Brand names

Common brand names and, if applicable, other names (synonyms) are listed.

Medication error potential

If the drug was included in the ISMP's *List of High-Alert Medications*, ISMP's *List of Confused Drug Names*, or the USP's *Findings of Look-alike and/or Sound-alike Drug Errors* at the time the monograph was written, it will be noted in this section. Tall man letters, per FDA and ISMP recommendations, will be used in this section, as well as in the monograph title and in the title in the references, if applicable.

Contraindications and warnings

While it may be noted in the monographs, it is understood that a drug would be contraindicated in a patient who has experienced a prior anaphylaxis or Type I hypersensitivity reaction. US boxed warnings, Contraindications, and Other warnings, if applicable, will be described under subheadings in this section. The Other warnings subheading will describe warnings deemed noteworthy and may not be the complete list of warnings included in the manufacturer's labeling. It is recommended to review the labeling for the most complete list.

Infusion related cautions

Warnings are provided where appropriate. If a drug requires premedication or if the administration of the drug necessitates the availability of another drug (i.e., to have on hand), information regarding premedication or the drug to have on hand will be provided in this section. If a drug should only be given via central access, this will be noted here. If a drug carries an increased risk of thrombophlebitis, infiltration, or extravasation, it will be noted in this section. Appendix E provides information regarding extravasation treatment for medications known to cause effects from infiltration or extravasation.

Dosage

Unless otherwise specified, dosages are for all age groups. These age groups are as follows: neonates (premature and term), up to 1 month; infants, 1–24 months; children, 2–12 years, and adolescents, 12–18 years. When applicable, adult dosing is also provided. While these age groups provide general guidelines for therapy in pediatric patients, it should be noted that changes in development, which affect drug pharmacokinetics and pharmacodynamics, and hence, dosing recommendations, are not confined to the limits of these defined age groups.

Dosage is often expressed as X mg/kg/day divided q Y–Z hours, where the total daily dose (X) is given in equally divided doses at evenly spaced intervals. Dosage may also be expressed as X mg/m^2/day divided q Y–Z hours, a calculation of body surface area (BSA) as determined from height and mass. See Appendix A for a BSA nomogram.

The presence of obesity may require the practitioner to estimate ideal body mass/weight and calculate an adjusted weight for the dosing of some medications. Appendix B provides a nomogram for estimating total body mass/weight.

Dosage adjustment in organ dysfunction

Drugs requiring dosage adjustment in patients with renal or hepatic dysfunction and serum drug concentration monitoring are indicated. The manufacturer's labeling and specialized references are provided when available. Information, if known, will also be included about dosage adjustment or therapeutic drug monitoring with dialysis, continuous renal replacement therapy, and with ECMO.

Maximum dosage

Maximum dosages are referenced to primary literature where available. However, maximum dosages for pediatric patients are often extrapolated from adult data because of a lack of documented experience with pediatric patients. Many manufacturers caution against exceeding the maximum recommended adult dosage (usually expressed as X g/day) in pediatric patients. In this reference, when the maximum dosage is expressed as "mg/kg/day, not to exceed X g/day," "X g/day" is typically the manufacturer's maximum recommended adult dosage and should be used only as an upper limit for pediatric dosing. It should not be inferred that use of these maximum dosages in pediatric patients is recommended and is without risk of toxicity. Readers should consult the references indicated for information on the use of these maximum dosages in the pediatric population.

Additives

Pertinent additives, including sodium and those with a potential for toxicity or adverse effects, are listed. Please see Appendix C for specific information on common additives with a potential for toxicity or adverse effects.

Suitable diluents

If a drug can be mixed or diluted with a fluid, the appropriate fluids will be listed here. Compatible drugs will NOT be listed.

Drug stability in some of the IV solutions listed is limited. The manufacturer's labeling and specialized references (e.g., Trissel LA. *Handbook on Injectable Drugs*. 15th ed. Bethesda, MD: American Society of Health-System Pharmacists; 2009) should be consulted for detailed stability information.

Maximum concentration

Generally, any concentration up to the maximum may be administered, taking into consideration the patient's fluid status (and potential for loss of vascular access), administration method (IV push vs. intermittent infusion), drug administration rate (and drug administration device flow rate range, if applicable), dose (and degree of accuracy required in dose measurement), and drug stability. However, some drugs, as indicated in these guidelines, should not be diluted.

For drugs available as solutions that may be administered undiluted, the maximum concentration is the commercially available concentration. For drugs that must be reconstituted prior to administration, the maximum concentration should serve as a guide for the minimum dilution required.

Concentrations listed are referenced to literature on drug use in pediatric patients to the extent possible. However, concentrations administered to adults are cited where documentation on use in pediatric patients is insufficient. The references should be consulted. The IV push, Intermittent infusion, Continuous infusion, and Other routes of administration sections all begin with information concerning the concentration or concentration range usual for that method or route of administration.

Preparation and delivery

When pertinent, issues related to preparation and delivery are included in this section and, if applicable, will be described under the following subheadings: Preparation, Delivery, Stability, Compatibility, and Photosensitivity. If a drug has information regarding compatibility with parenteral nutrition solutions, a statement will be included. Appendix D provides information regarding compatibility of medications with parenteral nutrition solutions.

IV push

This rate is generally expressed as a period of time over which the dose should be administered (seconds or minutes) or as a quantity of drug per unit of time. In the latter case, the size of the dose determines the administration time. For the purpose of this text, IV push was defined as ≤5 minutes. Drugs for which IV push administration is contraindicated are noted.

Intermittent infusion

The recommended infusion rate is expressed as a period of time over which the dose should be administered (minutes to hours) or as a quantity of drug per unit of time (size of dose determines administration time).

Introduction

Continuous infusion

The recommended infusion rate is usually expressed as a quantity of drug per unit of time; infusion is continued for 24 hours unless otherwise specified (e.g., until the desired therapeutic endpoint is achieved).

Other routes of administration

This section contains information on the appropriateness of other routes of administration, including IM, SC, ET, IT and IO administration and the best site for administration. The terms *contraindicated* and *not recommended* will be used. Contraindicated implies that you do not administer the drug in that manner. Not recommended implies that it may have been administered in that manner, but it is not recommended to administer it in that manner. Drugs for which other routes of administration are contraindicated are noted.

Comments

Miscellaneous information is included when pertinent. Information pertaining to adults is sometimes included because, in the absence of reports on pediatric use, adult data may be relevant and may be cautiously extrapolated to the pediatric population.

When applicable, the following subheadings may be included in the comments section: Significant adverse effects, Rare adverse effects, Monitoring, Drug interactions, Pharmacokinetic considerations, Pharmacodynamic considerations, Laboratory interference, Osmolality, and Other.

Abbreviations

Solutions:

ABS	Acrylonitrile, butadiene, and styrene
BW	Bacteriostatic water for injection
CVVH	Continuous venovenous hemofiltration
D-LR	Dextrose—Ringer's injection, lactated, combinations
D-R	Dextrose—Ringer's injection combinations
D-S	Dextrose—saline combinations
D10NS	Dextrose 10% in sodium chloride 0.9%
D10W	Dextrose 10% in water
D15W	Dextrose 15% in water
D20W	Dextrose 20% in water
D2.5W	Dextrose 2.5% in water
D2.5½NS	Dextrose 2.5% in sodium chloride 0.45%
D5LR	Dextrose 5% in Ringer's injection, lactated
D5NS	Dextrose 5% in sodium chloride 0.9%
D5¼NS	Dextrose 5% in sodium chloride 0.225%
D5⅓NS	Dextrose 5% in sodium chloride 0.3%
D5½NS	Dextrose 5% in sodium chloride 0.45%
D5R	Dextrose 5% in Ringer's injection
D5S	Dextrose 5% in sodium chloride 0.9%, 0.45%, 0.3% or 0.225%
D5W	Dextrose 5% in water
FE	Fat emulsion
HHV	Human herpes virus
HSV	Herpes simplex virus
IVFE	IV fat emulsion
LR	Ringer's injection, lactated
MAO	Monoamine oxidase
MAP	Mean arterial pressure
NS	Sodium chloride 0.9% (normal saline)
¼NS	Sodium chloride 0.225% (¼ normal saline)
⅓NS	Sodium chloride 0.3% (⅓ normal saline)
½NS	Sodium chloride 0.45% (½ normal saline)
PN	Parenteral nutrition
PVR	Pulmonary vascular resistance
R	Ringer's injection
SW	Sterile water for injection
TNA	Total nutrient admixtures

Terms:

AAP	American Academy of Pediatrics
ACT	Activated clotting time
ADH	Antidiuretic hormone
AHA	American Heart Association

AIDS	Acquired immunodeficiency syndrome
ALL	Acute lymphocytic leukemia
ALT (SGPT)	Alanine transaminase (may be referred to as SGPT)
ANA	Antinuclear antibody
ANC	Absolute neutrophil count
APAP	Acetaminophen
aPTT	Activated partial thromboplastin time
AST (SGOT)	Aspartate aminotransaminase (may be referred to as SGOT)
ATG	Antithymocyte globulin
AZT	Azidothymidine
BLC	Blood lead concentration
BMT	Bone marrow transplant
BSA	Body surface area
BUN	Blood urea nitrogen
CBC	Complete blood count
CDAD	*Clostridium difficile*–associated diarrhea
CDC	Centers for Disease Control and Prevention
CDP-1	Crystalline degradation products
CHD	Congenital heart disease
CHF	Congestive heart failure
CML	Chronic myelogenous leukemia
CMV	Cytomegalovirus
CNS	Central nervous system
CPK-MB	Serum creatine phosphokinase–MB isoenzyme
CPR	Cardiopulmonary resuscitation
CrCl	Creatinine clearance
CRRT	Continuous renal replacement therapy
CSF	Cerebral spinal fluid
CYP	Cytochrome P
CYP1A2	Cytochrome P450 isoenzyme 1A2
CYP2A4	Cytochrome P450 isoenzyme 2A4
CYP2B6	Cytochrome P450 isoenzyme 2B6
CYP2C19	Cytochrome P450 isoenzyme 2C19
CYP2C9/10	Cytochrome P450 isoenzymes 2C9 and 2C10
CYP2E1	Cytochrome P450 isoenzyme 2E1
CYP3A3/4	Cytochrome P450 isoenzymes 3A3 and 3A4
DEHP	Diethylhexyl phthalate
DKA	Diabetic ketoacidosis
DPT	Demerol, Phenergan, Thorazine
ECG	Electrocardiogram
ECMO	Extracorporeal membrane oxygenation
EEG	Electroencephalogram
EMIT	Enzyme multiplied immunoassay technique

Abbreviations

ESA	Erythropoiesis-stimulating agent
ET	Endotracheal
FAB	Digoxin immune Fab
FDA	Food and Drug Administration
FPIA	Fluorescence polarization immunoassay
FT4	Free thyroxine
GA	Gestational age
GI	Gastrointestinal
GM-CSF	Granulocyte-macrophage colony-stimulating factor
GVHD	Graft versus host disease
H1	Histamine-1 receptor antagonist
H2	Histamine-2 receptor antagonist
Hgb	Hemoglobin
HIV	Human immunodeficiency virus
HLA	Human leukocyte antigen
HPLC	High-performance liquid chromatography
IBW	Ideal body weight
ICP	Intracranial pressure
ICU	Intensive care unit
IM	Intramuscular
INR	International normalized ratio
IO	Intraosseous
IQ	Intelligence quotient
ISMP	Institute for Safe Medication Practices
IT	Intrathecal
ITP	Idiopathic thrombocytopenic purpura
IV	Intravenous
IVIG	Intravenous immune globulin
IVH	Intraventricular hemorrhage
LD	Loading dose
MAC	Mycobacterium avium complex
MRI	Magnetic resonance imaging
MTX	Methotrexate
NAC	N-acetylcysteine
NAPA	N-Acetylprocainamide
NEC	Necrotizing enterocolitis
NHL	Non-Hodgkin's lymphoma
NIH	National Institutes of Health
NMTT	N-methyl-thiotetrazole side chain
NSAIDs	Nonsteroidal anti-inflammatory drugs
PALS	Pediatric advanced life support
PCA	Postconceptional age
PDA	Patent ductus arteriosus

PE	Phenytoin equivalents
PID	Pelvic inflammatory disease
PMA	Postmenstrual age
PN	Parenteral nutrition
PNA	Postnatal age
PO	Orally
PTT	Partial thromboplastin time
PVC	Polyvinyl chloride
SC	Subcutaneous
SCr	Serum creatinine
SDC	Serum digitalis concentration
SLE	Systemic lupus erythematosus
TBW	Total body weight
THC	Tetrahydrocannabinol
TPA	Tissue plasminogen activator
TSH	Thyroid stimulating hormone
UGT	Uridine diphosphate-glucuronosyltransferase
UOP	Urine output
USP	United States Pharmacopeia
UTI	Urinary tract infection
Vitamin B12a	Hydroxocobalamin
Vitamin B12	Cyanocobalamin
WBC	White blood cell count

Monographs

Abatacept

Brand names	Orencia
Medication error potential	Look-alike, sound-alike error potential. USP reports potential for confusion between Orencia and Oracea.[1]
Contraindications and warnings	**Warnings:** Concomitant use with TNF antagonists is not recommended.[2] Hypersensitivity reactions may occur. Discontinue use if serious infection occurs. Screen for tuberculosis prior to starting therapy. Live vaccines should not be given during or until 3 months after abatacept discontinuation. Children's vaccination status should be current prior to beginning therapy.
Infusion related cautions	An acute hypersensitivity reaction occurred in one of 190 pediatric patients treated with abatacept.[2] Appropriate medical care should be available in the event this occurs.
Dosage	**Juvenile idiopathic arthritis ≤6 years**[2,3] **<75 kg:** 10 mg/kg repeated at 2 and 4 weeks after initial infusion and every 4 weeks thereafter. **75–100 kg:** 750 mg. **>100 kg:** 1000 mg. **Other uses:** One child with juvenile idiopathic arthritis-associated uveitis responded to treatment with abatacept after infliximab was discontinued due to adverse effects and etanercept and rituximab failed to elicit an improvement.[4]
Dosage adjustment in organ dysfunction	None recommended.
Maximum dosage	1000 mg.
Additives	Maltose. (See Laboratory interference in Comments section.)
Suitable diluents	SW to reconstitute. NS to dilute.[2]
Maximum concentration	10 mg/mL.[2]

Abatacept

Preparation and delivery	**Preparation:** Reconstitute by adding 10 mL SW with the silicone-free disposable syringe provided. Gently rotate the vial to dissolve. Do not shake. The vial should be vented to dissipate any foam that is present.[1]
	The reconstituted dose must be diluted in 100 mL of NS prior to infusion. Remove the volume of the dose from the 10-mL bag of NS and then using the silicone-free syringe slowly inject the dose into 100-mL NS. Gently mix.[2]
	Delivery system issues: Infuse through a sterile, nonpyrogenic 0.2 to 1.2-micron low protein-binding filter.[2]
	Stability: The vial contains no preservatives and once reconstituted must be used within 24 hours.[2]
IV push	Not indicated.
Intermittent infusion	Over 30 minutes.[2]
Continuous infusion	Not indicated.
Other routes of administration	Not indicated.
Comments	**Adverse events:** Serious infections have been reported in individuals receiving TNF-α blocker therapy and abatacept concurrently.[2]
	Laboratory interference: Because of the maltose additive, a falsely elevated blood glucose measurement may occur with some types of glucose monitors.[2]
	Juvenile idiopathic arthritis, juvenile rheumatoid arthritis, and juvenile chronic arthritis may be used interchangeably.

Acetazolamide

Brand names	Diamox
Medication error potential	ISMP's *Confused Drug Names* lists that Diamox may be confused with Diabinese.[1] USP reports confusion with acetaminophen, acetylcysteine, and methazolamide.[2] Confusion with acetohexamide has resulted in patient harm.[2]
Contraindications and warnings	Acetazolamide contains a sulfonamide moiety. Although rare, cross reactivity with other sulfonamides may be associated with severe dermatological reactions (e.g., Stevens-Johnson syndrome), which occurred due to sulfonamide structure.[3-5]
Infusion related cautions	None.
Dosage	Because of limited experience with acetazolamide, the doses and side effects have not been established. No pediatric-specific problems have been documented to date. **Acute glaucoma:** 20–40 mg/kg/day divided q 6 h.[3] **Edema/diuresis/urinary alkalinization:** 5 mg/kg/dose[3,6-8] or 150 mg/m²[8] once daily as required to achieve forced alkaline diuresis.[3] (See Comments section.) **Posthemorrhagic ventricular dilatation:** Studies have shown increased rates of shunt placement and greater neurological morbidity with maximum tolerale doses (100 mg/kg/day); therefore, use of acetazolamide is not recommended.[9-11] **Pseudotumor cerebri:** 40–120 mg/kg/day divided q 6–8 h up to 2 g/day.[12]
Dosage adjustment in organ dysfunction	Not effective at CrCl <20 mL/min.[3,4] If CrCl is 20–50 mL/min, give q 12 h.[13] Should not be used in with hepatic cirrhosis due to the risk of encephalopathy.[9]
Maximum dosage	100 mg/kg/day[3] up to 1–2 g/day.[4,7]
Additives	2.049 mEq of sodium/500 mg acetazolamide.[4,5]
Suitable diluents	D2.5W, D5W, D10W, NS, LR, or R.[14]
Maximum concentration	100 mg/mL.[5,14]
Preparation and delivery	**Compatibility:** See Appendix D for PN compatibility information.[15]
IV push	100 mg/mL at a rate not to exceed 500 mg/min.[4]
Intermittent infusion	100 mg/mL[14]
Continuous infusion	Not administered by this method.

Other routes of administration	IM administration not recommended; very painful due to alkaline pH of 9.2.[14]

Comments	**Rare adverse effects:** Acetazolamide is a carbonic anhydrase inhibitor that shares the pharmacological actions and toxic potentials of this class of medications.[5] May cause hypokalemia, paresthesia, and kidney stones.

Overdoses or too frequent dosing may cause a failure to produce diuresis. In these situations, acetazolamide should be withheld for 1–2 days to allow for kidney recovery.[5]

Laboratory interference: May cause false-positive results for urinary protein with Al-bustix, Labstix, Albutest, Bumintest; interferes with HPLC method for assaying Theophylline.[4]

Acetylcysteine (NAC)

Brand names	Acetadote
Medication error potential	ISMP's lists confusion between Mucomyst and Mucinex.[1] USP reports confusion with acetylcysteine and acetazolamide.[2]
Contraindications and warnings	**Warnings:** Caution in patients with asthma or history of bronchospasm. Acute flushing and erythema can occur 30–60 minutes after initiation of the infusion, with resolution despite continued infusion.[3]
Infusion related cautions	Anaphylactoid reactions and death have been reported causing some to recommend infusing the loading dose over 60 minutes.[3] Once the anaphylactoid reaction has been treated (e.g., antihistamines, H_2 blockers), NAC can be reinstituted cautiously, but it should be discontinued if anaphylactoid reaction recurs.[3]

Dosage

Acetaminophen overdose*: Use the Rumack-Matthew nomogram** to estimate the potential for hepatotoxicity due to acetaminophen overdose and guide therapy with NAC.[3] Ideally, administered within 8 hours of acetaminophen ingestion to prevent or lessen hepatic injury; however, may be effective when given 24 hours or longer after ingestion. Infuse loading dose of 150 mg/kg over 60 minutes, followed by 50 mg/kg over 4 hours, then 100 mg/kg over 16 hours (for a full course consisting of 300 mg/kg administered IV over 20.25 hours).[3] (See Comments section.)

* Despite low or undetectable acetaminophen serum concentrations, NAC should be given if any signs of hepatotoxicity are evident.[3]

** The nomogram is less predictive in a chronic ingestion or in an overdose with an extended release product. The nomogram also does not take into account patients at high risk of acetaminophen toxicity (e.g., alcoholics, malnourished patients) or individuals ingesting larger than recommended acetaminophen doses for extended periods of time.[3]

Advanced cerebral adrenoleukodystrophy (ALD): Administration of NAC (140 mg/kg/day followed by 70 mg/kg four times a day) before (54–67 days) and after (114–250 days) hematopoietic stem cell transplant (HSCT) was noted to protect from fulminant demyelination in three children.[4]

Prevention of acute renal failure associated with radiographic contrast media: Most reports involved oral dosing[5,6]; however, intravenous NAC has been given in *adults*.[7]

Prevention of BPD: When compared to placebo, there was no difference in the development of BPD or death in 194 infants (500–999 g) who received a 6-day continuous infusion of NAC (16–32 mg/kg/day beginning within 36 hours of birth).[8]

TPN-associate hepatic disease: NAC reduced liver biochemistries in three children with TPN-associated liver disease.[9] Each was begun on estimated maintenance requirements of cysteine (20–50 mg/kg/day of NAC). The NAC dose was increased by 10 mg/kg/day q 1–2 mo to maximum doses of 70, 120, 135 mg/kg/day. Doses were infused over 12 hours and continued for 3–18 months.

Dosage adjustment in organ dysfunction	No reduction recommended in hepatic or moderate/severe renal impairment.[3] Some suggest a 25% reduction in maintenance dose when the CrCl is <10 mL/min.[10]
Maximum dosage	Cummulative dose of 300 mg/kg per treatment course.[3] No adverse effects were noted following a mean rate of 4.2 mg/kg/h for 24 hours in preterm infants (gestational age of 25–31 weeks and weight of 500–1380 g)[11] or following infusion of 0.1–1.3 mg/kg/h for 6 days in six neonates (gestational age of 26–30 weeks and weight of 520–1335 g).[8]
Additives	Edetate disodium and sodium hydroxide and has a pH of 6–7.5.[3]

Acetylcysteine (NAC)

Suitable diluents	D5W, 0.45% sodium chloride, and SWI.[3]	
Maximum concentration	Up to 50 mg/mL for loading dose and 10 mg/mL for maintenance dose.[3] Adjust total volume as needed for patients' weight and those requiring fluid restriction.[3]	

Weight (kg)	Loading Dose (150 mg/kg over 60 min)		2nd Dose (50 mg/kg over 4 h)		3rd Dose (100 mg/kg over 16 h)	
	Acetadote (mL)	Diluent (mL)	Acetadote (mL)	Diluent (mL)	Acetadote (mL)	Diluent (mL)
10	7.5	30	2.5	70	5	140
15	11.25	45	3.75	105	7.5	210
20	15	60	5	140	10	280
25	18.75	100	6.25	250	12.5	500
30	22.5	100	7.5	250	15	500
40	30	200	10	500	20	1000
50	37.5		12.5		25	
60	45		15		30	
70	52.5		17.5		35	

Preparation and delivery	**Delivery system issues:** Contact with rubber, copper, iron, and cork may inactivate NAC.[12] **Stability:** Stable 24 hours after dilution at room temperature. Although solution may turn from colorless to slight pink or light purple color following puncture of stopper, this does not affect the activity of NAC.[3]
IV push	Not administered by this method.
Intermittent infusion	Loading dose should be given over 15 minutes.[8] Some clinicians recommend infusing the loading dose over 60 minutes to reduce the potential for a life-threatening anaphylactoid reaction.[2] (See Infusion related cautions section.)
Continuous infusion	First (50 mg/kg) and second (100 mg/kg) maintenance doses should be given over 4 hours and 16 hours, respectively.[2] Infusions of 0.3–4.6 mg/kg/h have been used safely in newborns.[9]
Other routes of administration	None.
Comments	**Monitoring:** Serum acetaminophen concentrations that are obtained within 4 hours of ingestion are not predictive of severity. Likewise, undetectable serum concentrations, in a patient who delayed seeking medical care, may not reflect the ingestion of a potentially lethal dose.[3] **Osmolality:** 2600 mOsm/L[3] **Other:** Contact a poison center at 1-800-222-1222 to obtain information about the clinical management of acetaminophen overdoses. NAC crossed the placenta when a mother was treated following an acetaminophen exposure.[13]

Acyclovir Sodium

Brand names	Zovirax, generic

Medication error potential

Look-alike, sound-alike error potential.

USP reports that acyclovir was confused with Retrovir and valacyclovir; no patient harm resulted.[1] USP reports that acyclovir was confused with ganciclovir; patient harm resulted.[1]

ISMP and USP report that Zovirax was confused with Zyvox and Zostrix; no patient harm resulted.[1,2] USP also reports that Zovirax was confused with Valtrex, Zithromax, and Zyloprim; no patient harm resulted.[1]

Contraindications and warnings

Contraindications: Hypersensitivity to acyclovir or valacyclovir.[3]

Warnings: Renal failure and thrombotic thrombocytopenic purpura (TTP)/hemolytic uremic syndrome (HUS) have both been reported with acyclovir. Deaths have occurred due to renal failure and TTP/HUS. Acyclovir should be used with caution in patients with underlying neurological abnormalities, as well as those with serious renal, hepatic, or electrolyte abnormalities or significant hypoxia.[3]

Infusion related cautions

To decrease the risk of nephrotoxicity, the patient should be adequately hydrated before and during the infusion.[3,4]

Extravasation may cause inflammation and phlebitis at the injection site.[3,5] See Appendix E for additional information regarding extravasation treatment.

Dosage

Doses generally range from 7.5–60 mg/kg/day or 750–1500 mg/m^2/day divided q 8 h depending on the infection.[1,6-16] Obese patients should be dosed using ideal body weight.[1]

Herpes simplex virus (HSV)

    Neonatal HSV: 60 mg/kg/day divided q 8 h for 14–21 days.[15,16]

    HSV encephalitis

        ≥3 months–12 years: 60 mg/kg/day divided q 8 h for 14–21 days; some experts recommend 45 mg/kg/day divided q 8 h for 14–21 days.[15,16]

        ≥12 years: 30 mg/kg/day divided q 8 h for 14–21 days.[15]

    Genital HSV (severe cases), ≥12 years: 15 mg/kg/day divided q 8 h for 5–7 days.[15]

    HSV in immunocompromised host (localized, progressive, or disseminated)

        <12 years: 30 mg/kg/day divided q 8 h for 7–14 days.[15]

        ≥12 years: 15 mg/kg/day divided q 8 h for 7–14 days.[15]

    HSV-seropositive patients: 15 mg/kg/day divided q 8 h during risk period.[15]

Varicella-zoster virus (VZV)

    Immunocompetent hosts ≥2 years: 30 mg/kg/day divided q 8 h or 1500 mg/m^2/day divided q 8 h for 7–10 days.[15]

    Immunocompromised hosts

        <1 year: 30 mg/kg/day divided q 8 h for 7–10 days.[15]

        ≥1 year: 1500 mg/m^2/day (or 30 mg/kg/day) divided q 8 h for 7–10 days.[11-15,17]

        Initiate therapy as soon as possible after rash appears. Early initiation therapy (<24–72 hours) is associated with more rapid improvement and less dissemination than late initiation therapy (>3–5 days).[12,13,17]

Acyclovir Sodium

Dosage *(cont.)*	Twenty-six children (1–13 years of age) receiving immunosuppressive therapy who developed VZV were given 1500 mg/m²/day divided q 8 h for 48 hours. If able to take oral medications, they were changed to oral therapy after 48 hours if there was no ongoing fever, no new skin lesions, and no evidence of systemic disease. Immunosuppressive drugs were discontinued or decreased by 50% during acyclovir treatment.[18]

Sixty-six pediatric renal transplant recipients with VZV were given 1500 mg/m²/day divided q 8 h. Azathioprine was temporarily discontinued until the lesions crusted over and no new lesions appeared; at that time, azathioprine was restarted at the usual dose. Three recipients experienced acute rejection that responded to prednisone. One patient died.[19]

Zoster

Zoster in immunocompetent host, all ages: Same as dosing for varicella in immunocompromised host.[15]

Zoster in immunocompromised host, all ages: 30 mg/kg/day divided q 8 h for 7–10 days.[15]

Prevention or suppression of cytomegalovirus infection in allogeneic bone marrow transplant recipients (this use has largely been replaced by ganciclovir): 1500 mg/m²/day divided q 8 h beginning 5 days before transplantation and continuing 30 days after.[8,20]

Aplastic anemia (use not established): 15 mg/kg/day (schedule not provided) for 10 days has been given to two patients (one, a 13-year-old girl) who had severe aplastic anemia refractory to standard treatment.[6] |
| **Dosage adjustment in organ dysfunction** | Adjust dosage in patients with renal dysfunction.[3,15,21-22] If CrCl is 25–50 mL/min, give normal dose q 12 h; if CrCl is 10–25 mL/min, give normal dose q 24 h, and if CrCl is <10 mL/min, give 50% of the dose q 24 h.[3]

Another source recommends the following dose adjustment based on GFR[23]:

GFR(mL/min/1.73m²)	Dose
30–50	10 mg/kg q 12 h
10–29	10 mg/kg q 24 h
<10	5 mg/kg q 24 h

Neonates with hepatic or renal dysfunction and young premature infants may also require dose adjustment.[22] |
| **Maximum dosage** | Do not exceed 20 mg/kg q 8 h.[3]

An 11-day-old neonate received a 258 mg/kg of IV acyclovir in a 24-hour period that was treated with NS hydration; the patient experienced only a transient increase in SCr.[24] |
Additives	Contains 49 mg sodium/500 mg acyclovir.[3]
Suitable diluents	D5W, NS, D5NS, LR.[3,25]
Maximum concentration	≤7 mg/mL.[3,25] Infusion of a solution ≥10 mg/mL increases the risk of phlebitis and extravasation.[3,26]

Acyclovir Sodium

Preparation and delivery	**Stability:** Vials should be reconstituted with SW for injection and should be used within 12 hours. Once diluted for administration, doses should be used within 24 hours.[3,25] Refrigeration may cause precipitation; however, the precipitate redissolves at room temperature and potency does not appear to be affected.[25] BW for injection containing parabens or benzyl alcohol should not be used to dilute acyclovir sodium powder because precipitation could occur.[25] **Compatibility:** For PN compatibility information, please see Appendix D.
IV push	Not recommended.[3] Rapid administration (<10 minutes) can cause crystalluria, elevations in serum urea and SCr, renal tubular damage, and acute renal failure.[3,4]
Intermittent infusion	Although acyclovir has been given over 30 minutes,[27] the dose should be infused over 1 hour to minimize renal dysfunction.[3,4,25]
Continuous infusion	No information available to support administration by this method.
Other routes of administration	Not recommended.[3,25]
Comments	**Significant adverse drug effects:** Nonherpetic vesicular eruptions occurred in a child receiving acyclovir for presumed herpes simplex encephalitis.[28] A 33-week-old infant with HSV encephalitis received IV acyclovir 30 mg/kg/day for 21 days followed by 30 mg/kg/day of oral acyclovir for 25 days. The infant developed neutropenia 5 days after starting a second course of acyclovir. Neutropenia corrected after switching to 30 mg/kg/day of vidarabine (no longer available in the United States) for 7 days and 10 mg/kg/day of oral acyclovir for 7 months.[29] A 9-year-old child with HSV encephalitis developed nonoliguric acute renal failure after 6 days of 30 mg/kg/day of IV acyclovir. Renal failure reversed following discontinuation of acyclovir.[30] If CrCl decreases by ≥20%, the authors recommended that acyclovir be discontinued. If the patient has a potentially life-threatening infection, the dosage should be adjusted and the drug continued. **Drug interactions:** Coadministration with probenecid has been shown to increase the mean half-life and the area-under-the-concentration time-curve for acyclovir.[3] Consult appropriate resources for dosing recommendations before combining probenecid with acyclovir. **Pharmacokinetic considerations:** A pharmacokinetic study of IV acyclovir and oral valacyclovir in patients 9 months to 20 years of age with malignancy showed that those with good renal function and/or lower body weight could possibly be underdosed based on current dosing guidelines.[31] **Other:** A 28-week premature infant was successfully treated with IV acyclovir for 21 days after the mother presented with eczema herpeticum at the time of delivery.[32] A full-term neonate was treated with IV acyclovir 60 mg/kg/day and other medications for neonatal herpes simplex type 1 infection that was complicated by hemophagocytic *Lymphohistiocytosis* and acute liver failure.[33]

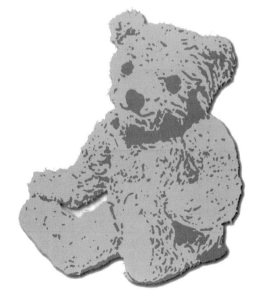

Adalimumab

Brand names	Humira
Medication error potential	None noted.
Contraindications and warnings	**US boxed warning:** Patients receiving adalimumab are at risk for developing serious infections. Those with active infections should not begin treatment. Those who develop infection while on treatment should be monitored closely.[1] Patients should be evaluated for latent tuberculosis infection with a tuberculin skin test. If the skin test is positive, treatment of tuberculosis should be started prior to beginning treatment with adalimumab.[1] (See Comments section.) **Other warnings:** Anaphylaxis has been reported.[2] Appropriate medical care should be available in the event this occurs. The needle cover of the prefilled syringes contains latex. Those with latex allergy should not handle the syringes.[1,2]
Infusion related cautions	None noted.

Dosage	**Juvenile idiopathic arthritis >4 years**[1-3]
	
	     15 kg to >30 kg: 20 mg SC every other week.
	
	     ≥30 kg: 40 mg SC every other week.
	
	     Alternatively: 24 mg/m² up to 40 mg.
	
	 Other uses: Refractory juvenile idiopathic arthritis associated uveitis.[4-6] Dosing has been based on improvement of uveitis and in one case required weekly dosing and in another dosing was every 3 weeks.[6]
	
	 Adults: Adalimumab is used to treat rheumatoid arthritis, Crohn's disease, and plaque psoriasis in *adults*.[1,2]

Dosage adjustment in organ dysfunction	No data available.[1]
Maximum dosage	40 mg.
Additives	None.
Suitable diluents	Not diluted.
Maximum concentration	50 mg/mL (commercially available).

Adalimumab

Preparation and delivery	Available as disposable prefilled syringes (20 mg/0.4 mL, 40 mg/0.8 mL) or as a prefilled injection pen (40 mg/0.8 mL). Must be refrigerated until use.[1,2] **Photosensitivity:** Protect from light exposure until ready to use.
IV push	Not indicated.
Intermittent infusion	Not indicated.
Continuous infusion	Not indicated.
Other routes of administration	Administer by SC injection.[1,2]
Comments	A negative skin test for tuberculosis does not rule out the possibility of disease since patients with immune diseases may exhibit cutaneous anergy.[7] **Drug interactions:** An increased incidence of infection was noted when used with anakinra or abatacept.[1,2] Live vaccines should not be given with adalimumab.[1,2] Methotrexate decreases clearance; however, no change in adalimumab dosage is recommended.[1]

Adenosine

Brand names	Adenocard

Medication error potential

Although ISMP considers adenosine (anti-arrhythmic) a high-alert medication,[1] the USP has no reports of errors.[2]

Contraindications and warnings

Contraindications: Known hypersensitivity to adenosine.[3]

Adenosine should not be given in second- and third-degree A-V block or sinus node disease (e.g., sick sinus syndrome, symptomatic bradycardia), unless a functioning artificial pacemaker is placed.[3] Use with extreme caution in heart transplant recipients as adenosine may cause prolonged asystole.[4] A reduction of initial adenosine dose is recommended in these patients.[4] Although the manufacturer does not list heart transplantation as a contraindicated, some have suggested it should be one.[5]

Warnings

> **Arrhythmias, postconversion:** A variety of new rhythms (e.g., premature ventricular contractions, atrial premature contractions, sinus bradycardia, sinus tachycardia, skipped beats, and varying degrees of A-V nodal block) may appear on the ECG at the time of conversion to normal sinus rhythm; however, these generally last only a few seconds and resolve without intervention.[3]

> **Bronchoconstriction:** Patients with a history of reactive airway disease may experience bronchospasm and respiratory failure.[3,6-8] Aminophylline has been used to relieve bronchospasm associated with adenosine.[8]

> **Heart block:** Adenosine decreases conduction through the A-V node and may produce first-, second-, or third-degree heart block, which is generally self-limiting due to adenosine's short half-life.[3] Additional doses should not be given if high-level block developed after one dose.[3] Transient or prolonged episodes of asystole have been fatal. Rarely, ventricular fibrillation has been reported following adenosine administration, including both resuscitated and fatal events.[3] (See Comments section.)

Infusion related cautions

None.

Dosage

Pulmonary hypertension: 0.05 mg/kg/min improved PaO2 in four of nine infants with persistent pulmonary hypertension without causing hypotension or tachycardia.[9]

Stress test in aortic valve disease: 0.14 mg/kg/min for 6 minutes.[10]

Supraventricular tachycardia

> **Initial dosing:** 0.05,[3-5] or 0.1[3-5,11-17] mg/kg. Infuse over 1–2 seconds, then flush catheter with saline.[3] One report noted that only 9% of infants responded to a dose of 0.05 mg/kg.[17] The maximum single initial dose is 0.5 mg/kg in children and 0.3 mg/kg in neonates.[18] Initial maximum dose in *adults* is 6 mg.[4]

> **Subsequent dosing:** If conversion does not occur in 1–2 minutes, increase dose by 0.1[3] or 0.2 mg/kg.[4] Follow each bolus with a saline flush. This process should continue until sinus rhythm is established or a maximum single dose of 0.3 mg/kg (maximum of 12 mg) is used.[3]

Dosage adjustment in organ dysfunction

No dosage adjustment necessary in renal dysfunction.[19]

Adenosine

Maximum dosage	The maximum single dose reported is 0.5 mg/kg in children and 0.3 mg/kg in neonates[18] up 12 mg.[3,4] A preterm neonate receiving theophylline required doses of 0.4–0.8 mg/kg to convert to normal sinus rhythm.[20] Over a 14.5-hour period, a 3-week-old was given 119 doses of 0.1–0.2 mg/kg.[21] A 14-year-old adolescent who failed to respond to an 18-mg dose was believed to have ventricular tachycardia.[12] (See Comments section.)
Additives	9 mg/mL of sodium.[22]
Suitable diluents	NS and RL.[22]
Maximum concentration	3 mg/mL (available commercially).[3]
Preparation and delivery	**Stability:** Store at room temperature. Do not refrigerate as crystallization may occur.[22] If crystallization occurs, dissolve crystals by warming to room temperature.[22] The solution must be clear at the time of use.[22]
IV push	Over 1–2 seconds, followed by a rapid saline flush.[3,4]
Intermittent infusion	Not given via this method.
Continuous infusion	Although concentration and solution type was not provided, one child received a continuous infusion.[23]
Other routes of administration	Has been administered intraosseously in emergencies.[4]
Comments	**Rare adverse effects:** Transient flushing, dyspnea, headache, complete atrioventricular block, sinus bradycardia, and other rhythm disorders have been reported.[3,4]
	Drug interactions: Although no causal relationship or drug-drug interaction has been established, adenosine should be used cautiously in patients receiving digoxin and less frequently with digoxin and verapamil since ventricular fibrillation, including resuscitated and fatal events, have occurred.[3]
	Adenosine effects are antagonized by methylxanthines (e.g., theophylline, caffeine); hence, larger dose of adenosine may be required.[3,14]
	The effects of adenosine are potentiated by dipyridamole.[24] Thus, smaller doses of adenosine may be effective in the presence of dipyridamole.[24]
	Because adenosine decreases conduction through the A-V node, higher degrees of heart block may be produced in the presence of carbamazepine.[3,4]

Albumin (Normal Human Serum)

Brand names	**50 mg/mL:** Albumarc, AlbuRx 5, Albumin (Human) 5% Solution, Albutein 5%, Buminate 5%, Plasbumin-5
	200 mg/mL: Human Albumin Grifols 20%, Plasbumin-20
	250 mg/mL: Albumarc 25%, Albuminar-25, Albumin (Human) 25% Solution, Albutein 25%, AlbuRx 25, Buminate 25%, Flexbumin 25%, Human Albumin Grifols 25%, Plasbumin-25
Medication error potential	None noted.
Contraindications and warnings	**Contraindications**[1]**:** Patients who should not be given albumin containing solutions include those who (1) are severely anemic, (2) have CHF with normal or increased intravascular volume, and (3) have known hypersensitivity to albumin products.
	Anaphylaxis has been reported in an *adult*.[2]
Infusion related cautions	Too rapid infusion may result in acute hypertension or vascular overload, causing pulmonary edema or cardiac failure.[1]
	Premature neonates are at risk for intraventricular hemorrhage from rapid intravascular volume expansion.[3]
	Allergic reactions may result in chills, fever, nausea, vomiting, or urticaria.[1]
Dosage	**Hypovolemia:** 0.5–1 g/kg.[1] 20 mL/kg of 4.5% (0.9 g/kg)[4] and 5% albumin (1 g/kg)[5] have been given over 20 minutes in premature neonates.
	Hypoalbuminemia: Albumin deficits have been replaced by intermittent infusions of up to 1 g/kg of albumin 25%.[6] The continuous infusion of albumin results in a more sustained increase in serum albumin concentration.[7] The albumin deficit can be estimated with the following equation:
	g albumin = weight (kg) $\times$ 3 dL/kg $\times$ (3.5 – observed serum albumin in g/dL)[8,9]
	Nephrotic syndrome (controversial): 0.25–1 g/kg of albumin 25% infused over $\geq$1–12 hours keeping in mind that rapid expansion of intravascular volume may increase the risk for CHF.[10-12] Infusion over a longer time decreases the risk for the development of CHF.[12] Furosemide (0.5 to 2-mg/kg)[10-12] infusion may accompany or follow the albumin infusion.
Dosage adjustment in organ dysfunction	None noted.[1]
Maximum dosage	125 g in 24 hours or 250 g in 48 hours have been given to *adults*.[1,12]
Additives	Contains 130–160 mEq sodium/L of albumin.[1,13] Aluminum is present as a contaminant.
	Contains no preservatives or antimicrobial.[1,13]

Albumin (Normal Human Serum)

Suitable diluents	D5W, D10W, or NS.[1,13] In patients who require sodium restriction, a 5% albumin solution that contains less sodium can be prepared by diluting each 1 mL of albumin 25% in 4 mL of D5W or D10W. However, infusion of large amounts of albumin diluted with D5W can result in hyponatremia; therefore, when using large volumes of albumin, dilution in NS is preferred.[1,13] Renal failure and fatal hemolysis may occur if SW is used as a diluent.[1,13,14,15]
Maximum concentration	Undiluted.
Preparation and delivery	**Compatibility:** See Appendix D for PN compatibility information. **Delivery:** Do not use if solution is turbid.[1,13] The infusion should begin within 4 hours of opening the bottle.[1] The institution specific protocol for blood product infusion should be used to guide infusion length from an opened bottle. Solutions containing >25 g/L of albumin are more likely to occlude 0.22-micron in-line filters; however, PN solutions containing as little as 10.8 g/L caused filter occlusion.[16,17]
IV push	When used as a plasma volume expander in the treatment of hypovolemic shock, the rate of administration should be adapted to the patient response.[1]
Intermittent infusion	Infuse over 30–60 minutes. In severe hypovolemia, faster rates may be required.[1] (See Infusion related cautions section.)
Continuous infusion	Can be infused continuously. (See Preparation and delivery section.)
Other routes of administration	Not indicated.
Comments	Albumin is derived from pooled human plasma that has the theoretical potential to contain infectious agents including the causative agent for Creutzfeldt-Jakob disease and West Nile virus.[1] Donor screening has greatly decreased the risk for transmission of hepatitis B, hepatitis C, and HIV.[1]

Alfentanil

Brand names	Alfenta, generic

Medication error potential

ISMP high-alert medication that has an increased risk of causing significant patient harm if it is used in error.[1]

Look-alike, sound-alike error potential.

USP reports that alfentanil has been confused with SUFentanil; no patient harm resulted.[2]

Contraindications and warnings

Contraindications: Alfentanil is contraindicated in patients with a hypersensitivity to the drug or known intolerance to opioid agonists.[3]

Warnings: Alfentanil should only be administered by persons specifically trained in the use of IV anesthetics.[3]

Infusion related cautions

Significant bradycardia, muscle or chest wall rigidity (dose-related), and apnea may occur early in administration of alfentanil or following rapid administration.[3-5] Pretreatment with atropine and a nondepolarizing neuromuscular blocking agent may aid in minimizing these adverse effects. Ventilatory support is indicated.

An opioid antagonist, resuscitation and intubation equipment and oxygen should be readily available when using alfentanil.[3]

Dosage

Alfentanil is not recommended in children <12 years.[3]

Dosages vary depending on the desired degree of analgesia/anesthesia and adjunctive therapies (e.g., halothane, propofol).

When dosing obese (>20% above ideal body weight) patients, use lean body weight.[3] (See Appendix B.)

Anesthesia (children >12 years and *adults*)[3,5,6]**:**

    Incremental injection of short duration (≤30 minutes)

        Spontaneously breathing or assisted ventilation when required: Induction 8–20 mcg/kg; maintenance 3–5 mcg/kg q 5–20 min or 0.5–1 mcg/kg/min (total dose 8–40 mcg/kg).

        Laryngoscopy and intubation (assisted or controlled ventilation required): Induction 20–50 mcg/kg; maintenance 5–15 mcg/kg q 5–20 min (total dose up to 75 mcg/kg).

    Continuous infusion (>45 minutes)

        Intubation and incision (assisted or controlled ventilation required): Induction 50–75 mcg/kg; maintenance 0.5–3 (average 1–1.5) mcg/kg/min; titrate to desired effect; total dose dependent on procedure.

    Anesthetic induction (>45 minutes)

        Assisted or controlled ventilation required: Induction 130–245 mcg/kg; maintenance 0.5–1.5 mcg/kg/min or general anesthetic; total dose dependent on procedure (administer slowly over 3 minutes; concentration of inhalation agents decreased by 30% to 50% for first hour).

Dosage (cont.)	**Monitored anesthesia care (MAC)** **For sedated and responsive, spontaneously breathing patients:** Induction 3–8 mcg/kg; maintenance 3–5 mcg/kg q 5–20 min or 0.25–1 mcg/kg/min (total dose 3–40 mcg/kg). **The following doses have been reported for anesthesia in children <12 years:** **Neonates (preterm and term) and infants:** Induction 20–25 mcg/kg over 30 minutes[4,7-9]; maintenance 3–5 mcg/kg/h.[7] **Children (<12 years):** Induction 20–100 mcg/kg (12.5–25 mcg/kg when combined with halothane)[9-12]; maintenance 2.5–5 mcg/kg/min.[12] **Infants and children on cardiac bypass (congenital heart repair):** 20 mcg/kg for induction followed by continuous infusion of 1 mcg/kg/min with supplemental doses of 5 mcg/kg as needed.[13]
Dosage adjustment in organ dysfunction	No dosage adjustment required in patients with renal dysfunction.[14] Patients with hepatic dysfunction may require smaller doses to achieve the same therapeutic effect.[3] Average doses may lead to medication accumulation; therefore, caution is warranted on administration of alfentanil to patients with liver dysfunction.[3]
Maximum dosage	Dosages are titrated to the desired level of sedation or analgesia.[3]
Additives	None.
Suitable diluents	D5W, D5NS, NS, LR.[15]
Maximum concentration	≤80 mcg/mL.[15]
Preparation and delivery	Dilute prior to administration.[3,15]
IV push	≤80 mcg/mL over 3–5 minutes.[3,15] Doses ≤100 mcg/kg have been given over 30 seconds.[11,12] (See Infusion related cautions section.)
Intermittent infusion	25–80 mcg/mL over 10–30 minutes.[4,8,10,15]
Continuous infusion	25–80 mcg/mL at a rate ≤5 mcg/kg/min.[7,11,12,15] (See Dosage section.) After the first hour, rates may need to be decreased by 30% to 50% in some patients.[3]
Other routes of administration	No information available to support administration by other routes.
Comments	**Significant adverse effects:** Delayed respiratory depression, respiratory arrest, bradycardia, asystole, arrhythmias, and hypotension have been reported with alfentanil use.[4] Epileptiform activity has occurred in patients receiving alfentanil during epilepsy surgery.[16,17]

Allopurinol Sodium

Brand names
Aloprim

Medication error potential
Look-alike, sound-alike error potential.

USP reports that allopurinol was confused with atenolol and enalapril. No patient harm resulted.[1]

Contraindications and warnings
Contraindications: Patients who experienced a severe reaction to a previous dose should not receive allopurinol.[2]

Discontinue at the first appearance of a rash.[2,3] (See Comments section.)

Hypersensitivity reactions are rare.[3]

Infusion related cautions
None noted.

Dosage
Prevention/treatment of hyperuricemia secondary to neoplastic disorders: Treatment is started 24–48 hours prior to chemotherapy.[2-5] Maintain adequate hydration to avoid potential formation of xanthine calculi and prevent renal precipitation of urates.[2,3]

> **<10 years of age:** 200 mg/m^2/day either as a single dose, in divided doses, or as a continuous infusion.[2-5]

> **10 years of age and older:** 200–400 mg/m^2/day (5–10 mg/kg/day) divided q 4–12 h[2-6] or as a continuous infusion.[3]

Inhibition of free radical production

> **Postasphyxial brain injury in newborns:** 20 mg/kg given within 4 hours of life and again 12 hours later.[7]

> **Severely hypoxic neonates on ECMO:** 10 mg/kg prior to cannulation followed by 5 mg/kg q 8 h for 72 hours after initiation of bypass.[8]

> **Congenital heart disease necessitating cardiopulmonary bypass (CPB):** No difference in pharmacokinetic parameters or decrease in uric acid concentration was noted in 12 neonates with hypoplastic left heart syndrome who received 5 or 10 mg/kg over 20 minutes.[9]

> 5 mg/kg given at least 16 hours preoperatively, 5 mg/kg given 8 hours preoperatively, 10 mg/kg given at 0700 the morning of surgery, 20 mg/kg intraoperatively via CPB circuit, and nine postoperative doses of 5 mg/kg q 8 h decreased morbidity in neonates with hypoplastic left-heart syndrome.[10]

Dosage adjustment in organ dysfunction
CrCl 10–20 mL/min: 50% of the usual dose.[2,3]

CrCl 3–10 mL/min: 25% of the usual dose.[2,3]

CrCl <3 mL/min: 25% of the usual dose and extend the interval.[2,3]

Maximum dosage
A 3-year-old with ALL received 410 mg/m^2/day for 11 days, and a 4-year-old with ALL received a cumulative dose of 8.8 g/m^2 over a 6-month period as an outpatient.[5]

600 mg/day in *adults*.[2]

Additives
Contains ~85 mg sodium/500-mg vial.

Allopurinol Sodium

Suitable diluents	SW to reconstitute, NS, or D5W to dilute.[2,3,10]
Maximum concentration	≤6 mg/mL.[2,3] Two pharmacokinetics studies evaluated six healthy *adult* volunteers in each study. One study infused a single 20-mg/mL dose over 2 minutes[12] and the other a single 10-mg/mL dose over 15 minutes.[13]
Preparation and delivery	**Preparation:** Reconstitute by adding 25 mL SW.[2,3] The pH of the reconstituted vial ranges from 11.1 to 11.8 and must be diluted with NS or D5W. [2,3] Do not refrigerate reconstituted or diluted product. **Stability:** Administer within 10 hours of reconstitution. Contains no preservatives.
IV push	Not recommended.
Intermittent infusion	Over 15–30 minutes.[4,5,8,9]
Continuous infusion	The daily dose can be given as a continuous infusion.[3,5]
Other routes of administration	Not indicated.
Comments	Ensure adequate urine flow by providing sufficient fluid intake.[2,3] **Adverse drug effects:** A 15-year-old boy with Williams syndrome receiving oral allopurinol for 6 weeks developed acute pure red-cell aplasia that resolved when the drug was discontinued.[14] **Drug interactions:** Azathioprine and mercaptopurine doses should be reduced by 25% to 33% and subsequent dosage based on patient response and occurrence of toxicity.[2,3] The dose may need to be increased with concomitant use of drugs that increase urate concentration.[2,3] The incidence of rash is increased with concomitant ampicillin or amoxicillin use.[2,3] Increased concentrations of cyclosporine have been reported with allopurinol use.[2,3]

Alprostadil

Brand names	Prostin VR Pediatric (Prostaglandin E1, PGE1)
Medication error potential	None.
Contraindications and warnings	**US boxed warning:** Apnea occurs in 10% to 12% of neonates with congenital heart defects and is seen most often in those weighing <2 kg at birth.[1] Signs and symptoms generally appear during the first hour of drug infusion.[1] The medication should only be used in places where ventilator support is available and respiratory status should be monitored. **Contraindications:** May cause gastric outlet obstruction in neonates secondary to antral hyperplasia.[1] The effect appears to be related to the duration of therapy (i.e., >120 hours) and cumulative dose.[1-3] Infuse alprostadil at lowest effective dose and for shortest period of time while weighing the risks of long-term effects versus benefits.
Infusion related cautions	Theoretically, intra-aortic or intra-arterial infusion should be the preferred route since it allows for the greatest concentration to the ductus; however, clinical studies have shown these routes to be no more effective than IV infusion.[1] Infusion rate should be slowed if fever or hypotension develops until resolution.[1] If apnea or bradycardia occur during the infusion, it is recommended to discontinue therapy and provide supportive therapy.[1] Cutaneous flushing usually results from improper catheter placement and rapidly reverses with repositioning of the intra-arterial catheter.[1] Extravasation may cause tissue sloughing and necrosis.[4]

Dosage	**Hepatic veno-occlusive disease:** 0.075 mcg/kg/h increasing q 12 h until the maximum tolerated dose of 0.5 mcg/kg/h has been reached.[5] Used in conjunction with 100 units/kg/day of heparin as a continuous infusion.[5]
	
	Patent ductus arteriosus (PDA): Short-term maintenance of PDA in neonates with ductal-dependent cyanotic and acyanotic congenital heart disease until surgery can be performed. 0.05–0.1 mcg/kg/min.[6-11] Although larger doses (0.4 mcg/kg/h) have been given, dosages exceeding 0.1 mcg/kg/min generally do not provide additional benefit.[12]
	
	Peripheral gangrene secondary to ischemia: 0.05 mcg/kg/min reversed acrocyanosis of the hands and feet within 4 days.[13,14]
	
	Pulmonary hypertension
	
	    Heart transplant: 0.05 mcg/kg/min during ECMO. After releasing aortic cross clamps, increase to 0.1–0.15 mcg/kg/min.[15,16]
	
	    Liver transplant: Prior to unclamping infuse 0.0125 mcg/kg/min. If hypotension occurs, double infusion to 0.025 mcg/kg/min.[17-21]

Dosage adjustment in organ dysfunction	No dosage adjustment required in renal dysfunction.
Maximum dosage	0.4–0.75 mcg/kg/min has been used without adverse effects, but doses of >0.1 mcg/kg/min have not improved efficacy in PDA.[1,6,22]
Additives	None.
Suitable diluents	Must be diluted before administration in D5W, D10W, or NS.[23]

Alprostadil

Maximum concentration	20 mcg/mL.[23]
Preparation and delivery	**Delivery system issues:** Direct contact of the concentrated alprostadil with the wall of the plastic volumetric infusion chamber should be avoided because the drug may interact with the plastic chamber to produce a hazy solution. If this occurs, the chamber and solution should be discarded.[1,23] **Stability:** Concentrated solution should be refrigerated.[23] Prepare fresh solution q 24 h.[23]
IV push	Not recommended because of short half-life.[1]
Intermittent infusion	Not recommended because of short half-life.[1]
Continuous infusion	The manufacturer suggests the following dilutions and infusion rates to provide a dose of 0.1 mcg/kg/min.[1]

Add 1 Ampule (500 mcg) to	Approximate Concentration of Resulting Solution	Infusion Rate (mL/kg/min)	Infusion Rate (mL/kg/h)
250	2 mcg/mL	0.05	3.0
100	5 mcg/mL	0.02	1.2
50	10 mcg/mL	0.01	0.6
25	20 mcg/mL	0.005	0.3

Other routes of administration	None.
Comments	**Significant adverse effects:** Because alprostadil inhibits platelet aggregation, it should be used cautiously in neonates with bleeding tendencies.[1] **Rare adverse effects:** Reports of an urticarial rash[24] and "harlequin color change"[25] have been documented during prostaglandin infusions in neonates with cardiac heart defects. The rash is erythematous, migratory, primarily limited to the upper torso, self-limiting, and resolves upon drug discontinuation.[24,25] Ectopic calcifications in the deep tissues of the axillae, thoracic inlet, and neck were noted on the chest x-ray of an infant who had received a cumulative alprostadil dose of 5654 mcg/kg for documented transposition. Brown fat necrosis was confirmed on autopsy.[26] A "pseudo-Barter syndrome" has been reported during infusions and is characterized by severe hyponatremia and polyuria, which resolves upon drug discontinuation.[1,27] Leukocytosis has been reported and resolves with discontinuation of therapy.[28] Cortical proliferation may develop as easily as 9 days into therapy (usually 4–6 weeks) and presents as soft tissue swelling, peripheral hard edema, and cortical hyperostosis.[1,29-32] The changes are reversible upon discontinuation of the infusion but have been reported to take up to 38 weeks to resolve completely.[29] It is believed that the effects are dose and duration dependent.[29-32] **Osmolality:** Undiluted solution is 23,250 mOsm/kg.[23]

Amikacin Sulfate

Brand names	Amikin

Medication error potential

Look a-like, sound-alike drug names.

ISMP's *Confused Drug Names* lists confusion with Kineret.[1]

USP reports confusion with Amicar.[2]

Contraindications and warnings

US boxed warning: Patients with impaired renal function and those receiving large doses or prolonged therapy have an increased risk for nephrotoxicity and ototoxicity (i.e., vestibular and auditory), both of which are generally reversible.[3-5] The risk of toxicity can also be increased by prolonged elevations in serum concentrations; concurrent use of medications known to be nephro-, neuro-, or oto-toxic; dehydration; and advancing age.[3-5] Observe closely for signs or symptoms of toxicity.[3] (See Rare adverse effects and Monitoring in Comments section.)

Aminoglycosides can cause fetal harm when administered to a pregnant woman.[3]

Contraindications: Known hypersensitivity to amikacin or other aminoglycosides.[3]

Other warnings: Aminoglycosides can cause neuromuscular blockade and potentiate the effects of neuromuscular blockers.[3,6,7] (See Appendix C for specific information.)

Infusion related cautions

None.

Dosage

In obese patients dosage should be based on the following equation in any obese patient.[8,9] Dosing weight = IBW + 0.4 (TBW − IBW). (See Appendix B.)

Neonates

Loading dose: Aminoglycoside loading doses have been advocated.[10-12,13] Some have advocated a loading dose of 10 mg/kg of amikacin in neonates.[10-13]

Maintenance dose

Based on age and weight

PNA	<1200 g	1200–2000 g	≥2000 g
<7 days	7.5 mg/kg q 18–24 h[14,15]	15 mg/kg/day divided q 12 h[14-21]	15–20 mg/kg/day divided q 12 h[14-21]
≥7 days	7.5 mg/kg q 18–24 h[14]*	15–20 mg/kg/day divided q 8–12 h[14,15]	30 mg/kg/day divided q 8 h[14]

*Until 4 weeks of age.

15 mg/kg once daily has also been used in neonates of all gestational ages with a postnatal age of ≥7 days.[13]

Based on gestational age[16]

Gestational Age	Dose
≤26 weeks	7.5 mg/kg q 24 h
27–34 weeks	7.5 mg/kg q 18 h
35–42 weeks	20 mg/kg/day divided q 12 h
≥43 weeks	30 mg/kg/day divided q 8 h

Dosage *(cont.)*	**Infants and children:** 22.5 mg/kg/day divided q 8 h[14,15] or 1260 mg/m^2/day divided q 8 h.[22]
	Several investigators have reported that once-daily dosing has comparable efficacy and perhaps less toxicity than dosing of 8–12 hours.[23-26] A single dose of 15–25 mg/kg has been given once daily (usually over 20–30 minutes) in critically ill infants and children with severe gram-negative infections,[13,27-29] bone marrow transplantation,[30] or in febrile neutropenic patients with cancer.[31-34] Once-daily therapy has also been used to treat UTI on an outpatient basis.[35] At this time, the use of once-daily dosing in infants and children is controversial.[36] The most recent edition of the *American Academy of Pediatrics Red Book: Report of the Committee on Infectious Diseases* continues to recommend that aminoglycosides be administered in multiple daily doses in all age groups.[14]
Dosage adjustment in organ dysfunction	If CrCl is >50 mL/min, give a normal dose q 12–24 h[37]; if CrCl is 10–50 mL/min, give q 24–48 h[26]; and if CrCl is <10 mL/min, give q 48–72 h.[37]
Maximum dosage	Larger doses or shorter dosing intervals of aminoglycosides are sometimes required in patients with cystic fibrosis, major thermal burns or dermal loss, or in patients with ascites.[37-41] Based on similarities between aminoglycosides, prolonged dosing interval may be required in those receiving ECMO.[42] Individualize dosage based on serum concentrations.
Additives	The 50-mg/mL and 250-mg/mL products contain 0.064 mEq/L and 0.319 mEq/mL of sodium bisulfate.[43] (See Appendix C for specific information about sulfite hypersensitivity.)
Suitable diluents	D5¼NS, D5½NS, D5W, LR, or NS.[3]
Maximum concentration	10 mg/mL.[45]
Preparation and delivery	**Delivery system issues:** The mixing of amikacin sulfate with an aminoglycoside in vitro can result in substantial inactivation of the aminoglycoside. (See Appendix C for more specific information.)
	Compatibility: See Appendix D for PN compatibility information.[44]
IV push	Although aminoglycosides have been given over 15 seconds,[46] 1 minute,[47] and 3–5 minutes,[48] rapid infusion is not recommended.
Intermittent infusion	Over 30–60 minutes. Infusion over 1–2 hours is recommended in infants.[3]
Continuous infusion	Not recommended. Has been given by continuous infusion.[49-51] Low serum concentrations[50] and nephrotoxicity may occur more frequently.[51]
Other routes of administration	Undiluted product for IM use.[23,18]

Amikacin Sulfate

Comments

Rare adverse effects: Aminoglycosides accumulate in renal cortical tissue and may damage proximal tubule cells leading to oliguric renal failure. Risk of nephrotoxicity may be influenced by type of aminoglycoside, dose, duration (cumulative dose), frequency of therapy, and elevated serum concentration.[3,4] It is also increased by advancing age, pre-existing renal or hepatic dysfunction, decrease renal perfusion, hypoalbuminemia, and dehydration.[3,4,23] Current administration of nephrotoxic medications may increase the risk of toxicity and should be avoided.[3]

Cochlear and/or vestibular ototoxicity has been associated with all aminoglycoside antibiotics.[5,6,23] Total AUC is a better indicator of ototoxic risk than either peak or trough serum concentration.[52,53] Use cautiously with other drugs (e.g., macrolide antibiotics, loop diuretics, platinum-based chemotherapeutic agents) known to cause ototoxicity.

Aminoglycosides may potentiate the curare-like effects on the neuromuscular junction and should be used with caution in patients with neuromuscular disorders since they may aggravate muscle weakness.[3,6,7] Aminoglycosides may enhance the respiratory depressant effect of neuromuscular-blocking agents and may prolonged blockade.[3,54,55]

Monitoring: Because large variability exists in patient response to therapy, individualize dosage based on serum concentrations, clinical response, and renal function. Recommended peak and trough serum amikacin concentration are ≤35 mg/L and ≤10 mg/L, respectively. Desired peak concentrations are dependent on the site of infection. Although serum concentration monitoring has become routine practice in many institutions, not all patients require monitoring.[56,57] Monitoring is indicated if the patient is not clinically responding, is ≤3 months of age, has disease that requires large doses or high concentrations (CNS infections, endocarditis, pneumonia, ascites, burns), has decreased or unstable renal function, or will be treated more than 10 days.

Drug interactions: Consult appropriate resources before combining any drug with gentamicin.

Laboratory interference: Serum concentrations may be falsely elevated when blood samples are collected through central venous Silastic catheters.[58]

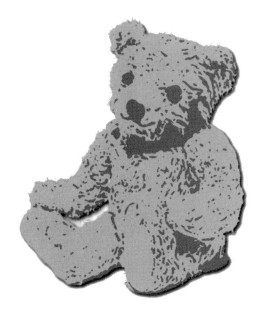

Aminocaproic Acid

Brand names	Amicar
Medication error potential	Look-alike, sound-alike error potential. USP reports that Amicar was confused with amikacin. No patient harm resulted. Amicar was confused with Omacor; patient harm resulted.[1]
Contraindications and warnings	Aminocaproic acid should not be used when there is a ongoing intravascular clotting process.[2,3]
Infusion related cautions	Hypotension, bradycardia, and cardiac arrhythmias may occur with rapid or undiluted administration.[2,3] Thrombophlebitis may occur.[2,3]
Dosage	**Continuous infusion:** Loading dose of 100–200 mg/kg not to exceed 5 g[2-9] followed by continuous infusion at 10–33.3 mg/kg/h or 1 g/m^2/h.[2-9] In high-risk infants on ECMO, aminocaproic acid infusion has been continued up to 72 hours during ECMO or until decannulation.[5] **Bolus dosing:** 100 mg/kg or 3 g/m^2 not to exceed 5 g every 4–6 hours or as needed.[2,3,10-14] In infants undergoing congenital diaphragmatic hernia repair during ECMO, 100 mg/kg was given 30–60 minutes prior to surgery and after surgery for 24–48 hours to maintain an ACT of 200–220 seconds.[14]
Dosage adjustment in organ dysfunction	Reduce dosage in patients with cardiac, renal, or hepatic disease.[3]
Maximum dosage	Total daily doses in children ≤18 g/m^2/day in children or in *adults* 30 g/day.[2,3] 36 g/day were given to a 12-year-old with ALL.[15]
Additives	Contains benzyl alcohol.[2,3] (See Appendix C for specific information about potential benzyl alcohol toxicity.)
Suitable diluents	NS, D5W, R.[16]
Maximum concentration	20 mg/mL.[2,3]
Preparation and delivery	250-mg multidose vial should be diluted in 250 mL.[2,3]
IV push	Not recommended.[2,3] (See Infusion related cautions section.)

Aminocaproic Acid

Intermittent infusion	Over 1 hour.[2,3] However, loading doses of 100 mg/kg were infused over 15–20 minutes in children 11–18 years of age.[4,9]
Continuous infusion	May be infused continuously.[2-9]
Other routes of administration	Not indicated.
Comments	Prophylactic aminocaproic acid in children undergoing cardiac surgery reduced intraoperative blood loss, but did not significantly decrease blood product transfusions.[8] Perioperative blood loss was reduced in patients during posterior spinal fusion and segmental spinal instrumentation.[4,9]

Reports on the ability of aminocaproic acid to decrease the incidence of intracranial hemorrhage and other hemorrhagic complications in neonates on ECMO are conflicting.[5-7]

Adverse events: A 12-year-old child with refractory thrombocytopenia after bone marrow transplantation developed myopathy after 98 days of treatment with doses ranging from 4 to 36 g/day.[15]

Serum creatine phosphokinase concentrations, particularly in patients with myalgia, may be a useful indicator of muscle injury. Myopathy is usually reversible on discontinuation of therapy.[2,3,15]

Pharmacokinetic considerations: In order to attain concentrations above the therapeutic threshold, children require larger loading and maintenance doses than *adults*.[17]

Aminophylline

Brand names	Various manufacturers
Medication error potential	Look-alike, sound-alike drug names. USP reports confusion with ampicillin and amitriptyline.[1]
Contraindications and warnings	**Contraindications:** In patients with a history of hypersensitivity to theophylline or other components in the product including ethylenediamine.[2] **Warnings:** Use with extreme caution as theophylline may exacerbate active peptic ulcer disease, seizure disorders, hyperthyroidism, and/or cardiac arrhythmias (not including bradyarrhythmias).[2,3]
Infusion related cautions	Rapid administration may result in toxic serum concentrations[4] and circulatory failure.[5]
Dosage	Aminophylline products contain varying amounts of theophylline (check manufacturers' information). All of the doses in this monograph are reported as **THEOPHYLLINE**. **Apnea and bradycardia of prematurity (usual therapeutic range 6–12 mg/L)** **Loading dose (LD):** 4–6 mg/kg over 20–30 minutes.[4-12] If the patient is already receiving theophylline, a serum concentration must be obtained and the LD based on that concentration[13] using the equation: LD (mg/kg) = (desired concentration – measured concentration)/2 (See Other in Comments section for more information about the equation.) **Initial maintenance dose:** 2–4 mg/kg/day divided q 12 h[4-7] or 3.3–7.5 mg/kg/day divided q 8 h.[8-12] **Severe acute asthma (usual therapeutic range 5–15 mg/L):** The role of IV aminophylline in acute asthma is controversial. Many *adult*[14-17] and pediatric[18-21] patients who respond to beta-agonist and systemic glucocorticoid experience no additional benefit from aminophylline. However, studies suggest that the addition of aminophylline may be beneficial in critically ill children with severe acute asthma and impending respiratory failure who are unresponsive to aggressive beta-agonist and systemic glucocorticoids.[22-24] *Loading*[25,26] *and maintenance*[27] *doses should be based on ideal body weight in children who are overweight or obese. (See Appendix B.)* **Loading dose (no theophylline in the past 24 hours):** 5–6 mg/kg over 20–30 minutes.[2,28,29] **Loading dose (theophylline in the past 24 hours):** A theophylline serum concentration must be obtained and the loading dose (LD) estimated based on the following equation: LD (mg/kg) = (desired concentration – measured concentration)/2[13] (See Comments section.)

Dosage *(cont.)*	**Maintenance dose (initial dose to achieve a target serum concentration of 10 mg/L)**
	Infants 6–52 weeks: $[0.008$ (age in weeks) $+ 0.21] = $ mg/kg/h.[29,30]
	Children 1–<9 years: 0.8 mg/kg/h.[29]
	Children 9–<12 years: 0.7 mg/kg/h.[29]
	Children 12–16 years (smoker): 0.7 mg/kg/h.[29]
	Children 12–16 years (nonsmoker): 0.5 mg/kg/h.[29]
	Not to exceed 900 mg/day unless a subtherapeutic serum concentration combined with an inadequate response indicate the need for larger doses.[29]

Dosage adjustment in organ dysfunction	Infants up to 3 months of age eliminate 50% of theophylline unchanged in the urine; hence, the dosage should be decreased in these infants.[6,29,31] The dose should also be reduced in patients with cardiac failure, hepatic dysfunction, acute hepatitis, or sustained high fever and asphyxiated neonates.[2,29,32,33]
Maximum dosage	Individualize dosage based on serum concentrations and clinical response.[2]
Additives	None.
Suitable diluents	D5W, D10W, D20W, LR, NS, R, ½NS, D5NS, D5½NS, D5¼NS, D–LR, D–R, D–S, D5LR. Stable in dextran 6% in D5W, dextran 6% in NS.[34]
Maximum concentration	25 mg/mL (commercially available)[34]
Preparation and delivery	**Compatibility:** For PN compatibility information, please see Appendix D.[35]
IV push	Not recommended.
Intermittent infusion	≤25 mg/mL (commercially available) over 15–30 minutes[2] not to exceed 0.36 mg/kg/min or 25 mg/min.[2,3]
Continuous infusion	≤25 mg/mL.[2] Normally diluted to 1 mg/mL.[3]
Other routes of administration	Should not be give IM.[2]

Aminophylline

Comments

Significant adverse effects: *Whenever a patient receiving theophylline develops nausea or vomiting, particularly repetitive vomiting, or other signs or symptoms consistent with theophylline toxicity, the infusion should be stopped and a serum theophylline concentration measured immediately.*

Death from theophylline toxicity is most often attributed to cardiorespiratory arrest and/or hypoxic encephalopathy that follows prolonged generalized seizures or intractable cardiac arrhythmias.[2,36,37] Generally, serum concentration above 30 mg/L are associated with a variety of signs and symptoms.[36,37] Toxicities may occur at lower serum concentrations following chronic toxicity when compared to those noted after an acute ingestion.[38] Anticonvulsants should be initiated with an intravenous benzodiazepine (e.g., lorazepam)[2] and repetitive seizures should be treated with a long- acting anticonvulsant. Reports in animal studies suggest that phenytoin is ineffective in terminating theophylline-induced seizures and that phenobarbital should be used.[39,40] (See Lorazepam and Phenobarbital monographs.)

Monitoring: Because large variability exists in patient response to initial and maintenance doses, individualize dosage based on attainment of a therapeutic serum concentration and clinical response.[29] The "therapeutic range" is generally considered 5–15 mg/L,[41] but concentrations up to 20 mg/L have been historically used.[42]

Drug interactions: Theophylline is a substrate of CYP1A2 (major), 2E1 (minor), and 3A4 (minor) and may be associated with many potentially fatal drug interactions.[3] Consult appropriate resources for dosing recommendations before combining any drug with theophylline.

Laboratory interference: When measured by the Bittner or colorimetric method, theophylline produces false-positive elevations of serum uric acid.[2] No inference is noted when other methods are employed.

Other: The equation to calculate loading dose (LD) is based on the following: LD = desired concentration × volume of distribution (assuming a normal volume of distribution of 0.5 L/kg). As a general rule, 1 mg/kg of theophylline will increase the serum theophylline concentration by 2 mg/L.[13]

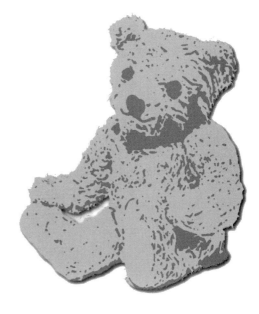

Amphotericin B

Brand names	Fungizone, Amphocin

Medication error potential

Look-alike, sound-alike error potential.

ISMP reports that amphotericin B has been confused with Abelcet and AmBisome.[1]

USP reports that amphotericin B has been confused with amphotericin B liposome; patient harm resulted. USP also reports that Fungizone has been confused with AmBisome; no patient harm resulted.[2]

Contraindications and warnings

US boxed warning: Reserve treatment with amphotericin B for progressive and potentially life-threatening fungal infections; do not use for noninvasive fungal infections in immunocompetent patients.[3]

Do not give a dose >1.5 mg/kg. Overdose may result in potentially fatal cardiac arrest or cardiopulmonary syndrome.[3]

Verify the product name, dosage and preadministration, especially if the dose >1.5 mg/kg.[3]

Contraindications: Amphotericin B therapy is complicated by many dangerous side effects. It is contraindicated in patients with hypersensitivity to amphotericin B or any of its components, unless benefit of treating life-threatening disease outweighs potential risk.[3]

Infusion related cautions

Hypersensitivity reactions, including anaphylaxis, have been reported.[4-6] Other infusion related symptoms include fever, chills, nausea, vomiting, headache, malaise, hypotension and arrhythmias.[7] Patients have been premedicated with acetaminophen, codeine, diazepam, diphenhydramine, hydroxyzine, meperidine, or prochlorperazine.[8-10]

Corticosteroids have been added to amphotericin B solutions to decrease the incidence and severity of febrile response during infusion.[8,11] However, congestive heart failure was reported in *adults* who received 25–40 mg/day of hydrocortisone with amphotericin B.[8]

Although amphotericin B is incompatible with FE,[12] it has been reconstituted in a small volume of D5W and then diluted in 20% IVFE in order to improve tolerance and decrease infusion-related side effects in *adults*.[13,14]

Thrombophlebitis and injection pain may also occur; adding 1 unit of heparin per mL of solution may reduce pain at the injection site and phlebitis.[15]

Arrhythmias have been reported during infusion in a neonate.[16]

Although cardiovascular collapse has occurred in animals after rapid injection,[17,18] it has been infused over 45–60 minutes without problems in *adults*.[19-21]

Dosage

Initial and maintenance: 0.25–0.5 mg/kg q 24 h infused over 2–6 hours. Increase daily dose as tolerated by 0.25–0.5 mg/kg up to 0.5–1.5 mg/kg q 24 h.[7,11,22-37]

Early studies, many administering amphotericin B in combination with flucytosine, used smaller initial doses and slower dose titration.[38-45] Recent data supports the use of larger doses initially (0.25–0.5 mg/kg q 24 h) followed by a more rapid dose titration to achieve the desired therapeutic dose.[7,23,26,28]

Test dose (to minimize anaphylactic response in susceptible individuals): Although one study in *adults*, who were frequently premedicated, failed to show that a test dose predicted anaphylactic reactions,[4] a single dose of 0.1 mg/kg, up to 1 mg, infused over 20–30 minutes is often used.[3,38,41,44,46] Vital signs should be monitored q 30 min for 2 hours. If a test dose is done, therapy should commence the same day with the remainder of a recommended therapeutic dose.[17]

Dosage *(cont.)*	Pharmacokinetic data suggest great variability in clearance, volume of distribution, and half-life in neonates, particularly premature neonates.[28,46,47] Some papers have advocated smaller and/or less frequent doses in neonates.[46,48,49] Doses of 0.5 mg/kg and dosing intervals >24 hours may be appropriate for these patients.[42,45,46] One study used an every-other-day dosing regimen with 0.5 mg/kg in neonates <1 kg or 1 mg/kg in neonates ≥1 kg.[50]
Dosage adjustment in organ dysfunction	Dose adjustment is not necessary in patients with renal insufficiency[7,51]; however, if renal insufficiency occurs during therapy, the dosing interval should be increased or alternate day dosing should be done prior to a decrease in the total daily dose.[7,51] Alternately, therapy may be changed to an amphotericin B lipid product.
Maximum dosage	Total daily dose should not exceed 1.5 mg/kg.[3,7] Doses of 1.5 mg/kg/day for an unspecified time[46] and 1.3 mg/kg/day for 31 days[36] have been used in children. Reported cumulative doses in pediatric patients have ranged from 2.5 to 52 mg/kg.[24,28-30,32-34,39,41-43,52]

Larger doses (>1 mg/kg) may be associated with increased risk of nephrotoxicity, which can present as oliguria, azotemia, increased SCr, potassium wasting, and renal tubular acidosis. Glomerular filtration rate was reduced permanently in *adults* who received >4 g over the course of therapy.[8,17,53] Pediatric patients have received total cumulative doses of 30–52 mg/kg without evidence of "permanent" nephrotoxicity.[30,32,33] Evidence does not support serum drug concentration or cumulative dose monitoring as a marker of toxicity.[54] (See Comments section.)

Three children who inadvertently received doses of 3.8, 4.6, or 5 mg/kg and two premature neonates who received 25 and 40.8 mg/kg experienced cardiac arrest during or shortly after the infusion. Only one child survived.[55] |
Additives	None.
Suitable diluents	D5W, D10W, D15W, or D20W.[12]
Maximum concentration	0.1 mg/mL.[3,12] The osmolality of this solution (0.1 mg/mL in D5W) is 256 mOsm/kg.[12] While one reference states that a concentration of 0.25 mg/mL may be given in fluid-restricted patients via a central catheter,[56] more concentrated solutions increase the risk of phlebitis.[57] Concentrations as high as 0.5–1 mg/mL have been found to be chemically stable for up to 120 hours when stored at 4°C.[58]
Preparation and delivery	**Filtration:** If in-line filtration is indicated, use filters with a pore size ≥1 micron.[12]

For PN compatibility information, please see Appendix D. |
IV push	No information available to support administration by this method.
Intermittent infusion	0.1 mg/mL in D5W, D10W, D15W, or D20W[12,59] over 2–6 hours.[12,17] Shorter infusion times (1–2 hours) have been tolerated in older children and *adults* and may improve drug delivery.[7]
Continuous infusion	No information available to support administration by this method.

Amphotericin B

Other routes of administration   Amphotericin B has also been given via IT route as well as intra-articularly, intrapleurally, and by irrigation.[12]

Comments   **Significant adverse effects:** Concomitant nephrotoxic drugs may increase the potential for nephrotoxicity.[49,51] Hydration and sodium repletion, either through sodium loading with NS over 30 minutes prior to administration or with sodium intakes of >4 mEq/kg/day, may reduce the risk of nephrotoxicity.[7,51,60] Because rifampin acts synergistically with amphotericin B, they have been given concomitantly to reduce the amphotericin B dose and, hence, the risk of nephrotoxicity.[61]

Hypokalemia and renal tubular acidosis may occur.[7]

Pharmacokinetic considerations: See Dosage section.

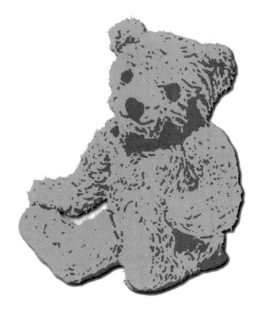

Amphotericin B Cholesteryl Sulfate Complex

Brand names	Amphotec
Medication error potential	ISMP high-alert medication that has an increased risk of causing significant patient harm if it is used in error (liposomal forms of drugs).[1] The product name and dosage should be verified prior to dispensing and administration.
Contraindications and warnings	Should not be used in patients with a hypersensitivity to any of the drug components.[2]
Infusion related cautions	Anaphylaxis has been reported.[2] Acute reactions (hypotension, fever, chills) may occur within 1–3 hours after administration. Infusion related reactions may be managed by decreasing the rate of infusion or by premedicating with antihistamines or corticosteroids.[2] Stop infusion immediately in cases of severe respiratory distress.[2]
Dosage	Amphotericin B cholesteryl sulfate complex has also been referred to as amphotericin B colloidal dispersion (ABCD) in clinical studies and case reports. **Systemic fungal infections (*Aspergillus* sp., *Candida* sp., and *Cryptococcus* sp.) in patients refractory or intolerant to conventional amphotericin B because of adverse effects, including nephrotoxicity** **Children and adolescents:** 3–6 mg/kg/day.[3-8] One study in premature neonates gave 3 mg/kg/day on day 1 followed by 5 mg/kg/day thereafter.[9] The manufacturer recommends administration of a test dose (10 mL of the final preparation containing between 1.6 and 8.3 mg) to be given over 15–30 minutes while observing the patient for tolerance.[2]
Dosage adjustment in organ dysfunction	No dosage adjustment recommended for hepatic or renal impairment (CrCl ≥35 mL/min). No information on dosage adjustment in more severe hepatic or renal disease.[2]
Maximum dosage	6 mg/kg/day.[3] However, doses as high as 7.5 mg/kg/day have been used.[2]
Additives	None.
Suitable diluents	Reconstitute with SW (5 mg/mL); dilute further with D5W.[2,10]
Maximum concentration	0.83 mg/mL.[2,10]

Amphotericin B Cholesteryl Sulfate Complex

Preparation and delivery	Do not mix lipid-based amphotericin B products with other IV medications or saline or coadminister with other parenteral solutions containing saline or electrolytes.[2,10]
	Do not filter or use an in-line filter during administration.[2,10]
IV push	Not recommended.[2]
Intermittent infusion	Dilute reconstituted drug with D5W to a final concentration of 0.6 mg/mL (range 0.16–0.83 mg/mL).[2,10] Infuse at a rate of 1 mg/kg/h.[2,10] May infuse over a minimum of 2 hours in patients exhibiting no adverse effects.[2,10]
Continuous infusion	No information available to support administration by this method.
Other routes of administration	No information available to support administration by other routes.
Comments	Hepatotoxicity has been reported.[2]
	There is some evidence that the colloidal dispersion formulation may be the least tolerable of the available amphotericin B lipid formulations.[11]

Amphotericin B Lipid Complex

Brand names	Abelcet
Medication error potential	ISMP high-alert medication that has an increased risk of causing significant patient harm if it is used in error (liposomal forms of drugs).[1]
	The product name and dosage should be verified prior to dispensing and administration.
	Look-alike, sound-alike error potential.
	USP reports that amphotericin B lipid complex has been confused with amphotericin B desoxycholate; no patient harm resulted.[2] ISMP reports that Abelcet has been confused with amphotericin B.[3] USP reports that Abelcet has been confused with Ambisome; patient harm and death resulted.[2]
Contraindications and warnings	Should not be used in patients with a hypersensitivity to any of the drug components.[4]
Infusion related cautions	Anaphylaxis has been reported.[4] Acute reactions (hypotension, fever, chills) may occur within 1–2 hours after administration.[4] Infusion related reactions may be managed by decreasing the rate of infusion or by premedicating with antihistamines or corticosteroids. Stop infusion immediately in cases of severe respiratory distress.[4]
	Chest discomfort has been reported.[5]
	Hypertension has been reported in an *adult*.[6]
Dosage	**Empiric treatment of febrile neutropenic patients:** 5 mg/kg/day has been studied in children 2–16 years of age.[5]
	Systemic fungal infections (*Aspergillus* sp., *Candida* sp., and *Cryptococcus* sp.) in patients refractory or intolerant to conventional amphotericin B because of adverse effects, including nephrotoxicity
	Neonates, infants, and children 2–17 years: 2.5–5 mg/kg/day.[4,7-11]
	One study in neonates gave up to 6.5 mg/kg/day.[12]
Dosage adjustment in organ dysfunction	The need for dosage adjustment with amphotericin B lipid complex in hepatic or renal impairment is not known.[4] Dosage adjustments have not been recommended for renal insufficiency.[13]
Maximum dosage	5 mg/kg/day.[4,7] However, doses as high as 6.5–13 mg/kg have been given to children and *adults*.[4,10,12,14,15]
Additives	Each mL contains 9 mg NaCl.[4,16]
Suitable diluents	D5W.[4,16]
Maximum concentration	2 mg/mL.[4,16]

Amphotericin B Lipid Complex

Preparation and delivery	Add desired dose of amphotericin B lipid complex, using the 5-micron filter needle supplied with each vial, to D5W to make a final concentration of 1–2 mg/mL (usual concentration is 1 mg/mL).[4,16]
	Do not mix lipid-based amphotericin B products with other IV medications, saline, or coadminister with other parenteral solutions containing saline or electrolytes.[4,16]
	Do not use an in-line filter during administration.[4,16]
	Shake bag thoroughly before infusion.[4,16]
IV push	Not recommended.[4,16]
Intermittent infusion	Infuse at a rate of 2.5 mg/kg/h. If >2 hours is required to administer a given dose, shake the bag to mix contents q 2 h.[4]
Continuous infusion	No information available to support administration by this method.
Other routes of administration	No information available to support administration by other routes.
Comments	Hepatotoxicity has been reported.[7]

Amphotericin B Liposomal

Brand names	AmBisome

Medication error potential

ISMP high-alert medication that has an increased risk of causing significant patient harm if it is used in error (liposomal forms of drugs).[1]

The product name and dosage should be verified prior to dispensing and administration.

Look-alike, sound-alike error potential.

USP reports that amphotericin B liposomal has been confused with amphotericin B; patient harm resulted.[2] ISMP reports that AmBisome has been confused with amphotericin B.[3] USP reports that AmBisome has been confused with Fungizone; no patient harm resulted.[2] USP also reports that AmBisome has been confused with Abelcet; patient harm resulted.[2]

Contraindications and warnings

Should not be used in patients with a hypersensitivity to any of the drug components.[4]

Infusion related cautions

Acute infusion related reactions (chest pain; dyspnea; hypoxia; severe abdomen, flank, or leg pain; and flushing and urticaria) may occur within the first 5 minutes of infusion and are not related to infusion rate. Use diphenhydramine and infusion interruption to manage these acute reactions. Acute reactions (hypotension, fever and chills) that occur with conventional amphotericin B may still occur within 1–2 hours after the administration of liposomal amphotericin B, but with decreased frequency.[4-6]

Anaphylaxis has been reported. Stop infusion immediately in cases of severe anaphylactic reaction.[4]

Dosage

Empiric treatment of febrile neutropenic patients

Children and adolescents: 3 mg/kg/day.[7,8]

Solid bone marrow transplant prophylaxis/treatment

Children and adolescents: 2–6 mg/kg/day over a mean of 25 days (range 5–90 days).[9-12]

10 mg/kg once weekly may provide useful prophylaxis against fungal infections as described in 14 children (4.5 months to 9 years of age) undergoing hematopoietic stem cell transplant.[13]

Systemic fungal infections (*Aspergillus* sp., *Candida* sp., and *Cryptococcus* sp.) in patients refractory or intolerant to conventional amphotericin B because of adverse effects, including nephrotoxicity

Neonates (term and preterm), infants, children, and adolescents: 3–5 mg/kg/day.[14-25]

Doses in neonates have been reported as high as 7 mg/kg/day.[20-22] Up to 10 mg/kg/day in pediatric patients and 15 mg/kg/day in *adults* has been found to be well-tolerated and effective for treatment of aspergillosis and other filamentous fungal infections.[4,26]

Visceral leishmaniasis

Immunocompetent children and adolescents[4,27-29]: 3 mg/kg/day on days 1–5 and on days 14 and 21 of therapy. Alternatively, 4 mg/kg has been given on days 1–5 and on day 10 of therapy. Mediterranean visceral leishmaniasis has been successfully treated with 20 mg/kg given either as 4 mg/kg for 5 days or 10 mg/kg for 2 days.[29]

Immunocompromised children and adolescents[4]: 4 mg/kg/day on days 1–5 and on days 10, 17, 24, 31, and 38 of therapy.

Amphotericin B Liposomal

Dosage adjustment in organ dysfunction	The need for dosage adjustment in hepatic impairment is not known. It has been given successfully to patients with pre-existing renal impairment.[4]
Maximum dosage	10 mg/kg/day in children; 15 mg/kg/day in *adults*.[4,26]
Additives	Each vial contains 0.64 mg alpha tocopherol.[4,30]
Suitable diluents	The manufacturer recommends dilution in D5W.[4] Another reference reports stability in D5W, D10W, D20W, and D25W.[30]
Maximum concentration	2 mg/mL.[4,30]
Preparation and delivery	**Preparation:** After reconstituting with SW and shaking vigorously, add desired dose of liposomal amphotericin B, using the 5-micron filter needle provided with each vial, to suitable diluent to make a final concentration of 1–2 mg/mL (more dilute concentrations of 0.2–0.5 mg/mL may also be used).[4,30] **Stability:** Administration should begin within 6 hours of dilution per the manufacturer.[4] **Delivery:** Do not mix lipid-based amphotericin B products with other IV medications or saline or coadminister with other parenteral solutions containing saline or electrolytes.[18] An in-line filter that is ≥1 micron may be used.[4,20]
IV push	Not recommended.[4]
Intermittent infusion	Infuse over 2 hours. May infuse over 1 hour in patients exhibiting no adverse effects.[4,30]
Continuous infusion	No information available to support administration by this method.
Other routes of administration	No information available to support administration by other routes.
Comments	Hepatotoxicity has been reported.[14] Hyperphosphatemia has been reported with liposomal amphotericin in patients receiving standard doses (5 mg/kg/day, n = 2) as well as high dose therapy (10–25 mg/kg/day, n = 3). Underlying renal insufficiency may play a role. The phospholipid carrier is the presumed source of the phosphate. Liposomal amphotericin B provides 37 mg inorganic phosphate per 50 mg amphotericin, whereas amphotericin B lipid complex, provides 6.8 mg per 50 mg drug.[31,32] Systemic liposomal amphotericin B in combination with liposomal amphotericin B central venous catheter lock therapy (3-mL solution of 8 mg drug in D5W with 200 units heparin) has successfully treated fungal central venous catheter infections in pediatric patients (6 months to 7 years of age).[33]

Ampicillin Sodium

Brand names	Multiple generics available

Medication error potential

Look-alike, sound-alike drug names.

USP reports confusion with aminophylline, augmentin, cefazolin, nafcillin, oxacillin, penicillin G sodium, piperacillin, and Unasyn.[1] Confusion with Unasyn has resulted in patient harm.[1]

Contraindications and warnings

Contraindications: Hypersensitivity to ampicillin or other penicillins or any component of the formulation.[2]

Warnings: Serious hypersensitivity and occasionally fatal anaphylactic reactions have been reported.[2] These are more likely in patients who are sensitive to multiple allergens (e.g., asthma) and in those with a history of Type I reaction to penicillin or cephalosporins. [2] (See Appendix C for specific information.)

Prolonged use may cause superinfection and/or *Clostridium difficile*–associated diarrhea (CDAD), which has been reported and may range in severity from mild diarrhea to fatal colitis.[2] If CDAD is suspected or confirmed, appropriate fluid and electrolyte management, protein supplementation, antibiotic treatment of *C. difficile,* and surgical evaluation should be instituted as clinically indicated.[2]

Infusion related cautions

If a decision is made to give this medication to a patient with known penicillin hypersensitivity, the patient should be closely observed for allergenicity. Although rare, anaphylactoid reactions may require immediate emergency treatment with epinephrine, oxygen, IV steroids, antihistamines, pressor amines, and airway management.

Dosage

Neonates

PNA	≤1200 g	1200–2000 g	≥2000 g
<7 days	25–50 mg/kg/day divided q 12 h[3,4]*	50–100 mg/kg/day divided q 12 h[4,5]	75–150 mg/kg/day divided q 8–12 h[4,5]
≥7 days		75–150 mg/kg/day divided q 8–12 h[4,5]	100–200 mg/kg/day divided q 6 h[4,5]

*Until 4 weeks of age.

Infants and children

    Mild-to-moderate infections: 100–150 mg/kg/day divided q 6 h up to 4 g/day.[4]

    Severe infections: 200–400 mg/kg/day divided q 6 h up to 12 g/day.[4]

Dosage *(cont.)*	**Bacterial endocarditis (prophylaxis)**

Dental, oral, respiratory tract, or esophageal procedures*: 50 mg/kg (up to 2 g) given as a single dose 30 minutes before a procedure.[6] Only for patients with underlying cardiac conditions associated with the highest risk of adverse outcome. (See Comments section.)

*that involve manipulation of gingival tissue or the periapical region of teeth or perforation of the oral mucosa[6]

Genitourinary and gastrointestinal procedures: Prophylactic antibiotics solely to prevent endocarditis is not recommended.[6] Patients with underlying cardiac conditions associated with the highest risk of adverse outcome (see Comments section), and who have *established* GI or GU tract infection or those receiving antibiotics to prevent wound infection or sepsis associated with a GI or GU procedure, may receive a single dose of antibiotic (e.g., penicillin, ampicillin, piperacillin, or vancomycin). The recommend ampicillin dose is 50 mg/kg (up to 2 g) within 30 minutes before a procedure.[6]

Bacterial endocarditis (treatment)

Enterococcal endocarditis (sensitive to penicillin, gentamicin and vancomycin): 300 mg/kg/day divided q 4–6 h plus gentamicin 3 mg/kg/day divided q 8 h.[7] If symptom ≤3 months treat for 4 weeks and if >3 months treat for 6 weeks.[7]

Enterococcus faecalis (resistant to penicillin, gentamicin and vancomycin): Imipenem/cilastatin 60–100 mg/kg/day divided q 6 h or ceftriaxone 100 mg/kg/day divided q 12 h plus ampicillin 300 mg/kg/day divided q 4–6 h for 4–6 weeks.[7]

Meningitis

≤1200 g: 100 mg/kg/day divided q 12 h.[3]

≤7 days and >1200 g: 100–300 mg/kg/day divided q 8–12 h.[4,8,9]

>7–28 days and ≥1200 g: 150–300 mg/kg/day divided q 6–8 h.[4,8,9]

Infants and children: 200–400 mg/kg/day divided q 6 h up to 6–12 g/day.[8-14]

Dosage adjustment in organ dysfunction	If CrCl is 10–29 mL/min, give normal dose q 8–12 h, and if CrCl <10 mL/min, give normal dose q 12 h.[15]
Maximum dosage	400 mg/kg/day,[2,16,17] not to exceed 8 g of ampicillin/day.[2,16,17]
Additives	2.9–3.1 mEq sodium/g of ampicillin.[18]
Suitable diluents	LR, NS, D5W, D5½NS, or SW.[2,18]
Maximum concentration	100 mg/mL in NS or 200 mg/mL in SW for central line administration[2,17,18] and 50 mg/mL[19] and up to 112 mg/mL in SW for peripheral line administration in fluid restricted patients.[17,18]

Ampicillin Sodium

Preparation and delivery	**Delivery system issues:** The mixing of ampicillin with an aminoglycoside in vitro can result in substantial inactivation of the aminoglycoside.[2] (See Appendix C for more specific information.) **Stability:** IM or direct IV products should be used within 1 hour; if dextrose is used as a diluent the resulting solution is only stable for 2 hours vs. 8 hours if prepared with NS.[17] **Compatibility:** For PN compatibility information, please see Appendix D.[20]
IV push	Has been given over 3–5 minutes.[2,17] More rapid administration is not recommended due to seizures.[2,17]
Intermittent infusion	≤30 mg/mL and dose >500 mg over 10–15 minutes.[17,18]
Continuous infusion	Not recommended.
Other routes of administration	≤250 mg/mL in SW or BW has been given IM but must be used within 1 hour.[17,18]
Comments	**Rare adverse events:** In a study of 14 very low birth weight neonates (<750 g and <28 weeks gestational age), the authors concluded that 50 mg/kg q 18–24 h sufficiently killed bacteria while reducing the risk of ampicillin-associated seizures.[21,22] Neurotoxic (e.g., lethargy, confusion, twitching, multifocal myoclonus, localized, or generalized epileptiform seizures) may occur with large doses, especially in patients with renal insufficiency.[2,23] A high percentage (43% to 100%) of patients with infectious mononucleosis develop a maculopapular, trunk skin rash that spreads while receiving ampicillin.[2,24] The rash generally appears 7–10 days after the start of ampicillin and persist for a few days to a week following drug discontinuation.[2] It is not known whether these patients are truly allergic to ampicillin, but the drug is not recommended in patients with mononucleosis. **Monitoring:** AST (SGOT) and ALT (SGPT) values should be obtained periodically during therapy to monitor for possible liver function abnormalities.[2] **Drug interactions:** Concurrent use of tetracycline should be avoided as it may antagonize the bactericidal effect of penicillin.[2] Probenecid may decrease the tubular secretion of ampicillin and increase its concentration in the serum. Consult appropriate resources for dosing recommendations before combining any drug with ampicillin. **Laboratory interference:** Ampicillin may cause false-positive urinary glucose results when cupric sulfate solution-based tests (Clinitest, Benedict's solution, Fehling's solution) are used.[2] It is recommended that glucose tests (Diastix, TEST-TAPE, Clinistix) based on enzymatic glucose oxidase reactions be used.[2] **Other:** Cardiac conditions associated with the highest risk of adverse outcome from endocarditis for which prophylaxis with dental procedures is reasonable: (1) prosthetic cardiac valve or prosthetic material used for cardiac valve repair; (2) previous IE; (3) congenital heart disease (CHD)* in a person with a) unrepaired cyanotic CHD, including palliative shunts and conduits, b) completely repaired congenital heart defect with prosthetic material or device, whether placed by surgery or by catheter intervention, during the first 6 months after the procedure,† or c) repaired CHD with residual defects at the site or adjacent to the site of a prosthetic patch or prosthetic device (which inhibit endothelialization); and (4) cardiac transplantation recipients who develop cardiac valvulopathy.[6]

---

*Except for the conditions listed above, antibiotic prophylaxis is no longer recommended for any other form of CHD.

†Prophylaxis is reasonable because endothelialization of prosthetic material occurs within 6 months after the procedure.

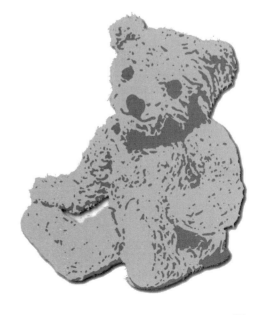

Ampicillin Sodium–Sulbactam Sodium

Brand names	Unasyn

Medication error potential

Look-alike, sound-alike drug names.

USP reports confusion of with aminophylline, ampicillin, Augmentin, cefazolin, nafcillin, oxacillin, penicillin G sodium, and piperacillin.[1] Unasyn has been confused with ampicillin, Levaquin, and Zosyn. Confusion with ampicillin has resulted in patient harm.[1]

Contraindications and warnings

Contraindications: Hypersensitivity to any of the penicillins.[2]

Warnings: Serious hypersensitivity and occasionally fatal anaphylactic reactions have been reported.[2] These are more likely in patients who are sensitive to multiple allergens (e.g., asthma) and in those with a history of Type I reaction to penicillin or cephalosporins.[2] (See Appendix C for specific information.)

Prolonged use may cause superinfection and/or *Clostridium difficile* associated diarrhea (CDAD), which has been reported and may range in severity from mild diarrhea to fatal colitis.[2] If CDAD is suspected or confirmed, appropriate fluid and electrolyte management, protein supplementation, antibiotic treatment of *C. difficile,* and surgical evaluation should be instituted as clinically indicated.[2]

Infusion related cautions

If a decision is made to give this medication to a patient with known penicillin hypersensitivity, the patient should be closely observed for allergenicity. Although rare, anaphylactoid reactions may require immediate emergency treatment with epinephrine, oxygen, IV steroids, antihistamines, pressor amines, and airway management.

Thrombophlebitis and pain at the injection site may occur.[2]

Dosage

Dosage based on *ampicillin* component.[2] 1.5 g contains 1 g of ampicillin and 0.5 g of sulbactam. Sulbactam is a beta-lactamase inhibitor that extends the spectrum of ampicillin but has little antibacterial activity.[2]

The American Academy of Pediatrics and manufacturer suggest that use be restricted to those >1 year of age.[2,3] Pediatric patients who weigh ≥40 kg may receive the usual *adult* dose.[2]

Mild-to-moderate infections: 100–150 mg/kg/day of ampicillin divided q 6 h.[3-6]

Severe infections: 200–400 mg/kg/day of ampicillin divided q 6 h.[3,7-13]

Bacterial endocarditis (treatment)

> **Culture negative and native valve:** 300 mg/kg/day of ampicillin divided q 4–6 h plus gentamicin (3 mg/kg/day divided q 8 h) for 4–6 weeks.[14]

> **Enterococcal endocarditis (resistant to penicillin and susceptible to aminoglycoside and vancomycin):** 300 mg/kg/day of ampicillin divided q 6 h plus gentamicin (3 mg/kg/day divided q 8 h) for 6 weeks.[14]

> **HACEK* microorganisms:** 300 mg/kg/day of ampicillin divided q 4–6 h.[14] Treat for 4 weeks unless prosthetic material is present then treat for 6 weeks.[14]

Ampicillin Sodium–Sulbactam Sodium

Dosage *(cont.)*	**Epiglottitis:** 100–200 mg/kg/day of ampicillin divided q 6 h.[15] **Meningitis:** 300–400 mg/kg/day of ampicillin divided q 4–6 h.[16,17] **Peritonsillar and retropharyngeal abscess:** 200 mg/kg/day of ampicillin divided q 6 h.[15] **Perioperative prophylaxis:** Although ampicillin–sulbactam has been used to reduce the incidence of infections in patients undergoing contaminated or potentially contaminated surgery,[18] other antibiotics are generally preferred.
Dosage adjustment in organ dysfunction	If CrCl is 10–29 mL/min give normal dose q 8–12 h, and if CrCl <10 mL/min, give normal dose q 12 h.[19]
Maximum dosage	400 mg/kg/day[3] up to 8 g/day of ampicillin.[2] Total daily sulbactam dose should not exceed 4 g.[2]
Additives	1.5 g ampicillin contains 115 mg (5 mEq) of sodium.[20]
Suitable diluents	D5½NS, D5W, NS, SW, LR.[18]
Maximum concentration	30 mg/mL for IV and 250 mg/mL for IM administration.[2]
Preparation and delivery	**Delivery system issues:** The mixing of ampicillin with an aminoglycoside in vitro can result in substantial inactivation of the aminoglycoside.[2] (See Appendix C for more specific information.) **Stability:** 20 mg/mL of ampicillin in D5W is stable at room temperature for 2 hours and 30 mg/mL in NS, SW, and LR is stable at room temperature for 8 hours.[2,20] 2 mg/mL in D5½NS is stable at room temperature for 4 hours.[2,20] 250 mg/mL of ampicillin in SW or lidocaine 0.5% to 2% for IM administration should be used within 1 hour.[2] **Compatibility:** See Appendix D for PN compatibility information.[21]
IV push	Ampicillin can be administered over 3–5 minutes, but more rapid administration is not recommended due to seizures.[2,15]
Intermittent infusion	≤30 mg/mL over 10–15 minutes[2,20] and larger dilutions of 50–100 mL given over 15–30 minutes.[2,20]
Continuous infusion	Not administered by this method.
Other routes of administration	250 mg/mL of ampicillin can be administered IM in SW or lidocaine 0.5% to 2% within 1 hour of reconstitution.[2,20] The safety and efficacy via IM administration in pediatric patients have not been established.[2]

Ampicillin Sodium–Sulbactam Sodium

Comments

Rare adverse events: Fourteen neonates (<750 g and <28 weeks gestational age) who received 50 mg/kg q 18–24 h had sufficient killing of bacteria while reducing the risk of ampicillin-associated seizures.[22] Neurotoxic (e.g., lethargy, confusion, twitching, multifocal myoclonus, localized or generalized epileptiform seizures) may occur with large doses, especially in patients with renal insufficiency.[2,23]

Urticaria, erythema multiforme, and an occasional case of exfoliative dermatitis have been reported. A high percentage (43% to 100%) of patients with infectious mononucleosis develop a maculopapular, trunk skin rash that spreads while receiving ampicillin.[2,24] The rash generally appears 7 to 10 days after the start of ampicillin and persists for a few days to a week after discontinuation.[2] It is not known whether these patients are truly allergic to ampicillin, but the drug is not recommended in patients with mononucleosis.

Monitoring: AST (SGOT) and ALT (SGPT) values should be obtained periodically during therapy to monitor for possible liver function abnormalities.[2]

Drug interactions: Concurrent use of tetracycline should be avoided as it may antagonize the bactericidal effect of penicillin.[2] Probenecid may decrease the tubular secretion of ampicillin and sulbactam and increase its concentration in the serum. Consult appropriate resources for dosing recommendations before combining any drug with ampicillin-sulbactam.

Laboratory interference: Ampicillin may cause false-positive urinary glucose results when cupric sulfate solution-based tests (Clinitest, Benedict's solution, Fehling's solution) are used.[2] It is recommended that glucose tests (Diastix, TEST-TAPE, Clinistix) based on enzymatic glucose oxidase reactions be used.[2] Some individuals have developed positive direct Coombs' test during treatment.[2]

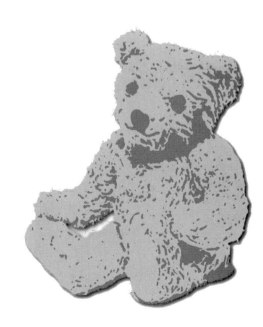

Anidulafungin

Brand names	Eraxis
Medication error potential	None reported by ISMP or USP.[1-3]
Contraindications and warnings	**Contraindications:** Patients with known hypersensitivity to the drug or any of its components.[4] **Warnings:** Clinically significant hepatic abnormalities (hepatic dysfunction, hepatitis and hepatic failure) may occur.[4]
Infusion related cautions	Histamine-mediated symptoms (rash, urticaria, flushing, pruritus, dyspnea, and hypotension) have been reported. These symptoms occur infrequently if infusion rate is ≤1 mg/min.[4] A 16-year-old developed moderate facial erythema and rash at the start of anidulafungin infusion that resolved within 1.5 hours of stopping the infusion. These symptoms did not recur with repeat infusion and continuation of therapy.[5]

Dosage	Experience with anidulafungin in children, particularly neonates, is limited[6]; currently there is no established dose range for pediatric patients.[7]
	
	Children 2–17 years (treatment/prophylaxis)
	
	    Loading dose[5,6]: 1.5 mg/kg (not to exceed 100 mg) or 3 mg/kg (not to exceed 200 mg).
	
	    Maintenance dose[5,6]: 0.75 mg/kg (not to exceed 50 mg) or 1.5 mg/kg (not to exceed 100 mg) given once daily.
	
	The above dosage regimens were found to produce similar concentrations as that seen in *adults* receiving maintenance therapy with 50 or 100 mg/day.[5]

Dosage adjustment in organ dysfunction	No dosage adjustment in renal or hepatic dysfunction.[4,8]
Maximum dosage	**Loading dose**[4,5]: 200 mg/day in children and *adults*. **Maintenance dose**[4,5]: 100 mg/day in children and *adults*.
Additives	None.
Suitable diluents	D5W or NS.[4,9]
Maximum concentration	0.43 mg/mL.[4,9]
Preparation and delivery	The anidulafungin powder is insoluble in water and slightly soluble in ethanol. Reconstitute with companion diluent (15 mL or 30 mL 20% w/w Dehydrated Alcohol in Water for Injection), then further dilute with D5W or NS to a concentration of 0.36–0.43 mg/mL.[4,9]

IV push	Not recommended.
Intermittent infusion	Infuse over 45 minutes to 3 hours at a rate not to exceed 1.1 mg/min.[4,5,9]
Continuous infusion	No information available to support administration via this method.
Other routes of administration	No information available to support administration by other routes.
Comments	Anidulafungin has been given empirically to neutropenic children (2–17 years) for 1–23 days (mean 8.7 days); none of the children developed a fungal infection.[5] The most common adverse drug effects were fever, feeling abnormal, rash/erythema, increased BUN, and hypotension. Most adverse effects in children receiving larger doses occurred in children <11 years of age.[5]

Argatroban

Brand names	Generic

Medication error potential	ISMP high-alert medication that has an increased risk of causing significant patient harm if it is used in error.[1]
	Look-alike, sound-alike error potential.
	ISMP and USP report that argatroban was confused with Aggrastat; no patient harm resulted.[2,3] ISMP also reports that argatroban was confused with Orgaran; no patient harm resulted.[2]

Contraindications and warnings	Use with caution in patients with diseases that have an increased risk for hemorrhage.[4,5]
	All parenteral anticoagulants should be discontinued before use of argatroban.[6]

Infusion related cautions	Allergic reactions have been reported, and they were primarily in patients receiving other antithrombotic therapy or contrast media.[4]

Dosage	**Children**[6-8]
	Prophylaxis or treatment of thrombosis: Infusion rates ranged from 0.1–12 mcg/kg/min (usually <6 mcg/kg/min) with doses titrated to aPTT >50 seconds (2 × baseline) (n = 14, six were <6 months of age).
	Hemodialysis or ECMO: Infusion rates ranged from 0.1–24 mcg/kg/min (usually <6 mcg/kg/min) titrated to ACT of ≥160 up to 200 seconds for anticoagulation during hemodialysis or ECMO (n = 17).
	Cardiac catheterization: 150 or 250 mcg/kg bolus followed by infusion rates of 7.5–15 mcg/kg/min titrated to an ACT of 300 (n = 5).
	Seriously ill children who required anticoagulation and who have heparin-induced thrombocytopenia (HIT) or suspected HIT[4]: 0.75 mcg/kg/min initially titrated by making incremental changes of 0.1–0.25 mcg/kg/min to aPTT of 1.5 – 3 × baseline.
	***Adults* with HIT**[4,5]
	Prophylaxis or treatment of thrombosis: 2 mcg/kg/min with the infusion adjusted up to 10 mcg/kg/min to steady-state aPTT of 1.5–3 × baseline value (≤100 seconds).

Dosage adjustment in organ dysfunction	No dosage adjustment is needed for impaired renal function.[4,5]
	Impaired hepatic function: 0.2 mcg/kg/min initially titrated to aPTT of 1.5 – 3 × baseline making incremental changes of ≤0.05 mcg/kg/minutes.[4,5]

Maximum dosage	In *adults,* 10 mcg/kg/min for HIT or 40 mcg/kg/min for percutaneous coronary interventions to maintain an ACT of ≥300 and ≤450 seconds.[5,6]
	A 5-month-old required 15 mcg/kg/min to reach a target ACT of 300 seconds during cardiac catheterization.[6] A 15-month-old on ECMO required 24 mcg/kg/min to attain an aPTT 2 × baseline; the rate subsequently stabilized at 13–15 mcg/kg/min.[9] (See Comments section.)

Additives	None.

Argatroban

Suitable diluents	NS, D5W, LR.[4,5,10]
Maximum concentration	1 mg/mL.[4,5,10]
Preparation and delivery	The IV solution may appear hazy after dilution. The solution should clear with continued mixing.[4,5,10]
IV push	Over 3–5 minutes (loading dose in *adults*).[4,5]
Intermittent infusion	Infused for the length of percutaneous coronary intervention or cardiac catheterization.[4,5]
Continuous infusion	May be infused continuously.[5,7,9]
Other routes of administration	Not indicated.
Comments	The eighth edition of the *Antithrombotic and Thrombolytic Therapy Guidelines* of the American College of Chest Physicians' notes that danaparoid sodium, hirudin, and argatroban are alternatives to heparin in the treatment of children with HIT.[11]

Arginine HCl

Brand names	R-Gene 10
Medication error potential	None noted.
Contraindications and warnings	**Older children (growth hormone reserve test):** Infuse via antecubital or other suitable vein.[1,4] **Infants (hyperammonemia):** Infuse via central venous line.[1] Do not use in patients with allergic tendencies. Antihistamines should be available in the event an allergic reaction occurs.[1] Anaphylactic reactions have been reported in two children.[2,3]
Infusion related cautions	Flushing, nausea, vomiting, numbness, headache, and local venous irritation are associated with rapid infusion.[1] (See Comments section.)

Dosage	**Growth hormone reserve test (pituitary function test):** 500 mg/kg not to exceed 30 g (*adult* dose = 300 mL or 30 g) over 30 minutes.[1,4-6]
	
	Hyperammonemia (inborn errors of urea synthesis): Arginine is used with sodium benzoate and sodium phenylacetate.[7-9]
	
	    Argininosuccinic acid lyase or argininosuccinic acid synthetase deficiency: Loading dose of 600 mg/kg (12 g/m^2) infused over 90 minutes followed by 600 mg/kg/day (12 g/m^2/day) as a continuous infusion.
	
	    Carbamyl phosphate synthetase or ornithine transcarbamylase deficiency: Loading dose of 200 mg/kg (4 g/m^2) followed by 200 mg/kg/day (4 g/m^2/day) as a continuous infusion.
	
	Other uses
	
	    Severe metabolic alkalosis: After sodium and potassium chloride supplementation have failed (serum pH >7.55).[1,10] Estimate deficit/dosage by
	
	    dose (g) = [desired decrease in plasma bicarbonate (mEq/L) × weight (kg)] ÷ 9.6.[1]
	
	    Pulmonary hypertension: 500 mg/kg over 30 minutes.[11-13]

Dosage adjustment in organ dysfunction	Arginine should be used with caution in patients with renal insufficiency.[1] (See Comments section.)
Maximum dosage	30 g.[1]
Additives	Contains 0.475 mEq/mL of chloride.[1] (See Comments section.)
Suitable diluents	**Hyperammonemia:** D10W.[16]
Maximum concentration	100 mg/mL (commercially available).[1] This solution is hypertonic (950 mOsm/L).[1]

Preparation and delivery	The dose (600 mg/kg) can be diluted in 25–35 mL D10W.[16]
IV push	Not recommended.[1] (See Infusion related cautions section.)
Intermittent infusion	**Growth hormone reserve test:** Over 30 minutes.[1,4,5] **Inborn errors of metabolism:** Over 90–120 minutes.[1,7,16]
Continuous infusion	Can be infused continuously for treatment of hyperammonemia.
Other routes of administration	Not indicated.
Comments	**Adverse effects:** Because of the high chloride content, those with electrolyte abnormalities may experience hyperkalemia.[1] Two patients with severe hepatic disease and moderate renal insufficiency developed hyperkalemia following treatment for metabolic alkalosis with L-arginine.[14] Despite aggressive treatment, one of these died.[14] Four *adults* with chronic renal failure on hemodialysis underwent an evaluation of growth hormone metabolism and developed significant hyperkalemia.[15] Those being treated for hyperammonemia may experience hyperchloremic metabolic acidosis. Serum concentrations of chloride and bicarbonate should be monitored to determine the need for bicarbonate therapy.[1] Extravasation, causing tissue necrosis, has been reported in three children (ages 3.5–7 years) who received a 10% solution.[17,18] Hypotension, within 10 minutes of drug administration, was reported in 11 children (9.4 ± 4.1 years) receiving 500 mg/kg of arginine for pituitary function testing. Blood pressure returned to normal within 30 minutes.[6] A 21-month-old girl inadvertently received 3.9 g/kg (300 mL of 10% arginine) over 30 minutes. She experienced gasping respirations and immediate cardiopulmonary arrest with acute metabolic acidosis and transient hyponatremia. Thirty-six hours later, she experienced fatal central pontine and extrapontine myelinolysis.[19]

Asparaginase

Brand names	Elspar

Medication error potential

ISMP high-alert medication that has an increased risk of causing significant patient harm if it is used in error.[1]

Look-alike, sound-alike error potential.

USP reports that asparaginase was confused with pegaspargase; no patient harm resulted.[2]

USP also reports that Elspar has been confused with Oncaspar; no patient harm resulted.[2]

Contraindications and warnings

US boxed warning: Asparaginase should be administered under the supervision of an experienced physician. The drug is highly toxic; special handling precautions should be in place.[3,4]

Contraindications: Asparaginase is contraindicated in patients with serious allergic reactions to asparaginase or other E-coli derived L-asparaginases, and serious thrombosis, pancreatitis, or serious hemorrhagic event with previous asparaginase use.[3]

Other warnings: Asparaginase carries a warning about the severity and incidence of anaphylaxis.[3] The following administration parameters are associated with an increased risk of hypersensitivity reactions: IV administration, dosages >6000–12,000 units/m^2, previous regimens containing asparaginase, and intermittent therapy.[5]

Asparaginase has also been associated with coagulopathy, hyperglycemia, pancreatitis, hepatic dysfunction, tumor lysis syndrome, and thrombosis.[3,4]

Infusion related cautions

Has been associated with serious anaphylaxis.[3] (See Contraindications and warnings section.)

When administering asparaginase, emergency treatment, including IV diphenhydramine, epinephrine, and hydrocortisone with a freely running IV in place, should be available.[4] Patients should be monitored for 30–60 minutes following administration and the drug should not be administered at night.[4]

Dosage

Consult institutional protocol for complete dosing information.

Asparaginase is used as a component of combination therapy to treat childhood acute lymphocytic leukemia (ALL).[3] To reduce the incidence of adverse effects, asparaginase should be administered after other chemotherapeutic agents, specifically vincristine and prednisone.

Test dose: Hypersensitivity reactions commonly occur and intradermal testing is recommended in all patients prior to asparaginase therapy.[4,5] Inject 0.1 mL of a 20-units/mL solution (2 units) intradermally and observe injection site for 1 hour.[4,5] A wheal or erythema represents a positive reaction; false negative reactions may occur.[4,5]

Patients with a positive skin test may undergo desensitization therapy if the benefits of therapy outweigh the risks. One desensitization protocol recommends 1 unit of asparaginase IV that is doubled q 10 min until the total amount of the daily total dosage has been met (provided no adverse events occur).[4]

Induction therapy (combination therapy)

> **IV:** 1000 units/kg/day for 10 days.[5-7]

> **IM:** 6000 units/m^2/dose given every third day for 3 weeks.[3,8,9] A high dose of 25,000 units/m^2 has also been administered once weekly for 9 weeks.[10]

Induction therapy (monotherapy—not recommended if patient can tolerate combination therapy): 200 units/kg/day for 28 days.[5,11]

Maintenance therapy: Not recommended.[3]

Asparaginase

Dosage adjustment in organ dysfunction	Asparaginase has been associated with hepatic dysfunction. However, no dosage adjustments have been recommended with any pre-existing organ dysfunction, including hepatic.[3]
Maximum dosage	Not established.
Additives	None.
Suitable diluents	Reconstitute with SW, NS; further dilute during administration with a running IV of D5W or NS.[3,12]
Maximum concentration	2000 units/mL (IV) and 5000 units/mL (IM).[3,12]
Preparation and delivery	**For IV administration:** The volume recommended for reconstitution is 5 mL suitable diluent to the 10,000 unit vial. Ordinary shaking during reconstitution does not inactivate the enzyme.[3] **For IM administration:** The volume recommended for reconstitution is 2 mL NS to the 10,000 unit vial.[3] Use within 8 hours and only if solution is clear.[3] Gelatinous fiber-like particles may develop after reconstitution; administration with a 5-micron filter will remove any particles without loss of potency.[3] When handling asparaginase (during preparation and administration), avoid inhaling aerosols or dust or contact with the mucous membranes or skin.[3]
IV push	Not recommended.[3,12]
Intermittent infusion	Administer over at least 30 minutes with a running infusion of D5W or NS.[3,12]
Continuous infusion	Intermittent infusion or IM administration are preferred routes of administration. Continuous infusions of asparaginase have been reported.[13]
Other routes of administration	May be given via IM administration. (See Preparation and delivery section.) Do not exceed 2 mL at each injection site.[3] Two injection sites should be used if the volume of required dose is >2 mL. IM administration is associated with a lower incidence of anaphylaxis compared to IV administration.[3,14] IT and intraventricular administration of asparaginase have been reported in patients with CNS lymphoblastic leukemia.[15,16] However, these routes have not demonstrated superiority over conventional treatments.
Comments	**Monitoring:** Vital signs during administration, CBC with platelets, urinalysis, liver function, coagulation, renal function, glucose level (urine and blood), and uric acid.[3,4] **Drug interactions:** Use caution when administering with dexamethasone as this may increase serum levels of dexamethasone.[3,4,17]

Asparaginase–pegylated (Pegaspargase)

Brand names	Oncaspar
Medication error potential	ISMP high-alert medication that has an increased risk of causing significant patient harm if it is used in error.[1] Look-alike, sound-alike error potential. USP reports that pegaspargase was confused with asparaginase; no patient harm resulted.[2] USP also reports that Oncaspar was confused with Elspar; no patient harm resulted.[2]
Contraindications and warnings	**Contraindications:** Pegaspargase is contraindicated in patients with serious allergic reactions to pegaspargase and in patients with serious thrombosis, pancreatitis, or serious hemorrhagic event with previous asparaginase therapy.[3] **Warnings:** May cause serious hypersensitivity reactions (see Infusion related cautions section) coagulopathy, glucose intolerance, pancreatitis, and thrombotic events.[3,4] Discontinue therapy if pancreatitis or thrombosis occur.[3]
Infusion related cautions	May cause anaphylaxis or serious allergic reactions; discontinue therapy if severe hypersensitivity occurs.[3] Due to risk of hypersensitivity reaction, IV diphenhydramine, epinephrine, hydrocortisone, and a freely running IV should be in place when administering pegaspargase.[4] Patients should be monitored for 60 minutes following administration and the drug should not be administered at night.
Dosage	Consult institutional protocol for complete dosing information. Pegaspargase is used as a component of combination therapy to treat first line acute lymphocytic leukemia (ALL) and to treat ALL in patients who are hypersensitive to the native forms of L-asparaginase (Elspar).[3] It may also be used in blast crisis of chronic lymphocytic leukemia (CLL) and salvage therapy of non-Hodgkin's lymphoma, although use has not been established.[4] A test dose is not required with pegaspargase as there is less risk for hypersensitivity reactions compared to L-asparaginase.[5] **Children >1 year and _adults_:** 2500 International Units/m^2/dose q 14 days.[3,5,6] Induction therapy with weekly doses of pegaspargase 2500 International Units/m^2 IM q 7 days, with or without intensification therapy (an additional 2500 International Units/m^2 IM dose), has also been studied, although the use of these regimens is not established.[7-9]
Dosage adjustment in organ dysfunction	Not established.
Maximum dosage	Not established. Three _adult_ patients received IV infusions of 10,000 International Units/m^2 with no major adverse events.[3]
Additives	Contains 8.5 mg NaCl per mL.[3]
Suitable diluents	D5W, NS.[3]

Asparaginase–pegylated (Pegaspargase)

Maximum concentration	Not established.
Preparation and delivery	**Preparation:** Pegaspargase may be a contact irritant. Professionals should wear gloves while handling and administering and should avoid inhalation of pegaspargase. If contact occurs with eyes, skin, or mucous membranes, wash with water for at least 15 minutes.[3,5,6] **Stability:** Freezing destroys the activity of pegaspargase; do not use if the product has been frozen.[3]
IV push	Not recommended.
Intermittent infusion	Administer over 1–2 hours in 100 mL of D5W or NS through an infusion already running.[3]
Continuous infusion	Not recommended.
Other routes of administration	IM administration is the preferred route of administration. Do not exceed 2 mL at each injection site. Two injection sites should be used if the volume of required dose is >2 mL.[3]
Comments	Monitor vital signs during administration, CBC with platelets, urinalysis, liver function, coagulation, renal function, glucose level (urine and blood), onset of abdominal pain, and uric acid concentrations.[3,5,6]

Atenolol

Brand names	Tenormin IV
Medication error potential	ISMP high-alert medication (adrenergic agonist) associated with an increased risk of significant patient harm if an error occurs.[1] USP reports confusion with Actonel, albuterol, Altenol, carvedilol, and labetalol.[2] Tenormin may be confused with Imuran, and tretinoin.[2]
Contraindications and warnings	**Contraindications:** Patients with pulmonary edema, cardiogenic shock, bradycardia, heart block, or uncompensated CHF.[3] Atenolol should not be administered to patients with untreated pheochromocytoma.[3] **Warnings:** Generally not used in patients with bronchospastic disease; however, when used the smallest effective dose should be given.[4] Atenolol may mask clinical signs of hyperthyroidism.[3] Abrupt withdrawal should be avoided; discontinue over 1–2 weeks.[3] Patients with a history of anaphylactic hypersensitivity reactions may be more reactive while receiving beta-blockers; these patients may not be responsive to the normal doses of epinephrine. (See Other in Comments section.)
Infusion related cautions	None.
Dosage	Little information on intravenous atenolol in pediatric patients. Labetalol is the most useful beta-blocker for treatment of severe hypertension.[3] (See Labetalol monograph.) 0.1 mg/kg/dose[3,7] up to 5 mg/dose in older adolescents and *adults*. If necessary, the dose may be repeated in 10 minutes.[3,7]
Dosage adjustment in organ dysfunction	If CrCl is 10–50 mL/min, give a normal dose q 48 h and if <10 mL/min, give q 96 h.[3,8]
Maximum dosage	Up to 15 mg/dose have been used in *adults*.[9,10]
Additives	None.
Suitable diluents	D5W or NS.[3,11]
Maximum concentration	0.5 mg/mL.[3]
Preparation and delivery	**Stability:** Stored at room temperature (i.e., 20°C to 25°C).[3] **Photosensitivity:** Protected from light.[3]
IV push	Over 5 minutes,[3,7] not to exceed 1 mg/min.[3]

Atenolol

Intermittent infusion	Not given by this method.
Continuous infusion	Not given by this method.
Other routes of administration	None.
Comments	**Monitoring:** Monitor heart rate, blood pressure, and ECG during infusion.[4]

Drug interactions: Drugs that slow AV conduction (i.e., hypotensive agents, diuretics, cardiac glycosides, amiodarone, calcium channel blockers) and general that depress the myocardium may have additive effects with beta-blockers. Nonsteroid anti-inflammatory drugs may decrease the antihypertensive effects of beta-blockers. Large doses of atenolol may reverse the effects of theophylline.

Other: Glucagon or ipratropium should be considered for treatment of anaphylaxis in patients receiving beta-adrenergic blocking agents.[3] Ipratropium also may be useful for the treatment of bronchospasm.[3]

Atracurium Besylate

Brand names	Tracrium, generic

Medication error potential	ISMP high-alert medication that has an increased risk of causing significant patient harm if it is used in error.[1]

Contraindications and warnings	**Contraindications:** Patients with a hypersensitivity to atracurium or any of its components.[2] **Warnings:** Use carefully under the supervision of experienced clinicians; personnel should also be skilled in airway management and respiratory support. Intubation and ventilatory support equipment (assisted or controlled), including positive pressure oxygen, should be readily available. Also should have anticholinesterase inhibitors readily available when giving atracurium.[2]

Infusion related cautions	Histamine release resulting in flushing, erythema, pruritus, urticaria, bronchospasm, hypotension, and changes in heart rate may occur.[2-6] Caution should be taken when administering this agent to patients who may be histamine sensitive (e.g., cardiovascular disease, previous anaphylactoid reactions, asthma).[2] Asystole has occurred in *adults*.[7]

Dosage	*Respiratory function must be supported and concurrent administration of a sedative is also necessary. Monitoring of neuromuscular transmission with a peripheral nerve stimulator is recommended during continuous infusion or with repeated dosing.*[2,8]
	
	Endotracheal intubation and maintenance of neuromuscular blockade
	
	   Initial dose
	
	      Neonates (≤1 month): 0.2–0.5 mg/kg.[9-11] (See Comments section.)
	
	      Infants and children (1 month–2 years): 0.3–0.4 mg/kg given as a single dose.[2,3,8,12-18] If the patient has a history of histamine sensitivity (anaphylactoid reactions or asthma), the dose should be given over 1 minute.[9] (See Infusion related cautions section.)
	
	      Children (≥2 years): 0.3–0.5 mg/kg given as a single dose.[2,3,9,12-18] If the patient has a history of histamine sensitivity (anaphylactic reactions or asthma), the dose should be divided over 1 minute.[9] (See Infusion related cautions section.)
	
	   Maintenance dose
	
	      Intermittent: 0.08–0.1 mg/kg as needed to maintain desired effects.[2,9] Children may require more frequent administration than *adults*.[9]
	
	      Continuous infusion: Not recommended in infants <2 years of age.[9] A continuous infusion (following initial dose) of 0.08–0.12 mg/kg/h (1.3–2 mcg/kg/min) has been safely used in neonates.[10] A continuous infusion of 0.15–1.2 mg/kg/h (2.5–20 mcg/kg/min) has been used in infants, children, and *adults*.[9,19-23] In a study with 20 children (1 month–13 years old), the dose of atracurium ranged from 0.44–2.4 mg/kg/h (7.3–40 mcg/kg/min).[22] (See Maximum dosage section.)
	
	      Larger doses have been required to facilitate mechanical ventilation in critically ill children.[23] Mean doses were 1.6–1.72 mg/kg/h (starting rate of 0.5 mg/kg/h) and increase until desired effect is achieved.[23] Infusion requirement may increase with prolonged administration.[24] (See Maximum dosage section.)

Dosage adjustment in organ dysfunction	No dosage adjustment required in renal[2,9,25] or hepatic dysfunction.[2,9]

Atracurium Besylate

Maximum dosage

0.6 mg/kg has been used safely in infants with severe hepatic dysfunction under halothane/nitrous oxide/oxygen anesthesia.[26] 0.53 ± 0.01 mg/kg/h (8.8 mcg/kg/min) has been used in those >1 month of age and 0.4 ± 0.01 mg/kg/h (6.7 mcg/kg/min) has been given to neonates.[27]

Occasionally, continuous infusion doses as large as 4.5 mg/kg/h (75 mcg/kg/min) may be required.[2,9,22,28] In one study, seven pediatric patients required a mean infusion of 1.72 mg/kg/h (28.7 mcg/kg/min) for up to 72 hours.[23] In other studies, a pediatric patient required 2.4 mg/kg/h,[22] and a 19-year-old received 4.5 mg/kg/h (75 mcg/kg/min).[28] (See Comments section.)

Additives

Multidose vials contain benzyl alcohol 0.9% as a preservative.[2,29]

See Appendix C for more specific information about potential adverse effects and/or benzyl alcohol toxicity in neonates.

Suitable diluents

D5W, D5NS, NS. Dilution in LR results in degradation of atracurium.[2]

Maximum concentration

10 mg/mL for IV push or 0.5 mg/mL for continuous infusion.[2,29]

Preparation and delivery

Atracurium is an acidic solution; do not administer with alkaline solutions.[2,29]

May be incompatible with propofol; however, the potential for incompatibility is concentration dependent and formulation specific.[29]

For PN compatibility information, please see Appendix D.

IV push

10 mg/mL given over 1 minute.[2,29]

Intermittent infusion

No information available to support administration by this method. Too slow of an injection may cause bradycardia.[2,3,9]

Continuous infusion

0.2–0.5 mg/mL.[2,29]

Other routes of administration

Should not be given IM due to tissue irritation.[2,9,29] No information available to support administration by other routes.

Comments

Significant adverse effects: Prolonged paralysis lasting 81 days was reported following atracurium infusion (20–75 mcg/kg/min) for 2 weeks in a 19-year-old patient.[28] The patient was also receiving corticosteroids, which may be a risk factor for this adverse effect. Prolonged paralysis has also been reported after long-term use of other neuromuscular blocking agents.[12,30] (See Drug interactions in Comments section.)

Prolonged administration of atracurium may also lead to the accumulation of its laudanosine metabolite. This metabolite has been associated with CNS irritation and seizures in animal models. Accumulation of laudanosine has been reported in patients with renal failure as well as those with hepatic failure, before and after liver transplantation, but generally at concentrations significantly lower than those associated with CNS excitation.[2,9,31,32]

Drug interactions: Enflurane and isoflurane anesthesia potentiate effects of atracurium; therefore, reduce atracurium dose by approximately 33% in these patients.[2,9,33] Also reduce atracurium dose in patients receiving succinylcholine or halothane.[2,9] Concomitant administration of atracurium with certain antibiotics (e.g., aminoglycosides, clindamycin, vancomycin) may prolong neuromuscular blockade.[2,9,14] Consult appropriate resources for additional information on drug interactions.

Other: Neonates and infants generally require smaller doses than children; however, they recover more rapidly.[10] One report noted a 25% smaller dose.[27]

Atropine Sulfate

Brand names	Generic, AtroPen (auto-injector)

Medication error potential	None noted.

Contraindications and warnings

Contraindications: In general, those with hypersensitivity to atropine, narrow-angle glaucoma, tachycardia, thyrotoxicosis, or obstruction in the gastrointestinal tract (i.e., pyloric stenosis) or urinary tract.[1]

In the event of life-threatening exposure to organophosphate insecticides or nerve agents, there are no absolute contraindications to treatment with AtroPen.[2] However, caution should be observed when used in individuals with the diseases listed above.[2]

Warnings: Children are at increased risk for increases in body temperature because of suppression of sweat.[1] Children who receive larger doses are at risk for paradoxical hyperexcitability.[1]

Infusion related cautions

Slow IV administration or doses <0.1 mg may cause paradoxical bradycardia.[1,3]

Dosage

Preanesthesia (to decrease secretions and block cardiac vagal reflexes during surgery)

Infants: 0.02–0.04 mg/kg 30–60 minutes preoperatively and then q 4–6 h as needed.[4-7]

Children: 0.01–0.02 mg/kg (0.1–0.4 mg) 30–60 minutes preoperatively and then q 4–6 h as needed.[6,8,9]

Other dosing recommendations include the following[1]

<20 kg: 0.1 mg for 3 kg, 0.2 mg for 7–9 kg, 0.3 mg for 12–16 kg given 30–60 minutes before anesthesia.

≥20 kg: 0.4 mg given 30–60 minutes before anesthesia.

CPR/bradycardia

Neonates: Atropine is not included in current neonatal resuscitation guidelines.[10]

Infants and children: 0.02 mg/kg (minimum 0.1 mg, maximum 0.5 mg) IV or IO; repeat if needed.[6]

Adolescents: 0.02 mg/kg (minimum 0.1 mg, maximum 1 mg) IV or IO; repeat if needed.[6]

Physostigmine toxicity: 0.5 mg for each 1 mg of the last dose of physostigmine administered.[5]

Organophosphate insecticide exposure in children: 0.05 mg/kg (2–5 mg in *adults*) slowly (IV); may be doubled and repeated q 10–20 min until desired response (e.g., drying of excessive secretions).[11,12]

Nerve agent poisoning with cholinergic symptoms in children: 0.05–0.1 mg/kg up to 4 mg repeated q 5–10 min until respiratory status improves or secretions resolve.[13,14]

AtroPen (auto-injector) IM dosing (only for use in insecticide or nerve agent exposure by trained individuals)[2]

10–20 kg: 0.5 mg.

20–40 kg: 1 mg.

≥ 40 kg: 2 mg.

Atropine Sulfate

Dosage adjustment in organ dysfunction

None noted for use in preanesthesia, CPR, or physostigmine toxicity.[1] However, caution should be used in those with significant renal insufficiency who require multiple doses as in organophosphate insecticide exposure or nerve agent poisoning.[2]

Maximum dosage

CPR/bradycardia: 0.4–0.5 mg (child), 1 mg (adolescent).[3,5]

Nerve agent exposure: 4 mg unless symptoms include apnea, convulsions, cardiopulmonary arrest, or rapid progression of symptoms.[13]

Organophosphate poisonings: Large doses may be required.[1,11] In a pediatric report, one patient received 86 doses and another patient received 61 doses (0.005–0.1 mg/kg/dose) in 24 hours. Another patient received 26 doses totaling 25 mg/kg over several days.[14]

Additives

Multiple-dose vials may contain methylparaben or benzyl alcohol.[1,15] (See Appendix C for specific information about potential adverse effects and toxicity.)

Suitable diluents

NS.[1,15] The auto-injector should not be diluted.[2]

Maximum concentration

1 mg/mL (available commercially).[1,15]

AtroPen doses are 0.5 mg, 1 mg, and 2 mg.[2]

Preparation and delivery

Available in prefilled syringes, multidose vials, and auto-injector formulations.

IV push

Infuse rapidly.[1,2] If administered into a peripheral vein during CPR, follow dose with a flush to facilitate drug delivery to the circulation.[1]

Intermittent infusion

Not recommended.[1]

Continuous infusion

Continuous infusion was used in a 68-year-old *adult* with intentional ingestion of an organophosphate insecticide.[16]

Other routes of administration

May be given IM, SC (preoperatively), or IO.[1] If injected in an extremity, it should be elevated for 10–20 seconds.[1] In preanesthesia induction, a faster onset of heart rate acceleration was reported following submental glossal injection than with deltoid or vastus lateralis injection.[17]

Comments

A 2-month-old given a 0.1-mg dose for bradycardia during ophthalmologic surgery subsequently had spontaneous extrusion of the lens and vitreous.[18]

Children with accidental wartime exposures who were given atropine doses ranging from 0.01–0.17 mg/kg had few adverse events that included dilated pupils, tachycardia, dry mucous membranes, flushed skin, temperature >37.8°C, and neurologic abnormalities.[13] There were no fatalities or life-threatening dysrhythmias.

Azithromycin

Brand names	Zithromax
Medication error potential	Look-alike, sound-alike drug names. USP reports confusion with azathioprine, aztreonam, erythromycin, and Zaroxolyn.[1] Zithromax has also been confused with Fosamax, Zoloft, Zyvox, Zinacef, Zovirox, and zinc sulfate.[1] Confusion with erythromycin has resulted in patient harm.[1]
Contraindications and warnings	**Contraindications:** Should not be used in patients with known hypersensitivity to azithromycin, erythromycin, any macrolide, or ketolide antibiotic.[2] **Warnings:** Serious allergic reactions, including angioedema, anaphylaxis, and dermatologic reactions (e.g., Stevens-Johnson syndrome and toxic epidermal necrolysis) have been reported.[2] If an allergic reaction occurs, the drug should be discontinued and appropriate therapy should be instituted. (See Infusion related cautions section.) Prolonged use may cause superinfection and/or *Clostridium difficile*–associated diarrhea (CDAD), which has been reported and may range in severity from mild diarrhea to fatal colitis.[2] If CDAD is suspected or confirmed, appropriate fluid and electrolyte management, protein supplementation, antibiotic treatment of *C. difficile*, and surgical evaluation should be instituted as clinically indicated.[2]
Infusion related cautions	Despite discontinuation of azithromycin and successful management of the allergic reaction, symptoms may recur after treatment is complete without further azithromycin exposure.[2] Patients required prolonged periods of observation and symptomatic treatment. Local IV site reactions have been reported.[2] The incidence and severity of these reactions were the same when 500 mg azithromycin were given over 1 hour (2 mg/mL as 250-mL infusion) or over 3 hours (1 mg/mL as 500-mL infusion).[2]
Dosage	Not recommended in patients <16 years of age.[3] **Community-acquired pneumonia (moderate to severe):** 500 mg IV q 24 h for a minimum of 2 days followed by 500 mg/day orally for a total of 7–10 days.[2-5] **Pelvic inflammatory disease (PID):** 500 mg IV for 1–2 days, followed by 250 mg/day orally to complete 7 days of therapy.[2,6,7] If anaerobic organisms are suspected, an antimicrobial agent with anaerobic activity should be given concurrently.[2]
Dosage adjustment in organ dysfunction	No recommendations available for patients with impaired hepatic function.[2] Caution should be exercised when administered in severe renal impairment (CrCL ≤10 mL/min).[2,8]
Maximum dosage	Little information is available, but generally 10 mg/kg/dose up to 500 mg.[2,9] Although serum concentrations persisted for >10 days, a large IV dose (4 g) was well-tolerated in healthy *adult* males.[10]
Additives	None.
Suitable diluents	D5W, NS, ½NS, LR, D5LR, D5⅓NS, D5½NS, or D5½NS + 20 mEq KCl, Normosol-M in D5 and Normosol-R in D5.[2,11]
Maximum concentrations	2 mg/mL.[2,11] Patients receiving azithromycin at higher concentrations have experienced pain and local inflammation at the site during administration.[2,10]

Azithromycin

Preparation and delivery	**Stability:** Stable for 24 hours at or below room temperature (30°C), or for 7 days under refrigeration (5°C).[2]
IV push	Not recommended.[2]
Intermittent infusion	1 mg/mL should be given over 3 hours.[2] Higher concentrations (2 mg/mL) and large doses (>500 mg) should be given over 1 hour.[2]
Continuous infusion	No information available.
Other routes of administration	Should not be given IM.[2,11]
Comments	**Rare adverse events:** One case of ototoxicity occurred in an *adult* receiving IV azithromycin for 8 days.[12] Macrolide antibiotics may prolonged cardiac repolarization and QT interval to cause cardiac arrhythmia and *torsades de pointes*.[2,14] A similar effect with azithromycin cannot be ruled out in patients at risk for prolonged cardiac repolarization.[2] Exacerbation of symptoms of myasthenia gravis and new onset of myasthenic syndrome have been reported.[2] **Drug interactions:** Azithromycin is a substrate for and inhibitor of CYP3A4 and is associated with numerous drug interactions.[13] Consult appropriate resources for dosing recommendations before combining any drug with azithromycin.

Aztreonam

Brand names	Azactam

Medication error potential

Look a-like, sound a-like drug names.

USP reports confusion with azithromycin.[1]

Contraindications and warnings

Contraindications: In patients with known hypersensitivity to aztreonam or any other component in the formulation.[2]

Warnings: Although the manufacturer recommends caution when aztreonam is given to patients with immediate hypersensitivity reactions to penicillins or cephalosporins,[2] the cross-reactivity between cephalosporins and penicillins does not appear to extend to the monobactams. Patients with penicillin hypersensitivity have been given aztreonam without incident.[3-6] Similarly, those who experience hypersensitivity to aztreonam may not be hypersensitive to other beta-lactam antibiotics.[7] There is some suggestion that cross-sensitivity may occur between ceftazidime and aztreonam due to similar side chains.[4,5]

Prolonged use may cause superinfection and/or *Clostridium difficile*–associated diarrhea (CDAD), which has been reported and may range in severity from mild diarrhea to fatal colitis.[2] If CDAD is suspected or confirmed, appropriate fluid and electrolyte management, protein supplementation, antibiotic treatment of *C. difficile*, and surgical evaluation should be instituted as clinically indicated.[2]

Infusion related cautions

Although rare, anaphylactoid reactions may require immediate emergency treatment with epinephrine, oxygen, IV steroids, antihistamines, pressor amines, and airway management. Local reactions such as phlebitis, thrombophlebitis, discomfort, and swelling at the injection site have been reported.[2]

Dosage

Safety and effectiveness have not been established in those <9 months of age.[2]

Neonates

PNA	≤1200 g	1200-2000 g	≥2000 g
<7 days	60 mg/kg/day divided q 12 h*[8]	60 mg/kg/day divided q 12 h[8-11]	90 mg/kg/day divided q 8 h[8-11]
≥7 days		90 mg/kg/day divided q 8 h[8,9,12]	120 mg/kg/day divided q 6 h[8,10]

*Until 4 weeks of age.

Infants and children

    Mild-to-moderate infections: 90 mg/kg/day divided q 8 h[2,8-13] up to 3 g/day.[8]

    Severe infections: 120 mg/kg/day divided q 6 h[2,8-13] up to 8 g/day.[8]

Cystic fibrosis (*P. aeruginosa*): 200 mg/kg/day divided q 6 h[10,11,14,15] up to 8 g/day.[8]

Dosage adjustment in organ dysfunction

If CrCl is 10–50 mL/min, give 50% of normal dose or 45–60 mg/kg/day divided q 8 h; if CrCl is <10 mL/min, give 25% of normal dose or 15–20 mg/kg/day divided q 12 h.[2,16] No adjustment in hepatic dysfunction.[2]

Maximum dosage

120 mg/kg/day[2] and 200 mg/kg/day (cystic fibrosis)[14,15] not to exceed 8 g/day.[2]

Additives

None.

Aztreonam

Suitable diluents	D5W, D10W, NS, LR, ¼NS, ½NS, D5¼NS, D5½NS, D5NS, D10¼NS, D10½NS, D10NS, and D5LR. Use SW or BW, NS, or bacteriostatic NS for IM administration.[2,17]
Maximum concentration	≤20 mg/mL for IV infusion, and 333 mg/mL for IM administration.[2,17]
Preparation and delivery	**Stability:** Following addition of diluent, contents should be shaken immediately and vigorously.[2] Solution may be colorless to light straw yellow and can develop a slight pink tint that does not affect potency.[2] Concentrations <20 mg/mL must be used within 48 hours if stored at room temperature (15° to 30° C) or within 7 days if refrigerated (2° to 8° C). Unused solutions >20 mg/mL must be discarded.[2] Solution may be frozen at <−2°C for up to 3 months. Thawed solution should be used within 24 hours, if thawed at room temperature, or within 72 hours, if thawed under refrigeration.[18] Do not refreeze.[18] **Compatibility:** See Appendix D for PN compatibility information.[19]
IV push	Over 3–5 minutes.[2,17]
Intermittent infusion	20–60 minutes.[2,17]
Continuous infusion	Not used.
Other routes of administration	May be given by deep injection into a large muscle in a concentration of <333 mg/mL.[11,12] (See Suitable diluents section.) The dose should be given IV in patients with septicemia, localized parenchymal abscess, peritonitis, or when doses >1 g are administered.[12] Commercially available frozen aztreonam injection in dextrose should only be used for IV infusion.[18] Aztreonam lysine is being investigated for inhalation administration in treatment of *Pseudomonal* infections in cystic fibrosis patients. *The IV form should not be inhaled as it contains arginine, which can cause airway inflammation when used long-term.* (See Other in Comments section.)
Comments	**Drug interactions:** Typhoid vaccine—Antibiotics may diminish the therapeutic effect of typhoid vaccine. Only the live attenuated Ty21a strain is affected.[18] **Laboratory interference:** May cause false-positive urinary glucose results when cupric sulfate solution-based tests (Clinitest, Benedict's solution, Fehling's solution) are used.[2] Glucose tests (Diastix, TEST-TAPE, Clinistix) based on enzymatic glucose oxidase reactions may be used. Positive direct Coombs' tests have been reported.[18] **Other:** Inhaled aztreonam lysine in a dosage of 75 mg 2–3 times/day has been shown to be effective in controlling *Pseudomonas* infections in patients with CF previously treated with tobramycin inhalation solution.[20,21] Inhaled aztreonam lysine delayed time to need for other antipseudomonal antibiotics and improved respiratory symptoms and pulmonary function. It was well tolerated.[20,21]

Baclofen

Brand names	Lioresal Intrathecal
Medication error potential	ISMP high-alert medication associated with significant patient harm should an error occur.[1] Baclofen may be confused with Bactroban, bethanechol, and Blocadren.[2] Lioresal may be confused with Lotensin.[2]
Contraindications and warnings	Not for IV, IM, SubQ, or epidural administration.[3] **US boxed warning:** Abrupt withdrawal has caused severe sequelae including high fever, altered mental status, exaggerated rebound spasticity, and muscle rigidity.[3] In rare cases, rhabdomyolysis, multiple organ system failure, and death has occurred.[3] (See Comments section.) **Other warnings:** Should not be used for spasticity to maintain posture or balance.[3]
Infusion related cautions	A sudden requirement for substantial dose escalation may indicate catheter complication (i.e., catheter kink, dislodgement, loss of patency).[3-6] Use extreme caution in filling implantable pump that allows direct access to the intrathecal catheter as direct injection through the catheter access port may cause a life-threatening overdose.[3]
Dosage	**Intrathecal Administration** **Severe spasticity (spinal cord or cerebral origin)** **Test dose for response to intrathecal baclofen:** 50 mcg into intrathecal space via barbotage over ≥1 minute.[3-14] Use 25 mcg in very small children.[3,13] If insufficient response within 4–8 hours, a second 75-mcg test dose can be given 24 hours after initial test dose.[3,7,9,11,13] If response continues to be inadequate, a third 100-mcg test dose[3,13,15] may be given 24 hours after the second test dose.[3,7] If an inadequate response continues, the patient is not a candidate for chronic intrathecal baclofen therapy.[3] A significant decrease in muscle tone and/or frequency and/or severity of spasms is considered a positive response.[3] **Maintenance therapy:** Initial daily dose is based on the effective test dose and duration of its effects.[16] If the test dose response lasted ≤8 hours, the initial daily dose should be twice the test dose.[3,13] If the response lasted >8 hours, the initial daily dose should equal the test dose.[3,13] The dose should be increased every 24 hours by 5% to 15% until desired results are achieved.[3] The infusion rate is the total daily dose divided by 24 hours. **≤12 years:** 100–300 mcg/day (4.2–12.5 mcg/h),[3,17] but doses as large as 1000–1500 mcg/day.[3,11,17] **>12 years:** 300–800 mcg/day (12.5–33.3 mcg/h).[3,12,17] If spasticity is of cerebral origin doses as large as 1000 mcg/day have been used.[3,9,16,17] Doses up to 1400 mcg/day have been given to children.[9,17] **Tetanus:** Intrathecal baclofen has also been used successfully in treating muscle rigidity associated with tetanus in *adults*.[18,19]
Dosage adjustment in organ dysfunction	Patients with renal impairment may require smaller doses.[17]
Maximum dosage	Although doses up to 1500 mcg/day have been given,[11] there is limited experience with dosages >1000 mcg/day.[3,17]

Baclofen

Additives	0.15 mEq sodium/mL. [3]
Suitable diluents	Sterile, preservative-free 0.9% NaCl injection. [3]
Maximum concentration	50 mcg/mL (commercially available) for test dose. For maintenance dosing the commercially available strengths (i.e., 0.5 or 2 mg/mL) *must* be diluted. [17] Intrathecal refill kit concentration 0.5 mg/mL in 20-mL ampules or 2 mg/mL in 5-mL ampules. [3]
Preparation and delivery	**Delivery system issues:** Catheter complication (i.e., catheter kink, dislodgement, loss of patency) may cause a sudden requirement for substantial increase in dose. [3-6] **Stability:** The concentrate contains no preservatives; hence, each vial is intended for single use only and any unused solution should be discarded. [3] It does not require refrigeration and is stable at 37°C; however, storage temperature should not exceed 30°C and it should not be frozen. [3]
IV push	Not intended for IV administration. [3]
Intermittent infusion	Not applicable.
Continuous infusion	Administered *intrathecally* via implantable pump device. Total daily dose in mcg divided by 24 hours = infusion rate. [1] Do not discontinue abruptly. [3] (See US boxed warning in Contraindications and warnings section and see Comments section.)
Other routes of administration	Not intended for IM, IV, SC, or epidural administration. [3]
Comments	**Significant adverse effects:** Baclofen withdrawal syndrome can develop quickly into an emergent, life-threatening situation if not recognized and treated. [20] It can be difficult to diagnose because symptoms can be similar to sepsis, [21] meningitis, autonomic dysreflexia, [4,20] and neuroleptic malignant syndrome. [22] Patients can present with fever, tachycardia, seizures, and spasticity. [20-24] Even with early diagnosis and treatment patients can become refractory to therapy, and withdrawal can lead to morbidity and mortality [23,24] including rhabdomyolysis, elevated plasma creatine kinase, elevated LFTs, organ failure, DIC, and death. [20,22,24,25] This syndrome has been reported in *adults* and pediatric patients. [22,26,27] Reinitiate baclofen as soon as possible if withdrawal syndrome occurs. [3,20,24] Other treatment options include oral baclofen replacement, [3,17] benzodiazepines, [20,24,27] dantrolene sodium, [28] and cyproheptadine. [29] Withdrawal symptoms have persisted despite oral baclofen replacement therapy. [30] **Monitoring:** If patient develops unexplained tolerance or symptoms of withdrawal despite continued infusion consider catheter leakage, [4,5,24] catheter dislodgement, [24] or pump failure. [6,24,31] One study recommends that CSF pressure should be measured prior to implantation to decrease risk of postoperative CSF leaks in patients with elevated CSF pressures. [32] **Rare adverse effects:** A study with *adult* patients found that intrathecal baclofen increased seizures in patients with multiple sclerosis. [33,34] A pediatric study reported no change in the incidence/frequency of seizures in patients with spasticity of cerebral origin receiving intrathecal baclofen. [9] The use of intrathecal baclofen pumps has also been associated with rapid progression of scoliosis in pediatric and *adult* patients. [35,36]

Bumetanide

Brand names	Bumex
Medication error potential	Look-alike, sound-alike error potential. USP reports that bumetanide was confused with budesonide. Bumex was confused with Demadex. No patient harm resulted.[1]
Contraindications and warnings	**Contraindications:** Patients with anuria.[2] (See Comments section.) **Warnings:** Patients with sulfonamide allergy may be hypersensitive to bumetanide.[2] Use cautiously in jaundiced neonates at risk for kernicterus. In vitro studies have shown bilirubin displacement in pooled cord blood samples from critically ill neonates.[3,4]
Infusion related cautions	None noted.
Dosage	0.01–0.1 mg/kg/dose (up to 2 mg) twice a day, daily, or every other day.[5-14] A dose of 0.035–0.04 mg/kg resulted in a maximum diuretic response in critically ill infants from 0–6 months of age.[6] Usual dose in *adults* is 0.5–1 mg q 2–3 h up to 10 mg/day.
Dosage adjustment in organ dysfunction	Larger doses (e.g., >2 mg in *adults*) may be needed in patients with CrCl <5 mL/min.[3] May need to reduce dosage in patients with hepatic impairment.[3] During neonatal ECMO, the elimination half-life was longer [10] than that reported in preterm infants not on ECMO.[8] (See Comments section.)
Maximum dosage	0.1 mg/kg up to 10 mg/day has been used in *adults* with normal renal function.[3] Up to 20 mg/day have been given to *adults* with renal dysfunction.[3]
Additives	Benzyl alcohol. (See Appendix C for specific information about potential benzyl alcohol toxicity.)
Suitable diluents	D5W, LR, or NS.[2,3,15]
Maximum concentration	0.25 mg/mL (available commercially).[2,3,15]
Preparation and delivery	**Compatibility:** See Appendix D for PN compatibility information. **Photosensitivity:** Discolors when exposed to light.[3,15]
IV push	0.25 mg/mL over 1–2 minutes.[3,11-15]

Intermittent infusion	May be infused over a longer time than with IV push.[16]
Continuous infusion	In *adults* with chronic renal insufficiency, a 1-mg loading dose followed by 0.912 mg/h for 12 hours was more effective than two 6-mg bolus doses given 6 hours apart.[16]
	Another study in *adults* reported onset of musculoskeletal symptoms within 8 to 48 hours of continuous infusions of doses ranging between 1 and 4 mg/h.[17]
Other routes of administration	May be given IM.[2,3,15]
Comments	**Pharmacokinetics:** Half-life in preterm neonates with bronchopulmonary dysplasia was 5.8 ± 0.7 hours[8] and in 11 term neonates on ECMO was 13.2 ± 3.8 hours.[5] Infants 2.2 ± 1.6 months of age with lung disease had a half-life of 1.74 ± 1 hours and those with heart disease had a half-life of 2.71 ± 1.59 hours.[6]
	Adverse effects: Electrolyte abnormalities, including hypokalemia, can occur; therefore, monitoring serum potassium concentration is important.[2,3]
	Ototoxicity may occur with large doses or prolonged IV therapy and may be additive when bumetanide is combined with aminoglycosides.[2,3]

Bupivacaine

Brand names	Marcaine, Sensorcaine, Sensorcaine-MPF

Medication error potential

ISMP high-alert medication that has an increased risk of causing significant patient harm if it is used in error.[1]

Look-alike, sound-alike error potential.

USP reports that bupivacaine has been confused with levobupivacaine, lidocaine, and ropivacaine; no patient harm resulted.[2]

USP reports that Marcaine has been confused with Sensorcaine; no patient harm resulted.[2] USP also reports that Sensorcaine has been confused with Marcaine; no patient harm resulted.[2]

Contraindications and warnings

US boxed warning: Convulsions followed by cardiac arrest with difficult resuscitation or death have occurred following the use of 0.75% bupivacaine for epidural anesthesia in obstetric patients; the 0.75% concentration of bupivacaine is not recommended for use in obstetrical anesthesia.[3]

Contraindications: Bupivacaine is contraindicated in obstetrical paracervical block anesthesia (has resulted in fetal bradycardia and death).[3] Also contraindicated in patients with a hypersensitivity to bupivacaine or any amide anesthetic.[3]

Other warnings: Bupivacaine should only be administered by persons specifically trained in the use of local anesthetics.[3]

The FDA notified healthcare professionals in November 2009 of the risk of chondrolysis following continuous intra-articular infusion of local anesthetics, including bupivacaine, via elastomeric infusion devices. The FDA has received 35 reports of chondrolysis, some were in previously healthy young *adults,* and most following shoulder surgery. The cases had received the local anesthetics for postoperative pain for periods of 48–72 hours. Chondrolysis symptoms (joint pain, stiffness, loss of motion) occurred as early as 2 (median 5) months following therapy with the local anesthetic.[4,5]

Infusion related cautions

Not for IV infusion or IM administration. Administer only by infiltration, or by epidural, spinal or peripheral or sympathetic nerve block as a single or repeat injections.[6]

Accidental IV injection may result in cardiac arrhythmia or cardiac arrest, seizures, coma, and respiratory arrest.[3,4]

Oxygen, cardiopulmonary resuscitation and intubation equipment and medications and trained personnel in emergency management should be immediately available when using bupivacaine.[3]

Dosage

Dose varies with the anesthetic procedure, the area to be anesthetized, the vascularity of the tissues, the number of neuronal segments to be blocked, the depth and duration of anesthesia required, as well as individual response.[3,4]

Once the catheter is placed, negative aspiration of blood or cerebrospinal fluid[7-10] with the absence of cardiovascular changes following a test dose indicates correct position of the catheter.[11-13]

The manufacturer does not recommend the use of bupivacaine with or without epinephrine in children <12 years and the solution for spinal anesthesia should not be used in those <18 year.[3] However, epinephrine containing solutions of bupivacaine have been used in neonates, infants, and children.[10,12,13]

Dosage *(cont.)*	**Caudal block (preservative-free solution only):** Children 1–2.5 mg/kg[3] or 0.5–1 mL/kg of the 0.25% solution (1.25 or 2.5 mg/kg).[7-11,14]
	
	Peripheral nerve block: 5 mL of 0.25% or 0.5% (12.5–25 mg).[4]
	
	Sympathetic nerve block: 20–50 mL of 0.25% solution (without epinephrine).[3,4]
	
	Continuous epidural (caudal or lumbar) infusion (preservative-free solution only)
	
	    Loading dose: 1.25–2.5 mg/kg (0.8–1 mL/kg) of the 0.25% bupivacaine.[4,12,14]
	
	    Infusion: 0.2–0.375 mg/kg/h (equivalent to 0.08–0.16 mL/kg/h of the 0.25% solution).[7-10] Use with caution in infants due to reduced levels of alpha$_1$-acid-glycoprotein leading to higher concentrations of unbound drug.[12,13]

Dosage adjustment in organ dysfunction	Reduce dosage and use with caution in patients with hepatic disease.[3,4] There is a potential for increased toxicity in patients with renal impairment, but no specific dosage adjustment is recommended.[3] Reduce dosage in patients with cardiac disease or in those who are acutely ill.[3,4]
Maximum dosage	In *adults*, do not exceed a maximum of 400 mg within a 24-hour period.[3,4]
Additives	Available with epinephrine 1:200,000. Products containing epinephrine should not be used for sympathetic nerve blocks.[4] Epinephrine containing solutions contain metabisulfite.[3] (See Appendix C for more specific information about potential adverse effects of sulfites.) Multidose vials contain paraben preservatives and should not be used for epidural or caudal blocks.[6] (See Appendix C for more specific information about potential adverse effects of parabens.)
Suitable diluents	Not diluted.
Maximum concentration	0.75% (7.5 mg/mL) is available. However, the maximum recommended concentration varies by indication.[3,4,13] (See Dosage section.)
Preparation and delivery	Epinephrine containing solutions should not be used if they are a pinkish color, darker than slightly yellow, or if there is visible precipitate.[6]
IV push	Do not administer IV.[3,4,6] (See Infusion related cautions section.)
Intermittent infusion	Do not administer IV.[3,4,6]
Continuous infusion	Do not administer IV.[3,4,6]

Bupivacaine

Other routes of administration	Do not administer IM.[3,4,6]

Comments	**Significant adverse effects:** Systemic absorption of local anesthetics may result in toxic plasma concentrations, resulting in cardiovascular adverse effects, including decreased cardiac output, heart block, hypotension, bradycardia, ventricular arrhythmias, and cardiac arrest. Patients should be carefully monitored during injection. Use with caution in patients with underlying cardiovascular disease.[4]
	Continuous infusions of bupivacaine in children has resulted in high plasma concentrations and seizures.[3]
	Other: Peripheral facial nerve paralysis lasting 8 hours has been reported after peritonsillar infiltration of bupivacaine in a 4-year-old.[15]
	Products containing epinephrine may produce an exaggerated vasoconstrictor response resulting in ischemic injury or necrosis. Use with caution in areas with restricted or limited blood flow, such as the fingers.[4]

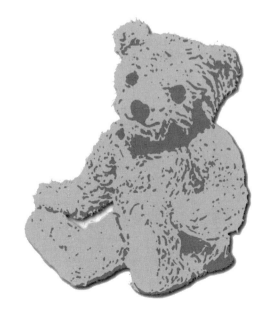

Caffeine Citrate

Brand names	Cafcit
Medication error potential	None.
Contraindications and warnings	**Contraindications:** Documented hypersensitivity to caffeine or any of its components.
	Warnings: Although no direct relationship has been established, necrotizing enterocolitis has been reported in newborns receiving caffeine.[1] (See Rare adverse effects in Comments section.)
	Use cautiously in patients with a history of peptic ulcer, impaired renal or hepatic function, seizure disorders, or cardiovascular disease.[1] Avoid in those with symptomatic cardiac arrhythmias.[1]
Infusion related cautions	None.
Dosage	*Do not interchange the caffeine citrate salt formulation with the caffeine sodium benzoate formulation as it contains benzyl alcohol.*
	Prior to initiation of caffeine citrate, baseline serum concentrations of caffeine should be measured in infants previously treated with theophylline and in infants born to mothers who consumed caffeine prior to delivery.[1]
	The dose of caffeine base is one half the dose of caffeine citrate (i.e., 20 mg of caffeine citrate is equivalent to 10 mg of caffeine base).[1]
	Apnea of prematurity[1-7]
	Loading dose: 10–40 mg/kg (as caffeine citrate) over 30 minutes.
	Maintenance dose: 5–8 mg/kg (as caffeine citrate) q 24 h. Begin maintenance dose 24 hours after loading dose.
	Facilitate extubation in neonatal apnea[2,5,6,7]
	Loading dose: 20–80 mg/kg (as caffeine citrate) 24 hours prior to planned extubation.
	Maintenance dose: 10–30 mg/kg q 24 h (as caffeine citrate). Begin maintenance dose 24 hours after loading dose.
	A loading dose of 80 mg/kg followed by 20 mg/kg/day resulted in a lower rate of extubation failure.[7]
Dosage adjustment in organ dysfunction	In neonates, approximately 86% of drug is excreted unchanged in the urine, with the remainder metabolized by the CYP1A2 hepatic enzyme system.[8] Dose adjustment may be required in neonates with renal/hepatic dysfunction or those suffering from birth asphyxia.
Maximum dosage	Individualize dosage based on serum concentration and clinical effect. Loading dose of 80 mg/kg and maintenance dose of 40 mg/kg have been used.[7]
Additives	None.

Caffeine Citrate

Suitable diluents	D5W, D5W¼NS, D5W¼NS with 20 mEq KCl/L.[9]
Maximum concentration	20 mg/mL (as citrate) (commercially available).[1]
Preparation and delivery	**Stability:** Caffeine citrate is stable for 24 hours at room temperature when diluted to 10 mg/mL with D5W, D50W, Aminosyn 8.5%, dopamine 0.6 mg/mL, calcium gluconate 10%, heparin sodium 1 unit/mL, or fentanyl citrate 10 mcg/mL.[9] Intact vials should be stored at room temperature.[9] **Compatibility:** See Appendix D for PN compatibility information.[10]
IV push	Not recommended.
Intermittent infusion	Loading dose should be given over 30 minutes.[1,3,5] The maintenance dose is usually infused over 10–15 minutes[1,3]; however, it has been infused over 3 minutes.[4]
Continuous infusion	None.
Other routes of administration	None.
Comments	**Rare adverse events:** During a randomized, double-blind, placebo-controlled trial, six cases of necrotizing enterocolitis were identified among 85 neonates studied (caffeine = 46, placebo = 39). Caffeine citrate 20-mg/kg loading dose followed by 5 mg/kg/day orally or intravenously, or placebo, was given to patients for up to 10 days. Four neonates receiving caffeine citrate and two infants receiving placebo developed necrotizing enterocolitis.[3] Caffeine is known to increase metabolic rate and oxygen consumption and may contribute to growth failure.[4] 2006 infants (500 to 1250 g) were randomly assigned to receive either caffeine or placebo for apnea of prematurity.[11] Treatment was continued until it was no longer required. Caffeine improved the rate of survival without causing neurodevelopmental disability at 18 to 21 months in infants with very low birth weight. **Monitoring:** Using standard dosage guidelines, a predicted concentration-time curve can be easily generated and routine monitoring of serum concentrations during treatment is probably not necessary unless a clinical problem arises.[5,12,13] If serum concentrations are monitored, the desired serum trough concentration ranges from 5–25 mcg/mL. Concentrations >50 mcg/mL are considered toxic.[1] **Drug interactions:** Caffeine is a substrate of CYP1A2.[1] It is an inhibitor of CYP1A2 and 3A4 (moderate).[8] Consult appropriate resources for dosing recommendations before combining any drug with caffeine citrate. **Pharmacokinetic considerations:** Caffeine exhibits single-compartment, linear pharmacokinetics where both weight and age influence caffeine clearance.[5,6] In young infants, the elimination of caffeine is much slower than that in *adults* due to immature hepatic and/or renal function. In neonates, the half-life is approximately 3–4 days. By 9 months of age, the metabolism of caffeine approximates that seen in *adults*. Interconversion between caffeine and theophylline has been reported in preterm neonates (3% to 8% of caffeine would be expected to be converted to theophylline).[1]

Calcitriol

Brand names	Calcijex

Medication error potential	Look-alike, sound-alike error potential. USP reported that calcitriol was confused with calcium carbonate, captopril, colestipol, paricalcitol, and ropinirole. No patient harm resulted.[1]

Contraindications and warnings	**Contraindications:** Patients with hypercalcemia or evidence of vitamin D toxicity.[2]

Infusion related cautions	None noted.

Dosage	**Secondary hyperparathyroidism in hemodialysis patients:** Initial dose based on PTH concentration.[2-4] Dose is given immediately after dialysis session. PTH and serum calcium concentration must be monitored closely. Serum Ca concentration should be ≤11 mg/dL and Ca × P product ≤75.

PTH Concentration	Dose
<500 pg/mL	0.5 mcg
500–1000 pg/mL	1.0 mcg
>1000 pg/mL	1.5 mcg

Dose can be increased by 0.25 mcg q 2 weeks until ≤30% decrease in PTH. Calcitriol should be discontinued if hypercalcemia develops and the dose reduced when the drug is restarted.

Maintenance doses[4]

2–12 years: 0.04 mcg/kg (range = 0.5–2 mcg).

13–18 years: 0.02 mcg/kg (range = 0.25–2.25 mcg).

Hyperparathyroidism in peritoneal dialysis patients: In a 12-month study, 16 patients (12.5 ± 1.1 years) had an initial dose of 1 mcg added to 50–100 mL residual dialysate volume that was instilled into the peritoneal cavity after overnight exchanges 3 × week.[5] Dose was increased by 0.5 mcg if Ca <10.0 mg/dL and P <6 mg/dL. If Ca was >11 mg/dL, the dose was held until Ca was <11 mg/dL at which time calcitriol was restarted at 50% of the previous dose. Average maintenance dose was 1.3 ± 0.08 mcg.

Other uses

Hypocalcemia: An 8-month-old African-American girl with hypocalcemic seizures and presumed rickets was given calcitriol 0.25 mcg two times a day (and calcium gluconate four times a day) for ≤2 days when she was changed to oral vitamin D and calcium.[6]

Of note: Hypocalcemic neonates ≤32 weeks GA (n = 19) failed to respond to large doses given IM.[7]

Dosage adjustment in organ dysfunction	None noted.

Maximum dosage	Usually ≤0.05 mcg/kg.[3] 0.06 mcg/kg was given as single dose to adolescents.[8]
Additives	Contains polysorbate 20 and sodium ascorbate.[9] Some products contain edetate disodium dihydrate.[9]
Suitable diluents	D5W, NS, SW.[9]
Maximum concentration	2 mcg/mL (available commercially).[2,3,9]
Preparation and delivery	**Stability:** Up to 50% of calcitriol was lost in 2 hours when calcitriol was placed in PVC, thus use of PVC bags and sets is not recommended.[10]
IV push	Over 15 seconds.[10] May be given the end of hemodialysis through venous catheter.[2,3]
Intermittent infusion	May be infused undiluted over 15 minutes.[11]
Continuous infusion	Not indicated.
Other routes of administration	1 or 2 mcg/mL has been added to a small volume of peritoneal dialysate and instilled intraperitoneally after nightly peritoneal dialysis.[5]
Comments	**Drug interactions:** Antacids containing magnesium should not be used during calcitriol treatment because of the potential for hypermagnesemia.[1] Hypercalcemia can cause cardiac arrhythmias in patients receiving digoxin; therefore, calcitriol should be used cautiously in these patients.[1] **Monitoring:** Hypercalcemia, hyperphosphatemia, and hypercalciuria can occur.[1,6] Monitor serum calcium and phosphorous concentrations once or twice a week during the first 12 weeks of treatment and during dose titration. If hypercalcemia occurs, discontinue therapy (including oral calcium phosphate binders) until serum calcium concentration normalizes.[2]

Calcium Chloride

Brand names	Various manufacturers
Medication error potential	Look-alike, sound-alike error potential.
	USP reports that calcium chloride was confused with calcium gluconate. No patient harm resulted.[1]

Contraindications and warnings

Contraindications: Calcium chloride should not be used during CPR when ventricular fibrillation is present.[2]

Neonates receiving ceftriaxone should not be given calcium containing fluids because of the risk for precipitation of calcium–ceftriaxone.[3] In older infants and children receiving ceftriaxone, the IV line should be flushed thoroughly before and after ceftriaxone infusion.[3]

Warnings: Several different salt forms of calcium are available. Attention must be paid to the salt during product ordering, selection, and administration.[4,5]

Infusion related cautions

Small veins (scalp, small hand or foot) should not be used for infusion.[4]

The infusion should be stopped if the patient complains of discomfort. Extravasation may cause tissue sloughing and necrosis.[6-9] (See Appendix E for management of extravasation.)

Dosage

10% (100 mg/mL) calcium chloride ($CaCl_2$) solution provides approximately 1.36 mEq/mL or 27.3 mg/mL of elemental calcium.[2,4-5] 1 mEq is equivalent to 20 mg elemental calcium.

Hypocalcemia in critically ill infants and children: 10–20 mg/kg q 4–6 h.[10] Base subsequent doses on calcium deficit.[2]

Hypocalcemia secondary to infusion of blood products

> **Neonatal exchange transfusion with citrated blood:** 0.45 mEq (0.33 mL 10% calcium chloride injection) per 100 mL blood exchanged.[4]

> **Citrated blood transfusion in *adults*:** 1.35 mEq (1 mL $CaCl_2$) per 100 mL blood infused.[2]

> $CaCl_2$ infusion during FFP administration decreased hypocalcemia in children with thermal injury.[11]

Cardiopulmonary resuscitation (Routine administration during CPR is no longer recommended.[12] When indicated, infusion should be through a central line.)

> **Infants and children:** 0.272 mEq (0.2 mL $CaCl_2$)/kg.[4,12]

> **Adolescents and *adults*:** 2–4 mg/kg.[4]

Dosage adjustment in organ dysfunction

Calcium is renally eliminated. Calcium concentrations should be monitored closely in patients with renal dysfunction who require calcium.

Calcium Chloride

Maximum dosage	1000 mg/dose in *adults*.[4]
Additives	Aluminum is present as a contaminant.[2]
Suitable diluents	Most standard dextrose and/or saline-containing IV fluids.[13]
Maximum concentration	Undiluted, 100 mg/mL.[1,2]
Preparation and delivery	**Compatibility:** Incompatible with bicarbonate or phosphate containing fluids. Calcium containing fluids should not be co-infused with ceftriaxone.[3] Calcium containing fluids should not be co-infused with PN because of the risk for precipitation with the phosphate component.
IV push	Slow, over 3–5 minutes.[2]
Intermittent infusion	Over 5–10 minutes during CPR.[12] 10% $CaCl_2$ (undiluted) at 1 mL (100 mg)/min in *adults*.[2]
Continuous infusion	May be given continuously.
Other routes of administration	IM or SC administration should not be used.[4] IO administration may be used during cardiopulmonary resuscitation.[12]
Comments	**Drug interactions:** IV calcium should be used cautiously in patients receiving cardiac glycosides because of the potential for development of arrhythmias.[2]

Calcium Gluconate

Brand names	Various manufacturers
Medication error potential	Look-alike, sound-alike error potential. USP reports calcium gluconate was confused with calcium chloride and calcium carbonate. No patient harm resulted.[1]
Contraindications and warnings	**Contraindications:** Calcium chloride should not be used during CPR when ventricular fibrillation is present.[2] Neonates receiving ceftriaxone should not be given calcium containing fluids because of the risk for precipitation of calcium–ceftriaxone.[3] In older infants and children receiving ceftriaxone, the IV line should be flushed thoroughly before and after ceftriaxone infusion.[3] **Warnings:** Several different salt forms of calcium are available. Attention must be paid to the salt during product ordering, selection, and administration.[4,5]
Infusion related cautions	Small veins (scalp, small hand or foot) should not be used for infusion.[4] The infusion should be stopped if the patient complains of discomfort. Extravasation may cause tissue sloughing and necrosis.[6-10] (See Appendix E for management of extravasation.) Should not be infused through an arterial catheter because of the potential for vasospasm.[6-11]

Dosage	10% calcium gluconate solution provides approximately 0.465 mEq/mL or 9.3 mg/mL of elemental calcium.[1,2] 1 mEq is equivalent to 20 mg elemental calcium.
	
	Hypocalcemia (dosing should be guided by monitoring serum calcium concentrations)
	
	    Neonates: 200 mg/kg[4,12,13] to 400 mg/kg/day as a continuous infusion or divided q 6-8 h.[14-17] Doses as large as 800 mg/kg have been used.[4,16]
	
	    Infants and children: 200–500 mg/kg/day as a continuous infusion or divided q 6 h.[4]
	
	    Adolescents and *adults*: 2–15 g/day as a continuous infusion or divided q 6 h.[4]
	
	Hypocalcemia secondary to infusion of blood products: 0.45 mEq per 100 mL of citrated blood.[4]
	
	Tetany
	
	    Neonates: 500 mg/kg/day divided q 6 h.[4]
	
	    Children: 100–200 mg/kg/dose given three to four times a day (maximum 500 mg/day) until tetany resolves.[13]

Dosage adjustment in organ dysfunction	Calcium is renally eliminated. Calcium concentrations should be monitored closely in patients with renal dysfunction who require calcium.
Maximum dosage	For term neonates, 800 mg/kg/day as a continuous infusion or in four divided doses.[9] For older infants and children, 500 mg/kg/day as continuous infusion or in four divided doses.[9]
Additives	Aluminum is present as a contaminant.[2]

Calcium Gluconate

Suitable diluents	D5NS, D5W, D10W, D20W, LR, NS.[18]
Maximum concentration	Undiluted, 100 mg/mL.[2]
Preparation and delivery	**Compatibility:** Calcium containing fluids should not be co-infused with ceftriaxone.[3] Calcium containing fluids should not be co-infused with PN because of the risk for precipitation with the phosphate component.
IV push	Slow, over 3–5 minutes.[4] In *adults*, 150 mg (1.5 mL) over 1 minute.[2]
Intermittent infusion	100–200 mg/kg over 5–10 minutes.[4]
Continuous infusion	May be given continuously.
Other routes of administration	IM or SC administration should not be used.[4]
Comments	**Drug interactions:** IV calcium should be used cautiously in patients receiving cardiac glycosides because of the potential for development of arrhythmias.[2] **Adverse effects:** Bradycardia, hypotension, and cardiac arrhythmias may occur.[2] Calcinosis cutis occurred in an 11-year-old boy within 3 weeks of calcium gluconate infusion.[19] Calcium gluconate bioavailability is considered to be less than that of calcium chloride. In 49 critically ill children an average age of 3.7 ± 5 years, ionized calcium concentrations were increased 30 minutes after calcium gluconate and calcium chloride infusions.[20] Serum calcium concentrations were greater in the calcium chloride group compared to the calcium gluconate group.[20] In stable burn patients 5.5 ± 4.4 years-old, ionized calcium concentrations were not different 10 minutes after infusion of either calcium chloride or calcium gluconate.[21] Polyethylene vials contains significantly less contaminant aluminum than calcium gluconate in glass vials.[22]

Caspofungin

Brand names	Cancidas
Medication error potential	None reported by ISMP or USP.[1,2]
Contraindications and warnings	**Contraindications:** Documented hypersensitivity to caspofungin or any of its components.[3] **Warnings:** Transient elevations in ALT and AST, as well as, isolated cases of clinically significant hepatic dysfunction, hepatitis, and hepatic failure have been reported.[3,4] (See Drug interactions in Comments section.) Caspofungin should be limited to patients for whom the potential benefit outweighs the potential risk.[3]
Infusion related cautions	Possible histamine-mediated symptoms (flushing, urticaria, pruritus and bronchospasm), including anaphylaxis, have been reported.[3]
Dosage	**Neonates (preterm and term) and infants <3 months of age:** Initial (i.e., loading) doses of 1.5–8 mg/kg/day on day 1 followed by 1–6 mg/kg/day have been reported.[5-7] A 6-week-old (24 weeks of gestation) neonate received a 50 mg/m²/day loading dose followed by a 35 mg/m²/day maintenance dose.[8] Other reports have given 1 mg/kg/day for 2 days followed by 2 mg/kg/day[9-11] and 5 mg/kg/day (50 mg/m²) for 3 days followed by 2.5 mg/kg/day (25 mg/m²).[12] **Neonates, infants, children (≥3 months up to 17 years of age):** It is recommended to use BSA (see Appendix A) for caspofungin dosing (see Pharmacokinetic considerations in Comments section). Loading dose of 70 mg/m²/day on day 1, followed by 50 mg/m²/day thereafter (maximum loading dose and maintenance dose should not exceed 70 mg).[3,11,13-18] ***Adults:*** 70 mg/day for 1 day followed by 50 mg/day.[3,11,13,19]
Dosage adjustment in organ dysfunction	No dosage adjustment is recommended with renal impairment or mild hepatic impairment. With moderate to severe hepatic impairment (Child Pugh score of >7–9), dose adjustment is recommended.[3,20]
Maximum dosage	70 mg/day.[3,13-15] 100 mg/day has been given to *adults* and a 13-year-old.[3,21]
Additives	May contain parabens or 0.9% benzyl alcohol if bacteriostatic water (BW) is used for reconstitution.[3] See Appendix C for more specific information about potential adverse effects of parabens and about potential adverse effects and/or benzyl alcohol toxicity in neonates.
Suitable diluents	SW, NS, BW (for reconstitution); NS, ½NS, ¼NS, LR for further dilution.[3,22] Do not use dextrose-containing solutions as diluents.[3,22]
Maximum concentration	0.5 mg/mL.[3]

Caspofungin

Preparation and delivery	Do not admix or infuse concomitantly with other drugs.[3,22]
IV push	Not recommended.
Intermittent infusion	Administer (0.1–0.5 mg/mL) over 1 hour.[3,22]
Continuous infusion	No information available to support administration by this method.
Other routes of administration	No information available to support administration by other routes.
Comments	**Drug interactions:** Caspofungin is a weak substrate for CYP450.[23] Drug interactions are possible when used with tacrolimus and cyclosporine and certain inducers or inhibitors of CYP450.[3] Concomitant use of inducers (rifampin, efavirenz, nevirapine, phenytoin, dexamethasone and carbamazepine) may decrease caspofungin concentrations, thus caspofungin doses may need to be increased up to 70 mg/m²/day (maximum: 70 mg/day).[3] Consult appropriate resources for dosing recommendations before combining any drug with caspofungin. Cyclosporine increases the AUC of caspofungin by approximately 35%.[3] Concomitant cyclosporine use has also been associated with increases in ALT (2–3 times the upper limit of normal) and AST.[3] **Pharmacokinetic considerations:** Caspofungin exhibits log-linear pharmacokinetics where both weight and age influence clearance. The beta (distribution) phase half-life is 30% to 40% lower in pediatric patients than in *adult* patients. The shorter caspofungin beta-phase half-life observed in children relative to that in *adults* is most likely due to an increase in the relative rate of plasma clearance as suggested by both the weight-normalized and BSA-normalized clearance. Caspofungin uptake into tissue cells is increased in children relative to *adults,* with highest concentrations seen in the liver. Minimal metabolism and excretion occur during the first 30 hours postdose.[3,14,15] Pharmacokinetic studies have found that BSA-based dosing regimens, compared to mg/kg/day based dosing regimens produce similar concentrations to those seen in *adults*.[14,15,23] 1 mg/kg/day resulted in suboptimal concentrations in a pharmacokinetic study of children and adolescents.[15] **Other:** 2 mg/kg/day for 1 day followed by 1.5 mg/kg/day has been used successfully in combination with liposomal amphotericin B in a 24-month-old.[24]

CeFAZolin Sodium

Brand names	Ancef, Kefzol

Medication error potential

ISMP recommends tall man lettering to decrease confusion between ceFAZolin and cefTRIAXone.[1] CeFAZolin may be confused with cefepime, cefotaxime, cefoxitin, cefprozil, ceftazidime, ceftizoxime, cefuroxime, cephalexin, cephalothin oxacillin, Rocephin, and Zosyn.[2] Kefzol may be confused with Cefzil.[2] Errors with Cefotan and cefotetan have resulted in harm.[2]

Contraindications and warnings

Contraindications: Do not use in patients with immediate-type hypersensitivity reactions to cephalosporins.[3]

Warnings: Individuals who have a Type I reaction to penicillin may have cross sensitivity to cephalosporins.[3] (See Appendix C for specific information.)

Prolonged use may cause superinfection and/or *Clostridium difficile*–associated diarrhea (CDAD), which has been reported and may range in severity from mild diarrhea to fatal colitis.[2] If CDAD is suspected or confirmed, appropriate fluid and electrolyte management, protein supplementation, antibiotic treatment of *C. difficile*, and surgical evaluation should be instituted as clinically indicated.[2]

Infusion related cautions

If given to a patient with known penicillin hypersensitivity, the patient should be closely observed for allergenicity. (See Appendix C.)

Dosage

Neonates: Safety in patients <1 month has not been established.[3] However, the following doses have been used:

PNA	≤2000 g	>2000 g
≤7 days	40 mg/kg/day divided q 12 h[4,5]	40 mg/kg/day divided q 12 h[4,5]
>7 days*		60 mg/kg/day q 8 h[4,5]

*Until 4 weeks of age.

Infants and children

Mild-to-moderate infections: 25–50 mg/kg/day divided q 6–8 h.[3,6-8]

Severe infections: 50–100 mg/kg/day divided q 6–8 h.[3,5,8,9]

Bacterial endocarditis

Prevention (for dental procedure*): 50 mg/kg not to exceed 2 g given 30–60 minutes prior to a procedure.[8,10] Only for patients with underlying cardiac conditions associated with the highest risk of adverse outcome. (See Comments section.)

*that involve manipulation of gingival tissue or the periapical region of teeth or perforation of the oral mucosa[10]

Treatment (oxacillin-susceptible staphylococci in nonanaphylactoid penicillin-allergic patient)

Absence of prosthetic material: 100 mg/kg/day divided q 8 h with or without gentamicin for 3–5 days.[11]

Prosthetic valve endocarditis: 100 mg/kg/day divided q 8 h plus rifampin for ≥6 weeks; plus gentamicin for 2 weeks.[11]

Perioperative prophylaxis: 20–30 mg/kg dose administered 30 minutes to 1 hour prior to the start of surgery. May need to redose during surgery for lengthy operative procedures longer than 2 hours.[3]

CeFAZolin Sodium

Dosage adjustment in organ dysfunction	If CrCl is 40–70 mL/min, give 60% of the normal daily dose divided doses q 12 h.[3,10] If CrCl is 20–40 mL/min, give 25% of the normal daily dose divided doses q 12 h.[3,12] If CrCl is 5–20 mL/min, give 10% of the normal daily dose q 24 h.[3,12]
Maximum dosage	100 mg/kg/day,[3,5,11] not to exceed 6 g/day in children and 12 g/day in *adults*.[3]
Additives	2.1 mEq (46 mg) sodium/g of cefazolin.[3]
Suitable diluents	D5LR, D5NS, D5½NS, D5¼NS, D5W, D10W, LR, NS, SW, or R.[3,13]
Maximum concentration	77 mg/mL (in D5W), 69 mg/mL (in NS), and 138 mg/mL in SW.[14] Concentrations of 225–330 mg/mL have been used for IM administration.[3]
Preparation and delivery	**Delivery system issues:** The mixing of cefazolin with an aminoglycoside in vitro can result in substantial inactivation of the aminoglycoside.[15-19] (See Appendix C for more specific information.) **Stability:** No change in potency when color is pale yellow to yellow.[3] Store intact vials at room temperature and protect from light.[3] Reconstituted solution is stable for 24 hours at room temperature or 10 days when refrigerated; thawed solutions of the commercially available, frozen cefazolin injections are stable for 48 hours at room temperature or 30 days when refrigerated.[3] Shake well before use.[3] **Compatibility:** See Appendix D for PN compatibility information.[20]
IV push	50–100 mg/mL over 3–5 minutes.[1,11] In fluid-restricted patients, 138 mg/mL has been administered.[14]
Intermittent infusion	5–20 mg/mL[1,11] over 10–60 minutes.[11,12]
Continuous infusion	Although no specific information is available, other beta-lactam antibiotics have been given by this method.[21] Manufacturer states that cefazolin may be administered by continuous infusion.[3]
Other routes of administration	Reconstitute in SW (225–330 mg/mL) and give by deep IM administration.[3]
Comments	**Rare adverse events:** Thrombophlebitis has been reported after 36–48 hours of intermittent infusion.[7] Cephalosporin-induced hepatitis can present as cholestatic hepatitis and eosinophilic hepatitis.[22] Interstitial nephritis has been reported.[23] Hemolytic anemia has been reported.[22]

CeFAZolin Sodium

Comments *(cont.)*

Laboratory interference: False-positive urinary glucose results when cupric sulfate solution-based tests (Clinitest, Benedict's solution, Fehling's solution) are used. Glucose oxidase methods (Diastix, TEST-TAPE, Clinistix) are not associated with false-positive test results.[3] May also cause false increase serum or urine creatinine.[3]

Positive direct and indirect Coombs' tests have been reported and may also occur in newborn infants whose mothers received cephalosporins before delivery.[3]

Drug interactions: Probenecid may decrease renal tubular secretion and increase serum concentrations of cefazolin.[3]

Other: Cardiac conditions associated with the highest risk of adverse outcome from endocarditis for which prophylaxis with dental procedures is reasonable: (1) prosthetic cardiac valve or prosthetic material used for cardiac valve repair; (2) previous IE; (3) congenital heart disease (CHD)* in a person with a) unrepaired cyanotic CHD including palliative shunts and conduits, b) completely repaired congenital heart defect with prosthetic material or device whether placed by surgery or by catheter intervention during the first 6 months after the procedure,† and c) repaired CHD with residual defects at the site or adjacent to the site of a prosthetic patch or prosthetic device (which inhibit endothelialization); and (4) cardiac transplantation recipients who develop cardiac valvulopathy.[10]

---

*Except for the conditions listed above, antibiotic prophylaxis is no longer recommended for any other form of CHD.

†Prophylaxis is reasonable because endothelialization of prosthetic material occurs within 6 months after the procedure.

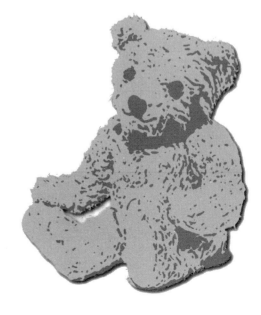

Cefepime

Brand names	Maxipime

Medication error potential

Look-alike, sound-alike drug names.

USP reports confusion with cefazolin, cefixime, cefotaxime, cefotetan, Cefotan, cefoxitin, ceftazidime, ceftriaxone, and ceftizoxime.[1] USP also reports confusion for Maxipime with cefotaxime and ceftazidime.[1]

Contraindications and warnings

Contraindications: Should not be used in those with a known allergy to cefepime or another cephalosporin antibiotic, penicillin, and other beta-lactam antibiotics.[2]

Warnings: Individuals who have a Type I reaction to penicillin may have cross sensitivity to cephalosporins (10%).[2] (See Appendix C for specific information.)

Adjust dosage in those with renal dysfunction (CrCL ≤60 mL/min).[2]

Prolonged use may cause superinfection and/or *Clostridium difficile*–associated diarrhea (CDAD), which has been reported and may range in severity from mild diarrhea to fatal colitis.[2] If CDAD is suspected or confirmed, appropriate fluid and electrolyte management, protein supplementation, antibiotic treatment of *C. difficile,* and surgical evaluation should be instituted as clinically indicated.[2]

Infusion related cautions

If a decision is made to give this medication to a patient with known penicillin hypersensitivity, the patient should be closely observed for allergenicity. Although rare, anaphylactoid reactions may require immediate emergency treatment with epinephrine, oxygen, IV steroids, antihistamines, pressor amines, and airway management.

Pain or phlebitis may occur at the injection site.[2]

Dosage

Neonates

≤14 days (term and preterm): 60 mg/kg/day divided q 12 h.[3]

>14 days: 100 mg/kg/day divided q 12 h.[3]

Infants and children (2 month–16 years)

Mild-to-moderate infection: 100–150 mg/kg/day divided q 8 h[4] or 12 h.[5]

Severe infections: 150 mg/kg/day divided q 8 h.[4]

Adolescents or patients >40 kg: 1–4 g/day divided q 12 h.[2]

Bacterial endocarditis (treatment of culture negative within 1 year of prosthetic valve infection): 150 mg/kg/day divided q 8 h for 6 weeks (plus gentamicin, vancomycin, and rifampin).[6]

Cystic fibrosis (acute pulmonary exacerbation): 150 mg/kg/day (up to 2 g/dose) divided q 8 h.[7,8]

Febrile neutropenia

Infants and children (2 months–16 years): 150 mg/kg/day divided q 8 h.[3,9-12]

Adolescents or those >40 kg: 6 g/day divided q 8 h.[3,12]

Meningitis: Although cefepime has been given to treat meningitis (150 mg/kg/day divided q 8 h),[13,14] the manufacturer recommends that patients with suspected or documented meningitis should receive an alternate antibiotic with demonstrated clinical efficacy.[4]

Skin and soft tissue infections, urinary tract infections (including pyelonephritis), pneumonia, and lower respiratory tract infections: Infants and children should receive 150 mg/kg/day divided q 8–12 h.[3,15-19]

Cefepime

Dosage adjustment in organ dysfunction	If CrCl is >50 mL/min give normal dose q 12 h; if 10–50 mL/min give q 16–24 h; and if <10 mL/min give q 24–48 h.[20] If not adjusted, serious adverse reactions, including life-threatening or fatal occurrences of encephalopathy, myoclonus, and seizures may occur.[2] No adjustment in impaired hepatic function.[2] Unlike other cephalosporins, no dosage adjustment is needed for burn patients.[21]
Maximum dosage	2 g/dose.[3]
Additives	None.
Suitable diluents	D5W, D10W, NS, D5NS, D5LR, Normosol-M in D5, or Normosol–R in D5.[3,22]
Maximum concentration	280 mg/mL for IM[3,20] and 160 mg/mL for IV administration.[3,22]
Preparation and delivery	**Stability:** Store at or below –20°C.[2] Thaw frozen container at room temperature (25°C) or under refrigeration (5°C).[2] Do not force thaw by immersion in water baths or by microwave irradiation.[2] The thawed solution is stable for 7 days if refrigerated (5°C) or for 24 hours at room temperature (25°C).[2] Do not refreeze.[2] **Compatibility:** See Appendix D for PN compatibility information.
IV push	Although not generally administered by this method, doses of 2 g have been given over 3–5 minutes in *adults*.[23]
Intermittent infusion	10–40 mg/mL over 30 minutes.[2,22]
Continuous infusion	3–4 g/day over 24 hours (125–167 mg/h) at a concentration of 3–4 mg/mL in *adults*.[24]
Other routes of administration	IM administration.[3] Diluted in D5W, 0.5 or 1% lidocaine, BW, SW, or NS to a maximum concentration of 280 mg/mL.[3,16]
Comments	**Rare adverse events:** Aminoglycosides may increase the potential of nephrotoxicity and ototoxicity.[2] Likewise, potent diuretics (e.g., furosemide) have been associated with nephrotoxicity.[2] Many cephalosporins can cause a decrease in prothrombin activity.[2,4,11] The drug may also suppress the gut flora that normally synthesizes these clotting factors. Patients with renal or hepatobiliary impairment or poor nutritional status, and those with cancer have an increased risk for this adverse effect.[2] Prothrombin time should be monitored in patients at risk and exogenous vitamin K administered as indicated. (See Appendix C for specific information.) **Monitor:** CBC, prothrombin time (especially if on warfarin); signs and symptoms of *Clostridium difficile*–associated diarrhea.

Cefepime

Drug interactions: Cephalosporins may enhance the anticoagulant effect of vitamin K antagonists (e.g., warfarin). Concomitant use of probenecid may increase the AUC of cefuroxime.[2] Consult appropriate resources for dosing recommendations before combining any drug with cefepime.

Laboratory interference: False-positive urinary glucose results when cupric sulfate solution-based tests (Clinitest, Benedict's solution, Fehling's solution) are used. It is recommended that glucose tests (Diastix, TEST-TAPE, Clinistix) based on enzymatic glucose oxidase reactions be used. Positive direct Coombs' tests have been reported during treatment with cefepime.[2]

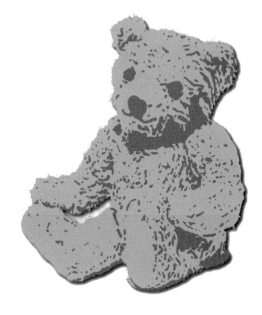

Cefotaxime Sodium

Brand names	Claforan

Medication error potential

Look-alike, sound-alike drug names.

USP reports confusion with cefazolin, cefepime, Cefotan, cefotetan, cefoxitin, ceftazidime, ceftizoxime, ceftriaxone, cefuroxime and Maxipime. Claforan has been confused with Cefotan and Cleocin.[1] Confusion with ceftriaxone has resulted in patient harm.[1]

Contraindications and warnings

Contraindications: Should not be used in those with a known allergy to cefotaxime or another cephalosporin antibiotics.[2] Solutions containing dextrose may be contraindicated in patients with hypersensitivity to corn products.[2]

Warnings: Individuals who have a Type I reaction to penicillin may have cross sensitivity to cephalosporins. Cefotaxime should be given cautiously to these patients.[2] (See Appendix C for specific information.)

A potentially life-threatening arrhythmia has been reported in six patients who received cefotaxime by rapid bolus injection (<60 seconds) through a central venous catheter.[2]

Prolonged use may cause superinfection and/or *Clostridium difficile*–associated diarrhea (CDAD), which has been reported and may range in severity from mild diarrhea to fatal colitis.[2] If CDAD is suspected or confirmed, appropriate fluid and electrolyte management, protein supplementation, antibiotic treatment of *C. difficile,* and surgical evaluation should be instituted as clinically indicated.[2]

Infusion related cautions

If a decision is made to give this medication to a patient with known penicillin hypersensitivity, the patient should be closely observed for allergenicity. Although rare, anaphylactoid reactions may require immediate emergency treatment with epinephrine, oxygen, IV steroids, antihistamines, pressor amines, and airway management.[2]

Dosage

Neonates: The manufacturer indicates that it is not necessary to differentiate between premature and normal-gestational age infants[2]; however, when dosing others recommend the following:

PNA	<1200 g	1200–2000 g	≥2000 g
<7 days	100 mg/kg/day divided q 12 h[2-4]*	100 mg/kg/day divided q 12 h[2-4]	100–150 mg/kg/day divided q 8–12 h[2-4]
≥7 days		150 mg/kg/day divided q 8 h[2-4]	150–200 mg/kg/day divided q 6–8 h[3-5]

*Until 4 weeks of age.

Doses as small as 50 mg/kg/day given as a single dose or divided q 12 h may provide effective serum concentrations for non-CNS infections in very low birth weight infants.[6,7]

Cefotaxime Sodium

Dosage *(cont.)*	**Infants and children**
	Mild-to-moderate infections: 75–100 mg/kg/day (up to 4–6 g/day) divided q 6–8 h.[4,8-10]
	Severe infections: 150–300 mg/kg/day (up to 8–10 g/day) divided q 6–8 h.[4]
	The manufacturer recommends 50–180 mg/kg/day divided q 4–6 h if <50 kg.[2]
	Adolescents and *adults*: Usual dose 2 g/day given as a single dose or divided q 12 h.[2] Depending on severity of infection, may be treated with 2 g/dose q 6, 8, or 12 h up to 12 g/day.[2]
	Meningitis: For neonates see maximum doses in above table. 225–300 mg/kg/day divided q 6–8 h[3,4,10-13] up to 8–12 g/day divided 4–6 hours.[11]
Dosage adjustment in organ dysfunction	If CrCl is 10–50 mL/min, give normal dose q 6–12 h; if <10 mL/min give q 24 h.[14,15] The manufacturer recommends halving the dose when CrCl is <20 mL/min.[2]
Maximum dosage	300 mg/kg/day in neonates, infants, and children with meningitis.[3,9,10] Total daily dose should not exceed 12 g/day.[2]
Additives	Contains 2.2 mEq sodium/g of cefotaxime.[2]
Suitable diluents	D5W, D10W, NS, LR, D5NS, D5¼NS, D5½NS, sodium lactate injection (M/6) and 10% invert sugar injection [2,16]
Maximum concentration	200 mg/mL in SW for IV push.[2] 86 mg/mL in D5W, 73 mg/mL in NS, and 147 mg/mL in SW results in a recommended osmolality for peripheral infusion in fluid-restricted patients.[16]
Preparation and delivery	**Delivery system issues:** The mixing of cefotaxime with an aminoglycoside in vitro can result in substantial inactivation of the aminoglycoside.[2] (See Appendix C for more specific information.)
	Stability: Satisfactory potency for 24 hours at or below 22°C, and at least 5 days under refrigeration (5°C).[2] Normal color is light yellow to amber; discoloration may suggest a loss of potency.[17]
	Compatibility: See Appendix D for PN compatibility information.[18]
	Photosensitivity: Protect from light.[17]
IV push	200 mg/mL via central catheter and 60 mg/mL via peripheral vein over 3–5 minutes.[2,4] A 25-mg/kg dose has been infused over 1 minute in neonates.[8] Rapid IV push (<1 minute) of a cephalosporin has caused potentially life-threatening arrhythmias.[2]
Intermittent infusion	10–60 mg/mL[2] over 10–30 minutes.[17]
Continuous infusion	May be used.[2]

Cefotaxime Sodium

Other routes of administration

230–330 mg/mL in BW may be given IM at same doses as IV.[2]

Comments

Rare adverse effects: Increased nephrotoxicity has been reported following concomitant administration of cephalosporins and aminoglycoside antibiotics[2]; however, the literature is conflicted on this adverse effect.[17,19]

Cephalosporins may inhibit vitamin K dependent clotting factors and may also suppress the gut flora that normally synthesize these clotting factors.[20] Patients with renal or hepatobiliary impairment or poor nutritional status, and those with cancer have an increased risk for this adverse effect.[2] (See Appendix C for specific information.)

Several cephalosporins have been implicated in triggering seizures, particularly in patients with renal impairment when the dosage was not reduced.[2,21] If seizures associated with drug therapy occur, the drug should be discontinued and anticonvulsants should be given as indicated.

Disulfiram-like reaction (flushing, sweating, headache, tachycardia) due to alcohol consumption have not been reported.[2]

Monitor: CBC, prothrombin time (especially if on warfarin); signs and symptoms of *Clostridium difficile*–associated diarrhea. Because of the potential for nephrotoxicity, renal function should be carefully monitored, especially if large doses of the aminoglycosides are administered or if therapy is prolonged.[2]

Drug interactions: Cephalosporins may enhance the anticoagulant effect of vitamin K antagonists (e.g., warfarin). Antibiotics may diminish the therapeutic effect of the live attenuated Ty21a strain Typhoid vaccine.[22] Uricosuric agents may decrease the excretion of cephalosporins.[22] Other interactions may occur; consult appropriate resources for dosing recommendations before combining any drug with cefotaxime.

Laboratory interference: False-positive urinary glucose results when cupric sulfate solution-based tests (Clinitest, Benedict's solution, Fehling's solution) are used.[2] It is recommended that glucose tests (Diastix, TEST-TAPE, Clinistix) based on enzymatic glucose oxidase reactions be used. Positive direct Coombs' tests have been reported during treatment with cefotaxime.[2]

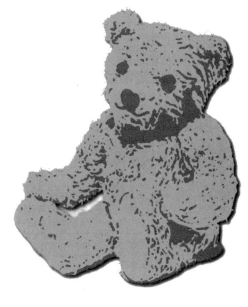

Cefotetan Disodium

Brand names	Cefotan

Medication error potential

Look-alike, sound-alike drug names.

USP reports confusion with cefamandole, cefazolin, cefotaxime, cefoxitin, ceftazidime and ceftriaxone.[1] Confusion with cefazolin has resulted in patient harm.[1] Cefotan may be confused with Ceftin.[1]

Contraindications and warnings

Contraindications: Should not be used in those with a known hypersensitivity reactions to cefotetan or another cephalosporin.[2] It is also contraindicated in those who have experienced cephalosporin-associated hemolytic anemia.[2]

Warnings: Individuals who have a Type I reaction to penicillin may have cross sensitivity to cephalosporins.[2] (See Appendix C for specific information.)

Although rare, an immune mediated hemolytic anemia, including fatalities, has been observed in patients receiving cephalosporins, especially cefotetan.[2] (See Comments section.)

Cefotetan contains the N-methyl-thiotetrazole (NMTT) side chain, which may inhibit vitamin K dependent clotting factors.[2,3] (See Comments section.)

Prolonged use may cause superinfection and/or *Clostridium difficile*–associated diarrhea (CDAD), which has been reported and may range in severity from mild diarrhea to fatal colitis.[2] If CDAD is suspected or confirmed, appropriate fluid and electrolyte management, protein supplementation, antibiotic treatment of *C. difficile,* and surgical evaluation should be instituted as clinically indicated.[2]

Infusion related cautions

Although rare, anaphylactoid reactions may require immediate emergency treatment with epinephrine, oxygen, IV steroids, antihistamines, pressor amines, and airway management.[2]

Dosage

Doses and side effects have not been established in neonates, infants, and children.

Neonates: No information.

Infants and children: Inappropriate for mild-to-moderate infections.[4] For severe infections, 40–80 mg/kg/day divided q 12 h up to 6 g/day.[4]

Adolescents and *adults*: 2–6 g/day divided q 12 h.[2]

Pelvic inflammatory disease: 4 g/day divided q 12 h (plus doxycycline 200 mg/day orally or IV divided q 12 h) for at least 48 hours after the patient clinically improves.[4-6]

Surgical prophylaxis: 20–40 mg/kg/dose (up to 1–2 g) 30–60 minutes prior to surgery.[2] May add 2 mg/kg of gentamicin if the viscus is ruptured.[4]

Dosage adjustment in organ dysfunction

Administer normal dose q 24 h if CrCl is 10–29 mL/min and q 48 h if CrCl is <10 mL/min.[7]

Maximum dosage

80 mg/kg/day; 40 mg/kg/dose up to 6 g/day in *adults*.[2]

Additives

3.5 mEq (80 mg) of sodium/g of cefotetan.[2,8]

Suitable diluents

D5W or NS.[8]

Cefotetan Disodium

Maximum concentration	182 mg/mL for IV infusion and 500 mg/mL for IM administration.[2,8]
Preparation and delivery	**Delivery system issues:** The mixing of cefotetan with an aminoglycoside in vitro can result in substantial inactivation of the aminoglycoside.[2,9-13] (See Appendix C for more specific information.) Cefotetan in Galaxy plastic containers should not be used for IM administration.[2] **Stability:** Thawed solutions of the commercially available frozen cefotetan injections are stable for 48 hours at room temperature or 21 days when refrigerated.[2] Do not refreeze.[2] **Compatibility:** See Appendix D for PN compatibility information.[14]
IV push	≤182 mg/mL over 3–5 minutes.[2,8]
Intermittent infusion	≤40 mg/mL over 20–60 minutes.[2]
Continuous infusion	No information available to support cefotetan administration by this method; however, other beta-lactams have been given by continuous infusion.[15]
Other routes of administration	500 mg/mL in SW, BW, NS, 0.5, or 1% lidocaine by deep IM injection.[2,8] Should not be given IM to patients with septicemia, bacteremia, or life-threatening infections.[2]
Comments	**Rare adverse effects:** The risk of cefotetan-induced hemolytic anemia is three times higher than that reported with cephalosporins.[2] If anemia develops anytime within 2–3 weeks of receiving cefotetan, the diagnosis of a cephalosporin-associated anemia should be considered.[2,3] Patients with renal or hepatobiliary impairment or poor nutritional status, and those with cancer have an increased risk for cefotetan inhibition of vitamin K dependent clotting factors.[2] **Monitoring:** CBC and prothrombin time (especially if on warfarin) and administer exogenous vitamin K as needed.[2] Monitor for signs and symptoms of hemolytic anemia and *Clostridium difficile*–associated diarrhea. **Drug interactions:** Cephalosporins may enhance the anticoagulant effect of vitamin K antagonists (e.g., warfarin).[2,16] Disulfiram-like reaction (flushing, sweating, headache, tachycardia) may occur when alcohol is consumed within 72 hours of administration of cefotetan.[2] Antibiotics may diminish the therapeutic effect of the Ty21a strain of the live attenuated Typhoid vaccine.[17] **Laboratory interference:** Cefotetan may cause false-positive urinary glucose results when cupric sulfate solution-based tests (Clinitest, Benedict's solution, or Fehling's solution) are used.[2] It is recommended that glucose tests (Diastix, TEST-TAPE, Clinistix) based on enzymatic glucose oxidase reactions be used. When the Jaffe reaction is used to determine creatinine, high concentrations of cefotetan may cause falsely elevated serum or urinary creatinine values.[2] **Osmolality:** 200 mg/mL has an osmolarity of 800 mOsm/L.[8] Concentrations used for IM injection are very hypertonic and have osmolarities >1500 mOsm/L.[8]

Cefoxitin Sodium

Brand names	Mefoxin
Medication error potential	USP reports confusion with cefazolin, cefepime, Cefotan, cefotaxime, cefotetan, ceftriaxone, and cefuroxime.[1]

Contraindications and warnings

Contraindications: In patients with known hypersensitivity to cefoxitin or to another cephalosporin antibiotic.[2] Individuals who have a Type I reaction to penicillin may have cross sensitivity to cephalosporins. (See Appendix C for specific information.)

Warnings: Prolonged use may cause superinfection and/or *Clostridium difficile*-associated diarrhea (CDAD), which has been reported and may range in severity from mild diarrhea to fatal colitis.[2] If CDAD is suspected or confirmed, appropriate fluid and electrolyte management, protein supplementation, antibiotic treatment of *C. difficile,* and surgical evaluation should be instituted as clinically indicated.[2] Antibiotic use that is not directed against *C. difficile* may need to be discontinued.[2]

Infusion related cautions

If a decision is made to give this medication to a patient with known cephalosporin or penicillin hypersensitivity, the patient should be closely observed for allergenicity.[2] (See Appendix C for specific information.)

Thrombophlebitis has been reported.[2]

Dosage

Neonates: Safety and efficacy in infants <3 months old have not been established.[2]

Doses of 75–90 mg/kg/day divided q 8 h have been reported.[3-5]

Infants and children

> **Mild-to-moderate infections:** 80–100 mg/kg/day (up to 3–4 g/day) divided q 4–6 h.[2,6-10]

> **Severe infections:** 80–160 mg/kg/day (up to 6–12 g/day) divided q 4–6 h.[2,6-10]

Adolescents and *adults*: 3–12 g/day divided q 6–8 h.[2] Dosage should be guided by susceptibility of organisms, severity of the infection, and clinical status of the patient. The larger dosages should be reserved for more severe or serious infections.

Pelvic inflammatory disease (PID): 8 g/day divided q 6 h (plus doxycycline 100 mg orally or IV q 12 g) for at least 48 hours after the patient clinically improves.[6,11]

Surgical prophylaxis: 30–40 mg/kg/dose (up to 1–2 g) given 30–60 minutes prior to surgery; followed by 120–160 mg/kg/day divided q 6 h for no longer than 24 hours.[2] One study gave 150 mg/kg/day divided q 8 h (first dose at anesthesia induction) for 5 days for acute appendicitis.[12]

Dosage adjustment in organ dysfunction

If CrCl is 30–50 mL/min, give normal dose q 8 h[13]; if CrCl is 10–29 mL/min, give normal dose q 12 h[13]; if CrCl is 5–10 mL/min, give 50% of a normal dose q 12–24 h[2]; if CrCl <5 mL/min, give 50% of a normal dose q 24–48 h.[2]

Maximum dosage

160 mg/kg/day, not to exceed 12 g/day.[2] (See Comments section.)

Additives

2.3 mEq sodium/g of cefoxitin.[2] Some products may contain benzyl alcohol. (See Appendix C for specific information about benzyl alcohol potential for toxicity.)

Suitable diluents

D5W, D10W, D5¼NS, D5½NS, D5NS, R, LR, D5LR, or NS.[14]

Cefoxitin Sodium

Maximum concentration	200 mg/mL for IV push, 40 mg/mL for IV infusion, and 400 mg/mL for IM administration.[14] 112 mg/mL in SW results in a maximum recommended osmolality for peripheral infusion in fluid-restricted patients.[15]
Preparation and delivery	**Delivery system issues:** The mixing of cefoxitin with an aminoglycoside in vitro can result in substantial inactivation of the aminoglycoside.[2] (See Appendix C for more specific information.)[16-20] **Compatibility:** See Appendix D for PN compatibility.[21]
IV push	180 mg/mL over 3–5 minutes via central catheter and 50 mg/mL via peripheral vein.[2,15,22]
Intermittent infusion	10–40 mg/mL over 15–40 minutes.[2,7,14]
Continuous infusion	10–40 mg/mL in D5W, NS, or D5NS.[2] Other beta-lactam antibiotics have been given by this method.[22]
Other routes of administration	None.
Comments	**Rare adverse effect:** Increased nephrotoxicity has been reported following concomitant administration of cephalosporins and aminoglycoside.[2] Large doses of cefoxitin have caused an increased incidence of eosinophilia and elevated SGOT.[2] Several cephalosporins may cause seizures, particularly in significant renal impairment when the dosage was not reduced.[2,23,24] **Laboratory interference:** A false-positive urinary glucose results when cupric sulfate solution-based tests (Clinitest, Benedict's solution, Fehling's solution) are used.[2] It is recommended that glucose tests (Diastix, TEST-TAPE, Clinistix) based on enzymatic glucose oxidase reactions be used. When the Jaffe reaction is used to determine creatinine, high concentrations of cefoxitin may falsely elevate serum or urinary creatinine values; hence, serum should not be analyzed for creatinine if withdrawn within 2 hours of cefoxitin administration.[2] A positive direct Coombs' test may occur, especially those with azotemia.[2] High concentrations in the urine may interfere with determination of urinary 17-hydroxy-corticosteroids by the Porter-Silber reaction and produce a false increase in the levels.[2] **Other:** The potential for toxic effects from chemicals that may leach from the single-dose IV preparation in plastic has not been determined.[2,25]

Ceftazidime

Brand names Ceptaz, Fortaz, Tazicef, Tazidime

Medication error potential

Look-alike, sound alike drug names.

USP reports confusion with cefazolin, cefepime, cefotaxime, cefotetan, ceftizoxime, ceftriaxone, cefuroxime and Maxipime. Confusion with ceftriaxone has resulted in patient harm.[1]

Contraindications and warnings

Contraindications: Should not be used in those with a known allergy to cefoperazone or another cephalosporin antibiotics.[2]

Warnings: Individuals who have a Type I reaction to penicillin may have cross sensitivity to cephalosporins. Ceftazidime should be given cautiously to these patients.[2] (See Appendix C for specific information.)

Prolonged use may cause superinfection and/or *Clostridium difficile*–associated diarrhea (CDAD), which has been reported and may range in severity from mild diarrhea to fatal colitis.[2] If CDAD is suspected or confirmed, appropriate fluid and electrolyte management, protein supplementation, antibiotic treatment of *C. difficile,* and surgical evaluation should be instituted as clinically indicated.[2]

Accumulation of ceftazidime in patients with renal insufficiency may lead to seizures, encephalopathy, coma, asterixis, neuromuscular excitability, and myoclonia.[2]

Infusion related cautions

If a decision is made to give this medication to a patient with known penicillin hypersensitivity, the patient should be closely observed for allergenicity. Although rare, anaphylactoid reactions may require immediate emergency treatment with epinephrine, oxygen, IV steroids, antihistamines, pressor amines, and airway management.[2]

Accidental intra-arterial administration has resulted in distal necrosis.[2]

Dosage

Neonates

PNA	<1200 g	≤2000 g	>2000 g
≤7 days	100 mg/kg/day divided q 12 h[3]*	50–100 mg/kg/day divided q 12–18 h[3-8]	100–150 mg/kg/day divided q 8–12 h[3,6,9-11]
>7 days		150 mg/kg/day divided q 8 h[3,10,11]	150 mg/kg/day divided q 8 h[3,4,10,11]

*Until 4 weeks of age.

The manufacturer recommends 60 mg/kg/day divided q 12 h for those 0–4 weeks of age.[2] 25 mg/kg q 24 h has also been recommended for those with a gestational age <32 weeks.[12,13]

Dosage *(cont.)*	**Infants and children**
	Mild-to-moderate infections: 75–100 mg/kg/day divided q 8 h up to 3 g/day.[2,3]
	Severe infections (including meningitis): 125–150 mg/kg/day divided q 8 h up to 6 g/day.[2,3,14-20]
	Adolescents and *adults*: 2–3 g/day divided q 8–12 h up to 6 g/day.[2,3] Dose is dependent on type and severity of infection.[2]
	The larger doses should be reserved for patients with cystic fibrosis, meningitis or those who are immunocompromised.
	Cystic fibrosis: 150–320 mg/kg/day divided q 6–8 h[21-26] or a loading dose of 100 mg/kg (up to 2 g) followed by 3.4–12.5 mg/kg/h.[27]
	Neutropenia and fever (empiric therapy): 100–150 mg/kg/day divided q 8–12 h as monotherapy.[17-19,28]
Dosage adjustment in organ dysfunction	If CrCl is 31–50 mL/min, give normal dose q 12 h and if CrCl is 16–30 mL/min, give q 24 h;[2] if 6–15 mL/min, give 50% of the normal dose q 24 h;[2] if CrCl is <5 mL/min, give 50% of the normal dose q 48 h.[2,29-31] Another reference recommends 50 mg/kg dose q 12 h if CrCl is 30–50 mL/min; 50 mg/kg dose q 24 h if CrCl is 10–29 mL/min; and 50 mg/kg dose q 48 h if CrCl is < 10 mL/min.[32] No dosage adjustment necessary in hepatic dysfunction.[2]
Maximum dosage	240 mg/kg/day in normal children[16,33] or 320 mg/kg/day in patients with cystic fibrosis,[23] not to exceed 6 g/day.[2,3,17,34]
Additives	Contains 2.3 mEq sodium/g of ceftazidime.[2]
Suitable diluents	D5W, D10W, LR, NS D5NS, D5⅓NS, D5¼NS, D5½NS, 1/6 M sodium lactate injection or Normosol-M.[2,35]
Maximum concentration	200 mg/mL for central catheter.[2,4] Although one reference noted a maximum concentration of 40 mg/mL for peripheral administration,[4] 126 mg/mL in SW results in a maximum recommended osmolality for peripheral infusion in fluid-restricted patients.[36]
Preparation and delivery	**Delivery system issues:** The mixing of ceftazidime with an aminoglycoside in vitro can result in substantial inactivation of the aminoglycoside.[2] (See Appendix C for more specific information.) When ceftazidime is reconstituted, carbon dioxide is produced, resulting in bubbles and positive pressure in the vial.[2] The pressure is reduced by removing air from the vial with a syringe.[2] Bubbles remaining in the solution must be expelled prior to infusion.[2]
	Stability: Variable stability based on diluents and storage conditions. See manufacturer information[2] or specialty reference.[35] Do not force thaw by immersion in water baths or by microwave irradiation.[2] Once thawed, solutions should not be refrozen.[2]
	Compatibility: See Appendix D for PN compatibility information.[37]
IV push	100–200 mg/mL in SW over 3–5 minutes.[2] A 25-mg/kg dose has been infused over 1–2 minutes in a neonate.[13] Generally, give at a rate ≤10 mg/kg/min.[6]

Ceftazidime

Intermittent infusion	1–40 mg/mL infused over 10–30 minutes.[2]
Continuous infusion	Although concentration and solution type are usually not specified, ceftazidime has been given by this method.[27,37,38] 200 mg/kg in 100 mL D5W has been given over 24 hours to febrile neutropenic children.[38]
Other routes of administration	May be given IM.
Comments	**Rare adverse effects:** Although nephrotoxicity has been reported following concomitant administration of aminoglycoside antibiotics, the literature is conflicted on this adverse effect.[39]

Many cephalosporins may decrease in prothrombin activity by suppressing the gut flora that normally synthesize these clotting factors.[2,4,11,40] Patients with renal or hepatobiliary impairment or poor nutritional status, and those with cancer have an increased risk for this adverse effect.[2] Prothrombin time should be monitored in patients at risk, and exogenous vitamin K administered as indicated.

Several cephalosporins have been implicated in triggering seizures, particularly in patients with renal impairment when the dosage was not reduced.[41] If seizures associated with drug therapy occur, the drug should be discontinued. Anticonvulsant therapy can be given if clinically indicated.

Monitor: CBC, prothrombin time (especially if on warfarin); signs and symptoms of *Clostridium difficile*–associated diarrhea. Because of the potential for nephrotoxicity, renal function should be carefully monitored, especially if large doses of the aminoglycosides are administered or if therapy is prolonged.[2]

Drug interactions: Cephalosporins may enhance the anticoagulant effect of vitamin K antagonists (e.g., warfarin).[2] May need to adjust dosage in premature neonates receiving indomethacin.[42] Concomitant administration of cephalosporins with an aminoglycoside or potent diuretics (e.g., furosemide) may increase the likelihood of nephrotoxicity.[2] Nephrotoxicity and ototoxicity were not noted when ceftazidime was given alone.[2] Other interactions may occur; consult appropriate resources for dosing recommendations before combining any drug with ceftazidime.

Laboratory interference: False-positive urinary glucose results when cupric sulfate solution-based tests (Clinitest, Benedict's solution, Fehling's solution) are used.[2] It is recommended that glucose tests (Diastix, TEST-TAPE, Clinistix) based on enzymatic glucose oxidase reactions be used. Positive direct Coombs' tests have been reported during treatment with cefepime.[2]

Other: Patients with a history of type I reactions to penicillin should not receive beta-lactam antibiotics. From 5% to 15% of patients allergic to penicillin will also be allergic to cephalosporins. Certain infections (e.g., syphilis) require penicillin for eradication. It is recommended that a desensitization protocol for penicillin-allergic individuals should be performed in a hospital setting. This can usually be completed in about 4 hours, at which time the first dose of penicillin can be given.[2]

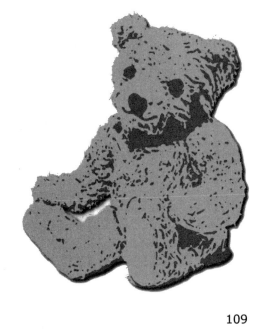

CefTRIAXone Sodium

Brand names	Rocephin

Medication error potential

ISMP recommends the following tall man letters (not FDA approved) to decrease confusion between ceFAZolin and cefTRIAXone.[1]

Look-alike, sound-alike drug names.

USP reports confusion with cefazolin, cefepime, Cefotan, cefotaxime, cefotetan, cefoxitin, ceftazidime, and cefuroxime.[2] Rocephin may be confused with cefazolin and Roferon.[2] Confusion with cefotaxime and ceftazidime have resulted in patient harm.[2]

Contraindications and warnings

Contraindications: Should not be used in those with a known allergy to ceftriaxone or another cephalosporin antibiotics.[3] Solutions containing dextrose may be contraindicated in patients with known allergy to corn or corn products.[3]

Ceftriaxone can displace bilirubin from its binding sites on serum albumin and may cause kernicterus and encephalopathy in hyperbilirubinemic neonates, especially premature neonates.[3]

Ceftriaxone must not be co-administered with calcium-containing IV solutions (e.g., Ringer's solution, Hartmann's solution, and parenteral nutrition formulations that contain calcium) in neonates because of the risk of precipitation of ceftriaxone–calcium salt.[3] Cases of fatal reactions with ceftriaxone–calcium precipitates in lungs and kidneys in neonates have been described.[3] In some cases the infusion lines and the times of administration of ceftriaxone and calcium-containing solutions differed.[3] There are no data on whether ceftriaxone might interact with calcium-containing products that are given orally and whether intramuscular ceftriaxone might interact with calcium-containing products, either IV or oral.[4] Ceftriaxone and products that contain calcium may be administered sequentially to patients older than 28 days of age, as long as the infusion lines are thoroughly flushed between infusions with a compatible fluid.[4] Ceftriaxone should not be administered simultaneously with any calcium-containing solution via Y-site in any patient.[4] Although the above information was current at the time this edition was printed, information related to the adverse effect is rapidly evolving and the reader is referred to the FDA website for the most up-to-date information.

Warnings: Individuals who have a Type I reaction to penicillin may have cross sensitivity to cephalosporins. Ceftriaxone should be given cautiously to these patients.[3] (See Appendix C for specific information.)

Prolonged use may cause superinfection and/or *Clostridium difficile*–associated diarrhea (CDAD), which has been reported and may range in severity from mild diarrhea to fatal colitis.[3] If CDAD is suspected or confirmed, appropriate fluid and electrolyte management, protein supplementation, antibiotic treatment of *C. difficile,* and surgical evaluation should be instituted as clinically indicated.[3]

Infusion related cautions

If a decision is made to give this medication to a patient with known penicillin hypersensitivity, the patient should be closely observed for allergenicity. Although rare, anaphylactoid reactions may require immediate emergency treatment with epinephrine, oxygen, IV steroids, antihistamines, pressor amines, and airway management.

CefTRIAXone Sodium

Dosage

Neonates: See Contraindications and warnings section.

PNA	<1200 g	≤2000 g	>2000 g
≤7 days	50 mg/kg q 24 h[5]*	50 mg/kg q 24 h[5]	50 mg/kg q 24 h[5]
>7 days		50 mg/kg q 24 h[5]	50–75 mg/kg q 24 h[5]

*Until 4 weeks of age.

Infants and children

>**Mild-to-moderate infections:** 50–75 mg/kg/day given as a single dose or divided q 12 h, up to 2 g/day.[5,6]

>**Severe infections (including meningitis):** 80–100 mg/kg/day given as a single dose or divided q 12 h, up to 4 g/day.[5,7-23]

Endocarditis (*enterococcus faecalis*): 2 g every 12 hours plus ampicillin (2 g every 4 hours) for 6 weeks.[24]

Gonococcal infection

>**Complicated:** 25–50 mg/kg/day (up to 1 g/day) as a single dose for 7 days.[5,25] If meningitis or endocarditis, give 50 mg/kg/day (up to 2 g/day) divided q 12 h for 10–14 days and 28 days, respectively, plus erythromycin.[5,25]

>**Ophthalmia:** Neonates born to mothers with known untreated gonorrhea should receive 25–50 mg/kg (up to 125 mg) as a single dose IV/IM.[5]

>**Prophylaxis:** Neonates born to mothers with gonococcal infections should be given 25–50 mg/kg (up to 125 mg) as a one-time dose.[5,25] Regardless of weight, children should receive 125 mg IM.[5] If providing prophylaxis after sexual victimization, add appropriate therapies for chlamydia trachomatis, hepatitis B, and trichomoniasis.[5,25]

>**Uncomplicated:** 125 mg as a single dose IM plus a macrolide antibiotic.[5,25]

Otitis media: 50 mg/kg (up to 1 g) as a single dose. Generally administered IM.[26-28]

Dosage adjustment in organ dysfunction

Most patients with renal dysfunction who receive ≤2 g/day do not require dosage adjustment.[3,29,30] However, some patients with end-stage renal disease receiving hemodialysis may accumulate ceftriaxone.[3,30] No adjustment in hepatic dysfunction; however, if both hepatic and renal dysfunction the dosage should not exceed 2 g/day.[3]

Maximum dosage

100 mg/kg/day,[3,5] not to exceed 4 g/day.[3,5]

Additives

Contains 3.6 mEq sodium/g of ceftriaxone.[3,31]

Suitable diluents

D5NS, D5½NS, D5W, D10W, NS, or S. Compatibility varies for dextrose-saline combinations. See more specific reference.[31]

Maximum concentration

40 mg/mL for IV administration and 350 mg/mL for IM use.[3]

CefTRIAXone Sodium

Preparation and delivery

Stability: Do not force thaw by immersion in water baths or by microwave irradiation.[3] 250-mg/mL reconstituted solutions are stable for 24 hours at room temperature and for 48 hours if refrigerated.[31] 100 mg/mL for 48 hours at room temperature and for 10 days if refrigerated.[31]

Compatibility: See Appendix D for PN compatibility information.[32]

Photosensitivity: Protect from light.[31]

IV push

10–40 mg/mL.[3,31] Doses have been given over 2–4 minutes in ambulatory patients >11 years of age[33] and over 5 minutes in children with meningitis.[34] However, 10 minutes after ceftriaxone was infused over 5 minutes, an *adult* being treated for presumed meningitis became diaphoretic, hypertensive, and tachycardic and developed palpitations.[35] Subsequent infusions over 30 minutes were uneventful.[35]

Intermittent infusion

10–40 mg/mL[3,31] infused over 10–30 minutes.[3,31]

Continuous infusion

Although no specific information is available to support administration by this route, other beta-lactam antibiotics have been given by this method.[36]

Other routes of administration

100–350 mg/mL in SW, NS, D5W, BW, or 1% lidocaine (without epinephrine) by deep IM injection.[6,31]

Comments

Rare adverse effects: Although nephrotoxicity has been reported following concomitant administration of aminoglycoside antibiotics, the literature is conflicted on this adverse effect.[37]

Ceftriaxone has been reported to cause primary cholelithiasis,[3,38] nephrolithiasis,[39] and hemolytic anemia.[40] Gallstones spontaneously resolved after discontinuation of the drug.[38] Cases of pancreatitis, possibly secondary to biliary obstruction, have been reported rarely in patients treated with ceftriaxone.[3]

Alterations in prothrombin times have occurred rarely in patients treated with ceftriaxone.[41] Patients with impaired vitamin K synthesis or low vitamin K stores (e.g., chronic hepatic disease and malnutrition) may require monitoring of prothrombin time during treatment. Vitamin K administration (10 mg weekly) may be necessary if the prothrombin time is prolonged before or during therapy.

Several cephalosporins have been implicated in triggering seizures, particularly in patients with renal impairment when the dosage was not reduced.[42] If seizures associated with drug therapy occur, the drug should be discontinued. Anticonvulsant therapy can be given if clinically indicated.

Monitor: CBC, prothrombin time (especially if on warfarin); signs and symptoms of *Clostridium difficile*–associated diarrhea. Because of the potential for nephrotoxicity, renal function should be carefully monitored, especially if large doses of the aminoglycosides are administered or if therapy is prolonged.[3]

Laboratory interference: Ceftriaxone false-positive urinary glucose results when cupric sulfate solution-based tests (Clinitest, Benedict's solution, Fehling's solution) are used.[3] It is recommended that glucose tests (Diastix, TEST-TAPE, Clinistix) based on enzymatic glucose oxidase reactions be used.[3] Positive direct Coombs' tests have been reported during treatment with ceftriaxone.[3]

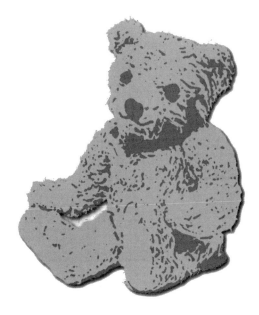

Cefuroxime Sodium

Brand names	Ceftin, Zinacef

Medication error potential

Look-alike, sound-alike drug names.

USP reports confusion with cefadroxil, cefazolin, cefepime, cefotaxime, cefoxitin, ceftazidime, ceftizoxime, ceftriaxone, and cephalexin.[1] USP reports confusion for Zinacef with Zithromax.[1]

Contraindications and warnings

Contraindications: Should not be used in those with a known allergy to cefuroxime or another cephalosporin antibiotics.[2]

Warnings: Individuals who have a Type I reaction to penicillin may have cross sensitivity to cephalosporins. Cefuroxime should be given cautiously to these patients.[2] (See Appendix C for specific information.)

Prolonged use may cause superinfection and/or *Clostridium difficile*–associated diarrhea (CDAD), which has been reported and may range in severity from mild diarrhea to fatal colitis.[2] If CDAD is suspected or confirmed, appropriate fluid and electrolyte management, protein supplementation, antibiotic treatment of *C. difficile,* and surgical evaluation should be instituted as clinically indicated.[2]

Infusion related cautions

If a decision is made to give this medication to a patient with known penicillin hypersensitivity, the patient should be closely observed for allergenicity. Although rare, anaphylactoid reactions may require immediate emergency treatment with epinephrine, oxygen, IV steroids, antihistamines, pressor amines, and airway management.[2]

Thrombophlebitis may occur.[2]

Dosage

Safety and efficacy in infants <3 months old have not been established.[2]

Neonates

PNA	<2000 g	>2000 g
<7 days	100 mg/kg/day divided q 12 h[3-5]	150 mg/kg/day divided q 8 h[3]
≥7 days	150 mg/kg/day divided q 8 h[3]*	150 mg/kg/day divided q 8 h[3]

*Until 4 weeks of age.

Infants ≥3 months and children

Mild-to-moderate infections: 50–100 mg/kg/day divided q 6–8 h.[2,6-11]

Severe infections: 100–150 mg/kg/day divided q 8 h.[6] Cefuroxime should not be used to treat bacterial meningitis. (See Comments section.)

Surgical prophylaxis (clean-contaminated or potentially contaminated procedures): In *adults* the manufacturer recommends that a 1.5-g dose be given 30–60 minutes before surgery to allow sufficient time to achieve effective antibiotic concentrations in the wound tissues during the procedure.[2] The dose should be repeated intraoperatively if the surgical procedure is lengthy (750 mg/dose q 8 h).[2]

Dosage adjustment in organ dysfunction

Adjust dosage in patients with renal dysfunction.[2] If CrCl is 10–20 mL/min, give a normal dose q 12 h and if CrCl is <10 mL/min, give q 24 h.[2]

Maximum dosage

300 mg/kg/day,[12,13] not to exceed 4 g/day in children[6] and 3 g/dose or 9 g/day in *adults* with meningitis.[2]

Cefuroxime Sodium

Additives	Contains 2.4 mEq sodium/g of cefuroxime.[2]
Suitable diluents	D5W, D10W, NS, LR, D5NS, D5¼NS, D5½NS.[2,14]
Maximum concentration	95 mg/mL for IV push and 225 mg/mL for IM administration.[2] 137 mg/mL in SW (489 mOsm/kg) resulted in a maximum recommended osmolality for peripheral infusion in fluid-restricted patients.[15]
Preparation and delivery	**Delivery system issues:** The mixing of cefuroxime with an aminoglycoside in vitro can result in substantial inactivation of the aminoglycoside. (See Appendix C for more specific information.) **Stability:** Stable for 24 hours at room temperature and 48 hours if refrigerated. **Compatibility:** See Appendix D for PN compatibility information.[16]
IV push	50–100 mg/mL over 3–5 minutes.[2]
Intermittent infusion	≤30 mg/mL over 15–60 minutes.[2,14]
Continuous infusion	7.5–15 mg/mL in D5W, D10W, NS, D5NS, D5½NS, or 1/6 M sodium lactate injection.[2]
Other routes of administration	220 mg/mL reconstituted with SW and administered into large muscle mass (gluteus or lateral thigh).[2,11,14]
Comments	**Rare adverse events:** Infants and children with meningitis who were treated with cefuroxime had an increased incidence of hearing loss[13,17] and an increased time to sterilization of their cerebrospinal fluid.[17] The AAP does not recommend cefuroxime for meningitis.[5] Although nephrotoxicity has been reported following concomitant administration of aminoglycoside antibiotics, the literature is conflicted on this adverse effect.[18] Several cephalosporins have been implicated in triggering seizures, particularly in patients with renal impairment when the dosage was not reduced.[19] If seizures associated with drug therapy occur, the drug should be discontinued. Anticonvulsant therapy can be given if clinically indicated. Cephalosporins may inhibit vitamin K dependent clotting factors and may also suppress the gut flora that normally synthesize these clotting factors.[20] Patients with renal or hepatobiliary impairment or poor nutritional status, and those with cancer have an increased risk for this adverse effect.[2] (See Appendix C for specific information.) **Monitor:** CBC, prothrombin time (especially if on warfarin); signs and symptoms of *Clostridium difficile*–associated diarrhea. Although rare cefuroxime may produce alterations in kidney function[2]; hence, evaluation of renal function is recommended, especially in seriously ill patients receiving large doses.

Cefuroxime Sodium

Comments *(cont.)*

Drug interactions: Cephalosporins may enhance the anticoagulant effect of vitamin K antagonists (e.g., warfarin).[20] Concomitant use of probenecid decreases tubular secretion and may increase serum concentrations of cefuroxime.[2]

Cephalosporins should be given with caution to patients receiving concurrent treatment with potent diuretics (e.g., furosemide) as these may negatively affect renal function.[2]

In common with other antibiotics, cefuroxime may affect the gut flora, leading to lower estrogen reabsorption and reduced efficacy of combined estrogen/progesterone oral contraceptives.

Laboratory interference: A false-positive urinary glucose results when cupric sulfate solution-based tests (Clinitest, Benedict's solution, Fehling's solution) are used.[2] It is recommended that glucose tests (Diastix, TEST-TAPE, Clinistix) based on enzymatic glucose oxidase reactions be used.[2] Positive direct Coombs' tests have been reported during treatment with cefuroxime.[2] Cefuroxime does not interfere with the assay of serum and urine creatinine by the alkaline picrate method.[2]

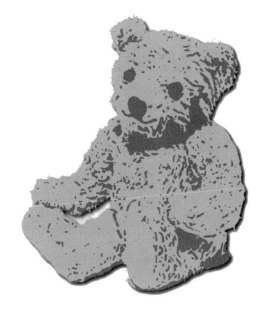

Chloramphenicol Sodium Succinate

Brand names	Chloromycetin

Medication error potential

None.

Contraindications and warnings

US boxed warning: Serious and fatal blood dyscrasias (aplastic anemia terminating in leukemia, hypoplastic anemia, thrombocytopenia, and granulocytopenia) have occurred with both short- and long-term use.[1]

Contraindications: Should not be used in individuals with a history of previous hypersensitivity and/or toxic reaction to chloramphenicol.[1] It must not be used in the treatment of trivial infections or where it is not indicated, as in colds, influenza, infections of the throat; or as a prophylactic agent to prevent bacterial infections.[1]

Other warnings: Prolonged use may cause superinfection and/or *Clostridium difficile*–associated diarrhea (CDAD), which has been reported and may range in severity from mild diarrhea to fatal colitis.[1] If CDAD is suspected or confirmed, appropriate fluid and electrolyte management, protein supplementation, antibiotic treatment of *C. difficile,* and surgical evaluation should be instituted as clinically indicated.[1]

Infusion related cautions

None.

Dosage

Inappropriate for mild-to-moderate infections.[1,2] Dosing should be optimized by measuring serum concentrations.[1-3]

Neonates (see Comments section)

> **Loading dose:** 20-mg/kg loading dose followed in 12 hours by maintenance doses.[4]

> **Maintenance dose:** Although the manufacturer recommends 25 mg/kg/day divided q 6 h,[1] most sources recommend more conservative dosing in neonate.[3-11]

>> **Premature, ≤1200 g:** 22 mg/kg given q 24 h.[6]

>> **Premature, ≤2000 g and ≤1 week:** 25 mg/kg given q 24 h.[6]

>> **Term, <2 weeks:** 25 mg/kg/day divided q 12 h.[3,5,7-11]

>> **Term, 2–4 weeks:** 25–50 mg/kg/day divided q 12 h.[3,5,7-11]

Infants and children: 50–100 mg/kg/day divided q 6–8 h.[1,2,5,8-21] Because of the emergence of vancomycin-resistant *Enterococcus*, some investigators have recommended 75–100 mg/kg/day divided q 6 h for the treatment of meningitis.[19-21] Other investigators noted that 100 mg/kg/day may be unnecessary and only increases the incidence of toxicity.[5,14,15]

Larger dosage that may be required for severe infections should only be given to maintain the serum concentration within a "therapeutic" range.[1]

Dosage adjustment in organ dysfunction

Adjust dosage in patients with hepatic[8-11] or renal[22,23] dysfunction. Dosage should be adjusted by on serum concentrations.[1]

Maximum dosage

100 mg/kg/day.[8-15] In neonates <2 weeks of age, 25 mg/kg/day[1,24] and 50 mg/kg/day in neonates <4 weeks of age.[1,25] Maximum *adult* dose should not exceed 2–4 g/day.[1] When large doses are used, serum concentration monitoring is imperative.

Additives

Contains 2.25 mEq sodium/g of chloramphenicol sodium succinate.[26]

Chloramphenicol Sodium Succinate

Suitable diluents	D2.5W, D5W, D10W, NS, ½NS, LR, D5LR, D5NS.[26]
Maximum concentration	100 mg/mL.[26]
Preparation and delivery	**Compatibility:** See Appendix D for PN compatibility information.[27]
IV push	100 mg/mL over ≥1 minute.[1]
Intermittent infusion	20–25 mg/mL over 15–60 minutes.[6,17,26]
Continuous infusion	Although concentration and solution type were not provided, chloramphenicol has been given by this method.[28]
Other routes of administration	Can be administered IM,[1,24,29] but the drug may be less effective.[24] Has been administered intraventricularly in an *adult.*[30]
Comments	**Significant adverse events:** Fatalities associated with gray syndrome (e.g., abdominal distension, progressive pallid cyanosis, circulatory collapse, acidosis, and myocardial depression) may result from drug accumulation in patients with immature or impaired hepatic or renal function.[31-36] Because it is generally associated with serum concentrations >50 mg/L, individualize dosage based on serum concentrations.[25-36]

Monitoring: Baseline blood studies and repeat test every 2 days are essential and may detect early peripheral blood changes.[1] The drug should be discontinued upon appearance of reticulocytopenia, leukopenia, thrombocytopenia, anemia or any other blood study findings attributable to chloramphenicol. However, normal blood tests do not exclude the possibility of later appearance of the irreversible type of bone marrow depression.[1]

Serum chloramphenicol concentrations should be collected 90 minutes after completion of the IV dose (peak) and immediately prior to the next dose (trough). Dose adjustments should be based on desired serum chloramphenicol concentrations (peak: 10–25 mg/L; trough: 5–15 mg/L).[37]

Drug interactions: Chloramphenicol inhibits the metabolism of several drugs (e.g., phenytoin, phenobarbital, tolbutamide, dicumarol, cyclosporine, and tacrolimus).[38-40] Likewise, many drugs (e.g., rifampin, phenobarbital, and phenytoin) decrease chloramphenicol concentrations. Consult appropriate resources for dosing recommendations before combining any drug with chloramphenicol. |

ChlorproMAZINE HCl

Brand names	Thorazine, generic

Medication error potential

Look-alike, sound-alike error potential.

ISMP reports that chlorproMAZINE has been confused with chlordiazepoxide and chlorpropamide. USP also reports that chlorproMAZINE has been confused with chlordiazepoxide (no patient harm resulted) and chlorpropamide (patient harm resulted).[1]

USP also reports that chlorproMAZINE has been confused with carbamazepine, chlorthalidone, clomipramine, Compazine, cyclobenzaprine, perphenazine, prochlorperazine, and thioridazine; no patient harm resulted.[2]

USP reports that Thorazine has been confused with thiamine, thioridazine, and trazodone; no patient harm resulted.[2]

Contraindications and warnings

US boxed warning: Chlorpromazine carries warnings for QT interval prolongation and increased mortality in elderly patients with dementia related psychosis.[3]

Contraindications: Known hypersensitivity to the drug, use in comatose patients, concomitant large doses of CNS depressants.[4]

Other warnings: Do not use in children <6 months of age, except where potential exists to save the child's life.[4]

Infusion related cautions

Systemic hypotension has occurred in neonates.[5] Because of the risk of hypotension, patients should continue to lie down for 30 minutes after the injection.[4]

Thrombophlebitis may occur.[6]

Dosage

Amphetamine-induced hyperactivity

Children (> 6 months of age): 1 mg/kg q 6 h as needed. If a barbiturate has been ingested, <4 mg/kg/day should be used.[7]

Adolescents: 25 mg q 6 h as needed.[7]

Hypoxia, neonatal: A loading dose of 0.13–0.88 mg/kg infused over 1 hour, followed by 0.03–0.21 mg/kg/h for up to 47 hours, has been used in severe hypoxia.[8]

Nausea and vomiting: 0.55 mg/kg IM q 6–8 h prn.[4,9]

During surgery

IM: 0.275 mg/kg; if nausea and vomiting persist after 30 minutes and hypotension has not occurred, the regimen may be repeated.[4,9]

IV: 1 mg at 2-minute intervals up to a total dose of 0.275 mg/kg; do not exceed IM dosage.[4,9]

Chemotherapy-induced: 1–3.3 mg/kg/day divided q 3–6 h[10-12] or 30 mg/m^2[13] infused over 15 minutes and given 30 minutes before chemotherapy.[12,13]

Neonatal abstinence syndrome/withdrawal: While phenobarbital is preferred, IM chlorpromazine has been used for this indication. If used, initial IM doses range from 0.5 to 0.7 mg/kg q 6 h.[14] Chlorpromazine 0.5 mg/kg q 6 h has been used to treat neonatal withdrawal after in utero SSRI exposure.[6]

Presurgical apprehension: 0.55 mg/kg IM 1–2 hours before surgery.[4,9]

Dosage *(cont.)*	**Sedation/hypnosis:** For infants and children, 0.2–0.5 mg/kg q 4–6 h.[15,16]
	Severe behavioral problems: 0.55 mg/kg IM q 6–8 h prn; for severe disorders, larger doses may be necessary; start low and increase gradually up to maximum doses (see Maximum dosage section); older patients may require 200 mg or more daily (further behavior improvement not seen with doses >500 mg/day).[4,9]
	Tetanus: 0.55 mg/kg IM/IV q 6–8 h.[4,9]
Dosage adjustment in organ dysfunction	Although one reference suggests that no dosage adjustment is necessary in renal dysfunction,[17] the manufacturer recommends chlorpromazine be administered cautiously in patients with renal disease.[4] It should also be used cautiously in patients with cardiovascular, liver, or chronic respiratory disease.[4]
Maximum dosage	**6 months–5 years or <23 kg:** 40 mg/day.[4,9]
	5–12 years or 23–45 kg: 75 mg/day.[4,9]
Additives	**1- and 2-mL ampules (25 mg/mL chlorpromazine) contain per mL:** 2 mg ascorbic acid, 1 mg sodium metabisulfite, 6 mg sodium chloride, and 1 mg sodium sulfite.[4,18]
	See Appendix C for more specific information about potential adverse effects of sulfites.
Suitable diluents	NS, ½NS, D2.5W, D5W, D10W, LR, R, D-LR combinations, D–R combinations, D-saline combinations.[4,18]
Maximum concentration	1 mg/mL.[18]
Preparation and delivery	See Appendix D for PN compatibility information.
IV push	Dilute to ≤1 mg/mL in NS[4,18] not to exceed 0.5 mg/min in children and 1 mg/min in *adults*.[4,18]
Intermittent infusion	Dilute to ≤1 mg/mL in NS[4,18] not to exceed 0.5 mg/min in children and 1 mg/min in *adults*.[4,18]
Continuous infusion	No information available to support administration by this method.
Other routes of administration	May be given via IM injection. Inject slowly, deep into large muscle.[1,13] If irritation is a problem, dilute with NS or 2% procaine.[4,18]
	SC injection not recommended.[4,18]

▸▸

ChlorproMAZINE HCl

Comments

Significant adverse effects: An association has been found between chlorpromazine use and acute and clinically relevant liver injury.[19]

Drug interactions: Because chlorpromazine is associated with several drug interactions, consult appropriate resources for dosing recommendations before combining any drug with chlorpromazine.[4]

Other: Meperidine, promethazine, and chlorpromazine have been used in combination (Demerol, Phenergan, Thorazine [DPT] cocktail) to sedate pediatric patients.[16,20-24] However, with the availability of safer and more effective agents,[22,25-26] this combination is no longer recommended.[24]

In one study in *adults*, incremental IV administration of 12.5 mg to a maximum of 37.5 mg was as effective as sumatriptan for the pain of acute migraine.[27]

Larger doses (4.6 ± 1.8 mg/kg) have been used for systemic vasodilation during cardio-pulmonary bypass in neonates.[28]

Chlorpromazine poisoning (17 mg/kg up to 100 mg/kg) has occurred in children; ingestions in children of ≤15 mg/kg producing clinical effects or >15 mg/kg should be referred to the hospital for therapy.[29]

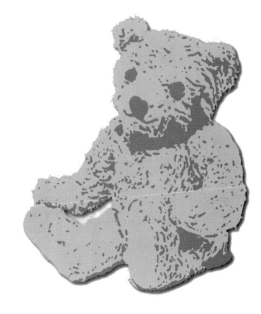

Cimetidine

Brand names	Tagamet, generic
Medication error potential	Look-alike, sound-alike error potential. USP reports that cimetidine has been confused with amantadine; no patient harm resulted.[1] USP reports that Tagamet has been confused with Tegretol; patient harm resulted.[1]
Contraindications and warnings	Known hypersensitivity to the drug.[2]
Infusion related cautions	In *adults*, rapid administration over 1–5 minutes has resulted in cardiac dysrhythmias,[3] hypotension,[4,5] and cardiac arrest,[6] particularly in individuals with myocardial disease.
Dosage	**Premature neonates:** 8–10 mg/kg/day divided q 6–12 h.[7-9] **Term neonates:** 8–24 mg/kg/day divided q 6–12 h.[7,8,10-13] **Infants and children:** 20–40 mg/kg/day up to 1.2 g divided q 4–6 h.[14-20] In *adults*, a loading dose of 150–300 mg infused over ≥5 minutes has been followed by a continuous infusion of 37.5–100 mg/h diluted in a compatible fluid.[21-23] (See Maximum dosage section.)
Dosage adjustment in organ dysfunction	Adjust dosage in patients with severe renal dysfunction.[2,24] If CrCl <30 mL/min, give 50% of normal dose.[2] Dosage adjustment may also be necessary in hepatic impairment.[2]
Maximum dosage	40 mg/kg/day,[14-17] not to exceed 2.4 g/day in *adults*.[2,25]
Additives	Multidose vials contain benzyl alcohol 0.9% as a preservative.[2,26] See Appendix C for more specific information about potential adverse effects and/or benzyl alcohol toxicity in neonates. Also available in a premixed solution in NS, which contains 7.7 mEq sodium per 50 mL.[26]
Suitable diluents	D5LR, D5NS, D5¼NS, D5½NS, D10NS, D5W, D10W, LR, NS, R, or sodium bicarbonate 5%.[26]
Maximum concentration	15 mg/mL for slow IV push, 6 mg/mL for IV infusion.[2,26] 150 mg/mL for IM injection.[2,26]
Preparation and delivery	Visually compatible with PN and stable in PN and TNA solutions for 24 hours at room temperature.[27,28] See Appendix D for additional PN compatibility information.
IV push	15 mg/mL[2] has been infused over no less than 5 minutes.[2,4,6,16,26,29] (See Infusion related cautions section.)

Cimetidine

Intermittent infusion	6 mg/mL[26] infused over 15–30 minutes.[15,17,29]
Continuous infusion	6 mg/mL in 100–1000 mL of suitable diluent.[26]
Other routes of administration	150 mg/mL (undiluted) may be given IM.[26]
Comments	**Significant adverse effects:** Reversible confusional states have been observed in *adults*.[2]

Comments

Significant adverse effects: Reversible confusional states have been observed in *adults*.[2]

Reversible cerebral toxicity (inattention, lack of spontaneous movements, no crying, and decreased ability to track objects or respond to verbal stimuli) has been reported in a 2-month-old infant receiving 40 mg/kg/day.[30] These effects did not reappear at doses of 25 mg/kg/day.

A 4-year-old child on 15 mg/kg/day of cimetidine in combination with two other CNS-active drugs was reported to have dysarthria, hallucinations, and was picking at bedclothes.[31]

Cimetidine has been associated with hypoxemia in a neonate receiving concomitant tolazoline therapy.[32]

Pharmacokinetic considerations: Clearance is increased in children with burns,[18,33] cystic fibrosis,[34] or critical illness.[15,17]

Drug interactions: Cimetidine inhibits a variety of CYP isoenzymes and is associated with numerous drug interactions.[2] Consult appropriate resources for dosing recommendations before combining any drug with cimetidine.

Other: The use of H2-blocker therapy has been associated with the incidence of necrotizing enterocolitis in very low birth weight infants.[35]

Ciprofloxacin Lactate

Brand names	Cipro IV

Medication error potential	Look a-like, sound a-like drug names.
	USP reports confusion with cephalexin, gatifloxacin, levofloxacin and moxifloxacin.[1] USP reports confusion for Cipro with Ceftin and Cleocin.[1]

Contraindications and warnings	**US boxed warning:** Fluoroquinolones are associated with an increased risk of tendinitis and tendon rupture in all ages.[2] This risk is further increased in older patients usually over 60 years of age, in patients taking corticosteroids, and in patients with kidney, heart, or lung transplants.[2]
	Contraindications: In persons with a history of hypersensitivity to ciprofloxacin, any member of the quinolone class of antimicrobials, or any of the product components.[2] Concomitant administration with tizanidine is contraindicated.[2]
	Because arthropathy have been noted in immature animals given ciprofloxacin, it should not be used in children <18 years.[2] (See Rare adverse effects in Comments section.)
	Other warnings: Rare cases of sensory or sensorimotor axonal polyneuropathy affecting small and/or large axons resulting in paresthesias, hypoesthesias, dysesthesias and weakness have been reported. Ciprofloxacin should be discontinued if (1) symptoms of neuropathy (e.g., pain, burning, tingling, numbness, and/or weakness) are present; and (2) the patient develops deficits in light touch, pain, temperature, position sense, vibratory sensation, and/or motor strength in order to prevent the development of an irreversible condition.[2]
	Prolonged use may cause superinfection and/or *Clostridium difficile*–associated diarrhea (CDAD), which has been reported and may range in severity from mild diarrhea to fatal colitis.[2] If CDAD is suspected or confirmed, appropriate fluid and electrolyte management, protein supplementation, antibiotic treatment of *C. difficile,* and surgical evaluation should be instituted as clinically indicated.[2]

Infusion related cautions	Anaphylaxis has occurred after the first dose[2-4] and may be accompanied by cardiovascular collapse, loss of consciousness, tingling, pharyngeal or facial edema, dyspnea, urticaria, and itching.[2] Serious anaphylactic reactions require immediate emergency treatment with epinephrine and other resuscitation measures, including oxygen, intravenous fluids, intravenous antihistamines, corticosteroids, pressor amines, and airway management, as clinically indicated.[2]
	Thrombophlebitis, burning, pain, erythema, and swelling occur more frequently when infusion time is <30 minutes.[2,5]

Dosage	The American Academy of Pediatrics recommends that ciprofloxacin is not appropriate in mild-to-moderate infections, and should be restricted to severe infections.[6]
	Neonates: Thirteen neonates with *Klebsiella pneumoniae* septicemia were treated with 10–40 mg/kg/day divided q 12 h for 10–20 days.[7]
	A neonate with multiple brain abscesses was given 10 mg/kg/day for 33 days.[8]
	This review notes that 28 preterm or low birth weight neonates received 4–40 mg/kg/day divided q 12 h for infections with multiresistant organisms (*Enterobacter cloacae, Pseudomonas aeruginosa, Klebsiella pneumoniae*).[9]
	Twelve cases of neonatal and infant nosocomial meningitis were treated with doses of 10–60 mg/kg/day for up to 28 days.[10]
	One hundred and sixteen septic neonates treated with ciprofloxacin (10 mg/kg/day divided q 12 h) showed no evidence of immediate hematologic, renal, or hepatic adverse events, and no evidence of arthropathy or growth impairment at 1 year of life.[11]

Ciprofloxacin Lactate

Dosage *(cont.)*	**Infants and children**

Mild-to-moderate infections: Inappropriate.[6]

Severe infections: 18–30 mg/kg/day divided q 8–12 h up to 400–800 mg q 12 h.[6] Some patients with sepsis may require 30 mg/kg/day divided q 8 h.[12]

An infant with ventriculitis was given 35 mg/kg/day divided q 12 h for four doses.[13] These doses resulted in an unacceptable increase in serum concentrations and the dosage was decreased (25 mg/kg/day divided q 12 h) and continued for 21 days.

Biologic warfare or bioterrorism: The CDC and other experts recommend that treatment of inhalational anthrax spores due to biologic warfare or bioterrorism should be started on a multiple-drug parenteral regimen that includes ciprofloxacin [(10 mg/kg/dose every 12 hours for 60 days; do not exceed 400 mg/dose (800 mg/day)] or doxycycline and one or two additional anti-infective agents (e.g., chloramphenicol, clindamycin, rifampin, vancomycin, clarithromycin, imipenem, penicillin, or ampicillin).[14,15]

Burns: Children with burn or burn-type wound infections have been given 20–30 mg/kg/day (interval not provided) for 7–10 days and had no radiographic evidence of arthropathy.[16]

Cystic fibrosis: 20–30 mg/kg/day divided q 8–12 h up to 1.2 g/day.[17] Two pharmacokinetic studies in children with cystic fibrosis recommend dosages of 20–30 mg/kg/day divided q 8–12 h.[18,19]

Typhoid fever: Eighteen children with severe typhoid fever were given 10 mg/kg/day divided q 12 h initially and then changed to oral therapy as tolerated.[20] The total duration of therapy was 7–14 days. In a separate study, 16 children received doses ranging from 7–24 mg/kg/day; all but one were eventually changed to oral therapy.[21]

Dosage adjustment in organ dysfunction	If CrCl is 10–50 mL/min, give 50% to 75% of a normal dose; if CrCl is <10 mL/min, give 50% of a normal dose.[22-24] No adjustment required for mild-moderate liver dysfunction.[25]
Maximum dosage	800 mg/day divided q 12 h in *adults*.[2] A 9-year-old child with cystic fibrosis received 76.9 mg/kg/day for 5 days; the only adverse effect noted was mild gastrointestinal distress.[26] A 5-year-old child with multidrug-resistant extrapulmonary tuberculosis received 16 mg/kg/day for 9 months without side effects, but the route of administration was not reported.[27]
Additives	None.
Suitable diluents	D5W, D10W, NS, R, RL, D5¼NS, D5½NS.[28]
Maximum concentration	2 mg/mL.[2]
Preparation and delivery	**Compatibility:** See Appendix D for PN compatibility information.[29]
IV push	Not recommended.[2]
Intermittent infusion	0.5–2 mg/mL over 60 minutes.[2,28] (See Infusion related cautions section.)

Ciprofloxacin Lactate

Continuous infusion	Not administered by this method.

Other routes of administration	None.

Comments	**Rare adverse events:** Several investigators were unable to prove ciprofloxacin-induced arthropathy in pediatric patients following IV or oral dosing.[30-34] Two retrospective safety studies of 1795[34] and >1700[35] children report arthralgia rates of 1.5% and 0%, respectively. An extensive review of the issue has been published.[36]

The Committee on Infectious Diseases of the American Academy of Pediatrics states that ciprofloxacin seems to be well tolerated and does not appear to cause arthropathy.[6] Use of ciprofloxacin in pediatric patients is justifiable if no other agent is available,[2] and infection is caused by multidrug-resistant, gram-negative, enteric, or one of several other pathogens.[30]

Serious and sometimes fatal hypersensitivity events have been reported.[2,3-5] These generally occur following multiple doses and manifestations as one or more of the following: (1) fever, rash, or severe dermatologic reactions (e.g., toxic epidermal necrolysis, Stevens-Johnson syndrome); (2) vasculitis, arthralgia, or myalgia; (3) serum sickness; (4) allergic pneumonitis; (5) interstitial nephritis, acute renal insufficiency or failure; (6) hepatitis, jaundice, acute hepatic necrosis or failure; and (7) anemia (including hemolytic and aplastic), thrombocytopenia (including thrombotic thrombocytopenic purpura), leukopenia, agranulocytosis, pancytopenia, and/or other hematologic abnormalities. There may be an increased risk of hypersensitivity reactions in HIV-seropositive patients.[4] The drug should be discontinued immediately at the first sign of a skin rash, jaundice, or any other sign of hypersensitivity. Two desensitization regimens have been described: one in a 29-month-old infant[37] and one in a 15-year-old patient with cystic fibrosis.[38]

A hypertensive reaction has been reported in an infant following IV ciprofloxacin 10 mg/kg/day.[39]

Convulsions, increased intracranial pressure, and toxic psychosis have been reported.[2,40-43] Should be used with caution in patients with known or suspected CNS disorders that may predispose to seizures or lower the seizure threshold, or in the presence of other risk factors that may predispose to seizures or lower the seizure threshold (e.g., certain drug therapy, renal dysfunction). Ciprofloxacin may also cause central nervous system (CNS) events including dizziness, confusion, tremors, hallucinations, depression, and, rarely, suicidal thoughts or acts.[2] These reactions may occur following the first dose. Ciprofloxacin should be discontinued and appropriate measures instituted.

Drug interactions: Ciprofloxacin is an inhibitor of CYP1A2.[2] Serious and fatal reactions have been reported in patients receiving concurrent administration of intravenous ciprofloxacin and theophylline.[2] These reactions have included cardiac arrest, seizure, status epilepticus, and respiratory failure. If concomitant use cannot be avoided, serum levels of theophylline should be monitored and dosage adjustments made as appropriate. Consult appropriate resources for dosing recommendations before combining any drug with ciprofloxacin.

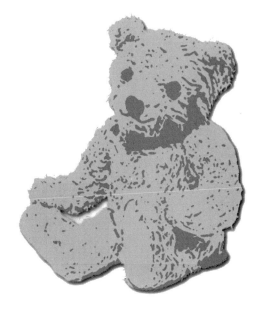

Cisatracurium Besylate

Brand names	Nimbex
Medication error potential	ISMP high-alert medication that has an increased risk of causing significant patient harm if it is used in error.[1]
Contraindications and warnings	**Contraindications:** Hypersensitivity to cisatracurium or any of its components.[2] **Warnings:** Use carefully under the supervision of experienced clinicians; personnel should also be skilled in airway management, resuscitation, and respiratory support.[2] Intubation and ventilatory support equipment, including oxygen therapy, should be readily available.[2] Also should have anticholinesterase inhibitors readily available when giving cisatracurium.[2]
Infusion related cautions	Hypersensitivity reactions, bronchospasm, and laryngospasm have been reported[3] but are rare.[2]
Dosage	*Respiratory function must be supported during use of this agent. Concurrent administration of a sedative is also necessary. Monitoring of neuromuscular transmission with a peripheral nerve stimulator is recommended during continuous infusion or with repeated dosing.*[2,4] **Continuous infusion:** 1–4 mcg/kg/min.[2,5-8] Clearance is higher in healthy pediatric patients compared to healthy *adult* patients.[2] **Intermittent dosing:** 0.1–0.15 mg/kg administered over 5 seconds followed by 0.03 mg/kg given as needed to maintain pharmacological paralysis.[2,5-8] Onset of action is faster and there is a longer duration of action in infants 1–23 months compared to children 2–12 years of age.[2]
Dosage adjustment in organ dysfunction	No dosage adjustment is required in patients with hepatic or renal dysfunction.[2,9]
Maximum dosage	The maximum dosage has not been established. In a study of 19 infants and children receiving cisatracurium, the maximum infusion rate was 10 mcg/kg/min.[8] Response may vary over time, resulting in the need for dosage adjustment.[2] Patients with burns may develop resistance to nondepolarizing neuromuscular blocking agents.[2] The extent of resistance is affected by the size of the burn and time since the burn injury.
Additives	The 2-mL concentration (10-mL vial) contains benzyl alcohol as a preservative.[2,10] See Appendix C for more specific information about potential adverse effects and/or benzyl alcohol toxicity in neonates.
Suitable diluents	D5W, D5NS, NS, D5LR may also be used as a diluent in final concentrations of 0.1–0.2 mg/mL only.[2,10] Do not use LR.[2,10]
Maximum concentration	2 mg/mL for IV push; 0.4 mg/mL for infusion.[2]

Cisatracurium Besylate

Preparation and delivery	Cisatracurium is an acidic solution; do not administer with alkaline solutions.[2,10]
	May be incompatible with propofol; however, the potential for incompatibility is concentration dependent and formulation specific.[10]
IV push	2 mg/mL administered over 5–10 seconds.[2]
Intermittent infusion	Not administered by this method.
Continuous infusion	0.1–0.4 mg/mL.[2,10]
Other routes of administration	IM administration is not recommended due to the potential for tissue irritation.[2,10] No information available to support administration by other routes.
Comments	**Significant adverse effects:** Prolonged paralysis has been reported after long-term infusion of neuromuscular blocking agents, including cisatracurium, and may be affected by concomitant therapies.[5,11,12] (See Drug interactions in Comments section.) Other factors that potentiate the duration of neuromuscular blockade include acidosis, hyponatremia, hypocalcemia, hypokalemia, and hypermagnesemia.[2,5]
	Patients with neurological diseases such as myasthenia gravis may exhibit increased sensitivity. Decreased sensitivity to cisatracurium may occur in patients with severe burns, muscle trauma, demyelinating lesions, peripheral neuropathies, or infection.[2]
	Drug interactions: Enflurane and isoflurane anesthesia may potentiate effects of cisatracurium; during long surgical procedures under enflurane and isoflurane anesthesia, up to 30% to 40% reduction in dose may be necessary.[2] Concomitant administration of corticosteroids with neuromuscular blockers is a risk factor for prolonged paralysis.[13] Likewise, concomitant administration with certain antibiotics (e.g., aminoglycosides, clindamycin, vancomycin) may prolong neuromuscular blockade.[2,5] Consult appropriate resources for additional information on drug interactions.
	Other: Cisatracurium, in weakening and incompletely paralyzing doses along with intermittent benzodiazepine therapy, has been used to facilitate isoflurane wean and treat withdrawal symptoms in a 4-year-old critically ill patient.[14]

CISplatin

Brand names	Platinol, generic

Medication error potential

ISMP high-alert medication that has an increased risk of causing significant patient harm if it is used in error.[1]

Look-alike, sound-alike error potential.

ISMP and USP report that CISplatin has been confused with CARBOplatin; patient harm resulted.[2,3] USP reports that CISplatin has been confused with Cytoxan; no patient harm resulted.[3]

ISMP reports that Platinol has been confused with Patanol.[2] USP also reports that Platinol has been confused with Plaquenil; no patient harm resulted.[3]

Contraindications and warnings

US boxed warning: Cisplatin should be administered under the supervision of a qualified physician. Use caution to prevent inadvertent overdose. (See Maximum dosage section.) Cisplatin is associated with severe renal toxicity. Also associated with other serious dose-related toxicities such as myelosuppression, nausea, and vomiting. Cisplatin can cause ototoxicity that is more pronounced in children. Cisplatin has been associated with serious anaphylactic-like reactions.[4,5] (See Infusion related cautions section.)

Contraindications: Cisplatin should not be used in patients with preexisting renal impairment, myelosuppression, or hearing impairment. Should also not be used in patients with known history of hypersensitivity to cisplatin or any components.[4,5]

Other warnings: Occasionally, fatal dosing errors have occurred when cisplatin has been inadvertently substituted for carboplatin. Can cause serious acute leukemia and neuropathies.[4,5]

Infusion related cautions

Anaphylactic-like reactions, including facial edema, bronchoconstriction, tachycardia, and hypotension, may occur within minutes of administration. Epinephrine, corticosteroids, and antihistamines have been used.[4]

Because extravasation may cause tissue sloughing and necrosis, the infusion should be stopped if the patient complains of discomfort.[5,6] If extravasation occurs, attempt to remove any residual drug from tissues. Because of extravasation and infiltration risk, small veins in the dorsum of the hand or foot and scalp veins should be avoided if at all possible. Severity of tissue damage appears to occur more often when concentration of solution is >0.5 mg/mL.[5] See Appendix E for additional information regarding extravasation treatment.

Dosage

Consult protocol for complete dosing information. Cisplatin should be administered with a regimen of hydration with or without mannitol and/or furosemide. (See Comments section.) Should not be given to patients with pre-existing renal or hearing impairment or myelosuppression.

The following dosing regimens have been used in pediatric patients

Intermittent dosing: 37–75 mg/m^2 q 2–3 weeks or 50–100 mg/m^2 q 3–4 weeks.[4,5]

Bone marrow transplantation: 55 mg/m^2/day for 72 hours by continuous infusion (165 mg/m^2).[4,5]

Brain tumor (recurrent): 60 mg/m^2/day for 2 days q 3–4 weeks.[4,5,7]

CISplatin

Dosage *(cont.)*	**Neuroblastoma:** 60–100 mg/m^2 once q 3–4 weeks[4,8,9] or 30 mg/m^2 every week.[4,5]
	Osteogenic sarcoma: 60–100 mg/m^2 once q 3–4 weeks[4,5,10-13] or 30 mg/m^2 every week.[4,5]
	A repeat course should not be given until the patient's renal, hematologic, and otic functions are within acceptable limits.[4]
	Daily dosing: 15–20 mg/m^2/day for 5 days q 3–4 weeks.[4,5,14,15]
Dosage adjustment in organ dysfunction	The manufacturer states that cisplatin is contraindicated in patients with pre-existing renal dysfunction.[4] Another reference recommends that if CrCl is 10–50 mL/min, administer 75% of the normal dose and if CrCl is <10 mL/min, administer 50% of the normal dose.[16] The manufacturer also recommends that repeat dosages be held until SCr <1.5 mg/dL, WBC ≥4000/mm^3, platelets ≥100,000/mm^3, and BUN <25.[4] Decrease dosage in infants <6 months of age due to decreased renal tubular secretion and decreased renal function.[17]
Maximum dosage	It is important to differentiate between daily doses and total dose per cycle or course of treatment. Verify any cisplatin dose exceeding 100 mg/m^2 per course.[4] Doses >100 mg/m^2 per course q 3–4 weeks are rarely used.[4]
Additives	None.
Suitable diluents	D5¼NS, D5½NS, D5NS, ¼NS, ⅓NS, ½NS, NS.[5,18]
Maximum concentration	Not established.
Preparation and delivery	**Preparation:** Skin reactions may occur following exposure; therefore, wear gloves when preparing and administering.[4] If exposure occurs, wash area with soap and water. Needles, syringes, catheters, or IV administration sets that contain aluminum parts that may come in contact with cisplatin should not be used for preparation or administration of the drug, because this may result in precipitate formation.[4,18] **Stability:** Do not infuse in solutions containing <¼NS; stable when combined with mannitol (12.5–50 g mannitol/L).[5] **Compatibility:** Incompatible with sodium bicarbonate and variable stability in D5W.[18] For PN compatibility information, please see Appendix D.
IV push	Although rapid administration over 1–5 minutes has been used, it is associated with an increased risk of ototoxicity and nephrotoxicity.[5,17]

CISplatin

Intermittent infusion	Concentration not specified. Diluted in compatible fluid, it has been given over 15–20 minutes without adverse effects.[5,7-15]
Continuous infusion	The manufacturer recommends diluting the dose in 2 L of D5W and sodium containing fluid (see Suitable diluents section) with 18.75 g mannitol/L and infusing over 6–8 hours.[4,5,18] Other studies have reported stability at concentrations of 20, 50, 200, and 500 mg/L.[18] Although cisplatin has been infused over 6–8 hours, 8–12 hours, or as a 24-hour infusion in order to decrease nephrotoxicity,[5] these various rates of administration have generally not been associated with a reduction in renal toxicity.[5]
Other routes of administration	Not administered IM. Has been given intra-arterial and intraperitoneal.[5]
Comments	**Significant adverse effects:** Aggressive hydration should be given to ensure good urinary output and reduce the likelihood of nephrotoxicity associated with cisplatin.[19] Several protocols have been advocated. One regimen consists of administration of 1–2 L of an NS-containing fluid over 8–12 hours before cisplatin.[18] The manufacturer recommends diluting the dose in 2 L of compatible fluid containing 37.5 mg of mannitol (18.75 g/L) and infusing over 6–8 hours.[4] Others have given infusion over 15–120 minutes and by continuous infusion over 1–5 days.[18]

Nephrotoxicity, neurotoxicity, and ototoxicity increase with cumulative doses.[19-27] Renal toxicity has been noted in 28% to 36% of patients treated with a single 50 mg/m^2/dose.[4]

Ototoxicity (high-frequency hearing loss) is especially pronounced in children and is related to a cumulative cisplatin dose >200 mg/m^2.[5] An audiometric test should be performed before therapy is initiated and prior to each subsequent dose of medication.[4]

Cisplatin is associated with a high (>90%) risk of emesis.[28] Patients should receive antiemetic therapy to prevent acute and delayed nausea and vomiting. The recommended therapy is a 5HT3 receptor antagonist in combination with dexamethasone on every day chemotherapy is administered.[28,29] These agents may be continued for up to 4 days after chemotherapy administration for the prevention of delayed nausea and vomiting. Breakthrough medications should also be offered, such as a phenothiazine (e.g., prochlorperazine), a butyrophenone (e.g., droperidol), a substituted benzamide (e.g., metoclopramide), or a benzodiazepine (e.g., lorazepam).[29]

Monitoring: Monitor renal function (e.g., SCr, BUN, CrCl), electrolytes (e.g., magnesium, calcium, and potassium), audiography, neurological tests, liver function tests, CBC with platelets, and urinalysis.[4,5] Electrolyte supplementation may be necessary.[4]

Drug interactions: Use caution with concomitant aminoglycoside use due to increased risk of nephrotoxicity.[4] |

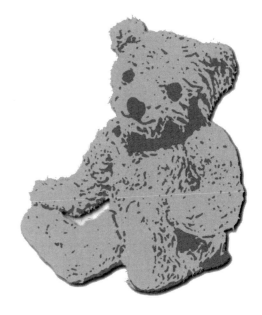

Clindamycin Phosphate

Brand names	Cleocin

Medication error potential

Look-alike, sound-alike drug names.

USP reports confusion with clarithromycin, Clinoril, vancomycin, and gentamicin. Confusion has also been noted between Cleocin and Cipro, Claforan, Cubicin, and oxycodone and acetaminophen.[1]

Contraindications and warnings

US boxed warning: Prolonged use may cause superinfection and/or *Clostridium difficile*–associated diarrhea (CDAD), which has been reported and may range in severity from mild diarrhea to fatal colitis.[2] Cleocin phosphate is highly associated with severe CDAD infections and should be reserved for the treatment of more severe infections. If CDAD is suspected or confirmed, appropriate fluid and electrolyte management, protein supplementation, antibiotic treatment of *C. difficile,* and surgical evaluation should be instituted as clinically indicated.[2]

Contraindications: Contraindicated in individuals with a history of hypersensitivity to preparations containing clindamycin or lincomycin.[2]

Other warnings: Clindamycin does not adequately penetrate into the cerebrospinal fluid and should not be used to treat meningitis.[2]

Infusion related cautions

If a decision is made to give this medication to a patient with known clindamycin hypersensitivity, the patient should be closely observed for allergenicity. Although rare, anaphylactoid reactions may require immediate emergency treatment with epinephrine, oxygen, IV steroids, antihistamines, pressor amines, and airway management.[2]

Thrombophlebitis, erythema, and pain may occur with infusion.[2]

Dosage

Neonates

Dose is based on postnatal age and weight or postmenstrual and postnatal age.

PNA	<1200 g	1200–2000 g	>2000 g
<7 days	10 mg/kg/day divided q 12 h[3,4]*	10 mg/kg/day divided q 12 h[3,4]	15 mg/kg/day divided q 8 h[3,4]
≥7 days		15 mg/kg/day divided q 8 h[3,4]*	20–30 mg/kg/day divided q 6–8 h[3-7]

*Until 4 weeks of age.

Infants and children

Pediatric patients >16 years may receive the usual *adult* dose (600–1200 mg/day divided q 6–12 h).[2]

Mild-to-moderate infection: 15–25 mg/kg/day (350 mg/m²/day) divided q 6–8 h.[2,3]

Severe infection: 25–40 mg/kg/day (450 mg/m²/day) divided q 6–8 h.[2,3, 8-10]

Bacterial endocarditis (prophylaxis)

Dental, oral, respiratory tract, or esophageal procedures*: Single 20 mg/kg/dose (up to 600 mg) given as single dose 30 minutes before a procedure.[11] Only for patients with underlying cardiac conditions associated with the highest risk of adverse outcome. (See Other in Comments section.)

*that involve manipulation of gingival tissue or the periapical region of teeth or perforation of the oral mucosa[11]

Dosage *(cont.)*	**Biochemical warfare or bioterrorism:** The CDC and other experts recommend treatment of inhalational anthrax spores due to biologic warfare or bioterrorism should be started on a multiple-drug parenteral regimen that includes ciprofloxacin or doxycycline and one or two additional anti-infective agents (i.e., chloramphenicol, clindamycin [30 mg/kg/day divided q 6 h], rifampin, vancomycin, clarithromycin, imipenem, penicillin, or ampicillin).[12,13] Strains of *Bacillus anthracis* associated with cases that occurred in the US during 2001, following bioterrorism-related anthrax exposures, were susceptible to clindamycin in vitro.[13] **Surgical (colorectal, appendectomy, incision through the oral mucosa, ruptured viscus):** 10 mg/kg/dose preoperative recommended.[3,14,15]
Dosage adjustment in organ dysfunction	No dose adjustment for renal dysfunction.[16] Dose adjustment has been recommended with severe hepatic impairment, no dose specific recommendation is available.[2,3]
Maximum dosage	20 mg/kg not to exceed 4.8 g/day in *adults*,[2,3] not to exceed 1200 mg in a single, 1-hour infusion.[2] 600 mg IM is the maximum dose.[2]
Additives	9.45 mg/mL benzyl alcohol.[2] (See Appendix C for specific information about benzyl alcohol and potential for toxicity.)
Suitable diluents	NS, LR, D5W, D10W, D5NS, D5R, D5½NS.[17] Stability varies depending on the concentration, diluents, and storage conditions. See appropriate resource.
Maximum concentration	18 mg/mL.[2]
Preparation and delivery	**Delivery system issues:** Premade IV preparations are in special plastic containers that can leach out very small amounts of chemicals when in contact with solutions. Toxicity from the leached chemicals has not been evaluated in pediatrics.[18] **Stability:** Do not refrigerate because crystallization may occur.[17] Bulk package preparations should not be directly infused and should be prepared with single entry use. Discard any unused portion within 24 hours after initial entry.[17] **Compatibility:** See Appendix D for PN compatibility information.[19]
IV push	Not recommended.[2] Hypotension and cardiopulmonary arrest may occur following rapid IV administration.[2,20]
Intermittent infusion	Infuse over 10–60 minutes, not to exceed a rate of 1800 mg/h.[2]
Continuous infusion	Concentration was not specified, 0.75–1.25 mg/min has been given.[2]
Other routes of administration	IM not to exceed 600 mg.[2] Pain induration and sterile abscess may occur with IM injections.[2]

Clindamycin Phosphate

Comments

Rare adverse events: Rare cases of erythema multiforme, resembling Stevens-Johnson syndrome,[21] and anaphylactoid reactions[2,22] have been reported in *adults.*

Leukopenia and eosinophilia have been reported.[2]

Monitoring: Intravenous clindamycin or vancomycin are recommended for treatment of community acquired MRSA. In addition to MIC testing, a D-test should be performed by the clinical laboratory. A negative D-test suggests that the methicillin/oxacillin-resistant organism will not induce resistance to clindamycin therapy during therapy; hence, the patient can be managed with clindamycin.[23] During prolonged therapy periodic liver and kidney function tests and blood counts should be performed.

Drug interactions: Clindamycin can potentiate the effects of neuromuscular blockers.[24,25] Clindamycin may antagonize the activity of erythromycin and should not be used concurrently.[2,26] Because succinylcholine is associated with numerous drug interactions, consult appropriate resources for dosing recommendations before combining any drug with succinylcholine.

Other: Cardiac conditions associated with the highest risk of adverse outcome from endocarditis for which prophylaxis with dental procedures is reasonable: (1) prosthetic cardiac valve or prosthetic material used for cardiac valve repair; (2) previous IE; (3) congenital heart disease (CHD)* in a person with a) unrepaired cyanotic CHD, including palliative shunts and conduits, b) completely repaired congenital heart defect with prosthetic material or device, whether placed by surgery or by catheter intervention, during the first 6 months after the procedure,† c) repaired CHD with residual defects at the site or adjacent to the site of a prosthetic patch or prosthetic device (which inhibit endothelialization); and (4) cardiac transplantation recipients who develop cardiac valvulopathy.[11]

---

*Except for the conditions listed above, antibiotic prophylaxis is no longer recommended for any other form of CHD.

†Prophylaxis is reasonable because endothelialization of prosthetic material occurs within 6 months after the procedure.

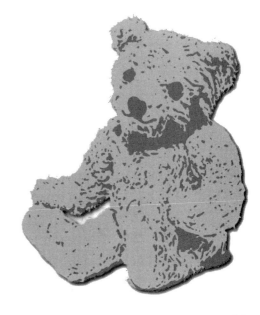

Co-Trimoxazole
(Trimethoprim-Sulfamethoxazole)

Brand names	Generic

Medication error potential

USP reports confusion with Bactroban.[1]

Contraindications and warnings

Contraindications: In those (1) with known hypersensitivity to sulfa drug, trimethoprim, or any component of the formulation; (2) with documented megaloblastic anemia due to folate deficiency; (3) <2 months of age*; and (4) who are breast-feeding since sulfonamides are excreted in the milk and may cause kernicterus in the infant.[2]

*except for *Pneumocystis carinii prophylaxis* in neonates born to HIV infected mothers[3]

Warnings: Fatalities have occurred due to severe dermatologic reactions (i.e., Stevens-Johnson syndrome and toxic epidermal necrolysis). Sulfonamides should be discontinued at the first appearance of skin rash.[2] Fulminant hepatic necrosis and a variety of blood dyscrasias (e.g., agranulocytosis, aplastic anemia) have been reported.[2] Dose-dependent hemolysis may occur in patients with G6PD-deficiency.[2] (See Rare adverse effects in Comments Section.)

Because folate depletion may worsen the psychomotor regression associated with the fragile X chromosome disorder, co-trimoxazole should be used with caution in these children.[2]

Cough, shortness of breath, and pulmonary infiltrates are hypersensitivity reactions of the respiratory tract that have been reported.[2]

Prolonged use may cause superinfection and/or *Clostridium difficile*–associated diarrhea (CDAD), which has been reported and may range in severity from mild diarrhea to fatal colitis.[2] If CDAD is suspected or confirmed, appropriate fluid and electrolyte management, protein supplementation, antibiotic treatment of *C. difficile,* and surgical evaluation should be instituted as clinically indicated.[2]

Infusion related cautions

Skin necrosis may occur following extravasation.[2] Pain, local irritation, inflammation, and rarely thrombophlebitis may occur.[2,3]

Dosage

Dosage is based on trimethoprim component.

Neonates: Not recommended for those <2 months of age since sulfonamides may cause kernicterus by displacing bilirubin from plasma protein binding sites[2]; however, may be used for *Pneumocystis carinii* prophylaxis in neonates born to HIV-infected mothers.[3]

Infants and children

Mild-to-moderate infections: 6–12 mg/kg/day divided q 6–12 h.[2,4] Give up to 14 days for severe UTI and 5 days for shigellosis.[2]

Severe infections: 8–12 mg/kg/day divided q 6 h.[2,4]

Meningitis (not first-line; alternative therapy for *Listeria monocytogenes*): 15–20 mg/kg/day divided q 6–12 h.[2,5-9]

***Pneumocystis carinii* pneumonia:** 15–20 mg/kg/day divided q 6–8 h for 14–21 days.[2-4,10-17]

Co-Trimoxazole
(Trimethoprim-Sulfamethoxazole)

Dosage adjustment in organ dysfunction	If CrCl is 15–30 mL/min, give 50% the normal dose.[2,18] Not recommended if CrCl is <15 mL/min,[2,18-21] but if required give 5–10 mg/kg q 24 h.[18]
Maximum dosage	20 mg/kg/day for *P. carinii* pneumonia[2,10-12] up to 4 g/day.[2]
Additives	Contains sodium metabisulfite, 400 mg/mL propylene glycol and 1% benzyl alcohol.[2] (See Appendix C for specific information about sulfite hypersensitivity, benzyl alcohol and propylene glycol toxicity.)
Suitable diluents	D5W.[2,22]
Maximum concentration	5 mL of the concentrate in 125 mL of D5W,[2,22] or 5 mL of concentrate in 75 mL of D5W in fluid-restricted patients.[2,22,23] May add 5 mL of concentrate to 50 mL of D5W but observe for precipitation.[3]
Preparation and delivery	**Stability:** Do not refrigerate concentrate for injection.[2] Stability at room temperature is 5 mL concentrate in 125 mL D5W is stable for 6 hours; 5 mL concentrate in 100 mL D5W is stable for 4 hours; 5 mL concentrate in 75 mL D5W is stable for 2 hours; 5 mL in 50 mL D5W may precipitate in 1–2 hours.[2,3,22] **Compatibility:** See Appendix D for PN compatibility information.[24] **Photosensitivity:** Protect from light exposure until ready to use.[2]
IV push	Not recommended.[2]
Intermittent infusion	Over 60–90 minutes.[2]
Continuous infusion	Not used.
Other routes of administration	None.
Comments	**Significant adverse effects:** Stevens–Johnson syndrome and toxic epidermal necrolysis may occur with sulfonamide therapy.[2] One to three days before the appearance of a rash, patients develop a prodrome of fever, stinging eyes, and sore throat.[25] The initial lesions are erythematous to purpuric macules, which first appear on the trunk and spreading to the face and proximal extremities.[25] Lesions may then progress to full-thickness necrosis with flaccid blisters. Most patients (90%) develop buccal, oral, and genital mucosal involvement with erythema and erosions.[25] Sulfonamide should be discontinued immediately at first sign of rash.[2] Agranulocytosis, aplastic anemia, thrombocytopenia, leukopenia, neutropenia, hemolytic anemia, megaloblastic anemia, hypoprothrombinemia, methemoglobinemia, and eosinophilia have been reported.[2] Hemolysis has been reported in individuals with G6PD deficiency.[2] Administration of folic acid will reverse methemoglobinemia and will not affect the antibacterial effects of co-trimoxazole.[3] Hepatitis, including cholestatic jaundice and hepatic necrosis, and liver failure that required transplantation have occurred.[2,26,27]

Co-Trimoxazole
(Trimethoprim-Sulfamethoxazole)

Comments *(cont.)*

Rare adverse effects: Trimethoprim can cause hyperkalemia by reducing renal potassium excretion through competitive inhibition of epithelial sodium channels in the distal nephron.[2] This can occur with both large and standard dosages of trimethoprim but generally occurs in those with renal impairment, hypoaldosteronism, or concurrent medications known to impair renal potassium excretion.[28] Management frequently requires discontinuation of trimethoprim, volume repletion with isotonic fluids, and administration of therapies specific to hyperkalemia.

Monitoring: Serum potassium, serum transaminases and bilirubin. Coagulation time should be monitored in those on warfarin.

Drug interactions: Sulfamethoxazole and trimethoprim are both substrates of CYP2C9 (major) and 3A4.[3] Sulfamethoxazole is an inhibitor of CYP2C9 and trimethoprim moderately inhibits CYP2C8 and 2C9.[3] Trimethoprim is 45% and sulfamethoxazole is 68% bound to plasma protein.[2] Because co-trimoxazole is associated with numerous drug interactions, consult appropriate resources for dosing recommendations before combining any drug with co-trimoxazole.

Laboratory interference: The presence of trimethoprim and sulfamethoxazole may interfere with the Jaffe assay for creatinine, resulting in about 10% overestimation.[2] The trimethoprim component can interfere with determination of serum methotrexate concentrations.[2] This occurs if a bacterial dihydrofolate reductase is used as the binding protein source in the competitive binding protein technique, but does not occur if a radioimmunoassay is used.[2]

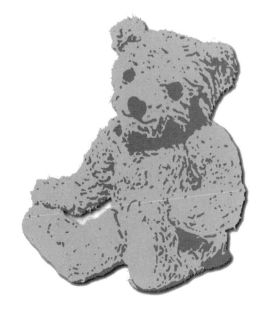

Coagulation Factor VIIa (Recombinant) (rFVIIa)

Brand names	NovoSeven RT
Medication error potential	None noted.
Contraindications and warnings	**Warnings:** Use caution when administering to individuals with known hypersensitivity to NovoSeven, its components, or who have hypersensitivity reactions to mouse, hamster, or bovine proteins.[1] Use of rFVIIa in patients without hemophilia may be associated with an increased risk for development of thrombosis.[1,2]
Infusion related cautions	Thrombophlebitis occurred during continuous infusion via peripheral vein.[3] (See Preparation and delivery section and Continuous infusion section.)
Dosage	**Hemophilia A or B with inhibitors to Factor VIII or IX**[1]

Prophylaxis for invasive procedures: 90 mcg/kg prior to surgery with doses repeated at 2-hour intervals during the procedure.

    Minor procedures postoperatively: 90 mcg/kg q 2 h for 48 hours followed by q 2–6 hours until healing.

    Major procedures postoperatively: 90 mcg/kg q 2 h for 5 days after surgery followed by q 4 h intervals until healing. Alternatively, continuous infusion with Factor VII concentration monitoring (target concentration 10 International Units/mL) to determine maintenance infusion rate has been used.[3] Others report infusing 50 mcg/kg/h for 5 days then 25 mcg/kg/h for 5 days.[4]

Treatment: 90 mcg/kg (35–120 mcg/kg) q 2 h until hemostasis occurs or treatment is felt to be ineffective. The dosing interval may be adjusted according to bleeding severity. Also, continuous infusion has been used.[5]

Congenital factor VII deficiency (prophylaxis for invasive procedures): 15–30 mcg/kg q 4–6 h until hemostasis.[1,6] A 3-year-old with cleft palate received 15 mcg/kg beginning 20 minutes prior to surgery for repair and q 12 h for 3 days after without any bleeding events.[6]

Surgery related bleeding

    Cardiac surgery with cardiopulmonary bypass (CPB): Eight children 5 days to 8 years of age received 30 or 60 mcg/kg repeated in 15 minutes and again in 2 hours if bleeding continued.[7] A single 70-mcg/kg dose was effective in a 4-month-old with bleeding after atrial septal defect repair.[8] A 9-month-old received two 90 mcg/kg doses for intraoperative bleeding.[9] On the other hand, a randomized, double-blind, placebo controlled trial found no benefit and time to chest closure was prolonged in 42 infants receiving rFVIIa compared to 40 infants receiving standard treatment.[10]

    Bleeding during ECMO: An 11-year-old and a 13-year-old were given 90 mcg/kg q 4 h for three doses or q 2 h for 10 doses to control bleeding.[11] Four children from age 6 days to 33 months were given two doses of 90–120 mcg/kg 4 hours apart.[12] All except the 13-year-old were on ECMO after open heart surgery. Of interest, an infant who failed to be weaned from CPB after a Ross procedure for aortic stenosis was placed on ECMO and developed thrombotic occlusions of both subclavian arteries and truncus brachiocephalicus after receiving rFVIIa for uncontrollable bleeding.[13]

    Miscellaneous bleeding: Four days after cardiac surgery, a 10-month-old male with Noonan's syndrome developed gastrointestinal (GI) bleeding unresponsive to standard treatment.[14] He initially responded to a 90-mcg/kg dose but began bleeding again after about 8 hours. Two more doses were given and the bleeding stopped. Another 16-month-old being treated for acute megakaryoblastic leukemia developed severe GI bleeding that responded to 100 mcg/kg given at 0, 2, and 12 hours.[15]

Coagulation Factor VIIa (Recombinant) (rFVIIa)

Dosage *(cont.)*	**Liver failure coagulopathy**

Bleeding management: Twenty-two children with liver disease received doses ranging from 36–118 mcg/kg to treat a variety of bleeding episodes.[16,17] A 3-month-old, a 9-year-old, and an 11-year-old received 67 mcg/kg × 3, 130 mcg/kg × 2, and 200 mcg/kg to control bleeding from various sources.[18] Following a right hepatectomy, a 5-month-old boy with internal bleeding was given a single 90-mcg/kg dose.[19]

Prior to invasive procedure: Six children (2 months to 15 years) received doses of 34–163 mcg/kg prior to liver biopsy and other invasive procedures.[17]

Transplant: A 2½-year-old and a 7-year-old received 100 mcg/kg prior to transplant, and one of them received a second dose 2 hours later during transplant.[20] A 7-month-old with an INR of 3 and multiple bleeding sites received 300 mcg/kg prior to transplant.[21] Seven children with bleeding after liver graft reperfusion received 37–168 mcg/kg that resulted in improved hemostasis.[21] No postoperative thrombotic events were noted in these children. On the other hand, four *adults* undergoing liver transplantation received 90 mcg/kg preoperatively and intraoperatively. One developed portal vein thrombosis and another myocardial ischemia leading the authors to express concern over the potential for thrombotic complications.[22]

Congenital platelet disorders: A 15-year-old girl with Bernard-Soulier syndrome received 98 mcg/kg × 2 that controlled severe menorrhagia. On a separate occasion she received two doses of 98 and 122.5 mcg/kg that controlled severe epistaxis and mild menorrhagia.[23] Four children with Glanzmann thrombasthenia received 89–116 mcg/kg q 2 h until bleeding stopped.[24] Thirty-three uses of rFVIIa (100 mcg/kg q 90 min × 3 doses) were evaluated in seven children with Bernard-Soulier syndrome or Glanzmann thrombasthenia.[25] When rFVIIa was started 30–45 minutes prior to a planned surgical intervention (seven procedures in five children), no bleeding occurred postoperatively; however, efficacy in treating an established bleed was variable.

Preterm neonates

Intraventricular hemorrhage (IVH): The incidence of IVH was not different in 10 infants who received rVIIa compared to those who did not, and the two with umbilical artery catheters developed thrombi at the catheter tip.[26] Another neonate with IVH was given rVIIa, and while the bleeding stopped, the infant did not survive the grade IV bleed.[27]

Necrotizing enterocolitis (NEC): During surgical management of NEC, four very low birth weight infants with intraoperative bleeding received rVIIa.[28] Bleeding was controlled in three of the four; however, one infant developed a brachial artery thrombus necessitating thrombectomy and arterial reconstruction, and another had transient ischemia of the distal phalanges.

Pulmonary hemorrhage: Four very low birth weight infants were treated for 2 or 3 days.[27,29,30] After treatment, all had stabilization of coagulation parameters. However, one developed pulmonary hemorrhage 8 hours after the dose.[27]

Dosage adjustment in organ dysfunction	None noted.

Maximum dosage	Not established. Accidental overdoses of 246–986 mcg/kg have been reported without thrombotic complications.[1] Antibodies against rFVIIa were detected in a newborn with congenital factor VII deficiency who received 800 mcg/kg rFVIIa.[1]

Additives	Contains polysorbate 80, mannitol, and sucrose.[1]

Suitable diluents	Histidine diluent (provided with lyophilized powder).[1]

Coagulation Factor VIIa (Recombinant) (rFVIIa)

Maximum concentration	1000 mcg/mL (reconstituted).[1]
Preparation and delivery	Reconstitute with provided diluent. Reconstituted solution must be administered within 3 hours.[1] **Compatibility:** The addition of heparin to reduce thrombophlebitis results in a 20% to 30% loss of activity unless the pH is adjusted from 5.5 to 7.4.[3]
IV push	Over 3–5 minutes.[1]
Intermittent infusion	Not indicated.
Continuous infusion	A parallel infusion of saline (20 mL/h in *adults*) into same vein as undiluted rFVIIa may minimize the thrombophlebitis.[5] Selection of infusion pump devices appeared to be important to the success of continuous infusion.[5]
Other routes of administration	Not indicated.
Comments	**Pharmacokinetics:** Children have a shorter half-life, more rapid clearance, and larger volume of distribution at steady state than *adults*.[31]

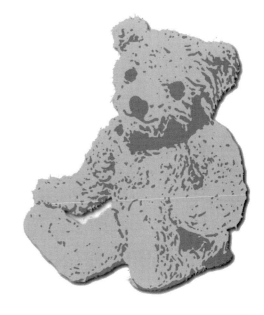

Conivaptan

Brand names	Vaprisol
Medication error potential	None reported by ISMP or USP.[1-3]
Contraindications and warnings	**Contraindications:** Hypersensitivity to any component, hypovolemic hyponatremia, and in patients receiving other medications that are potent CYP3A4 inhibitors.[4-8] (See Drug interactions in Comments section.)
	Warnings: Conivaptan is not indicated for treatment of congestive heart failure and should only be used for treatment of hyponatremia in patients with heart failure when the benefit of raising serum sodium outweighs the risk of adverse effects.[4,5,8]
	Avoid rapid correction of serum sodium (>12 mEq/L in 24 hours) due to the risk of osmotic demyelination syndrome. Discontinue therapy if the patient develops a rapid rise in serum sodium. If hyponatremia persists, conivaptan may be resumed at a lower dose if there is no evidence of neurologic sequelae from rapid rise in sodium.[4,7,8]
Infusion related cautions	Conivaptan has been associated with infusion site reactions. Administer via large veins and rotate infusion site q 24 h to minimize risk of irritation.[4,6,8] See Appendix E for information regarding infiltration.
Dosage	Conivaptan has not been extensively studied in pediatric patients. Currently there is no established dosage range for pediatric patients.
	One report describes conivaptan use for aggressive hydration to prevent tumor lysis syndrome in a 13-year-old with lymphoma and SIADH as follows[9]:
	Loading dose: 10 mg IV infused over 30 minutes.
	Maintenance dose: 10 mg/day infused over 24 hours titrated up to 30 mg/day infused over 24 hours.
	This treatment regimen was successful and the patient experienced no adverse effects.[9]
	The following doses are recommended in *adults*[4-8]:
	Loading dose: 20 mg IV infused over 30 minutes.
	Maintenance dose: 20–40 mg/day via continuous infusion over 24 hours (0.83–1.7 mg/h).
Dosage adjustment in organ dysfunction	Conivaptan use in patients with hepatic and/or renal disease has not been adequately evaluated. However, increased systemic exposure in patients with hepatic impairment and increased AUC in patients with renal impairment has occurred following administration of *oral* conivaptan.[4,8] Use caution when administering to patients with hepatic or renal impairment.
	Not currently recommended for use in patients with cirrhosis as safety profile likely not favorable.[4]
Maximum dosage	In *adults*, after giving loading dose, do not exceed 40 mg/day for 4 days of therapy.[4,6-8]

Conivaptan

Additives

Contains 1.2 g propylene glycol and 0.4 g ethanol and water for injection per ampule.[4] See Appendix C for more specific information about potential adverse effects of propylene glycol.

Suitable diluents

D5W.[4,7,8]

Maximum concentration

0.2 mg/mL.[4,7,8]

Preparation and delivery

Conivaptan is available in 20-mg and 40-mg ampules for dilution in 250 mL D5W and as a premixed solution in D5W (20 mg/100 mL).[4,7,8]

IV push

Not indicated.

Intermittent infusion

Loading dose is given over 30 minutes.[4,6-8]

Continuous infusion

Maintenance doses are to be administered via continuous infusion.[4,6-8]

Other routes of administration

No information to support administration by other routes.[4]

Comments

Monitoring: Serum sodium, vital signs, and fluid status.[4,6-8]

Drug interactions: Conivaptan is a substrate for CYP3A4 and is also a potent inhibitor of CYP3A4. Concomitant use with potent CYP3A4 inhibitors is contraindicated and caution should be used if co-administering drugs that are substrates for CYP3A4.[4,6-8] Consult appropriate resources for dosing recommendations before combining any drug with conivaptan.

Pharmacokinetic considerations: Nonlinear metabolism likely due to inhibition of its own metabolism.[4,6]

Pharmacodynamic considerations: Net result is increased free water excretion.[4]

Cyclophosphamide

Brand names	Cytoxan, generic
Medication error potential	ISMP high-alert medication that has an increased risk of causing significant patient harm if it is used in error.[1] Look-alike, sound-alike error potential. USP reports that cyclophosphamide has been confused with cyclosporine; no patient harm resulted.[2] USP reports that Cytoxan has been confused with cisplatin and Cytarabine; no patient harm resulted. USP also reports that Cytoxan has been confused with Cytosar-U; patient harm resulted.[2]
Contraindications and warnings	**Contraindications:** Cyclophosphamide is contraindicated in patients with known hypersensitivity to the drug and patients with severely depressed bone marrow.[3] **Warnings:** Secondary malignancies, hemorrhagic cystitis, and acute cardiac toxicity have developed (see Comments section). Cyclophosphamide also carries an increased risk of infection.[3]
Infusion related cautions	Anaphylaxis, including fatal hypersensitivity reactions, have occurred.[3]
Dosage	Consult institutional protocol for complete dosing information. Cyclophosphamide is used as a component of combination therapy to treat both oncologic and nononcologic diseases. Specifically, the FDA approves it for the oncologic treatment of lymphomas, Hodgkin's disease, multiple myeloma, leukemias, mycosis fungoides, neuroblastoma, ovarian adenocarcinoma, retinoblastoma, and breast cancer.[3] Nononcologic FDA indications include pediatric minimal change nephrotic syndrome.[3] It may also be used in SLE, rheumatoid arthritis, vasculitis, and in consolidation therapy prior to autologous BMT, although its use here is not established.[4] Selected dosage regimens include the following: **Pediatric solid tumors:** 40–50 mg/kg IV (1.5–1.8 g/m^2) in divided doses over 2–5 days. [3-5] Other regimens include 10–15 mg/kg (350–550 mg/m^2) given q 7–10 days or 3–5 mg/kg (110–185 mg/m^2) twice weekly.[3-6] **SLE:** 500–750 mg/m^2 every month (maximum dose 1 g/m^2).[5,7] Continuous daily doses of 60–120 mg/m^2 (1–2.5 mg/kg) have been given every day.[4,8] **BMT conditioning regimen:** 50 mg/kg IV once daily for 3–4 days.[5,9]
Dosage adjustment in organ dysfunction	If CrCl is <10 mL/min, administer 75% of the usual dosage.[3,10]
Maximum dosage	Not established.
Additives	None.
Suitable diluents	D5W, D5NS, D5R, LR, NS, ½NS, sodium lactate injection ⅙M.[3,10]

Cyclophosphamide

Maximum concentration

20 mg/mL.[3,10]

Preparation and delivery

Preparation: Reconstitute cyclophosphamide with NS. May also use SW; however, cyclophosphamide reconstituted with SW is hypotonic and should not be administered by direct IV injection; dilute with suitable diluents prior to IV administration.[3,10] Shake the vial vigorously after adding diluents to dissolve all the powder; allow vial to stand for a few minutes if powder still apparent.[3]

Compatibility: See Appendix D for PN compatibility information.

IV push

Dilute with NS for direct injection/IV push.[3]

Intermittent infusion

Most infusions occur over 30–60 minutes.[5] If the dosage is >1800 mg/m^2, the infusion should last 4–6 hours.

Continuous infusion

Although cyclophosphamide may be administered continuously,[4,8,10] its use is not established.

Other routes of administration

Cyclophosphamide has been administered IM,[10] but use is not established. IM administration may be less effective as this route bypasses the liver.[4] May also be given intraperitoneally or intrapleurally.[10] Reconstitute with NS if administering via IM, intraperitoneal, or intrapleural route.[3]

Comments

Significant adverse effects: Cyclophosphamide is associated with hemorrhagic cystitis.[3] Patients should be encouraged to drink excess fluids and void frequently starting 24 hours before therapy and continuing 24 hours after therapy.[3,4] Mesna therapy has also been used with high dosages of cyclophosphamide (i.e., dosages >1 g/m^2/day).[3] The urine should be examined for the presence of red blood cells, an indicator of hemorrhagic cystitis.

Cyclophosphamide is associated with long-term gonadal function damage and infertility in pediatric patients.[3,4]

Cyclophosphamide is associated with a high (>90%) risk of emesis in IV dosages >1500 mg/m^2 and a moderate (30% to 90%) risk of emesis with IV dosages ≤1500 mg/m^2.[12] Patients should receive antiemetic therapy to prevent acute and delayed nausea and vomiting. The recommended therapy is a 5HT3 receptor antagonist in combination with dexamethasone on each day chemotherapy is administered.[12,13] These agents may be continued for up to 4 days after chemotherapy administration for the prevention of delayed nausea and vomiting. Breakthrough medications should also be offered, such as a phenothiazine (e.g., prochlorperazine), a butyrophenone (e.g., droperidol), a substituted benzamide (e.g., metoclopramide), or a benzodiazepine (e.g., lorazepam).

Rare adverse effects: Cardiac toxicity has been reported at dosages ranging from 2.4–26 g/m^2.[3]

Monitoring: Renal function, electrolytes, BUN, CBC with platelets, and urinalysis.[3,4]

Drug interactions: Cyclophosphamide is a major substrate for CYP2B6 and 3A4 and a minor substrate for CYP2A6, 2C9, and 2C19; it is associated with numerous drug interactions. Consult appropriate resources for dosing recommendations before combining any drug with cyclophosphamide.[3,5]

Concomitant allopurinol use may enhance toxicity, particularly bone marrow suppression.[3,5]

CycloSPORINE

Brand names	Sandimmune

Medication error potential

Look-alike, sound-alike error potential.

USP reports Sandimmune was confused with Sandostatin. CycloSPORINE was confused with cyclophosphamide and has potential for confusion with cephalexin.[1]

Contraindications and warnings

US boxed warning: Cyclosporine should only be prescribed by physicians with experience in immunosuppressive therapies. Patients undergoing immunosuppressive therapies are at increased risk for infection and the development of lymphoma. See product literature for complete information.

Contraindications: Patients with hypersensitivity to cyclosporine or Cremophor EL.[2] (See Comments section.)

Other warnings: Anaphylactic reactions have occurred.[2] In phase I/II trials of high-dose cyclosporine for multidrug-resistant tumors in 21 children, anaphylactoid reactions occurred in five patients due to improper mixing of the Cremophor EL vehicle.[3] With high-dose cyclosporine, it was recommended that a homogenous mixture be achieved and premedication with antihistamine and corticosteroid be administered.[3,4] Anaphylaxis requires immediate discontinuation of the infusion and emergency treatment with epinephrine and oxygen.[2]

Infusion related cautions

Patients should be under continuous observation for signs of hypersensitivity reaction during the first 30 minutes of the infusion.[2]

Dosage

Children have required and tolerated larger doses than *adults*.[2] Change to oral therapy as soon as possible. The IV dose is approximately one third of the oral dose.[2]

Transplant immunosuppression (bone marrow transplant (BMT), cardiac, liver, and renal): 5–6 mg/kg prior to transplant[2] then 2–10 mg/kg/day divided q 8–24 h[5-12] or via continuous infusion.[13-18]

Recurrent nephrotic syndrome post-transplant: Continuous infusion of 3 mg/kg/day titrated to maintain desired serum concentrations.[19]

Prevention of graft vs. host disease: 1–5 mg/kg/day either continuously or in two divided doses beginning up to 7 days before transplant with or without titration to desired trough concentrations.[20-25]

Acute myeloid leukemia: 10 mg/kg followed by a continuous infusion of 30 mg/kg/day for a period of 98 hours as part of a mitoxantrone, etoposide, and cyclosporine (MEC) induction regimen.[26]

Inflammatory bowel disease refractory to steroids: 1.3–4 mg/kg/day by continuous infusion or 5 mg/kg/day by intermittent infusion.[27-32]

Atypical sprue: Diarrhea resolved and histology improved in a 23-month-old started on 2 mg/kg q 12 h that was increased to 4 mg/kg q 12 h.[33]

Dosage adjustment in organ dysfunction

No dosage adjustment required in renal dysfunction.[2] However, nephrotoxicity occurs in 25% to 38% of patients.[2] This may be associated with larger accumulated doses or persistently high trough concentrations.[2] (See Comments section.)

Maximum dosage

Not established.

Additives

Contains polyoxyethylated castor oil 650 mg (Cremophor EL) and 32.9% alcohol by volume.[2]

152

CycloSPORINE

Suitable diluents	NS, D5W.[2]
Maximum concentration	2.5 mg/mL.[2]
Preparation and delivery	**Stability:** The extent of cyclosporine sorption in PVC is greater when mixed with NS compared to D5W.[34] NS admixtures are considered usable for 6 hours in PVC and 12 hours in glass containers.[35] Storage in glass containers has been recommended.[36] Reconstituted product should be discarded after 24 hours.[2] **Drug delivery system issues:** The Cremophor EL vehicle may leach DEHP, a known hepatotoxin, from PVC bags and tubing.[33] If PVC bags are used, solutions should be infused immediately to minimize DEHP exposure.[37] A solution with 0.5–2.5 mg/mL of cyclosporine had detectable DEHP after >4.5 hours of contact with PVC.[38] **Compatibility:** See Appendix D for PN compatibility information.
IV push	Contraindicated.[2]
Intermittent infusion	Over 2–8 hours.[2,3,4,11,27-32]
Continuous infusion	1.2–4.5 mg/kg have been given over 24 hours.[13-18]
Other routes of administration	Not indicated.
Comments	Anaphylaxis may be a result of the Cremophor EL vehicle.[2,3,39-41] **Monitoring:** Serum concentration monitoring is essential to determining the appropriate dosage. Trough concentrations should be maintained within therapeutic range for the specific assay and transplant type.[38-40] Trough concentration monitoring is being replaced by a 2-hour postdose concentration because it better approximates $AUC^{(0-4)}$ that correlates with the risk of rejection.[41,42] Use the same analytical methodology and sample matrix (i.e., whole blood vs. plasma) consistently. HPLC assays are specific for cyclosporine. Cyclosporine metabolites cross-react with polyclonal radioimmunoassay[47] and FPIA and may result in an overestimation of serum concentrations compared to other methods.[42,43,47,48] The FPIA assay may not be reliable in liver dysfunction.[42,44] Concentrations drawn through a second catheter lumen may be falsely increased when the patient is receiving cyclosporine as a continuous infusion through the other lumen.[49] Cyclosporine is adsorbed to silicone; blood samples drawn through central venous lines made from silicone may be falsely increased if cyclosporine has been infused through them.[50,51] **Drug interactions:** Cyclosporine is principally metabolized by the CYP3A4 isoenzyme and is associated with numerous important drug interactions.[2] Consult appropriate resources for dosing recommendations before combining any drug with cyclosporine. **Adverse effects:** Nephrotoxicity, hypertension, tremor, hirsutism, and gum hyperplasia.[2] In renal transplant patients, it is often difficult to determine if a decrease in renal function is due to nephrotoxicity or allograft rejection.[2] Nephrotoxicity: increased trough concentrations, gradual increases in SCr, and a BUN/SCr ≥20. Rejection: lower trough concentrations, more dramatic increase in SCr, and BUN/SCr <20.

Cytomegalovirus Immunoglobulin

Brand names	CytoGam

Medication error potential

None reported by ISMP and USP.[1,2]

Contraindications and warnings

US boxed warning: Human immune globulin products have been associated with renal dysfunction, acute renal failure, osmotic nephrosis, proximal tubular nephropathy, and death. These renal effects have been most commonly associated with immune globulin products that contain sucrose as a stabilizer (such as cytomegalovirus immunoglobulin) and daily immune globulin doses of 400 mg/kg or higher. Administer immune globulin products in the lowest concentration and rate of infusion for patients with renal disease, diabetes mellitus, volume depletion, sepsis, paraproteinemia; for patients ≥65 years; and for those receiving other nephrotoxic drugs.[3]

Contraindications: Known hypersensitivity to the drug, selective immunoglobulin deficiency.[4]

Other warnings: Carries the possibility for transmission of blood-borne viral agents, including a theoretical risk of Creutzfeldt-Jakob disease, since it is made from human plasma.[4] Hemolysis, thrombotic events, aseptic meningitis syndrome, and transfusion-related acute lung injury have also been reported with the use of immune globulin products.[4]

Infusion related cautions

Monitor vital signs before, during, and after infusion, and before any rate increases.[4] Flushing, chills, muscle cramps, back pain, fever, vomiting, arthralgias, and wheezing are usually related to infusion rate and may be managed by interrupting the infusion temporarily and restarting at a lower rate. If anaphylaxis or a decrease in blood pressure occurs, the infusion should be discontinued. Epinephrine should be available in case of anaphylaxis.[4]

Dosage

Renal function should be assessed before beginning therapy, as well as at appropriate intervals thereafter, and discontinuation should be considered if renal function deteriorates. Patients should be well hydrated prior to beginning therapy.[4] (See Dosage adjustment in organ dysfunction section.)

HIV-infected patients: 200 mg/kg alternating biweekly with IV immune globulin.[5]

Transfusions (multiple) in neonates: 150 mg/kg.[6]

Transplantation

> **Bone marrow:** 200 mg/kg given 6 and 8 days prior to transplant and on days 1, 7, 14, 21, 28, 42, 56, and 70 after transplant.[7]

> **Heart, liver, lung, and pancreas:** 150 mg/kg within 72 hours of transplant, 150 mg/kg at 2, 4, 6, and 8 weeks after transplant, and 100 mg/kg at 12 and 16 weeks after transplant.[4,8,9]

> **Liver and intestine:** 100 mg/kg (on alternating day from ganciclovir) followed by 150 mg/kg at weeks 6 and 8 followed by 100 mg/kg at 12 and 18 weeks after transplant.[9]

> **Renal:** 150 mg/kg within 72 hours of transplant, 100 mg/kg at 2, 4, 6, and 8 weeks after transplant, and 50 mg/kg at 12 and 16 weeks after transplant.[4,10,11]

Infantile cytomegalovirus-associated autoimmune hemolytic anemia: One dose of 500 mg/kg.[12]

Dosage adjustment in organ dysfunction

Use with caution in patients with renal insufficiency or in those at risk for developing renal insufficiency.[4] In order to decrease the risk of renal dysfunction, patients should be well hydrated prior to administration.[4]

Cytomegalovirus Immunoglobulin

Maximum dosage

For transplant patients, the manufacturer recommends a maximum dose of 150 mg/kg. 200 mg/kg has been given in HIV infection and multiple transfusions in neonates.[5,7] 500 mg/kg has been administered to two infants for autoimmune hemolytic anemia.[12]

Additives

Each mL contains 50 mg sucrose and 10 mg human serum albumin. Sodium content is 20–30 mEq/L.[4]

Suitable diluents

Predilution is not recommended.[4]

Maximum concentration

50 mg/mL.[4]

Preparation and delivery

Delivery: The product should be infused through an in-line filter with a pore size of 15 microns. A 0.2-micron filter is also acceptable. Should be administered through an IV line with a constant infusion pump.[4]

Stability: Do not shake vial; avoid foaming. Does not contain any preservatives; thus, the infusion should be initiated within 6 hours of entering the vial and be completed within 12 hours of entering the vial.[4]

IV push

Not recommended.[4]

Intermittent infusion

May piggyback into existing infusions of NS or D2.5W, D5W, D10W, D20W (all with or without NaCl) and deliver via an infusion device at no more than 1:2 dilution.[4]

Initial dose[4]: 15 mg/kg/h for 30 minutes. If no adverse effects are noted, increase to 30 mg/kg/h for 30 minutes and then to maximum rate of 60 mg/kg/h.

Subsequent infusions[4]: 15 mg/kg/h for 15 minutes. If no adverse effects are noted, increase to 30 mg/kg/h for 15 minutes and then to a maximum rate of 60 mg/kg/h.

Volume should not exceed 75 mL/h.[4]

Continuous infusion

No information available.

Other routes of administration

Not recommended.[4]

Comments

Vaccinations with live virus vaccines (measles, mumps, rubella, varicella) should be deferred for 3 months after infusion.[4]

DACTINomycin

Brand names	Cosmegen

Medication error potential

ISMP high-alert medication that has an increased risk of causing significant patient harm if it is used in error.[1]

Look-alike, sound-alike error potential.

ISMP and USP report that DACTINomycin has been confused with DAPTOmycin; no patient harm resulted.[2,3]

Contraindications and warnings

US boxed warning: Dactinomycin should be administered under the supervision of an experienced physician. The drug is highly toxic; both the powder and solution should be handled with care. Inhalation of vapors or dust and contact with skin and mucous membranes should be avoided. Do not use or handle during pregnancy. Special precautions should be in place and reviewed prior to handling due to the toxic properties of dactinomycin (corrosivity, carcinogenicity, mutagenicity, and teratogenicity). Dactinomycin is highly corrosive and will damage soft tissue if extravasation occurs (see Infusion related cautions section); dactinomycin extravasation has resulted in contracture of the arm in at least one case.[4]

Contraindications: Known hypersensitivity to the drug or to any component of this product. Should not be administered around the time of infection with chicken pox or herpes zoster.[4]

Other warnings: Veno-occlusive disease (especially in children less than 48 months), myelosuppression, dermatological reactions, emesis, and secondary malignancies.[4,5] Dactinomycin should not be used in infants <6 months based on a higher incidence of side effects.[4] (See Comments section.)

Infusion related cautions

Extravasation will result in severe soft tissue damage. If extravasation occurs, ice should be applied to the affected area immediately for 30–60 minutes.[4] It has been suggested to ice 15 minutes four times daily for 3 days. See Appendix E for additional information regarding extravasation treatment.

Dosage

Consult institutional protocol for complete dosing information.

Dactinomycin is used as a component of combination therapy for several malignant pediatric solid tumors. Dactinomycin has also been used in patients with nephroblastoma, malignant melanoma, and osteosarcoma.

Dosage should be based on body surface area (BSA) for obese or edematous patients.[4] (See Appendix A.)

Suggested regimens for different disease states include the following:

Wilms' tumor, rhabdomyosarcoma, Ewing's sarcoma: 15 mcg/kg/day IV for 5 days in combination with chemotherapeutic agents.[4-10]

Metastatic nonseminatous testicular cancer: 1000 mcg/m²/day IV on day 1 with cyclophosphamide, bleomycin, vinblastine, and cisplatin.[4,11]

Gestational trophoblastic neoplasia: 12 mcg/kg/day IV for 5 days as monotherapy or 500 mcg IV on days 1 and 2 as part of a combination regimen with etoposide, methotrexate, folinic acid, vincristine, cyclophosphamide, and cisplatin.[4,12,13]

Regional perfusion in locally recurrent and locoregional solid malignancies: 50 mcg/kg for lower extremity or pelvis; 35 mcg/kg for upper extremity.[4]

Dosage adjustment in organ dysfunction

Not established.

DACTINomycin

Maximum dosage	The manufacturer recommends that dosages should not exceed 15 mcg/kg/day or 400–600 mg/m^2/day for 5 days per 2-week cycle.[4]
Additives	None.
Suitable diluents	Reconstitute with SW; further dilution with D5W, NS.[4,14]
Maximum concentration	500 mcg/mL.[4,14]
Preparation and delivery	**Preparation:** Both the powder and solution can cause severe damage when in direct contact with the skin or through inhalation. Use caution when preparing. Reconstitute by adding 1.1 mL of SW (without preservative). Use of SW containing preservatives is not recommended as it results in precipitation formation.[4,14] Once reconstituted the solution (500 mcg/mL) can be added to a suitable infusion solution.[4] **Delivery:** Binds to cellulose filters; therefore, avoid in-line filtration. Adsorbs to glass and plastic so dactinomycin should not be given by continuous infusion.[4,14]
IV push	The desired dose of reconstituted drug may be injected into the tubing of a running infusion of D5W or NS.[4,14]
Intermittent infusion	The desired dose of reconstituted drug may be further diluted with D5W or NS or may be injected into the tubing of a running infusion of D5W or NS.[4,14]
Continuous infusion	No information available to support administration by this method.
Other routes of administration	Dactinomycin is highly corrosive and will damage soft tissue. Do not administer as IM or SC injection.[14]
Comments	**Significant adverse effects:** Dactinomycin has been associated with the development of hepatic veno-occlusive disease in children <48 months.[4,15] Dactinomycin has been associated with an increased risk of dermatological adverse effects when used concomitantly with or after radiation.[4] Risks may be increased when radiation involves mucous membranes or when dactinomycin is administered within 2 months of radiation for right-sided Wilms' tumors. Dactinomycin is associated with a moderate (30% to 90%) risk of emesis.[16] Patients should receive antiemetic therapy to prevent acute and delayed nausea and vomiting. The recommended therapy is a 5HT3 receptor antagonist in combination with dexamethasone every day chemotherapy is administered.[16,17] These agents may be continued for up to 4 days after chemotherapy administration for the prevention of delayed nausea and vomiting. Breakthrough medications should also be offered, such as a phenothiazine (e.g., prochlorperazine), a butyrophenone (e.g., droperidol), a substituted benzamide (e.g., metoclopramide), or a benzodiazepine (e.g., lorazepam). **Monitoring:** Monitor CBC with platelets, liver function tests, and renal function tests.[4,5] **Laboratory interference:** May interact with the bioassay for determination of antibacterial drug levels.[4]

Darbepoetin

Brand names	Aranesp

Medication error potential

Look-alike, sound-alike error potential.

USP reports that darbepoetin has been confused with dalteparin; no patient harm resulted. USP reports that Aranesp has been confused with Aralast and Aricept; no patient harm resulted.[1]

Contraindications and warnings

US boxed warning: Erythropoiesis-stimulating agents (ESAs) carry boxed warnings for increased mortality, serious cardiovascular and thromboembolic events, and increased risk of tumor progression or recurrence. In patients with renal failure, ESAs should be given to achieve and maintain hemoglobin concentrations of 10–12 g/dL, as increased mortality and serious cardiovascular events have occurred in two clinical trials when targeting higher hemoglobin concentrations (i.e., 13–14 g/dL).[2]

ESAs shortened survival and/or increased tumor progression in clinical cancer trials (breast, head and neck, lymphoid, non-small cell lung, and cervical cancers). Use the lowest dose possible to avoid transfusions, use only for anemia in combination with chemotherapy, and discontinue when chemotherapy is completed. ESAs should not be given to patients on myelosuppressive therapy if the anticipated outcome is cure.[2]

Contraindications: Uncontrolled hypertension and known hypersensitivity to the drug or any of its components.[2]

Other warnings: Hypertension and seizures have occurred in patients with chronic renal failure receiving darbepoetin. Pure red cell aplasia and severe anemia have also occurred. Antibody-mediated pure red cell aplasia occurred in patients with hepatitis C infection receiving ESA in combination with antiviral therapy. ESA therapy should be withheld in any patients with antibody-mediated anemia.[2]

Infusion related cautions

Rare serious allergic reactions, including rash and urticaria, have been reported.[2]

In patients with latex allergy, be aware that the needle cover of the prefilled syringe contains dry natural rubber (a latex derivative).[2]

Dosage

To ensure the erythropoietic response, iron status should be evaluated and supplemental iron prescribed if stores are low. Transferrin saturation should be ≥20% and ferritin should be ≥100 ng/mL.[2]

Target hemoglobin range should be 10–12 g/dL.[2]

Anemia in (nonmyeloid or solid tumor) cancer[3-6]: Safety and efficacy of darbepoetin in anemia of childhood cancer has not been established. The following dosages have been used in *adults:*

> 1–4.5 mcg/kg SC once weekly[3,4]

> 3–9 mcg/kg SC q 2 weeks[5]

> 4.5–15 mcg/kg q 3 weeks[6]

Do not treat if Hb >10 g/dL. If Hb has increased by <1 g/dL during initial 6 weeks of therapy (with adequate iron stores), then increase dose by 25% every week (up to 4.5 mcg/kg/dose) until at target Hb concentration. If Hb has increased >1 g/dL over a 2-week period or the Hb concentration reaches a level needed to avoid transfusion, then decrease dose by 40%. If Hb exceeds level needed to avoid transfusion, then temporarily hold therapy.[2]

One pharmacokinetic study in pediatric cancer patients gave 2.25 mcg/kg SC once weekly for up to six doses.[7]

Darbepoetin

Dosage *(cont.)*	**Anemia of chronic renal insufficiency**[2,8-12] **1–18 years:** 0.25–0.75 mcg/kg IV or SC once weekly or once every 2 weeks.[2,8-10,13,14] (See Comments section.) Adjust dosage (monthly) to achieve and maintain a target Hb concentration of 10–12 g/dL.[2] If Hb has increased <1 g/dL during initial 4 weeks of therapy (with adequate iron stores), then increase dose by 25% q 4 weeks until at target Hb. If the Hb increases by more than 1 g/dL in 2 weeks or the Hb is increasing and approaching 12 g/dL, then decrease dose by 25%.[2] **<8 kg (use not established):** 0.5 mcg/kg once weekly was given to six infants with renal dysplasia, three on peritoneal dialysis.[11] Doses were increased or decreased by 25% to maintain Hb concentrations 10–11 g/dL. After 20 weeks, in three stable patients (one on peritoneal dialysis), Hb ranged from 11.7–13.5 g/dL, and doses were 0.17 or 0.25 mcg/kg q 4 weeks or 0.34 mcg/kg q 3 weeks. In three medically unstable patients, Hb ranged from 8.5–9.7 g/dL, and doses were 1.06–1.24 mcg/kg weekly. Investigators concluded that individualized dosing was warranted. **Peritoneal dialysis, 0–17 years (use not established):** 0.45 mcg/kg once weekly given intraperitoneally at the end of peritoneal dialysis session.[15] **Anemia of prematurity (use not established):** Erythroid progenitor cells in cord blood, fetal marrow, and fetal liver were equally stimulated by erythropoietin and darbepoetin.[16] In a pharmacokinetics study, a single dose of 1 or 4 mcg/kg SC increased erythropoiesis in preterm infants <1500 g.[17] Another pharmacokinetic study evaluated a 4-mcg/kg IV dose in 10 neonates 704–3025 g and found a shorter half-life and more rapid clearance than has been noted in children.[18] In addition, both the immature reticulocyte count and the absolute reticulocyte count increased.[18]
Dosage adjustment in organ dysfunction	Patients with chronic renal insufficiency who are not on dialysis may require lower maintenance doses.[2]
Maximum dosage	Not established. Doses up to 8 mcg/kg once weekly and 15 mcg/kg q 3 weeks have been used in *adults* with cancer.[5,6]
Additives	Available in two formulations. The albumin solution contains 2.5 mg human albumin and 8.18 mg sodium chloride in water for injection per mL.[2] The polysorbate solution contains 0.05 mg polysorbate and 8.18 mg sodium chloride in water for injection per mL.[2]
Suitable diluents	Darbepoetin should not be diluted.[2]
Maximum concentration	500 mcg/mL.[2]
Preparation and delivery	Vigorous shaking and/or exposure to light may physically denature the glycoprotein and inactivate the molecule.[2] Do not administer with any other IV drug.[2]
IV push	Rapid, within 15 seconds.[8]

Darbepoetin

Intermittent infusion	No information to support this method of administration.
Continuous infusion	No information to support this method of administration.
Other routes of administration	SC route is preferred except in patients on hemodialysis when IV administration is preferred.[2] IM is not indicated.
Comments	**Monitoring:** Monitor Hb weekly until target is achieved, then monthly.[2] **Other:** One study in children with chronic renal insufficiency based the initial dose on current recombinant human erythropoietin dosing (rHuEPO dose/200 = darbepoetin weekly dose).[10] Investigators noted an excessive increase in Hb in six of seven children evaluated. The two youngest received 3.6 and 2.79 mcg/kg weekly and developed hypertension (Hb was >13 g/dL). The dose was held for 2 weeks and restarted at half the previous dose. At the end of 6 months, doses in all seven patients ranged from 0.37–0.69 mcg/kg weekly. This is consistent with the manufacturers' current recommendations.[2] Another study used a conversion ratio of 100 units rHuEPO to 0.42 mcg darbepoetin.[13] The manufacturer recommends giving darbepoetin once weekly if the patient was receiving rHuEPO two to three times per week and once every 2 weeks if the patient was receiving rHuEPO once per week.[2] Darbepoetin (0.42–0.66 mcg/kg SC weekly in combination with ferric gluconate or iron dextran over 4–18 months) has been given to four pediatric patients (age 10–16 years) with anemia associated with recessive dystrophic epidermolysis bullosa.[19] Inform patients of risks associated with ESA therapy. Medication guides, available from the manufacturer, should be given to all patients receiving ESA therapy at home.[2]

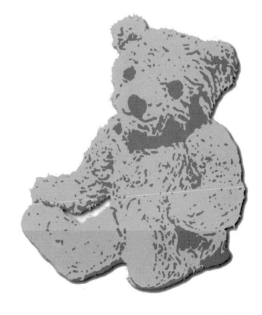

Deferoxamine Mesylate

Brand names	Desferal Mesylate

Medication error potential	Look-alike, sound-alike error potential.
	USP reports that Desferal has been confused with DexFerrum; no patient harm resulted.[1]

Contraindications and warnings	Contraindicated in severe renal disease or anuria (both deferoxamine and iron chelate are renally excreted).[2]

Infusion related cautions	Flushing, urticaria, hypotension, and shock may occur, particularly with rapid IV administration.[2-5]
	Anaphylaxis may occur.[2]

Dosage	**Iron exposure**

Acute iron ingestion: While the manufacturer states that IM administration is the preferred route and should be used for all patients not in shock,[2] toxicology literature supports the IV administration of deferoxamine for acute iron poisoning.[3]

15 mg/kg/h by continuous infusion[2,3,6-8] until urine is a normal color for 24 hours[7-8] or until clinical status and laboratory values normalize. Alternatively, an initial dose of 20 mg/kg or 600 mg/m^2 (IM or slow IV infusion) followed by 10 mg/kg or 300 mg/m^2 q 4 h for two doses.[9] Subsequent doses of 10 mg/kg or 300 mg/m^2 q 4–12 h are given as clinically needed.[9]

Chronic iron overload due to transfusion-dependent anemias: 14–98 mg/kg/day over 8–12 hours.[10-12] Individualize dose based on the degree of iron overload. Doses that exceed a "therapeutic index" (ratio of mean daily dose in mg/kg divided by serum ferritin) >0.025 increase the risk for sensorineural hearing loss.[12]

Aluminum-related disorders in kidney disease (use not established): To avoid deferoxamine induced adverse effects (neurotoxicity), it should not be given to patients with an initial serum aluminum >200 mcg/L. Treat these patients with intensive high flux dialysis until serum aluminum <200 mcg/L.[13]

Deferoxamine test: 5 mg/kg given during last hour of dialysis session. Measure serum aluminum before infusion and 2 days later (before next dialysis session). Doses as low as 0.5 mg/kg have also been used.[13]

Aluminum rise <300 mcg/L and no side effects after test: 5 mg/kg IV over last hour of hemodialysis, once per week for 2 months; high flux hemodialysis 44 hours after dose.

Aluminum rise >300 mcg/L or side effects after test: 5 mg/kg IV over 1 hour; give 5 hours before hemodialysis, once per week for 4 months; high flux hemodialysis after deferoxamine.

Dosage adjustment in organ dysfunction	Product labeling states that deferoxamine is contraindicated in patients with severe renal dysfunction or anuria because the drug and the iron chelate are renally eliminated.[2] Another reference states that therapy should continue in renal failure; however, the infusion rate should be adjusted. No guidelines for adjusting rate are given.[3] Another reference recommends in *adults* to decrease dose by 25% to 50% with GFR between 10 and 50 mL/min and to avoid use with GFR <10 mL/min.[14]

Deferoxamine Mesylate

Maximum dosage

Although the labeling recommends that total amounts should not exceed 6 g/24 h,[2] these doses have been exceeded in clinical practice.[3]

16 g was infused to an *adult* with transfusion-related iron overload over 24 hours without apparent adverse effects.[15] While doses >50 mg/kg/day (up to 235 mg/kg/day) have been used,[10-12, 16-18] doses <50–60 mg/kg/day are recommended to avoid neurotoxicity.[19] (See Comments section.)

2520 mg or 210 mg/kg/day (15 mg/kg/h over 14 hours) has been given to an 18-month-old with acute iron intoxication (serum iron concentration 447 mcg/dL). No adverse effects were seen.[20]

Additives

None.[21]

Suitable diluents

SW (for reconstitution). NS, ½NS, D5W, LR (for dilution).[2, 21]

Maximum concentration

250 mg/mL.[2]

Preparation and delivery

Reconstitution recommended with SW; other diluents may cause precipitation.[21] Turbid solutions should not be used.[2]

IV push

Not recommended.[2] (See Infusion related cautions section.)

Intermittent infusion

Dilute with suitable diluent. Do not exceed 15 mg/kg/h.[2]

Continuous infusion

Dilute with suitable diluent. Do not to exceed 15 mg/kg/h.[2]

Other routes of administration

IM is preferred route of administration in acute iron ingestion in patients not in shock.[2]

May be given via SC infusion with a portable controlled-infusion device.[21]

Comments

Significant adverse effects: Vision and hearing impairment has been attributed to chronic chelation treatment with deferoxamine.[4,6,10,12,16,18,19,22] Cessation of chelation therapy and/or dosage reduction frequently leads to improvement.[4,10,18,22]

A pulmonary syndrome has been associated with prolonged continuous infusion[17,23-27] and total daily doses >6 g.[28] Another study suggests that the pulmonary abnormalities are related to inadequate chelation.[29] Intermittent infusions for <24 hours have been recommended[25,30] but are investigational.

Nephrotoxicity has also been reported.[31] Adequate hydration decreases the incidence of this adverse effect.[31]

Neurotoxicity has been reported.[4,10-12,16,18,19,22] Large doses may exacerbate neurologic dysfunction (i.e., seizures) in patients with aluminum-related encephalopathy.[2]

Growth retardation has occurred in patients with low ferritin concentrations who receive large doses of deferoxamine. Following reduction in the deferoxamine dose, growth velocity may partially return to pretreatment rate. Pediatric patients should be monitored for body weight and growth every 3 months.[2]

Deferoxamine Mesylate

Comments *(cont.)*

Rare adverse effects: Deferoxamine has been associated with an increased risk of infection. This is particularly true for *Yersinia enterocolitica* and *Yersinia pseudotuberculosis*. Mucormycosis has also been reported, particularly in dialysis patients.[2,13] The drug should be discontinued until any suspected or documented infection resolves.[2]

Other: Patients with chronic iron overload usually become vitamin-C deficient. *Adults* with chronic iron overload have developed cardiac impairment following concomitant treatment with deferoxamine and high doses of vitamin C. The abnormalities reversed when vitamin C was discontinued.[2] Recommended daily vitamin C doses should not be exceeded.

Urine may not always be vin rosé color with administration of deferoxamine, even when iron overload is present.[32]

5 mg/kg/h by continuous infusion, in combination with aggressive fluid resuscitation and inotropic support, successfully lowered serum iron concentrations in a 7-week-old preterm (27 weeks GA) neonate. The dose was not able to be increased due to hypotension.[33]

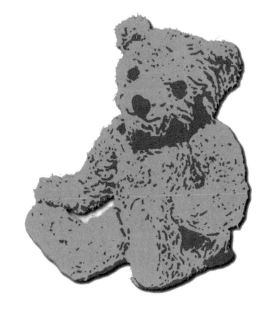

Dexamethasone Sodium Phosphate

Brand names	Decadron, Dexasone, Solurex, generic

Medication error potential

Look-alike, sound-alike error potential.

USP reported that dexamethasone was confused with betamethasone, doxazosin, methadone, and methylprednisolone and patient harm did not occur. Dexamethasone was confused with dexmedetomidine and patient harm occurred. Decadron was confused with Depacon and Dexedrine, and patient harm did not occur.[1]

Contraindications and warnings

Contraindications: Patients with systemic fungal infections except in the management of drug reactions to amphotericin B.[2]

Patients with hypersensitivity to any component in the product.[2]

Live virus (MMR, varicella, rotavirus, smallpox) vaccinations should not be given during treatment with immunosuppressive doses of glucocorticoids.[2] (See Comments section.)

Warnings: Anaphylactoid reactions have been reported and those with a prior history of such reactions require appropriate precautions.[2]

Patients on chronic steroid therapy may require increased doses during stressful situations.[2]

Supraphysiologic doses of corticosteroids may result in suppressed pituitary-adrenal function, so therapy of more than a few days should be decreased gradually.[2,3]

Immunosuppression and an increased risk for infection are possible during steroid therapy.[2]

Infusion related cautions

None noted.

Dosage

Prevention of chronic lung disease (CLD) in very low birth weight (VLBW) infants: 0.25–0.5 mg/kg/day tapered over 14–42 days.[4,5] Alternatively, 0.5 mg/kg/day for 3 days followed by 0.25 mg/kg/day for 3 days and then 0.1 mg/kg/day on day 7.[6] Of note, a multicenter study was stopped early because of concerns over side effects in the steroid group.[7] The AAP recommends limited use of dexamethasone in this group because of the association with serious complications.[8] (See Comments section.)

Extubation (dexamethasone given prior to extubation was not beneficial during uncomplicated airway management[9])

Preterm infants: 0.25 mg/kg q 8 h for three doses[10] or 0.15 mg/kg/day for 3 days followed by 0.1 mg/kg/day for 3 days and then 0.05 mg/kg/day for 2 days.[11] (See Comments section.)

Infants and children: 0.5 mg/kg (≤10 mg) q 6 h for six doses beginning 6–12 hours before anticipated extubation.[12] (See Comments section.)

Dexamethasone Sodium Phosphate

Dosage *(cont.)*	**Nausea and vomiting prevention** **Prevention of chemotherapy induced nausea and vomiting (in addition to 5-hydroxytryptamine 3 antagonists):** 10 mg/m² q 12 h on chemotherapy days[13] or 8 mg/m² prior to chemotherapy and again 4 and 8 hours after.[14] For highly emetogenic chemotherapy, dexamethasone should be given on days 1, 2, and 3.[15] For moderate to low emetogenic chemotherapy, dexamethasone is used once prior to chemotherapy.[15] **Prevention of postoperative nausea and vomiting:** In children undergoing surgery for strabismus, 0.25 mg/kg was as effective as 0.5 and 1 mg/kg given during induction.[16] In another study in 135 children undergoing strabismus surgery, 0.5 mg dexamethasone (maximum of 25 mg) was as effective as ondansetron.[17] For tonsillectomy, single preoperative doses of 0.5 mg/kg (≤8 mg)[18,19] and 1 mg/kg (≤50 mg) have been effective.[20] **Acute laryngotracheitis (croup):** For those who are unable to take po, 0.6 mg/kg IM or IV as a single dose has been used.[21-25] In children with moderate to severe croup, 0.15 mg/kg (n = 20; maximum dose 3 mg) was as effective as 0.6 mg/kg (n = 21; maximum dose 12 mg).[25] **Meningitis, bacterial:** 0.15 mg/kg q 6 h for 2–4 days of antibiotic therapy was effective in reducing hearing loss in those with *Haemophilus influenza* type b (Hib) disease. However, the outcome in patients with pneumococcal meningitis treated with dexamethasone has been either worse or no different than controls.[26,27] With the use of Hib and pneumococcal conjugate vaccines, both Hib and pneumococcal meningitis have decreased. Where dexamethasone fits in the treatment of meningitis is unclear.[28,29] **Asthma:** Methylprednisolone sodium succinate is the recommended parenteral glucocorticoid for asthma.[30] **Cerebral edema/elevated ICP:** Not recommended for traumatic brain injury in pediatric patients.[31]
Dosage adjustment in organ dysfunction	Those with cirrhosis of the liver or who are hypothyroid may have an exaggerated response.[2]
Maximum dosage	Not established.[2]
Additives	Contains sodium sulfite or sodium metabisulfite. Vials with preservative contain benzyl alcohol.[2,32] See Appendix C for more specific information about potential adverse effects and/or benzyl alcohol toxicity in neonates.
Suitable diluents	D5W, NS.[2]
Maximum concentration	Undiluted (10 mg/mL).[2,32]
Preparation and delivery	**Compatibility:** See Appendix D for PN compatibility information.
IV push	Over 1 to several minutes.[2]

Dexamethasone Sodium Phosphate

Intermittent infusion	The dose can be infused intermittently.
Continuous infusion	Not indicated.
Other routes of administration	4 or 10 mg/mL may be used IM or IV.[2,23,24] 4 mg/mL can be given intra-articular, intrasynovial, intralesional, or as a soft tissue injection.[33]
Comments	Live virus vaccines may be given 1 month after ending a ≥2-week course of high-dose systemic corticosteroids (2 mg/kg/day of prednisone or its equivalent; or 20 mg/day if >10 kg).[34]

While early dexamethasone facilitates extubation in VLBW infants, the Vermont Oxford Network Steroid Study Group concluded that neither CLD nor mortality was favorably affected.[7] Additionally, exposure is associated with a worsened neurological outcome[5] and poor weight gain.[7] On the other hand, 15 years after treatment, a group of ventilator-dependent VLBW infants given a 42-day course beginning at 2 weeks of age (n = 9) had improved neurological outcome compared to infants who received an 18-day treatment (n = 9) or a control group (n = 5).[4] This investigator speculated that steroids might be of benefit in some situations.

Extremely low birth weight infants who received dexamethasone were more likely to have decreased growth and intestinal perforation and no decrease in mortality or chronic lung disease than controls.[35]

Avoiding dexamethasone in the first 10 days of life has been suggested.[36] If it must be used, recommendations were 0.2–0.3 mg/kg/day divided q 12 h for 48 hours; if treatment is extended beyond 48 hours, the dose should be halved q 48 h with a maximum treatment length of 10 days.[36]

Adverse effects: Musculoskeletal effects, fluid and electrolyte abnormalities, cataracts, and hyperglycemia.[2] Patients with diabetes may be at particular risk for hyperglycemia.

Drug interactions: Drugs that enhance hepatic clearance (e.g., phenytoin, phenobarbital, ephedrine, rifampin) may decrease blood levels and lessen physiologic activity. Drugs that inhibit hepatic clearance may increase dexamethasone concentrations.[2]

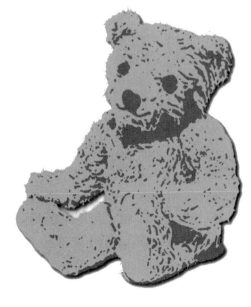

Dexmedetomidine HCl

Brand names	Precedex

Medication error potential

Look-alike, sound-alike error potential.

USP reported that dexmedetomidine was confused with dexamethasone and patient harm occurred. Precedex has the potential to be confused with Cerebyx.[1]

Contraindications and warnings

Warnings: Because of known cardiovascular effects, including bradycardia, sinus arrest, and hypotension, patients should be continuously monitored.[2,3] Slowing the rate of the infusion may modify the cardiovascular effects.[2] Transient hypertension has been noted during loading dose infusion.[2] During infusion, some patients may be arousable and alert when stimulated and this alone should not be considered lack of efficacy.[2] Abrupt withdrawal symptoms include nervousness, agitation, and headaches with increased blood pressure can occur following a continuous infusion over 24 hours.[2] (See Comments section.)

Infusion related cautions

See Contraindications and warnings section.

Dosage

Little information is available on the use of dexmedetomidine in children.

Procedural sedation: Children (n = 48; 5 months–16 years) received a loading dose of 0.92 ± 0.36 mcg/kg (range, 0.3–1.9 mcg/kg) over 10.3 ± 4.7 minutes followed by continuous infusion of 0.69 ± 0.32 mcg/kg/h (range: 0.25–1.14 mcg/kg/h) for noninvasive procedures lasting 47 ± 16 minutes.[3] Thirty-two of 40 children given a loading dose of 1 mcg/kg over 10 minutes followed by 0.5 mcg/kg/h for 45 ± 11.7 minutes achieved adequate sedation for MRI compared to eight of 40 children given midazolam.[4] Propofol alone (n = 20) or dexmedetomidine (1 mcg/kg over 10 minutes followed by 0.5 mcg/kg/h) and a single midazolam dose (n = 20) for sedation during MRI produced similar anesthesia but recovery was prolonged, heart rate slower, and blood pressure higher in the dexmedetomidine group.[5]

Critically ill children requiring mechanical ventilation: Three groups of 10 children per group received continuous infusion midazolam, a 0.25 mcg dexmedetomidine/kg bolus (n = 10) over 5 minutes followed by 0.25 mcg/h, or 0.5 mcg dexmedetomidine/kg over 5 minutes followed by 0.5 mcg/kg/h (n = 10). The dexmedetomidine or midazolam infusions were increased if three to four doses of morphine were required within 8 hours.[6] Less morphine and fewer infusion rate changes were required by either of the dexmedetomidine groups than the midazolam comparator.[6] To minimize midazolam use and to facilitate weaning from mechanical ventilation, an initial continuous infusion of 0.2 ± 0.2 increased to 0.5 ± 0.2 mcg/kg/h (used with fentanyl or morphine) based on adequacy of sedation was used for 3 to 75 hours in 17 infants and children.[7] None experienced significant changes in blood pressure or heart rate.[7]

Following cardiothoracic surgery: An average infusion rate of 0.3 ± 0.05 mcg/kg/h (range, 0.2–0.75) for 14.7 ± 5.5 h (range 3–26 hours) was used in 38 children; a loading dose was not used.[8] Of the six children who developed hypotension, three responded to a dose reduction; however, three required drug discontinuation.[8]

Facilitate opioid weaning in cardiac transplant: A 6-month-old infant and a 7-year-old child sedated for 8 weeks and 15 days prior to transplant and for 4 weeks and 3 days after, respectively, were given 1 mcg/kg over 10 minutes followed by 0.8–1 mcg/kg/h and 0.5–1 mcg/kg/h for 10 and 8 days, respectively.[9] Doses were then weaned as tolerated over 6 days and 24 hours.[9]

Dosage adjustment in organ dysfunction

Dose reduction should be considered in patients with hepatic impairment.[2]

Dexmedetomidine HCl

Maximum dosage	The maximum loading dose was 1.92 mcg/kg over 10 minutes and the maximum infusion rate reported was 1.14 mcg/kg/h. This was used for short-term (~45 minutes) procedural sedation.[3]
Additives	Contains 9 mg sodium chloride/mL.[2]
Suitable diluents	D5W, NS, R, RL, mannitol 20%.[10]
Maximum concentration	4 mcg/mL.[2]
Preparation and delivery	The 100 mcg/mL vial must be diluted in NS for infusion.[2]
IV push	Not indicated.[2]
Intermittent infusion	An initial loading dose of 0.92 ± 0.36 mcg/kg administered over 5 minutes has been used.[3] 1 mcg/kg over 10 minutes is usual.[2,4]
Continuous infusion	May be infused continuously for 24 hours.[2]
Other routes of administration	Not indicated. However, dexmedetomidine has been combined with bupivacaine and given via caudal block in boys from 1–6 years of age in Cairo, Egypt.[11] Intranasal dexmedetomidine produced more sedation than oral midazolam in children undergoing a minor surgical procedure in Hong Kong.[12]
Comments	Dexmedetomidine appears to have less effectiveness in infants <1 year.[6,8]

Adverse effects: Bradycardia (high 40s–low 50s) was reported in a 5-week-old girl with trisomy 21, who had a large atrioventricular septal defect and was also receiving digoxin.[13]

Twelve children with supraventricular tachycardia who underwent cardiac electrophysiology study and ablation under anesthesia were given 1 mcg/kg over 10 minutes followed by a continuous infusion of 0.7 mcg/kg/h for 10 minutes. During the infusion, sinus and atrioventricular nodal function were significantly depressed and heart rate and arterial blood pressure were increased.[14]

A severe rash was noted within 4 hours of beginning a continuous infusion in a critically ill, intubated *adult*. The infusion was discontinued and by 48 hours the rash had disappeared. According to the Naranjo adverse drug reaction probability scale, the relationship with dexmedetomidine was probable.[15]

Pharmacokinetics: The terminal half-life in 24 children from 2–12 years of age was 1.8 hours.[16] In 10 postsurgical, critically ill children from 0.4–7.9 years of age, the terminal half-life was 2.65 ± 0.88 hours (range: 1.59–4.27 hours).[17] A study evaluating population pharmacokinetics in children from 4 days–14 years found that clearance in neonates was about one third that of *adults* and reached 87% of *adult* values at 1 year of age.[18] The terminal half-life in *adults* is ~ 2 hours.[2] |

Dextrose

Brand names	Various manufacturers
Medication error potential	ISMP high-alert medication that has an increased risk of causing significant patient harm if it is used in error.[1]
Contraindications and warnings	**Contraindications:** Concentrated dextrose solutions should not be used when intracranial hemorrhage is present.[2] Dextrose injection should not be infused with blood through the same infusion set because red cell pseudoagglutination may occur.[2] **Warnings:** Significant hyperglycemia and hyperosmolality may occur with rapid infusion of concentrated dextrose solutions.[2]
Infusion related cautions	Infusion of hypertonic dextrose solutions is irritating to veins and can cause phlebitis when infused via peripheral vein.[3] Usually, the concentration infused peripherally is limited to 11.5% to 12.5% dextrose.[3] Abrupt withdrawal of concentrated dextrose solutions may result in hypoglycemia. This may be avoided by gradual decreases in the rate of infusion.[2] If an IV line infusing concentrated dextrose becomes nonfunctional, a peripheral IV can be used to infuse a lower concentration of dextrose (i.e., D5W, D10W).

Dosage	**Hypoglycemia** (neonatal hypoglycemia is a metabolic emergency; serious neurological injury can occur if normal blood glucose is not established)
	
	    Preterm neonates: 0.1–0.2 g/kg (1–2 mL/kg of 10% dextrose) followed by 6 mg/kg/min.[4-6] (See Comments section.)
	
	    Term neonates and infants ≤6 months: 0.2–0.5 g/kg (2–5 mL/kg of 10% dextrose or 1–2 mL/kg of 25% dextrose) administered slowly followed by 6–12 mg/kg/min.[3,4,6-11] Neonates with persistent hypoglycemia may require >12–15 mg/kg/min.[6,11]
	
	    Infants >6 months and children: 0.5–1 g/kg (5–10 mL/kg of 10% dextrose or 2–4 mL/kg of 25% dextrose)[4] administered slowly followed by 3–7.5 mg/kg/min.
	
	    Titrate dose to serum glucose concentration >40[3,5,7] or >50 mg/dL.[6]
	
	    Pediatric resuscitation: 10% dextrose, 5–10 mL/kg; 25% dextrose, 2–4 mL/kg; 50% dextrose, 1–2 mL/kg[12]
	
	Hyperkalemia (with insulin): 0.2–1 g/kg (3.2–16 mg/kg/min) initially in combination with insulin dosed at 4–5 g dextrose for every 1 unit of regular insulin.[4,13]

Dosage adjustment in organ dysfunction	In liver failure the glucose requirement may be increased due to depletion of glycogen stores.
Maximum dosage	1 g/kg not to exceed 0.8 g/kg/h in *adults*.[2] 15–25 mg/kg/min (0.9–1.5 g/kg/h) has been given to hyperinsulinemic neonates.[3,13,14]
Additives	Contains contaminant aluminum.[2]

Dextrose

Suitable diluents	Concentrated dextrose should be diluted in compatible parenteral fluids including PN.
Maximum concentration	**Peripheral:** 12.5% dextrose (except for emergency situations). **Central venous lines:** Usually 25% dextrose, 30% dextrose has also been used.[15] **Resuscitation:** 25% in neonates, infants, and children. 50% has been used in adolescents and *adults*.[12]
Preparation and delivery	Dilute to desired concentration in compatible electrolyte solution or PN.
IV push	0.2 g/kg over 1 minute.[4,10] Too rapid infusion may result in hyperglycemia.[2] (See Comments section.)
Intermittent infusion	Over 30 minutes–2 hours (treatment of hyperkalemia).[4,12]
Continuous infusion	≤30% dextrose, depending on indication and venous access.[8,10,15] 4.5–15 mg/kg/min.[3,7-10,14]
Other routes of administration	Not for SC or IM administration.[2] May be given IO during neonatal resuscitation.[12]
Comments	**Monitoring:** Blood glucose concentrations should be monitored often during treatment for hypoglycemia and hyperkalemia. Hyperglycemia causes osmotic fluid shifts that may result in rapid dehydration and intraventricular hemorrhage in neonates.[5,10] Following hyperglycemia, rebound hypoglycemia can occur because of stimulation of insulin secretion.[3,5] The osmolality of body fluids is about 310 mOsm/L. The osmolality of 10% dextrose is 505 mOsm/L, and 25% dextrose is 1330 mOsm/L.[4]

Diazepam

Brand names	Valium, Zetran

Medication error potential

ISMP high-alert medication (moderate sedation) that has an increased risk of causing significant patient harm if it is used in error.[1]

Look-alike, sound-alike drug names.

USP reports confusion with alprazolam, clonazepam, DiaBeta, Ditropan, doxepin, lorazepam, midazolam, oxazepam and temazepam.[2] USP reports confusion for Valium with Vicodin.[2] Confusion with diltiazem has resulted in patient harm.[2]

Contraindications and warnings

Contraindications: Should not be used in patients with a known hypersensitivity to this drug or other benzodiazepines.[3] Contraindicated in those with acute narrow angle glaucoma and in open angle glaucoma unless patient is receiving appropriate therapy.[3]

Warnings: Administer cautiously to very ill patients and to those with limited pulmonary reserve due to the possibility of apnea and/or cardiac arrest.[3] Should not be administered to patients in shock, coma, or in acute alcoholic intoxication with depression of vital signs.[3] When used with a narcotic analgesic, the dosage of the narcotic should be reduced by at least one third and given incrementally.[3] Tonic status epilepticus may be precipitated in patients receiving diazepam for absence (petit mal) status or absence (petit mal) variant status.[3] Withdrawal symptoms (e.g., convulsions, tremor, abdominal and muscle cramps, vomiting, and sweats) have occurred following abrupt discontinuation. The more severe symptoms are usually seen in patients who received excessive doses over an extended period of time.[3] (See Infusion related cautions section.)

Infusion related cautions

Resuscitative equipment including ones necessary to support respiration should be readily available.[3] Thrombophlebitis may occur,[3] and tissue necrosis may develop following infiltration.[4,5] To reduce the possibility of venous thrombosis, phlebitis, local irritation, and (rarely) vascular impairment, inject slowly into a large vein.[3] (See IV push section.)

Dosage

Flumazenil should be readily available for reversal. (See Comments section, Other routes of administration section, and Flumazenil monograph.)

Procedural sedation: *Midazolam* is the preferred benzodiazepine because of its rapid onset and short duration.[6-8] (See Midazolam monograph.)

0.05–0.1 mg/kg slowly titrated q 15–30 min for desired effect (to a cumulative dose of 0.25 mg/kg).[6,8] The lowest effective dose should be used.

Status epilepticus (convulsive): *Lorazepam* is the preferred benzodiazepine for use in the pediatric population.[10-12] (See Lorazepam monograph.)

> **Neonates:** Not recommended due to benzyl alcohol content in product, prolonged sedation, and decreased ability to metabolize.[3] (See Additives section and Comments section.)

> **Infants and children:** 0.1–0.4 mg/kg (up to 10 mg/dose) repeat q 5–10 min for two to three doses.[10-18] Although continuous infusion diazepam has been used, midazolam or lorazepam are preferred for continuous administration. (See Continuous infusion section and Midazolam and Lorazepam monographs.)

Tetanus (muscle spasms): A series of 19 neonates received 20–40 mg/kg/day (0.83–1.67 mg/kg/h) as continuous infusion accompanied by intermittent bolus doses of 5–10 mg.[19] Three neonates (7–10 days) were given 48–50 mg/kg/day divided into 2-hour intervals.[20] Three children (6–12 years) received 7.5–15 mg/kg/day divided into 2-hour intervals.[20] The manufacturer recommends 1–2 mg/dose q 3–4 h if >30 days and <5 years of age and 5–10 mg/dose q 3–4 h if ≥5 years of age.[3] (See Pharmacodynamics in Comments section.)

Diazepam

Dosage adjustment in organ dysfunction	No dosage adjustment required in renal dysfunction[3,21]; however, prolonged administration may result in propylene glycol toxicity.[22,23] Use cautiously in hepatic dysfunction.
Maximum dosage	1 mg/kg, not to exceed a total dose of 5 mg in children <5 years or 10 mg in children ≥5 years.[3] 2.7 mg/kg was given without adverse effects to a neonate[24] and 1.7 mg/kg/h was given via continuous infusion.[25] Neonates should not receive doses larger than 1 mg/kg/h because of benzyl alcohol toxicity.[26] (See Additives section.)
Additives	Each 1 mL contains 1.5% benzyl alcohol and 40% propylene glycol.[27] (See Appendix C for specific information about benzyl alcohol and propylene glycol potential for toxicity.)
Suitable diluents	D5W, LR, or NS.[26] (See Preparation and delivery section.)
Maximum concentration	5 mg/mL for IV push.[17,22]
Preparation and delivery	**Stability:** Variable stability in D5W, LR, or NS.[27] Consult appropriate reference for specific information about compatibility and stability. **Photosensitivity:** The commercial product should be protected from light exposure until ready to use.[27]
IV push	5 mg/mL (available commercially) infused ≥3 minutes.[27] Rate should not exceed 2 mg/min in infants and children.[28] The manufacturer recommends 5 mg/min in *adults* and that doses in children be given over at least 3 minutes.[3] Apnea may occur if given too rapidly.[18]
Intermittent infusion	No information available.
Continuous infusion	Although a review on continuous infusion diazepam has been published,[29] this administration method is rarely used. 0.01 mg/kg/min increased by 0.005 mg/kg/min q 15 min to a maximum dosage of 0.03 mg/kg/min.[26] Doses in neonates should not exceed 1 mg/kg/h because of benzyl alcohol toxicity.[21]
Other routes of administration	Although undiluted (5 mg/mL) diazepam can be given deep into a muscle, the alkaline product is prone to cause tissue damage,[4,5] and its bioavailability is erratic. For these reasons, *midazolam* is the benzodiazepine of choice for IM administration. (See Midazolam monograph.)
Comments	**Rare adverse effects:** Abnormal movements of limbs (e.g., myoclonus or seizures) have been described in premature and full-term neonates given benzodiazepines.[30-32] The movements began a few minutes after a bolus injection and continued for several hours.[31,32] **Drug interactions:** Diazepam is a substrate of CYP1A2, 2B6, 2C9, 2C19 (major), and 3A4 (major).[33] It is a weak inhibitor of CYP2C19 and CYP3A4.[33] Consult appropriate resources for dosing recommendations before combining any drug with diazepam. **Pharmacodynamics:** Use in neonates is controversial since benzodiazepines may decrease blood pressure and cerebral blood flow velocity.[34] Neonates may also experience prolonged CNS depression because of an inability to biotransform diazepam to an inactive metabolite.[3] Some recommend the initial dose should be reduced by 50% in infants <2 months of age[35]; regardless, diazepam should be used cautiously in neonates.

Diazepam

Laboratory interference: False-positive urinary glucose results when cupric sulfate solution-based tests (Clinitest, Benedict's solution, Fehling's solution) are used.[3] It is recommended that glucose tests (Diastix, TEST-TAPE, Clinistix) based on enzymatic glucose oxidase reactions be used.[3]

Other: Flumazenil, a specific benzodiazepine-receptor antagonist, is indicated for complete or partial reversal of benzodiazepine toxicity.[36] (See Flumazenil monograph.) Although rare (1% to 2%) who receive flumazenil experience seizure activity.[37] Activity has ranged from simple twitching and jerking, to single or multiple seizure events, to status epilepticus.[35] Seizures responded to reintroduction of a benzodiazepine or use of an anticonvulsant.[35,36] Because of the presence of flumazenil, larger than normal doses of benzodiazepines may be required.

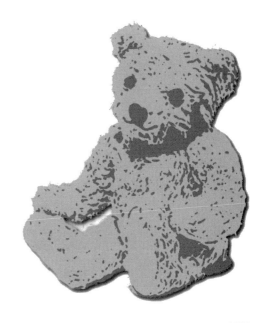

Digoxin

Brand names	Lanoxin

Medication error potential

ISMP high-alert medication that has an increased risk of causing significant patient harm if it is used in error.[1]

Look-alike, sound-alike drug names.

USP reports confusion digoxin and doxepin and Digibind.[2] Lanoxin has also been confused with levothyroxine, Inapsine, Lasix, Lomotil, Levoxyl, Levsin, Lonox, Lovenox, and Xanax.[2]

ISMP's *Confused Drug Names* lists confusion with Lanoxin and levothyroxine.[3]

Contraindications and warnings

Contraindications: Known hypersensitivity to digoxin or other digitalis preparations or ventricular fibrillation.[4]

Warnings: Caution is advised in patients with the following: acute myocarditis or amyloid cardiomyopathy, AV block, chronic constrictive pericarditis, electrical cardioversion (low voltage), electrolyte imbalance, hypo- or hyperthyroidism, hypoxia, renal disease, severe bradycardia, severe heart failure, severe pulmonary disease, sick sinus syndrome, ventricular tachycardia, ventricular premature contractions, Wolff-Parkinson-White syndrome.[4]

Infusion related cautions

Inadvertent over administration may occur if a tuberculin syringe is used to measure very small doses.[5,6] Do not aspirate fluid or blood into the syringe containing digoxin because administration of residual drug left in the syringe hub may cause an overdose.[5,6]

Dosage

Dosage based on lean body weight and normal renal function.[4] Administer one half of total digitalizing dose (TDD) initially, one fourth 8–12 hours after the first dose, and the remaining one fourth 8–12 hours after the second dose.[7-10] Assess clinical response before administering each dose.[4]

Age	TDD (mcg/kg)	Maintenance Dose (mcg/kg/day)
Premature neonates	15–30[4,8-10,6-10]	5–10 divided q 12 h[8,10-16]
Full-term neonates	10–30[4,8-10]	8–10 divided q 12 h[4,10,16]
Infants <2 y	30–50[7,10,11]	10–12 divided q 12 h[4,10,16]
Children 2–10 y	20–35[4,8,10]	8–10 divided q 12 h[10,16]
Children >10 y	8–12[4]	2–3 divided q 12 h[4,17] or given once daily[18]

Because large variability exists in patient response to initial and maintenance doses, individualize dosage based on serum concentration and clinical response.

Dosage adjustment in organ dysfunction

If CrCl is 30–50 mL/min, give 75% of the dose; If 10–29 mL/min, give 50% of normal dose q 36 h; and if CrCl is <10 mL/min, give 25% of a normal dose q 48 h.[19] Dosing should be optimized by measuring serum concentrations.

Digoxin

Maximum dosage	TDD should not exceed 1 mg.[20] Maintenance dose generally approximates 30% of TDD. Maintenance doses rarely exceed 10 mcg/kg/day or 0.25 mg/day.[2-16]
Additives	Pediatric (100 mcg/mL) and *adult* (250 mcg/mL) injection contains propylene glycol 40% and alcohol 10%.[4] (See Appendix C for specific information about propylene glycol potential for toxicity.)
Suitable diluents	D5W, NS, ½NS, D5½NS, or LR.[21]
Maximum concentration	100 mcg/mL for pediatric patients and 250 mcg/mL for *adults*.[4]
Preparation and delivery	**Preparation:** For dose volumes <0.1 mL, prepare a 1:10 dilution to improve measurement accuracy. Dilute 0.1 mL of digoxin (100 mcg/mL) with 0.9 mL of saline to make a 10-mcg/mL concentration. Use the two-syringe technique to make the dilution: draw up the drug in one syringe and the diluent in another. Inject drug into diluent syringe and mix well. This technique avoids "syringe dead space overdose," which can occur when additional fluid is drawn into a drug-containing syringe. Failure to use the two-syringe technique causes drug in the dead space to be drawn up also, and it can result in a significantly larger dose than intended (5 mcg vs. 8–12 mcg for digoxin).[5,6,13] Dilute at least fourfold (25 mcg/mL).[4,21] Use of less than a fourfold volume of diluent may result in precipitation.[4]
	Stability: It is recommended to use digoxin immediately after diluting.[4] Stable in LR and ½NS for 4–6 hours at 23°C.[21]
	Compatibility: See Appendix D for PN compatibility information.[22]
	Photosensitivity: Protect from light exposure until ready to use.[4]
IV push	Undiluted (100 mcg/mL) over at least 5 minutes or longer.[4] Rapid IV infusion causes systemic and coronary arteriolar vasoconstriction.[4]
Intermittent infusion	≥25 mcg/mL[4,21] and infuse over >5 minutes.[4] (See Comments section.)
Continuous infusion	No information available.
Other routes of administration	IM administration is not recommended because of local pain, irritation, and tissue damage.[21] If it must be given IM, it should be given by deep injection followed by massage of the area.[4] Inject no more than 2 mL (200 mcg) at any one site.[21]
Comments	**Significant adverse effects:** Virtually every arrhythmia including sinus bradycardia, A-V block, S-A block, atrial or nodal ectopic beats, ventricular arrhythmias, bigeminy, trigeminy, atrial tachycardia with A-V block.[4]
	Monitoring: Serum electrolytes and renal function should be monitored. Hypercalcemia may increase the risk of toxicity.[4] Toxicity may also occur with hypokalemia and hypomagnesemia despite serum drug concentrations within therapeutic range.[4] ECG may assist in the diagnosis of digoxin-associated toxicity.

Digoxin

Serum digoxin concentrations will be falsely elevated if drawn during the predistribution phase (i.e., within 6 hours of digoxin dose).[10] Serum concentrations for clinical use should be at least 6–8 hours after the last dose, regardless of the route of administration or formulation used.[4] "Therapeutic" serum concentrations generally range between 0.8–2 ng/mL. Although toxicity is usually accompanied by values >2 ng/mL, serum concentration must be used in conjunction with clinical symptoms and ECG to confirm diagnosis of digoxin toxicity.

Drug interactions: The metabolism of digoxin is not dependent on the cytochrome P-450 system, and it is not known to induce or inhibit the cytochrome P-450 system.[4] Digoxin is a substrate of P-glycoprotein and should be used with caution when administered concomitantly with drugs known to inhibit glycoprotein (e.g., quinidine, verapamil, amiodarone, ketoconazole, and itraconazole).[23] Macrolides (erythromycin and clarithromycin) can increase digoxin bioavailability via inhibition of intestinal flora, which metabolizes digoxin in the gut while simultaneously inhibiting P-glycoprotein. Consult appropriate resources for dosing recommendations before combining any drug with digoxin.

Laboratory interference: Depending on the assay used, serum digitalis concentrations may be falsely elevated because of endogenous digoxin-like immunoreactive substances in patients with renal or hepatic dysfunction, neonates, infants, and children.[24-29] Spironolactone may interfere with digoxin radioimmunoassay.[30]

Digoxin immune FAB has been shown to interfere with many radioimmunoassays of digoxin.[31,32] This interference results in a significant overestimation of digoxin serum concentrations. To determine the degree of interference, review the manufacturer specification for the assay used at your institution.

Other: In patients experiencing serious cardiac effects due to digitalis toxicity, patients may receive digoxin-immune Fab.[4] See Digoxin Immune Fab monograph for more information.

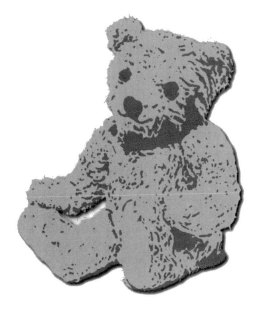

Digoxin Immune Fab

Brand names	Digibind, DigiFab

Medication error potential

Look-alike and sound-alike drug names.

USP reports confusion with digoxin.[1]

Contraindications and warnings

Contraindications: Hypersensitivity to digoxin immune Fab, sheep products, or any component of the formulation.[2]

Warnings: If digoxin has been used to treat heart failure, exacerbation of symptoms may appear as serum digoxin concentrations fall.[2] (See Comments section.)

Patients allergic to papain, chymopapain, or papaya extracts may be allergic to Fab.[2] Likewise, those with known allergies to dust mite and latex may experience a cross allergy.[2] Use cautiously in those with hypokalemia, poor heart function (withdrawal of inotropic effect), and/or renal failure.[2]

Infusion related cautions

Anaphylactoid, hypersensitivity, and febrile reactions have occurred.[2-4] Individuals at high risk for allergy should receive a test dose.[2] Give a 1:100 dilution by mixing 0.1 mL of reconstituted Fab (9.5 mg/mL) in 9.9 mL NS (95 mcg/mL). Inject 0.1 mL of the dilution through 0.22-micron filter intradermally or place one drop on skin and make a ¼ scratch through drop with a sterile needle.[2] Evaluate test site for 20–30 minutes.[2-4] Epinephrine should be immediately available.

Dosage

For manifestations of severe digitalis toxicity unresponsive to other therapies.[1]

Dose should be based on amount of digoxin or digitoxin ingested or on serum digitalis concentration.[2-4] 38 mg (one vial Digibind) or 40 mg (one vial DigiFab) binds 0.5 mg of digoxin or digitoxin.[2,11] To calculate the total body load of digitalis, use either[2-11]:

Dosing method based on estimated amount ingested

For digoxin tablets, oral solution, or IM injection[10]

$$\text{Dose in mg} = \frac{(\text{dose ingested (mg)} \times 0.8) \times 38}{0.5}$$

For digitoxin tablets, digoxin capsules, IV digoxin, or IV digitoxin[10]

$$\text{Dose in mg} = \frac{\text{dose ingested (mg)}}{0.5} \times 38$$

Digibind dosing based on measured serum *digoxin* concentration[2,10]

Weight (kg)	SDC† 1 ng/mL	SDC† 2 ng/mL	SDC† 4 ng/mL	SDC† 8 ng/mL	SDC† 12 ng/mL	SDC† 16 ng/mL	SDC† 20 ng/mL
1	0.4 mg*	1 mg*	1.5 mg*	3 mg	5 mg	6 mg	8 mg
3	1 mg	2 mg	5 mg	9 mg	14 mg	18 mg	23 mg
5	2 mg	4 mg	8 mg	15 mg	23 mg	30 mg	38 mg
10	4 mg	8 mg	15 mg	30 mg	46 mg	61 mg	76 mg
20	8 mg	15 mg	30 mg	61 mg	91 mg	122 mg	152 mg
40	0.5 vial	1 vial	2 vials	3 vials	5 vials	7 vials	8 vials
60	0.5 vial	1 vial	3 vials	5 vials	7 vials	10 vials	12 vials
70	1 vial	2 vials	3 vials	6 vials	9 vials	11 vials	14 vials
80	1 vial	2 vials	3 vials	7 vials	10 vials	13 vials	16 vials
100	1 vial	2 vials	4 vials	8 vials	12 vials	16 vials	20 vials

*Dilution of reconstituted vial to 1 mg/mL may be desirable.
†SDC = serum digoxin concentration.

Digoxin Immune Fab

Dosage *(cont.)*

DigiFab dosing based on measured serum *digoxin* concentration[2,10]

Weight (kg)	SDC† 1 ng/mL	SDC† 2 ng/mL	SDC† 4 ng/mL	SDC† 8 ng/mL	SDC† 12 ng/mL	SDC† 16 ng/mL	SDC† 20 ng/mL
1	0.4 mg*	1 mg*	1.5 mg*	3 mg	5 mg	6.5 mg	8 mg
3	1 mg	2.5 mg	5 mg	10 mg	14 mg	19 mg	24 mg
5	2 mg	4 mg	8 mg	16 mg	24 mg	32 mg	40 mg
10	4 mg	8 mg	16 mg	32 mg	48 mg	64 mg	80 mg
20	8 mg	16 mg	32 mg	64 mg	96 mg	128 mg	160 mg

*Dilution of reconstituted vial to 1 mg/mL may be desirable.

†SDC = serum digoxin concentration.

or

$$\text{Dose in mg} = \frac{\text{serum } digoxin \text{ concentration (ng/mL)} \times \text{weight (kg)} \times 38}{100}$$

Dosing method based on measured serum *digitoxin* concentration[10]

$$\text{Dose in mg} = \frac{\text{serum } digitoxin \text{ concentration (ng/mL)} \times \text{weight (kg)} \times 38}{1000}$$

Amount ingested unknown or SDC unavailable[2,10]**:** Give 760 mg (twenty 38-mg vials).

Chronic toxicity and SDC unavailable: Infants and children ≤20 kg, 1 vial is adequate to reverse most cases of toxicity.[11] If ≥20 kg give 6 vials.[12]

Dosage adjustment in organ dysfunction

Fab fragments may be eliminated more slowly in patients with renal failure.[2-4]

Maximum dosage

Not established. Following acute ingestion, 760 mg should be sufficient. For chronic ingestion, a single vial (38 mg) should be sufficient for infants and small children (<20 kg) and 228 mg (six vials) should be sufficient for children ≥20 kg and *adults*.[12]

Additives

Processed with papain, which may cause hypersensitivity reactions in patients allergic to papaya, other papaya extracts, papain, chymopapain, or the pineapple enzyme bromelain.[2]

Suitable diluents

SW, NS.[2,11]

Maximum concentration

9.5 mg/mL.[2]

Preparation and delivery

Stability: Store reconstituted drug at 2°C to 8°C for up to 4 hours.[2,11]

IV push

In one study, an 1800-g infant received 160 mg over 5 minutes.[7] May give dose more rapidly in cases of impending cardiac arrest.[2]

Digoxin Immune Fab

Intermittent infusion

1–9.5 mg/mL over 20–60 minutes[2,6,9,13] through a 0.22-micron filter to remove protein aggregate.[2,11] After reconstitution, no additional dilution is needed prior to administration.[2,3,11] For very small doses, a reconstituted vial can be diluted to 1 mg/mL with 34 mL of NS (Digibind) and 36 mL of NS (DigiFab).[2,11]

Continuous infusion

No information available.

Other routes of administration

No information available.

Comments

Monitoring: Clinical improvement in signs and symptoms associated with digitalis toxicity generally occur in ≤30 minutes following administration of Fab.[2] Complete reversal of cardiac and noncardiac manifestations of toxicity generally occur 3 to 4 hours after completion infusion.[14]

Serum potassium should be monitored closely as concentrations may fall rapidly (i.e., within 30 minutes) after initiation of Digibind.[2,3,9] ECG. should be monitored for evidence of conduction disturbances.[2]

Laboratory interference: Digoxin immune Fab in human serum interferes with many radioimmunoassays for digoxin to produce a significant overestimation of concentration.[4,15-19] This interference precludes the use of serum digoxin concentrations in monitoring response in patients treated with digoxin immune Fab. To determine the degree of interference, review the manufacturer specification for the assay used at your institution.

Other: Digoxin should not be initiated until Fab fragments have been eliminated from the body.[2,4] This may take several days in those with normal renal function and may take more than a week in patients with impaired renal function.[2,4]

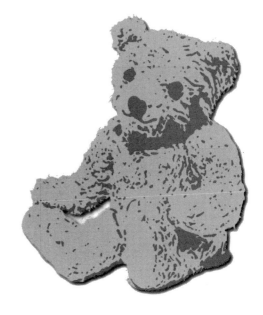

Dihydroergotamine Mesylate

Brand names	D.H.E 45, and generics

Medication error potential

None.[1,2]

Contraindications and warnings

Contraindications: Co-administration of ergot alkaloids with potent CYP3A4 inhibitors (e.g., protease inhibitors, macrolide antibiotics) may elevate the serum levels of dihydroergotamine, which has resulted in vasospasm that causes serious and/or life-threatening peripheral and cerebral ischemia.[3] Cases of amputation have been reported. (See Drug interactions in the Comments section.)

Should not be used with peripheral and central vasoconstrictors because the combination may result in additive or synergistic elevation of blood pressure.[3]

Do not use within 24 hours of sumatriptan, zolmitriptan, other serotonin agonists, or ergot-like agents; do not use during or within 2 weeks of discontinuing MAO inhibitors.[3]

Do not use in patients with (1) uncontrolled hypertension; (2) ischemic heart disease, angina pectoris, history of MI, silent ischemia, or coronary artery vasospasm including Prinzmetal's angina; (3) hemiplegic or basilar migraine; (4) patients with peripheral vascular disease, sepsis, severe hepatic or renal dysfunction; and (5) following vascular surgery.[3]

Warnings: Rare reports of increased blood pressure in patients without a history of hypertension.[3] Although rare, there have been reports of pleural and retroperitoneal fibrosis and cardiac valvular fibrosis following prolonged daily use of injectable dihydroergotamine mesylate.[3] Patients who developed cardiac valvular fibrosis also received drugs associated with cardiac valvular fibrosis.[3]

Infusion related cautions

None.

Dosage

IV dihydroergotamine, given in conjunction with an antiemetic, is an appropriate choice for treatment of severe migraine; however, it should be reserved for patients who do not respond to other drug therapy, including 5-HT$_1$ selective receptor agonists.[1]

Safety and efficacy of dihydroergotamine not established in children.[3] 1 mg at the first sign of headache; repeat hourly to a maximum total dose of 2 mg in a 24-hour period.[1] One report, in a 4-year-old, gave 0.1 mg q 8 h.[4] (See Other routes of administration section.)

Dosage adjustment in organ dysfunction

Although no studies have been conducted on the effect of renal or hepatic impairment, the manufacturer notes that the drug is contraindicated in patients with severely impaired hepatic or renal function.[3]

Maximum dosage

2 mg in a 24-hour period in *adults* if given IV and 3 mg in a 24-hour period in *adults* if given IM or SC.[3] Total weekly IM, subcutaneous, or IV dosage should not exceed 6 mg.[3]

Additives

6.2% ethanol.[3]

Suitable diluents

Administered without dilution.[3]

Maximum concentration

1 mg/mL (commercially available).[3]

Dihydroergotamine Mesylate

Preparation and delivery	**Photosensitivity:** Protect the ampules from light and heat and only administer if the solution is clear and colorless.[3]
IV push	Over 1–2 minutes.[3]
Intermittent infusion	Not applicable.
Continuous infusion	3 mg of dihydroergotamine in 1000 mL NS has been administered at a constant rate over 24 hours in *adults*.[5]
Other routes of administration	May be administered IM or SC.[3]
Comments	**Rare adverse effects:** Cases of acute myocardial infarction and arrhythmias have occurred in *adults*.[3] A 4-year-old with cyclic vomiting syndrome developed intestinal ischemia after receiving 0.1 mg q 8 h (total eight doses).[4] **Drug interactions:** The concurrent administration of potent CYP3A4 inhibitors with dihydroergotamine should be avoided.[3] Potent CYP3A4 inhibitors include antifungals (e.g., ketoconazole and itraconazole), the protease inhibitors (e.g., ritonavir, nelfinavir, and indinavir), and macrolide antibiotics (e.g., erythromycin, clarithromycin, and troleandomycin). Other less potent inhibitors (e.g., saquinavir, nefazodone, fluconazole, grapefruit juice, fluoxetine, fluvoxamine, zileuton, and clotrimazole) should be administered with caution.[3] These lists are not exhaustive; therefore, consult appropriate resources before combining any drug with dihydroergotamine mesylate. **Other:** Metoclopramide (0.2 mg/kg) may be administered 30 minutes prior to dihydroergotamine to reduce the incidence of abdominal discomfort.[3] Concomitant antiemetics may not be needed with IM administration.[6]

Diltiazem HCl

Brand names	Cardizem injectable

Medication error potential

Look-alike, sound-alike error potential.

USP reports that diltiazem was confused with Calan and dilantin and no patient harm resulted.[1] Diltiazem was confused with diazepam and patient harm occurred. Cardizem was confused with Cardene, Cardizem SR, and cortisone and no patient harm occurred.

Contraindications and warnings

Contraindications[2]: Patients with sick sinus syndrome who do not have a ventricular pacemaker, patients with 2nd or 3rd degree AV block who do not have a ventricular pacemaker, patients with severe hypotension or cardiogenic shock, patients with atrial fibrillation or atrial flutter who have an accessory bypass tract, patients with ventricular tachycardia, and patients who have hypersensitivity to the drug. IV diltiazem and IV beta-blockers should not be infused together or within a few hours of each other.

Warnings[2]: Cardiac conduction may be affected during infusion. Use with caution in patients with impaired ventricular function. Hypotension may occur with infusion. Acute hepatic injury has been reported after oral diltiazem, thus, IV diltiazem has potential to cause this injury. Transient ventricular premature beats have been noted on conversion of paroxysmal supraventricular tachycardia to normal sinus rhythm and are usually considered to be benign.

Infusion related cautions

Monitor ECG and blood pressure during infusion.[2]

In the event of diltiazem overdose or exaggerated response the following are recommended by the manufacturer[2]:

Bradycardia: Atropine.

High-degree AV block: Atropine (for bradycardia); fixed-degree block should be treated with pacing.

Cardiac failure: Inotropes.

Hypotension: Vasopressors.

While some have recommended that IV calcium be available should hypotension occur,[3,4] the manufacturer states that the response to calcium is inconsistent.[2]

Dosage

Intravenous diltiazem is not considered first line treatment of dysrhythmias or hypertension in children.[5] Only a few reports of IV diltiazem use in children have been published.[3,6,7]

Atrial tachycardias: Seven children from 0.6–13 years old were given 0.25 mg/kg over 5 minutes followed by a continuous infusion of 0.05–0.15 mg/kg/h for up to 126 hours as a bridge to definitive treatment.[3]

In *adults*, 0.25 mg/kg (≤20 mg) over 2 minutes. If the response is inadequate after 15 minutes, a second bolus of 0.35 mg/kg (≤25 mg) can be given.[2] In *adults* with atrial fibrillation or atrial flutter, the bolus dose may be followed by a continuous infusion of 5- to 15-mg/h for up to 24 hours.[2]

Pulmonary hypertension: Five neonates on ECMO were given 1–2 mg twice daily that was titrated upwards to 3–7 mg given four times daily.[6]

Dosage adjustment in organ dysfunction

Cautious use is recommended in patients with renal or hepatic disease, in particular those taking other drugs metabolized by the CYP P450 3A4 enzyme system.[2]

Diltiazem HCl

Maximum dosage	In *adults*, 25 mg (0.35 mg/kg).[2]
Additives	Cardizem Lyo-Ject includes a diluent that contains benzyl alcohol.[2] See Appendix C for specific information about benzyl alcohol toxicity in neonates.
Suitable diluents	D5W, NS, D5½NS.[2]
Maximum concentration	5 mg/mL.[2]
Preparation and delivery	Dilutions for continuous infusion must be used within 24 hours.[2]
IV push	5 mg/mL (undiluted) over 2 minutes.[2]
Intermittent infusion	Not indicated.
Continuous infusion	Has been used in *adults* with atrial fibrillation or atrial flutter.[2] (See Dosage section.)
Other routes of administration	Not indicated.
Comments	**Drug interactions:** Diltiazem is metabolized by the cytochrome P450 isozymes and moderately inhibits the 3A4 isozyme.[2] Other drugs that are substrates, inhibitors, or inducers of this enzyme system may have an impact on the side effect profile and efficacy of diltiazem. Drugs with interactions noted by the manufacturer include anesthetics, benzodiazepines, beta-blockers, buspirone, carbamazepine, cyclosporine, digitalis, lovastatin, quinidine, and rifampin.[2] Consult appropriate resources before combining any drug with diltiazem.

DiphenhydrAMINE HCl

Brand names	Benadryl
Medication error potential	ISMP and USP report that diphenhydrAMINE has been confused with dimenhydrinate; no patient harm resulted.[1,2] USP reports that diphenhydrAMINE has been confused with dipyridamole; no patient harm resulted.[2] USP also reports that diphenhydrAMINE has been confused with dicyclomine; patient harm resulted.[2] ISMP and USP report that Benadryl has been confused with benazepril; no patient harm resulted.[1,2] USP reports that Benadryl has been confused with Benicar; no patient harm resulted.[2] USP also reports that Benadryl has been confused with Bentyl; patient harm resulted.[2]
Contraindications and warnings	Do not use in patients with a previous hypersensitivity to the drug.[3] Contraindicated in neonates and preterm infants.[3]
Infusion related cautions	Local necrosis has been associated with the administration of IV diphenhydramine by the SC or intradermal routes.[3]

Dosage	**Acute hypersensitivity or dystonic reactions**
	
	    Neonates: Contraindicated because of potential CNS effects.[3]
	
	    Infants and children: 1–2 mg/kg/dose[4-9] up to 5 mg/kg/day or 150 mg/m^2/day divided q 6 h.[3]

Dosage adjustment in organ dysfunction	No adjustment is necessary in patients with renal dysfunction.[10]
Maximum dosage	50 mg/dose,[4] not to exceed 300 mg/day.[3] In *adults*, the maximum is 100 mg/dose, not to exceed 400 mg/day.[3,11]
Additives	The multidose vial contains 0.1 mg/mL benzethonium chloride.[3,12]
Suitable diluents	D5W, D10W, LR, NS, ½NS, or R.[12]
Maximum concentration	50 mg/mL (available commercially).[3,12]
Preparation and delivery	For PN compatibility information, please see Appendix D.
IV push	May give (≤50 mg/mL)[3,12] slowly over 5 minutes.[4,5,7,8]
Intermittent infusion	May give via intermittent infusion (≤50 mg/mL) not to exceed 25 mg/min.[3,12]

DiphenhydrAMINE HCl

Continuous infusion

May give via continuous infusion (≤50 mg/mL).[3,12]

Other routes of administration

50 mg/mL may be given by deep IM injection.[3,12] Avoid SC or intradermal injection.[3,12]

Comments

Significant adverse effects: Overdose may result in hallucinations, convulsions, respiratory arrest, arrhythmias, or death.[3]

Although antihistamines may diminish mental alertness, paradoxical hyperactivity may occur in pediatric patients.[3,14]

Other: One paper describes adjuvant analgesic therapy with diphenhydramine 25 mg IV q 4 h in addition to fentanyl PCA in an 8-year-old patient with end stage oncologic pain.[15]

DOBUTamine HCl

Brand names	Dobutrex, generic
Medication error potential	ISMP high-alert medication that has an increased risk of causing significant patient harm if it is used in error.[1] ISMP and USP report that DOBUTamine has been confused with DOPamine; patient harm resulted.[2,3] USP also reports that Dobutrex has been confused with DOPamine; patient harm resulted.
Contraindications and warnings	**Contraindications:** Dobutamine is contraindicated in patients with idiopathic hypertrophic subaortic stenosis and patients with previous hypersensitivity to dobutamine.[4] **Warnings:** Dobutamine may increase heart rate or blood pressure (especially systolic blood pressure).[4] Dobutamine use in patients with atrial fibrillation increases risk of rapid ventricular response; use of digoxin prior to dobutamine should be used in patients with atrial fibrillation and a rapid ventricular response.[4] Patients with hypertension are at increased risk of exaggerated pressor response with dobutamine. Dobutamine may also cause ventricular ectopic activity.[4]
Infusion related cautions	Infiltration or extravasation results in local inflammation and pain. Isolated cases of skin necrosis have been reported.[5,6] Aliquots of phentolamine mesylate (0.1–0.2 mg/kg up to 10 mg in 10 mL NS) should be injected intradermally into the ischemic area.[6] See Appendix E for additional information regarding extravasation treatment. Tachycardia, arrhythmias (PVCs), and hypertension may occur, especially at greater infusion rates.[4] The tachycardia produced by dobutamine may make it unacceptable for use in children after cardiopulmonary bypass.[7]
Dosage	Correct hypovolemia prior to dobutamine administration.[4] **Shock, heart failure:** 2–20 mcg/kg/min, titrated to desired clinical effect.[6,8] Other references have recommended initial doses of 2.5–10 mcg/kg/min increased by 2.5–5 mcg/kg/min q 20–40 minutes up to 25 mcg/kg/min.[4,5,7,9-21] Given the wide variability in clearance, doses must be individualized.[16,22,23] (See Pharmacokinetic considerations in Comments section.)
Dosage adjustment in organ dysfunction	No dosage adjustment required in renal dysfunction.[24]
Maximum dosage	40 mcg/kg/min has been used in *adults*[4,5]; however, this dose is associated with increased toxicity.[5]
Additives	Some products contain sodium bisulfite.[4,25] See Appendix C for more specific information about potential adverse effects of sulfites.
Suitable diluents	D5W, D5NS, D5½NS, D10W, Isolyte M with dextrose 5%, LR, D5LR, Normosol-M in D5W, 20% Osmitrol in Water for Injection, NS, or sodium lactate injection.[4,25] Not compatible with strongly alkaline solutions such as sodium bicarbonate or diluents containing both sodium bisulfite and ethanol.[4]
Maximum concentration	5 mg/mL.[4,25] The concentration used depends on the patient size and/or fluid requirements. For example, a patient who requires a large amount of dobutamine or a fluid-restricted patient may require a more concentrated fluid.

DOBUTamine HCl

Preparation and delivery	Hemodynamic instability may be attributed to significant variability between the ordered dosage and the actual solution concentration of dobutamine.[26]

May be filtered through a 0.2-micron filter without significant dobutamine loss.[25]

For PN compatibility information, please see Appendix D. |
| **IV push** | Not indicated. |
| **Intermittent infusion** | Not indicated. |
| **Continuous infusion** | Usually 0.25–1 mg/mL.[12,25]

The following formula has been recommended for preparation of the infusion: 6 × weight (kg) = mg of drug to be added to IV solution for a total volume of 100 mL. An infusion rate of 1 mL/h provides 1 mcg/kg/min.[20,21] This formula estimates initial concentration. Ultimately, the concentration of the drug should consider the patient's fluid requirements.

Despite widespread use of the above formula, recent Joint Commission guidelines recommend the implementation of standardized concentrations of vasoactive medications.[27] |
| **Other routes of administration** | Not indicated. Intraosseous administration may be used in post-resuscitation stabilization.[6,8,21,28] |
| **Comments** | **Monitoring:** Blood pressure and ECG monitoring should occur continuously throughout therapy.[4]

Pharmacokinetic considerations: Pediatric pharmacokinetic studies have shown large variability in dobutamine clearance; changes in clearance do not appear to be associated with age, weight, underlying disease state, or addition of dopamine infusion.[16,22,23]

Pharmacodynamic considerations: Long-term infusion (i.e., 3–4 days) has produced tolerance to hemodynamic effects and necessitated dosage increases in *adults*.[29] |

Dolasetron Mesylate

Brand names	Anzemet

Medication error potential

Look-alike, sound-alike error potential.

USP reports that dolasetron was confused with ondansetron and that Anzemet was confused with Antivert.[1]

ISMP reports that Anzemet was confused with Avandamet.[2]

Contraindications and warnings

Contraindications: Patients with known hypersensitivity to the drug.[3]

Warnings: ECG changes can occur and are directly related to blood concentrations of the active metabolite, hydrodolasetron.[3]

Use with caution in children with congenital QT syndrome or in children receiving concomitant medications that prolong the QT interval.[3]

Infusion related cautions

Local pain or burning can occur with infusion.[3]

Dosage

Information is available for children 2 years of age and older.[3]

Prevention of chemotherapy induced nausea and vomiting: 1.8 mg/kg up to 100 mg given 30 minutes before chemotherapy.[3-5] While smaller (0.6 mg/kg) and larger (2.4 mg/kg) doses have been studied, doses of 1.2 and 1.8 mg/kg were more effective.[4] The inclusion of dexamethasone is recommended.[6]

Prevention of postoperative nausea and vomiting: Usually, 0.35 mg/kg up to 12.5 mg given 15 minutes prior to surgery.[3,5,7] 0.5 mg/kg up to 25 mg given at the time of intubation for tonsillectomy was also effective.[8]

Dosage adjustment in organ dysfunction

None required.[3]

Maximum dosage

100 mg.[3]

Additives

Contains 38.2 mg of mannitol/mL.[3]

Suitable diluents

NS, D5W, D5½NS, D5LR, LR.[9]

Maximum concentration

20 mg/mL (undiluted).[3]

Preparation and delivery

0.25–2 mg/mL.

IV push

100 mg over 30 seconds in *adults* (undiluted).[3]

Dolasetron Mesylate

Intermittent infusion	Over 15 minutes.[3]
Continuous infusion	Not indicated.[3]
Other routes of administration	Not indicated.[3]
Comments	None.

DOPamine HCl

Brand names	Generic

Medication error potential

ISMP high-alert medication that has an increased risk of causing significant patient harm if it is used in error.[1]

ISMP and USP report that DOPamine has been confused with DOBUTamine; patient harm resulted.[2,3] USP also reports that DOPamine has been confused with Dobutrex; patient harm resulted.

Contraindications and warnings

US boxed warning: Extravasation may cause local ischemia and tissue necrosis.[4,5] Aliquots of phentolamine mesylate (0.1–0.2 mg/kg up to 10 mg in 10–15 mL NS) should be injected using a fine hypodermic needle into the ischemic area.[4] This should be done as soon as possible and within the first 12 hours of noting the extravasation.[4] (See Infusion related cautions section.)

Contraindications: Do not use in patients with pheochromocytoma or in patients with uncorrected tachyarrhythmias or ventricular fibrillation.[4]

Other warnings: Patients who have received an MAO inhibitor prior to use of dopamine will require lower dopamine doses.[4]

Infusion related cautions

Administer high concentrations and large volume infusions via a central venous catheter.[6]

A 65-year-old patient receiving dopamine and dobutamine experienced swelling at the infusion site that resolved with local injection of 3 mL of terbutaline (1 mg in 10 mL NS) given SC.[7]

Two case reports of distal extremity gangrene have been related to dopamine infusion, and in one infant the catheter had good blood return and no signs of infiltration or extravasation were present.[8,9] Digital ischemia with sudden onset of extremity cyanosis (without evidence of infiltration) was observed in a 2-week-old neonate after infusing dopamine via a peripheral line into the left saphenous vein and right hand. The authors suggested that dopamine be infused through a central line.[10]

Infusion through an umbilical artery catheter is not recommended.[11]

See Appendix E for additional information regarding extravasation treatment.

Dosage

The intravascular volume should be corrected before starting dopamine.[4,12,13]

Shock: 2–20 mcg/kg/min.[6,14]

0.5–10 mcg/kg/min[4,12,15-22] increased by 1–10 mcg/kg/min q 10–40 min up to 25 mcg/kg/min.[4,12,15,16,19,23,24] In certain cases, larger doses may be required (see Maximum dosage section). Because doses >20 mcg/kg/min may decrease renal blood flow,[15] either epinephrine, norepinephrine, or dobutamine should be used concomitantly if continued ionotropic support is needed.[25]

Hypotensive preterm neonates: 5–20 mcg/kg/min is usual.[23,24,26-28] If doses >10–15 mcg/kg/min are required to maintain blood pressure or cardiac output, then epinephrine, norepinephrine or dobutamine should be added.[25]

Dosage *(cont.)*	**Other:** "Low-dose" dopamine (<5 mcg/kg/min) does not appear to prevent or reduce the incidence of acute oliguric renal failure in critically ill patients and is no longer recommended. Furthermore, low doses of dopamine may suppress respiratory drive, increase myocardial oxygen demand, worsen splanchnic oxygenation, impair GI function and impair endocrine and immunologic systems.[29] Doses of 5–10 mcg/kg/min affect beta-receptors and are used for inotropic response; and doses >10 mcg/kg/min affect alpha-receptors and are used to increase blood pressure, heart rate, and peripheral vascular resistance.[30] Infusions >20 mcg/kg/min are associated with an increased risk for dysrhythmias.[31] They may also result in peripheral, renal, and splanchnic vasoconstriction and ischemia.[6]
Dosage adjustment in organ dysfunction	Dopamine clearance is decreased in critically ill children with renal or hepatic dysfunction.[32]
Maximum dosage	Usually 50 mcg/kg/min.[4] 75 mcg/kg/min has been used in children with advanced circulatory decompensation.[25,31] Doses as large as 125 mcg/kg/min have been given to neonates.[25]
Additives	Contains sodium metabisulfite.[4,33] See Appendix C for more specific information about potential adverse effects of sulfites.
Suitable diluents	D5LR, D5NS, D5½NS, D2.5W, D5W, D10W, LR, mannitol 20%, NS, or sodium lactate ⅙M.[33] Not compatible with strongly alkaline solutions such as sodium bicarbonate (dopamine inactivated).[4,6,33]
Maximum concentration	3.2 mg/mL.[33] Concentrations up to 6 mg/mL have been infused into large veins (i.e., central vein) of extremely fluid-restricted patients.[34]
Preparation and delivery	**Preparation:** Significant variability between the ordered dosage and the actual solution concentration of dopamine may occur and account for hemodynamic changes when infusates are replaced. Failure to consider the HCl salt in the stock drug accounts for some of the inaccuracy in preparation.[35] **Compatibility:** For PN compatibility information, please see Appendix D. **Delivery:** May be filtered through a 0.2-micron filter without significant dopamine loss.[33]
IV push	Not indicated.
Intermittent infusion	Not indicated.

DOPamine HCl

Continuous infusion	400–800 mcg/mL.[4,33]

The following formula has been recommended for preparation of the infusion: 6 × weight (kg) = mg of drug to be added to IV solution for a total volume of 100 mL. An infusion rate of 1 mL/h provides 1 mcg/kg/min.[12] This formula estimates an initial concentration. Ultimately, the concentration of the drug should consider the patient's fluid requirements or fluid limitations.

Despite widespread use of the above formula, recent Joint Commission guidelines recommend the implementation of standardized concentrations of vasoactive medications.[36] |
| **Other routes of administration** | Not indicated. Intraosseous administration may be used in post-resuscitation stabilization.[6,12,14,37] |
| **Comments** | **Significant adverse effects:** A 16-year-old patient with pulmonary vascular obstructive disease developed suprasystemic pressure in the right ventricle during dopamine infusion. It was suggested that dopamine may be contraindicated in patients with this underlying disease.[38] In a blinded, cross-over trial in 19 children (2–54 months of age) requiring inotropic support after cardiac surgery, dopamine in doses >7 mcg/kg/min caused pulmonary vasoconstriction. The authors concluded that dopamine should not be used in infants with increased PVR secondary to pulmonary hypertension.[39]

An evaluation of 629 children undergoing cardiovascular surgery found that a younger age, longer cardiopulmonary bypass time and infusion of dopamine or milrinone were associated with the development of junctional ectopic tachycardia.[40] The authors suggest that dopamine be discontinued in those who develop this condition.

Monitoring: Blood pressure and ECG monitoring should occur continuously throughout therapy.

Pharmacokinetic considerations: Studies using a first-order kinetic model were unable to relate clearance to age.[32,41] Using a nonlinear model, clearance varied according to concentration, and increased weight (but not age) was related to a decreased clearance.[42] Still another study reported that clearance is almost two times greater in those <2 years old.[43]

Other: A prospective study in 20 preterm infants with arterial hypotension refractory to volume therapy noted that dobutamine or dopamine (10 mcg/kg/min) increased MAP and decreased superior mesenteric artery resistance and proposed that the risk for developing NEC during infusion would be reduced.[18]

Prolonged use may inhibit TSH release.[6] |

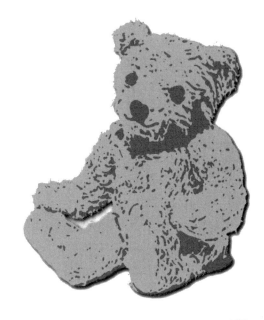

Doxapram HCl

Brand names	Dopram
Medication error potential	None noted.
Contraindications and warnings	**Contraindications:** Seizure disorders; possible pulmonary embolism; mechanical disorders of ventilation; evidence of head injury, cerebral vascular accident, or cerebral edema; and in cardiovascular disorders including those associated with hyperthyroidism.[1]
Infusion related cautions	Monitor blood pressure closely for evidence of hypertension.[1-3] Extravasation should be avoided because of the potential for thrombophlebitis or local skin irritation.[1]
Dosage	Reserve for neonates unresponsive to theophylline or caffeine. (See Additives section and Comments section.) **Neonatal apnea:** Loading dose of 2.5–3 mg/kg[4,5] followed by continuous infusion of 0.2 mg/kg/h.[2,5-7] Alternatively, a continuous infusion of 0.5 mg/kg/h with increases of 0.5 mg/kg/h up to a maximum of 2.5 mg/kg/h for a total length of infusion of 48 hours.[7] Then decrease dose to lowest that controls apnea.[7] In one study, 0.2 mg/kg/h was as effective as 1–2.5 mg/kg/h when used with a methylxanthine.[5] **Neonatal extubation:** A small study in premature neonates began with an infusion of 0.5–1 mg/kg/h and titrated to ≤2.5 mg/kg/h for 48 hours.[8] In another larger study, 27 preterm infants who received a 3.5 mg/kg infusion over 20 minutes followed by 1 mg/kg/h for 48 hours after extubation had no greater likelihood of remaining extubated than the control group.[9] In addition, an intervention review concluded that the routine use of doxapram to facilitate extubation in preterm neonates was not warranted.[10] ***Adults* with postanesthesia respiratory depression, drug-induced respiratory depression, chronic obstructive pulmonary disease**[1]**:** 0.5–1 mg/kg q 5 min up to a maximum dose of 2 mg/kg. Alternatively, 5 mg/min until a satisfactory response is obtained and maintained at an infusion of 1–3 mg/min up to a total dose of 4 mg/kg (maximum 300 mg). The regimen may be repeated if relapse occurs.
Dosage adjustment in organ dysfunction	Use with caution in patients with significantly impaired renal or hepatic function.[1]
Maximum dosage	2.5 mg/kg/h for 48 hours in neonates.[2,6-8] 3 g/day in *adults*.[1]
Additives	Contains benzyl alcohol 0.9% as a preservative.[1] (See Appendix C for specific information about benzyl alcohol toxicity in neonates.)
Suitable diluents	D5W, D10W, NS.[1]
Maximum concentration	2 mg/mL.[1,11]

Doxapram HCl

Preparation and delivery	**Compatibility:** Incompatible with alkaline solutions such as aminophylline, furosemide, sodium bicarbonate, and thiopental.[1,11]
IV push	Not recommended. Rapid infusion may result in hemolysis.[1]
Intermittent infusion	For loading dose dilute in D5W, D10W, or NS (1 mg/mL) and infuse no faster than 5 mg/min in *adults*.[1]
Continuous infusion	Continuous infusion may be used.[1]
Other routes of administration	Not indicated.[1]
Comments	**Adverse effects:** A group of preterm infants with mental delay was compared to a control group matched for gestational age, birth weight, sex, intraventricular hemorrhage grade, and socioeconomic status.[12] Steroid use and methylxanthine use was similar; however, both oxygen supplementation and doxapram therapy were longer in the group with mental delay compared to controls.[12] This led investigators to speculate about the possible role of benzyl alcohol. Subsequently, investigators evaluated 20 preterm neonates during escalating doxapram doses using cerebral Doppler ultrasonography and near-infrared spectroscopy.[13] Doxapram increased oxygen consumption and requirements and at the same time decreased oxygen delivery. Investigators proposed that these effects are caused by decreased cerebral blood flow.
	QTc interval prolongation has been reported in premature infants receiving 0.5–1 mg/kg/h for 72 hours.[14]
	Monitoring: Heart rate, blood pressure, and deep tendon reflexes.[1]

Doxycycline Hyclate

Brand names	Doxy, Doxychel Hyclate, Vibramycin IV
Medication error potential	USP reports confusion with Declomycin, dicloxacillin, dicyclomine, doxazosin, doxepin, minocycline, and tetracycline.[1]
Contraindications and warnings	**Contraindications:** Persons who have shown hypersensitivity to any of the tetracyclines.[2] **Warnings:** Use during tooth development (last half of pregnancy, infancy, and childhood to the age of 8 years) may cause permanent tooth discoloration (yellow-gray-brown).[2,3] This is more common during long-term use but has been observed following repeated short-term courses.[2,3] Tetracycline drugs should not be used in this age group, except for postexposure to anthrax.[2,4,5] Tetracyclines may cause an increase in BUN; however, this does *not* occur with the use of doxycycline in patients with impaired renal function.[2]
Infusion related cautions	Avoid extravasation.[4] (See Appendix E for treatment of extravasation.) Phlebitis occurs frequently.[4,6,7]
Dosage	**Children <8 years of age:** See Contraindications and warnings section.[2,3] **Children ≥8 years of age** **≤45 kg (100 lb):** 4.4 mg/kg/day (given in one or two divided doses) on day 1 followed by 2.2–4.4 mg/kg/day given once daily or divided q 12 h.[2,4,5] **>45 kg (100 lb):** 200 mg/day (given in one or two divided doses) on day 1 followed by 100–200 mg/day given once daily or 200 mg/day divided q 12 h.[2,4,5] **Pelvic inflammatory disease (PID):** 200 mg/day divided q 12 h.[5] **Postexposure inhaled anthrax:** If oral therapy is not possible, use doses recommended above.[2,5] Oral therapy must be continued for 60 days.[2,5]
Dosage adjustment in organ dysfunction	One reference suggests doxycycline accumulates in chronic renal failure[8] and another suggests if CrCl <10 mL/min the dose should be reduced to 2.2 mg/kg/day divided every 12 hours.[9] Others have found little to no accumulation.[10,11]
Maximum dosage	200 mg/day for children ≥8 years of age and >45 kg.[2,5]
Additives	100- and 200-mg vials contain 480 and 960 mg of ascorbic acid, respectively.[12] Mannitol is also present in some preparations.[12]
Suitable diluents	D5LR, D5W, LR, NS, or R.[2,12]
Maximum concentration	1 mg/mL.[12] Concentrations <0.1 mg/mL are not recommended.[2]

Doxycycline Hyclate

Preparation and delivery	**Compatibility:** See Appendix D for PN compatibility information.[13] **Photosensitivity:** Protect from light exposure until ready to use. Cover during infusion is recommend if solution is exposed to sunlight.[12] Stable for 48 hours if exposed to fluorescent light only.[2]
IV push	Not recommended.[2,12]
Intermittent infusion	0.1–1 mg/mL[2,12] over 1–4 hours.[2,4] A recommended minimum infusion time for a 100 mg dose (0.5 mg/mL) is 1 hour.[2]
Continuous infusion	Not given by this method.[2]
Other routes of administration	None.
Comments	**Rare adverse effects:** Nail discoloration has occurred in an 11-year-old receiving oral doxycycline 200 mg on day 1 followed by 100 mg daily for 10 days.[14] Doxycycline can form stable calcium complex in any bone-forming tissue. A decrease in the fibula growth rate has been observed in premature neonates who receive tetracyclines.[3,5] **Laboratory interference:** Doxycycline may cause false-positive urinary glucose results when cupric sulfate solution–based tests (Clinitest, Benedict's, or Fehling's solution) are used.[4] Glucose oxidase methods (Clinistix) may be associated with false-negative test results.[4] **Osmolality:** 1 mg/mL in D5 and in NS was 292 mOsm/kg and 310 mOsm/kg, respectively.[12] **Other:** Recent concerns regarding both Rocky Mountain spotted fever, ehrlichiosis, cholera, and anthrax have caused the American Academy of Pediatrics to recommend doxycycline 4.4 mg/kg/day (maximum 100 mg/dose) divided q 12 h if these infections are suspected.[5]

Droperidol

Brand names	Inapsine, generic
Medication error potential	Look-alike, sound-alike error potential.
	USP reports that Inapsine has been confused with Imitrex; no patient harm resulted.[1]
Contraindications and warnings	**US boxed warning:** QT prolongation and torsades de pointes have been reported in patients treated with droperidol at or below recommended doses. Cases have occurred in patients with no known risk factors for QT prolongation and some have been fatal.[2]
	Droperidol should only be used in patients who fail to respond to other therapies and risks of administration must be weighed against any potential benefit.[2] Prior to administration, all patients should have a 12 lead ECG to assess for QT interval prolongation.[2]
	Contraindications: Contraindicated in those with known or suspected QT prolongation including those with congenital long QT syndrome.[2] Contraindicated in patients with known hypersensitivity to droperidol.[2]
	Other warnings: Droperidol should be administered cautiously in patients at risk for prolonged QT interval (congestive heart failure, cardiac hypertrophy, significant bradycardia, significant cardiac disease, low potassium or magnesium concentrations, concomitant drug therapy that prolongs the QT interval, concomitant Class I and III antiarrhythmics or monoamine oxidase inhibitors, concomitant diuretic use). Administer cautiously in patients >65 years of age and in those with alcohol abuse, benzodiazepine use, or opiate use.[2]
Infusion related cautions	Fluids and other agents used to manage hypotension should be available when giving droperidol.[2]
	Elevated blood pressure has occurred when given concomitantly with fentanyl and other parenteral analgesics.[2]
Dosage	Not recommended for any use other than perioperative nausea and vomiting unresponsive to other therapies.[2]
	Postoperative nausea/vomiting
	Prophylaxis: 0.015–0.075 mg/kg/dose[3-10] concomitantly with anesthesia induction,[4,8,10] immediately after induction,[3,7] 30 minutes before end of procedure,[6] or at end of procedure.[5]
	Treatment: 0.1 mg/kg/dose.[9] Administer additional doses with caution and only if benefit clearly outweighs risk.[2]
Dosage adjustment in organ dysfunction	Use cautiously in patients with impaired hepatic or renal function.[2]
Maximum dosage	Maximum initial dose is 0.1 mg/kg in children (2–12 years) and 2.5 mg/dose in *adults*.[2]
Additives	None.
Suitable diluents	D5W, LR, NS.[11]

Droperidol

Maximum concentration	2.5 mg/mL.[2,11]
Preparation and delivery	For PN compatibility information, please see Appendix D.
IV push	2.5 mg/mL given by slow IV injection, over 2–5 minutes.[2,11] (See Infusion related cautions section.)
Intermittent infusion	No information is available to support administration by this method.
Continuous infusion	No information is available to support administration by this method.
Other routes of administration	2.5-mg/mL solutions may be given IM.[2,11]
Comments	**Significant adverse effects:** Acute dystonia has been reported in two patients (ages 14 and 16 years) receiving droperidol (0.04 and 0.08 mg/kg) with patient controlled analgesia.[12]
	Drug interactions: Droperidol should not be given concomitantly with other agents known to prolong the QT interval, agents that cause electrolyte imbalances, or CNS depressant agents.[2]

Edetate Calcium Disodium

Brand names
Edetate Calcium Disodium (Calcium Disodium Versenate), has also been referred to as Calcium EDTA (see Contraindications and warnings section)

Medication error potential
Look-alike, sound-alike error potential.

ISMP and USP report that edetate calcium disodium (calcium EDTA) has been confused with edetate disodium (disodium EDTA); patient death resulted.[1,2]

Contraindications and warnings
US boxed warning: Mortality from lead encephalopathy in pediatric patients has been high. Patients with lead encephalopathy and cerebral edema may experience a lethal increase in intracranial pressure following IV infusion. IM administration is the preferred route in these patients.[7,8]

When giving intravenously, avoid rapid infusion. Do not exceed the recommended daily dose.[9]

Other warnings: In January 2008, the FDA issued an advisory regarding patient deaths, including the death of at least one child (see Comments section), that have occurred when edetate disodium was mistakenly given instead of edetate calcium disodium.[3,4] The FDA recommends that hospitals evaluate the need to keep edetate disodium on stock and that only edetate calcium disodium be used for treatment of lead poisoning in children and *adults*.[3] The FDA also recommends using the full product name, and not using the abbreviation EDTA, when prescribing and dispensing edetate calcium disodium, and to consider including the indication for the drug on the prescribing order.[3]

Edetate disodium (disodium EDTA) should never be used to treat lead poisoning because it chelates calcium and induces tetany and potential fatal hypocalcemia.[5,6]

Infusion related cautions
Rapid infusion may result in thrombophlebitis or precipitation of encephalopathy.[7,9] Diluted solutions ($\leq$5 mg/mL) infused over at least 4 hours may decrease the risk of thrombophlebitis.[10]

Dosage
Treatment of lead poisoning (dosing is based on blood lead concentration [BLC] and clinical presentation). Continuation of therapy should also be based on BLC. Patients who require >5 days of therapy should have a 2–4 day, drug-free period between courses.[5,8,10]

Measure BLC 7–21 days after therapy to determine if retreatment is necessary.[5]

Acute lead encephalopathy: 1500 mg/m^2/day for 5 days.[5,8] IM administration is the preferred route in patients with lead encephalopathy and cerebral edema.[7,10] (See Contraindications and warnings sections.)

Combine with dimercaprol (British anti-lewisite or BAL); second course may be required after a 2–4 day interval; give third course if BLC $\geq$50 mcg/dL within 48 hours (wait 5–7 days before third course).[5,8,10]

Symptomatic and/or BLC $\geq$70 mcg/dL (symptomatic or asymptomatic): 1500 mg/m^2/day[5] or 50 mg/kg/day[8] for 5 days via an 8–24 hour infusion.[5,7,8,10] One reference recommends 1000 mg/m^2/day if BLC $\geq$70 mcg/dL and patient is asymptomatic.[8]

Combination therapy with BAL until BLC is $\leq$50 mcg/dL.[8] Second and third courses may be given depending on BLC and severity of symptoms.[5,7,8,10]

BLC of 45–69 mcg/dL (asymptomatic): 1000 mg/m^2/day[5] or 25 mg/kg/day[10] for 5 days via an 8–24 hour infusion[5,7,8,10] or in divided doses q 8–12 h (IV/IM)[5,11]; a second course may be required if BLC rebounds.[5]

Edetate Calcium Disodium

Dosage *(cont.)*	**BLC 25–44 mcg/dL:** Chelation therapy not routinely given.[5,10]

Provocative chelation test: *No longer recommended by the AAP.*[10] After patient empties bladder, infuse 500 mg/m² in D5W over 1 hour[5,8,12] and collect urine for the following 8 hours. Dose may also be given IM. Urinary excretion ≥200 mcg of lead or a ratio of urinary lead (mcg) to edetate calcium disodium dose (mg) of ≥0.6 (children <36 months) or ≥0.7 (children >36 months) identifies patients who will respond to chelation therapy.[8,13] A 5-hour lead mobilization test has also been validated.[14] With IM therapy, infusing IV fluids after administration ensures a greater diuresis.[15] |
| **Dosage adjustment in organ dysfunction** | Reduce dose with pre-existing renal disease.[7] Stop therapy if anuria or severe oliguria develop.[7] Avoid in patients with inadequate urine flow.[5,8] |
| **Maximum dosage** | 75 mg/kg/day (reserved for severely symptomatic patients) not to exceed 1 g/24 h.[16]

Five times the recommended dose infused over 24 hours in a 16-month-old without adverse effects.[7] |
Additives	Contains 5.3 mEq sodium/g of edetate calcium disodium.[11]
Suitable diluents	NS, D5W.[11]
Maximum concentration	0.5% or 5 mg/mL.[5,8,10-11]
Preparation and delivery	Supplied from the manufacturer as a 200-mg/mL solution; must be diluted prior to administration.[11]
IV push	Not recommended.[7,10-11]
Intermittent infusion	Dilute to a concentration of <0.5%[5] or 2–4 mg/mL.[11] Although 15- to 60-minute infusions have been used,[5,8,11] 4 hours or greater is recommended[10] and usually given over 8–12 hours; however, continuous infusion is preferred.[8,10-11]
Continuous infusion	Preferred method of administration in hospitalized patients.[5,8] Dilute to a concentration of <0.5%[5] or 2–4 mg/mL.[11]
Other routes of administration	IM administration is extremely painful; must be given with procaine or lidocaine (final anesthetic concentration = 0.5%) at 8- to 12-hour intervals.[5,7,8,11]
Comments	**Significant adverse effects:** Renal toxicity is dose-related and reversible, and it rarely occurs at daily doses <1500 mg/m² if the patient is adequately hydrated.[5,7,8] Edetate calcium disodium is renally excreted; adequate hydration and urine output must be maintained to reduce nephrotoxicity.[5,7,8,10] Beginning 1–2 days after 5 days of edetate calcium disodium and BAL therapy, about 16% of children developed increased SCr lasting for ≤22 days and oliguria lasting for 2–4 days.[17]

Hypercalcemia has been reported in children treated with edetate calcium disodium.[18] |

Edetate Calcium Disodium

Comments *(cont.)*

Laboratory interference: A falsely elevated lead concentration may occur if blood is drawn during a continuous infusion of edetate calcium disodium; therefore, the infusion should be stopped at least 1 hour before a test is performed.[19]

Other: Animal studies found a redistribution of lead from bone to target organs (e.g., brain and kidneys) following edetate calcium disodium administration.[20]

Neonatal lead poisoning has been treated with edetate calcium disodium in combination with BAL, with and without exchange transfusion within the first week of life.[21,22]

A 5-year-old autistic child died from cardiac arrest due to hypocalcemia during his third chelation treatment when edetate disodium was given instead of edetate calcium disodium.[4]

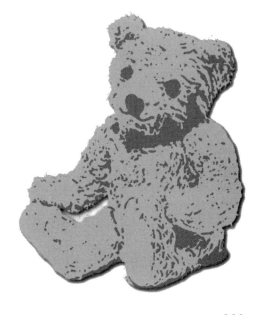

Edrophonium Chloride

Brand names Enlon, Reversol, Tensilon

Medication error potential

Look-alike, sound-alike error potential.

USP reports that Tensilon has been confused with tamsulosin; no patient harm resulted.[1]

Contraindications and warnings

Contraindications: Edrophonium is contraindicated in patients with known hypersensitivity to anticholinesterase agents and in patients with mechanical intestinal or urinary obstructions.[2]

Warnings: Use with caution in patients with asthma or with cardiac dysrhythmias or cardiovascular disease (especially those taking digoxin or quinidine).[2,3]

Infusion related cautions

Hypersensitivity, arrhythmias, bronchospasm, and laryngospasm have been reported.[2,3] Rare cases of cardiac and respiratory arrest have occurred with edrophonium administration.[2]

Atropine sulfate injection should be available to reverse signs and symptoms of life-threatening cholinergic reaction.[2,3]

Dosage

Anti-arrhythmic: Edrophonium has been used to terminate supraventricular tachycardia but has generally been replaced by other antiarrhythmic agents.

Myasthenia gravis (diagnosis): Edrophonium establishes the diagnosis in 90% to 95% of patients suspected of having the disease.[2,3] If a cholinergic reaction occurs after the initial dose, the test should be discontinued.

> **Infants:** Manufacturer recommends a dose of 0.5 mg.[2] Another reference recommends 0.04 mg/kg over 1 minute followed by 0.16 mg/kg if no response.[4]
>
> **Children:** Initial dose of 1 mg (≤34 kg) or 2 mg (>34 kg) over 1 minute.[2,3] If no response within 45 seconds, repeat dose q 30–45 sec up to a maximum cumulative dose of 5 mg for children ≤34 kg and up to 10 mg for heavier children and adolescents.[2,3]
>
> Alternatively, some recommend that children receive a total of 0.2 mg/kg or 6 mg/m². [3] One fifth of the dose should be given over 1 minute. If no response occurs in 45 seconds, the remainder should be given.

Myasthenia gravis (assessment of anticholinesterase therapy): Edrophonium is used to determine the adequacy of chronic dosing of another anticholinesterase medication in a patient with myasthenia gravis.

0.04 mg/kg (up to 1–2 mg) given 1 hour after administration of the oral drug being used to chronically treat myasthenia gravis.[3] If the patient's muscle strength or forced vital capacity improves following edrophonium, the dose of the chronic therapy should be increased.[4,5]

Because it requires several days for results to occur following changes in chronic oral dosage, the patient should be tested with edrophonium every 1–3 days after dosage adjustment of the chronic medication.[3]

Postsurgical reversal of nondepolarizing neuromuscular blocking agents: 0.4–1 mg/kg administered IV over 30–45 seconds and repeated q 5–10 min as needed.[5-9] If a larger dose of edrophonium is required, it should be preceded by IV atropine sulfate (0.01 mg/kg; minimum 0.1 mg and maximum 2 mg).[3,4]

Edrophonium Chloride

Dosage adjustment in organ dysfunction	No information available.
Maximum dosage	Maximum cumulative dose is 5 mg for children ≤34 kg and up to 10 mg for heavier children and *adults*.[2]
Additives	May contain 0.2% sodium sulfite.[2] See Appendix C for more specific information about potential adverse effects of sulfites.
Suitable diluents	Not diluted prior to administration.[2]
Maximum concentration	10 mg/mL.[2,10]
Preparation and delivery	No specific comments; see product labeling.
IV push	10 mg/mL given over 1 minute.[2,10]
Intermittent infusion	Not recommended.
Continuous infusion	Not recommended.
Other routes of administration	Edrophonium is usually given IV but may also be given IM or SC.[2,3] Children weighing up to 34 kg should receive 2 mg IM for the diagnosis of myasthenia gravis, and children weighing more than 34 kg should receive 5 mg IM. There is a delay of 2–10 minutes before a reaction is noted following IM administration.[2]
Comments	**Drug interactions:** Administration of edrophonium may prolong the effect of succinylcholine.[2,3] **Other:** While edrophonium reverses the effects of most nondepolarizing neuromuscular blocking agents, it is less effective in reversing depolarizing agents such as mivacurium, decamethonium, and succinylcholine.[3,9]

Enalaprilat

Brand names	Vasotec IV
Medication error potential	None.[1,2]
Contraindications and warnings	**US boxed warning:** May cause injury and death to the developing fetus when used during pregnancy.[3] Refer to package insert for more complete information about the boxed warning. **Contraindications:** Patients with known hypersensitivity to any component of this product, those with a history of angioedema related to previous treatment with an angiotensin converting enzyme inhibitor, and individuals with hereditary or idiopathic angioedema.[3] **Other warnings:** Anaphylactoid reactions and angioedema with laryngeal edema have occurred.[3] Immediate airway management and treatment with epinephrine, oxygen, IV steroids may be required.
Infusion related cautions	Monitor for hypotension, especially in volume-depleted patients for 1–3 hours after the first dose or following an increase in dosage.[3]
Dosage	*There are significant differences between IV and oral dosing.* **Hypertensive or congestive heart failure (left-right ventricular shunt)** **Neonates:** 5–10 mcg/kg/dose,[4] 5–30 mcg/kg/day divided q 8–24 h.[5,6] Doses as large as 120 mcg/kg/day divided q 6 h have been used.[7] Premature infants may require extended dosing intervals due to decreased glomerular filtration rates.[5] **Infants and children:** 5–10 mcg/kg/dose up to 1.25 mg/dose.[8-13] Clinical response should occur in <15 minutes and therapy should be titrated according to blood pressure. Peak effect after first dose should occur by 4 hours.[3] **Adolescents and *adults*:** 0.625–1.25 mg/dose repeated q 6 h as needed.[3]
Dosage adjustment in organ dysfunction	Administer 75% of a dose when CrCl is 10–50 mL/min and 50% of a dose if CrCl is <10 mL/min in children.[14] Initial doses of *adult* patients with creatinine clearance >30 mL/min (serum creatinine ≥3 mg/dL is 0.625 mg.[3]
Maximum dosage	120 mcg/kg/day divided q 6 h[4] or 150 mcg/kg/day divided q 8 h.[1] In hypertensive emergencies, 320 mcg/kg q 6 h has been used.[6] Although 20 mg/day divided q 6 h has been tolerated in *adults*,[3,10,15] no data have clearly demonstrated these large doses to be more effective in treating hypertension than 1.25 mg every 6 hours.
Additives	0.9% benzyl alcohol.[3] (See Appendix C for specific information about benzyl alcohol toxicity.)
Suitable diluents	D5LR, D5NS, D5W, or NS.[3,15]
Maximum concentration	1.25 mg/mL (commercially available).[3]

Enalaprilat

Preparation and delivery	**Compatibility:** See Appendix D for PN compatibility information.
IV push	Not recommended.[3] However, an infusion over 60 seconds was given without adverse effects.[5,10,11]
Intermittent infusion	Over 5 minutes.[3]
Continuous infusion	None.[3]
Other routes of administration	None.[3]
Comments	**Rare adverse effects:** Transient hyperkalemia (>5.7 mEq/L)[3] was reported in about 1% of hypertensive *adults* in clinical trials. In most cases hyperkalemia resolved despite continued therapy.
	Drug interactions: A variety of drug interactions have been reported. Consult appropriate resources for dosing recommendations before combining any drug with enalaprilat.
	Pharmacokinetics: Neonates have decreased elimination and extended duration of action; hence, they may experience prolonged hypotension and acute renal failure.[5,8]

Enoxaparin Sodium

Brand names	Lovenox

Medication error potential

ISMP high-alert medication that has an increased risk of causing significant patient harm if it is used in error.[1]

USP reported that enoxaparin was confused with dalteparin and Fragmin, and no patient harm occurred. Enoxaparin was confused with Fluvoxamine and patient harm occurred. Lovenox was confused with Lanoxin, Lasix, Levaquin, and Lovastatin, and no patient harm occurred. Lovenox was confused with Luvox and patient harm occurred.[2]

Contraindications and warnings

US boxed warning: Patients receiving enoxaparin who undergo spinal/epidural anesthesia are at increased risk for the development of an epidural or spinal hematoma.[3]

Contraindications: Major bleeding, thrombocytopenia with positive in vitro anti-platelet antibodies, hypersensitivity to enoxaparin or any component, or hypersensitivity to porcine, heparin, or benzyl alcohol.[3]

Infusion related cautions

None noted.

Dosage

Prophylaxis[4,5]**:** Therapeutic anti-factor Xa (anti-Xa) concentrations for prophylaxis range from 0.1–0.4 units/mL.[4,6]

> **<2 months of age:** 0.75 mg/kg SC q 12 h.

> **>2 months of age:** 0.5 mg/kg SC q 12 h.

Treatment[4-9]**:** Therapeutic anti-Xa concentrations for treatment range from 0.5–1 unit/mL.[6]

> **<2 months of age:** 1.5 mg/kg SC q 12 h.

> **>2 months of age:** 1 mg/kg SC q 12 h.

Compared to infants ≥37 weeks gestational age (GA), those <37 weeks GA required larger doses both to achieve (1.9 ± 0.6 mg/kg q 12 h vs. 1.6 ± 0.3) and to maintain (2.1 ± 0.6 mg/kg q 12 h vs. 1.7 ± 0.3) target anti-Xa concentrations.(10) Similarly, 10 preterm infants (24–34 weeks GA) required an average dose of 2.27 mg/kg (2–3.5) q 12 h to maintain the target anti-Xa concentrations.[6]

Doses from 0.94–2.36 mg/kg (mean 1.69) q 12 h in infants ≤2 months old and from 0.56–1.6 mg/kg (mean 1.06) q 12 h in patients >2 months old were needed to achieve therapeutic anti-Xa concentrations.[8] Still another study reported that 12 preterm infants <2 months old required 1.94 ± 0.39 mg/kg q 12 h to achieve therapeutic concentrations compared to term infants who achieved therapeutic concentrations with 1.65 ± 0.14 mg/kg q 12.[12]

Thus, infants <2 months old may require larger doses than are currently recommended.[13]

Enoxaparin Sodium

Dosage *(cont.)*	Concentrations should be drawn 4–6 hours after a SC dose.[14,15] The following recommendations are made for dosage adjustment[14,15]:

Anti-Xa (units/mL)	<0.35	0.35–0.49	0.5–1	1.1–1.5	1.6–2	>2
Dose adjust	Increase dose 25%	Increase dose 10%	No change	Decrease dose 20%	Decrease dose 30%	Decrease dose 40%
Re-dose	On time	On time	On time	On time	Delay dose 3 h	Delay dose until anti-Xa <0.5
Measure anti-Xa	4 h after next dose	4 h after next dose	Every other day	4 h after next dose	4 h after next dose	q 12 h until <0.5

Dosing in *adults*[3]

Abdominal surgery, thromboembolic prophylaxis: 40 mg SC once daily.

Hip or knee replacement surgery prophylaxis: 30 mg SC q 12 h.

Unstable angina or myocardial infarction: 1 mg/kg SC q 12 h.

Treatment of deep vein thrombosis with or without pulmonary embolus: 1 mg/kg SC q 12 h or 1.5 mg/kg SC once daily.

Dosage adjustment in organ dysfunction	In *adults* with CrCl <30 mL/min, decrease dose to 30 mg SC once daily.[3] Use caution in patients with hepatic failure. Doses may need to be reduced in pediatric patients with cardiac conditions or impaired renal or liver function.[10,11]

Maximum dosage	1.5 mg/kg in *adults*.[4] One group reported that 3.5 mg/kg q 12 h was required to produce therapeutic anti-Xa concentrations in a preterm neonate.[6]

Additives	Prefilled syringes and graduated prefilled syringes are preservative-free.[3] Each multiple-dose vial (300 mg/mL) contains benzyl alcohol 15 mg/mL.[3] See Appendix C for specific information about benzyl alcohol toxicity in neonates.

Suitable diluents	Not indicated.

Maximum concentration	150 mg/mL (commercially available).[3]

Preparation and delivery	A tuberculin syringe should be used for administration.[3]

IV push	Not indicated.

Enoxaparin Sodium

Intermittent infusion	Not indicated.
Continuous infusion	Not indicated.
Other routes of administration	Administered SC, not IM.[3] (See Comments section.)

Comments

Enoxaparin diluted to 20 mg/mL with preservative-free SW did not lose significant anticoagulant activity for 4 weeks.[16]

One 29-week, GA preterm infant (normal cranial ultrasound) with a suspected radial artery thrombus and discolored fingers was given 1 mg/kg IV q 8 h for 7 days.[17] Perfusion improved and only the tip of one finger was ultimately affected. There was no bleeding associated and no future thromboses were noted. Seven infants and children with congenital heart defects (2 months to 3 years) who were in the ICU received enoxaparin IV every 8 hours.[18] The therapeutic dose for those <1 year was 2.4 ± 0.58 mg/kg/dose and for those ≥1 year it was 1.11 ± 0.13 mg/kg/dose.

Adverse effects: Enoxaparin has been associated with the development of heparin-induced thrombocytopenia in a pediatric patient.[19]

Monitoring: CBC including platelet count during treatment. Anti-Factor Xa concentrations should be measured 4–6 hours after a dose.

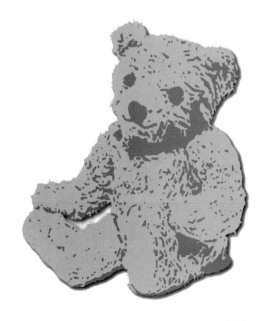

EPINEPHrine HCl

Brand names	Adrenalin Chloride

Medication error potential

ISMP high-alert medication that has an increased risk of causing significant patient harm if it is used in error.[1]

Look-alike, sound-alike error potential.

ISMP and USP report that EPINEPHrine has been confused with ePHEDrine; no patient harm resulted.[2,3] USP reports that EPINEPHrine has been confused with Neo-Synephrine, norepinephrine and phenylephrine; no patient harm resulted.[3]

USP reports that Adrenalin has been confused with ePHEDrine; no patient harm resulted.[3] EPINEPHrine is available in two concentrations (1:1000 or 1 mg/mL dilution and 1:10,000 or 0.1 mg/mL dilution). Medication errors have occurred when the concentrations have been confused.[4] (See Dosage section.)

Contraindications and warnings

Contraindications: Hypersensitivity to epinephrine or any of its components, cardiac arrhythmias, angle-closure glaucoma, and in patients receiving chloroform, trichloroethylene, or cyclopropane anesthetics.[4,5]

Warnings: Use with caution, if at all, in patients receiving halogenated hydrocarbon anesthetics (e.g., halothane). Use cautiously in patients with diabetes, thyroid disease, cardiovascular disease, and cerebral arteriosclerosis.[4,5]

Infusion related cautions

Bradycardia, tachycardia, dysrhythmias, myocardial ischemia, syncope, weakness, renal failure, and hypertension have occurred.[6-9]

Extravasation may cause local ischemia and tissue necrosis.[9-11] Therefore, infusion should be via a secure peripheral catheter or, preferably, a central route.[9] To prevent necrosis, the area should be infiltrated with a solution containing 0.1–0.2 mg/kg up to 10 mg phentolamine mesylate in 10 mL NS.[12]

A series of case reports on a 13-year-old, a 31-year-old, and a 39-year-old who accidentally discharged an epinephrine autoinjector into their thumbs reported that local injection of 1 or 3 mL of SC terbutaline (1 mg in 10 mL NS) was an effective alternative to phentolamine.[13]

See Appendix E for additional information regarding extravasation treatment.

Dosage

Clinicians should be aware that epinephrine is available in two concentrations (1:1000 or 1 mg/mL dilution and 1:10,000 or 0.1 mg/mL dilution).[4,12]

Dilution anaphylaxis: The airway should be maintained and oxygen should be administered in severe, life-threatening anaphylaxis.

Mild symptoms (e.g., pruritus, erythema, urticaria, angioedema): 0.01 mg/kg (0.01 mL/kg of the 1:1000 aqueous dilution) given IM. This may be followed by administration of antihistamines.[5,9,14] The epinephrine dose can be repeated q 10–20 min for up to three doses if symptoms continue or recur. The patient should be observed for 4 hours.[14] SC administration is no longer recommended as higher concentrations are more rapidly achieved with IM administration.[14]

Life-threatening symptoms (e.g., severe bronchospasm, laryngeal edema, other airway compromise, shock, cardiovascular collapse): 0.01 mg/kg (0.1 mL/kg of the 1:10,000 dilution) by IV repeated q 10–20 min as required.[9,14] Continuous infusion should be started if repeated doses are required. Add 1 mL (1 mg) of 1:1000 dilution to 250 mL of D5W (4 mcg/mL) and infuse at 0.1 mcg/kg/min that is increased gradually to 1.5 mcg/kg/min to maintain blood pressure.[9,14]

Patients previously on beta-adrenergic blocking agents may be less responsive to epinephrine and may require more aggressive therapy.[14] Likewise, some anaphylactic reactions (e.g., latex allergy) require large doses.[12]

Dosage *(cont.)*	**Asthma:** *The National Asthma Education and Prevention Program Expert Panel Report 3* [15] states that there is no proven advantage of systemic beta-agonist therapy over aerosol. However, it lists a dose of 0.01 mg/kg (0.01 mL/kg of 1:1000 dilution) administered SC up to 0.3–0.5 mg every 20 minutes for 3 doses. [9,15]
	Cardiopulmonary resuscitation
	Asystole: 0.01 mg/kg (0.1 mL/kg of 1:10,000 dilution) up to 1 mg IV or intraosseously (IO) or 0.1 mg/kg (0.1 mL/kg of 1:1000 dilution) endotracheally (ET) up to 10 mg. [9] Repeat q 3–5 min as needed. [9]
	No survival benefit from routine high-dose epinephrine 0.2 mg/kg (0.2 mL/kg of 1:1000 dilution) IV, IO, or ET has been found, and it may be harmful, particularly in asphyxia. [16-20] High-dose epinephrine may be considered in exceptional circumstances such as beta-blocker overdose. [16]
	Bradycardia
	Neonates: 0.01–0.03 mg/kg (0.1–0.3 mL/kg of 1:10,000 dilution) given IV or IO. IV is the preferred route of administration. [21] Repeat q 3–5 min as needed. [21] Alternatively, 0.1 mg/kg through ET followed by 1 mL NS until IV/IO access established. Safety and efficacy of the ET route of administration have not been evaluated. [21]
	Infants and children, initial doses: 0.01 mg/kg (0.1 mL/kg of 1:10,000 dilution) given IV or IO. [9] If given ET, administer 0.1 mg/kg (0.1 mL/kg of the 1:1000 dilution) followed by a 1–5 mL saline flush. [9,12] Repeat q 3–5 min as needed. [9]
	Persistent shock after volume resuscitation: 0.1 mcg/kg/min increased by 0.1 mcg/kg/min to desired response (up to 5 mcg/kg/min). [12]
	Toxins/overdose (e.g., beta blockers, calcium channel blockers): 0.01 mg/kg (0.1 mL/kg of 1:10,000 dilution) up to 1 mg given IV or IO. [9] If no response, may give higher doses up to 0.1 mg/kg (0.1 mL/kg of 1:1000 dilution) IV or IO. [9] Alternately, may infuse 0.1–1 mcg/kg/min; consider higher doses if refractory hypotension to the dose. [9]
Dosage adjustment in organ dysfunction	No dosage adjustment required.
Maximum dosage	The recommended maximum IV/IO dose is 0.03 mg/kg for neonates and 0.01 mg/kg for infants and children. [9,12,21] Continuous infusion of ≤5 mcg/kg/min may be used after resuscitation in children with persistent shock. [12]
	Although IV/ET/IO doses of 0.2 mg/kg (0.2 mL/kg of 1:1000 dilution) were safely given as high-dose therapy to patients who failed standard therapy, [22-24] no survival benefit from routine high-dose epinephrine has been found, and it may be harmful. [16-20]
Additives	Some products contain metabisulfite. See Appendix C for more specific information about potential adverse effects of sulfites.
Suitable diluents	D–LR, D–R, D–S, D5LR, D5NS, D5W, D10W, LR, NS, or R. [25]
Maximum concentration	0.1 mg/mL (1:10,000 dilution) for IV push and IO or ET administration. [9] The EpiPen, Jr delivers a dose of 0.15 mg in a concentration of 0.5 mg/mL (1:2000 dilution) and the EpiPen delivers a dose of 0.3 mg in a concentration of 1 mg/mL (1:1000 dilution). [4] For continuous infusion, 64 mcg/mL has been recommended as a maximum. [4]

EPINEPHrine HCl

Preparation and delivery	**Preparation:** Hemodynamic instability may be attributed to significant variability between the ordered dosage and the actual solution concentration of epinephrine. Failure to consider the HCl salt in the stock drug accounted for some, but not all, of the inaccuracy in preparation.[26] Epinephrine is easily destroyed by oxidants and in alkaline solutions; therefore, solutions should be protected from light.[25] Do not infuse if solution is pinkish, darker than slightly yellow, or if it contains a precipitate.[25] ET doses are 2–2½ times larger than IV doses. The dose should be diluted in 1–5 mL saline, depending on patient size, prior to ET tube instillation.[5] **Compatibility:** For PN compatibility information, please see Appendix D.
IV push	0.1 mg/mL (1:10,000 dilution) in NS over seconds.[4,12,27] The 1-mg/mL (1:1000 dilution) solution should be used for high-dose therapy only, not for initial therapy. Because standard and high-dose therapies require different dilutions, take caution to avoid errors in product selection and dosing.
Intermittent infusion	Not indicated.
Continuous infusion	May be given via continuous infusion. (See Dosage section and Maximum dosage section.) The following formula has been recommended for preparation of the infusion: 0.6 × weight (kg) = mg of drug to add to IV solution for a total volume of 100 mL. An infusion rate of 1 mL/h provides 0.1 mcg/kg/min.[28] This formula estimates an initial concentration. Ultimately, the concentration of the drug should consider the patient's fluid requirements or fluid limitations. Despite widespread use of the above formula, recent Joint Commission guidelines recommend the implementation of "standardized concentrations" of vasoactive medications.[29]
Other routes of administration	The IV and IM routes are the preferred methods of administration in pediatric patients. In children, the IM dose should be injected into the anterolateral aspect of the thigh; administration in the buttock should be avoided.[9,25] In life-threatening situations, may also be given IO (0.1 mL/kg of a 1:10,000 dilution) or ET (0.1 mL/kg of a 1:1000 dilution) route.[9,12] SC route has been used in asthma.[9,15]
Comments	A 13-month-old infant (8.6 kg) inadvertently given 327 mcg/kg of epinephrine IV developed metabolic acidosis and hypertension followed by tachycardia and pulmonary edema requiring mechanical ventilation.[30]

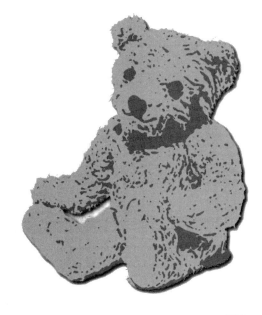

Epoetin Alfa

Brand names	Epogen, Procrit

Medication error potential	Look-alike, sound-alike error potential.
	USP reports that Epogen has been confused with Neupogen; no patient harm resulted.[1]

Contraindications and warnings	**US boxed warning:** Erythropoiesis-stimulating agents (ESAs) carry boxed warnings for increased mortality, serious cardiovascular and thromboembolic events, and increased risk of tumor progression or recurrence. In patients with renal failure, ESAs should be given to achieve and maintain hemoglobin concentrations of 10–12 g/dL, as increased mortality and serious cardiovascular events have occurred in two clinical trials when targeting higher hemoglobin concentrations (i.e., 13–14 g/dL).[2]
	ESAs shortened survival and/or increased tumor progression in clinical cancer trials (breast, head and neck, lymphoid, non-small cell lung, and cervical cancer). Use the lowest dose possible to avoid transfusions, use only for anemia in combination with chemotherapy, and discontinue when chemotherapy is completed. ESAs should not be given to patients on myelosuppressive therapy if the anticipated outcome is cure.[2]
	Due to increased thrombotic events in patients receiving epoetin, deep vein thrombosis prophylaxis should be considered in any patients receiving epoetin and undergoing surgery.[2]
	Contraindications: Uncontrolled hypertension and known hypersensitivity to mammalian cell-derived products, and known hypersensitivity to albumin.[2]
	Other warnings: Hypertension and seizures have occurred in patients with chronic renal failure receiving epoetin. Pure red cell aplasia and severe anemia have also occurred. ESA therapy should be withheld in any patients with antibody-mediated anemia.[2]

Infusion related cautions	Do not administer through same IV line as other drugs.[3]

Dosage	To ensure the erythropoietic response, iron status should be evaluated and supplemental iron prescribed if stores are low. Transferrin saturation should be ≥20% and ferritin should be ≥100 ng/mL.[2]

Anemias (a target hemoglobin (Hb) of 12 g/dL is usual)

End-stage renal disease: 10–150 units/kg three times weekly after dialysis through venous line in patients on hemodialysis.[4-9] In patients receiving continuous ambulatory or cycling peritoneal dialysis, SC injection is preferred, but 300 units/kg IV once a week have been used.[10]

HIV-infected children, zidovudine-treated: 40 and 90 units/kg three times weekly for 1 and 1.5 months were used in a 4- and 14-year-old child. Failure of adequate response in the 4-year-old child was attributed to use of a low dose for a short length of time.[11]

Children on chemotherapy: In children 5–18 years of age, an initial dose of 600 units/kg IV (maximum 40,000 units) weekly for 16 weeks has been used.[12,13] If Hb did not increase by 1 g/dL after 4–5 weeks, the dose was increased to 900 units/kg (maximum 60,000 units). Sixty percent of patients required the increased dose.[12] In 37 children (1–18 years) with solid tumors, 300 units/kg was given IV or SC three times weekly if the Hb was <12 g/dL, and 150 units/kg was given three times weekly if the Hb was ≥12 g/dL and ≤16 g/dL.[14] Epoetin was not given if the Hb was ≥16 g/dL.[14] 450 units/kg SC given once weekly for 12 weeks has also been studied.[15]

Dosage *(cont.)*

Prematurity: 100–400 units/kg either two to three times a week up to 10 weeks,[16-21] daily for 10–14 days,[22-24] or five times a week for 2 weeks.[25] Generally, the initiation of treatment varies from within 72 hours of life to 5 weeks of age.

Epidermolysis bullosa: 150 or 350 units/kg three times a week.[26]

Adjust dosage monthly to achieve and maintain an Hb concentration of ≤12 g/dL. If Hb has increased by <1 g/dL during initial 4 weeks of therapy (with adequate iron stores), then increase dose by 25% q 4 weeks until at target Hb. If the Hb increases by >1 g/dL in 2 weeks or the Hb reaches a concentration that will avoid transfusion, then decrease dose by 25%.[2,27]

Preoperative surgery (to reduce the need for blood transfusion): In cardiac surgery, 150 or 300 units/kg given two or three times approximately 1 week prior to surgery and postoperatively for two doses or until the hematocrit is increased to the preoperative value.[28,29]

In infants undergoing elective cranial vault remodeling, 600 units/kg SC given at 3 weeks, 2 weeks, and 1 week prior to surgery, combined with the use of recycled blood with Cell Saver technology, decreased transfusion requirements compared to control infants.[30]

Dosage adjustment in organ dysfunction

No dosage adjustment required.[2]

Maximum dosage

Not established. 900 units/kg/week have been given to children with cancer.[2] Doses of 1200[17] and 5000[31] units/kg/week have been given to neonates.

Additives

1-mL single-use (preservative-free) vials also contain 2.5 mg human albumin and 5.8 mg NaCl.[2,3]

1-mL and 2-mL multidose (containing preservative) vials also contain 2.5 mg human albumin, 8.2 mg NaCl, and benzyl alcohol 1% in SW.[2,3]

See Appendix C for more specific information about potential adverse effects and/or benzyl alcohol toxicity in neonates.

Suitable diluents

Dilution not recommended, except in cases of SC administration with preservative-free drug.[2,3] (See Other routes of administration section.)

Maximum concentration

40,000 units/mL.[2]

Preparation and delivery

Avoid vigorous shaking as it can denature glycoprotein.[2] Protect solution from light.[2]

For PN compatibility information, please see Appendix D.

IV push

Rapid.

Intermittent infusion

Dilute dose in 2 mL of protein-containing parenteral nutrition fluid or 2 mL of 5% albumin and infuse over 4 hours (to mimic the pharmacokinetics of SC dosing).[20]

Continuous infusion

Can be mixed in IV fluids containing at least 0.05% protein (amino acids).[22,32,33]

Epoetin Alfa

Other routes of administration

SC route is preferred except in patients on hemodialysis when IV administration is preferred.[2,27] For SC administration the dose can be diluted 1:1 with bacteriostatic 0.9% sodium chloride injection, USP, with benzyl alcohol 0.9%. The benzyl alcohol in the bacteriostatic saline decreases the discomfort from SC injection. This is not necessary when using the multidose product that contains benzyl alcohol.[2] (See Additives section.) IM is not indicated.

Comments

Significant adverse effects: Hypertension[2,5,7,10] and blood vessel[6] or vascular access occlusion[4,7] have occurred in children with renal failure. A 12-year-old boy with end-stage renal disease developed hypertension with encephalopathy, which resolved with discontinuation of phenytoin and erythropoietin.[34]

Transient neutropenia was associated with larger erythropoietin doses in preterm neonates.[35]

Rare adverse effects: Pure red cell aplasia, in association with neutralizing antibodies to erythropoietin (anti-EPO antibodies), has been reported as a rare yet important reaction in *adults* and children, particularly those with chronic renal failure.[2,36] Any child with a loss of response to erythropoietin should be evaluated.

Other: Failure to respond may be a result of iron deficiency.[2,16,17,27] Following the erythropoietin infusion, IV ferrous gluconate,[7] or iron dextran[20,37] may be given to patients who have inadequate iron stores and who are unable to tolerate oral iron.

Inform patients of risks associated with ESA therapy. Medication guides, available from the manufacturer, should be given to all patients receiving ESA therapy at home.[2]

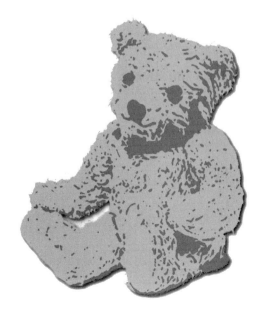

Ertapenem

Brand names	Invanz
Medication error potential	ISMP recommends the following tall man letters (not FDA approved): INVanz and AVINza. [1] Look-alike, sound- alike drug names. ISMP's *Confused Drug Names* lists confusion for Invanz with Avinza. [2] USP reports confusion with imipenem, cilastatin, and meropenem. [3]
Contraindications and warnings	**Contraindications:** In patients with a known hypersensitivity to any component of this product or to other carbapenems or in patients who have demonstrated anaphylactic reactions to beta-lactams. [4] **Warnings** **Allergic reactions:** Serious hypersensitivity and occasionally fatal anaphylactic reactions have been reported. [4] These are more likely in patients who are sensitive to multiple allergens and in those with a history of penicillin, cephalosporins, or other beta-lactam hypersensitivity. [4] **Seizures:** Neurotoxicity of the carbapenem antibiotics has been reported. [4] Seizures occur most commonly in patients with renal impairment and/or underlying neurologic disorders. (See Comments section.) **Superinfection:** Prolonged use may cause superinfection and/or *Clostridium difficile*-associated diarrhea (CDAD), which has been reported and may range in severity from mild diarrhea to fatal colitis. [2] If CDAD is suspected or confirmed, appropriate fluid and electrolyte management, protein supplementation, antibiotic treatment of *C. difficile,* and surgical evaluation should be instituted as clinically indicated. [2] Antibiotic use that is not directed against *C. difficile* may be discontinued. [2]
Infusion related cautions	If a decision is made to give ertapenem to a patient with known penicillin, cephalosporins, or other beta-lactam hypersensitivity, the patient should be closely observed for allergenicity. [4] Serious anaphylactic reactions require immediate emergency treatment with epinephrine, oxygen, intravenous steroids, and airway management, including intubation. Other therapy may also be administered as indicated.
Dosage	Because ertapenem has been administered to a limited number of pediatric patients, the doses and side effects have not been established in this age group. **3 months to 12 years:** 30 mg/kg/day divided q 12 h up to 1 g/day. [4-7] **13 to 17 years of age:** 20 mg/kg q 24 h up to 1 g/day. [4-7] Duration of therapy varies depending on the type and severity of infection, as well as causative organism.
Dosage adjustment in organ dysfunction	If CrCl is ≤30 mL/min, decrease dose by 50%. [4]
Maximum dosage	1 g/day. [1]
Additives	Contains approximately 137 mg (6 mEq) of sodium/g of ertapenem. [1]
Suitable diluents	NS.
Maximum concentration	20 mg/mL. [1]

Ertapenem

Preparation and delivery	**Stability:** Immediately dilute reconstituted solution in NS.[4] Reconstituted solution can be stored at room temperature (25°C) and used within 6 hours or may be stored for 24 hours under refrigeration (5°C).[4] Should be used within 4 hours after removal from refrigeration.[4] **Compatibility:** Do not dilute in dextrose containing solutions.[4]
IV push	Not administered by this method.
Intermittent infusion	15–20 mg/kg over 30 minutes.[1]
Continuous infusion	Not administered by this method.
Other routes of administration	May be administered IM following reconstitution with 1% lidocaine HCl injection, USP (in saline without epinephrine).[4,9] Maximum duration of IM therapy is 7 days.[4]
Comments	**Rare adverse effects:** Neurotoxicity of the carbapenem antibiotics has been reported.[10,11] In *adults*, seizures most often occur after 7 days and appear to be related to an underlying CNS disorder, impaired renal function, and/or large doses.[11] Because of the risk of seizures, the drug should be used cautiously in patients with CNS infections or renal dysfunction, patients with history of seizure disorders, and when used in combination with drugs that lower the seizure threshold.[12] If seizures occur, the need for ertapenem should be considered and the dosage should be assessed. **Drug interactions:** Oral probenecid may increase serum concentrations of ertapenem.[4,7] Carbapenems may reduce serum concentrations of valproic acid, which can result in a loss of seizure control.[13] Serum valproic acid concentrations should be monitored frequently after beginning or increasing the dose of a carbapenem. Alternative antibiotics or anticonvulsant therapy should be considered if serum valproic acid concentrations drop below the therapeutic range or a seizure occurs.

Erythromycin Gluceptate/Lactobionate

Brand names
Erythrocin Lactobionate-IV, Ilotycin Gluceptate

Medication error potential
Look-alike, sound alike drug names.

USP reports confusion with azithromycin, which has resulted in patient harm.[1]

Contraindications and warnings

Contraindications: In patients with known hypersensitivity to erythromycin.[2] It should not be given to patients taking terfenadine or astemizole.[2]

Warnings: Hepatic dysfunction, with or without jaundice, has been reported.[2]

Prolonged use may cause superinfection and/or *Clostridium difficile*–associated diarrhea (CDAD), which has been reported and may range in severity from mild diarrhea to fatal colitis.[2] If CDAD is suspected or confirmed, appropriate fluid and electrolyte management, protein supplementation, antibiotic treatment of *C. difficile,* and surgical evaluation should be instituted as clinically indicated.[2]

Infusion related cautions
Thrombophlebitis frequently occurs.[3]

Dosage

Neonates: Little information available. Seventeen neonates ≤15 days of age with birth weights ≤1500 g were given 40 mg/kg/day divided every 8 hours.[4] Fourteen infants (30.6 ± 5.4 weeks gestational age and birth weight: 1466 ± 825 g) were given 3–6 mg/kg/day divided q 8 h.[5] Fourteen neonates ≤1500 g and ≤15 days of age received 25 or 40 mg/kg/day divided q 6 h for a total of 10 days.[6]

Evidence from studies with a small sample size have not demonstrated a reduction in chronic lung disease or death when erythromycin (prophylaxis or treatment) was given to intubated preterm infants with suspected or confirmed *Ureaplasma urealyticum*.[7]

Infants and children

    Mild-to-moderate infections: Not appropriate.[8]

    Severe infections: 15–20 mg/kg/day (up to 4 g/day) divided q 6 h or given by continuous infusion.[2]

Pelvic inflammatory disease: Although the manufacturer recommends 500 mg q 6 h for at least 3 days followed by 7 days of oral therapy,[2] the CDC guidelines do not include erythromycin as first-line therapy for PID due to *N. gonorrhoeae*.[9]

Prokinetic agent: Doses of 10–48 mg/kg/day divided q 6–8 h,[10-15] 3 mg/kg/h continuous infusion,[12] and 1 mg/kg infused over 30 minutes followed by octreotide[13] have been used in children. At this time, there is insufficient evidence to recommend small or large dose erythromycin for preterm infants at risk of feeding intolerance.[15]

Dosage adjustment in organ dysfunction
If CrCl is <10 mL/min, administer 50% to 75% of normal dose q 6 h.[16] Use cautiously in hepatic dysfunction.[2,17]

Maximum dosage
50 mg/kg/day[8] not to exceed 4 g/day.[2]

Additives
Vials containing the equivalent of 1 g of erythromycin have 180 mg of benzyl alcohol as a preservative; vials containing the equivalent of 500 mg of erythromycin have 90 mg of benzyl alcohol.[2] (See Appendix C for specific information about benzyl alcohol potential for toxicity.)

Erythromycin Gluceptate/Lactobionate

Suitable diluents	D5W, NS.[2,18]
Maximum concentration	5 mg/mL.[2] 10 mg/mL has been recommended for administration via a central venous line.[19]
Preparation and delivery	**Stability:** If added to D5 use within 2 hours and if added to NS use within 8 hours.[2] **Compatibility:** See Appendix D for PN compatibility information.[20]
IV push	Not recommended due to local irritation and risk of cardiovascular effects.[2,18]
Intermittent infusion	1–5 mg/mL over 20–120 minutes.[2,18]
Continuous infusion	Preferred to intermittent delivery.[2]
Other routes of administration	None.
Comments	**Rare adverse effects:** Although high-frequency sensorineural deafness occurred in a 17-year-old with renal failure,[21] this complication usually occurs in older patients.[21-23] Macrolide antibiotics may prolonged cardiac repolarization and QT interval to cause cardiac arrhythmia and *torsades de pointes*.[2,24] Treatment includes discontinuing erythromycin and administering magnesium.[24] Ventricular arrhythmias (in individuals with pre-existing myocardial disease), nausea, vomiting, and abdominal cramps have occurred.[2,25-27] Bradycardia and hypotension have been reported in neonates[27-29] and in a child.[30] Prolonging the infusion to ≥60 minutes has been recommended to decrease potential direct cardiotoxicity.[29,30] Exacerbation of symptoms of myasthenia gravis and new onset of myasthenic syndrome have been reported.[2] **Drug interactions:** Erythromycin is a substrate of CYP2B6 and CYP3A4.[30] It is an inhibitor CYP1A2 and 3A4.[30] Because erythromycin is associated with numerous drug interactions that may result in loss of efficacy or significant toxicity, consult appropriate resources for dosing recommendations before combining any drug with erythromycin. **Laboratory interference:** Erythromycin interferes with the fluorometric determination of urinary catecholamines.[2] **Osmolality:** 5 mg/mL in D5W and NS is 265 and 291 mOsm/kg, respectively.[18]

Esmolol HCl

Brand names	Brevibloc

Medication error potential

ISMP high-alert medication (adrenergic antagonist and antiarrhythmic) that has an increased risk of causing significant patient harm if it is used in error.[1]

Look-alike, sound-alike drug names.

USP reports confusion for Brevibloc with Brevital.[2]

Contraindications and warnings

Contraindications: Hypersensitivity to esmolol or any component of the formulation.[3] Should not be used in those with sinus bradycardia, heart block greater than first degree (unless functional pacemaker), cardiogenic shock, or overt heart failure.[3]

Warnings: Use cautiously in patients with diabetes mellitus as esmolol may block hypoglycemia-induced tachycardia and blood pressure changes.[3] Use lowest dose possible in patients with a history of bronchospasm (e.g., asthma) and discontinue infusion if bronchospasm occurs.[3] Should not be used to treat hypertension due to the vasoconstriction associated with hypothermia.[3]

Infusion related cautions

Extravasation may result in serious local reactions, including tissue necrosis.[3] The use of butterfly needles should be avoided.[3]

Dosage

Anti-arrhythmias (supraventricular tachycardia): Initiate dose of 500–600 mcg/kg over 1–2 minutes.[3,4] If response is inadequate, a second loading dose of 500 mcg/kg has been given.[5] The loading dose should be followed by 200 mcg/kg/min.[4,5] If no response in 4 minutes, increase infusion by 25 mcg/kg/min[5] or 50–100 mcg/kg/min[4] q 4 min until >10% decrease in heart rate or blood pressure occurs.[4] The mean dose for control in one study was 550 mcg/kg/min but ranged from 400–1000 mcg/kg/min.[4] Maintenance doses >200 mcg/kg/min have not been shown to have significantly increased benefits and are not recommended.[3] An 8-day-old with severe tachycardia secondary to neonatal tetanus received a loading dose of 1000 mcg/kg over 1 minute followed by a continuous infusion of 120 mcg/kg/min.[6]

Hypertensive crisis

> **Loading dose:** 500–600 mcg/kg over 1 minute.[7-9]

> **Maintenance dose:** 100–500 mcg/kg/min initially.[8-10] Increase rate by 50–100 mcg/kg/min[7,10] q 5–10 min until heart rate or mean blood pressure decreases by at least 10%.

Postoperative tachycardia/hypertension: Loading doses of 125, 200, and 500 mcg/kg have been given over 10–20 seconds.[11] Doses of 200[12] and 750[12] mcg/kg were used in an 18-month-old and a 15-year-old, respectively. Loading dose should be followed by an initial dose of 200 mg/kg/min.[11] One study reported that postoperative cardiac patients required a mean dose of 700 mcg/kg/min to normalize blood pressure and that patients having coarctation repair required larger doses.[1] While some studies have noted that larger doses might be necessary when esmolol was used as a single antihypertensive in postoperative tachycardia/hypertension,[1,12] others did not report a difference between three doses (125, 250, and 500 mcg/kg/min) in the treatment of postoperative hypertension after coarctation of aorta repair.[11]

Dosage adjustment in organ dysfunction

No dosage adjustment required in renal dysfunction[13]; however, the half-life of the active metabolite may be increased 10-fold.[3]

Esmolol HCl

Maximum dosage	1000 mcg/kg as a single dose over 1 minute in a neonate.[6] Although the safety of dosages above 300 mcg/kg/min has not been studied,[3] a 6-year-old received 1000 mcg/kg/min.[4]
Additives	Each mL of the concentrate (2500 mg/10 mL) product contains 25% propylene glycol.[3] (See Appendix C for specific information about propylene glycol potential for toxicity.)
Suitable diluents	D5W, LR, NS, ½NS, D5LR, D5NS, D5½NS, D5R, or D5W with KCl 40 mEq/L.[14]
Maximum concentration	20 mg/mL (commercially available).[1,14] The 2500-mg ampule is not for direct injection.[3] Concentrations >10 mg/mL are associated with more severe vein irritation and phlebitis.[3]
Preparation and delivery	**Stability:** Clear, colorless to light yellow solution.[3,14] Stored at controlled room temperature (25°C). Protect from excessive heat and do not freeze.[3,14]
IV push	10 mg/mL given over 1–2 minutes.[3]
Intermittent infusion	Not administered by this route.
Continuous infusion	10–20 mg/mL.[3,14]
Other routes of administration	None.
Comments	**Rare adverse effects:** Although abrupt withdrawal of beta-blockers may cause acute tachycardia, hypertension, and/or ischemia, these effects have not been reported following abrupt discontinuation of esmolol.[3] Regardless, caution should be used when abruptly discontinuing esmolol.

Monitor: Heart and respiratory rate, blood pressure, and ECG should be continuously assessed during therapy.[3] Titrate doses to achieve beta blockade (usually defined as a 10% decrease in heart rate or mean blood pressure).[3,11] If hypotension occurs, decrease the infusion rate or discontinue esmolol. Once esmolol is discontinued, effects last approximately 2–16 minutes.[4,5]

Drug interactions: Concomitant use of morphine may increase esmolol serum concentration up to 50%.[15] A variety of drug interactions have been reported. Consult appropriate resources for dosing recommendations before combining any drug with esmolol.

Laboratory test interference: Increases cholesterol (S) and glucose.[16]

Other: Once a stable heart rate is achieved, transition to alternative anti-arrhythmic agents (e.g., propranolol, digoxin, or verapamil). Thirty minutes following the first dose of the alternative agent, reduce the infusion rate of esmolol by 50%. Following the second dose of the alternative agent, monitor the patient's response and if satisfactory control is maintained for the first hour, discontinue esmolol.[3] |

Esomeprazole

Brand names	Nexium

Medication error potential

Look-alike, sound-alike error potential.

USP reports that esomeprazole has been confused with lansoprazole; no patient harm resulted. USP also reports that Nexium has been confused with Nexavar (a high-alert chemotherapy agent), Fexium and Norvasc; no patient harm resulted.[1]

Contraindications and warnings

Esomeprazole is contraindicated in patients with a hypersensitivity to esomeprazole, substituted benzimidazoles, or any of the constituents in the formulation.[2]

Infusion related cautions

None.

Dosage

In *adults*, oral and IV dosage have been found to be similar in gastric acid suppression.[2] While a randomized, open-label, multinational phase I study is currently being conducted by the manufacturer to examine the pharmacokinetics of once daily IV esomeprazole in hospitalized children ages 0–17 years old,[3] no studies of IV esomeprazole have been published to date in pediatric patients. General ranges from pediatric oral dosing studies are as follows:

Infants and children: ≤2 years, gastroesophageal reflux: 0.25–1 mg/kg/day.[4]

Children 1–11 years: The safety and efficacy of doses >1 mg/kg/day and/or treatment duration >8 weeks have not been determined.

> **Gastroesophageal reflux**[5,6]
>
> > **<20 kg (or 1–5 years):** 5 or 10 mg every day for 8 weeks.
> >
> > **>20 kg (or 6–11 years):** 10 or 20 mg every day for 8 weeks.

Adolescents 12–17 years, gastroesophageal reflux[7,8]**:** 20–40 mg every day for up to 8 weeks.

***Adults,* gastroesophageal reflux:** 20–40 mg every day for 4–8 weeks; treatment may be continued for additional 4–8 weeks if incomplete healing.[2]

Dosage adjustment in organ dysfunction

No dosage adjustment required in renal dysfunction or in mild-to-moderate hepatic impairment. Do not exceed 20 mg/day in patients with severe hepatic disease (Child Pugh Class C).[2]

Maximum dosage

The manufacturer states 40 mg/day in *adults*; single doses of 80 mg have not been associated with adverse effects.[2]

Additives

Edetate disodium.[2]

Suitable diluents

D5W, LR, NS.[2,9]

Maximum concentration

8 mg/mL.[2]

Esomeprazole

Preparation and delivery	**Delivery:** No other medications should be given through the same IV site or tubing as esomeprazole. The IV line should be flushed with D5W, NS, or LR, before and after esomeprazole administration.[2]
	Stability: The manufacturer states that esomeprazole sodium is stable in either NS or LR for 12 hours and is stable in D5W for 6 hours.[2] Another study has found solutions of esomeprazole 0.4 and 0.8 mg/mL to be physically and chemically stable in D5W, LR, and NS for a minimum of 2 days at room temperature and 5 days refrigerated. Samples stored at room temperature and refrigerated samples reconstituted with D5W developed a yellow tint within 24 hours; this discoloration was associated with <10% loss of activity.[9]
IV push	4–8 mg/mL over at least 3 minutes.[2]
Intermittent infusion	Dilute reconstituted drug (4 mg/mL or 8 mg/mL) to a total volume of 50 mL with suitable diluent and infuse over 10–30 minutes.[2]
Continuous infusion	Not indicated.
Other routes of administration	No information available to support administration by other routes.
Comments	**Significant adverse effects:** Respiratory distress with chest retraction, wheezing, and facial edema occurred in an infant receiving esomeprazole; symptoms resolved with discontinuation of the esomeprazole.[10]
	Common adverse effects include abdominal pain, constipation, flatulence, dyspepsia, and headache.[2]
	Administration of proton pump inhibitors has been associated with increased risk of developing gastroenteritis and pneumonia in children.[11]
	Prolonged use (>3 years) may lead to impaired absorption of cyanocobalamin (vitamin B12) due to achlorhydria.[12]
	Drug interactions: Metabolized to inactive metabolites mainly by CYP2C19 and to lesser extent by CYP3A4. Esomeprazole should not be given concomitantly with Reyataz (atazanavir and nelfinavir) because it substantially lowers atazanavir plasma concentrations and decreases efficacy.[2]
	A known interaction exists between esomeprazole and clopidogrel. Since clopidogrel is metabolized to its active metabolite primarily via CYP2C19, and to a lesser extent, via CYP3A4 and CYP2C9, its use with esomeprazole may decrease the formation of the active metabolite and decrease antiplatelet effects.[13] Consult appropriate resources for dosing recommendations before combining any drug with lansoprazole.

Etanercept

Brand names	Enbrel

Medication error potential	Look-alike, sound-alike error potential. ISMP reports Enbrel was confused with Levbid.[1]

Contraindications and warnings

US boxed warning

> **Risk of serious infections:** Patients receiving etanercept are at risk for developing serious infections. Those with active infections should not begin treatment. Those who develop infection while on treatment should be monitored closely.[2]

> Patients should be evaluated for latent tuberculosis (TB) infection with a tuberculin skin test. If the skin test is positive, TB treatment should be started prior to beginning treatment with etanercept.[2] (See Comments section.)

> **FDA alert:** On August 4, 2009, the FDA announced that it is requiring those who manufacture TNF blockers to update the box warning to include an increased risk of lymphoma and other cancers in children and adolescents treated with TNF blockers.[3]

> **Contraindications:** Patients who have sepsis should not be given etanercept.[2] Those who have had a previous severe hypersensitivity reaction to etanercept should not receive any additional doses.[2]

> **Other warnings:** Anaphylactic type reactions have been reported.[3] Appropriate medical care should be available in the event this occurs.

> The needle cover of the prefilled syringes and auto-injector contains latex. Those with latex allergy should not handle the syringes.[2,4]

Infusion related cautions	Not intended for IV use.

Dosage

Polyarticular-course juvenile idiopathic arthritis (JIA) in children ≥2 years[2,4-6]: 0.4 mg/kg up to 25 mg twice weekly or 0.8 mg/kg up to 50 mg once a week. <31 kg should be dosed from the multidose vial and not a prefilled syringe. ≥63 kg may use the 50-mg prefilled syringe.

Psoriasis[7-9]: 0.4 mg/kg twice weekly or 0.8 mg/kg (up to 50 mg) once a week.

Chronic uveitis[10-12]: 0.4 mg/kg up to 25 mg twice weekly. Infliximab may be more effective in preventing uveitis than etanercept.[12,13] (See Comments section.)

Dosage adjustment in organ dysfunction	No data available.

Maximum dosage	50 mg once a week.

Additives	Multidose vials contain benzyl alcohol.[2,4] (See Appendix D for specific information about potential benzyl alcohol toxicity in neonates.)

Suitable diluents	Not diluted.

Maximum concentration	50 mg/mL.

Etanercept

Preparation and delivery	**Preparation:** The multidose vial is reconstituted with 1-mL BW that is included. The product literature should be consulted for detailed instructions. Available as disposable, prefilled syringes, or prefilled SureClick autoinjector (25 mg/0.5 mL, 50 mg/mL). Must be refrigerated until use.[2] **Delivery system issues:** Allow to come to room temperature (~15–20 minutes) prior to injection. Do not remove the needle cover until ready to inject. **Stability:** Etanercept reconstituted from the multidose vial must be discarded after 14 days.
IV push	Not indicated.
Intermittent infusion	Not indicated.
Continuous infusion	Not indicated.
Other routes of administration	Administer by SC injection.
Comments	A negative skin test for TB does not rule out the possibility of disease since patients with immune diseases may exhibit cutaneous anergy.[14] Etanercept treatment improved longitudinal growth in prepubertal children with JIA.[15] Juvenile idiopathic arthritis, juvenile rheumatoid arthritis, and juvenile chronic arthritis may be used interchangeably. **Adverse effects:** Injection site reactions include erythema and/or itching, pain or swelling. These usually decrease in frequency with continued treatment.[2]

Ethacrynate Sodium

Brand names	Sodium Edecrin
Medication error potential	None noted.
Contraindications and warnings	**Contraindications:** Infants, patients with anuria, and those with hypersensitivity to ethacrynate.[1,2] **Warnings:** Ethacrynic acid is a potent diuretic that may lead to significant water and electrolyte loss.[2]
Infusion related cautions	Rapid administration has been associated with reversible deafness, acute vertigo, and tinnitus.[3] (See Comments section.)
Dosage	0.5–1 mg/kg, repeat if needed q 8–12 h.[4-10]
Dosage adjustment in organ dysfunction	No dosage decrease required in patients with renal dysfunction. Use with caution in patients with advanced cirrhosis.[1,2]
Maximum dosage	2 mg/kg/dose,[7] not to exceed 100 mg/dose in *adults*.[1,2]
Additives	Contains 0.165 mEq sodium/50 mg of ethacrynic acid equivalent.[11,12]
Suitable diluents	D5W, NS, R, LR.[11] Reconstitution with D5W products with a pH <5 results in hazy or opalescent solutions. These should not be used.[2,11]
Maximum concentration	2 mg/mL.[7]
Preparation and delivery	Reconstitute to 1 mg/mL[1,2]
IV push	Not recommended.[1,2]
Intermittent infusion	Slowly, over several minutes through a running IV infusion solution.[1,2] (See Comments section.)
Continuous infusion	Not indicated.

236

Ethacrynate Sodium

Other routes of administration	Should not be given IM or SC because of local pain and irritation.[1,2]

Comments

Ethacrynate sodium may be used to manage edema in patients with impaired renal function.[1,2]

Alternating doses of ethacrynic acid with furosemide may not overcome diuretic resistance.[8]

Adverse effects: Local pain and irritation at the infusion site have occurred.[1,2]

The duration of treatment is directly related to the development of sensorineural hearing loss in neonates with persistent pulmonary hypertension.[13] Investigators point out that this may be transient; however, they suggest that infusion over at least 5–10 minutes may be protective.[13]

In *adults*, irreversible deafness[14] and upper GI bleeding[15] have occurred following infusion.

Electrolyte abnormalities, including hypokalemia, occur.

Monitoring: Serum potassium concentration monitoring is important.[1,2]

Etomidate

Brand names	Amidate
Medication error potential	ISMP high-alert medication that has an increased risk of causing significant patient harm if it is used in error.[1]
	Look-alike, sound-alike drug names.
	USP reports confusion with Trandate.[2]
Contraindications and warnings	**Contraindications:** Should not be used in a person with known hypersensitivity to etomidate.[3]
	Warnings: Should only be given by persons trained in the administration of general anesthetics and management of their complications.[3]
	May cause suppression of endogenous cortisol and aldosterone and is *not* intended for prolonged infusion.[3] (See Significant adverse effects in Comments section.)
Infusion related cautions	Avoid administration into small vessels.[3] Transient pain at the injection site may be managed by preadministration with lidocaine.[3]
Dosage	Etomidate should not be used in children <10 years of age because of lack of sufficient safety and efficacy data.[3] Current evidence suggests etomidate should be avoided in children with known or suspected septic shock. (See Significant adverse effects in Comments section.)
	Sedation: 0.3 mg/kg given over 30–60 seconds[3]; however, usual doses range between 0.2–0.6 mg/kg.[1-8] Loss of consciousness generally occurs within 60 seconds of administration.[3]
	Etomidate has been given via continuous infusion (0.3–1.2 mg/kg/h)[9]; however, the manufacturer recommends against administering etomidate for prolonged periods as a continuous infusion due to the potential for adrenal suppression,[3,10] and propylene glycol toxicity.[11] If given longer than 24 hours, consider the need for cortisol replacement.
	Severe hypercortisolemia: 0.03–0.1 mg/kg/h.[12-16]
Dosage adjustment in organ dysfunction	No dosage adjustment is necessary in renal or hepatic dysfunction[10]; however, renal dysfunction may increase the likelihood of propylene glycol toxicity. (See Additives section.)
Maximum dosage	1.1 mg/kg as a single dose.[8]
Additives	Contains propylene glycol 35%.[3] (See Appendix C for specific information about propylene glycol's potential for toxicity.)
Suitable diluents	Administered undiluted.
Maximum concentration	2 mg/mL (commercially available).[3]

Preparation and delivery	**Stability:** Do not administer unless solution is clear.[3]
IV push	Over 30–60 seconds.[3]
Intermittent infusion	No information.
Continuous infusion	Has been administered as a continuous infusion, 0.02 mg/kg/min; however, it should not be given for prolonged periods.[11] (See Significant adverse effects in Comments section.)
Other routes of administration	None.
Comments	**Significant adverse effects:** Etomidate inhibits 11-B-hydroxylase, an enzyme necessary for the production of cortisol, aldosterone, and corticosterone. This suppression does not appear to be dose related and has been noted after a single dose.[18] An increase in adrenal insufficiency and mortality was reported among critically-ill and multitrauma patients receiving etomidate infusions.[10,19] Until the risk for developing adrenal insufficiency has been assessed in a large randomized, controlled trial, alternative agents (e.g., midazolam, thiopental, pentobarbital, and ketamine) should be used for sedation. **Rare adverse effects:** Etomidate can increase EEG activation with epileptiform spikes and large doses have caused EEG slowing and isoelectricity.[4] Transient skeletal muscle movements occur in 30% to 50% of patients.[3] While the movements are usually bilateral and predominately myoclonic,[20,21] tonic, ocular, and averting movements have been reported. Movements appear to be more frequent in patients who also manifest venous pain on injection.[3] Administration of a benzodiazepine or fentanyl may decrease movements.[3] One report noted successful termination with dantrolene.[20]

Etoposide

Brand names	Toposar, VePesid, generic
Medication error potential	ISMP high-alert medication that has an increased risk of causing significant patient harm if it is used in error.[1]
Contraindications and warnings	**US boxed warning:** Etoposide should be administered under the supervision of a qualified physician. Severe myelosuppression with resulting infection of bleeding may occur.[2] **Contraindications:** Etoposide is contraindicated in patients who have a hypersensitivity to etoposide or any of the components of the formulation.[2] **Other warnings:** May cause myelosuppression, hypotension, severe emesis (see Significant adverse effects section in Comments section) and anaphylaxis.[2,3]
Infusion related cautions	Hypotension has been reported with rapid administration of etoposide.[2] Stop or slow the rate of the infusion, and administer IV fluids if necessary.[3] Infusing etoposide at a rate slower than 100 mg/m²/h (or 3.3 mg/kg/h) has been shown to minimize hypotensive effects.[4] Anaphylactic reactions have been seen with etoposide administration, manifesting as bronchospasm, tachycardia, dyspnea, and hypotension. Higher rates of anaphylaxis have been seen in children that receive higher than recommended concentrations of etoposide.[2] Extravasation has occurred but has rarely been associated with necrosis.[2] See Appendix E for additional information regarding extravasation treatment.
Dosage	Consult institutional protocol for complete dosing information. Etoposide is used as a component of combination therapy or as single agent therapy in multiple pediatric and hematologic neoplasms. A general dosage regimen has included 60–150 mg/m²/day IV for 2–5 days q 3–6 weeks.[4,5] Specific regimens include the following: **AML remission induction:** 150 mg/m² for 2–3 days starting with course 2.[4-6] **Brain tumor:** 150 mg/m² on days 1–3 or days 2–3 of treatment course.[4,7] **Neuroblastoma or osteosarcoma:** 100 mg/m² over 1 hour on days 1–5 of cycle or 75 mg/m² over 1 hour on days 1–4 of weeks 4–9 in combination with other chemotherapeutic agents.[4,8-10] **High dose conditioning regimen for BMT:** 60 mg/kg as a single dose in combination chemotherapy.[4,11,12]
Dosage adjustment in organ dysfunction	The manufacturer recommends to reduce the dose by 25% in patients with a CrCl of 15–50 mL/min and that no data exists on patients with CrCl <15 mL/min but that further dosage reductions are likely to be necessary.[2] Another reference recommends a dose reduction of 25% in patients with CrCl of 10–50 mL/min and a 50% dose reduction in patients with a CrCl <10 mL/min.[13] Use caution in patients with hepatic dysfunction.[3] Specifically, a 50% dosage reduction is recommended for patients with a serum bilirubin of 1.5–3 mg/dL and a 75% dosage reduction for a serum bilirubin >3 mg/dL.[3] Another source recommends that if the serum bilirubin is 1.5–3 mg/dL or the AST is 60–180 units/L, the dosage should be reduced by 50%; if the bilirubin is 3–5 mg/dL or AST >180, reduce the dosage by 75%; and if bilirubin is >5 mg/dL, do not administer.[14]
Maximum dosage	Not established.

Additives	Each mL contains 30 mg benzyl alcohol.[2,15] See Appendix C for more specific information about potential adverse effects and/or benzyl alcohol toxicity in neonates.
Suitable diluents	D5W or NS.[2]
Maximum concentration	0.2–0.4 mg/mL.[2,15] Precipitation has developed with concentrations >0.4 mg/mL.[15]
Preparation and delivery	The surfactant component may alter drop size. Administration with infusion devices that do not operate via drop size is recommended.[15]
	Administration devices made up of acrylic or acrylonitrile, butadiene, and styrene (ABS) should be avoided, as they have cracked and leaked when used with etoposide.[2]
IV push	Not recommended.[2,15] Rapid administration has been associated with the development of hypotension (see Infusion related cautions section).
Intermittent infusion	0.2–0.4 mg/mL may be infused over at least 30–60 minutes.[2,15] If volume is a concern, it may be infused over a longer time period, up to 210 minutes.[2,3]
Continuous infusion	Has been administered as a continuous infusion over 5 days.[3] No therapeutic benefit exists and use is not established. High-dose etoposide administered as a continuous infusion has been associated with more nonhematological toxicities compared to intermittent infusions.[16]
Other routes of administration	IT, intraperitoneal, and intrapleural administration not recommended.
Comments	**Significant adverse effects:** Etoposide is associated with a low (10% to 30%) risk of emesis.[17] Patients should receive antiemetic therapy to prevent acute and delayed nausea and vomiting. The recommended therapy is a corticosteroid on every day chemotherapy is administered; alternatives are a phenothiazine (e.g., prochlorperazine) or a butyrophenone (e.g., droperidol).[17,18] Therapy for delayed nausea and vomiting is generally not needed. Breakthrough medications should also be offered, such as a phenothiazine (e.g., prochlorperazine), a butyrophenone (e.g., droperidol), a substituted benzamide (e.g., metoclopramide), or a benzodiazepine (e.g., lorazepam). Selection should be based on what the patient is currently receiving for acute emesis prophylaxis.
	Monitoring: CBC with platelets, vital signs, renal function, bilirubin, and hemoglobin.[2,3]
	Drug interactions: Etoposide is a major substrate for CYP3A4, a minor substrate for CYP1A2 and 2E1, and a weak inhibitor for CYP2C9 and 3A4. The potential for drug interactions exists. Cyclosporine may substantially increase exposure to etoposide by decreasing metabolism.[3,4] Consult appropriate resources for dosing recommendations before combining any drug with etoposide.

Famotidine

Brand names	Pepcid, generic
Medication error potential	Look-alike, sound-alike error potential.
	USP reports that famotidine has been confused with fluoxetine, furosemide, lisinopril and paroxetine; no patient harm resulted.[1] USP reports that Pepcid has been confused with Prevacid and Prinivil; no patient harm resulted.[1]
Contraindications and warnings	Known hypersensitivity to the drug or its additives. Cross sensitivity with other H2-blockers may occur.[2]
Infusion related cautions	None known.
Dosage	**Neonates:** 0.5 mg/kg q 24 h.[3]
	Infants and children: 0.5–2.4 mg/kg/day divided q 8–12 h.[2,4-11]
Dosage adjustment in organ dysfunction	Adjust dosage in patients with severe renal dysfunction.[2,12,13]
	CrCl 30–50 mL/min: 0.5 mg/kg/day q 24 h.[13]
	CrCl 10–29 mL/min: 0.25 mg/kg/day q 24 h.[13]
	CrCl <10 mL/min: 0.125 mg/kg/day q 24 h.[13]
	Supplement doses above for hemodialysis and peritoneal dialysis (0.125 mg/kg/day q 24 h) and continuous renal replacement therapy (0.5 mg/kg/day q 24 h).[13]
	Another source recommends the following dose adjustment: CrCl >50 mL/min, 0.5 mg/kg (maximum 20 mg) q 12–24 h[12]; CrCl 10–50 mL/min, increase interval to q 36–48 h[12]; CrCl <10 mL/min, increase interval to q 72–96 h or give 0.25 mg/kg (maximum 10 mg) q 36–48 h.[12]
Maximum dosage	Usually 40 mg/day.[2] In one study, children who failed to respond to lower doses were given two 1.6-mg/kg doses (≤40 mg) 8 hours apart.[6] 160 mg q 6 h orally has been given with no serious adverse effects to *adults* with hypersecretory conditions.[2]
Additives	Each mL of the concentrated injection contains 4 mg L-aspartic acid and 20 mg mannitol; each 50 mL of the premixed injection contains 6.8 mg L-aspartic acid and 450 mg sodium chloride (7.8 mEq sodium).[2,14]
	Multidose vials contain benzyl alcohol 0.9% as a preservative.[2,14]
	See Appendix C for more specific information about potential adverse effects and/or benzyl alcohol toxicity in neonates.
Suitable diluents	NS, D5W, D10W, LR, or SW.[2,14]
	May be diluted (0.2 mg/mL) with sodium bicarbonate 5%; concentrations >0.2 mg/mL may form precipitates.[2]
Maximum concentration	4 mg/mL.[2,14]

Famotidine

Preparation and delivery	Stable in PN[15] and TNA[16] solutions for 24 hours at room temperature. See Appendix D for additional PN compatibility information.
IV push	Infuse (2–4 mg/mL) over ≥2 minutes[2] and ≤10 mg/min.[14]
Intermittent infusion	Infuse (0.2 mg/mL) over 15–30 minutes.[2,14]
Continuous infusion	In *adults*, the total daily dose has been added to a compatible fluid and infused over 24 hours.[17]
Other routes of administration	No information available to support administration by other routes.
Comments	**Significant adverse effects:** Cardiovascular adverse effects (negative inotropic effect) have occurred in *adults* on famotidine.[18] **Pharmacokinetic considerations:** Clearance is decreased and half-life increased in infants up to 3 months of age compared to infants >3 months, children, and *adults*.[2] **Pharmacodynamic considerations:** Duration of acid suppression is longer in infants up to 3 months of age compared to older infants, children, and *adults*.[2] Two of 18 critically ill children failed to respond to two 1.6-mg/kg doses (≤40 mg) given 8 hours apart.[6] Prolonged dosing has been associated with decreased duration of effect.[6] **Other:** H2-blocker therapy has been associated with the incidence of necrotizing enterocolitis in very low birth weight infants.[19]

Fenoldopam

Brand names	Corlopam
Medication error potential	None known.
Contraindications and warnings	None known.
Infusion related cautions	Rapid titration of dose may cause hypotension.[1] Reflex tachycardia occurs with larger doses.[1,2] Tachycardia in pediatric patients receiving doses >0.8 mcg/kg/min lasted for at least 4 hours.[1]
Dosage	**Controlled hypotension during surgery (children)[1-3]:** 0.3–0.5 mcg/kg/min increased by 0.3–0.5 mcg/kg/min q 20–30 min. In one study, 0.8 mcg/kg/min (range 0.05–3.2 mcg/kg/min) was the most effective dose; no effect on blood pressure <0.2 mcg/kg/min while larger doses (>1–1.2 mcg/kg/min) produced no additional benefit in decreasing blood pressure; heart rate was significantly elevated at 3.2 mcg/kg/min.[2]
	Diuresis during/after cardiopulmonary bypass in neonates[4,5]: 0.05–0.3 mcg/kg/min titrated over 24 hours to a maximum dose of 1 mcg/kg/min has been given for 1–15 days in neonates unresponsive to conventional therapy; urine output increased from 3.6 to 5.8 mL/kg/h resulting in an additional 158 mL/day urine.[4] Another study gave 0.1 mcg/kg/min during surgery and continued for 72 hours and found no effect on urine output.[5]
	Severe hypertension (children 1–17 years)[6]: 0.2–0.8 mcg/kg/min.
	Acute kidney injury in children[7]: 0.2 mcg/kg/min titrated up to 0.4 and 1.5 mcg/kg/min has been reported in two children with severe cardiomyopathy and acute kidney injury on ventricular assist devices; in one patient, urine output increased, BUN and SCr decreased, and renal replacement therapy was avoided on 0.4 mcg/kg/min. In the other patient, no effect was seen with doses up to 1.5 mcg/kg/min.
Dosage adjustment in organ dysfunction	No dosage adjustment necessary for renal or hepatic dysfunction.[1]
Maximum dosage	Doses up to 4 mcg/kg/min have been given to children and up to 1.6 mcg/kg/min have been given to *adults*.[1]
Additives	Contains 1 mg sodium metabisulfite/mL.[1,8] See Appendix C for more specific information about potential adverse effects of sulfites.
	Contains 518 mg/mL propylene glycol.[1,8] See Appendix C for more specific information about potential adverse effects of propylene glycol.
Suitable diluents	D5W, NS.[8]
Maximum concentration	60 mcg/mL.[1]

Fenoldopam

Preparation and delivery	Contents of ampules must be diluted prior to administration.[1]
IV push	Not recommended.[8]
Intermittent infusion	Not recommended.[8]
Continuous infusion	Dilute to a concentration of 40 mcg/mL.[8] Infuse via continuous infusion pump appropriate for delivery of low infusion rates.[8] May begin at 0.2 mcg/kg/min with increases of 0.3–0.5 mcg/kg/min q 20–30 min; titrate to desired effect.[1] In volume-restricted patients, fenoldopam may be diluted to a final concentration of 60 mcg/mL.[1]
Other routes of administration	No information available to support other routes of administration.
Comments	**Significant adverse effects:** Tachycardia and hypotension are the most commonly observed adverse events in pediatric patients.[1] Increased intraocular pressure and hypokalemia have also been reported in *adults*.[1] **Drug interactions:** Beta-blockers inhibit the sympathetic reflex response to fenoldopam and can cause unexpected hypotension; if possible, avoid concomitant use.[1] **Monitoring:** Blood pressure should be monitored continuously during therapy with fenoldopam.[1] **Other:** One neonate receiving fenoldopam for 48 hours after Norwood procedure acutely clotted the Blalock-Taussig shunt and required ECMO therapy for resuscitation; this event was thought to be potentially related to the brisk diuresis achieved (451 mL).[4] A 3-year-old with glomerulonephritis status post renal transplantation who developed severe hypertension secondary to renal failure/renal graft rejection failed to respond to 1.5 mcg/kg/min.[9]

FentaNYL Citrate

Brand names	Sublimaze, generic
Medication error potential	USP and ISMP reported that fentaNYL citrate was confused with SUFentanil citrate.[1,2] USP also reported that patient harm occurred.[2]
Contraindications and warnings	**Contraindications:** Patients with known intolerance to the drug.[3] **Warnings:** Only individuals trained in the use of IV anesthetics and the management of opioid respiratory effects should administer fentanyl citrate.[3] An opioid antagonist, intubation equipment, and oxygen should be available.
Infusion related cautions	Apnea may occur with rapid bolus injection or with large doses. Peak respiratory depression occurs 5–15 minutes after dosing.[3] Chest wall rigidity is related to high doses and rapid escalation to moderate doses.[4-6] Neonates may be more sensitive to respiratory depressant effects and chest wall rigidity than *adults*.[7-9] Respiratory depression and rigidity is reversible with naloxone.[3]

Dosage	**Anesthesia:** 10–50 mcg/kg/dose.[4,7,10-14]
	
	Sedation/analgesia: In all cases, fentanyl doses should be titrated to clinical effect.[3,15]
	
	    Intermittent dosing
	
	        Neonates: 1–4 mcg/kg q 2–4 h.[15]
	
	        Infants and children: 1–3 mcg/kg q 30–60 min.[15]
	
	Continuous infusion: Loading dose of 1–5 mcg/kg[6,17] followed by continuous infusion of 1–20 mcg/kg/h (normal starting dose of 1 mcg/kg/h)[15-18]; the infusion rate should be titrated by increments of 0.5-mcg/kg/h until desired effect occurs (usually 1–3 mcg/kg/h).[19] For adequate sedation in the intensive care setting, larger doses may be required.[20] Tolerance to sedation may develop with continuous infusion.[15,18] Premature neonates with hyaline membrane disease have been given 0.5–2 mcg/kg/h (mean, 1.1 mcg/kg/h) during mechanical ventilation.[21]

Dosage adjustment in organ dysfunction	**CrCl 10–50 mL/min:** 75% of usual dose.[15] **CrCl <10 mL/min:** 50% of usual dose.[15] Use with caution in hepatic impairment.[3] During ECMO fentanyl is sequestered by the circuit, primarily the membrane oxygenator, which may become saturated over time.[22] Therefore, much larger doses may be required during early ECMO.[15,22]
Maximum dosage	75–100 mcg/kg/dose for anesthesia.[12,23]
Additives	None.

FentaNYL Citrate

Suitable diluents	D5W, NS.[3,24]
Maximum concentration	50 mcg/mL.[3,25]
Preparation and delivery	**Compatibility:** See Appendix D for PN compatibility information.
IV push	Over 1–3 minutes.[7,8,12,14,26] Apnea may occur with rapid injection.[3]
Intermittent infusion	Usually given IV push (slow) or continuously.
Continuous infusion	May be given by continuous infusion.[3,15,19,25] Has been given as a continuous infusion by the SC route in children weaning from prolonged sedation.[25]
Other routes of administration	IM,[3,25] SC.[25]
Comments	**Adverse effects:** Withdrawal syndrome is associated with both dose and duration of therapy.[27,28] Acute dystonia occurred following combined treatment with fentanyl and propofol.[29] Emergence agitation following sevoflurane or desflurane anesthesia was greater with fentanyl than with use of a preoperative caudal block or preoperative midazolam with thiopental induction.[30,31] **Drug interactions:** Other CNS depressants will potentiate the effects of fentanyl citrate.[3]

Ferric Gluconate

Brand names	Ferrlecit
Medication error potential	None noted.
Contraindications and warnings	**Contraindications:** Anemias not associated with iron deficiency, hypersensitivity to ferric gluconate or its components, evidence of iron overload.[1,2]
Infusion related cautions	Acute and delayed hypersensitivity reactions have been reported at a much lower rate with ferric gluconate than with iron dextran products.[3-7] Typical reactions during infusions include flushing, hypotension, nausea, vomiting, and diarrhea,[3-7] which may be related to release of free iron. Premedication may not decrease the incidence of reactions.[8]
Dosage	An erythropoiesis stimulating agent should be used concurrently. **Iron deficiency in hemodialysis (chronic renal failure):** 1.5 mg/kg (≤125 mg/dose) × eight dialysis sessions is recommended.[1,2,9] Doses of 1–5 mg/kg have been evaluated and doses >3 mg/kg have shown limited additional efficacy and potential for added toxicity.[12] **Test dosing:** No longer recommended because reactions to 25-mg doses are no more frequent or severe than to usual doses in *adults*.[1]
Dosage adjustment in organ dysfunction	No information available; however, considering the distribution characteristics of iron, there should be no dose adjustment necessary relative to liver or kidney function.
Maximum dosage	While doses >3 mg/kg have been used, they are associated with increased adverse effects.[11,12] Maximum total dose is 125 mg.[1,2]
Additives	Contains 9 mg benzyl alcohol/mL.[1] See Appendix C for more specific information about benzyl alcohol toxicity in neonates.
Suitable diluents	NS.[1] Stability in other solutions has not been evaluated and is not recommended.[1]
Maximum concentration	12.5 mg/mL.[1,2]
Preparation and delivery	Dilution in dextrose results in infusion-related phlebitis and pain.[2]
IV push	Up to 12.5 mg/min. Higher infusion rates may be associated with increased adverse effects.[1]

Ferric Gluconate

Intermittent infusion	Over 1 hour.[1]
Continuous infusion	Not indicated.[1]
Other routes of administration	Not indicated.[1]
Comments	A reaction to one parenteral iron product does not predict a similar response to a different product nor does the lack of a reaction to a test dose predict that a hypersensitivity reaction will not occur during infusion of subsequent doses.[1]

Monitoring: Goal serum ferritin >100 ng/mL, transferrin saturation >20%, and hemoglobin 11–12 g/dL.[9]

Pharmacokinetics: A study in pediatric hemodialysis patients determined that the area under the concentration-time curve (mg • h/L) was greater in children than a comparative group of *adults*. Clearance was slower in children and volume of distribution was also lower.[14]

Filgrastim

Brand names	Neupogen, Granulocyte Colony-Stimulating Factor

Medication error potential

Look-alike, sound-alike error potential.

USP reported that filgrastim was confused with sargramostim.[1] USP reported that Neupogen was confused with Epogen, Neulasta, and Neurontin.[1] ISMP reported that Neupogen was confused with Neumega.[2]

Contraindications and warnings

Contraindications: Individuals with known hypersensitivity to *Escherichia coli*–derived proteins, filgrastim, or any product components.[3]

Warnings: Rare cases of splenic rupture have been reported; some were fatal. Abdominal pain or shoulder tip pain that occurs during infusion should be evaluated.[3]

Infusion related cautions

Allergic reactions occur more frequently with IV infusion and usually within 30 minutes of infusion.[3] Epinephrine, antihistamines, corticosteroids, and/or bronchodilators are usually effective in alleviating symptoms.[3]

Dosage

Aplastic anemia: 400 mcg/m^2/day IV for 2 weeks[4] or 90 days.[5]

Bone marrow transplantation: 5–10 mcg/kg/day administered ≥24 hours after chemotherapy and ≥24 hours after bone marrow infusion until neutrophil recovery.[3] The table depicts dosing based on neutrophil response.[3]

Absolute Neutrophil Count (ANC)	Filgrastim Adjustment
If ANC >1000/mm^3 × 3 day	Reduce dose to 5 mcg/kg/day
If ANC remains >1000/mm^3 for 3 more days	Discontinue filgrastim
If ANC decreases to <1000/mm^3	Resume 5 mcg/kg/day
If ANC decreases to <1000/mm^3 while receiving 5 mcg/kg/day	Increase dose to 10 mcg/kg/day

Neutropenia following chemotherapy for ALL, non-Hodgkin's lymphoma, Wilms' tumor, advanced-stage neuroblastoma, rhabdomyosarcoma, CNS tumors, acute myelogenous leukemia: 5–17 mcg/kg/day SC or IV for up to 10 days.[6-10]

Congenital neutropenia or agranulocytosis: 3–15 mcg/kg/day SC as a single dose or divided and given twice a day[11] or 10–30 mcg/kg/day as an intermittent infusion up to 60 mcg/kg/day as a continuous infusion.[12]

Neutropenia and sepsis in neonates: 5–10 mcg/kg once[12-15] or twice[13,16] a day for 3–6 days.

Neutropenia/neutrophil dysfunction due to glycogen storage disease type 1b: 3–8 mcg/kg/day for up to 290 days[17] or 3–7.5 mcg/kg/day (SC) for 6–12 months.[18]

Mobilization of peripheral blood progenitor cells (PBPCs): 10–24 mcg/kg/day SC for 3 to 5 days before PBPC apheresis.[19-21]

Dosage adjustment in organ dysfunction

None noted.

Filgrastim

Maximum dosage	Not established. Children with severe chronic neutropenia (19 months–14 years) have received 3–8 mcg/kg/day for up to 290 days.[18] Five of 20 children with severe aplastic anemia who failed to respond to 400 mcg/m²/day were given 800 mcg/m²/day or 1200 mcg/m²/day for up to 2 weeks.[4]			

Additives

Additive	300 mcg per 1-mL Vial	480 mcg per 1.6-mL Vial	300 mcg per 0.5-mL Syringe	480 mcg per 0.8-mL Syringe
Acetate	0.59 mg	0.94 mg	0.295 mg	0.472 mg
Sorbitol	50 mg	80 mg	25 mg	40 mg
Polysorbate 80	0.04 mg	0.064 mg	0.02 mg	0.032 mg
Sodium	0.035 mg	0.056 mg	0.0175 mg	0.028 mg

Suitable diluents

D5W.[3]

Maximum concentration

600 mcg/mL[3]

Preparation and delivery

Important Correction Notice *see bottom of page*

Pediatric Injectable Drugs Ninth Edition (The Teddy Bear Book) [23]

The publisher wishes to inform you of the following corrections.

IV push

Not indicated.

Intermittent infusion

Over 15–60 minutes.[3,5,11-14]

Continuous infusion

The total daily dose may be diluted in 10–50 mL D5W and infused continuously over 24 hours by SC infusion at a rate not to exceed 10 mL/24 h.[3,12,22] (See Comments section.)

Other routes of administration

SC as a bolus injection or continuous infusion IV.[3] Not administered IM.[3]

Comments

The use of colony-stimulating factors decreased febrile neutropenia, length of hospitalization, and number of infectious episodes but did not shorten the duration of neutropenia nor lessen treatment delays in children with ALL.[23]

Monitoring: A CBC including a platelet count should be obtained before initiation therapy with filgrastim and should be repeated at least twice a week during treatment.[3] When the ANC if >10,000/mm³ after the expected neutrophil nadir following chemotherapy filgrastim should be discontinued.[3]

In the monograph for **Filgrastim** (pages 250-251)

"Preparation and delivery" section – second and third line should read:

"normal human serum albumin should be added at a final concentration of 2 mg/mL".

Fluconazole

Brand names	Diflucan

Medication error potential

Look-alike, sound-alike error potential.

USP reports that fluconazole has been confused with flucytosine, fluoxetine, furosemide, itraconazole, metronidazole and phenytoin sodium; no patient harm resulted.[1]

ISMP reports that Diflucan has been confused with Diprivan.[2] USP reports that Diflucan has been confused with diclofenac sodium, diflunisal, and Dilantin; no patient harm resulted.[1]

Contraindications and warnings

Contraindications: Concomitant administration with cisapride is contraindicated; concomitant administration with terfenadine is contraindicated in *adults* receiving multiple fluconazole doses of 400 mg or greater.[3] (See Drug interactions in Comments section.)

Fluconazole is contraindicated in patients with a hypersensitivity to the drug or any of its components.[3]

Warnings: Fluconazole has been associated with rare cases of hepatotoxicity, including liver failure and death, exfoliative skin disorders that have rarely resulted in death, and rare cases of QT prolongation and torsades de pointes.[3]

Infusion related cautions

Anaphylaxis has been reported rarely.[3]

Dosage

Daily dose varies according to infecting organism and response to therapy. Duration of therapy is generally 4 weeks for systemic infections and 10–12 weeks following sterilization of cerebrospinal fluid in patients with cryptococcal meningitis.[3]

Neonates

Treatment: 5–6 mg/kg/dose, per following schedule for dosing interval.[3-13]

>**≤7 days:** q 72 h.
>
>**7–14 days:** q 48 h.
>
>**>14 days:** q 24 h.

Although one study reported doses as large as 12 mg/kg/day given as a single dose in 20 patients (0–17 years of age), the authors did not specify whether any neonates received this dose.[10]

Prophylaxis: 3–6 mg/kg/dose; various schedules have been used, as follows[14-17]:

q 72 h for 14 days, then q 48 h for 14 days, then daily for a total of 6 weeks of prophylaxis

q 72 h for 14 days, then q 48 h for a total of up to 4–6 weeks of prophylaxis

q 72 h for 7 days then daily for a total of 28 days of prophylaxis

Fluconazole

Dosage *(cont.)*	**Infants and children:** In general, 3–6 mg/kg/day is given in a single dose; may give up to 12 mg/kg/day for serious infections.[18] **Cryptococcal meningitis:** Initial dose of 12 mg/kg (up to 400 mg) followed by 6–12 mg/kg (up to 200–400 mg) given once daily.[3,6,18-22] **Immunocompromised (e.g., leukemia, bone marrow transplant):** 6–12 mg/kg given once daily.[18-20] **Oropharyngeal/esophageal candidiasis:** Initial dose of 6 mg/kg followed by 3 mg/kg given once daily.[3,18] **Systemic candidiasis:** Initial dose of 12 mg/kg (up to 400 mg) followed by 6–12 mg/kg (up to 200–400 mg) given once daily.[3,6,18-21]
Dosage adjustment in organ dysfunction	Adjust dosage in patients with renal dysfunction.[3,13,23,24] If CrCl is 10–50 mL/min, administer 50% of normal dose; and if CrCl is <10 mL/min, administer 50% of normal dose and administer q 48 h.[3,25] Following hemodialysis, patients should be given the recommended dose based on CrCl.[3,25] With continuous renal replacement therapy, give 6 mg/kg q 24 h.[25] During continuous arteriovenous hemodiafiltration in an *adult*, total body clearance was similar to normal healthy volunteers.[26]
Maximum dosage	12 mg/kg/day[3,18,19] not to exceed 600 mg/day in older children and *adults*.[3] A 6-month-old with hydrocephalus and mycotic ventriculitis received 22 mg/kg/day with concomitant intraventricular administration (4 mg/24 h).[27]
Additives	Available in glass or plastic containers in either sodium chloride or dextrose. Each mL of solution contains either 9-mg NaCl or 56-mg dextrose, depending on the diluent.[3,28] The plastic containers contain DEHP.[3]
Suitable diluents	D5W, LR.[3,28]
Maximum concentration	2 mg/mL.[3,28]
Preparation and delivery	For PN compatibility information, please see Appendix D.
IV push	Not recommended.[3]
Intermittent infusion	≤2 mg/mL in D5W or LR.[3,28] Doses ≤6 mg/kg may be given over 1 hour[9,11,29] while doses >6 mg/kg should be given over 2 hours in pediatric patients.[11,20] Not to exceed 200 mg/h in *adults*.[3,28]
Continuous infusion	No information available to support administration by this method.
Other routes of administration	Has been administered intraventricularly (4 mg/24 h in an infant and 5 and 7.5 mg/24 h and 7.5 and 10 mg/12 h in an 18-year-old).[27]

Fluconazole

Comments

Significant adverse effects: Prolonged QT interval and torsades de pointes have been reported in an 11-year-old receiving fluconazole.[29]

Drug interactions: Fluconazole, a strong inhibitor for CYP2C9 and CYP2C19, a moderator inhibitor of CYP3A4, and a weak inhibitor of CYP1A2, is associated with numerous drug interactions.[3,30,31] Consult appropriate resources for dosing recommendations before combining any drug with fluconazole.

Pharmacokinetic considerations: One pharmacokinetic study reported increased fluconazole clearance in children; the authors suggested q 12 h dosing may be required in children 3–12 years of age in order to achieve therapeutic serum concentrations.[32] Fluconazole pharmacokinetics have also been evaluated in young infants using a simulated model.[33]

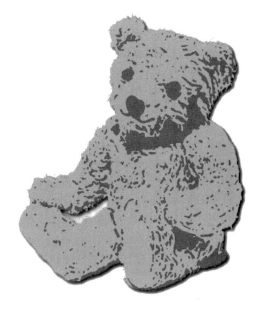

Flumazenil

Brand names	Romazicon

Medication error potential

Look-alike, sound-alike drug names.

USP reports confusion for Romazicon with rocuronium.[1]

Contraindications and warnings

US boxed warning: Flumazenil has been associated with seizures.[2] These occur most frequently when (1) a benzodiazepine have been used for long-term sedation; (2) in association with a tricyclic antidepressant overdose; (3) concurrent major sedative-hypnotic drug withdrawal; (4) recent therapy with repeated doses of parenteral benzodiazepines; and/or (5) myoclonic jerking or seizure activity prior to flumazenil administration.[2] Practitioners should individualize the dosage of flumazenil and be prepared to manage seizures.[2] (See Rare adverse effects in Comments section.)

Contraindications: In those with a known hypersensitivity to flumazenil or benzodiazepines[2] and in those receiving a benzodiazepine for control of a life-threatening condition (e.g., ICP or status epilepticus).[2] Flumazenil should not be used in those with symptoms of serious tricyclic antidepressant overdosage.[2] (See other in Comments section.)

Other warnings: The use of flumazenil is not recommended in patients with epilepsy who have received benzodiazepine therapy for a prolonged period.[2] It should be used cautiously in the ICU setting because of the increased risk of unrecognized benzodiazepine dependence.[2] Administration to diagnose benzodiazepine-induced sedation in the ICU is not recommended due to the risk of adverse events.[2] Flumazenil should not be used until the effects of neuromuscular blockade have been fully reversed.[2] Use cautiously in cases of mixed drug overdosage because their toxic effects (e.g., convulsions and cardiac dysrhythmias) may emerge.

Infusion related cautions

To minimize pain or local inflammation, infuse through a freely running IV into a large vein.[2] Extravasation may cause local irritation.[2]

Dosage

The safety and effectiveness of flumazenil has not been established in patients <1 year of age.[2] The dose should be individualized based on patient response.

Reversal of

Benzodiazepine-induced anesthesia or conscious sedation: 0.01 mg/kg (up to 0.2 mg) over 15 seconds.[2-10] If the desired clinical response is not achieved within 45 seconds, give 0.01 mg/kg (up to 0.2 mg) and repeated at 60-second intervals to a maximum total dose of 0.05 mg/kg or 1 mg, whichever is smaller.[2,8] About 50% of patients require five doses.[2,8]

A single, large dose of 0.1–0.2 mg has been used successfully.[10-12] Conversely, one study used smaller doses (0.002 mg/kg).[13] Another study used a loading dose of 10 mcg/kg followed by 5 mcg/kg/min until the patient awoke or until a maximum of 1 mg had been infused.[5] Some patients who regain complete consciousness may develop resedation within 19–50 minutes.[2] (See Other in Comments section.)

Benzodiazepine overdose or ingestion: 0.01 mg/kg; if no effect in 1–2 minutes; repeat dose q 2 min until patient responds or a total of 1 mg is given. A single dose of 0.2 mg (0.017 mg/kg) was used in a 12-kg child.[14] Initial doses have been followed by infusions of 0.004–0.005 mg/kg/h for 2–6 hours to prevent resedation.[15,16] Infusions as large as 0.3 mg/kg/h have been used.[5]

Neonatal apnea due to prenatal benzodiazepine exposure: 0.02 mg/kg followed by 0.05 mg/kg/h for 6 hours.[17]

Dosage *(cont.)*	**Diagnostic potential**
	Coma of unknown origin: Several studies have reported successful use of flumazenil in this situation.[18-20] Forty percent of patients could provide information regarding their ingestion within about 10 minutes, which resulted in a 30% decrease in gastric lavage, urinary catheterization, and intubation.
	Diagnose of benzodiazepine-induced sedation in the ICU: Not recommended due to the risk of adverse events.[2] The prognostic significance of a patient's failure to respond in cases confounded by metabolic disorder, traumatic injury, drugs other than benzodiazepines, or any other reasons not associated with benzodiazepine receptor occupancy is unknown.[2]
Dosage adjustment in organ dysfunction	No adjustment in renal dysfunction.[21] Flumazenil clearance is reduced to 40% to 60% in mild-to-moderate hepatic disease and to 25% in severe hepatic dysfunction.[2] The initial dose should not be reduced, but repeat doses should be reduced or the interval prolonged in hepatic dysfunction.[2]
Maximum dosage	0.2 mg/dose up to a cumulative dose of 1 mg in infants and children.[2,11] Seventy-five percent of *adults* respond to 3 mg.[2] Doses above 3 mg do not produce additional effects.[2]
Additives	Contains 1.8 mg methylparabens, 0.2 mg propylparabens/mL.[22] (See Appendix C for specific information about parabens potential for toxicity.)
Suitable diluents	D5W, LR, or NS.[2]
Maximum concentration	0.1 mg/mL (commercially available).[2]
Preparation and delivery	**Stability:** Store at 15°C to 30°C.[22] Should be used within 24 hours following removal from vial.[22]
IV push	0.1 mg/mL over 15 seconds (conscious sedation) to 30 (general anesthesia) seconds.[2,22] Not to exceed 0.2 mg/min.[2]
Intermittent infusion	None.
Continuous infusion	Has been given by this method to prevent/minimize resedation; however, the final concentration and solution type was not provided.[5,15,16]
Other routes of administration	Undiluted flumazenil has been given rectally to seven children.[23,24] Doses ranged from 0.02–0.033 mg/kg and time to regain consciousness ranged from 3–15 minutes. No resedation was reported.

Flumazenil

Rare adverse effects

Seizures: Although rare (1% to 2%), seizure activity may occur in patients (1) dependent on benzodiazepines for seizure control; (2) with severe hepatic impairment, who are physically dependent on benzodiazepines; and (3) who have ingested large doses of other drugs (mixed-drug overdose).[2] Activity has ranged from simple twitching and jerking, to single or multiple seizure events, to status epilepticus.[3] Seizures responded to reintroduction of a benzodiazepine or use of an anticonvulsant.[2,3] Because of the presence of flumazenil, larger than normal doses of benzodiazepines may be required.

Resedation: Due to the short duration of flumazenil, compared to some benzodiazepines, resedation may occur. This is especially true in the pediatric population. The use of flumazenil to reverse the effects of benzodiazepines used for conscious sedation was evaluated in one uncontrolled trial involving 107 pediatric patients (1–17 years).[8] Although 7 patients (1–5 years) experienced resedation between 19 and 50 minutes (mean 25 minutes) after the start of flumazenil administration, none return to the baseline level of sedation.[8] Patients experiencing resedation may require repeat bolus doses or continuous infusion.

Elevation in intracranial pressure (ICP): Has been noted to increase intracranial pressure (ICP) and decrease cerebral perfusion pressure in those who already have an elevated ICP; hence, should be used cautiously in those with head trauma.[3]

Monitoring: Monitor patient for return of sedation or respiratory depression for 2 hours after administration of last dose of flumazenil.[2,6,9] (See Rare adverse effects in Comments section.)

Other: Symptoms of tricyclic antidepressant overdosage include motor abnormalities (e.g., twitching, rigidity, focal seizures), arrhythmias (e.g., wide QRS complexes, ventricular arrhythmias, heart block), anticholinergic effects (e.g., mydriasis, dry mucosa, hypoperistalsis), or cardiovascular collapse.[2]

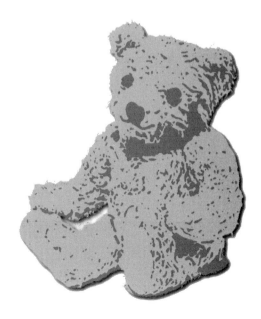

Fomepizole

Brand names	Antizol

Medication error potential

Look-alike, sound- alike drug names.

ISMP's *Confused Drug Names* lists confusion with omeprazole.[1]

Contraindications and warnings

Contraindications: Should not be administered to patients with a documented serious hypersensitivity reaction to fomepizole or other pyrazoles.[2]

Warnings: Should not be given undiluted or by bolus injection.[2] (See Infusion related cautions section.)

Infusion related cautions

Vein irritation and phlebosclerosis can occur following rapid administration ($\leq$5 minutes) of a 25-mg/mL solution.[2]

Dosage

Fomepizole is indicated if ethylene glycol or methanol ingestion is suspected based on patient history and/or anion gap metabolic acidosis, increased osmolar gap, visual disturbances, oxalate crystals in the urine, or a documented serum ethylene glycol or methanol concentration >20 mg/dL.[2]

Fomepizole is safer than ethanol or hemodialysis for suspected or confirmed ethylene glycol or methanol poisoning and is considered first-line therapy by the American Academy of Clinical Toxicology.[3,4] (See Comments section.)

Although safety and efficacy in pediatric patients has not been established,[2] fomepizole has been given to infants,[6-9] children,[9-12] and adolescents.[9]

Loading dose of 15 mg/kg over 30 minutes[2,5-8,10-12] followed by 10 mg/kg q 12 h for four doses.[2,5,8] then increased to 15 mg/kg q 12 h.[2,5] Fomepizole may be discontinued at any time when ethylene glycol or methanol concentrations are <20 mg/dL and the patient is asymptomatic with a normal pH.[2,5]

If used during hemodialysis, the interval should be decreased to q 4 h.[2,5] (See Dosage adjustment in organ dysfunction section and Comments section.)

Although little information is available, some advocate concurrent administration of thiamine (ethylene glycol),[11,13] pyridoxine (ethylene glycol),[5,11,13] and folic acid or folinic acid (methanol).[5,14] (See Comments section.)

Dosage adjustment in organ dysfunction

Extensively metabolized by the liver, with metabolites excreted renally.[2] Dosage adjustments in organ dysfunction has not been studied. Recommendations relative to hemodialysis are[2,5]

Beginning of hemodialysis	<6 h since last dose: do not administer $\geq$6 h since last dose: give next scheduled dose
During hemodialysis	normal dose q 4 h
At completion of hemodialysis	<1 h: do not administer dose 1–3 h: 50% of next scheduled dose >3 h: give next scheduled dose
Off hemodialysis	Administer next scheduled dose 12 h after the last dose that was administered

Some advocate a continuous infusion of 1–1.5 mg/kg/h during hemodialysis.[15-17]

Fomepizole

Maximum dosage	15 mg/kg/dose.[2] Some have advocated 20 mg/kg dosing.[18]
Additives	None.
Suitable diluents	<25 mg/mL in NS or D5W.[2]
Maximum concentration	<25 mg/mL.[2]
Preparation and delivery	**Stability:** Solidifies in the vial at temperatures <25°C. If solid, running the vial under warm water or holding in the hand will liquefy. Solidification does not affect the stability or efficacy. Dilutes solution is stable and sterile for at least 24 hours when refrigerated or at room temperature.[2]
IV push	Not recommended.[3]
Intermittent infusion	All doses (including loading dose) over 30 minutes.[2,5]
Continuous infusion	1–1.5 mg/kg/h during hemodialysis.[15-17]
Other routes of administration	Although IV is preferred, one group of authors notes that about one third of their patients receive the antidote orally.[15,19,20]
Comments	**Rare adverse effects:** Vertical nystagmus, lasting 60 minutes, has been reported within 2 hours of a single dose of 15 mg/kg of fomepizole in a 6-year-old child.[11] This adverse effect has not been reported in any other patient. Although adverse effects are rare,[21] transient elevations in ALT and AST have been reported.[2,5] **Monitoring:** Serum concentrations of fomepizole should be monitored. Concentrations of 8.2–24.6 mg/L are normally seen following dosing; however, concentrations of 0.8 mg/L are required to inhibit alcohol dehydrogenase in most patients.[5] Acidosis and electrolyte imbalances can affect cardiac function; hence, ECG should be monitored.[2] If comatose an EEG may be required. Hepatic enzymes and white blood cell counts should be monitored during treatment.[2] Plasma/urinary ethylene glycol or methanol levels, urinary oxalate (ethylene glycol), plasma/urinary osmolality, renal/hepatic function, serum electrolytes, arterial blood gases; anion and osmolar gaps.[2] Clinical signs and symptoms of ethylene glycol or methanol intoxication should be assessed. **Pharmacokinetics:** Unknown if the pharmacokinetics in infants and children differs from *adults* due to insufficient studies. Elimination is best characterized by Michaelis-Menten kinetics after acute doses, with saturable elimination occurring at therapeutic blood concentrations (8.2–24.6 mg/L).[2,18] It is thought that fomepizole rapidly induces its own metabolism; however, little evidence supports autoinduction.[18] After enzyme induction, elimination follows first-order kinetics. **Other:** Fomepizole does not affect existing acid but works by halting further acid production. It promotes the breakdown of formic acid (metabolite of methanol); therefore, supplemental intravenous 1 mg/kg q 6 h of either folate or folinic acid (leucovorin) should be considered in those poisoned with methanol.[5,14] Thiamine (100 mg q 6 h) and pyridoxine (1 mg/kg up to 50 mg q 6 h) may be administered to prevent the formation of oxalic acid in those who have ingested ethylene glycol.[5,11,13]

Foscarnet Sodium

Brand names	Foscavir, generic
Medication error potential	None reported by ISMP or USP.[1,2]
Contraindications and warnings	**US boxed warning:** Renal impairment is the major toxicity of foscarnet injection and frequent monitoring of renal function and hydration, accompanied by dose adjustment for renal function, is imperative.[3]
	Seizures related to alterations in electrolytes have been reported, and patients must be monitored for these changes and any potential sequelae.[3]
	Foscarnet is only indicated for use in immunocompromised patients with CMV retinitis and mucocutaneous acyclovir-resistant HSV infections.[3]
	Contraindications: Clinically significant hypersensitivity to foscarnet.[3]
	Other warnings: Anemia and granulocytopenia have been reported.[3]
Infusion related cautions	Patients should be adequately hydrated prior to receiving foscarnet. Diuresis should be established prior to the first dose by administering NS or D5W; administer fluid concurrently with subsequent doses of foscarnet.[3]
	To avoid local irritation, administer via a vein that provides adequate blood flow for rapid dilution and distribution.[3]
Dosage	**CMV retinitis:** 180 mg/kg/day in two to three divided doses for 14–21 days, followed by 90–120 mg/kg once daily as maintenance.[3-7]
	HSV infection resistant to acyclovir: 80–120 mg/kg/day in two to three divided doses until the infection has resolved.[3,4,8,9]
	Varicella infection resistant to acyclovir: 80–120 mg/kg/day in two to three divided doses until the infection has resolved.[10,11] One case reported the use of 165 mg/kg/day for acyclovir-resistant Oka strain varicella infection while on chemotherapy.[12]
Dosage adjustment in organ dysfunction	Dosage adjustments are recommended for renal dysfunction.[3,4] Data is limited regarding use in patients with baseline CrCl <50 mL/min or SCr >2.8 mg/dL, or in patients receiving hemodialysis or peritoneal dialysis; the manufacturer does not recommend use in these patients.[3,13]
	One reference suggests administering 60–80 mg/kg q 48 h for CrCl 30–50 mL/min, 50–65 mg/kg q 48 h for CrCl 10–29 mL/min, and use not recommended for CrCl <10 mL/min.[13]
Maximum dosage	180 mg/kg/day during induction therapy.[3,4,5-7]
Additives	None.[3,14]
Suitable diluents	D5W, NS.[3,14]
Maximum concentration	12 mg/mL in NS or D5W for peripheral infusion and 24 mg/mL for central administration.[3,14]

Foscarnet Sodium

Preparation and delivery	**Stability:** Solutions prepared using D5W or NS should be stored under refrigeration and used within 24 hours.[3,14]
	Compatibility: No other drugs or supplements should be infused in the same catheter as foscarnet.[3,14] D30W, LR, and many other drugs and solutions (including PN solutions) are incompatible with foscarnet.[3,14] For additional PN compatibility information, please see Appendix D.
IV push	Not recommended.[3,14]
Intermittent infusion	For peripheral administration, dilute with D5W or NS to a concentration of 12 mg/mL. For infusion via a central line, the 24-mg/mL solution may be used and no dilution is required. Infuse at a rate not to exceed 60 mg/kg over 1 hour or 120 mg/kg over 2 hours.[3,14]
Continuous infusion	No information.
Other routes of administration	Not recommended.[3]
Comments	Foscarnet deposits in teeth and bone have been documented in animal studies, especially during early growth and development; deposits in bone have been reported in humans.[3]
	One report described successful HIV rescue therapy over 4 weeks in a 4-year-old with 90 mg/kg IV q 12 h foscarnet in combination with IV zidovudine and oral nelfinavir and nevirapine.[15]
	One report described the use of ganciclovir and foscarnet concomitantly in a 9-year-old HIV patient who presented with CMV polyradiculopathy.[16]
	One report described the course of a 24-week premature infant with CMV-associated haemophagocytic lymphohistiocytosis being treated with 100 mg/kg/day of foscarnet after ganciclovir therapy failed.[17]

Fosphenytoin

Brand names	Cerebyx

Medication error potential

Look-alike, sound-alike drug names.

USP reports confusion with phenytoin resulted in patient harm.[1] Cerebyx has been confused with Avelox, Celebrex, cetirizine, and Precedex.[1]

Confusion between the **mg/mL concentration** of fosphenytoin (50 mg PE/mL) and **total drug content per vial** (either 100 mg PE/2 mL vial or 500 mg PE/10 mL vial) has resulted in overdose and death.[2] To avoid confusion, the total drug content per container should be used (instead of the concentration in mg per mL) and pediatric hospitals should stock only the 2 mL vial.[3] ISMP recommends that no order for fosphenytoin should be accepted if "PE" is omitted.[4]

Confusion with phenytoin has resulted in patient harm.[1]

Contraindications and warnings

Contraindications: Patients with a known hypersensitivity to Cerebyx or its ingredients or to other hydantoins (e.g., phenytoin) should not receive fosphenytoin.[5] Parenteral phenytoin effects ventricular automaticity and is contraindicated in patients with sinus bradycardia, sino-atrial block, second and third degree A-V block, and Adams-Stokes syndrome.[5]

Warnings: Fosphenytoin should *always* be prescribed and dispensed in phenytoin sodium equivalents (PE) since doses of Cerebyx are expressed as their phenytoin sodium equivalents (PE=phenytoin sodium equivalent). Do *not* make any adjustment in the recommended doses, concentration in solutions or rate of administration when substituting Cerebyx for phenytoin sodium or vice versa.[5]

Abrupt discontinuation of fosphenytoin may increase seizure frequency and/or precipitate status epilepticus.[5] If an allergic or hypersensitivity reaction or if a life-threatening adverse effect occurs, rapid substitution of alternative anticonvulsant may be necessary.[5] If a rash is present, an anticonvulsant *not* belonging to the hydantoin family and one structurally dissimilar should be used.[5,6-8] (See Comments section.)

The FDA is investigating the possibility of an increased risk of serious skin reactions (e.g., Stevens-Johnson syndrome and toxic epidermal necrolysis) in patients given phenytoin who have the human leukocyte antigen allele HLA-B*1502.[5] This allele occurs almost exclusively in individuals with ancestry across broad areas of Asia, including Han Chinese, Filipinos, Malaysians, South Asian Indians, and Thais.[5] Until the FDA evaluation is finalized, fosphenytoin should be avoided as an alternative for carbamazepine in patients who test positive for HLA-B*1502.[5] (See Comments section.)

Infusion related cautions

Administration of >3 mg PE/kg/min (150 mg PE/min) or doses larger than 15 mg PE/kg may lead to hypotension, bradycardia, and/or arrhythmias.[5] Vomiting, transient pruritus (groin and neck areas) tinnitus, nystagmus, somnolence, and ataxia have also occurred when faster rates or larger doses have been given.[5,9]

Dosage

Doses of fosphenytoin are expressed in phenytoin sodium equivalents (PEs); therefore, fosphenytoin and phenytoin products can be converted directly (1 mg PE = 1 mg phenytoin).[5]

Larger doses may be required in obese patients.[10] (See Comments section.)

Fosphenytoin

Dosage *(cont.)*	**Acute seizure or status epilepticus**
	Loading doses (assumes no previous fosphenytoin/phenytoin)
	Neonates (few published reports in newborns; may prefer to use phenobarbital or a benzodiazepine): 15–24 mg PE/kg at a rate not to exceed 1–3 mg PE/kg/min[3] have resulted in total phenytoin concentrations of 10.5–34.5 mg/L (mean 21.6 mg/L) 8–12 hours after a dose.[11,12]
	Infants and children: 15–20 mg PE/kg.[5,13,14] at a rate not to exceed 1–3 mg PE/kg/min[3] or 150 mg PE/min.[5]
	Maintenance doses: 4–8 mg PE/kg/day given as two to three doses.[5,13,14] Final maintenance dose should be individualized. Some reports have noted a failure to obtain "therapeutic" serum concentration despite adequate doses.[14-16]
	Post-traumatic epilepsy (see status epilepticus for dosing): Although prophylactic phenytoin for the prevention of epilepsy following head trauma is controversial, some have reported that it reduces early post-traumatic epilepsy.[17-19] It should not be used for the prevention of late epilepsy.[19] (See Comments section.)
Dosage adjustment in organ dysfunction	Decreases in protein binding, increases in volume of distribution, and altered clearance in hepatic or renal dysfunction require dosage adjustment and unique monitoring.[5] (See Comments section.) Although several equations have been used to predict free phenytoin serum concentrations in those with low albumin or renal failure, they may over predict concentrations and are not recommended for use in children.[20]
Maximum dosage	Typically patients require <8 mg PE/kg/day from chronic dosing. One study in infants suggests that larger fosphenytoin maintenance doses (10 mg PE/kg/day) and more frequent dosing may be required.[15,21] Patients receiving medications known to increase the clearance of phenytoin may require larger doses.
Additives	There are approximately 0.0037 mmol of phosphate in 1 PE of fosphenytoin.[3] (See Other in Comments section.)
Suitable diluents	D5W, D10W, LR, NS, ½NS, D5LR, D5½NS.[22]
Maximum concentration	25 PE/mL.[5]
Preparation and delivery	**Stability:** Do not store at room temperature for more than 48 hours. Refrigerate at 2°C to 8°C. Do not use if particulate matter is visible.[5]
IV push	Not recommended.[3]
Intermittent infusion	≤25 mg PE/mL[5] at a rate of 1–3 PE/kg/min (maximum of 150 mg PE/min).[3,5] (See Infusion related caution section.)
Continuous infusion	Not given via this method.

265

Fosphenytoin

Other routes of administration	Rapidly absorbed via the IM route.[23] Doses of 15–18.7 mg PE/kg have been given to patients >6 months. Total injection volumes: infants 1–6.1 mL, children 2.6–8.7 mL, adolescents 5–12 mL.[24] Maintenance doses have been given IM for up to 4 days in volumes of 0.3–6 mL.[24] For IM administration, the quadriceps have been recommended. Although irritation may occur at the site of injection, the incidence is less than that noted with phenytoin sodium.[9,25] To minimize irritation, rotate the injection site and use multiple injection sites for large medication volumes. Has been given intraosseously.

Comments	**Rare adverse effects:** Anticonvulsant hypersensitivity syndrome is an acute, life-threatening, idiosyncratic reaction that has been reported in patients receiving phenytoin, phenobarbital, carbamazepine, primidone, and lamotrigine.[6-8] Symptoms generally develop within 1–12 weeks following initiation and include a classic triad of fever, rash, and lymphadenopathy.[6-8] Peripheral blood leucocytosis and eosinophilia and internal organ involvement may also be noted. Immediate discontinuation of the suspected anticonvulsant is essential for good outcome.[6-8] Cross-reactivity among the aromatic anticonvulsants has been noted; hence, these should not be used as alternative agents.[6-8]

Suicidal behavior/ideation: The incidence of this adverse effect has been noted to be greater than placebo (0.43% vs 0.24% risk) in patients receiving 11 anticonvulsants (carbamazepine, divalproex sodium, felbamate, gabapentin, lamotrigine, levetiracetam, oxcarbazepine, pregabalin, tiagabine, topiramate, zonisamide) as either monotherapy or as adjuvant therapy for the treatment of epilepsy, psychiatric disorders, and other conditions.[26] The FDA will require that the product labeling of the entire class of antiepileptics include a warning concerning the risk of suicide.

Hyperphosphatemia has been attributed to fosphenytoin in a 17-year-old patient with renal failure.[27]

Monitoring: Continuous monitoring of blood pressure, respiratory function, and ECG during IV loading doses and for approximately 10–20 minutes after the end of an infusion.[5]

Due to an increased fraction of unbound phenytoin in patients with renal or hepatic disease, or in those with hypoalbuminemia, the interpretation of total phenytoin plasma concentrations should be made with caution and unbound phenytoin concentrations may be more useful.

Free phenytoin serum concentrations should be measured in newborns, in patients with renal dysfunction, or in those who are hypoalbuminemic because of decreases in protein binding, increases in volume of distribution, and altered clearance.[5,28,29] Phenytoin serum concentrations should not be measured until at least 2 hours after an IV dose and for 4 hours after an IM dose of fosphenytoin.[8,9,12]

The FDA does not recommend testing for the presence of *HLA-B*1502* prior to initiating phenytoin.[5]

Pharmacokinetics: In obese patients the loading doses should be calculated on adjusted body weight using the following equation[10]:

Dosing weight (kg) = ideal body weight (IBW) + 1.33 (measured weight − IBW). (See Appendix B.)

Children with severe, acute neurotrauma have markedly altered protein binding and phenytoin metabolism and may require larger doses and more frequent dosing.[21] Free serum phenytoin concentration should be monitored.

Drug interactions: No drugs are known to interfere with conversion of fosphenytoin to phenytoin.[5] Because phenytoin is a substrate for CYP2C9, CYP2C19 and CYP2A4, is an inducer of CYP2C9, CYP2C19, CYP2B6 and CYP3A families, and UGT, and is highly protein bound, it is associated with numerous drug interactions.[20] Consult appropriate resources for dosing recommendations before combining any drug with fosphenytoin or phenytoin.

Comments *(cont.)*

Laboratory interference: Fosphenytoin may cross react with phenytoin in fluorescence polarization immunoassay (e.g., TDx/TDxFLx) and enzyme multiplied (e.g., EMIT) assays to falsely overestimate fosphenytoin concentrations if measured too soon after a dose of fosphenytoin. The error is dependent on serum concentrations of phenytoin/fosphenytoin, which is influenced by dose, route, rate of administration, and time of sampling relative to dosing.[5] It is recommended that phenytoin concentrations not be measured until at least 2 hours after an IV dose and 4 hours after an IM dose of fosphenytoin.[30] Blood samples should be collected in tubes containing EDTA, which is an anticoagulant that minimize ex vivo conversion from fosphenytoin to phenytoin.[5]

Phenytoin may decrease serum concentrations of T4; produce artifactually low results in dexamethasone or metyrapone tests; and cause increased in serum concentrations of glucose, alkaline phosphatase, and gamma glutamyl transpeptidase (GGT).[5]

Other: Formaldehyde is produced on conversion to phenytoin. No accumulation has been noted in *adults* and children during short-term use; however, caution is warranted in those with renal impairment.[5]

Furosemide

Brand names	Lasix

Medication error potential

Look-alike, sound-alike error potential.

ISMP reports that Lasix was confused with Luvox.[1]

USP reports that Lasix was confused with Lovenox and Lanoxin. Furosemide was confused with famotidine, finasteride, fluconazole, fluoxetine, fosinopril, loperamide, and torsemide. No patient harm resulted.[2]

Contraindications and warnings

Contraindications: Patients with anuria or hypersensitivity to furosemide.[3]

Warnings: Loop diuretics used in excessive amounts may lead to profound diuresis with fluid and electrolyte losses.[3]

Patients with sulfonamide allergy may be hypersensitive to furosemide.[3]

Infusion related cautions

Transient and permanent ototoxicity has been associated with administration rates >4 mg/min or >0.5 mg/kg/min.[4-6] (See Comments section.)

Dosage

Diuresis

    Intermittent dosing

        Neonates

           <29 weeks postconceptional age: 1 mg/kg q 24 h.[7]

           >32 weeks postconceptional age: 1 mg/kg q 12 h.[7]

        Infants and children: 0.5–2 mg/kg q 4,[8,9] 6,[10] or 24 hours.[8,11-22] Dose may be increased by 1 mg/kg to achieve desired response.[11-14]

        Continuous infusion dosing: 0.1 mg/kg bolus (≥1 mg in those >10 kg) followed by continuous infusion of 0.05–0.4 mg/kg/h.[8-10,22] A 24-hour study in infants found that continuous infusion resulted in a similar urine output at a lower dose than intermittent bolus doses (2.5 ± 0.3 mg/kg [n = 11] vs 6.8 ± 1.2 mg/kg [n = 15]).[9]

Alternating furosemide with ethacrynic acid may not overcome diuretic resistance.[23]

Nephrotic syndrome: 0.5–2 mg/kg after albumin 25% infusion.[24-29]

Dosage adjustment in organ dysfunction

Larger doses may be required in patients with renal dysfunction.[3]

During ECMO, 63% to 87% of the dose was adsorbed to the circuit. Saturation occurred by 30 minutes.[30]

Maximum dosage

4[6] or 6 mg/kg have been suggested in children.[11] In *adults* with acute renal failure, an initial dose of up to 2 g has been used.[3]

Additives

Contains 0.162 mEq sodium/10 mg furosemide.[31]

Suitable diluents

D5W, NS, LR.[31]

Furosemide

Maximum concentration	10 mg/mL (undiluted).[9,31]
Preparation and delivery	**Stability:** The final pH of diluted furosemide must be slightly alkaline or in the neutral pH range or precipitation of furosemide may occur.[31] **Compatibility:** See Appendix D for PN compatibility information. **Photosensitivity:** Light exposure may cause discoloration. Discolored products should not be used.[31]
IV push	Over 1–2 minutes, not to exceed 4 mg/min in *adults*.[3,31] Not to exceed 0.5 mg/kg/min in infants and children.[12,13,16] (See Comments section.)
Intermittent infusion	Infusion over at least 5–10 minutes may provide protection against otoxicity in infants.[32]
Continuous infusion	Dilute to 1–2 mg/mL[3] in D5W, LR, or NS for continuous infusion.[31]
Other routes of administration	IM.[3]
Comments	**Adverse events:** Electrolyte abnormalities including hypokalemia can occur. The duration of treatment is directly related to the development of sensorineural hearing loss in neonates with persistent pulmonary hypertension.[32] Investigators point out that this may be transient; however, they suggest that infusion over at least 5–10 minutes may be protective.[32] Premature neonates with respiratory distress syndrome may have an increased risk of persistent patent ductus arteriosus secondary to furosemide stimulation of renal production of prostaglandin E2.[33] Up to 65% of premature infants develop nephrocalcinosis following prolonged use.[6,34] About 50% of these resolve within 5–6 months of drug discontinuation[35]; however, obstructive nephrolithiasis can occur.[36] In these patients, renal ultrasonography is warranted a few months after initiation of therapy.[37] **Monitoring:** Serum potassium concentration monitoring is important.[3] **Drug interactions:** Aminoglycosides potentiate the ototoxicity of loop diuretics.[3,38-41] **Pharmacokinetics:** Furosemide is 91% to 99% protein bound. Use cautiously in jaundiced neonates at risk for kernicterus. In vitro studies have shown bilirubin displacement in pooled cord blood samples from critically ill neonates receiving furosemide.[42]

Ganciclovir Sodium

Brand names	Cytovene

Medication error potential

Look-alike, sound-alike error potential.

USP reports that ganciclovir has been confused with valacyclovir; no patient harm resulted. USP also reports that ganciclovir has been confused with acyclovir; patient harm resulted.[1]

Contraindications and warnings

US boxed warning: Granulocytopenia, anemia, and thrombocytopenia are possible with ganciclovir therapy. IV ganciclovir is indicated for use only in the treatment of CMV retinitis in immunocompromised patients and for the prevention of CMV disease in transplant patients at risk for CMV disease.[2]

Contraindications: Patients with hypersensitivity to ganciclovir or acyclovir.[2]

Other warnings: Do not administer if ANC <500 cells/μL or platelet count is <25,000 cells/μL. Ganciclovir has been shown to impair fertility in animal studies. Because of the possible teratogenic potential, contraception should be used for an appropriate timeframe during and after therapy.[2]

Infusion related cautions

After initial reconstitution, the solution has a pH of 11. Despite further dilution, phlebitis and/or pain may occur at infusion site, and it should be administered only into veins with adequate blood flow to permit rapid dilution and distribution.[2]

Dosage

Adequate hydration is recommended during therapy.[2]

CMV prophylaxis in high-risk hosts

> **Bone marrow, liver, kidney transplantation:** 10 mg/kg/day divided q 12 h for 1–2 weeks, then 5 mg/kg given once daily or 6 mg/kg/day for 5 days/week for 100 days.[3-9] Maintenance doses of 5 mg/kg/day for 3–5 days per week were well tolerated but did not prevent reactivation of CMV.[10]
>
> One reference recommends 6 mg/kg/day for 1 month, followed by 6 mg/kg/day for 5 days per week for a total of 100 days of treatment for liver transplantation patients.[11]
>
> **Cardiac transplantation:** One reference recommends 10 mg/kg/day divided q 12 h for 2 weeks followed by 6 mg/kg/day for 2 weeks, combined with CMV immunoglobulin therapy at 0, 2, 4, 6, 8, 12, and 16 weeks.[12]
>
> **Lung transplantation:** One reference gave 10 mg/kg/day divided q 12 h for 2 weeks followed by 5 mg/kg/day for up to 5 months.[13] Another reference gave 10 mg/kg/day divided q 12 h for 21 days, followed by 5 mg/kg/day to complete 12 weeks of therapy.[14]

CMV retinitis: 10 mg/kg/day divided q 12 h for 14–21 days, then 5 mg/kg/day given 7 days/week or 6 mg/kg/day given 5 days/week.[2,7]

CMV infection in allograft recipients: 7.5–10 mg/kg/day divided q 8–12 h for 14–47 days.[15-18]

Congenital (symptomatic) CMV infections: 5–15 mg/kg/day divided q 12 h in neonates and infants.[19-27]

Dosage (cont.)

CMV/HIV coinfection (use not established): One infant received 10 mg/kg/day divided q 12 h for 2 weeks, then 5 mg/kg/day as maintenance.[28]

CMV infection in immunocompetent host: One child (30 months old) received 10 mg/kg/day in two divided doses for 21 days due to a deteriorating case of primary CMV.[29]

Human herpesvirus-6 in BMT patients (use not established)

Prophylaxis: 10 mg/kg/day divided q 12 h for 1 week prior to transplantation followed by 5 mg/kg/day for 120 days after transplant.[30]

Treatment: 10 mg/kg/day divided q 12 h for 2 weeks followed by 5 mg/kg given daily or three times/week for 4 weeks.[30] One 7-year-old received ganciclovir up to 24 mg/kg/day divided into three doses for treatment of HHV-6 encephalitis.[31] (See Maximum dosage section.)

Dosage adjustment in organ dysfunction

Adjust dosage in patients with renal dysfunction.[2]

CrCl (mL/min)	Induction	Maintenance
≥70	5 mg/kg q 12 h	5 mg/kg q 24 h
50–69	2.5 mg/kg q 12 h	2.5 mg/kg q 24 h
25–49	2.5 mg/kg q 24 h	1.25 mg/kg q 24 h
10–24	1.25 mg/kg q 24 h	0.625 mg/kg q 24 h
<10	1.25 mg/kg three times/week following hemodialysis	0.625 mg/kg three times/week following hemodialysis

Another reference suggests the following dosing in renal dysfunction[32]

GFR (mL/min/1.73m²)	Induction	Maintenance
30–50	2.5 mg/kg q 24 h	1.25 mg/kg q 24 h
10–29	1.25 mg/kg q 24 h	0.625 mg/kg q 24 h
<10	1.25 mg/kg three times/week	0.625 mg/kg three times/week

Dose adjustments should also be considered in patients with hematologic toxicity. No dose adjustment is necessary with hepatic dysfunction.

Maximum dosage

15 mg/kg/day has been given to infants[25]; recommended maximum dose per labeling is 10 mg/kg/day.[2] There is a published report of a 7-year-old receiving up to 24 mg/kg/day for HHV-6, with very close therapeutic drug monitoring and renal function monitoring.[31]

Additives

46 mg sodium/500 mg ganciclovir.[2,33]

Suitable diluents

D5W, NS, R, LR.[2,33]

Maximum concentration

10 mg/mL.[2,33]

Ganciclovir Sodium

Preparation and delivery	**Preparation:** Reconstituted solution has a pH of 11. Therefore, avoid direct contact with skin or mucous membranes. If contact occurs, wash skin thoroughly with soap and water and rinse eyes thoroughly with plain water. Use safe handling techniques (latex gloves, protective eyewear, and other protective equipment); ganciclovir is carcinogenic and mutagenic.[2]
	Stability: Reconstitute 500 mg in 10 mL of SW and then dilute to ≤10 mg/mL in suitable diluents.[2,33] BW (containing parabens) is incompatible with ganciclovir; reconstitution with BW may cause precipitation.[2,33]
	Reconstituted solution in the vial is stable for 12 hours at room temp. The further diluted solution for infusion should be refrigerated and used within 24 hours to prevent bacterial contamination.[2,33]
	Compatibility: For PN compatibility information, please see Appendix D.
IV push	Contraindicated.[2,33]
Intermittent infusion	Infuse over 1 hour.[2,33]
Continuous infusion	No information available to support administration by this method.
Other routes of administration	IM or SC injection not recommended and may result in severe tissue irritation due to high pH.[2,33]
Comments	**Significant adverse effects:** Morphological changes to the neutrophils of a 13-year-old allogeneic BMT patient were attributed to twice-daily infusions of ganciclovir. The changes resolved within 48 hours of discontinuing the drug.[34]
	Decreased renal function and myelosuppression have been reported in children; renal function improved with a dose decrease.[17]
	Drug interactions: Because ganciclovir is associated with numerous drug interactions,[2] consult appropriate resources for dosing recommendations before combining any drug with ganciclovir.
	Other: IV ganciclovir may be beneficial in infants with CMV associated cholestasis.[35,36] In one study, 10 mg/kg/day divided in two doses for 21 days led to improvement in the clinical course of infants with neonatal cholestatic CMV hepatitis.[35]
	Ganciclovir has been used to treat CMV enterocolitis in an 8-week-old and protein-losing enteropathy and retinitis due to CMV in a 6-week-old.[37,38] It was also successfully used for CMV colitis in a 12-week-old.[39]
	Ganciclovir 10 mg/kg/day divided q 12 h for 14 days was used to successfully treat an immunocompetent child with CMV infection and isolated abducens nerve palsy.[40]
	Ganciclovir has been used in the treatment of CMV polyradiculopathy with an induction dose of 10 mg/kg/day divided q 12 h for 10–14 days, followed by maintenance therapy of 5 mg/kg/day, 5 days per week.[41]
	In vivo placental transfer of ganciclovir has occurred in a premature neonate born to a woman with AIDS receiving ganciclovir therapy for CMV retinitis and pneumonitis.[42]

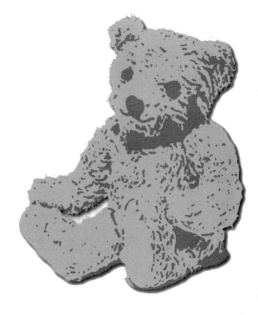

Gentamicin Sulfate

Brand names	Garamycin

Medication error potential

Look a-like, sound-alike drug names.

ISMP's *Confused Drug Names* lists confusion with gentian violet.[1]

USP reports confusion with clindamycin, GenTeal, tobramycin, and vancomycin.[2]

Contraindications and warnings

US boxed warning: Patients with impaired renal function and those receiving large doses or prolonged therapy have an increased risk for nephrotoxicity and ototoxicity (i.e., vestibular and auditory), both of which are generally irreversible.[3-5] The risk of toxicity can also be increased by prolonged elevations in serum concentrations, concurrent use of medications known to be nephro-, neuro-, or oto-toxic, dehydration, and advancing age.[3-5] Observe closely for signs or symptoms of toxicity.[3] (See Rare adverse effects, Monitoring, and Drug interactions in Comments section.)

Aminoglycosides can cause fetal harm when administered to a pregnant woman.[3]

Contraindications: Known hypersensitivity reaction to gentamicin or other aminoglycosides.[3]

Other warnings: Aminoglycosides can cause neuromuscular blockade and potentiate the effects of neuromuscular blockers.[3,6-8] If neuromuscular blockade occurs, calcium salts may reverse it.[3] (See Appendix C for specific information.)

Infusion related cautions

Chills, fever, tachycardia, and decreased systolic blood pressure have been associated with a pyrogenic, endotoxin-like reaction following once-daily administration of gentamicin.[9,10]

Dosage

In obese patients dosage should be based on the following equation[11]:

Dosing weight = IBW + 0.4 (TBW − IBW). (See Appendix B.)

Loading dose: Although limited data are available, some advocate an initial 3–5 mg/kg dose in neonates and infants.[12-14]

Maintenance dose

Neonates: Dose is estimated using age and weight,[15-17] or gestational age.[18-30].

Based on age and weight[15-17]

PNA	<1200 g	1200-2000 g	≥2000 g
<7 days	2.5 mg/kg q 18–24 h[15,16]*	5 mg/kg/day divided q 12 h[16,17]	5 mg/kg/day divided q 12 h[16,17]
≥7 days		5–7.5 mg/kg/day divided q 8–12 h[16,17]	7.5 mg/kg/day divided q 8 h[16,17]

*Until 4 weeks of age.

Dosage *(cont.)*

Based on gestational age[18-30]

Gestational Age	Dose
≤7 days	
<28 weeks	2.5 mg/kg q 24 h
28–34 weeks	2.5 mg/kg q 18 h
>7 days	
<28 weeks	2.5 mg/kg q 18 h
28–34 weeks	2.5 mg/kg q 12 h

Gestational Age	Postnatal Age	Dose
≤30 weeks	≤7 days	5 mg/kg q 48 h[31]
30–34 weeks	≤7 days	4.5 mg/kg q 36 h[31]
≥35 weeks	≤7 days	4 mg/kg q 24 h[31-36]

*Until 4 weeks of age.

Although the above dosing is used by some practitioners, the most recent edition of the *American Academy of Pediatrics Red Book: Report of the Committee on Infectious Diseases* continues to recommend 2.5 mg/kg/dose administered in multiple daily doses for newborns of all body weights.[16]

Infants and children

Mild-to-moderate infections: Not appropriate.[16]

Severe infections: 7.5 mg/kg/day divided q 8 h.[14,16,20,37-40]

Once-daily dosing: Several investigators have reported that once-daily dosing has comparable efficacy and perhaps less toxicity than classical 8–12 hour dosing.[41-51] A single dose of *aminoglycoside* has been given once daily (over 20–30 minutes) in critically ill infants and children with severe gram-negative infections,[42-44] severe pneumonia,[52] urinary tract infections,[53] bone marrow transplantation,[45] or in febrile neutropenic patients with cancer.[46-50] At this time, the use of once-daily dosing in infants and children is controversial.[51,54] The most recent edition of the *American Academy of Pediatrics Red Book: Report of the Committee on Infectious Diseases* continues to recommend 2.5 mg/kg/dose administered in multiple daily doses in all age groups and states that once daily dosing is investigational in children.[16]

Bacterial endocarditis (prophylaxis): In contrast to the 2005 AHA guidelines, prophylactic antibiotics solely to prevent endocarditis is no longer recommended for patients who undergo GU or GI tract procedures, including diagnostic procedures.[55]

Bacterial endocarditis (treatment): Patients with endocarditis will receive a variety of primary antibiotics (e.g., cephalosporins, ampicillin, penicillin, gentamicin, vancomycin) that are given with or without 3 mg/kg/day of gentamicin as a single dose or divided as multiple daily doses.[39] Duration of gentamicin varies and depends on organism sensitivity and the infection of either a native or prosthetic valve. See guideline for specific recommendations.[56]

Dosage adjustment in organ dysfunction

If CrCl is between 30–50 mL/min, give a normal dose q 12–18 h; if CrCl is 10–29 mL/min, give a normal dose q 18–24 h, and if <10 mL/min, give a normal dose q 48–72 h.[57] Individualize dose based on serum concentrations, pharmacokinetic parameters, and pharmacodynamic response.

Gentamicin Sulfate

Maximum dosage	Larger doses or shorter dosing intervals are sometimes required in patients with cystic fibrosis,[58-61] major thermal burns or dermal loss,[62] ascites, or in patients with febrile granulocytopenia.[46-50] Based on similarities between aminoglycosides, prolonged dosing interval may be required in those receiving ECMO.[63]
Additives	May contain sulfites and parabens.[64] (See Appendix C for specific information about sulfite hypersensitivity and parabens potential for toxicity.)
Suitable diluents	D5W, D10W, NS, LR.[64]
Maximum concentration	40 mg/mL[17]; however, the volume must allow for accurate measurement and administration over 30–60 minutes.
Preparation and delivery	**Delivery system issues:** The mixing of gentamicin sulfate with an aminoglycoside in vitro can result in substantial inactivation of the aminoglycoside. (See Appendix C for more specific information.) **Compatibility:** See Appendix D for PN compatibility information.[65]
IV push	Not recommended. Aminoglycosides have been safely administered by rapid IV push (over 3–5 minutes)[66-68]; however, ototoxicity has been associated with elevated peak serum concentrations following bolus administration in *adults*.[69]
Intermittent infusion	10 mg/mL or 40 mg/mL (commercially available) over 20–30 minutes.[3]
Continuous infusion	Not recommended. Toxicity occurs more frequently, and the value of this administration method compared to intermittent infusion has not been established.[69-71]
Other routes of administration	May be administered IM.[3]
Comments	**Rare adverse effects:** Aminoglycosides accumulate in renal cortical tissue and may damage proximal tubule cells leading to oliguric renal failure. Risk of nephrotoxicity may be influenced by type of aminoglycoside, dose, duration (cumulative dose), frequency of therapy and elevated serum concentration.[3,4] It is also increased by advancing age, pre-existing renal or hepatic dysfunction, decrease renal perfusion, hypoalbuminemia, and dehydration.[3,4,8] Current administration of nephrotoxic drugs (e.g., cisplatin, cephaloridine, kanamycin, amikacin, neomycin, polymyxin B, colistin, streptomycin, tobramycin, vancomycin) and ototoxic medications (e.g., ethacrynic acid, furosemide) may increase the risk of toxicity and should be avoided.[3] Cochlear and/or vestibular ototoxicity has been associated with all aminoglycoside antibiotics.[5,8] Total AUC is a better indicator of ototoxic risk than either peak or trough serum concentration.[72,73] Use cautiously with other drugs (e.g., macrolide antibiotics, loop diuretics, platinum-based chemotherapeutic agents) known to cause ototoxicity.

Gentamicin Sulfate

Comments (cont.)

Aminoglycosides may potentiate the curare-like effects on the neuromuscular junction and should be used with caution in patients with neuromuscular disorders since they may aggravate muscle weakness.[3,6] During or following gentamicin therapy, paresthesias, tetany, positive Chvostek, and Trousseau signs and mental confusion have been described in patients with hypomagnesemia, hypocalcemia, and hypokalemia.[3] Tetany and muscle weakness have been described in infants. Aminoglycosides may enhance the respiratory depressant effect of neuromuscular-blocking agents and may prolonged blockade.[3,74,75] Appropriate corrective electrolyte therapy should be initiated. Neuromuscular blockade may be reversed by administration of calcium salts.[3]

Monitoring: Because large variability exists in patient response to therapy, individualize dosage based on serum concentrations, clinical response, and renal function. Recommended peak and trough serum gentamicin concentration are 4–12 mg/L and <2 mg/L, respectively. Desired peak concentrations are dependent on the site of infection.

Although serum concentration monitoring has become routine practice in many institutions, not all patients require monitoring.[76,77] Monitoring is indicated if the patient is not clinically responding, is ≤3 months of age, has disease that requires large doses or high concentrations (CNS infections, endocarditis, pneumonia, ascites, burns), has decreased or unstable renal function, or will be treated more than 10 days.

Drug interactions: Consult appropriate resources before combining any drug with gentamicin.

Laboratory interference: Serum concentrations may be falsely elevated when blood samples are collected through central venous Silastic catheters.[78]

Glycopyrrolate

Brand names	Robinul, generic
Medication error potential	Look-alike, sound-alike error potential. ISMP reported that Robinul was confused with Reminyl.[1]
Contraindications and warnings	**Contraindications:** Known hypersensitivity to glycopyrrolate or product components.[2] **Warnings:** Glycopyrrolate causes decreased sweating and children with fever, who are in environments with high temperatures, or who undergo physical exercise are at risk for development of heat prostration.[2]
Infusion related cautions	Dysrhythmias have been reported in children.[2]
Dosage	**Preanesthetic:** Given 30–60 minutes prior to anesthesia induction or when preanesthetic narcotic and/or sedatives are given.[2-7]
	Neonates: 3–5 mcg/kg.[6]
	Infants and children: 4 mcg/kg; up to 9 mcg/kg may be needed for infants 1 month–2 years old.[2] One group evaluating the effects of ondansetron on vomiting associated with ketamine sedation used 5 mcg/kg (maximum 250 mcg) for an emergency department procedure.[8]
	Intraoperative arrhythmias (secondary to drugs or vagal reflexes): 4 mcg/kg[2-5] but ≤0.1 mg as a single dose.[2] May be repeated at 2- to 3-minute intervals as needed.[1]
	Reversal of neuromuscular blockade: Glycopyrrolate may be mixed with neostigmine or pyridostigmine to minimize cardiac side effects.[2]
	5–10 mcg/kg[9-11] (0.2 mg of glycopyrrolate for every 1 mg of neostigmine or 5 mg of pyridostigmine[2])
Dosage adjustment in organ dysfunction	Patients with renal impairment have delayed elimination.[2]
Maximum dosage	The maximum intraoperative dose is 0.1 mg.[2]
Additives	Contains benzyl alcohol 0.9% as a preservative.[2] See Appendix C for more specific information about benzyl alcohol toxicity in neonates.
Suitable diluents	D5W, D5½NS, D5NS, D10W, NS, R.[2]
Maximum concentration	0.2 mg/mL (undiluted).[2]

Glycopyrrolate

Preparation and delivery	**Compatibility:** Incompatible in LR.[2]
IV push	Slowly.[2]
Intermittent infusion	Over 15–20 minutes.
Continuous infusion	Not indicated.[2]
Other routes of administration	IM.[2,12]
Comments	**Adverse effects:** A paradoxical reaction, hyperexcitability, has been noted in children who receive large doses of anticholinergics.[2] Pretreatment with glycopyrrolate did not alter the incidence of ventricular arrhythmias during halothane anesthesia.[2] One group found that glycopyrrolate at 6 mcg/kg prevented the bradycardia usually seen with sevoflurane-remifentanil-based anesthesia for cardiac catheterization of children (1–36 months of age) with congenital heart disease.[13]

Granisetron HCl

Brand names	Kytril

Medication error potential	Look-alike, sound-alike error potential. USP reported that granisetron was confused with ondansetron.[1]

Contraindications and warnings	**Contraindications:** Patients with hypersensitivity to the drug or its components.[2] **Warnings:** Hypersensitivity reactions may occur in patients with hypersensitivity to other 5-hydroxytryptamine 3 (5-HT3) antagonists.[2]

Infusion related cautions	The data on the effect of granisetron on ECG is inconsistent. One study in 22 children receiving 40 mcg/kg infused over 30 seconds following chemotherapy for ALL demonstrated transient changes on ECG but no clinical symptoms.[3] In *adults*, a 30-second or 5-minute infusion of 10 mcg/kg resulted in a statistically significant prolongation in the QTc interval; however, no clinical symptoms were reported.[4] In four of 12 *adults*, bradycardia, integral change of P-waves, junctional escape beat, and atrioventricular block occurred.[5] Doses of 80 mcg/kg or 120 mcg/kg, in single or split doses, produced no clinically significant effects on ECG, pulse rate, or blood pressure in *adults*.[6]

Dosage	**Prevention of chemotherapy-induced nausea and vomiting:** 10, 20, or 40 mcg/kg,[2,7-16] given 5[10,11]–30[7-9,12,13,17] minutes prior to chemotherapy. For breakthrough nausea and vomiting in the first 24 hours of chemotherapy, the dose can be repeated.[18] The inclusion of dexamethasone is recommended.[19] **Prevention of postoperative nausea and vomiting (PONV):** 10, 20, 40, 80, or 100 mcg/kg doses have been compared in children.[20-23] The 40-mcg/kg dose was more effective than the 10-mcg/kg dose.[20] The 80- or 100-mcg/kg doses were no more effective than 40 mcg/kg.[20,21] The combination of granisetron and dexamethasone was more effective than granisetron alone.[24,25] In *adults*, doses of 0.1, 1, and 3 mg were studied and 3 mg was no more effective than 1 mg.[2]

Dosage adjustment in organ dysfunction	No dosage adjustment is needed for renal or hepatic dysfunction.[2] Clearance is significantly decreased in hepatic impairment; however, the pharmacokinetics of granisetron are highly variable and larger doses are well tolerated.[2]

Maximum dosage	Although doses of 100 mcg/kg have been studied,[23] 40 mcg/kg is the usual maximum dose.[2,7,8]

Additives	The 4-mL multidose vials (1 mg/mL) contain benzyl alcohol.[2] See Appendix C for specific information about benzyl alcohol toxicity in neonates.

Suitable diluents	D5W, D5¼ NS, D5½ NS, NS.[2,26]

Maximum concentration	Undiluted [0.1 mg/mL (preservative free) or 1 mg/mL (multidose vial)].

Preparation and delivery	**Stability:** Once the multidose vial has been entered, it should be used or discarded in 30 days.[2] **Compatibility:** See Appendix D for PN compatibility information.
IV push	Over 30 seconds (undiluted) or over 2–5 minutes.[2,10,21] A 40-mcg/kg dose (concentration unspecified) was infused over 30 seconds in children.[3]
Intermittent infusion	Over 30 minutes.[8,9,12]
Continuous infusion	Although continuous infusion has been used in *adults*,[27] continuous infusion has not been reported in pediatric patients.
Other routes of administration	Has been given IM in *adults*.[28,29]
Comments	A decrease in effectiveness was noted with prolonged use.[13] Response appears to be best in children <6 years of age[12] and is least in girls.[13] **Pharmacokinetics:** Pharmacokinetic parameters were significantly more variable in children with ALL who were given 1–3 mg (48.6–85.7 mcg/kg) compared to *adults* with lung cancer who were given 3 mg (41.7–53.6 mcg/kg).[30]

Haloperidol Lactate

Brand names	Haldol
Medication error potential	Look-alike, sound-alike error potential. USP reported that haloperidol was confused with hydralazine, hydromorphone, and nadolol. Haldol was confused with Halcion, Hytrin, and nadolol. Confusion with Stadol resulted in patient harm.[1]
Contraindications and warnings	**US boxed warning:** Elderly patients with dementia-psychoses that are treated with antipsychotic drugs are at increased risk for mortality.[2] **Contraindications:** Hypersensitivity to haloperidol, Parkinson's disease, patients with toxic CNS depression or who are comatose from any cause. **Other warnings:** Both QT prolongation and torsades de pointes were reported with IV administration in *adults*[2,3] and were more likely to occur with larger doses.[3] If haloperidol is administered IV, ECG should be monitored at baseline and periodically during treatment and the dosage should be reduced or drug should be discontinued if prolongation of the QT interval occurs.[2,4]
Infusion related cautions	Extrapyramidal symptoms, dystonia, and hyperpyrexia were reported in children with burns who received IV therapy.[5] Do not infuse the decanoate product IV.
Dosage	**Agitation and delirium in critically ill children:** Doses have ranged from 0.013–0.28 mg/kg.[4-8] (See Infusion related cautions section.)
Dosage adjustment in organ dysfunction	None noted.[2]
Maximum dosage	Usually 0.1 mg/kg not to exceed 5 mg.[6]
Additives	Contains methylparaben and propylparaben.[2] See Appendix C for specific information about potential adverse effects.
Suitable diluents	D5W.[9]
Maximum concentration	5 mg/mL (undiluted).
Preparation and delivery	**Photosensitivity:** Protect from light during storage. **Compatibility:** See Appendix D for PN compatibility information.
IV push	Slowly.[8] ECG should be monitored if the drug is infused IV.[2]

Haloperidol Lactate

Intermittent infusion	ECG should be monitored if the drug is infused IV.[2]
Continuous infusion	Has been infused continuously in *adults*.[10]
Other routes of administration	IM is the preferred route of administration.[2]
Comments	**Adverse effects:** Hypotension and dystonic reactions may occur.[2,5,6]
	Haloperidol may lower the seizure threshold.[2] Use cautiously in patients with a history of epilepsy or in those receiving antiepileptic medications.[2]
	One child developed hypertension after ingesting 1.15–1.54 mg/kg haloperidol.[11] A 29-month-old girl developed bradycardia and arrhythmia and an 11-month-old boy developed bradycardia and hypotension after ingestion.[12]

Heparin Sodium

Brand names	Various manufacturers

Medication error potential

ISMP high-alert medication that has an increased risk of causing significant patient harm if it is used in error.

ISMP reported that heparin was confused with Hespan.[2]

Contraindications and warnings

Contraindications: Severe thrombocytopenia, lack of appropriate monitoring techniques (full-dose heparin), and uncontrolled active bleeding except when due to disseminated intravascular coagulation.[3]

Warnings: Heparin sodium is available in a variety of concentrations including 1000 units/mL, 5000 units/mL, 10,000 units/mL, and 20,000 units/mL.[3] Medication errors from using a concentrated heparin solution as a catheter lock solution have resulted in fatalities in pediatric patients.[3]

Bleeding may result from overdosage.[3] Neonates may be at increased risk for intracranial hemorrhage.[4]

Heparin-induced thrombocytopenia (HIT), a potentially serious side effect, may occur and is not dose related.[5,6]

Infusion related cautions

Confirm the choice of the correct heparin concentration on the vial prior to use.[3]

Dosage

FDA alert: On October 1, 2009 the FDA alerted healthcare professionals that the USP adopted new manufacturing controls for heparin. On October 8, 2009, the reference standard for heparin products changed to the World Health Organization's International Standards (IS) unit dose definition. This is about 10% less potent than the previous USP unit. Thus the potency of heparin products has decreased.[7]

Systemic heparinization for thromboembolic disease* (see Infusion related cautions section)[8,9]

Loading dose: 75 units/kg IV over 10 minutes; obtain blood for aPTT 4 hours after loading dose.

Initial maintenance dose

Infants <1 year: 28 units/kg/h.

Childrens >1 year: 20 units/kg/h.

Monitoring: Measure aPTT 4 hours after every change in rate. When aPTT is in the therapeutic range, perform daily CBC and aPTT measurements.

Dosage *(cont.)*

Adjustments in infusion rate

aPTT, sec	Bolus, units/kg	Hold, min	Rate Change, %	Repeat aPTT
<50	50	0	+10%	4 h
50–59	0	0	+10%	4 h
60–85	0	0	0	next day
86–95	0	0	−10%	4 h
96–120	0	30	−10%	4 h
>120	0	60	−15%	4 h

*Reproduced with permission from *Chest*.[9]

Neonates: Loading dose of 50 units/kg of preservative-free heparin followed by 20–35 units/kg/h, titrated to desired aPTT.[10]

Infants and children: Loading dose of 50–100 units/kg followed by 10–25 units/kg/h, titrated to desired aPTT.[11,12]

Cardiac catheterization: 100–150 units/kg bolus to achieve ACT >200 seconds.[2,13] Monitor ACT q 1–2 h and administer additional heparin as needed.[1]

Catheter patency

Arterial lines: 0.5–2 units/mL.[14] 0.5 unit/mL in premature or low birth weight infants and patients with multiple lines.[14] Alternatively, a 5-unit/mL continuous infusion at 1 mL/h has also been recommended for peripheral arterial catheters.[7]

Peripheral IV catheter infusing PN: 0.5–1 unit/mL (final concentration).[14-19] May need to decrease to 0.5 unit/mL in small neonates receiving large volumes. (See Comments section.)

Peripheral IV lock irrigation: Usually 1 mL of 10 units/mL instilled q 8 h.[20-22] However, concentrations (10–100 units/mL), volumes (2–5 mL), and dosing intervals vary widely depending on institutional protocols.[14,22] Some studies suggest there is no clinical difference between 2 units/mL, 10 units/mL, and saline.[23,24]

Peripherally inserted central catheter (PICC): In preterm neonates (28 ± 4 weeks gestational age), continuous infusion of heparin at 0.5 units/kg/h (in D5W or D10W, n = 100) compared to placebo (D5W or D10W, n = 101) resulted in fewer occlusions (6% vs 31%, respectively) and more completed therapies (63% vs 42%, respectively).[25] No difference in thrombosis (20% vs 21%) or infection (10% vs 6%) was noted.

Tunneled central venous catheter (flush): In children with hematologic or oncologic disease who were up to 17 years of age, a 3 mL, 200 unit/mL flush twice a week resulted in fewer complications than a NS flush once a week in those with a positive-pressure-valve cap device.[26] Investigators could not rule out the possibility that more frequent flushing in the heparin group was also important.

Umbilical artery catheter: 0.5–2 units/mL of infusate as continuous infusion.[14,27-32] (See Comments section.)

Continuous arteriovenous hemofiltration: Loading dose of 100 units/kg followed by 5–7 units/kg/h was successfully used in neonates.[33]

ECMO: 75–100 units/kg followed by 25–35 units/kg/h usually titrated to ACT of 180–225 seconds.[34] (See Dosage adjustment in organ dysfunction section.)

Promotion of fat emulsion clearance: 1 unit/mL of infusate as continuous infusion.[35,36]

Heparin Sodium

Dosage adjustment in organ dysfunction

Dosage should be titrated to the appropriate aPTT.[3] Patients with renal dysfunction may be at greater risk for hemorrhage.

During ECMO, heparin adsorbs onto the circuit. Up to one half of the heparin administered may be inactivated by the circuit.[37]

Maximum dosage

Individualize dosage based on aPTT,[3] or in some neonatal cases, ACT.[12]

≤35 units/kg/h have been used in neonates with major vessel thrombosis.[11]

Additives

While some products are preservative- and antioxidant-free, many heparin products contain sodium metabisulfite, benzyl alcohol, or parabens.[38] See Appendix C for specific information about adverse effects and potential toxicity from benzyl alcohol in neonates.

Suitable diluents

D–LR, D–R, D–S, D5NS, D5½NS, D5W, D10W, fat emulsion 10%, LR, NS, ½NS, PN, R.[38]

Maximum concentration

Undiluted solutions may be used.[3] In order to infuse the correct dose safely, the product concentration must be considered; using a less concentrated product for lower doses results in a dosage that is more accurate.

Preparation and delivery

Preparation: The addition of heparin to infusates requires adequate mixing to ensure that pooling of heparin does not occur.[3,38] One manufacturer recommends inverting the container ≥6 times.[3]

Compatibility: See Appendix D for PN compatibility information.

IV push

Not indicated.

Intermittent infusion

Over 10 minutes.[3]

Continuous infusion

Usual method of delivery.

Other routes of administration

Deep SC.[3] Not for IM use.[3]

Comments

Protamine sulfate reverses the effects of heparin. (See Protamine Sulfate monograph.)

Neonates have demonstrated both resistance and sensitivity to heparin.[15]

One group of investigators concluded that the addition of heparin to fluids infused to neonates peripherally did not affect catheter life significantly.[19] Similarly, a systematic review of 10 studies that met review criteria could not support the use of heparin in neonates receiving peripheral infusions.[39]

Very low birth weight infants may receive pharmacologic doses with frequent IV line flushes.[3]

There have been anecdotal reports of precipitation when certain heparin premixed products that contain phosphate are co-infused with calcium chloride.

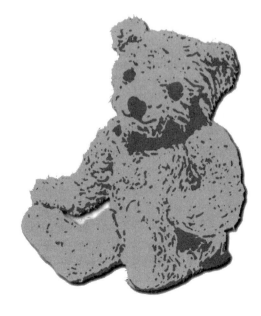

HydrALAZINE HCl

Brand names	Apresoline, generic
Medication error potential	Look-alike, sound-alike error potential. ISMP and USP report that hydrALAZINE has been confused with hydroxyzine; no patient harm resulted.[1,2] USP also reports that hydrALAZINE has been confused with haloperidol, hydrochlorothiazide and hydrocortisone; no patient harm resulted.[2] ISMP reports that Apresoline has been confused with Priscoline.[1] USP reports that Apresoline has been confused with Aldactone and atropine; no patient harm resulted.[2]
Contraindications and warnings	Contraindicated in patients with hypersensitivity to hydralazine, coronary artery disease, and mitral valvular rheumatic heart disease.[3] May cause SLE and syndromes associated with it, including glomerulonephritis.[3] More commonly occurs in slow acetylators and patients with renal dysfunction.[4] If SLE or similar symptoms develop, hydralazine should be discontinued unless benefit of continued therapy outweighs potential risk.[3] Use with caution in patients with several renal disease or cerebrovascular accident.[3]
Infusion related cautions	May cause reflex tachycardia, headaches, flushing, and fluid retention.[5] May use adjuvant beta-blocker and/or diuretic to combat these effects.[4,6] Combination with beta-blocker may reduce hydralazine dose requirements.[6] Average maximum decrease in blood pressure should occur within 10–80 minutes.[3] Monitor blood pressure and heart rate during and after infusion.[3,4] When combined with other potent IV antihypertensive agents, such as diazoxide, hypotensive episodes can be prolonged; monitor patients for several hours after an precipitous decrease in blood pressure.[3]
Dosage	...g q 3–6 h[5,7-17], 1.7–3.5 mg/kg/day divided ... 4–6 h.[4]

> **Important Correction Notice**
>
> *Pediatric Injectable Drugs Ninth Edition (The Teddy Bear Book) – P2432*
>
> The publisher wishes to inform you of the following corrections.
>
> 1. In the monograph for **HydrALAZINE HCl (pages 288-289)**
>
> "Dosage" section – Hypertension/heart failure second line should read:
>
> **50-100 mg/m²/day**
>
> slow acetylators and q 8–16 h in fast acetylators.[20,21]

Dosage in org...	...isure pres- rs, a ease 25% f the ...inister ... h in
Maximum dosage	1.5 mcg/kg/min,[8,12] 2 mg/kg q 3–6 h[8,12,17] up to 9 mg/kg/day[22] or a 20[23]–25[14,16] mg dose.
Additives	Contains 103.6 mg propylene glycol/mL.[24] See Appendix C for more specific information about potential adverse effects of propylene glycol. Contains 0.65 mg methylparaben and 0.35 mg polyparaben/mL.[24] See Appendix C for more specific information about potential adverse effects of parabens.

HydrALAZINE HCl

Suitable diluents	The manufacturer does not recommend adding to infusion solutions.[24] Hydralazine should not be diluted in dextrose or other sugar-containing solutions because of the formation of hydrazones, which are associated with toxicity (e.g., headache, nausea, vomiting).[25]
Maximum concentration	20 mg/mL.[24]
Preparation and delivery	Use immediately after vial is opened. Do not add to infusion solutions.[3] Color change occurs after dilution with most IV solutions. Color changes within 8–12 hours after admixture do not indicate loss of potency when stored at 30°C.[24]
IV push	20 mg/mL over 1–2 minutes in infants.[7,13,24] A 12-year-old child received 0.32 mg/kg over 2 minutes.[9]
Intermittent infusion	No information to support administration by this method.
Continuous infusion	Not recommended to be added to infusion solutions.[24]
Other routes of administration	0.2–0.6 mg/kg/dose may be given IM.[4,26]
Comments	**Significant adverse effects:** Peripheral neuritis (paresthesias, numbness, tingling) may occur; use concomitantly with pyridoxine if symptoms develop.[3] Blood dyscrasias may occur.[3] **Monitoring:** Complete blood counts and antinuclear antibodies (ANA) should be measured before and periodically during therapy. Benefit over risk should be determined when beginning or continuing therapy in a patient with a positive ANA titer.[3] **Pharmacokinetic considerations:** Acetylation is a major route of elimination. The metabolism of hydralazine will be variable in fast and slow acetylators.[4] Most patients developing SLE symptoms will be slow acetylators.[4] If symptoms occur, consider performing appropriate laboratory studies. If tests confirmatory, discontinue use of hydralazine unless potential benefit outweighs risk.[4] **Drug interactions:** May paradoxically reduce pressor response to epinephrine.[3,4] Use MAO inhibitors with caution in patients receiving hydralazine due to potentiation of hypotensive effects.[3,4] Many other drugs may potentiate the hypotensive effects of hydralazine. Consult appropriate resources for recommendations before combining any drug with hydralazine. **Other:** Reduce dosage when converting from oral to IV therapy. One study established that 20–25 mg of IV hydralazine hydrochloride was estimated to equal 75–100 mg of oral hydralazine.[4] In patients with normal renal function prior to therapy, hydralazine may increase renal blood flow.[3]

Hydrochloric Acid (HCl)

Brand names	Various manufacturers
Medication error potential	None noted.
Contraindications and warnings	**Warnings:** HCl has sclerosing potential if used incorrectly.
Infusion related cautions	Infusion of 0.1 N HCl through a peripheral line results in pain at the injection site and may cause thrombophlebitis.[1] Infusion via a large vein or central venous line is preferred.[2,3]

Dosage

Central venous catheter occlusion: Using a 3-mL or larger syringe, instill a volume of 0.1 N HCl equal to the catheter volume (0.2–2 mL) and allow it to dwell for at least 20 minutes.[4-8] (See Comments section.) Then withdraw and discard HCl, and flush the catheter with an appropriate solution. If unsuccessful, the procedure can be repeated.[4-7] (See Comments section.)

Severe metabolic alkalosis (not first line treatment; see Comments section): 0.1–0.2 mmol/kg/h until alkalosis is corrected.[9] A 16-day-old infant with refractory metabolic alkalosis received 0.5 mmol/kg/h for 5.5 hours, then 0.75 mmol/kg/h for 4.5 hours, and 1 mmol/kg/h for 4 hours.[10] 0.1 N HCl has been added to an amino acid and lipid solution and infused via peripheral vein in infants with alkalosis.[1]

The amount of HCl to correct the alkalosis can be calculated using[11]:

Chloride deficit
mEq HCl = 0.2 L/kg × weight (kg) × [103 − observed serum Cl (mEq/L)]

Bicarbonate excess[2,3]
mEq (mmol) HCl = 0.5 L/kg × weight (kg) × [observed serum HCO_3 (mEq/L) − 24]

Base-excess
mEq HCl = 0.3 L/kg × weight (kg) × measured base excess (mEq/L)

The chloride-deficit method usually results in a lower dose than the other two. The dose calculated using the chloride deficit should be infused over ≥12 hours, and the dose calculated using the bicarbonate excess or base-excess method over ≥24 hours.[11] Arterial blood gas and electrolytes should be measured q 4 h during the infusion and therapy adjusted as needed.[2,11]

Dosage adjustment in organ dysfunction	No information available.
Maximum dosage	0.2 mmol/kg/h has been recommended.[3] Rates up to 25 mEq/h in *adults* have been reported.[2] Monitor arterial pH closely during therapy and discontinue HCl when alkalosis has been corrected.
Additives	None. 0.1 N HCl provides 0.1 mEq/mL of hydrogen and chloride ion and has a pH of 1–1.5.

Hydrochloric Acid (HCl)

Suitable diluents	0.1 N HCl is ready for catheter instillation.
Maximum concentration	**Catheter instillation:** Usually 0.1 N HCl. In Australia, a more concentrated HCl product that is commercially available has been used as part of a protocol to treated infected catheters in children with cancer.[12] **Infusion:** Usually 0.2 N HCl[2,3]; however, a 0.5 N HCl solution has been used via central line.[10] (See Comments section.)
Preparation and delivery	**Compatibility:** See Appendix D for PN compatibility information.
IV push	Not indicated.
Intermittent infusion	Not indicated.
Continuous infusion	Because of the sclerosing potential, the rate of infusion should not exceed 0.2 mmol/kg/h.[3]
Other routes of administration	Contraindicated.
Comments	The diameter of the syringe tip is inversely related to the pressure generated when pushing fluid through. Therefore, larger syringes are used to instill dwell therapies to avoid catheter rupture.[6] HCl is indicated for hypochloremic metabolic alkalosis if NaCl or KCl are contraindicated or if correction is required quickly such as with an arterial pH >7.55, during hepatic encephalopathy, cardiac arrhythmia, digitalis cardiotoxicity.[3] In an in vitro study, the surface and interior of pulmonary artery catheters infused with 0.2, 0.3, or 0.4 N HCl showed degenerative changes.[13] A subsequent in vitro study found no catheter changes following daily infusions of 0.1 N HCl for 8 weeks.[14]

Hydrocortisone Sodium Succinate

Brand names	A-HydroCort, Solu-Cortef

Medication error potential

Look-alike, sound-alike error potential.

USP reported that hydrocortisone sodium succinate was confused with hydroxyzine hydrochloride, hydroxyzine pamoate, and methylprednisolone sodium succinate. Solu-Cortef was confused with Solu-Medrol.[1]

Contraindications and warnings

Contraindications: Neonates (products with benzyl alcohol), patients with systemic fungal infections, and patients with hypersensitivity to any component in the product.[2]

Live virus (MMR, varicella, rotavirus, smallpox) vaccinations should not be given during treatment with immunosuppressive doses of glucocorticoids.[2] (See Comments section.)

Warnings: Anaphylactoid reactions have been reported and those with a prior history of such reactions require appropriate precautions.[2,3]

Patients on chronic steroid therapy may require increased doses during stress.[2]

Supraphysiologic doses of corticosteroids may result in suppressed pituitary-adrenal function, so therapy of more than a few days should be decreased gradually.[2,4,5]

Immunosuppression and an increased risk for infection are possible during steroid therapy.[2] (See Comments section.)

Infusion related cautions

None noted.

Dosage

Doses are based on severity of disease and patient response.[2,6] The lowest dose that results in the desired effect should be used.[2,6] (See Comments section.)

Adrenal insufficiency

Acute

Infants and young children: 1–2 mg/kg IV bolus followed by 25–150 mg/day divided q 6–8 h.[6]

Older children: 1–2 mg/kg IV bolus followed by 150–250 mg/day divided q 6–8 h.[6]

Physiologic replacement: 0.25–0.35 mg/kg/day IM as a single dose.[6]

Anti-inflammatory/immunosuppressive therapy: 1–5 mg/kg/day[6] or 30–150 mg/m^2 given once a day or divided q 12 h.[6] Children (n = 19) from 3 to 18 years of age with refractory rheumatoid disease were given four doses of 500 mg in 24 hours.[7]

Congenital adrenal hyperplasia (emergency treatment): 1–2 mg/kg followed by 2 mg/kg q 8 h until po can be resumed[8]; po treatment is usual.[9,10]

Neonatal uses (preservative-free)

Hypoglycemia: 5 mg/kg/day divided q 12 h.[9]

Hypotension: 2–6 mg/kg/day divided q 6, 12, or 24 hours depending on response.[11,12]

Asthma: Methylprednisolone sodium succinate is the recommended parenteral glucocorticoid for asthma.[13] The National Asthma Education and Prevention Program recommends that asthmatics (*adult*) who have received systemic corticosteroids in the past 6 months and who will undergo surgery be given 100 mg hydrocortisone q 8 h during surgery with rapid weaning postoperatively.[13] (See Comments section.)

Hydrocortisone Sodium Succinate

Dosage *(cont.)*	**Cystic fibrosis:** 10 mg/kg/day divided q 6 h for 10 days added to standard treatment of infants hospitalized for lower respiratory illness resulted in a greater and more sustained improvement in lung function following hospitalization.[14]
Dosage adjustment in organ dysfunction	Those with cirrhosis of the liver or who are hypothyroid may have an exaggerated response.[2]
Maximum dosage	Not established. Use of high doses for >48–72 hours may result in hypernatremia.[2]
Additives	Contains 2.066 mEq of sodium/g.[15] May contain benzyl alcohol.[2] See Appendix C for specific information about potential benzyl alcohol toxicity in neonates.
Suitable diluents	D5W, D5NS, NS.[2,15]
Maximum concentration	Usually 1 mg/mL. However, 5 mg/mL in D5W was administered to 19 children without apparent adverse effects.[7]
Preparation and delivery	**Compatibility:** See Appendix D for PN compatibility information.
IV push	Over ≥30 seconds.[2,3]
Intermittent infusion	Over 10 minutes[2] up to 30 minutes.[7]
Continuous infusion	May be given by continuous infusion.[6]
Other routes of administration	May be given IM.[2]
Comments	Live virus vaccines may be given 1 month after ending a ≥2-week course of high-dose systemic corticosteroids (2 mg/kg/day of prednisone or its equivalent; or 20 mg/day if >10 kg).[16] **Adverse effects**: Musculoskeletal effects, fluid and electrolyte abnormalities, cataracts, and hyperglycemia.[2] Patients with diabetes may be at particular risk for hyperglycemia. Increased risk for immunosuppression and infection.[2] In one report, neonates who received IV hydrocortisone for refractory hypotension were more likely to develop disseminated candidal infection than those who did not.[17] In a study to evaluate hydrocortisone in preventing bronchopulmonary dysplasia associated with adrenal insufficiency, extremely low birth weight neonates (500–999 g) receiving indomethacin were randomized to placebo or 0.5 mg/kg q 12 h for 12 days followed by 0.5 mg/kg/day for 3 days. Compared to placebo, the treated group had a greater incidence of gastrointestinal perforation leading to early study termination.[18] **Drug interactions**: Drugs that enhance hepatic clearance (e.g., phenytoin, phenobarbital, ephedrine, rifampin) may decrease blood levels and lessen physiologic activity.[2]

Hydroxocobalamin

Brand names	Cyanokit, generic
Medication error potential	None reported by ISMP or USP.[1,2]

Contraindications and warnings

Contraindications: Should not be used in patients with hypersensitivity to the drug or any of its components.[3]

Warnings: Treatment of cyanide poisoning must also include supportive emergency care, including airway management, oxygenation, hydration, cardiovascular support and control of seizure activity.[4]

Use with caution in patients with known anaphylactic reactions to hydroxocobalamin or cyanocobalamin.[4] (See Infusion related cautions section.)

Use will result in red discoloration of the skin and urine. Patients have also reported photosensitivity. Patient should be instructed to avoid sun exposure until the red discoloration disappears (up to 2 weeks).[4] Urine discoloration may persist for up to 5 weeks.[4]

The use of folic acid alone in megaloblastic anemia due to vitamin B12 deficiency may result in irreversible neurologic damage.[3] The use of vitamin B12 alone in megaloblastic anemia due to folic acid deficiency may prevent the correct diagnosis since it will improve symptoms of folic acid deficiency.[3]

Infusion related cautions

Allergic reactions, which may include anaphylaxis, chest tightness, edema, urticaria, pruritus, dyspnea, rash, and angioneurotic edema have occurred with hydroxocobalamin administration.[4]

Increased blood pressure has occurred after initiation of the infusion, with the greatest increase occurring toward the end of the infusion.[4] Increased blood pressure was transient; a return to baseline should be expected within 4 hours of completing the infusion.[4]

Dosage

Hydroxocobalamin (vitamin B12a) is a precursor to cyanocobalamin (vitamin B12).[5] Two hydroxocobalamin products are available, a lyophilized powder for IV administration (25 mg/mL when reconstituted) to be used for cyanide poisoning and a sterile 1000-mcg/mL solution for IM administration to be used for anemias and vitamin B12 deficiency.[3,4]

Cyanide poisoning (hydroxocobalamin product for IV injection)[4,5]

   Adults: 2.5 g over 7.5 minutes repeated once; another dose of 5 g may be given if the first doses are ineffective.

   Pediatric patients: 70 mg/kg (up to 5 g) over 30 minutes as a single infusion.

Anemia, vitamin B12 (hydroxocobalamin product for IM administration)[3,5]

Cyanocobalamin preferred over hydroxocobalamin due to potential for antibody formation to the hydroxycobalamin-transcobalamin complex.[5]

   Children with vitamin B12 deficiency: 100 mcg/day for 10–15 days (total dose of 1–5 mg), then 30–60 mcg/month maintenance has been cited.[3,5]

   Schilling test: 1000 mcg once.[5]

Dosage adjustment in organ dysfunction

No information available.

Maximum dosage

5 g in pediatric patients and 10 g in *adults*.[4] Ten *adult* patients with smoke inhalation from fire or cyanide poisoning by ingestion or inhalation have received total doses of up to 20 g; only one of the ten survived with unspecified neurologic sequelae.[4]

Hydroxocobalamin

Additives

Hydroxocobalamin for IM administration contains 4.34% cobalt, 1.5 mg/mL methylparaben and 0.2 mg/mL propylparaben.[3] See Appendix C for more specific information about potential adverse effects of parabens.

Suitable diluents

NS, D5W, LR (hydroxocobalamin product for IV injection).[4] Hydroxocobalamin for IM administration should not be further diluted.

Maximum concentration

25 mg/mL.[4]

Preparation and delivery

Hydroxocobalamin product for IV injection: Each carton comes with 2 vials containing 2.5 g each of lyophilized hydroxocobalamin. Reconstitute vial with 100 mL NS (D5W or LR may be used if NS not available) using transfer spike provided in carton. Rock or rotate vial for 30 seconds to mix solution (do not shake). Use vented IV tubing provided in carton for infusion to patient.[4]

Do not administer blood products or other drugs through the same infusion line with hydroxocobalamin.[4]

Do not administer the IM product via the IV route.[3]

IV push

Not indicated.

Intermittent infusion

Infuse the IV product over 30 minutes in pediatric patients and over 7.5 minutes in *adults*.[4]

Continuous infusion

Not indicated.

Other routes of administration

Hydroxocobalamin for IM administration should only be administered via the IM route.[3]

Comments

Significant adverse effects: An acneiform rash may occur anywhere on the body within 7 to 28 days of administration; the rash should resolve on its own within several weeks.[4]

Monitoring: A blood cyanide concentration is recommended by the manufacturer; however, collection of blood cyanide sample should not delay treatment.[4]

Hypokalemia and thrombocytosis may occur when severe megaloblastic anemia is reversed to normal erythropoiesis by B12 administration; monitor potassium and platelet count closely.[3]

Laboratory interference: Hydroxocobalamin has a dark red color, and its use may interfere with laboratory analysis with colorimetric assays (chemistry panels, hematologic and coagulation tests, and urinalysis).[4] The interference may result in increased, decreased or unpredictable concentrations and duration of interference may occur for up to 48 hours after hydroxocobalamin administration.[4] Please see manufacturer's labeling for more specific information on tests that may be affected.[4]

Other: For cyanide poisoning, hydroxocobalamin may be advantageous over other antidotes (amyl nitrate, sodium nitrile, and sodium thiosulfate) in that it requires administration of a single antidote and does not result in methemoglobinemia. In patients with concomitant carbon monoxide poisoning, sodium thiosulfate should be added to treat the carbon monoxide poisoning.[6,7]

Ibuprofen Lysine

Brand names	NeoProfen
Medication error potential	None.

Contraindications and warnings

Contraindications: Hypersensitivity to ibuprofen, any component, aspirin, or other NSAIDs.[1] Neonates with (1) active bleeds (especially intracranial or gastrointestinal), thrombocytopenia, or coagulation defects; (2) proven or suspected infections that are untreated; (3) impaired renal function; (4) existing or suspected necrotizing enterocolitis; and (5) congenital heart disease in whom patency of the ductus arteriosus is necessary for satisfactory pulmonary or systemic blood flow (e.g., pulmonary atresia, severe tetralogy of Fallot, severe coarctation of the aorta).[1]

Warnings: Increasing BUN, creatinine, decreased glomerular filtration rate, and a small reduction in urine output (UOP) may be seen in neonates.[1] These effects are generally transient and resolve upon discontinuation of ibuprofen.[1] Ibuprofen may cause acute kidney injury especially in neonates.[1] It should be withheld in any patient with significant decreases in UOP until output returns to normal.

Infusion related cautions

Avoid extravasation.[1]

Dosage

Patent ductus arteriosus (closure of the ductus arteriosus): In premature infants (500–1500 g) ≤32 weeks gestational age.[1] Dose should be based on birth weight. The initial dose of 10 mg/kg should be followed by two doses of 5 mg/kg at 24 and 48 hours.[1-7] UOP should be assessed prior to each dose. If <0.6 mL/kg/h or anuria occurs, no dose should be given until renal function normalizes.[1] A second course of treatment, alternative pharmacologic therapy, or surgery may be needed if the ductus arteriosus fails to close or reopens following the initial course of therapy.

The prophylactic use of ibuprofen is not currently indicated nor recommended.[8,9]

Dosage adjustment in organ dysfunction

Should be withheld if oliguria (<0.6 mL/kg/h) or anuria.[1] Avoid use in severe hepatic impairment.[10]

Maximum dosage

10 mg/kg.[1]

Additives

None.[1]

Suitable diluents

NS, D5W.[1]

Maximum concentration

17.1 mg/mL (commercially available).[1]

Preparation and delivery

Stability: Use within 30 minutes of preparation. Unused contents must be discarded after first withdrawal.[1]

Compatibility: Should not be administered concurrently with TPN. Stop TPN for 15 minutes before and after ibuprofen lysine administration[1]

Ibuprofen Lysine

IV push	Not used.
Intermittent infusion	Over 15 minutes.[1]
Continuous infusion	Not used.
Other routes of administration	None.

Comments

Rare adverse effects: Spontaneous intraventricular hemorrhage (IVH) is a known complication of prematurity. Because ibuprofen may cause a transient reduction in cerebral blood flow[11,12] and is neuroprotective in animals,[3] some hypothesized that it might reduce the incidence or severity of IVH. In a large prospective study of 415 infants, 8% given ibuprofen developed severe IVH compared to 9% receiving placebo.[8] In a second study of 155 infants, grade 2 to 4 IVH developed for 16% of the ibuprofen-treated infants and 13% of the infants in the placebo group.[13]

Although nonsteroidal anti-inflammatory drugs (NSAIDs) have the ability to reduce mesenteric blood flow,[14-17] one study reported that ibuprofen did not significantly reduce mesenteric blood-flow velocity in infants.[18] The ability of NSAIDs to affect mesenteric blood flow raised concerns about its association with GI bleeding, isolated bowel perforation, and necrotizing enterocolitis (NEC) in infants. While an isolated case has been reported,[19] the incidence of NEC is similar between those given ibuprofen and indomethacin.[3,4,20,21] The incidence of NEC was significantly greater in those with (21%) compared to those without (5%) oliguria.[3]

Like other NSAIDs, ibuprofen also affects renal blood flow; however, the incidence is lower than that noted with indomethacin.[3,20-22] Preterm infants treated with ibuprofen experience lower serum creatinine values, higher urine output, and less undesirable decreased organ blood flow and vasoconstrictive adverse effects than those given indomethacin.[3,20] In a separate study, oliguria was commonly seen with both agents within the first 3 days of treatment, but resolved sooner in the ibuprofen group first.[3]

Ibuprofen lysine is about 99% is bound to albumin.[1] Intravenous ibuprofen lysine was found to be 94% to 95% protein bound in preterm newborns.[23] Ibuprofen should be used cautiously in infants with elevated total bilirubin concentrations since it may displace bilirubin from high-affinity albumin-binding sites.[1,24] One report noted possible ibuprofen-induced kernicterus in a preterm infant with hyperbilirubinemia.[25]

One case of pulmonary hypertension has been reported.[26]

NSAID therapy in *adults* has led to reports of liver disease.[27,28] If signs or symptoms develop, ibuprofen should be discontinued.

Monitoring: Renal function (serum creatinine and BUN), urine output, CBC and platelets, liver function, electrolytes (especially K and Na).

Drug interactions: Ibuprofen is a minor substrate of CYP2C9, 2C19, and a major inhibitor of CYP2C9.[1] It is also highly protein bound to albumin. Consult appropriate resources for dosing recommendations before combining any drug with ibuprofen.

Ifosfamide

Brand names	Ifex, generic
Medication error potential	ISMP high-alert medication that has an increased risk of causing significant patient harm if it is used in error.[1]
Contraindications and warnings	**US boxed warning:** Ifosfamide should be administered under the supervision of a qualified physician. It may cause serious urotoxic effects (hemorrhagic cystitis), CNS toxicity, and severe myelosuppression.[2] (See Significant adverse effects in Comments section.) **Contraindications:** Ifosfamide is contraindicated in patients with hypersensitivity to the drug and patients with severely depressed bone marrow.[2]
Infusion related cautions	Hydration should accompany ifosfamide administration.[2] (See Significant adverse effects in Comments section.)
Dosage	Consult institutional protocols for complete dosing information. Ifosfamide is used for pediatric bone and soft tissue sarcomas, as well as Wilms' tumor, neuroblastoma, and germ cell tumors. Common pediatric regimens include 1.2–1.8 g/m^2/day for 5 days q 21–28 days or 5 g/m^2/dose as a single 24-hour infusion or 3 g/m^2/day for 2 days.[3-7] High-dose therapy with 3.5 g/m^2/day for 5 days has also been used.[8]
Dosage adjustment in organ dysfunction	The dose of etoposide should be reduced by 25% in patients with CrCl <10 mL/min.[9] No specific guidelines exist on ifosfamide use in patients with hepatic insufficiency. However, one investigator recommended a decrease in the ifosfamide dosage by 75% in patients with an AST >300 units/L or a bilirubin >3 mg/dL.[10]
Maximum dosage	Not established.
Additives	None.
Suitable diluents	D2.5W, D5W, D5NS, NS, ½NS, LR.[2,11]
Maximum concentration	Manufacturer recommends 20 mg/mL, while another reference lists 40 mg/mL.[2,3]
Preparation and delivery	For PN compatibility information, please see Appendix D.
IV push	Not recommended.

Ifosfamide

Intermittent infusion	Dilute with SW to 50 mg/mL, then further dilute solution to a final concentration of 0.6–20 mg/mL with suitable diluents and infuse over a minimum of 30 minutes.[2,11]
Continuous infusion	Ifosfamide has been administered as a continuous infusion.[12] Compared to intermittent administration, this route is associated with greater nephrotoxicity.[13] One paper suggested no mechanistic reason for this effect.[12]
Other routes of administration	No information available to support administration by other routes.
Comments	**Significant adverse effects:** Ifosfamide is a known bladder irritant. Clinical trials have shown the development of hemorrhagic cystitis in 50% of patients receiving 1.2 g/m^2 of ifosfamide.[2] Therefore, vigorous hydration (i.e., a minimum of 2 L of IV or PO fluids per day) and the uroprotectant, Mesna, are recommended in conjunction with ifosfamide administration.
	Ifosfamide has been associated with severe nephrotoxicity.[3,14] Risk factors include age <5 years, history of cisplatin therapy, nephrectomy, renal impairment, or cumulative doses of ifosfamide >50–60 g/m^2.
	Ifosfamide is associated with a moderate (30% to 90%) risk of emesis.[15] Patients should receive antiemetic therapy to prevent acute and delayed nausea and vomiting. The recommended therapy is a 5HT3 receptor antagonist in combination with dexamethasone every day chemotherapy is administered.[15,16] These agents may be continued for up to 4 days after chemotherapy administration for the prevention of delayed nausea and vomiting. Breakthrough medications should also be offered, such as a phenothiazine (e.g., prochlorperazine), a butyrophenone (e.g., droperidol), a substituted benzamide (e.g., metoclopramide), or a benzodiazepine (e.g., lorazepam).
	Monitoring: CBC with neutrophils and platelets, urinalysis, liver function, and renal function.[2,3]
	Drug interactions: Ifosfamide is major substrate for CYP2A6, 2C19, and 3A4, and a minor substrate for CYP2B6, 2C8, and 2C9; concomitant use with inhibitors or inducers of these CYP isoenzymes may result in drug interactions.[2,3] Consult appropriate resources for dosing recommendations before combining any drug with ifosfamide.

Imipenem–Cilastatin Sodium

Brand names	Primaxin IM, Primaxin IV

Medication error potential

Look-alike, sound-alike drug names.

USP reports confusion with ertapenem as well as confusion between Primaxin and Prevacid and Protonix.[1]

Contraindications and warnings

Contraindications: In patients with a known hypersensitivity to any component of this product or to other carbapenems or in patients who have demonstrated anaphylactic reactions to beta-lactams.[2]

Warnings

Allergic reactions: Serious hypersensitivity and occasionally fatal anaphylactic reactions have been reported.[2] These are more likely in patients who are sensitive to multiple allergens and in those with a history of penicillin, cephalosporins, or other beta-lactam hypersensitivity.[2]

Seizures: Neurotoxicity of the carbapenem antibiotics has been reported.[2] Seizures occur most commonly in patients with renal impairment and/or underlying neurologic disorders. Not recommended in pediatric patients with CNS infections because of the risk of seizures.[2] (See Rare adverse effects in Comments section.)

Superinfection: Prolonged use may cause superinfection and/or *Clostridium difficile*–associated diarrhea (CDAD), which has been reported and may range in severity from mild diarrhea to fatal colitis.[2] If CDAD is suspected or confirmed, appropriate fluid and electrolyte management, protein supplementation, antibiotic treatment of *C. difficile*, and surgical evaluation should be instituted as clinically indicated.[2] Antibiotic use that is not directed against *C. difficile* may need to be discontinued.[2]

Infusion related cautions

If a decision is made to give this medication to a patient with known hypersensitivity to penicillins, cephalosporins, other beta-lactams, the patient should be closely observed for allergenicity. Epinephrine, oxygen, intravenous steroids, and airway management may be required.

IM suspensions should *not* be given intravenously.[2]

Decrease administration rate in those who develop nausea during infusion.[2]

May cause pain at the injection site, phlebitis/thrombophlebitis, and erythema.[2]

Dosage

Neonates (limited data are available)

PNA	<1200 g	>1500 g
<7 days	40 mg/kg/day divided q 12 h[2,3]*	50 mg/kg/day divided q 12 h[2,4]
≥7 days		75 mg/kg/day divided q 8 h[2,4]

*Although no reference is provided, one handbook recommends 20 mg/kg/dose q 18–24 h for infants 0–4 weeks who weigh <1200 g.[3]

Imipenem–Cilastatin Sodium

Dosage *(cont.)*	**Infants and children**
	4 weeks to 3 months: 100 mg/kg/day divided q 6 h.[2,4]
	>3 months: 60–100 mg/kg/day divided q 6 h.[2,4]
	Up to 2 g/day[2] for mild-to-moderate infections and 4 g/day[2,5-9] for severe infections or moderately-susceptible organisms.[2]
	Doses ≤500 mg may be given over 15–30 minutes, while doses >500 mg should be infused over 40–60 minutes.[2]
	Biologic warfare or bioterrorism: The CDC and other experts recommend that treatment of inhalational anthrax spores due to biologic warfare or bioterrorism should be started on a multiple-drug parenteral regimen that includes ciprofloxacin or doxycycline and one or two additional anti-infective agents (e.g., chloramphenicol, clindamycin, rifampin, vancomycin, clarithromycin, imipenem, penicillin, or ampicillin).[10,11]
Dosage adjustment in organ dysfunction	If CrCl is 30–50 mL/min, give 20–40 mg/kg/day divided q 8 h[12]; if CrCl is 10–29 mL/min, give 15–25 mg/kg/day divided q 12 h.[12] One reference suggest if the CrCl is <10 mL/min, give 7.5–12.5 mg/kg q 24 h[12]; however, the manufacturer recommends the drug be withheld if CrCl is ≤5 mL/min unless the patient is undergoing dialysis.[2]
Maximum dosage	100 mg/kg/day.[1,2,4] Up to 2 g/day in mild-to-moderate infections[2] and 4 g/day in severe infections.[2] IM dosages >1500 mg/day are not recommended.[2]
Additives	The 250- and 500-mg intravenous vials contain 0.8 mEq (18.8 mg) and 1.6 mEq (37.5 mg) of sodium, respectively.[13] The 500- and 750-mg intramuscular vials contain 1.4 mEq (32 mg) and 2.1 mEq (48 mg) of sodium, respectively.[13]
Suitable diluents	D5W, D10W, NS, D5¼NS, D5½NS, D5NS, D5LR.[13]
Maximum concentration	5 mg/mL.[2]
Preparation and delivery	**Compatibility:** See Appendix D for PN compatibility information.[14]
IV push	Not recommended.[2]
Intermittent infusion	2.5–5 mg/mL over 20–60 minutes.[2] The manufacturer recommends that smaller doses be infused over 20–30 minutes and that doses >500 mg be infused over 40–60 minutes.[2] Doses ≤500 mg have been infused over 15 minutes in children.[15] (See Infusion related cautions section.)
Continuous infusion	Not recommended.[2]

Imipenem–Cilastatin Sodium

Other routes of administration	Suspension for IM administration should be reconstituted with 1% lidocaine HCl without epinephrine.[2] IM administration should not given IV and should not be used for severe or life-threatening infections (e.g., sepsis, endocarditis).[2]

Comments

Rare adverse effects: Neurotoxicity of the carbapenem antibiotics has been reported.[16,17] Two neonates who received 20 mg/kg/day and 80 mg/kg/day of imipenem experienced seizures.[18] Seizures as early as the first day of therapy or after 3 days have been reported in children with meningitis. Three of 82 pediatric patients with cancer developed seizures attributed to imipenem/cilastatin.[19] In *adults*, seizures most often occur after 7 days and appear to be related to an underlying CNS disorder, impaired renal function, and/or large doses.[20] Because of the risk of seizures, the drug should not be used in patients with CNS infections and in patients with a history of seizure disorders.[1] Use cautiously in combination with drugs that lower the seizure threshold and in patients with renal dysfunction.

Drug interactions: Carbapenems may reduce serum valproic acid concentrations to sub-therapeutic levels, resulting in loss of seizure control.[21] Serum valproic acid concentrations should be monitored frequently after beginning or increasing the dose of a carbapenem. Alternative antibiotics or anticonvulsant therapy should be considered if serum valproic acid concentrations drop below the therapeutic range or a seizure occurs. Because imipenem is associated with numerous drug interactions, consult appropriate resources for dosing recommendations before combining any drug with imipenem.

Laboratory interference: May cause false-positive urinary glucose results when cupric sulfate solution-based tests (Clinitest, Benedict's, or Fehling's solutions) are used.[22]

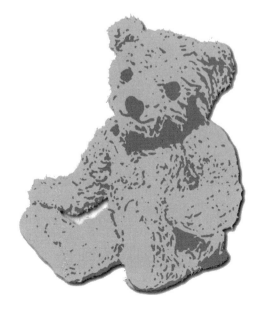

Immune Globulin Intravenous

Brand names	Carimune NF, Flebogamma, GAMMAGARD LIQUID, GAMMAGARD S/D, Gamunex, Octagam, Privigen
Medication error potential	Look-alike, sound-alike error potential.
	USP reported that IGIV was confused with hepatitis B immune globulin.[1]
Contraindications and warnings	**US boxed warning:** Acute renal dysfunction, acute renal failure, and death in predisposed patients have been associated with IGIV administration.[2-8] (See Comments section.)
	Contraindications: Previous severe hypersensitivity reaction to immune globulin.[2-8] Those with selective IgA deficiency and antibodies to IgA are at risk for developing severe hypersensitivity and anaphylactic reactions.
	Other warnings: Aseptic meningitis, hemolysis, transfusion related acute lung injury, osmotic nephrosis, and thrombotic events have been reported.[2-8]
Infusion related cautions	Epinephrine should be available during infusion.[2-8] Patients should not be volume depleted prior to infusion.[2-8]
	Infusion reactions including facial flushing, chest tightness, chills, fever, dizziness, nausea, vomiting, diaphoresis, and hypotension beginning 30 minutes to 1 hour may occur.[2] Decreasing the infusion rate or stopping the infusion until the reaction subsides; then restarting at a slower rate usually decreases the severity.[2-7] One large British study found that infusion reactions occurred at a rate of 0.7% in children <10 years, which is not significantly different from the *adult* rate of 0.8%.[9]
	Changing brands of IVIG may result in an increase in infusion related reactions. Use a slower rate of infusion than usually tolerated when a change in IVIG brand is necessary. The infusion rate may be increased as the patient tolerates the change.
Dosage	**Primary immunodeficiency:** 200–800 mg/kg/day q 3–4 weeks to maintain serum IgG concentrations ≥400–500 mg/dL.[2-8,10,11]
	ITP: 1–2 g/kg/day for 1–7 days initially and then as needed to maintain platelet count >30,000/mm^3.[2,5,6,10,12-15]
	Kawasaki disease: A single dose of 2 g/kg[15-21] is recommended over 400 mg/kg/day for four consecutive days.[5,17,19,22] Patients who have persistent fever or who have recrudescent fever after treatment may be retreated.[16,22,23]
	Chronic lymphocytic leukemia: 400 mg/kg every 3–4 weeks.[5]
	Chronic inflammatory demyelinating polyneuropathy: Loading dose of 2 g/kg in divided doses given over 2–4 days with maintenance doses of 1 g/kg given over 1–2 days every 3 weeks. [6]
	Hematopoietic stem cell transplantation with severe hypogammaglobulinemia (IgG <400 mg/dL): 400 mg/kg monthly to maintain IgG ≥400 mg/dL.[24] Because the half-life is shorter in severe hypogammaglobulinemia, patients may need larger than usual doses to maintain the desired IgG concentrations.[25]
	Guillain-Barré syndrome: 1 g/kg/day for 2 days or 400 mg/kg/day for 5–7 days.[15,26,27]

Immune Globulin Intravenous

Dosage *(cont.)*	**Other uses**

Advanced HIV infection: 300–400 mg/kg q 4 weeks.[28,29]

Hemolytic disease of the newborn: 500 mg/kg/day for 1–3 days was associated with a decreased need for exchange transfusion and a shorter duration of photo-therapy.[30,31]

Obsessive-compulsive and tic disorder associated with pediatric autoimmune neuropsychiatric disorders associated with streptococcal infection (PANDAS): 1 g/kg/day for 2 days resulted in significant improvements in neuropsychiatric symp-toms within 1 month compared to placebo.[32]

Sepsis prevention in premature neonates: 0.5[33-35]–1[33-37] g/kg at varying intervals to achieve an IgG concentration ≥700 mg/dL.[36,37]

Sydenham's chorea: In four children who received 1 g/kg/day for 2 days, a 72% improvement in chorea severity scores was noted 1 month after treatment. The long-term response was similar to that seen with prednisone, but the response occurred more rapidly with IVIG.[38]

Toxic epidermal necrolysis/Stevens-Johnson syndrome: Seven children received a total of 1.2–4 g/kg over up to 4 days depending on symptom improvement.[39] In a separate multicenter retrospective review that included eight children 4–16 years old, a total of 1.8–5.8 g/kg was given over 1–5 days.[40] These investigators recom-mended early IVIG treatment of 1 g/kg/day for 3 days.[40]

Dosage adjustment in organ dysfunction	No dosage adjustment may be required in renal dysfunction. However, in patients with pre-existing renal insufficiency or at risk for renal insufficiency, recommended doses should not be exceeded, the dilution should be at the minimum concentration possible, and the rate of infusion should be as slow as is practical.[24]

Maximum dosage	2 g/kg.[17]

Additives	Carimune NF contains sucrose.[2]

Flebogamma contains polyethylene glycol and D-sorbitol.[3]

GAMMAGARD LIQUID contains glycine.[4]

GAMMAGARD S/D contains glycine, polyethylene glycol, polysorbate 80, and 8.5 mg NaCl/L.[5]

Gamunex contains glycine.[6]

Octagam contains ≤30 mmol Na/L and maltose.[7]

Privigen contains proline.[8]

IgA concentrations range from <2.3 mcg/mL (GAMMAGARD S/D) to ≤0.2 mg/mL (Octagam).[2-8]

See Appendix C for more specific information about potential polyethylene glycol toxicity.

Suitable diluents	GAMMAGARD LIQUID, Gamunex, and Privigen may be diluted in D5W.[4,6,8]

Lyophilized and dried concentrate products are reconstituted according to manufacturer's recommendations.[2,5]

Immune Globulin Intravenous

Maximum concentration

12% (Carimune NF).[2]

Preparation and delivery

Filtration requirements for constitution and administration vary among products. Refer to manufacturer's recommendations for specific details.[2-8]

Stability: See Appendix D for PN compatibility information.

IV push

Not indicated.[2-8,24]

Intermittent infusion

The rate of the infusion depends on patient tolerance.[2-8] Infusion reactions are more likely with the first dose; as the patient continues receiving IVIG reactions usually subside and the infusion rate may increase. (See Comments section.)

According to patient tolerance, doses of 400 mg/kg are usually infused over 2 hours[19,33] and doses of 2 g/kg over 8–12 hours.[19]

Continuous infusion

Not indicated.

Other routes of administration

Not indicated. Only for IV use.

Comments

Significant adverse effects: Those at risk for acute renal dysfunction and death include those with pre-existing renal insufficiency, diabetes mellitus, >65 years of age, volume depletion, sepsis, paraproteinemia, and those receiving other nephrotoxic drugs.[2-8] Products that include sucrose are more likely to develop this toxicity.[2,3,7,8] Using the lowest concentration and the slowest infusion rate should be used in these individuals.[24]

Transient neutropenia can occur after IVIG in children with ITP.[41] A severe hemolytic anemia has been reported following infusion of high-dose IGIV for Kawasaki disease.[42]

Monitoring: Urine output, SCr, BUN prior to initial infusion and periodically after.[2-8]

Laboratory interference: Use of products containing maltose may result in false interpretations of blood glucose readings when glucose dehydrogenase pyrroloquinoline quinone or glucose-dye-oxidoreductase based testing methods are used.[7]

Osmolality: Carimune NF reconstituted to 3% in SW is 192 mOsm/kg and to 12% in NS is 1074.[2] Most other products range from 240–440 mOsm/kg.[3,4,6-8]

Other: The length of time between IVIG infusion and measles, mumps, and rubella (MMR) vaccination varies according to dose as follows[43]:

IVIG Dose	Interval before Vaccination
300–400 mg/kg	8 mo
1000 mg/kg	10 mo
1600–2000 mg/kg	11 mo

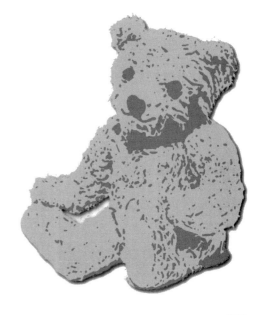

Inamrinone Lactate*

Brand names	Inocor
Medication error potential	ISMP high-alert medication (antiarrhythmic) that has an increased risk of causing significant patient harm if it is used in error.[1] USP reports confusion with amiodarone.[2]
Contraindications and warnings	**Contraindications:** Patients with a known hypersensitive to inamrinone or bisulfites.[3] **Warnings:** Allergic-type reactions to sulfites, including anaphylactic symptoms and life-threatening or less severe asthmatic episodes, may occur in susceptible people.[3] Sulfite sensitivity is seen more frequently in individuals with asthma compared to those without asthma.[3] (See Appendix C for specific information about sulfite hypersensitivity.)
Infusion related cautions	If hypotension occurs during loading dose, administer 5–10 mL/kg of NS or other appropriate fluid and position patient flat or with head down (if possible). If hypotension persist administer a vasopressor and discontinue further inamrinone.[3,4]

Dosage	Because inamrinone lactate has been administered to only a limited number of pediatric patients, the doses and side effects have not been established.[3] Although it has been used successfully to treat myocardial dysfunction and increased systemic or pulmonary vascular resistance, it has generally been replaced by milrinone.
	
	Loading dose: Usually 0.75–1 mg/kg over 2–3 minutes.[3,5-9] May repeat two to four times q 15 min to a total loading dose of 3 mg/kg.[3-8] Total loading doses have ranged from 0.75–4.5 mg/kg.[3,6,10-12]
	
	Maintenance infusion: It is difficult to predict the optimal infusion rate due to as much as a sixfold variation in the pharmacokinetics of inamrinone lactate in children[3]; hence, dose should be titrated to effect.
	
	    Neonates: 3–7.5 mcg/kg/min.[12,13]
	
	    Infants and children: 2–20 mcg/kg/min.[4]

Dosage adjustment in organ dysfunction	If CrCl is 10–29 mL/min, give 50% of the dose and if CrCl is <10 mL/min, give 25% of the dose.[14]
Maximum dosage	Not established. The PALS guidelines recommends up to 20 mcg/kg/min.[4] One group administered doses up to 40 mcg/kg/min for 30 minutes in seven children who had undergone cardiac surgery.[15] This study did not show statistically significant increases in stroke volume or cardiac index at the larger doses. Total dosage (initial, supplemental doses and cumulative infused dose) should not generally exceed 10 mg/kg/day in *adults*,[3] but doses up to 18 mg/kg/day have been infused for short periods in *adults*.[3] A 2.5-month-old infant died from accidental infusion of 180–198 mcg/kg/min.[16]
Additives	0.25 mg sodium metabisulfite per mL of inamrinone.[3] (See Appendix C for specific information about sulfite hypersensitivity.)
Suitable diluents	½NS, NS.[17]
Maximum concentration	5 mg/mL (commercially available).[3]

---

*Previously amrinone.

Inamrinone Lactate

Preparation and delivery	**Stability:** Use diluted solutions (1–3 mg/mL) within 24 hours.[3] **Compatibility:** Should not be diluted with solutions containing dextrose prior to injection[3] but may be administered into running dextrose infusions through a Y-Connector or directly into the tubing where preferable.[17] Furosemide should not be administered in intravenous lines containing inamrinone as a precipitate will form.[3] Incompatible with sodium bicarbonate.[17]
IV push	5 mg/mL (commercially available) over 2–3 minutes.[3] The 2005 PALS Guidelines recommend infusing bolus dose over 5 minutes.[4] One group of investigators infused 0.75 mg/kg over 30 seconds.[9] Another group noted that hypotension was related to the infusion rate and recommended dividing any loading dose larger than 0.75 mg/kg into two or three smaller doses.[5]
Intermittent infusion	Although concentration and solution type were not specified, a loading dose of 4.5 mg/kg has been infused over 2 hours.[11]
Continuous infusion	1–3 mg/mL in ½NS or NS.[3]
Other routes of administration	May be given IO.[4]
Comments	**Rare adverse effects:** Thrombocytopenia has been reported. In one study involving 16 children (1–134 months of age), eight developed thrombocytopenia within 19–71 hours after initiation of inamrinone lactate. When inamrinone lactate was discontinued, thrombocytopenia resolved after 54 ± 15 hours.[8] **Drug interactions:** Because inamrinone lactate is associated with several drug-drug interactions, consult appropriate resources for dosing recommendations before combining any drug with inamrinone lactate.

Indomethacin Sodium Trihydrate

Brand names	Indocin IV

Medication error potential

Look-alike, sound-alike drug names.

USP reports confusion with indapamide.[1]

Contraindications and warnings

US boxed warning: May increase the risk of cardiovascular thrombotic events, including potentially fatal MI and stroke.[2,3] Risk may be increased in patients with existing cardiovascular disease and following prolonged use.[2,3] Is contraindicated for perioperative pain following coronary artery bypass graft (CABG) surgery.[3]

Spontaneous bleeding, ulceration, and perforation of stomach or intestines may occur without warning and could be fatal.[3] (See Rare adverse effects in Comments section.)

Contraindications: Hypersensitivity to indomethacin, any component, aspirin, or other NSAIDs.[4] Neonates with (1) active bleeds (especially intracranial or gastrointestinal), thrombocytopenia, or coagulation defects; (2) proven or suspected infections that are untreated; (3) impaired renal function; (4) existing or suspected necrotizing enterocolitis; and (5) congenital heart disease in whom patency of the ductus arteriosus is necessary for satisfactory pulmonary or systemic blood flow (e.g., pulmonary atresia, severe tetralogy of Fallot, severe coarctation of the aorta).[2]

Other warnings: May cause increasing BUN, creatinine, decreased glomerular filtration rate, and ≥50% reduction in urine output (UOP).[2]

These effects are generally transient and resolve upon discontinuation of indomethacin.[2] However, indomethacin may precipitate renal insufficiency, including acute renal failure. This is especially evident in neonates with other conditions capable of adversely affecting renal function (e.g., extracellular volume depletion from any cause, congestive heart failure, sepsis, concomitant administration of nephrotoxic drugs, hepatic dysfunction).[2] Indomethacin should be withheld in any patient with significant decreases in UOP until output returns to normal.

Spontaneous intraventricular hemorrhage (IVH) is a known complication of prematurity. Because indomethacin causes platelet inhibition, it may increase the risk for IVH.[2] (See Rare adverse effects in Comments section.)

Infusion related cautions

Avoid extravasation.[2]

Dosage

Patent ductus arteriosus (closure of the ductus arteriosus)

Prophylaxis (used for subclinical PDA and routine prophylaxis within 24 hours of life in very low birth weight newborns): 0.1 mg/kg q 24 h for 5 days.[5-7] Continuous infusion has been used (0.004 mg/kg/h) from 6–12 hours postnatal age until ductus closure.[8]

Prophylaxis has not been found to improve survival without neurosensory impairment.[9,10]

Indomethacin Sodium Trihydrate

Dosage *(cont.)*

Conventional treatment[2,11,12]

PNA at First Dose	Dose 1	Dose 2	Dose 3
<2 days	0.2 mg/kg	0.1 mg/kg	0.1 mg/kg
2–7 days	0.2 mg/kg	0.2 mg/kg	0.2 mg/kg
>7 days	0.2 mg/kg	0.25 mg/kg	0.25 mg/kg

Assess UOP after first and second dose to determine dosing interval. If UOP is >1 mL/kg/h, dose q 12 h; if 0.6–1 mL/kg/h, dose q 24 h; if <0.6 mL/kg/h, no dose should be given until renal function normalizes.

In a study of ventilated neonates with respiratory distress syndrome conventional doses were given q 12–18 h.[13]

Reopening of the ductus arteriosus, after a successful course of indomethacin, may require a second course of one to three doses using the above recommendations. If unresponsive, surgical correction may be needed.[2]

Continuous infusion: 0.004–0.011 mg/kg/h over 36 hours has been reported to reduce alterations in renal, cerebral, and mesenteric blood flow compared to bolus administration.[8,14,15]

Prevention of intraventricular hemorrhage: 0.1 mg/kg q 24 h for three doses beginning at 6–12 hours of age.[16-18]

Dosage adjustment in organ dysfunction

Should be withheld if oliguria (<0.6 mL/kg/h) or anuria.[4]

Maximum dosage

0.25–0.4 mg/kg/dose[11,19] or cumulative 0.9–1 mg/kg in 3 days.[20,21]

Additives

None.

Suitable diluents

Preservative free SW or NS.[22]

Maximum concentration

1 mg/mL.[2, 22]

Preparation and delivery

Stability: Reconstitute with 1 or 2 mL of preservative-free diluent just prior to administration. Portions not used should be immediately discarded.[2,22]

Compatibility: See Appendix D for PN compatibility information.[23]

IV push

Although indomethacin has been given over 5–10 seconds,[24,25] rapid administration causes a significant decrease in mesenteric artery[26] and cerebral blood flow that may contribute to the development of necrotizing enterocolitis[26] or cerebral ischemia.[26-28]

Indomethacin Sodium Trihydrate

Intermittent infusion	0.5–1 mg/mL over IV over 20–30 minutes.[2,22]
Continuous infusion	Not recommended.[2]
Other routes of administration	IM administration not recommended.[2]
Comments	**Rare adverse events:** Indomethacin may cause a transient reduction in cerebral and mesenteric blood flow.[2] In a large multicenter study, the incidence of intraventricular hemorrhage in neonates was not significantly different in neonates given indomethacin and placebo.[18] Others have reported that indomethacin may decrease the incidence and severity of IVH.[29,30]

Bleeding, with a focus on GI or NEC, has been reported with IV indomethacin regimens that consisted of six doses.[21,31-33] Although major gastrointestinal bleeding was no more common in neonates receiving indomethacin than in those given placebo, minor gastrointestinal bleeding (i.e., chemical detection of blood in the stool) was more commonly noted in those receiving.[2]

Hypoglycemia that developed during indomethacin therapy persisted for up to 72 hours.[34-36]

Neurological effects (dizziness, headache, and somnolence) may be attributed to the variable absorption into the CNS and rapid concentrations found in the CSF.[37]

Nonsteroidal therapy in *adults* has caused liver disease.[2,38,39] If signs or symptoms develop therapy should be discontinue.

Monitoring: Renal function (serum creatinine and BUN), UOP, CBC and platelets, serum transaminases, electrolytes (especially K and Na), and glucose.

Drug interactions: Digoxin is dependent on renal function for elimination, and that could be reduced with the use of indomethacin. Additional monitoring with ECGs or serum digoxin levels may be needed to detect digoxin toxicity.[2,33,40] Concurrent aminoglycoside and indomethacin (standard course was given q 8 h) produced elevation in aminoglycoside peak and trough.[2,41] Indomethacin is a minor substrate of CYP2C9, 2C19 and is a strong inhibitor of CYP 2C9.[4] It is also bound to albumin and could displace bilirubin from albumin binding sites.[42] Consult appropriate resources for dosing recommendations before combining any drug with indomethacin.

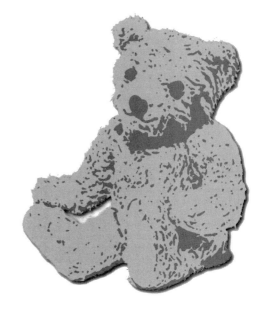

Infliximab

Brand names	Remicade

Medication error potential

Look-alike, sound-alike error potential.

ISMP and USP report that rituximab was confused with infliximab.[1,2] USP reports that this error caused patient harm.[2]

Contraindications and warnings

US boxed warning

Risk of serious infections: Patients receiving infliximab are at risk for developing serious infections. Those with active infections should not begin treatment. Those who develop infection while on treatment should be monitored closely.[3,4]

Patients should be evaluated for latent tuberculosis infection with a tuberculin skin test. If the skin test is positive, treatment of tuberculosis should be started prior to beginning treatment with infliximab.[3,4] (See Comments section.)

Hepatosplenic T-cell lymphomas: These have been reported in adolescents and young *adults* receiving infliximab. Usually patients who develop this are being treated concurrently with 6-mercaptopurine or azathioprine.[3,4]

FDA alert: On August 4, 2009 the FDA announced that it is requiring those who manufacture TNF blockers to update the boxed warning to include an increased risk of lymphoma and other cancers in children and adolescents treated with TNF blockers.[5]

Contraindications: Patients who have had a previous severe hypersensitivity reaction to infliximab should not receive any additional doses.[3]

Other warnings: Anaphylactic type reactions have been reported.[3] Appropriate medical care should be available in the event this occurs.

Infusion related cautions

Flushing, chest pain, and shortness of breath have occurred during infusion in up to 38.6% of pediatric patients.[6-9] Acetaminophen, antihistamines, corticosteroids, and epinephrine, or by slowing the rate of infusion aids in symptom management.[3,4,8] The infusion should be stopped if this regimen symptoms do not improve or if epinephrine is required. Infusion reactions can occur with the first or any subsequent dose[6] but are most likely to occur after the second or third infusion.[4,6] A history of an infusion reaction is not predictive of future infusion-related reactions.

A delayed infusion reaction may be experienced 3–5 days after treatment. The physician should be notified if this occurs. Longer intervals between treatments (more than a year) increase the risk of delayed infusion reactions.[3,4]

Dosage

Crohn's disease: Usual doses are 5 mg/kg repeated as needed.[10-19] Regimens include 5 mg/kg every 8 weeks for a year if showing a favorable response,[15] 5 mg/kg at 0, 2, and 6 weeks followed by 5 mg/kg every 8 weeks,[15-18] and 5 mg/kg administered on days 0, 15, and 45.[19] Doses of 1 mg/kg are less effective.[20]

Ulcerative colitis: 5 mg/kg[21-24] initially followed by 5–10 mg/kg in 2 weeks[22] or 5 mg/kg as induction therapy at 0, 2, and 6 weeks with maintenance treatment every 6–8 weeks.[12,23,24]

Refractory juvenile idiopathic arthritis (JIA): 3–4 mg/kg initially or at weeks 0, 2, and 6 weeks followed by up to 10 mg/kg every 4–8 weeks.[25,26] One study in 122 children who were receiving methotrexate found that infusion reactions were greater in the group receiving 3 mg/kg than those receiving 6 mg/kg.[27]

Infliximab

Dosage *(cont.)*	**JIA uveitis:** 5–10 mg/kg at weeks 0, 2, and 4 followed by infusions every 6–8 weeks with a more rapid infusion rate based on tolerance (stable vital signs).[28] In a case series of pediatric uveitis patients with or without associated JIA, all patients responded to infliximab at 5–10 mg/kg at 2–8 week intervals.[29] (See Comments section.) **Refractory Kawasaki syndrome:** Limited data suggests that a single infusion of 5–10 mg/kg may be beneficial in patients who have not responded to two doses of IVIG and high-dose daily aspirin therapy.[30]
Dosage adjustment in organ dysfunction	Information not available.
Maximum dosage	Doses up to 20 mg/kg have been used in *adults*[3] and one case series reported successful treatment of a 15-year-old patient receiving an 18-mg/kg dose.[29]
Additives	None.[3,4]
Suitable diluents	SWI to reconstitute, NS to dilute.[3,4]
Maximum concentration	4 mg/mL.[3,4]
Preparation and delivery	**Preparation:** Reconstitute a 100-mg vial by adding 10 mL SWI via a 21 gauge or small needle with the stream directed to the glass wall of the vial. Gently rotate the vial to dissolve. Do not shake. The reconstituted vial should be allowed to sit for 5 minutes prior to dilution.[3,4] After the total dose (which may include multiple vials) has been reconstituted, withdraw an equivalent dose volume of NS from a 250-mL bag or bottle. Slowly add the total volume of reconstituted infliximab to the 250-mL bag or bottle. Gently mix.[3,4] **Delivery:** Administer the infusion using an in-line, low-protein-binding filter with a pore diameter ≤1.2 microns.[3,4] **Stability:** The vial contains no preservatives and once reconstituted the infusion must begin within 3 hours.[3,4]
IV push	Not indicated.[3,4]
Intermittent infusion	The infusion rate was increased after 15 minutes from 15 mL/h to 30 mL/h for 15 minutes to 60 mL/h for 30 minutes to 90 mL/h to complete the infusion[4,15] or was increased q 15 min from 10 mL/h to 20 mL/h to 40 mL/h to 80 mL/h to a maximum of 125 mL/h based on the stability of vital signs.[4,6] The infusion should be administered over ≥2 hours.[3,4]
Continuous infusion	Not indicated.
Other routes of administration	Not indicated.

Infliximab

Juvenile idiopathic arthritis, juvenile rheumatoid arthritis, and juvenile chronic arthritis may be used interchangeably.

A negative skin test for tuberculosis does not rule out the possibility of disease since patients with immune diseases may exhibit cutaneous anergy.[31]

Infusion related reactions are believed to be caused by the production of antibodies to infliximab. The concomitant administration of immunomodulating medications (or use within the preceding 4 months) is believed to be protective.[3]

Infliximab was a more effective therapy for JIA uveitis than etanercept.[32,33]

Drug interactions: Patients receiving anakinra should not receive infliximab due to a possible increased risk for infection.[3]

Live virus vaccines (measles-mumps-rubella, varicella, rotavirus) should be avoided during treatment.[3,4]

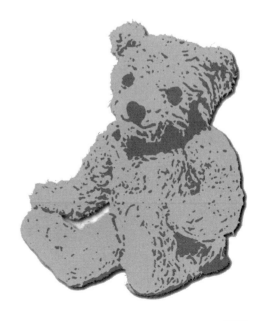

Insulin

Brand names	Humulin R, Novolin R, Humulin R (concentrated U-500)

Medication error potential

ISMP high-alert medication that has an increased risk of causing significant patient harm if it is used in error.[1]

Look-alike, sound-alike error potential.

ISMP reported that Humulin R was confused with Humalog.[2]

USP reported that Humulin R was confused with Humulin 70/30, Novolin 70/30, Novolin R, and NovoLog.[3] Patient harm resulted when Humulin R was confused with Humalog.

USP reported that Novolin R was confused with Humulin R. Patient harm resulted with Novolin R was confused with Novolin 70/30, Novolin GE NPH, and NovoLog.

Contraindications and warnings

FDA alert: On March 19, 2009 the FDA reminded healthcare providers and patients that insulin pens must not be shared due to the potential of transmission of viruses (including HIV and hepatitis C) and other blood borne pathogens.

Contraindications: Hypersensitivity to regular insulin or any of its components, hypoglycemia.[4]

Warnings: Hypoglycemia is the most common adverse effect.[4] Serum glucose concentrations must be monitored closely to detect hypoglycemia early.

Accurate choice of product is critical since many different types of insulin preparations are available. Availability and use of concentrated insulin should be restricted.

Infusion related cautions

Regular insulin products can be infused IV.[5]

Dosage

Hyperglycemic crises in diabetes (DKA and hyperosmolar hyperglycemic state [HHS]): Biochemical evidence of DKA includes HCO_3 <15 mmol/L and pH <7.25 and an increased blood glucose (BG).[6] Baseline electrolytes must be obtained and rehydration with NS should be done prior to beginning insulin as BG concentrations will begin to decrease with rehydration.[6] Institutional protocols for fluid and electrolyte replacement, monitoring and use of insulin should be followed.

Initially, 0.05–0.1 unit/kg/h.[6-11] A loading dose is no longer recommended.[6] BG should be measured hourly to ensure that the decrease in BG is 50–90 mg/dL/h.[6] Too rapid a decrease in BG may cause cerebral edema and may require the addition of a glucose infusion even before glucose is <300 mg/dL. If the biochemical parameters of DKA do not improve, the insulin infusion may be increased. SC dosing can be started when the HCO_3 ≥18 mmol/L, pH >7.3, and plasma glucose is <200 mg/dL.[6]

Hyperkalemia (after therapy with NaHCO₃ and calcium gluconate): 0.05–0.1 unit/kg/h infused with 400 mg dextrose/kg or 1 unit insulin/4 g dextrose.[8] Alternatively, 0.5–1 g/kg dextrose with 1 unit insulin/4–5 g/dextrose infused over 2 hours has been suggested.[8] A systematic review included two unblinded studies in preterm neonates.[12] One of these reported that 20 infants who received 1 unit insulin/10–15 g dextrose had shorter duration of hyperkalemia and fewer episodes of intraventricular hemorrhage than those (n = 20) receiving Kayexalate.[12] However, authors of the review concluded that no firm practice recommendations could be made for preterm neonates.[12]

Hyperglycemia: The optimum target BG range and best method to attain this BG and avoid hypoglycemia is unknown.[13]

Critically ill children: A survey found that pediatric ICU practitioners initiated insulin at a BG of 150 mg/dL while *adult* practitioners began insulin at a BG of 120 mg/dL.[14] Of pediatric practitioners, 33% used a starting dose of 0.1 unit/kg/h. Most *adult* and pediatric practitioners defined hypoglycemia as a BG of <60 mg/dL.

Dosage *(cont.)*	A retrospective study of pediatric burn patients found that initiating insulin at a BG of 140 mg/dL titrated to a BG of 90–120 mg/dL resulted in a lower amount of insulin delivered per day but a longer duration of therapy (mean of 1.9 ± 1.6 units/kg/day for 38.1 ± 48 days) than those who started insulin at a BG of 200 mg/dL titrated to a BG <200 mg/dL (3.7 ± 5.3 units/kg/day for 8.9 ± 6.8 days).[15] Of note, infections and mortality were lower in the group who attained the lower BG concentrations. Critically ill children in Belgium had insulin titrated to a normal age-related BG measurement (intensive insulin therapy; n = 349) or received a conventional therapy (n = 351).[15] Starting doses in the intensive group was 0.1 unit/kg/h in those with a BG above normal and 0.2 unit/kg/h in those with BG twice the normal BG concentration. Conventional dosing began insulin after the second BG >11.9 mmol/L (~214 mg/dL) that was titrated to 10–11.9 mmol/L (~180–214 mg/dL). While short term outcomes were improved in the intensive group, hypoglycemia occurred in 25%.
	Glucose intolerance in low birth weight (LBW) infants: A 2008 multicenter trial compared early insulin treatment in 195 LBW infants (0.05 unit/kg/h with D20W to maintain euglycemia) within 24 hours of age to conventional therapy in 194 infants (titrate dextrose to avoid hyperglycemia (glucose of 180 mg/dL) and hypoglycemia (47 mg/dL) or manage hyperglycemia with insulin).[17] The trial was ended early because of increased mortality at 28 days of life in the early group (11.9% vs 5.7%, respectively; odds ratio 0.45, confidence interval 0.21–0.96). Earlier studies evaluated 0.03–0.08 unit/kg/h with the dose titrated to desired BG concentration.[18-23] (See Maximum dosage, Preparation and delivery, and Comments sections.)
Dosage adjustment in organ dysfunction	CrCl 10–50 mL/min, give 75% of the normal dose.[4] CrCl <10 mL/min, give 50% of normal dose.[4] Use cautiously in patients with hepatic impairment.[4]
Maximum dosage	Up to 4.2 units/kg/h were required occasionally in hyperglycemic very LBW neonates (<1000 g) during first 2 weeks of life.[22,23] It has been speculated that the increased requirement in these infants was due to insulin resistance, inappropriate insulin secretion, or decreased sensitivity of the liver to insulin effects.[20,24] In DKA, some endocrinologists do not use more than 3 units/h in children.[7]
Additives	100 units contain 10–40 mcg Zn. Novolin R contains glycerin and metacresol. Humulin R contains glycerin and cresol.[4]
Suitable diluents	NS.[4,5,16]
Maximum concentration	Depends on the dose to be delivered. 0.1–1 unit/mL has been reported.[16] 100 units/mL (commercially available) for IM or SC dosing.[5]
Preparation and delivery	Insulin binds to glass bottles, plastic IV bags, syringes, and tubing and results in decreased delivery of insulin. IV tubing may be primed with an insulin solution to saturate insulin-binding sites and prevent further absorption.[5,9,10,21,25,26] Alternatively, human serum albumin occupies binding sites on glass[27] and plastic and has been added to insulin-containing solutions[6,19,22] to increase insulin delivery. **Compatibility:** See Appendix D for PN compatibility information.
IV push	A loading dose has been used in DKA and HHS[23] but is no longer recommended.[6]

Insulin

Intermittent infusion	Not indicated.
Continuous infusion	Commonly used.[9,24] (See Dosage section.)
Other routes of administration	IM and SC. IM administration results in faster absorption than SC.[11] However, in DKA and HHS these routes of administration may require hourly dosing of insulin. IM and SC dosing should not be used in patients with hypovolemic shock, hyperosmolar hyperglycemia, or hyperkalemia.
	A 5-year-old with DKA and dehydration received insulin via IO infusion.[28]

Comments

Blood glucose measurements: 120 mg/dL = 6.7 mmol/L.

In LBW infants, a 12–14 hour delay in response was noted when IV tubing was not primed with insulin.[21] Whether this was due to lack of priming or insulin resistance was not evaluated.

Monitoring: It is essential that BG concentrations be measured regularly during insulin therapy to avoid hypoglycemia. Bedside measurements should be periodically compared to plasma samples performed in the laboratory to insure their accuracy.

DKA[6]**:** Electrolytes, magnesium, phosphorous, and blood gas must be measured every 2–4 hours or more frequently if clinically indicated. BUN, SCr, and hematocrit should be measured every 6–8 hours. Intake and output should be measured hourly and are neurological assessments and vital signs.

Hyperkalemia: Serum potassium concentrations and BG. Treatment should be discontinued when potassium concentrations are normalized.

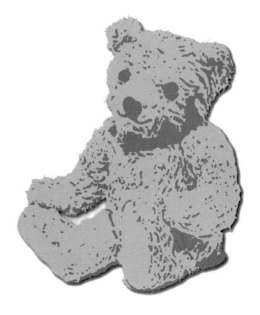

Interferon Alfa-2b

Brand names	Intron A for Injection

Medication error potential	Look-alike, sound-alike error potential.
	USP reported that interferon alfa-2a has been confused with interferon alfa-2b.[1]

Contraindications and warnings	**US boxed warning:** Alpha interferons cause or aggravate fatal or life-threatening neuropsychiatric, autoimmune, ischemic, and infectious disorders. Patients should be monitored closely, and periodic clinical and laboratory valuations should be performed. Treatment should be stopped in patients with persistently severe or worsening signs or symptoms of these conditions. In many cases, but not all, these disorders resolve after therapy is discontinued.[2]
	Contraindications: Hypersensitivity to interferon alfa-2b or product components, autoimmune hepatitis, and decompensated liver disease.[2]

Infusion related cautions	The solution vials for injection and the multidose pens for injection are not indicated for IV use.[2]
	Injection site reactions occur in 5% of pediatric patients with chronic hepatitis B.[2]

Dosage	**Chronic hepatitis B with compensated liver disease:** 3 million units/m² SC or IM three times/week for 1 week, then increased to 6 million units/m² SC three times/week for 16–24 weeks.[2] Children from 3–15 years of age have been treated with 3–10 million units/m² SC or IM[3-9] three times/week for up to 1 year, alone or in combination with lamivudine.[10,11] Larger doses are associated with higher rates of viral clearance.[4] (See Comments section.)
	Chronic hepatitis C: Children ≥2 years of age have received 3–5 million units/m² SC three times/week[12-15] or 0.1 million unit/kg/day for 2 weeks then three times/week for 26 weeks.[16] (See Comments section.)
	Melanoma: In a small tolerability study, 15 children from 1.5–17 years old received induction therapy with 20 million units/m² IV five times/week for 4 weeks. This was followed by 10 million units/m² SC times/week for 48 weeks.[17]
	Hemangiomas or Kasabach-Merritt syndrome: 100,000–6 million units/m²/day SC for ≥9 weeks.[18-21] One group treated 39 children from 1.5 to 158 months of age with 3 million units/m²/day SC for 6 months.[21] Treatment continued for another 6 months, and in those who responded the interval was changed to three times/week; however, in those without hemangioma regression, the dose was increased to 6 million units/m²/day SC.[21] In Kasabach-Merritt syndrome (an aggressive vascular tumor), six of eight children responded to 3 million units/day that was given for up to 12 months.[22]
	Relapsed T-cell acute lymphoblastic leukemia (ALL) or non-Hodgkin's lymphoma (NHL): Twenty children from 3–18 years of age were given 30 million units/m²/day to three times/week IV or SC; two of these developed congestive heart failure.[23] Doses from 3–50 million units/m² for 10 doses in 2 weeks were used in a limited number of pediatric patients with ALL, NHL, and Philadelphia chromosome–positive chronic myelogenous leukemia.[24]

Interferon Alfa-2b

Dosage adjustment in organ dysfunction

Recommendations for dosage decreases are according to hematologic indices, liver, and renal function. In addition, recommended dosage changes vary according to disease being treated. (See Comments section.)

Interferon alfa-2b may be used in combination with ribavirin for the treatment of hepatitis C and hepatitis B. This combination should not be used in patients with CrCl <50 mL/min.

Chronic hepatitis B

Dose	WBC	Granulocytes	Platelets
Decrease 50%	$<1.5 \times 10^9$/L	$<0.75 \times 10^9$/L	$<50 \times 10^9$/L
Discontinue	$<1 \times 10^9$/L	$<0.5 \times 10^9$/L	$<25 \times 10^9$/L

Malignant melanoma (during induction or maintenance therapy)[2]

   Withhold doses: Granulocytes >250 mm³ but <500 mm³; SGPT/SGOT >5 to ≤10 × upper limit of normal (restart at 50% of initial dose once normal).

   Permanently discontinue: Granulocytes <250 mm³ or SGPT/SGOT >10 × upper limit of normal.

Follicular lymphoma[2]

   Withhold doses: Neutrophil count <1000/mm³ or platelet count <50,000/mm³.

   Decrease dose 50%: Neutrophil count >1000/mm³ but <1500/mm³.

   Permanently discontinue: SCr >2 mg/dL or SGOT> 5 × upper limit of normal.

Maximum dosage

Children with chronic hepatitis B: 10 million units three times/week.

***Adults* with chronic hepatitis B:** 35 million units IM or SC/week for 16 weeks.[1]

Additives

When the lyophilized powder is reconstituted with the provided diluent (SW), each mL contains 20 mg glycine, 2.3 mg sodium phosphate dibasic, 0.55 mg sodium phosphate monobasic, and 1 mg albumin (human).[1]

Each mL of the solution vials for injection (given IM, SC, intralesional) and the multidose pens for injection (given SC) contain 7.5 mg sodium chloride, 1.8 mg sodium phosphate dibasic, 1.3 mg sodium phosphate monobasic, 0.1 mg edetate disodium, 0.1 mg polysorbate 80, and 1.5 mg *m*-cresol.[2]

Suitable diluents

NS.

Maximum concentration

≥10 million units/100 mL for IV infusion.[2]

Concentrations for SC and IM use range from 6–50 million units/mL depending on the product and indication.[2]

Interferon Alfa-2b

Preparation and delivery	The lyophilized powder is reconstituted with the provided diluent (SW).[2] After the diluent is added, swirl the vial gently to dissolve the powder, do not shake. The reconstituted powder is suitable for IM or SC administration. For IV infusion, the reconstituted dose should be withdrawn and added to 100 mL of NS. The final concentration for IV infusion should be ≥10 million units/100 mL. This contains no preservative and should be discarded after the first dose is withdrawn. Multidose vials (IM, SC) and pens (SC) are available in a variety of concentrations that are ready to use.[2]
IV push	Not indicated.
Intermittent infusion	Over 20 minutes.[2]
Continuous infusion	Not indicated.
Other routes of administration	IM, SC.[2]
Comments	**Adverse effects:** A flu-like syndrome of fever, fatigue, malaise, myalgia, chills, headache, arthralgia, and rigors occurs frequently.[2,3,7,18,25] Severity of this increases with higher dosages.[2,3,7,18] Fevers peak within 6 hours and may persist for up to 12 hours. Pretreatment with antipyretics (e.g., APAP or NSAIDs) may be beneficial. Dosing at night may decrease the flu-like adverse effects.[2] Children may experience a decrease in linear growth and weight gain.[2] Interferon alfa-2b used in combination with ribavirin for the treatment of hepatitis C and hepatitis B resulted in hemolytic anemia in 10% of patients. **Monitoring:** CBC pretreatment and routinely during therapy.[2] **Drug interactions:** Interferon decreases theophylline clearance.[2,26] Theophylline serum concentrations should be monitored during treatment.

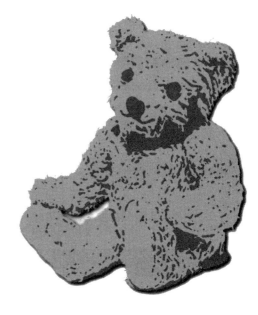

Irinotecan HCl

Brand names	Camptosar, generic
Medication error potential	ISMP high-alert medication that has an increased risk of causing significant patient harm if it is used in error.[1] Look-alike, sound-alike error potential. USP reports that irinotecan has been confused with topotecan; no patient harm resulted.[2]
Contraindications and warnings	**US boxed warning:** Irinotecan must be administered under the supervision of physician experienced with chemotherapeutic agents. Irinotecan can induce both late and early forms of diarrhea and severe myelosuppression can occur.[3] (See Significant adverse effects in Comments section.) **Contraindications:** Irinotecan is contraindicated in patients with known hypersensitivity to the drug or any of its components.[3] **Other warnings:** May cause severe diarrhea, neutropenia, hypersensitivity, colitis/ileus, renal impairment, severe emesis, and risk of thromboembolism.[3,4] (See Significant adverse effects in Comments section.)
Infusion related cautions	A higher incidence of cholinergic side effects has been reported with shorter infusion times.[5] Extravasation should be avoided. If extravasation occurs, flush site with sterile water and apply ice.[3]
Dosage	Consult institutional protocol for complete dosing information. Irinotecan is used as a component of combination therapy or as a single agent to treat multiple pediatric tumors, including neuroblastoma, hepatocellular tumors, Wilms' tumor, osteosarcoma, rhabdomyosarcoma, and CNS tumors, including medulloblastoma, ependymomas, brain stem gliomas, and astrocytomas.[5] **Refractory solid tumors (low-dose, protracted schedule):** 20 mg/m²/day for 5 days for 2 consecutive weeks repeated q 21 days.[5-7] **Refractory solid tumors or CNS tumors:** 50 mg/m²/day for 5 days repeated q 21 days.[5,8-10] **Heavily pretreated refractory solid tumors or CNS tumors:** 125 mg/m²/dose once weekly for 4 weeks, repeated q 6 weeks.[5,11] **Less heavily pretreated refractory solid tumors or CNS tumors:** 160 mg/m²/dose once weekly for 4 weeks, repeated q 6 weeks.[5,11]
Dosage adjustment in organ dysfunction	No information to guide administration of irinotecan in patients with hepatic (i.e., serum bilirubin >2 mg/dL) or renal dysfunction.[3] Some studies suggest that patients with moderate hepatic dysfunction (i.e., serum bilirubin of 1–2 mg/dL) and a prior history of abdominal or pelvic radiation may be at increased risk of developing neutropenia.[12] Some clinicians reduce dose in this scenario.

Irinotecan HCl

Maximum dosage	Not established. In clinical trials, single dosages up to 345–750 mg/m^2 have been administered to *adult* cancer patients.[3] No antidotes for overdoses are known. Patients should receive supportive care to prevent neutropenia and diarrhea.
Additives	None.
Suitable diluents	D5W, NS.[3,13]
Maximum concentration	2.8 mg/mL.[3,13]
Preparation and delivery	**Preparation:** Irinotecan must be diluted prior to infusion. Most clinical trials have used 250–500 mL of D5W as a diluent, as the relatively acidic pH of irinotecan favors dilution with D5W over NS.[3,12,13] **Stability:** Do not refrigerate solutions mixed in NS since visible particulates may develop.[4]
IV push	Not recommended.
Intermittent infusion	Dilute with suitable diluent to a final concentration of 0.12–2.8 mg/mL and infuse over 60–90 minutes.[3]
Continuous infusion	Hepatic arterial continuous infusions have been explored in *adult* colorectal cancer patients with metastases to the liver.[14]
Other routes of administration	No information available to support administration by other routes.
Comments	**Significant adverse effects:** Irinotecan is associated with both acute (within first several hours) and delayed (24 hours after drug administration) diarrhea, both of which can be dose-limiting.[3] Patients should be premedicated with 0.01 mg/kg of IV atropine (maximum dose: 0.4 mg) to prevent acute diarrhea and should receive a prescription for loperamide to prevent delayed diarrhea. Acute diarrhea is usually transient and patients may develop cholinergic symptoms such as rhinitis, miosis, flushing, or lacrimation. However, delayed diarrhea can have life-threatening consequences, such as dehydration, electrolyte disturbances, fever, or severe neutropenia.[3] If patients develop late diarrhea, loperamide should be administered q 3 h while the patient is awake and q 4 h while the patient is asleep for up to 24 hours after complete resolution of loose stools. Please note that this loperamide regimen differs from what is listed on the package insert for OTC cases of diarrhea. The table below lists the suggested doses based on weight of the child.[5]

Irinotecan HCl

Comments *(cont.)*

Dose of Loperamide Based on Weight of Patient

Weight (kg)	Immediate Dose	Daytime Dose (q 3 h)*	Nighttime Dose (q 4 h)
8–10	1 mg	0.5 mg	0.75 mg
10.1–20	1 mg	1 mg	1 mg
20.1–30	2 mg	1 mg	2 mg
30.1–43	2 mg	1 mg q 2 h	2 mg
>43	4 mg	2 mg q 2 h	4 mg

*Unless noted.

Patients that develop severe neutropenia and/or diarrhea while on normal dosages of irinotecan may need pharmacogenetic testing to evaluate if they are homozygous for the UGT1A1 allele that has been associated with increased irinotecan side effects.[3] Homozygous patients may require a dosage reduction.

Patients should have a baseline absolute neutrophil count >1500 cells/mm^3 and a platelet count >100,000 cells/mm^3 before drug administration.[3] The manufacturer has outlined dosage reductions for diarrhea, neutropenia, and neutropenic fever in the labeling.[3]

Irinotecan is associated with a moderate (30% to 90%) risk of emesis.[15] Patients should receive antiemetic therapy to prevent acute and delayed nausea and vomiting. The recommended therapy is a 5HT3 receptor antagonist in combination with dexamethasone on every day chemotherapy is administered.[15,16] These agents may be continued for up to 4 days after chemotherapy administration for the prevention of delayed nausea and vomiting. Breakthrough medications should also be offered, such as a phenothiazine (e.g., prochlorperazine), a butyrophenone (e.g., droperidol), a substituted benzamide (e.g., metoclopramide), or a benzodiazepine (e.g., lorazepam).

Monitoring: Patients should be monitored for signs of diarrhea and dehydration, electrolytes, BUN and SCr, CBC and platelet counts, and liver enzymes. Infusion site should also be monitored for signs of inflammation.[3,4]

Drug interactions: Irinotecan is a major substrate for CYP2B6 and CYP3A4 and thus concomitant administration with other medications that interact with similar isoenzymes should be approached with caution.[3,5] Consult appropriate resources for dosing recommendations before combining any drug with irinotecan.

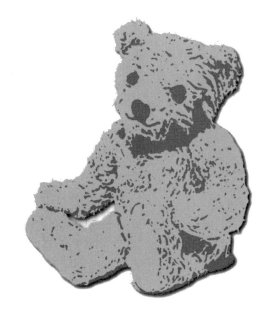

Iron Dextran

Brand names	INFeD, DexFerrum

Medication error potential

Look-alike, sound-alike error potential.

USP reports that DexFerrum has been confused with Desferal; no patient harm resulted.[1]

Contraindications and warnings

US boxed warning: Parenteral iron products carry boxed warnings for the risk of anaphylactic type reactions with deaths reported.[2] Reserve parenteral iron therapy for patients with iron deficiency who are unable to take oral iron products.[2]

Administer parenteral iron products only when resuscitation equipment and personnel trained to detect and treat anaphylactic reactions are readily available.[2]

A test dose should be administered prior to the first therapeutic dose.[2] During parenteral iron infusion (test and therapeutic doses), patients should be monitored for signs and symptoms of anaphylactic reaction.[2] Deaths have occurred following a test dose, as well as during administration of therapeutic doses after a test dose was tolerated.[2] Patients with drug allergies may be at increased risk of anaphylactic-type reactions.[2]

Infusion related cautions

Acute and delayed hypersensitivity reactions have been reported at a higher rate with iron dextran than other parenteral iron products in large *adult* studies.[3-6] One study reported a higher rate of hypersensitivity reactions with the high molecular weight dextran (Dexferrum) than the lower molecular weight (InFeD).[4] Use particular caution in patients with multiple drug allergies.[2]

Successful receipt of test doses or prior therapeutic doses does not ensure safety. Most patients who develop severe reactions have received prior doses without incident.[7]

Acute reactions include hypotension, bronchospasm, pharyngeal/angioedema, urticaria, and pruritus.[3-6] Premedication does not appear to decrease the incidence of acute reactions. Delayed reactions such as arthralgias, myalgias, headache, fever, and lymphadenopathy may appear 24–48 hours after infusion.

Dosage

Test dosing: A one-time test dose should be administered prior to initiating therapy. Guidelines for the use of parenteral iron for children with renal disease recommend a weight adjusted test regimen of [8]:

Weight	Test Dose
<10 kg	10 mg
10–20 kg	15 mg
>20 kg	25 mg

Others have recommended the use of the standard *adult* test dose of 25 mg.[9-12] Test doses should be administered slowly over ≤50 mg/min followed by the administration of the remainder of the initial dose 1 hour after the test dosing is complete.[2,8,13] Anaphylactic reactions occur with the first few minutes of infusion; therefore, immediate access to emergency medications (i.e., epinephrine) and trained personnel should be available.[2,8]

Some practitioners suggest that the daily dose be added to PN solutions, and heart rate, blood pressure, respiration, and temperature can be monitored q 15 min for the first hour of the initial dose.[10] (See Infusion related cautions section.)

Anemia of prematurity: In conjunction with erythropoietin therapy, 0.2–1 mg/kg/day[14,15] or 5 mg/kg/week has been added to PN solutions or infused over 4–6 hours.[16] Doses up to 10 mg/kg/week[16] of iron dextran have been used to maintain serum ferritin levels.

Dosage *(cont.)*

Studies utilizing alternative forms of parenteral iron (iron sucrose) with erythropoietin have utilized doses of 2 mg/kg/day and up to 20 mg/kg/week.[17-19]

Iron-deficiency anemia: The deficit (mL of iron dextran) can be calculated based on hemoglobin (Hgb)[2]:

5–15 kg

$$\text{Total iron dose (mL)*} =$$
$$0.0442 \text{ (Desired Hgb}\dagger - \text{Observed Hgb)} \times \text{wt (kg)} + (0.26 \times \text{wt [kg])}$$

*50 mg/mL, undiluted product.
†Desired Hgb for children is usually 12 g/dL.

>15 kg

The same equation is used. However, the individual's lean body mass (LBM) in kg is substituted for weight in obese individuals. LBM can be calculated in those >5 feet tall as follows:

LBM (males): 50 kg + 2.3 kg for each inch over 5 feet.

LBM (females): 45.5 kg + 2.3 kg for each inch over 5 feet.

≤100 mg (up to 2 mL) may be administered daily until the calculated amount to correct the deficit is achieved.[2]

Correction secondary to blood loss[2]**:** The deficit can be calculated based on hematocrit (Hct).

Total iron dose (mL)* = 0.02 × Blood loss (mL) × Hct (as decimal fraction)

*50 mg/mL, undiluted product.

Long-term PN: Maintenance dose of 0.11–0.15 mg/kg/day[20-22] or monthly infusion of estimated requirements. (See Continuous infusion section.)

Iron deficiency in hemodialysis (HD) patients (chronic renal failure): *The National Kidney Foundation Guidelines for Chronic Anemia* recommend weight adjusted dosing of iron dextran in children[8,23]:

Patient Weight	<10 kg	10–20 kg	>20 kg
Each dose or dialysis × 10 doses	0.5 mL (25 mg)	1 mL (50 mg)	2 mL (100 mg)

Alternatively, 2–4 mg/kg (≤100 mg) three times per week for 10 doses during erythropoietin therapy.[12,24]

Iron deficiency in peritoneal dialysis patients (chronic renal failure): *The National Kidney Foundation Guidelines for Chronic Anemia* recommend weight adjusted dosing of iron dextran in children.[8] This dose can be repeated to maintain adequate iron stores.

Patient Weight	<10 kg	10–20 kg	>20 kg
Iron dose	125 mg	250 mg	500 mg
Volume of saline for infusion	75 mL	125 mL	250 mL

Iron Dextran

Dosage adjustment in organ dysfunction

No information available; however, considering the distribution characteristics of iron, there should be no dose adjustment necessary relative to liver or kidney function.

Maximum dosage

In most cases, daily doses should not exceed the following weight based doses.[2]

Patient Weight	Dose (mg)
<5 kg	25 mg
≥5 kg–≤10 kg	50 mg
>10 kg	100 mg

Additives

Each mL contains NS.[13]

Suitable diluents

Dilution is not recommended by the manufacturer since product was originally developed for IM use. However, IV administration is preferred via dilution with NS.[9,12,13] Dextrose solutions may be employed but may increase the incidence of phlebitis.[13]

Maximum concentration

50 mg/mL.[2,8,25]

Preparation and delivery

Although not recommended by the manufacturer, iron dextran has been administered in PN formulations. Results of studies evaluating iron dextran stability and compatibility in PN solutions are inconsistent.[26,27] To ensure compatibility, the PN solution should contain at least 2% amino acids (10 mg iron dextran/L was visually compatible in neonatal PN solutions containing at least 2% amino acids).[25] For additional PN compatibility information, please see Appendix D.

IV push

May be administered undiluted (50 mg/mL) at a rate of <50 mg/min.[2,13] Administration by this method is not recommended. (See Infusion related cautions section.)

Intermittent infusion

Dilute in 50–1000 mL NS and infuse over 4–6 hours.[2,9,12,13]

Continuous infusion

The iron deficit can be replaced over several days by adding iron to PN solutions in daily amounts not exceeding maximum daily recommendations.[20-22,28] (See Maximum dosage section.)

Other routes of administration

Although the IV route is preferred, iron dextran has been administered IM using Z-track technique into upper quadrant of buttock.[2,8,13] May be associated with pain, staining of skin, tissue necrosis or abscess, and sarcoma development at the injection site.[29]

Comments

Monitoring: Serum ferritin monitoring is recommended to prevent potential iron overload.[2,7,8]

Other: A hypersensitivity reaction to one parenteral iron product does not predict a similar response to a different product.

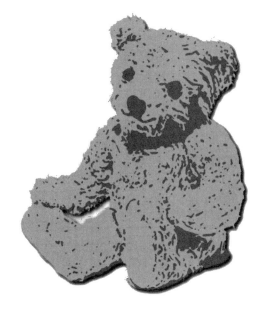

Isoproterenol HCl

Brand names	Isuprel
Medication error potential	ISMP high-alert medication that has an increased risk of causing significant patient harm if it is used in error.[1] Look-alike, sound-alike error potential. USP reports that isoproterenol has been confused with isosorbide mononitrate; no patient harm resulted. USP reports that Isuprel has been confused with Inderal; no patient harm resulted.[2]
Contraindications and warnings	Contraindicated in patients with tachyarrhythmias, tachycardia, or heart block due to cardiac glycoside digoxin toxicity, ventricular arrhythmias requiring inotropics, and angina pectoris.[3]
Infusion related cautions	Cardiac dysrhythmias,[4,5] ECG changes suggestive of transient myocardial ischemia,[6] and abnormal ECG and enzymatic findings suggestive of myocardial dysfunction have been reported in pediatric patients.[7,8] Although rare in pediatric patients, myocardial ischemia may occur.[7-10] Two adolescents with severe asthma who were treated with isoproterenol had myocardial necrosis at autopsy.[9,10]
Dosage	Doses in children range from 0.03–2 mcg/kg/min, usually starting at a lower dose and titrated up to desired response.[3,4,7,8,11-16] In *adults*, IV bolus doses range from 0.02–0.06 mg and increase to 0.01–0.2 mg; continuous infusion starts at 5 mcg/min and is titrated up to 20 mcg/min.[3,17] ECG monitoring during infusion is essential.[3] Adequate oxygenation and fluid status should be maintained during infusion to minimize risk of ventricular arrhythmias and myocardial ischemia.[18] In *adults*, heart rate >110 beats/min or ECG changes warrant a decrease in dose or discontinuation.[3] **Asthma:** Not recommended.[19] Newer therapies have largely replaced its use in the treatment of shock and pulmonary hypertension.[20,21] **Cardiac arrhythmias and CPR:** No longer considered a drug of choice. **Head-up tilt testing for syncope:** 0.02–0.08 mcg/kg in escalating doses every 2 minutes, or 1–3 mcg/min for ≤20 minutes, targeting a heart rate of 150 beats/min.[22,23]
Dosage adjustment in organ dysfunction	None reported.
Maximum dosage	Critically ill children from 2 days to 14 years of age received doses ≤5.5 mcg/kg/min.[14] (See Comments section.) In *adults* with advanced shock, >30 mcg/min adjusted according to heart rate, blood pressure, urine output, and central venous pressure has been used.[3]
Additives	Each mL also contains 7 mg sodium chloride and 1 mg sodium metabisulfite.[3,24] See Appendix C for more specific information about potential adverse effects of sulfites.
Suitable diluents	NS, D5W.[24]
Maximum concentration	20 mcg/mL.[3,4,24]

Isoproterenol HCl

Preparation and delivery	For PN compatibility information, please see Appendix D.

IV push	0.2 mg in *adults*.[3]

Intermittent infusion	Not indicated.

Continuous infusion	Usually 0.4–4 mcg/mL in D–LR, D–R, D–S, D5LR, D5NS, D5W, D10W, LR, NS, or ½NS for IV infusion.[3,24] The following formula has been recommended for preparation of the infusion: 0.6 × weight (kg) = mg of drug to add to IV solution for a total volume of 100 mL. An infusion rate of 1 mL/h provides 0.1 mcg/kg/min.[18] This formula estimates an initial concentration. Ultimately, the concentration of the drug should consider the patient's fluid requirements or fluid limitations. Despite widespread use of the above formula, Joint Commission guidelines recommend the implementation of "standardized concentrations" of vasoactive medications.[25]

Other routes of administration	In *adults*, IM or SC administration is recommended as initial therapy if time is not critical.[3] One reference states that intracardiac injection may be used in extreme emergencies.[24]

Comments	**Significant adverse effects:** Risk factors for the development of arrhythmias include severe asthma, acidosis, and concomitant use of theophylline or corticosteroids.[3] **Pharmacokinetic considerations:** Ten postoperative cardiac pediatric patients received doses of 0.029 ± 0.002 mcg/kg/min while nine with reactive airway disease received 0.5 ± 0.1 mcg/kg/min. Clearance was lower in the postoperative cardiac patients compared to those with reactive airway disease.[14] **Pharmacodynamic considerations:** Tolerance may occur following prolonged use.[17] **Other:** May be safer than isosorbide dinitrate or nitroglycerin for use during tilt table testing for syncope.[22,23]

Itraconazole

Brand names	Sporanox

Medication error potential

Look-alike, sound-alike error potential.

USP reports that itraconazole has been confused with fluconazole; no patient harm resulted.[1] USP also reports that Sporanox has been confused with Topamax; no patient harm resulted.[1]

Contraindications and warnings

US boxed warning: Itraconazole carries a boxed warning describing the potential risk of negative inotropic effects.[2] The use of itraconazole should be reassessed in patients exhibiting signs and symptoms of congestive heart failure.[2]

Itraconazole carries a boxed warning regarding drug interactions and the potential for serious cardiovascular events, including QT prolongation, torsades de pointes, ventricular tachycardia, cardiac arrest and/or sudden death.[2] (See Drug interactions in Comments section.)

Contraindications: Concomitant administration with cisapride, oral midazolam, pimozide, quinidine, dofetilide, triazolam, levacetylmethadol (levomethadyl), HMG CoA-reductase inhibitors, and ergot alkaloids metabolized by CYP3A4 is contraindicated.[2] (See US boxed warning in Contraindications and warnings section and Drug interactions in Comments section.)

Itraconazole is contraindicated in patients with a hypersensitivity to the drug or any of its components.[2]

Other warnings: Contains hydroxypropyl-beta-cyclodextrin.[2] (See Dosage adjustment in organ dysfunction section and Additives section.)

Itraconazole has been associated with rare cases of hepatotoxicity, including liver failure and death.[2]

Itraconazole has also been associated with cardiac dysrhythmias and sudden death. It should not be used in patients with underlying ventricular dysfunction unless the benefits outweigh the risks of therapy.[2]

Infusion related cautions

Anaphylaxis and Stevens-Johnson syndrome have been reported very rarely.[2]

Dosage

Experience with itraconazole in children is limited[3]; currently there is no established dosage range for pediatric patients.

Children: 5–10 mg/kg/day given as a single dose or divided into two doses.[3,4]

Doses given to *adults* are 200–400 mg/day given as a single dose or divided into two doses.[3]

Dosage adjustment in organ dysfunction

Contains cyclodextrin as a solubilizer; cyclodextrin is rapidly eliminated via glomerular filtration.[5] Therefore, itraconazole should not be used in patients with CrCl <30 mL/min and should be used with caution in patients with CrCl between 30 and 50 mL/min or in patients receiving renal replacement therapy.[2,6-7]

Use with caution in patients with hepatic impairment.[2]

Maximum dosage

400 mg/day in *adults*.[2,3]

Itraconazole

Additives

Each mL contains 400 mg hydroxypropyl-beta-cyclodextrin.[2] Hydroxypropyl-beta-cyclodextrin has produced pancreatic adenocarcinomas in rats.[2] The clinical significance to humans is unknown. (See Dosage adjustment in organ dysfunction section.)

Each mL also contains 25 microliters of propylene glycol.[2] See Appendix C for more specific information about potential adverse effects of propylene glycol.

Suitable diluents

NS.[2] Incompatible with D5W or LR.[2]

Maximum concentration

3.33 mg/mL.[2]

Preparation and delivery

A dedicated infusion line should be used for administration; do not introduce concomitant medications in the same bag or same line.[2]

IV push

Not recommended.[2]

Intermittent infusion

Infuse over 1 hour.[2]

Continuous infusion

No information available to support administration by this method.

Other routes of administration

No information available to support administration by other routes.

Comments

Drug interactions: Itraconazole is a potent inhibitor of CYP3A4 and is associated with numerous serious and potentially life threatening drug interactions.[2] (See Contraindications and warnings section.) Consult appropriate resources for dosing recommendations before combining any drug with itraconazole.

Other: Bone defects have occurred in rats receiving itraconazole.[2]

Kanamycin Sulfate

Brand names	Kantrex
Medication error potential	None.
Contraindications and warnings	Aminoglycosides can cause neuromuscular blockade and potentiate the effects of neuromuscular blockers.[1,2] (See Appendix C for specific information.)
Infusion related cautions	None.

Dosage

Inappropriate for mild-to-moderate infections.[3]

Except in neonates, dosage for the aminoglycosides should be based on the following equation[4,5]: Dosing weight = IBW + 0.4 (TBW – IBW). (See Appendix B.)

Neonates

PNA	<1200 g	1200–2000 g	≥2000 g
<7 days	15 mg/kg/day divided q 12 h[6]*	15 mg/kg/day divided q 12 h[6,7]	15–20 mg/kg/day divided q 12 h[6,7]
≥7 days		22.5–30 mg/kg/day q 8–12 h[6,7]	30 mg/kg/day divided q 8 h[6-8]

*Until 4 weeks of age.

Infants and children: 15–30 mg/kg/day divided q 8–12 h.[3,5,9] No information exists for once-daily kanamycin dosing.

Dosage adjustment in organ dysfunction

If CrCl is 10–50 mL/min, give normal dose q 24–72 h; if CrCl is <10 mL/min, give q 48–72 h.[10]

Maximum dosage

40–50 mg/kg/day, 500 mg/kg per course of therapy.[11] Daily *adult* dose is 1–1.5 g.[2,9] Larger doses or shorter dosing intervals of aminoglycosides are sometimes required in patients with cystic fibrosis, major thermal burns or dermal loss, ascites, or in patients with febrile granulocytopenia.[12-14] As with other aminoglycosides, individualize dosage based on serum concentrations.[15]

Additives

Contains 0.45% sodium bisulfite.[16] (See Appendix C for specific information about sulfite hypersensitivity.)

Suitable diluents

D5NS, D5W, D10W, LR, or NS.[16]

Maximum concentration

5 mg/mL.[15] The amount of diluent should be sufficient to infuse the drug over 20–30 minutes.[15]

Preparation and delivery	**Delivery system issues:** The mixing of kanamycin with an aminoglycoside in vitro can result in substantial inactivation of the aminoglycoside.[9] (See Appendix C for more specific information.)
	Compatibility: See Appendix D for PN compatibility information.[22]

IV push	Although aminoglycosides have been safely administered over 15 seconds,[23] 1 minute,[24] and 3–5 minutes,[25] rapid infusion is not used.

Intermittent infusion	2.5–5 mg/mL[16] infused over 20–30 minutes.[14,15]

Continuous infusion	Although aminoglycosides have been given by continuous infusion,[26-28] this method is not recommended.[15] Administration of a normal daily dose over 24 hours results in low serum concentrations[27] and more frequent nephrotoxicity.[26]

Other routes of administration	May be given IM.[3,9,29,30]

Comments	**Rare adverse effects:** Cochlear and/or vestibular ototoxicity has been associated with all aminoglycoside antibiotics.[9] Either total dose (>500 mg/kg)[11] or total AUC are better indicators of ototoxic risk than either peak or trough.[33,34]
	Aminoglycosides accumulate in renal cortical tissue and may damage proximal tubule cells leading to oliguric renal failure. This has been associated with elevated trough serum concentrations. Risk of nephrotoxicity may increase if aminoglycosides are combined with other potentially nephrotoxic drugs.[9] Use with caution when other drugs (e.g., macrolide antibiotics, loop diuretics, platinum-based chemotherapeutic agents) known to cause ototoxicity.
	Monitoring: Because large variability exists in patient response to therapy, individualize dosage based on serum concentrations, clinical response, and renal function. Recommended peak and trough serum kanamycin concentrations are 15–30 mg/L and 5–10 mg/L, respectively.[15] Although serum concentration monitoring has become routine practice in many institutions, not all patients require monitoring.[31,32] Monitoring is indicated if the patient is not clinically responding, is ≤3 months of age, has disease that requires large doses or high concentrations (CNS infections, endocarditis, pneumonia, ascites, burns), has decreased or unstable renal function, or will be treated more than 10 days.
	Laboratory interference: Serum concentrations may be falsely elevated when samples are collected through central venous Silastic catheters.[35]
	Osmolality: The osmolality of 250-mg/mL solution ranged from 858–952 mOsm/kg depending on the testing method used.[16]

Ketamine HCl

Brand names	Ketalar, generic

Medication error potential	Look-alike, sound-alike error potential.
	ISMP reported that Ketalar was confused with ketorolac.[1]

Contraindications and warnings	**Contraindications:** Those in whom a significant increase in blood pressure would result in harm and those with a known hypersensitivity reaction.[2]
	Does not impair laryngeal reflexes or independent airway maintenance; however, transient laryngospasm, apnea, and respiratory arrest have occurred.[3-5]

Infusion related cautions	Rapid administration (<60 seconds) may result in increased pressor response and/or increased apnea and respiratory depression.[2]
	Oxygen saturation should be monitored, and resuscitation and intubation equipment should be readily available for respiratory support.[2,6,7]
	Use with caution in patients at risk for increasing intracranial pressure.[2]
	Infants ≤3 months have a higher incidence of airway complications, and some recommend that ketamine be avoided in this age group.[3]
	Emergence reactions (e.g., dream-like states, hallucinations, delirium) occur in ~12% of *adults*.[2] Of children who were premedicated with midazolam prior to ketamine, 1% of those <10 years of age and 4.2% of those ≥10 years of age experienced a severe emergence reaction.[8] Minimizing verbal, tactile, and visual stimulation after dosing decreases the likelihood of these reactions.[2] Short- or ultra-short acting barbiturates may be used as treatment.[2]

Dosage	Pretreatment with atropine or other drying agent prevents vagal-mediated bradycardia and decreases secretions.[2,6,7,9]
	Anesthesia
	Induction
	IV: 1–4.5 mg/kg.[2]
	IM: 5–13 mg/kg.[2,10]
	Maintenance: One-half to full induction dose repeated as needed[2] or 1–5 mg/kg/h.[2,11]
	Adjunct to intubation: 1–2 mg/kg IV.[6]
	Procedural sedation/analgesia: Usually IV doses of 0.25–5 mg/kg and IM doses of 0.5–13 mg/kg are used for nonsurgical procedures.[3,6,12,13] In 32 children undergoing muscle biopsy, 2 mg/kg IV repeated in 10 minutes if needed or 10 mg/kg IM was used.[14] In the emergency department, 3–4 mg/kg IM has been used.[9,15-17] For emergencies, the AAP recommends 1–2 mg/kg IM or 0.5–1 mg/kg IV.[6] One group reported using a 1 mg/kg IV bolus followed by 51.4 ± 3.54 mcg/kg/min for the procedure's duration.[4]

Dosage *(cont.)* **Other uses**

Sedation in the intensive care unit: After cardiac surgery, 10 children were given 1 or 2 mg/kg/h for 24 hours.[18] Others report doses of 0.5–1 mg/kg followed by 10 mcg/kg/min for 48–72 hours.[19]

Severe bronchospasm: An 8-month-old received two doses of 1.4 mg/kg 10 minutes apart followed by 0.2 mg/kg/h that was weaned over 40 hours.[20] The other cases reviewed also improved with bolus doses of 0.5–4.8 mg/kg and three of these also received a continuous infusion of 1 or 2.5 mg/kg/h for 8–24 hours.[20] A separate retrospective review identified 17 mechanically ventilated children who improved with bolus doses of 2 mg/kg followed by a continuous infusion of 20–60 mcg/kg/min (1.2–3.6 mg/kg/h) for 12–96 hours.[21] Mechanical ventilation was avoided in two children with severe asthma who were given 2 mg/kg followed by 2–3 mg/kg/h.[22]

Opioid withdrawal: A 9.5-kg toddler who failed traditional fentanyl weaning strategies was started on ketamine at 10 mg/h. The fentanyl was successfully weaned off and then the ketamine was weaned.[23]

Dosage adjustment in organ dysfunction

No dosage adjustment required in renal insufficiency.[24,25]

Prolonged effects may be observed in patients with liver disease. Consider dose reductions in patients with hepatic impairment.[9]

Maximum dosage

Not established. Large doses prolong recovery and increase the risk of adverse events. IV doses up to 11 mg/kg and IM doses up to 17 mg/kg have been used during surgery.[3]

Additives

None.

Suitable diluents

1 or 2 mg/mL in SW, D5W, or NS.[2,26]

Maximum concentration

50 mg/mL for IV push.[2] The 100-mg/mL vial must be diluted prior to IV infusion.[2,26]

Preparation and delivery

Compatibility: Incompatible with barbiturates and diazepam.[2]

IV push

Over 60 seconds not to exceed 2 mg/min in *adults*.[2] The dose may be repeated to maintain anesthesia.

Intermittent infusion

Not indicated.

Continuous infusion

May be given by continuous infusion.[2,26]

A 12-year-old female with severe pain due to a cervical spinal tumor received a 7.5-mg test dose of ketamine followed by a continuous infusion ranging from 26–410 mg/24 h. She received long-term therapy for 67 days in a home-care setting.[27]

Ketamine HCl

Other routes of administration

IM.[2,15,16,28,29] Laryngospasm was more common with IM compared to IV ketamine.[29]

Comments

Adverse effects: The vomiting associated with ketamine is not related to the initial dose but may be increased in those receiving greater cumulative doses.[30] In one study, vomiting incidence in 128 children receiving ketamine alone was 12.6% and in 127 children receiving concomitant ondansetron was 4.7%.[13] Ketamine used with midazolam resulted in fewer respiratory adverse events but more vomiting than midazolam and fentanyl.[31] Similarly, combining ketamine with propofol resulted in fewer episodes of hypotension and bradycardia but more agitation than propofol alone.[12]

A previously healthy 8-year-old female developed severe neurogenic pulmonary edema following a 6.25-mg/kg IM dose for dressing changes for first-degree burns.[32]

Drug interactions: Substrate for CYP 450 isoenzymes 2B6, 2C9, and 3A4.

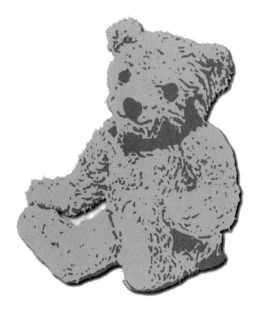

Ketorolac Tromethamine

Brand names	Generic

Medication error potential	Look-alike, sound-alike error potential.

USP reported that ketorolac was confused with Kenalog and has the potential to be confused with Kerlone.[1] USP reported that Toradol (no longer in the US) was confused with Nizoral, Tofranil, and Tridil and has the potential to be confused with Stadol.

ISMP reported that ketorolac was confused with Ketalar and Tordol was confused with Foradil.[2]

Contraindications and warnings	**US boxed warning**[3]

Gastrointestinal: Contraindicated in patients with active peptic ulcer disease, recent GI bleeding/perforation, or history of peptic ulcer disease or GI bleeding.

Renal: Contraindicated in patients with advanced renal impairment and in patients with risk for renal impairment due to hypovolemia.

Bleeding: Contraindicated in patients with suspected/confirmed cerebrovascular bleeding, hemorrhagic diathesis, incomplete hemostasis, before any major surgery and intraoperatively, and others at high risk of bleeding.

Hypersensitivity: Contraindicated in patients with previous hypersensitivity to ketorolac or aspirin or other NSAID.

Other contraindications: IT or epidural administration (alcohol content), labor and delivery, nursing mothers, concomitant aspirin, or other NSAID use.

Infusion related cautions	Anaphylactic reactions may occur in patients with a history of hypersensitivity to other nonsteroidal anti-inflammatory agents, including aspirin, or in patients with nasal polyps, asthma, angioedema, or bronchospastic reactions of the histamine-dependent type.[3,4]

Dosage	The manufacturer recommends single-dose therapy ($\leq$30 mg IM or 15 mg IV) for pediatric patients.[3] Therapy (parenteral and oral) should not exceed 5 days in *adults*.

Analgesia/pain management

Surgery/procedures: The use of a lower dose of 0.5 mg/kg has been recommended.[5-7] 0.5–1 mg/kg have been given to infants $\geq$1 month and children after induction of general anesthesia or at beginning of procedure, 30 minutes before the end of surgery/procedure, or immediately postoperative.[5-19] One study in neonates gave 1 mg/kg.[20]

Multidose therapy: 0.5 mg/kg q 6 h.[4,6,15,21] May give a loading dose of 1 mg/kg prior to beginning scheduled dosing.[4,21] One study in neonates, infants, and children supported the postsurgical use of 0.5 mg/kg q 8 h for 1–2 days.[22]

While the manufacturer's labeling limits therapy to $\leq$5 days,[3] early clinical experience with ketorolac in children reported the use of 0.17–1 mg/kg q 4–6 h for an average length of 3.4 days (range 1–12) and up to 31 doses.[21]

Antipyretic: 0.5–1 mg/kg as a single dose.[21,23]

Other uses

Postoperative bladder spasms (after ureteral reimplantation): 0.5 mg/kg q 6 h for 48 h reduced the frequency and severity of spasms.[24]

Migraine headaches: 0.5 mg/kg was inferior to prochlorperazine.[25]

Sickle cell vaso-occlusive pain crisis: 0.9 mg/kg did not reduce the total morphine dose required.[26]

Complex regional pain syndrome: IV regional anesthesia using 0.5 mg/kg (and lidocaine) in an 11-year-old and 15-year-old.[27]

Ketorolac Tromethamine

Dosage adjustment in organ dysfunction	**CrCl 10–29 mL/min:** 50% of the usual dose.[28] **CrCl <10 mL/min:** 25% to 50% of the usual dose.
Maximum dosage	30 mg IM or 15 mg IV in children.[3] A single 60-mg loading dose was administered to a 16-year-old adolescent.[21] 120 mg in healthy *adults*, ≤60 mg/day in those ≥65 years of age, <50 kg, or with moderately elevated SCr.[3]
Additives	**15 mg/mL (IV or IM use):** 10% (w/v) ethanol, 6.68 mg/mL NaCl.[3] **30 mg/mL (IV or IM use):** 10% (w/v) ethanol, 4.35 mg/mL NaCl.[3] **60 mg/2 mL (IM use only):** 10% (w/v) ethanol, 8.7 mg/mL NaCl.[3]
Suitable diluents	D5NS, D5W, LR, R, NS.[29]
Maximum concentration	30 mg/mL for IV infusion.[3] The 60-mg/2 mL product is intended for IM use only.[3]
Preparation and delivery	Incompatible in a syringe with morphine, meperidine, promethazine, and hydroxyzine.[3]
IV push	Over ≥15 seconds[3] to over 1–5 minutes in children.[21]
Intermittent infusion	Not indicated.
Continuous infusion	May be given by continuous infusion.[4]
Other routes of administration	IM.[3] Because of pain associated with IM administration, IV is preferred in children.[21]
Comments	**Adverse effects:** Ketorolac was considered a contributing factor to hematuria in a 16-year-old adolescent and to incision-site bleeding in an 11-year-old child.[21] While post-tonsillectomy patients receiving 1 mg/kg ketorolac had fewer emetic episodes than those given 0.1 mg/kg/dose of morphine, they had more major bleeding.[18] More measures to control bleeding were also noted post-tonsillectomy in children receiving ketorolac (1 mg/kg) compared to those receiving 35 mg acetaminophen/kg rectally.[19] **Pharmacokinetics:** A study in 36 children found that a 0.5 mg/kg dose IV resulted in similar concentrations over a 6-hour period as that reported for *adults*.[5] The pharmacokinetic parameters were not different among ages 1–3 years, 4–7 years, 8–11 years, and 12–16 years.[5] IV and IM bioavailability and efficacy are comparable.[30]

L-Cysteine HCl

Brand names	Various manufacturers
Medication error potential	None noted.
Contraindications and warnings	**Contraindications:** Patients with hepatic coma or metabolic disorders that impair nitrogen metabolism.[1]
Infusion related cautions	Peripheral infusion of amino acids may result in local reactions and phlebitis.[1]
Dosage	30–40 mg/g pediatric amino acid[1-3] or 0.4–1 mmol/kg (~48–121 mg/kg).[4,5]
Dosage adjustment in organ dysfunction	In hepatic and renal dysfunction, the overall amino acid dose should be decreased. In these cases, dosing using mg L-cysteine/g pediatric amino acids is appropriate because it is based on the grams of amino acids provided and not on patient weight.
Maximum dosage	**Based on mg/g pediatric amino acids:** 30 mg/g in those prescribed 3 g/kg and 40 mg/g in those prescribed 2.5 g/kg results in a 90- or 100-mg/kg dose, respectively.[1-3] Doses of 121 mg/kg have also been used.[4,5]
Additives	L-cysteine hydrochloride monohydrate contains 5.7 mEq Cl/g of L-cysteine HCl. Contains contaminant aluminum.[1]
Suitable diluents	PN solutions.
Maximum concentration	Dependent on volume of PN solution.
Preparation and delivery	**Stability:** L-cysteine HCl should be added to PN solutions just prior to infusion.[1]
IV push	Not indicated.
Intermittent infusion	Not indicated.
Continuous infusion	Given via PN solution.
Other routes of administration	Not indicated.

L-Cysteine HCl

Comments

L-cysteine HCl addition to PN solutions formulated with pediatric amino acids results in normalization of plasma amino acid patterns in infants.[2,4]

Acidosis, primarily in neonates, has been reported.[4,5]

The pH of L-cysteine HCl is about 1–2.5.[1] It has been added to solutions formulated with standard amino acid solutions to acidify the solution and enhance calcium and phosphorous solubility.[6]

L-cysteine exists in equilibrium with its dimer, cystine, and the extent of dimerization depends on pH. 1 mmol = 121 mg of cysteine/cystine.

Labetalol HCl

Brand names	Normodyne, Trandate
Medication error potential	ISMP high-alert medication (adrenergic antagonist) that has an increased risk of causing significant patient harm if it is used in error.[1] USP reports confusion with albuterol, atenolol, Carbatrol, Felbatol, Lipitor, and Tegretol. Confusion with Lamictal, lamotrigine, Lopressor, and metoprolol tartrate has resulted in patient harm.[2]
Contraindications and warnings	Because labetalol has negative inotropic and dromotropic activity, it is contraindicated in patients with asthma, chronic lung disease, overt cardiac failure, greater than first degree heart block, cardiogenic shock, or severe bradycardia.[3]
Infusion related cautions	Patients must be kept in a supine position during administration because a substantial fall in blood pressure may occur upon standing.[3]
Dosage	There are significant differences between IV and oral dosing. **Intermittent infusion:** 0.25–1 mg/kg[4-6] over 2 minutes up to 40 mg.[3] The dose can be repeated at 10-minute intervals to a maximum of 3–4 mg/kg up to a total dose of 300 mg.[4] The maximum hypotensive effect usually occurs within 5–15 minutes after injection.[3] **Continuous infusion:** 0.5–3 mg/kg/h titrated to blood pressure.[4-7] In a study of 13 children (3.6–15.3 years of age), the mean initial dose was 0.55 mg/kg (range of 0.2–1 mg/kg) and was followed by 0.78 mg/kg/h (range of 0.25–1.5 mg/kg/h).[6] In a retrospective study involving 25 children with hypertensive emergencies, doses of 1–3 mg/kg/h were used safely and effectively.[7]
Dosage adjustment in organ dysfunction	If CrCl is <10 mL/min, adequate blood-pressure control may be achieved with once-daily dosing.[3] While it is effective in severe renal dysfunction, it may have limited efficacy if mean arterial pressure is significantly elevated.[8,9]
Maximum dosage	1 mg/kg/dose[4-6] up to 40 mg.[5] A cumulative dose of 3–4 mg/kg per event and up to 300 mg per event.[4] Continuous infusion up to 3 mg/kg/h have been used.[7]
Additives	Some products contain methyl and/or propyl parabens.[3] (See Appendix C for specific information about parabens, potential for toxicity.)
Suitable diluents	D5LR, D2.5½NS , D5NS, D5¼NS, D5⅓NS , D5½NS, D5W, LR, or NS.[10]
Maximum concentration	5 mg/mL for IV injection and 1 mg/mL for continuous infusion.[8,10]
Preparation and delivery	**Compatibility:** Incompatible with sodium bicarbonate.[10]
IV push	5 mg/mL (commercially available) not to exceed 2 mg/min.[3,10]

Labetalol HCl

Intermittent infusion	Not administered by this method.
Continuous infusion	1 mg/mL.[8,10]
Other routes of administration	None.

Comments

Laboratory interference: Labetalol metabolites in the urine may cause falsely elevated concentrations of urinary catecholamines (e.g., metanephrine, normetanephrine, vanillylmandelic acid) when measured by fluorimetric or photometric methods.[3] When screening labetalol-treated patients suspected of having pheochromocytoma or when evaluating those with the tumor, specific assay methods such as high-performance liquid chromatography with solid phase extraction should be used.[3]

Labetalol may produce a false-positive amphetamine test when urine is screened using the Toxi-Lab A or Emit-d.a.u. assays.[3]

Lansoprazole

Brand names	Prevacid

Medication error potential

Look-alike, sound-alike error potential.

USP reports that lansoprazole has been confused with omeprazole; patient harm resulted.[1] USP also reports that lansoprazole has been confused with aripiprazole, esomeprazole, latanoprost, and rabeprazole and that Prevacid has been confused with prednisone and Prilosec, Pepcid, Percocet, Pravachol, Primaxin, Prinivil, and Procardia XL; no patient harm resulted.[1]

Contraindications and warnings

Lansoprazole is contraindicated in patients with known hypersensitivity to the formulation.[2]

Infusion related cautions

None.

Dosage

In *adults*, oral and IV dosage have been found to be similar in gastric acid suppression.[3] No studies of IV lansoprazole have been published to date in pediatric patients. General ranges from pediatric oral dosing studies are as follows:

Gastroesophageal reflux and esophagitis: 0.7–1.5 mg/kg/day.[4-7] Optimal starting dose of 1.4–1.5 mg/kg/day has been suggested.[4,5]

Neonates and infants: 14.3–23.8 mg/m^2/day for up to 14 days.[8] Doses of 0.5–1 mg/kg/day for neonates and 1–2 mg/kg/day for infants have also been reported.[9,10] Another study gave 15 mg/day or 7.5 mg q 12 h to infants for reflux.[11]

One study dosed lansoprazole based on age. Infants ≤10 weeks received 0.2–0.3 mg/kg/day while infants >10 weeks received 1–1.5 mg/kg/day (see Pharmacokinetic considerations in Comments section). There was no difference in efficacy between lansoprazole and placebo in this study.[12]

Children 1–11 years

> **<10 kg:** 7.5 mg/day.[13]

> **10 kg–≤30 kg:** 15 mg/day for 8–12 weeks.[14-19]

> **>30 kg:** 30 mg/day for 8–12 weeks; may increase up to 30 mg q 12 h if symptomatic after ≥2 weeks.[14-19]

Children 12–17 years of age[2,17,20]

> **Nonerosive gastroesophageal reflux:** 15 mg/day for 8–12 weeks.

> **Erosive esophagitis:** 30 mg/day for 8–12 weeks.

Dosage adjustment in organ dysfunction

No dosage adjustment necessary with renal dysfunction[2,13]; however, should consider dose adjustment in patients with severe hepatic dysfunction.[2]

Maximum dosage

60 mg/day.[2,21]

Additives

60 mg mannitol per 30 mg lansoprazole.[2]

Suitable diluents

Reconstitute with SW; solution may be further diluted in D5W, LR, NS.[2]

Lansoprazole

Maximum concentration	Reconstituted drug (6 mg/mL) in a minimum of 50 mL of diluent.[2]
Preparation and delivery	Reconstitution with diluents other than SW may cause precipitation.[2]
	Use in-line filter provided and observe closely for precipitation which may form when reconstituted drug is mixed with IV solutions. While holding filter below the level of the solution, connect luer adapter of administration set to filter using a twisting motion. Open the administration set clamp and slowly prime filter (0.7 mL), then close the administration set clamp and check for air bubbles.[2]
IV push	No information available to support administration by this method.
Intermittent infusion	Dilute reconstituted drug (6 mg/mL) in 50 mL of suitable diluent and infuse over 30 minutes using in-line filter provided.[2]
Continuous infusion	90–120 mg IV load followed by 6–9 mg/h has been given for 24 hours in *adults*.[22]
Other routes of administration	No information available to support administration by other routes.
Comments	**Significant adverse effects:** Common adverse effects include headache, constipation, and elevated serum gastrin levels.[15]
	Anemia, flushing, and elevated AST levels have been reported in pediatric patients <1 year of age treated with oral lansoprazole.[10]
	An 8½-year-old patient developed skin flushing and transient hypertension with oral lansoprazole.[8]
	Administration of proton pump inhibitors has been associated with increased risk of developing gastroenteritis and pneumonia in children.[23]
	Prolonged use (>3 years) may lead to impaired absorption of cyanocobalamin (vitamin B12) due to achlorhydria.[24]
	Drug interactions: Lansoprazole is metabolized by CYP3A4 and CYP2C19. Lansoprazole does not have clinically significant drug interactions with most drugs metabolized through the CYP system.[2] Dosage adjustments may be necessary with concomitant administration of theophylline or warfarin.[2]
	A known interaction exists between lansoprazole and clopidogrel. Since clopidogrel is metabolized to its active metabolite primarily via CYP2C19, and to a lesser extent, via CYP3A4 and CYP2C9, its use with lansoprazole may decrease the formation of the active metabolite and decrease antiplatelet effects.[25] Consult appropriate resources for dosing recommendations before combining any drug with lansoprazole.
	Pharmacokinetic considerations: Infants ≤10 weeks of age exhibit higher plasma concentrations and decreased clearance compared to infants >10 weeks of age; lower doses may be warranted in these patients.[9]

Levetiracetam

Brand names	Keppra
Medication error potential	Look-alike, sound-alike drug names. USP reports confusion with lamotrigine, levocarnitine and levofloxacin. Confusion with levofloxacin has resulted in patient harm.[1]
Contraindications and warnings	**Contraindications:** Hypersensitivity to levetiracetam or any component of the formulation.[2] **Warnings:** Anticonvulsants should not be discontinued abruptly because of the possibility of increasing seizure frequency.[3]
Infusion related cautions	None.

Dosage	Labeled as replacement therapy for patients >16 years of age who have been on oral therapy, but cannot temporarily tolerate oral medications.[3] There is very little information available on use in infants[4-7] and children.[4-6] IV levetiracetam has been given to patients as young as 3 weeks,[6] 1 month,[7,8] 2 months,[5] and 3 months.[4]
	
	Naive patient (no previous levetiracetam)
	
	    Loading dose: 8.8 mg/kg (mean; n=7),[4] 22 mg/kg (mean, n=10),[8] and 50 mg/kg (n=9).[5]
	
	    Maintenance dose: 36.1 mg/kg/day (mean; range: 5–92 mg/kg/day) divided q 12 h (n=7),[4] and 50 mg/kg/day divided q 12 h.[5]
	
	Replacement therapy (prior levetiracetam)[4-7]: The initial total daily IV dosage should equal the total daily dosage and frequency of oral levetiracetam.[3] Although mean doses have ranged from 5–120 mg/kg/day,[4-7] most patients received 50–60 mg/kg/day divided q 12 h.[5-7] One study gave q 8 h in infants.[6]
	
	The patient may be switched to oral levetiracetam at the same daily dosage and frequency as that administered intravenously.[3]

Dosage adjustment in organ dysfunction	If CrCl is <50 mL/min give 50% of normal dose[9]; in *adults* with moderate renal dysfunction (30–50 mL/min) give 250–750 mg q 12 h and 250–500 mg q 12 h if CrCl <30 mg/mL.[3] No dose adjustment is needed for patients with hepatic impairment.[3] (See Other in Comments section.)
Maximum dosage	70-mg/kg loading dose[5] 120 mg/kg/day[6] up to 3 g/day.[3]
Additives	None.
Suitable diluents	NS, LR, or D5W.[3]

Levetiracetam

Maximum concentration	1500 mg (3 × 5 mL vials) injection should be diluted in 100 mL of compatible diluents.[3]
Preparation and delivery	**Stability:** Any unused portion of a vial should be discarded.[3] At least 24 hours when stored in polyvinyl chloride bags at room temperature (15°C to 30°C).[3] Product with particulate matter or discoloration should not be used.[3]
IV push	No used.
Intermittent infusion	Over 15 minutes.[3]
Continuous infusion	Not used.
Other routes of administration	None.
Comments	**Rare adverse effects:** Neuropsychiatric adverse events including somnolence, fatigue, coordination difficulties, behavioral abnormalities (e.g., aggression, agitation, anxiety, anger, hostility, irritability, depression) and psychotic symptoms (e.g., psychosis, hallucinations) may occur.[3] Behavioral abnormalities may occur more frequently in children and may required dosage reductions.[2]
	The incidence of suicidal behavior/ideation has been noted to be greater than placebo (0.43% vs 0.24% risk) in patients receiving 11 anticonvulsants (carbamazepine, divalproex sodium, felbamate, gabapentin, lamotrigine, levetiracetam, oxcarbazepine, pregabalin, tiagabine, topiramate, zonisamide) as either monotherapy or as adjuvant therapy for the treatment of epilepsy, psychiatric disorders, and other conditions.[10] The FDA will require that the product labeling of the entire class of antiepileptics include a warning concerning the risk of suicide.
	Monitoring: Virtually no laboratory tests are altered.[3] Although abnormalities have been noted in hematologic parameters (e.g., decreases in red blood cell counts, hemoglobin, hematocrit, white blood cell counts and neutrophils) and serum transaminases (increased), the values remained within the normal range.[11,12]
	Drug interactions: Levetiracetam is not a substrate for any CYP-isozyme, is not highly protein bound, and does not interfere with the metabolism of other anticonvulsants.[13] No clinically significant drug interactions have been reported.[3]
	Other: Pharmacokinetics parameters were unchanged in mild (Child-Pugh A) to moderate (Child-Pugh B) hepatic impairment.[3] Total body clearance was half that of normal subjects compared to those with severe hepatic impairment (Child-Pugh C).[3] Most of the change was attributed to a decrease in renal clearance.

Levocarnitine

Brand names	Carnitor, generic

Medication error potential	Look-alike, sound-alike error potential.
	USP reports that levocarnitine has been confused with levetiracetam; no patient harm resulted.[1]

Contraindications and warnings	L-carnitine (oral and IV) has been noted to cause seizures in patients with and without pre-existing seizure disorder.[2] Children and infants experiencing reported seizures have had other risk factors, including microcephaly, large doses of carnitine, and metabolic acidosis.[3]

Infusion related cautions	None known.

Dosage	**Hemodialysis:** 10–40 mg/kg/dose following dialysis.[2,4,5] Other papers support the use of considerably lower doses of 2–5 mg/kg/dose following dialysis.[6-8] The clinical practice recommendations for anemia in chronic kidney disease in children state there is no firm evidence to support its use.[9]
	Primary carnitine deficiency/metabolic disorders: A loading dose of 50 mg/kg followed by 50–60 mg/kg/day divided q 3–6 h or given continuously.[2,10]
	PN supplementation in neonates/infants with little or no enteral intake: 10–30 mg/kg/day.[11-18]
	Valproate-associated hepatotoxicity
	Active hepatotoxicity/overdose: 150–500 mg/kg/day, up to 3 g/day.[19,20]
	Prophylaxis against valproate or other anticonvulsant-associated hepatotoxicity: 15–100 mg/kg/day has been used in children with or without hyperammonemia.[20] Decreased ammonia levels were seen after 9 days of treatment with 1000 mg/m²/day divided in two equal doses.[21]

Dosage adjustment in organ dysfunction	No dose adjustment recommended. However, carnitine is excreted renally and renal insufficiency may lead to the accumulation of potentially toxic metabolites.[2,9]

Maximum dosage	**PN supplementation:** 48 mg/kg/day has been given.[22] (See Comments section.)
	Metabolic disorders: 300 mg/kg/dose (age not specified).[2]
	Valproate induced hepatotoxicity: 3 g/day.[19,20]
	VPA/anticonvulsant therapy: 100 mg/kg/day or 1000 mg/m²/day.[20]

Additives	None

Suitable diluents	NS, LR.[2]

Maximum concentration	1 g/5 mL (200 mg/mL).[2]

Levocarnitine

Preparation and delivery	**Preparation:** Mix with suitable diluents to concentrations of 0.5–8 mg/mL.[2]
	Stability: May be stored at room temperature for up to 24 hours in PVC plastic bags.[2]
	Compatibility: May be added to PN solutions and infused over 24 hours or during a PN cycling schedule.[11-13,15,16,18] One study documented stability of carnitine via PN and TNA with Y-site administration of 20% fat emulsion at all study points (IV bag, distal to filter, after mixing with fat emulsion) for up to 24 hours at room temperature and up to 30 days when stored at 4°C to 5°C.[23] Another study evaluated stability with carnitine in TNA and observed creaming.[24]
IV push	200 mg/mL over 2–3 minutes.[2]
Intermittent infusion	May give by intermittent infusion.[2]
Continuous infusion	May be given by continuous infusion.[2]
Other routes of administration	No information available to support administration by other routes.
Comments	Higher metabolic rate, greater nitrogen excretion, and lower weight gain were associated with 48 mg/kg/day given via PN in 12 preterm neonates.[22]
	IV carnitine has been shown to be beneficial in childhood cardiomyopathy.[25]
	Life-threatening lactic acidosis associated with reverse transcriptase inhibitors was corrected in an HIV-positive 10-year-old patient with 12–50 mg/kg/day L-carnitine.[26]

Levothyroxine Sodium

Brand names   Synthroid, generic

Medication error potential

Look-alike, sound-alike error potential.

ISMP and USP report that levothyroxine has been confused with lamotrigine and Lanoxin; no patient harm resulted.[1,2] USP also reports that levothyroxine has been confused with amantadine, digoxin, leucovorin, Levaquin, levofloxacin, levonorgestrel, levorphanol and liothyronine; no patient harm resulted.[2]

USP reports that Synthroid has been confused with Symmetrel and thyroid; no patient harm resulted.[2]

Contraindications and warnings

US boxed warning: Should not be used for weight loss or the treatment of obesity. Large doses of levothyroxine needed for weight loss in euthyroid patients produce serious and life threatening toxicity, particularly when given in combination with sympathomimetic agents.[3]

Other warnings: Recommend cautious initiation of therapy in patients with cardiovascular disease, endocrine disorders, and thyrotoxicosis.[3]

Infusion related cautions

Large, sudden doses of IV levothyroxine may have cardiovascular risks.[3,4]

Dosage

Congenital or acquired hypothyroidism: 5–8 mcg/kg q 24 h[5] or[4]

Age	IV Dose is 50% to 75% of the Oral Doses Listed Below
0–3 mo	10–15 mcg/kg/day
3–6 mo	8–10 mcg/kg/day
6–12 mo	6–8 mcg/kg/day
1–5 y	5–6 mcg/kg/day
6–12 y	4–5 mcg/kg/day
>12 y	2–3 mcg/kg/day
Growth and puberty complete	1.6–1.7 mcg/kg/day

The AAP recommends an initial oral dosage of 10–15 mcg/kg/day for infants with hypothyroidism.[6] IV dose should be 50% to 75% of oral doses.[3,4]

The goal of therapy is to normalize T4 within 2 weeks and TSH within 1 month.[6] Neonates and infants with very low or undetectable serum T4 concentrations (<5 mcg/dL) should be started at the higher end of the dosage range.[4,6] Patients with evidence of cardiac disease or long-standing or severe hypothyroidism should receive a lower starting dose.[3,4] Adjust dosage based on clinical response and serum free T4 and TSH.[3,6]

Dosage adjustment in organ dysfunction

No information available.

Levothyroxine Sodium

Maximum dosage	Not established. In *adults* with myxedema coma or stupor, without concomitant severe heart disease, may give doses of 200–500 mcg.[3]
Additives	10 mg mannitol per vial.[3]
Suitable diluents	Use only NS for reconstitution.[7]
Maximum concentration	100 mcg/mL[3]; however, one reference recommends a final concentration of 20 mcg/mL.[5]
Preparation and delivery	Reconstitute with NS only. Use immediately.[3]
IV push	40–100 mcg/mL in NS[3,4] over 2–3 minutes.[8]
Intermittent infusion	No information available to support administration by this method. Should not be mixed with IV infusion solutions.[3,4]
Continuous infusion	No information available to support administration by this method. Should not be mixed with IV infusion solutions.[3,4]
Other routes of administration	May be administered by IM injection; however, because absorption is variable following IM administration, IV is preferred.[4]
Comments	**Adverse effects:** Pseudotumor cerebri has been reported to follow levothyroxine therapy in both *adults* and infants and children.[9]
	Drug interactions: Because levothyroxine is associated with numerous drug interactions,[4] consult appropriate resources for dosing recommendations before combining any drug with levothyroxine.
	Other: The aim of therapy is to ensure normal growth and development.[6]
	Early, high-dose levothyroxine therapy has been shown to eliminate the negative impact that congenital hypothyroidism has on IQ and CNS development.[6,10,11]
	One study documented improved hemodynamic stability, which may translate into improved donor organ viability, with thyroxine (loading dose followed by continuous infusion) in critically ill children with documented brain death.[12]

Lidocaine HCl

Brand names	Xylocaine
Medication error potential	ISMP high-alert medication (anesthetic agent and antiarrhythmic) that has an increased risk of causing significant patient harm if it is used in error.[1] Look-alike, sound-alike drug names. USP reports confusion with bupivacaine and linezolid.[2]
Contraindications and warnings	**Contraindications:** In patients with a known history of hypersensitivity to local anesthetics of the amide type.[3] It should not be used in patients with Stokes-Adams syndrome, Wolff-Parkinson-White syndrome, or with severe degrees of sinoatrial, atrioventricular, or intraventricular block.[3] **Warnings:** Emergency resuscitative equipment and drugs should be immediately available to manage adverse reactions involving cardiovascular, respiratory, or central nervous systems.[3]
Infusion related cautions	Bronchospasm has been reported.[3] (See Rare adverse effects in Comments section.)

Dosage	**Arrhythmias (ventricular-resistant to electrical cardioversion or in pulseless ventricular tachycardia):** Lidocaine solutions that contain epinephrine must *not* be used to treat arrhythmias. See Other routes of administration section for information related to endotracheal and intraosseous administration in those without IV access.
	
	    Initial: 0.5–1 mg/kg (maximum single dose 100 mg) q 5–10 min until desired effect or maximum total dose of 3–5 mg/kg.[4-7] Decrease loading dose by 50% in patients with moderate to severe congestive heart failure.
	
	    Maintenance: 0.5–3 mg/kg/h (10–50 mcg/kg/min).[4-7] If more than 15 minutes has lapsed between initial dose and start of infusion, give 0.5–1 mg/kg.[6]
	
	Epilepsy (refractory status): Initial dose of 1–3 mg/kg over 2 minutes.[7-16] If seizures do not stop in 2 minutes give an additional dose of 0.5 mg/kg.[6] A continuous infusion of 2–6 mg/kg/h effectively controlled severe intractable seizures in neonates,[9,10,15] infants,[11,12,16] and children.[13,16] A dose of 1.5–3.5 mg/kg/h has been used in *adults*.[14]
	
	Intracranial pressure (acute increases due to procedures): 1–1.5 mg/kg given 30 seconds prior to intubation or endotracheal suctioning to reduce airway reflexes.[5,17,18]
	
	Pain associated with Anti-GD2 antibody therapy: A loading dose of 2 mg/kg infused over 30 minutes before antibody therapy, followed by a continuous infusion of 1 mg/kg/h.[19] The infusion should be discontinued 2 hours after antibody therapy is stopped.

Dosage adjustment in organ dysfunction	Doses should not exceed 20 mcg/kg/min in patients with shock, congestive heart failure, liver failure, or decreased liver blood flow.[3,20,21] No adjustment in renal dysfunction.[3,22]
Maximum dosage	1 mg/kg (maximum single dose 100 mg) until desired effect or maximum total dose of 5 mg/kg[4-6] or <300 mg in 1 hour.[3] Administration of ≤88 mcg/kg/min (50 mg/min) by continuous infusion has been proposed.[23] Dosage should be titrated using serum concentration monitoring. (See Monitoring in Comments section.)

Lidocaine HCl

Additives

Some multidose vials may contain sulfites and parabens.[24] (See Appendix C for specific information about sulfite hypersensitivity and paraben potential for toxicity.)

Suitable diluents

D5W, LR, NS, ½NS, D5-LR, D5¼NS, and D5½NS.[24]

Maximum concentration

20 mg/mL for IV push[6,24] and 8 mg/mL for infusion in fluid-restricted patients.[24]

Preparation and delivery

The 10% and 20% concentrated solutions must not be administered without proper dilution.[3]

Stability: Do not use if solution is discolored or cloudy.[3]

Compatibility: See Appendix D for PN compatibility information.[25]

IV push

Generally over 2–3 minutes, not to exceed 0.7 mg/kg/min or 50 mg/min, whichever is less.[3]

Intermittent infusion

Not recommended due to short half-life.[3]

Continuous infusion

Usually 1–2 mg/mL; however, 8 mg/mL in D5W has been used in fluid-restricted patients.[3]

Other routes of administration

Generally not given via other methods. Can be given IM into the deltoid muscle provided bradycardia is not present[2]; however, a formulation specific for IM delivery is no longer available in the US. For endotracheal administration give 2–3 mg[3] and for IO administration give 1 mg/kg.[5]

Comments

Rare adverse effects: Transient mydriasis has been reported in a neonate treated with lidocaine for seizures.[26]

Transient bronchospasm was noted in a 17-month-old with mild intermittent asthma.[27]

Monitoring: Because large variability exists in patient response to initial and maintenance doses, individualize dosage based on serum concentration and clinical response. Reference range: 1.5–5 mg/L for antiarrhythmic effect and toxicity.[3] The reference range for the management of status epilepticus has not been established.

Monitor for bradycardia and hypotension. Widening of the QRS interval by >0.02 seconds prolongation of the PR interval, significant ventricular slowing, or the appearance or aggravation of arrhythmias suggests toxicity.[3] Excessive serum concentrations may also produce CNS symptoms (e.g., drowsiness, nausea, vomiting, disorientation, seizures, and muscle twitching).[3]

Drug interactions: Should be used with caution in patients with digitalis toxicity accompanied by atrioventricular block.[3] Beta-blocking agents and cimetidine may reduce hepatic blood flow, decrease lidocaine clearance which increase serum lidocaine concentrations to cause an increased incidence of adverse reactions. Consult appropriate resources for dosing recommendations before combining any drug with lidocaine.

Linezolid

Brand names	Zyvox

Medication error potential	Look-alike, sound-alike drug names. USP reports confusion with lidocaine and lisinopril.[1] Confusion also reported between Zyvox and Avelox, Vioxx, Zithromax, Zosyn, Zovirax, and Zyflo.[1]

Contraindications and warnings	**Contraindications:** In those with a known hypersensitivity reaction to linezolid or its components.[2] Linezolid should not be used within 2 weeks of or in combination with a MAOI inhibitor.[2] Serotonin syndrome could occur in patients receiving concurrent serotonergic agent (e.g., SSRI).[2] Linezolid should not be administered to patients with Carcinoid syndrome or to those currently taking: serotonin reuptake inhibitors, tricyclic antidepressants, buspirone, meperidine, or serotonin (5-HT1) receptor agonists.[2] (See Rare adverse effects in Comments section.) Unless patients are monitored for potential increases in blood pressure, linezolid should not be given to those with uncontrolled hypertension, thyrotoxicosis, pheochromocytoma, and/or patients with medicines that are direct or indirect acting sympathomimetics, vasopressive agents or dopaminergic agents.[2] **Warnings:** Transient myelosuppression has been reported, especially when therapy last >2 weeks. CBC should be monitored more closely if (1) there is a known history of myelosuppression; (2) other bone marrow suppressing drugs are given; or (3) used in those with chronic infection who have received previous concomitant antibiotics.[2] Prolonged use may cause superinfection and/or *Clostridium difficile*–associated diarrhea (CDAD), which has been reported and may range in severity from mild diarrhea to fatal colitis.[2] If CDAD is suspected or confirmed, appropriate fluid and electrolyte management, protein supplementation, antibiotic treatment of *C. difficile*, and surgical evaluation should be instituted as clinically indicated.

Infusion related cautions	If a decision is made to give this medication to a patient with known linezolid hypersensitivity, the patient should be closely observed for allergenicity. Although rare, anaphylactoid reactions may require immediate emergency treatment with epinephrine, oxygen, IV steroids, antihistamines, pressor amines, and airway management.

Dosage	**Neonates**

PNA	≤1200 g	1200–2000 g	≥2000 g
<7 days	20–30 mg/kg/day divided q 8–12 h[3,4]	20–30 mg/kg/day divided q 8–12 h[3-5]	20–30 mg/kg/day divided q 8–12 h[3-5]
≥7 days		30 mg/kg/day divided q 8 h[3, 5-7]	30 mg/kg/day divided q 8 h[3,5-7]

*Until 4 weeks of age.

Linezolid

Dosage *(cont.)*	**Infants and children (<12 y):** 30 mg/kg/day divided q 8 h.[3,5,6,8-10] **Adolescents (≥12 y):** 20 mg/kg/day divided q 12 h (up to 1200 mg/day divided q 12 h.[3,10,11] The manufacturer does not recommend the use of linezolid for empiric treatment of pediatric CNS infections.[2] Limited data, as *adult* and pediatric case reports, suggest that linezolid may be used to treat gram-positive CNS infections that failed to respond to other treatment.[12,13] **Bacterial endocarditis (treatment):** Treatment of *E faecium* endocarditis of native or prosthetic valve that is resistant to penicillin, aminoglycoside, and vancomycin: 30 mg/kg/day divided q 8 h (not to exceed normal dosing of adolescents) for ≥8 weeks.[14-16] **Central line infections:** 2 mg/mL plus 100 units of heparin as an 8-hour catheter lock.[17] May be used in combination with 30 mg/kg/day divided q 8 h of systematic linezolid. Another method instilled 3 mL of a linezolid solution (2 g/L) into the lumen of the catheter for 16 hours without the use of heparin.[18] (See Other in Comments section.)
Dosage adjustment in organ dysfunction	No adjustment in renal impairment.[19] Although metabolites may accumulate in renal insufficiency, the clinical significance is unknown.[2] No adjustment in mild-to-moderate hepatic impairment; caution should be used in severe hepatic impairment.[2]
Maximum dosage	45 mg/kg/day divided q 8 h was given to a 7-week-old infant.[15] 1200 mg/day if >12 years of age.[2,3]
Additives	100 mL contains 1.7 mEq sodium, 200 mL contain 3.3 mEq of sodium, and 300 mL contains 5 mEq of sodium.[20]
Suitable diluents	May be given undiluted.[20]
Maximum concentration	2 mg/mL (commercially available).[2,20]
Preparation and delivery	**Stability:** Do not freeze. The solution is a yellow color that can intensify with no affect on potency. **Compatibility:** See Appendix D for PN compatibility information.[21]
IV push	Not recommended.[2]
Intermittent infusion	2 mg/mL over 30–120 minutes.[2,20]
Continuous infusion	No information.

Linezolid

| **Other routes of administration** | None. |

Comments

Rare adverse events: Lactic acidosis has been reported in some patients that experience repeat nausea and vomiting.[2,22] Death has been reported; however, most patients' serum lactate levels return to normal after discontinuation of linezolid.[21] Nonspecific clinical symptoms make it difficult to detect; therefore, serum bicarbonate levels should be monitored.[23]

Peripheral and optic neuropathy has occurred with treatment >28 days; however, it can manifest within days to months. Linezolid should be discontinued if neuropathy is attributed to linezolid. Recovery is variable.[23]

An infant receiving linezolid for sepsis, developed auditory nerve neuropathy and permanent hearing deficiencies.[24]

Serotonin syndrome has been reported in patients given concurrent serotonergic agents.[25-27] A 4-year-old burn victim who received linezolid and fluoxetine became agitated and developed myoclonic movement in limbs.[28] Symptoms resolved following discontinuation of linezolid.

Brownish tooth and tongue discoloration has been reported in pediatric patients receiving IV linezolid.[29] The discoloration desists with discontinuation of linezolid and with manual removal by a dentist.[29,30]

Convulsions have been reported in pediatric patients receiving linezolid.[2,9] One report described a patient with known epilepsy who experienced an increased frequency and worsened control of seizures while on IV linezolid therapy that occurred again with re-challenge.[31]

In a 2-year-old boy receiving linezolid for treatment of infective endocarditis, progressive fatigue and anemia developed 2 weeks post-linezolid initiation. Four days after discontinuation of linezolid Hgb, Hct and reticulocyte increased.[32]

Monitoring: Serum bicarbonate, serum transaminases, CBC and platelet, blood pressure, and signs or symptoms of serotonin syndrome (e.g., hyperreflexia, clonus, hyperthermia, etc.) Although transient thrombocytopenia may occur,[2,33] one study found no significant difference in the platelet count for linezolid (n=215) vs. vancomycin (n=101) treated pediatric patients.[11]

Drug interactions: Consult appropriate resources for dosing recommendations before combining any drug with linezolid.

Other: Use of linezolid for catheter-related bloodstream infections is an off-label indication. One study showed a mortality imbalance [Linezolid (21.5%) vs. comparator (16.0%); odds ratio 1.426, 95% CI 0.970, 2.098] on the linezolid side in patients with mixed gram-positive and gram-negative pathogens, gram-positive pathogens, or cases without pathogen identification.[2,33]

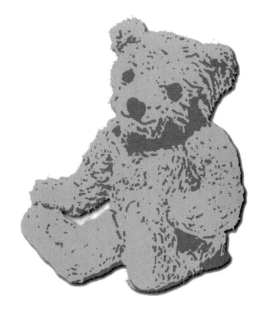

LORazepam

Brand names	Ativan

Medication error potential

ISMP high-alert medication (moderate sedation) that has an increased risk of causing significant patient harm if it is used in error.[1]

ISMP recommends the following tall man letters (not FDA approved): ALPRAZolam–LORazepam and clonazePAM–LORazepam.[2]

Look-alike, sound-alike drug name.

USP reports confusion with alprazolam, clonazepam, diazepam, loperamide, loratadine, midazolam, oxazepam, temazepam and zolpidem. USP reports confusion for Ativan with alprazolam, Ambien, Antivert, Artane, Atarax, and clonazepam. Confusion with alprazolam has resulted in patient harm.[3]

Contraindications and warnings

Contraindications: Should not be used in patients with (1) a known sensitivity to benzodiazepines or its vehicle (polyethylene glycol, propylene glycol, and benzyl alcohol); (2) acute narrow-angle glaucoma; (3) sleep apnea syndrome; and (4) severe respiratory insufficiency (except in those patients requiring relief of anxiety and/or diminished recall of events while being mechanically ventilated).[4] (See Infusion related cautions section.)

Infusion related cautions

Respiratory depression may occur; hence, artificial ventilation equipment should be available. Inadvertent intra-arterial injection can cause vasospasm that may produce gangrene and subsequent amputation.[4] If a patient complains of pain during injection, the infusion should be stopped and the site should be inspected.

Dosage

Flumazenil should be readily available for reversal. (See Other in Comments section and see Flumazenil monograph.)

Adjunct to antiemetic therapy: Single doses of 0.01 mg/kg have been used preoperatively for nausea associated with strabismus surgery[5]; however, single doses of at least 0.04 mg/kg (maximum 3 mg/dose) were required for emesis associated with chemotherapy.[6,7] Multiple doses of 0.04–0.08 mg/kg (maximum 2 mg/dose) may be given q 6 h as needed.[6]

Adjunct for procedural sedation[8,9]: Many consider midazolam the benzodiazepine of choice for procedural sedation.[10-12] (See Midazolam monograph.) 0.05 mg/kg (0.01–0.1 mg/kg) q 4–8 h[9] not to exceed 2 mg/dose.[4,8] For premedication therapy, give first *intravenous* dose 15–20 minutes before procedure and first *intramuscular* dose 2 hours before procedure.

Sedation with mechanical ventilation: Use lowest effective dose. 0.025–0.05 mg/kg (maximum initial dose of 2 mg) given as intermittent infusion q 2–4 h or by continuous infusion, at a rate of 0.025 mg/kg/h (up to 2 mg/h).[13] (See Additives section.)

Seizures

Prophylaxis (busulfan-associated seizures)[14-16]: 0.02–0.05 mg/kg (up to 2 mg/dose) given 30 minutes before each dose of busulfan.[15] Give 0.02 mg/kg if <2-years-old over 30 minutes. Continued every 6 hours for four additional doses after the last dose of busulfan.[15] 0.1 mg/kg/day (up to 2 mg/day) has been given by continuous infusion.[16] The infusion was started 12 hours before busulfan and was discontinued 24 hours after the last dose of busulfan.[16] Duration of infusion was 5.5 days.[16]

Dosage *(cont.)*	**Treatment**
	Neonates: In a recent survey of neonatologist, 82% (n=480) of neonates were given phenobarbital as the preferred anticonvulsant.[17] 0.05–0.1 mg/kg.[18-21] If seizures continue after 10–15 minutes, repeat 0.05 mg/kg; if no response after 10–15 minutes, repeat 0.05 mg/kg to a maximum of 0.15 mg/kg.[19] (See Pharmacokinetic considerations and Pharmacodynamic considerations in Comments section.)
	Infants and children: 0.1 mg/kg[18-25] up to 4 mg/dose.[23] If seizures continue after 10–15 minutes, repeat 0.05 mg/kg; if no response after 10–15 minutes, repeat 0.05 mg/kg.[23-25]
Dosage adjustment in organ dysfunction	No adjustment in renal dysfunction[4,26]; however, use cautiously when giving multiple doses.[4] Not metabolized by cytochrome oxidation; hence, liver disease should not have an effect on metabolic clearance.[4] Use cautiously in patients with combined renal and hepatic dysfunction.[4]
Maximum dosage	4 mg/dose.[12,23] Doses as large as 0.4 mg/kg have been safely administered.[5,27] A 14-year-old with refractory seizures who had been on chronic lorazepam was given 0.25 mg/kg/dose to a cumulative dose of 186 mg (4.3 mg/kg) over 24 hours.[28]
Additives	Contains benzyl alcohol 2% and 40% propylene glycol.[29] (See Appendix C for specific information about benzyl alcohol and propylene glycol potential for toxicity.)
Suitable diluents	Variability stability in D5W, NS, SW[4,29]; hence, the reader is referred to more specific references. Although the manufacturer recommends diluting the commercially available solution 1:1 in D5W, NS, or SW,[4] undiluted 2-[22] and 4-mg/mL[23] solutions have been given.
Maximum concentration	Although 4 mg/mL[23] has been given, the manufacturer recommends dilution to ≤1 mg/mL.[4]
Preparation and delivery	**Stability:** Store in refrigerator.[4]
	Compatibility: See Appendix D for PN compatibility information.[30]
	Photosensitivity: The commercial product should be protected from light exposure until ready to use.[4]
IV push	Not to exceed 2 mg/min[4,22] or 0.05 mg/kg over 2–5 minutes.[18]
Intermittent infusion	Not administered by this method.
Continuous infusion	0.2 mg/mL has been administered in *adults*[31-35]; however, little information is available in pediatric patients.[13,16]
Other routes of administration	Although undiluted lorazepam can be given deep into a muscle, it may cause pain at the injection site, a sensation of burning, or observed redness.[4] Should *not* be given IM for status epilepticus.[4] *Midazolam is the benzodiazepine of choice for IM administration. (See Midazolam monograph.)*

LORazepam

Rare adverse effects: An *adult* patient developed severe lactic acidosis as a result of propylene glycol from large-dose, continuous infusion of lorazepam.[36,37] Continuous infusions of lorazepam have also been correlated with propylene glycol-associated renal toxicity in *adults*.[38,39]

Paradoxical reactions (i.e., anxiety, excitation, hostility, aggression, rage, etc.) may occur in children and have been reported in 10% to 30% of those <8 years of age.[4] Brief tonic-clonic seizures have occurred in patients with atypical absence (petit mal) status epileptics who receive a benzodiazepine.[4] Seizure activity and myoclonus have also been reported following administration, especially in very low birth weight neonates.[4,40-42] The movements began a few minutes after a bolus injection and continued for several hours.[41,42]

Drug interactions: Consult appropriate resources for dosing recommendations before combining any drug with lorazepam.

Pharmacokinetic considerations: Mean total clearance normalized to bodyweight was reduced by 80% in neonates (≥37 weeks of gestational age) compared to normal *adults*.[4] Terminal half-life was prolonged threefold, and volume of distribution was decreased by 40% in neonates with asphyxia neonatorum compared to normal *adults*.[4]

Pharmacodynamic considerations: Use in neonates is controversial because other benzodiazepines may decrease blood pressure and cerebral blood flow velocity.[43] Some recommend the initial dose should be reduced by 50% in infants <2 months of age[13]; regardless, lorazepam should be used cautiously in neonates.

Other: Flumazenil, a specific benzodiazepine-receptor antagonist, is indicated for complete or partial reversal of benzodiazepine toxicity.[44,45] (See Flumazenil monograph.)

Larger doses may be required in patients on ECMO since 50% of a dose may be extracted by the PVC tubing and the membrane oxygenator during bypass.[46]

Rebound or withdrawal symptoms may occur following abrupt discontinuation or large decreases in dose.[4] Use caution when reducing dose or withdrawing therapy; decrease slowly and monitor for withdrawal symptoms.

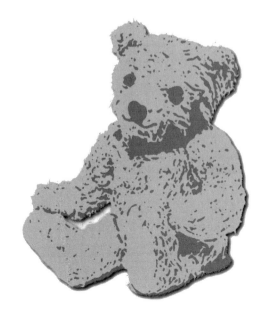

Lymphocyte Immune Globulin–Antithymocyte Globulin (equine)

Brand names	Atgam

Medication error potential	None noted.

Contraindications and warnings

US boxed warning: Only physicians experienced in immunosuppressive therapy for renal transplant or aplastic anemia patients should use lymphocyte immune globulin–antithymocyte globulin (equine).[1]

Patients receiving lymphocyte immune globulin–antithymocyte globulin (equine) should be treated in facilities equipped and staffed with adequate laboratory and supportive medical resources.[1]

Contraindications: Patients who have a severe systemic reaction including a generalized rash, tachycardia, dyspnea, hypotension, or anaphylaxis to a previous Atgam infusion or any other equine gamma globulin product.[1]

Infusion related cautions

The manufacturer recommends that patients be tested with an intradermal injection of 0.1 mL of 1:1000 dilution and a contralateral saline control. Sites should be observed q 15 min for 1 hour. A wheal or erythema ≥10 mm or marked local swelling should be considered a positive test. In the event of a positive test, alternative therapies should be considered and the risk benefit ratio weighed. A negative test dose does not preclude the possibility of an anaphylactic reaction.[1]

Chills, fever, itching, and erythema can be controlled with antipyretics, antihistamines or corticosteroids.[1,2] Many centers have developed premedication protocols to minimize these reactions.

Dosage

Transplant

Renal: 5–25 mg/kg/day for 5–14 days[1,3-7] followed by 10–20 mg/kg as a single dose every other day for ≤2 weeks after transplant.[3] Duration of therapy may be longer in cadaveric allograft recipients.[6]

Bone marrow: 30–40 mg/kg/day over 12 h for 3–4 days prior to transplantation[8-11] or 20 mg/kg every other day for eight doses beginning the day before transplantation.[12]

Lung and/or cardiac transplant: 15–25 mg/kg/day for 3–7 days after transplant.[2,13,14]

Cord blood transplant in infant leukemia: 30 mg/kg/day for 3 days before transplantation.[15]

Aplastic anemia: 15 mg/kg/day for 10 days,[16] 10 mg/kg/day for 5 days,[17] or 40 mg/kg/day over 4 hours for 4 days.[18-21]

Graft-versus-host disease: 30 mg/kg/day for six doses[22] or 15 mg/kg over 3 hours twice a day for 10 days for steroid-resistant disease.[23]

Dosage adjustment in organ dysfunction	None noted. (See Comments section.)

Lymphocyte Immune Globulin–Antithymocyte Globulin (equine)

Maximum dosage	Not established. The largest reported dose was 7 g in an *adult*.[1]
Additives	Contains 0.3 M glycine.[1]
Suitable diluents	D5¼NS, D5½NS, or NS.[1]
Maximum concentration	4 mg/mL.[1]
Preparation and delivery	Store refrigerated. Add Atgam to an inverted container of the sterile diluent to avoid contact with the air; swirl or rotate to mix. Do not shake. The diluted infusate should be at room temperature prior to infusion. **Compatibility:** Addition to dextrose injection is not recommended because low-salt concentrations can cause precipitation.[1]
IV push	Not indicated.[1]
Intermittent infusion	Over ≥6 hours into a high-flow vein.[1] A 0.2–1 micron in-line filter should be used. Resuscitative equipment should be at the bedside during infusion.
Continuous infusion	Not indicated.
Other routes of administration	Not indicated.
Comments	**Adverse effects:** Phlebitis occurred in 46% of children given the drug through a peripheral vein.[5] One study, including six pediatric patients from 7–16 years of age, reported that infusion of Atgam (15 mg/kg) plus 1000 units heparin and 20-mg Solu-Cortef per 250–500 mL of ½NS was associated with a peripheral IV site complication rate of 3.2%.[24] Hence, the study concluded that Atgam could be safely administered via a peripheral vein. Thrombocytopenia, neutropenia,[5,25] and serum sickness[1,5,25] have occurred. Treatment of serum sickness with corticosteroids has generally resulted in resolution of symptoms.[1] Treatment should be discontinued if severe and unremitting thrombocytopenia and leukopenia occurs.[1] This product is made using both human and equine blood components; thus, there is a risk of the transmission of infectious agents, including viruses and the prion that causes Creutzfeldt-Jakob disease.[22] **Monitoring:** Monitoring for bacterial and viral infections during therapy is important.[1,13] Antimicrobial prophylaxis may be included as a part of the treatment regimen.[6,13] Antibiotics can be discontinued if fever persists <48 hours and cultures are negative.[26]

Lymphocyte Immune Globulin–Antithymocyte Globulin (rabbit)

Brand names	Thymoglobulin
Medication error potential	None noted.

Contraindications and warnings

US boxed warning: Only physicians experienced in immunosuppressive therapy for renal transplant patients should use lymphocyte immune globulin-antithymocyte globulin (rabbit).[1]

Contraindications: Patients who have a history of allergy or anaphylaxis to rabbit proteins or product excipients. Patients who have active infections that contraindicate additional immunosuppression.[1]

Infusion related cautions

Fever, chills, dyspnea, hypotension or hypertension, rash, nausea/vomiting may occur during the infusion. Premedication with corticosteroids, acetaminophen, and an antihistamine or decreasing the infusion rate may lessen the incidence and duration of the reaction.[1]

Infusion site reactions include pain, swelling, and erythema.[1]

Dosage

Transplant

Renal: 1.5 mg/kg intra-operatively followed by 1.5 mg/kg/day for 4 to 14 days[1,2] or 1.5–2 mg/kg/day for up to 15 days during induction therapy.[3,4] Others reported administering 0.5–2.5 mg/kg/day for up to 14 doses.[5] More recently, 5 mg/kg was given q 24 h for two doses followed by 2.5 mg/kg/day for six to 10 doses.[6]

Liver and/or intestinal: 5 mg/kg divided in two doses and infused just prior to and soon after transplantation.[7-9]

Bone marrow: 2–2.5 mg/kg/day infused over 1 hour for 3 to 5 days before transplantation (cumulative dose up to 10 mg/kg).[10,11]

Cardiac: 1–2 mg/kg/day or every other day infused over 12 hours as induction therapy for a total of five doses.[12] 1–2.5 mg/kg/day for 1 to 7 days as induction therapy has also been used.[13]

Aplastic anemia: 2.5–3.5 mg/kg/day infused over 6–8 hours for 5 days either as initial treatment or following relapse.[14-16]

Dosage adjustment in organ dysfunction

None noted.

Maximum dosage

150 mg/day.[5]

Additives

Contains 50 mg of glycine, 50 mg of mannitol, 10 mg of sodium chloride, and no preservatives.[1]

Lymphocyte Immune Globulin–Antithymocyte Globulin (rabbit)

Suitable diluents	NS, D5W.[1,17]
Maximum concentration	0.5 mg/mL.[1,17]
Preparation and delivery	**Reconstitution:** The lyophilized powder should reach room temperature prior to reconstitution with SW.[1] **Photosensitivity:** Protect from light during storage.[1]
IV push	Not indicated.
Intermittent infusion	Over ≥6 hours into a high-flow vein for the first dose.[1] Subsequent doses can be infused over 4 hours according to patient tolerance. A 0.22 micron in-line filter should be used.
Continuous infusion	Not indicated.
Other routes of administration	Not indicated.
Comments	**Adverse effects:** If the WBC is ≥2000–3000/mm^3 or if platelets are ≥50,000–75,000/mm^3, the dose should be decreased by half. The drug should be stopped if the WBC is <2000/mm^3 or platelets are <50,000/mm^3.[1] Patients are at an increased risk for infectious complications. The use of anti-infective prophylaxis is recommended.[1] **Monitoring:** Measurement of T-cell counts (absolute and/or subsets) helps assess T-cell depletion.[1] WBC and platelets should be monitored during therapy.[1]

Magnesium Sulfate

Brand names	Various manufacturers, concentrations of 50%, 12.5%, 10%, 8%, 4%, 2%, and 1% are available.
Medication error potential	ISMP high-alert medication that has an increased risk of causing significant patient harm if it is used in error.[1]
Contraindications and warnings	Contraindicated in patients with heart block or with myocardial damage.[2]
Infusion related cautions	Magnesium is available in several different salt forms and magnesium sulfate is available in seven concentrations. Choose products carefully.

Dosage

1 g magnesium sulfate = 8.12 mEq magnesium = 98.6 mg elemental magnesium.[2]

Hypomagnesemia

> **Neonates:** 25–50 mg magnesium sulfate/kg 8–12 hours for two or three doses.[3-5] (See Comments section.)

> **Infants and children:** 25–50 mg magnesium sulfate/kg (maximum 2 g/dose) q 6 h for three or four doses.[5] One 9-year-old, 19-kg child receiving a 21-day course of tobramycin developed tetany, hypomagnesemia (serum magnesium 1 mg/dL), and hypocalcemia and was treated with 950 mg magnesium sulfate and 2 g calcium gluconate and had symptom improvement within hours.[6]

PALS (torsades de pointes, resuscitation with hypomagnesemia): 25–50 mg magnesium sulfate/kg up to a maximum of 2 g. A more rapid infusion rate may be needed in torsades de pointes.[7]

Asthma: 25–75 mg magnesium sulfate/kg up to a maximum of 2 g.[5,8-12]

Epilepsy: 20–100 mg magnesium sulfate/kg q 4–6 h.[5] Doses up to 200 mg/kg have been used.

Following cardiopulmonary bypass (CPB): In one study, the development of arrhythmias was compared in those given 30 mg magnesium sulfate/kg (n = 13) or saline control (n = 15) after CPB.[13] If serum Mg concentration decreased to <1.6–2.3 mg/dL at any time during the ICU stay, 10 mg/kg was given. Junctional ectopic tachycardia occurred in 27% of the saline control group (n = 15) compared to none of the treatment group.

Persistent pulmonary hypertension of the newborn: Seven of nine infants who received 200 mg magnesium sulfate/kg followed by 20–50 mg/kg/h for up to 8 hours survived.[14] Predicted mortality in these patients was 100%.

Dosage adjustment in organ dysfunction	Use with caution in severe renal insufficiency.[2] The manufacturer recommends that in severe renal insufficiency doses not exceed 20 g in 48 hours and serum magnesium concentration be obtained often.
Maximum dosage	In children with hypomagnesemia, 2 g/dose.[5,7] Up to 40 g/day has been used in *adults* with pre-eclampsia to treat or prevent seizures.[2]
Additives	Contains contaminant aluminum.[2]

Magnesium Sulfate

Suitable diluents	D5W, NS, LR.[2,15]
Maximum concentration	200 mg/mL or 1.6 mEq/mL (20%) for IV infusion in children or *adults*.[2] 20% for IM administration in infants and children, 50% for IM administration in *adults*.[2]
Preparation and delivery	**Compatibility:** See Appendix D for PN compatibility information.
IV push	Infrequently used due to the potential for increased adverse effects.[2] (See Comments section.)
Intermittent infusion	Usually over 10–20 minutes in infants and children. ≤150 mg/min in *adults*.[2]
Continuous infusion	May be infused continuously.[2,15]
Other routes of administration	IM.[2]
Comments	**Monitoring:** Monitor for cardiac dysrhythmias, hypotension, respiratory depression, and CNS depression during intermittent infusion.[3] In neonates, infusion of 250 mg magnesium sulfate/kg over 10 minutes was associated with respiratory depression and infusion of 400 mg/kg over 10–30 minutes was associated with an unacceptable rate of hypotension.[16] **Drug interactions:** Drug interactions between magnesium and CNS depressants and neuromuscular blockers can occur.[2] Treatment of hypermagnesemia with calcium in patients receiving digoxin can result in heart block.[2]

Mannitol

Brand names	Osmitrol, generic
Medication error potential	None noted.
Contraindications and warnings	**Contraindications:** Well-established anuria due to severe renal disease, severe pulmonary congestion or frank pulmonary edema, active intracranial bleeding except during craniotomy, severe dehydration, and progressive renal dysfunction. After mannitol is started if progressive heart failure or pulmonary congestion develops, mannitol should be stopped.[1] **Warnings:** Excessive fluid and electrolyte losses can occur; serum electrolytes, especially sodium and potassium, should be monitored.
Infusion related cautions	Rapid administration can result in hypotension, hyperosmolality, and elevations in ICP.[2]
Dosage	**Oliguria test dose (renal function assessment):** 0.2 g/kg to a maximum of 12.5 g over 3–5 minutes to produce a urine output of ≥1 mL/kg/h or 30–50 mL/h in *adults* for 1–3 hours.[1,3] This may be repeated after 2 hours if the response is inadequate. **Cerebral edema/elevated ICP:** 0.25–1 g/kg over 15 minutes.[2-8] The AAP recommends 0.25 g/kg given over 5–15 minutes repeated as needed and 0.5 g/kg given over 15 minutes for an acute increase in ICP.[2] (See Comments section.) **Nephrotic syndrome:** Three children (ages 4, 7, and 9 years) with nephrotic syndrome and diuretic-resistant edema responded to furosemide (2 mg/kg) and 5 mL/kg/day of 20% mannitol infused over 1 hour for 5–7 days.[8]
Dosage adjustment in organ dysfunction	Mannitol should not be used in patients with severe renal disease and well-established anuria.[1]
Maximum dosage	2.5 g/kg has been used in *adults*.[7] However, there does not appear to be a therapeutic advantage to doses >1 g/kg.[7]
Additives	None.
Suitable diluents	D5W.[1]
Maximum concentration	25% solution.[1,9]
Preparation and delivery	Mannitol may crystallize at lower temperatures if concentrations are ≥15%.[9] To avoid crystal formation, store the solutions in a warming chamber or if crystals are present, warm the vial using a dry heat cabinet and vigorous shaking. Be sure the solution is at body temperature prior to infusion. Supersaturated mannitol solutions in PVC bags develop a heavy flocculent precipitate within minutes.[9] Heating the bag may temporarily dissolve the crystals, but they quickly reappear. Solutions containing ≥20% mannitol should be infused through an in-line filter.[1,9] **Compatibility:** See Appendix D for PN compatibility information.

Mannitol

IV push	3–5 minutes in oliguria.[1]
Intermittent infusion	Over 15–60 minutes for cerebral edema, elevated ICP, or preoperative in neuro-surgery.[2-8]
Continuous infusion	Sixty patients from age 1–73 were given a continuous infusion over 6–100 hours (total dose 2–20 g/kg).[7]
Other routes of administration	Dry powder mannitol has been given via inhalation to children with cystic fibrosis.[10]
Comments	**Adverse effects:** Mannitol increases the intravascular volume and can worsen hyponatremia.

Comments

Adverse effects: Mannitol increases the intravascular volume and can worsen hyponatremia.

Use furosemide for increased ICP in patients with pre-existing cardiac disease because mannitol increases the intravascular volume and may exacerbate CHF and pulmonary edema.[11]

A 16-year-old and a 28-year-old with increased ICP and normal renal function developed reversible acute renal failure after receiving 2 and 4 days of doses ranging from 50 and 900 g/day.[12]

Monitoring: The resultant diuresis can lead to sodium and potassium losses. Electrolytes should be monitored.[1] Monitor serum osmolality during mannitol therapy for elevated ICP.

Osmolality: 25% mannitol has an osmolarity of 1372 mOsmol/L.[1]

Other: Whether saline or mannitol is more beneficial in treating increased ICP is not established.[3]

Meperidine HCl

Brand names	Demerol, generic
Medication error potential	ISMP high-alert medication that has an increased risk of causing significant patient harm if it is used in error.[1]

Look-alike, sound-alike error potential.

USP reported that meperidine was confused with methadone.[2] Meperidine was confused with morphine and patient harm resulted. Demerol was confused with Demadex and Dilaudid. |
| **Contraindications and warnings** | **Contraindications:** Those with hypersensitivity to meperidine and those on monoamine oxidase (MAO) inhibitors or who have recently received MAO inhibitors.[3]

Warnings: Use with caution in those receiving other CNS depressants. Meperidine may elevate cerebrospinal fluid pressure and, if possible, an alternative agent should be used in patients with head injury.[3] |
| **Infusion related cautions** | For IV infusion the patient should be lying down.[3] Rapid injection may cause severe respiratory depression, apnea, hypotension, peripheral circulatory collapse, and cardiac arrest. For this use, the patient should be in a facility with appropriate supportive measures and a narcotic antagonist must be available.

Anaphylaxis has been reported.[4] |
| **Dosage** | Because of the potential for adverse effects, meperidine has largely been replaced by other analgesics.[5] Doses should be titrated to desired analgesic effect.

Demerol, Phenergan, Thorazine [DPT] cocktail has been used to sedate children.[6-9] However, safer and more effective agents are available,[6,8,10] and this combination is no longer recommended.[9]

Analgesia: 0.5–2 mg/kg (usually IM or SC) q 3–4 h as needed.[3,11-14] A loading dose of 0.3–1 mg/kg followed by continuous infusion, beginning at 0.3 mg/kg/h and titrating to desired response up to 0.7 mg/kg/h has been used in severe sickle cell pain crisis.[15] (See Comments section.)

Preoperative sedation: 0.25–1.5 mg/kg (usually IM or SC) and ≤100 mg given 30–90 minutes prior to procedure.[10,16,17] 2 mg/kg and ≤100 mg has been used IV.[18] |
| **Dosage adjustment in organ dysfunction** | **CrCl 10–50 mL/min/1.73 m²:** 75% of the usual dose.[19]

CrCl <10 mL/min/1.73 m²: 50% of the usual dose.[19]

Avoid repeated or high doses in patients with renal impairment.[3]

The dose or frequency of dosing should be decreased in hepatic disease.[3] Those with renal and hepatic disease are at risk for accumulation of normeperidine, an active metabolite.[20] (See Comments section.) |
| **Maximum dosage** | 2 mg/kg[14,15,17,18] and ≤100 mg/dose.[3,18] A continuous infusion of 1.5 mg/kg/h has been used in children with sickle-cell disease.[15] (See Comments section.) |

Meperidine HCl

Additives

Products may contain sodium metabisulfite and/or phenol and *m*-cresol as preservatives.[21] See Appendix C for specific information about adverse effects.

Suitable diluents

D–LR, D–R, D–S, D5W, D10W, LR, NS, or ½NS.[3,21]

Maximum concentration

10 mg/mL for IV injection. 1 mg/mL for IV infusion.[3]

Preparation and delivery

Compatibility: Meperidine is incompatible with heparin[21,22] and barbiturates.[3,21] To avoid precipitation with heparin, flush heparinized IV catheters with NS before and after meperidine injection.[21,22]

See Appendix D for PN compatibility information.

IV push

Not indicated. Rapid injection increases risk for adverse reactions (e.g., respiratory depression, apnea, hypotension, cardiac arrest).[3] One group reported that five of 154 children undergoing endoscopy required supplemental oxygen for a short time after receiving 2 mg/kg infused over 1–2 minutes.[18]

Intermittent infusion

Over >5 minutes.[3]

Continuous infusion

Maybe be used as continuous infusion.[3]

Other routes of administration

Usually given IM. SC can be used occasionally.[3,10,16] Local tissue irritation and induration are more common with SC administration.[3]

Comments

Adverse effects: The meperidine metabolite, normeperidine, may cause a variety of CNS effects including excitability, twitches, tremors, or seizures.[23,24]

When pain management was inadequate with morphine, a 32-month-old febrile and hyponatremic boy with 90% BSA burns was changed to a meperidine infusion.[25] One hour after the dose had been gradually increased to 25 mg/kg/h, he began having intermittent seizures and became comatose. The meperidine was stopped, phenobarbital was started, and the seizures stopped after 6 hours. While there were confounding factors, it was felt that the seizures were due to the large dose of meperidine.

A 6-week-old infant received two 1-mg/kg doses IV during rigid bronchoscopy and developed acute orofacial dyskinesias (e.g., tongue thrusting, pursing or puckering, facial grimacing) that were unresponsive to 0.1 mg/kg of naloxone.[26] This lasted about 36 hours; he had no residual effects.

Monitoring: Vital signs, oxygen saturation, pain relief.[14]

Pharmacokinetics: The pharmacokinetics of meperidine are highly variable in neonates and infants. Half-life ranged from 3.3–59.4 hours in 21 infants.[11] Clearance increased with increasing BSA; however, half-life was not different among term infants <1 week of age, term infants >3 weeks of age (26–150 days of age), and preterm neonates (3.6–65 days of age).

Meropenem

Brand names	Merrem

Medication error potential

Look-alike, sound-alike drug names.

USP reports confusion with ertapenem, metronidazole, and midazolam.[1]

Contraindications and warnings

Contraindications: In patients with a known hypersensitivity to any component of this product or to other drugs in the same class or in patients who have demonstrated anaphylactic reactions to beta-lactams.[2]

Warnings

Allergic reactions: Serious hypersensitivity and occasionally fatal anaphylactic reactions have been reported.[2] These are more likely in patients who are sensitive to multiple allergens and in those with a history of hypersensitivity to a penicillin, cephalosporin, or other beta-lactam.[2]

Seizures: Neurotoxicity of the carbapenem antibiotics has been reported.[2] Seizures occur most commonly in patients with renal impairment and/or underlying neurologic disorders. (See Rare adverse effects in Comments section.)

Superinfection: Prolonged use may cause superinfection and/or *Clostridium difficile*–associated diarrhea (CDAD), which has been reported and may range in severity from mild diarrhea to fatal colitis.[2] If CDAD is suspected or confirmed, appropriate fluid and electrolyte management, protein supplementation, antibiotic treatment of *C. difficile*, and surgical evaluation should be instituted as clinically indicated.[2] Antibiotic use that is not directed against *C. difficile* may need to be discontinued.[2]

Infusion related cautions

If a decision is made to give meropenem to a patient with known penicillin, cephalosporins or beta-lactam hypersensitivity, the patient should be closely observed for allergenicity.[2] Serious anaphylactic reactions require immediate emergency treatment with epinephrine, oxygen, intravenous steroids, and airway management, including intubation. Other therapy may also be administered as indicated.[2]

May cause phlebitis at the injection site.[2]

Dosage

Neonates *(Safety and effectiveness have not been established for patients <3 months of age.[2] Little dosing information is available in this age group.)*

≤7 days: 30–40 mg/kg/day divided q 12 h over 15–30 minutes.[3,4]

>7 days: 40 mg/kg/day divided q 8 h over 15–30 minutes.[4]

A 15-day-old premature neonate (33 weeks gestational age; 1.59 kg) was given 120 mg/kg/day divided q 8 h for 8 weeks as treatment for a brain abscess.[5]

Infants and children

Mild infection (e.g., skin): 10 mg/kg/day divided q 8 h up to 1.5 g/day.[2]

Moderate infections (e.g., intra-abdominal): 60 mg/kg/day divided q 8 h up to 3 g/day.[2]

Serious infections (e.g., meningitis): 120 mg/kg/day divided q 8 h up to 6 g/day.[2,5,7-9]

Meropenem

Dosage adjustment in organ dysfunction

If CrCl is 30–50 mL/min, give 20–40 mg/kg/day divided every 12 hours; if CrCl is 10–29 mL/min, give 10–20 mg/kg/day divided every 12 hours; if CrCl is <10 mL/min, give 10–20 mg/kg every 24 hours.[9]

Maximum dosage

120 mg/kg/day up to 6 g/day.[2,7-9]

Additives

Contains 3.92 mEq sodium/g of meropenem.[10]

Suitable diluents

D5W, D10W, NS, ½NS, D5NS, D5½NS, D5¼NS, D5LR, LR. Mannitol 2.5%, mannitol 10%, 5% sodium bicarbonate.[10]

Maximum concentration

50 mg/mL.[10]

Preparation and delivery

Stability: 4 hours in NS at controlled room temperature and up to 24 hours if refrigerated.[10] Variable stability based on storage conditions; hence, consult appropriate reference for detailed information).

Compatibility: See Appendix D for PN compatibility information.[11]

IV push

50 mg/mL over 3–5 minutes.[2,10]

Intermittent infusion

50 mg/mL over 15–30 minutes.[2,10]

Continuous infusion

Not generally done. Meropenem has been administered as a 3-hour infusion for the treatment of CNS infections.[12] Additionally, a 24-hour continuous infusion, divided into three 8-hour infusions, has been used in the treatment of critically ill *adults*.[13]

Other routes of administration

IM administration has been used in the treatment of urinary tract infections and pneumonia in *adults*.[14]

Comments

Rare adverse effects: Neurotoxicity of the carbapenem antibiotics has been reported.[15,16] In *adults*, seizures most often occur after 7 days and appear to be related to an underlying CNS disorder, impaired renal function, and/or large doses.[2] If seizures occur, the need for meropenem should be considered and the dosage should be assessed.

Thrombocytopenia has been reported in patients with renal dysfunction who are receiving meropenem.[2]

An increase in alkaline phosphatase occurred in cystic fibrosis patients.[18]

Drug interactions: Carbapenems may reduce serum concentrations of valproic acid, which can result in a loss of seizure control.[19] Serum valproic acid concentrations should be monitored frequently after beginning or increasing the dose of a carbapenem. Alternative antibiotics or anticonvulsant therapy should be considered if serum valproic acid concentrations drop below the therapeutic range or a seizure occurs.

Laboratory interference: Positive direct and indirect Coombs' tests have been reported.[20]

Methotrexate

Brand names	Folex, generic

Medication error potential

ISMP high-alert medication that has an increased risk of causing significant patient harm if it is used in error.[1]

Look-alike, sound-alike error potential.

USP reports that methotrexate (MTX) was confused with methylprednisolone sodium succinate, metolazone, metronidazole, mercaptopurine and mitoxantrone; no patient harm resulted. USP also reports that MTX was confused with minoxidil; patient harm resulted.[2]

ISMP reports that Folex has been confused with Foltx.[3]

Contraindications and warnings

US boxed warning: Administer under the supervision of a physician with experience in antimetabolite therapy. Because of the toxic and potentially life-threatening toxicity associated with MTX, it should only be used in life-threatening neoplastic disease or in patients with severe, recalcitrant psoriasis or rheumatoid arthritis unresponsive to other therapies.[4]

MTX may cause serious neoplastic disease (malignant lymphoma) and increased risk of death. It has also been associated with tumor lysis syndrome and serious immune suppression, bone marrow suppression, and liver, lung, and kidney toxicities. May cause fetal death or congenital abnormalities when given to pregnant women. MTX also associated with life-threatening diarrhea/stomatitis, dermatologic reactions, and opportunistic infections.[4,5]

Use caution when administering MTX concurrently with other hepatotoxic and nephrotoxic agents. Concurrent use with NSAIDs may cause serious adverse events (bone marrow suppression, aplastic anemia, and GI toxicity).[4,5]

Use with radiotherapy may increase risk of soft tissue necrosis and osteonecrosis.[4]

MTX elimination is decreased in patients with renal insufficiency, ascites, or pleural effusions; use cautiously with increased monitoring for toxicity in these patients.[4]

High-dose regimens for osteosarcoma require considerable caution. (See Infusion related cautions section.) Other high dose therapies should be considered investigational.[4]

MTX formulations containing preservatives must be not be used intrathecally or as high-dose therapy.[4,5]

Contraindications: Hypersensitivity to MTX or any component of the formulation, severe renal or hepatic impairment, pre-existing profound bone marrow suppression, alcoholic liver disease, AIDS, and pre-existing blood dyscrasias.[4,5]

Other warnings: Neurotoxicity leading to seizures has been reported in pediatric ALL patients.[4,5]

Infusion related cautions

Aggressive hydration should accompany administration. (See Significant adverse effects in Comments section.)

Two patients experienced anaphylactoid reactions to high-dose MTX and BCG injections for osteosarcoma.[6]

Methotrexate

Dosage

Consult protocol for complete information regarding MTX and leucovorin dosages, hydration, and alkalinization.

MTX is used for a variety of neoplastic disease states.

Cancer

Acute lymphocytic leukemia (ALL)

High-dose therapy: Loading dose of 200 mg/m².[7,8] This is generally followed by 0.8–5 g/m²/day infused over 2–24 hours for 2–3 weeks.[7-10] Although doses as large as 33.6 g/m² have been infused over 4–48 hours,[11-13] outcomes were not substantially improved over those noted with lower doses (1.2 g/m²).[7]

Maintenance therapy: 20–50 mg/m² IV weekly.[7,14] Adjust dose to maintain a specific WBC count.

Lymphoma: 30 mg/m² IV push,[15] 300 mg/m² IV infusion over 4 hours,[16] 1 g/m²[17] up to 10 g/m² administered over 3–24 hours,[18] 3–30 mg/kg[16] up to 50–200 mg/kg infused over 3–6 hours.[19]

Meningeal leukemia: Doses administered q 2–5 days until CSF normal, followed by weekly dose for 2 weeks, followed by monthly dose. IT doses in pediatric patients should be based on age (not BSA) as follows[20]:

Age (years)	IT Dose (mg)
<1	6
1	8
2	10
≥3	12

Only preservative-free MTX should be used for IT administration.[21]

Osteosarcoma: 1.25–15 g/m² infused over 4–6 hours.[22-25]

Juvenile rheumatoid arthritis: 0.8–1.1 mg/kg/week,[26] 15 mg/m²/week,[27] up to 40 mg/m²/week.[28] Generally given orally or IM.

Dosage adjustment in organ dysfunction

Adjust dosage in patients with renal dysfunction. If CrCl is 10–50 mL/min, give 50% of a normal dose; if CrCl is <10 mL/min, do not administer.[29]

Patients with renal dysfunction or those demonstrating toxicity with previous doses of IT MTX may require leucovorin rescue in small doses.[30,31] Hemodialysis has limited usefulness in lowering plasma MTX in patients with renal failure,[32] but hemodialysis in combination with charcoal hemoperfusion has been successful in managing a patient with severe renal failure following high-dose MTX.[33] Oral administration of activated charcoal may be effective in lowering plasma MTX concentrations.[34]

Maximum dosage

Doses >100 mg/m² should be administered with leucovorin.[35] When given with leucovorin rescue, MTX may be escalated to the dosage that yields the best therapeutic effect.[35] Maximum IT dosage is 15 mg.[20]

Methotrexate

Additives

MTX sodium for injection contains 0.43, 0.86, and 2.15 mEq sodium in the 2, 4, and 10 mL sizes, respectively. The lyophilized product contains 7 mEq sodium per 1-g vial.[4,21]

May contain benzyl alcohol.[4,21] See Appendix C for more specific information about potential adverse effects and/or benzyl alcohol toxicity in neonates.

Suitable diluents

D5NS, D5W NS.[4,21]

Maximum concentration

<25 mg/mL for IV or IM administration; 1 mg/mL for IT administration.[21]

Preparation and delivery

Incompatible with fluorouracil, cytarabine, prednisolone, and sodium phosphate.[5]

For PN compatibility information, please see Appendix C.

IV push

<25 mg/mL. May be administered by this method.[4,5,21]

Intermittent infusion

<25 mg/mL. May be administered by this method.[4,5,16-18,21]

Continuous infusion

<25 mg/mL. Doses >100–300 mg/m^2 are generally administered by continuous infusion.[4,5,11-13,18,21]

Other routes of administration

May be administered IM, intra-arterial, and IT.[4,5,21] IT doses should be with a preservative-free product diluted to 1 mg/mL using an appropriate sterile preservative-free diluent such as sodium chloride injection.[21]

Comments

Significant adverse effects: The administration of MTX has been associated with fatal pulmonary toxicity,[36] erythema and desquamation,[37] and death related to high doses.[25,38] Pulmonary toxicity may occur with low doses and be rapidly progressive.[4]

Aggressive hydration from 100 mL/m^2/h to 200 mL/m^2/h during and after MTX must be administered in patients receiving intermediate to high doses of MTX to improve clearance and minimize toxicity.[9,13,35,39-43]

Urinary alkalinization (pH >6.5) should be maintained during high-dose infusions of MTX and for 48 hours after infusion.[9,35,39-44]

Leucovorin should be administered with MTX when doses are ≥100 mg/m^2 and should be dosed according to the patient's protocol and the amount of MTX given.[35,39] Leucovorin dosages should be modified if MTX clearance is delayed.[35,39]

Clinical features known to place patients at risk for increased MTX toxicity include renal dysfunction,[41] dehydration,[25] vomiting,[13,41,45] diarrhea,[45] decreased urine flow,[46] urine pH below 6.5,[13,41,46] pleural effusions,[47,48] GI obstruction,[49] ascites,[47,48] concomitant use of nephrotoxic medications (e.g., amphotericin B and acyclovir),[13] previous history of cisplatin use,[50] Down syndrome,[51] and drug interactions decreasing elimination of MTX (e.g., salicylates,[52] omeprazole,[53] NSAIDs,[54-56] sulfamethoxazole/trimethoprim,[57] probenecid,[52,58] and penicillins).[59]

Comments (cont.)

MTX (250–1000 mg/m²) is associated with a moderate (30% to 90%) risk of emesis.[60] Patients should receive antiemetic therapy to prevent acute and delayed nausea and vomiting. The recommended therapy is a 5HT3 receptor antagonist in combination with dexamethasone on every day chemotherapy is administered.[60,61] These agents may be continued for up to 4 days after chemotherapy for the prevention of delayed nausea and vomiting.

MTX (50 mg/m² to <250 mg/m²) is associated with a low (10% to 30%) risk of emesis.[60] Patients should receive antiemetic therapy to prevent acute nausea and vomiting. The recommended therapy is a corticosteroid on every day chemotherapy is administered; alternatives are a phenothiazine (e.g., prochlorperazine) or a butyro-phenone (e.g., droperidol).[60,61] Therapy for delayed nausea and vomiting is generally not needed.

MTX (<50 mg/m²) is associated with a minimal (<10%) risk of emesis.[60] Generally, prophylaxis for acute and delayed emesis is not needed. Patients may receive one-time prophylaxis with a phenothiazine (e.g., prochlorperazine) or a butyrophenone (e.g., droperidol).[60,61]

Breakthrough medications for nausea and vomiting should be offered to patients receiving any dose of MTX. Appropriate medications include a phenothiazine (e.g., prochlorperazine), a butyrophenone (e.g., droperidol), a substituted benzamide (e.g., metoclopramide), or a benzodiazepine (e.g., lorazepam). Selection should be based on what the patient is currently receiving for acute anti-emesis prophylaxis.[60,61]

Monitoring: Monitoring should include liver function tests, CBC with platelets, renal function tests, and chest x-ray.[4,5]

MTX serum concentrations should be monitored when administering large doses of drug. The relationship between serum concentration and toxicity is well established.[25,35,40,44] Recommended procedure is to monitor concentrations at 23 hours and 44 hours, and until concentrations decrease to <0.05 micromol/L.

Drug interactions: Because MTX is associated with numerous drug interactions,[4,5] consult appropriate resources for dosing recommendations before combining any drug with MTX.

Methyldopate HCl

Brand names	Aldomet, generic
Medication error potential	Look-alike, sound-alike error potential.
	USP reports that Aldomet has been confused with Aldactone; no patient harm resulted.[1]
Contraindications and warnings	**Contraindications:** Active hepatic disease (hepatitis, cirrhosis), liver disorders previously associated with methyldopate, hypersensitivity to methyldopate or any of its components, including sulfites, and therapy with MAO inhibitors.[2]
	Warnings: Methyldopate therapy has been associated with a positive Coombs' test, hemolytic anemia, and liver disorders; these may be fatal if not identified and managed appropriately.[2] (See Comments section.)
Infusion related cautions	The injectable product contains sodium bisulfite and anaphylaxis may occur.[2] (See Additives section.)
Dosage	A decrease in blood pressure generally occurs within 4–6 hours and lasts 10–16 hours.[2,3]
	Hypertensive crisis or emergency
	Initial dose: 2–4 mg/kg/dose; if no effect observed within 4–6 hours, double the dose.[4]
	Maintenance dose: 5–50 mg/kg/day (usually 20–40 mg/kg/day) divided q 6 h[3,5] or 0.6–1.2 g/m²/day divided q 6 h.[3]
	In hypertensive emergencies, blood pressure should be frequently monitored to ensure that it does not decrease too quickly.[3,6] One group recommended that the blood pressure decrease by one third of the desired total blood pressure decrease within 6 hours, a further one-third decrease within the next 24–36 hours, with the final one-third decrease achieved over the next 48–72 hours.[7] Alternatively, a blood pressure decrease of <25% within minutes to 1 hour followed by further decreases over the next 2–6 hours if the patient is stable has been suggested.[3]
Dosage adjustment in organ dysfunction	Adjust dosage in patients with renal dysfunction.[8] Active metabolite may accumulate in uremia.[3] If CrCl is 10–50 mL/min, administer normal dose q 8–12 h; if CrCl is <10 mL/min, give normal dose q 12–24 h.[8]
Maximum dosage	65 mg/kg/day, not to exceed 3 g/day or 2 g/m²/day [2,3] or 1 g/dose.[9] The maximum *adult* dose recommended by the manufacturer is 1 g q 6 h.[3]
Additives	Each mL contains 3.2 mg sodium bisulfite.[2] See Appendix C for more specific information about potential adverse effects of sulfites.
	Each mL contains 1.5 mg methylparaben and 0.2 mg propylparaben.[2] See Appendix C for more specific information about potential adverse effects of parabens.
Suitable diluents	D5W.[10]
Maximum concentration	10 mg/mL.[2,3,10]

Methyldopate HCl

Preparation and delivery	For PN compatibility information, please see Appendix D.
IV push	Not recommended.[3]
Intermittent infusion	To avoid a paradoxical pressor effect, dilute in 50–100 mL D5W ($\leq$10 mg/mL) and infuse slowly over 30–60 minutes.[3,4,10]
Continuous infusion	No information available to support administration by this method.
Other routes of administration	IM and SC administration are not recommended due to erratic absorption.[3,10]
Comments	**Significant adverse effects:** May cause hemolysis in patients with glucose-6-phosphate dehydrogenase deficiency.[3] May cause positive Coombs' test; if evidence of hemolytic anemia, the drug should be discontinued.[3] **Monitoring:** Complete blood count at baseline and periodically during therapy; Coombs' test at baseline and at 6 and 12 months of therapy; liver function tests at baseline, and over the first 6–12 weeks of therapy, and any time there is unexplained fever.[2] **Other:** May cause urine to be discolored (pink/red to darkened).[2,3] A paradoxical pressor response has been reported.[4]

MethylPREDNISolone Sodium Succinate

| **Brand names** | A-METHAPRED, Solu-Medrol, generic |

Medication error potential

ISMP's *Confused Drug Names* reports that Solu-Medrol has been confused with Depo-Medrol.[1]

USP reported that methylPREDNISolone sodium succinate was confused with hydrocortisone sodium succinate, methotrexate, metoclopramide, metronidazole, prednisolone sodium phosphate and no patient harm occurred. MethylPREDNISolone sodium succinate was confused with methylprednisolone acetate and patient harm resulted.[2]

USP reported that Solu-Medrol was confused with salmeterol and Solu-Cortef and no patient harm occurred. Solu-Medrol was confused with DepoMetrol and patient harm resulted.[2]

Contraindications and warnings

Contraindications: Neonates (products with benzyl alcohol), patients with systemic fungal infections, and patients with hypersensitivity to any component in the product.[3]

Live virus (MMR, varicella, rotavirus, smallpox) vaccinations should not be given during treatment with immunosuppressive doses of glucocorticoids.[3] (See Comments section.)

Warnings: Anaphylactoid reactions have been reported and those with a prior history of such reactions require appropriate precautions.[3-7]

Patients on chronic steroid therapy may require increased doses during stress.[3]

Supraphysiologic doses of corticosteroids may result in suppressed pituitary-adrenal function, so therapy of more than a few days should be decreased gradually.[2,8,9]

Immunosuppression and an increased risk for infection are possible during steroid therapy.[3] (See Comments section.)

Based on trials in *adults,* corticosteroids are contraindicated in sepsis syndrome and septic shock.[10,11] Although there is no primary literature to support this, some neonatal and pediatric intensive care centers administer steroids to a subset of pediatric patients who are unresponsive to conventional therapies.

Infusion related cautions

Large doses should be infused slowly. Cardiac arrhythmias and cardiac arrest has been reported within minutes or hours of infusion in *adults* receiving ≥500 mg over <10 minutes.[12-14]

Dosage

Doses are based on severity of disease and patient response.[3,12] The lowest dose that results in the desired effect should be used.[3,12]

Anti-inflammatory/immunosuppressive "pulse" therapy: 10–30 mg/kg/day either daily for 3–4 days or every other day for three to four doses [15-20] or 600 mg/m² for 3 days.[21]

Asthma

Status: 2 mg/kg as a loading dose, followed by 0.5–1 mg/kg q 6 h.[22]

Exacerbation: 1–2 mg/kg divided q 12 h (maximum of 60 mg/day × 3 – 10 days).[12,22]

Idiopathic thrombocytopenic purpura: 30 mg/kg/day for 3 days.[23]

Pneumocystis carinii pneumonia

≤13 years: 4–8 mg/kg/day divided q 6–12 h for 5–7 days followed by oral prednisone.[24-26]

>13 years: 30 mg q 12 h for 5 days, then 30 mg as single dose for 5 days,[27] and then 15 mg as single dose for 7 days,[27] to 11 days (or until antibiotic therapy is complete).

MethylPREDNISolone Sodium Succinate

Dosage *(cont.)*

Spinal-cord injury: A loading dose of 30 mg/kg over 15 minutes followed in 45 minutes by a continuous infusion of 5.4 mg/kg/h × 23 hours (if started within 3 hours of injury) or × 48 hours (if started 3–8 hours after injury).[28,29] Although the National Acute Spinal Cord Injury trial did not include any patients <13 years old,[29] many pediatric clinicians have adopted this practice.[30,31]

Other uses

Ventricular tachycardia/silent lymphocytic myocarditis: 30 mg/kg/day for 3 days.[32]

Chronic interstitial lung disease: 300 mg/m²/day for 3 days, repeated q 4–6 weeks.[33]

Lupus nephritis: 30 mg/kg every other day for six doses.[12]

Periocular hemangiomas of infancy: 2 mg/kg divided q 12 h for 2 days, then transitioned to oral corticosteroid to taper resulted in rapid hemangioma shrinkage and visual improvement in 15 infants.[34] Recently, oral prednisolone (n = 10) was as effective as IV methylprednisolone (n = 10) in problematic infantile hemangiomas.[35]

Dosage adjustment in organ dysfunction

Those with cirrhosis of the liver or who are hypothyroid may have an exaggerated response.[3]

Maximum dosage

Usually 500 mg.[12] However, 30 mg/kg[18] 30 mg/kg rounded to 500 mg, 1 g, or 2 g,[15] or up to 3 g/dose[17] has been used as pulse therapy for severe glomerulonephritis, systemic lupus erythematosus, and renal transplant rejection.

Additives

Contains benzyl alcohol. See Appendix C for more specific information about potential benzyl alcohol toxicity in neonates.[3]

Contains 2.01 mEq sodium/g of methylprednisolone sodium succinate.[36]

Suitable diluents

D5W, D5NS, D5½NS, LR, NS.[37]

Maximum concentration

125 mg/mL for IV push and 2.5 mg/mL for intermittent infusion.[12]

Preparation and delivery

Compatibility: See Appendix D for PN compatibility information.

IV push

Over 1 to several minutes.[3,12] High-dose (15 mg/kg; 500 mg) therapy should be infused over ≥30 minutes.[3,12] (See Comments section.)

Intermittent infusion

Over 20–60 minutes.[3]

Continuous infusion

May be infused continuously.[12,28,29]

Other routes of administration

May be administered IM.[3,12]

MethylPREDNISolone Sodium Succinate

Comments

An early study found 30 mg/kg methylprednisolone as an initial treatment of Kawasaki disease (in combination with IVIG and aspirin) resulted in faster resolution of fever, improvement in inflammatory markers, and shorter hospital stay.[38] A more recent study did not support the use of methylprednisolone in Kawasaki disease because coronary-artery outcomes were not different between the active and placebo treated groups.[39] One child with Kawasaki disease who had a severe rash similar to Stevens-Johnson syndrome but without mucosal involvement was felt to respond to the third 30 mg/kg methylprednisolone dose.[40]

Adverse effects: Intractable hiccups, palpitations, and anaphylaxis have been reported.[6,7,41]

Children with a history of drug-induced cutaneous reactions are more likely to have an adverse reaction to IV corticosteroids.[42]

Corticosteroid-induced bronchospasm with methylprednisolone in an *adult* with severe asthma was reported. The author recommended considering corticosteroids as a contributing factor in asthmatics who do not improve on IV steroids (especially if aspirin allergy also present). Skin testing may help guide safe alternative corticosteroids.[43]

Atrial fibrillation,[44] seizures, transient blindness,[45] and fatal varicella[46] have occurred after methylprednisolone administration.

A pediatric study looking at effects of short-term (3 days) methylprednisolone 2 mg/kg/day on bone metabolism in infants and children reported significant, but reversible, inhibition of bone formation markers.[47]

A 14-year-old male with nephrotic syndrome being treated with oral prednisolone developed Stevens-Johnson syndrome. The boy was changed to IV methylprednisolone 20 mg/kg/dose every other day. By day 2 of treatment, fever subsided and by day 4 the bullae began to subside.[48]

Drug interactions: Drugs that enhance hepatic clearance (e.g., phenytoin, phenobarbital, ephedrine, rifampin) may decrease blood levels and lessen physiologic activity.[3]

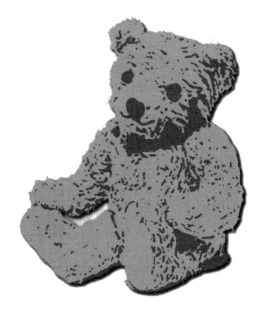

Metoclopramide HCl

Brand names　　　Reglan, generic

Medication error potential

Look-alike, sound-alike error potential.

USP reports that metoclopramide has been confused with methocarbamol, methylprednisolone sodium succinate, metolazone, metoprolol tartrate and trimethobenzamide; no patient harm resulted. USP also reports that metoclopramide has been confused with metronidazole; patient harm resulted.[1]

USP reports that Reglan has been confused with Regitine, Regonol, Relafen, Renagel, Requip, Robaxin, and Zofran; no patient harm resulted.[1]

Contraindications and warnings

US boxed warning: Effective February 2009, metoclopramide carries a boxed warning about the use of high-dose or long-term therapy and the risk of tardive dyskinesia. Therapy with metoclopramide should not continue beyond 12 weeks, unless benefits of continued therapy clearly outweigh the risk of tardive dyskinesia.[2]

Contraindications: Known hypersensitivity to the drug, patients with pheochromocytoma, patients with epilepsy or patients on medications that cause extrapyramidal symptoms, and when gastrointestinal motility would be dangerous.[3]

Other warnings: Extrapyramidal symptoms, tardive dyskinesia and neuroleptic malignant syndrome may develop during metoclopramide therapy. Dystonias and other extrapyramidal symptoms more commonly develop in pediatric patients.[3]

Infusion related cautions

Rapid administration may result in anxiety, restlessness, and drowsiness.[3]

Dosage

Emetogenic cancer chemotherapy: 1–3 mg/kg 30 minutes prior to chemotherapy, with repeat doses q 2–3 h for 8–12 hours.[3,4,5] Pretreatment with diphenhydramine may decrease the likelihood of extrapyramidal side effects seen with this dose.[3]

One study used 0.4 mg/kg/h for 6 hours in a 2-year-old boy.[6] (See Comments section.)

In *adults*, a 0.6- to 3.5-mg/kg bolus 30 minutes prior to cisplatin infusion followed by 0.5 mg/kg/h for 8 hours has been used.[7,8]

Gastroesophageal reflux: 0.4–0.8 mg/kg/day divided q 6–8 h.[9,10]

Hypomotility: 0.1 mg/kg q 4–6 h up to 0.5 mg/kg/day.[11]

Postsurgical nausea and vomiting prophylaxis: 0.15–0.5 mg/kg up to 10 mg as a single dose infused after anesthesia induction or on arrival in the recovery room.[12-14] Repeat q 6–8 h as needed.

Studies comparing metoclopramide to ondansetron for postoperative emesis after strabismus surgery[15,16] and post-tonsillectomy/adenotonsillectomy[17,18] have found ondansetron to be more effective.

Small bowel intubation (single dose only)[3]

　　　<6 years: 0.1 mg/kg.[3]

　　　6–14 years: 2.5–5 mg.[3]

　　　>14 years: 10 mg.[3]

Metoclopramide HCl

Dosage adjustment in organ dysfunction

The labeling recommends a 50% decrease in dose if CrCl <40 mL/min.[3]

Another reference recommends adjustment of dose in patients with renal dysfunction as follows[19]:

CrCl 30–50 mL/min: give 75% of a normal dose.[19]

CrCl 10–29 mL/min: give 50% of a normal dose.[19]

CrCl <10 mL/min: give 25% of a normal dose.[19]

Supplement doses above for hemodialysis and peritoneal dialysis (25% of a normal dose) and continuous renal replacement therapy (75% of a normal dose).[19]

Maximum dosage

Emetogenic cancer chemotherapy: 2 mg/kg when chemotherapy is started followed by 2-mg/kg doses 2, 6, and 12 hours later.[4]

In *adults*, 4 mg/kg as single dose[20] or 2 mg/kg q 2–3 h for a total of 10 mg/kg over 8.5 hours[21] has been used for emetogenic cancer chemotherapy.

Reflux/motility: 0.8 mg/kg/day.[10]

Additives

Each mL contains 8.5 mg NaCl.[22]

Suitable diluents

D5W, D5½NS, NS, LR, R.[3,22]

Maximum concentration

5 mg/mL.[22]

Preparation and delivery

For PN compatibility information, please see Appendix D.

IV push

5 mg/mL over 1–2 minutes in *adults* receiving a 10-mg dose.[3,22]

Intermittent infusion

Dilute doses >10 mg in 50 mL of a compatible fluid and infuse over ≥15 minutes.[3,22]

Continuous infusion

Dilute doses >10 mg in at least 50 mL of a compatible fluid.[3,22] NS is the preferred diluent due to the stability of the solution.[3]

Other routes of administration

5-mg/mL solution may be given via IM administration.[3]

Metoclopramide HCl

Comments

Significant adverse effects: Neonates are more susceptible to methemoglobinemia during metoclopramide use.[3,9] Children are also more likely than *adults* to experience acute dystonic reactions; these reactions occur more frequently at larger doses.[3,5,23,24]

2.5 mg/kg as a bolus followed by 0.4-mg/kg/h continuous infusion resulted in a dystonic reaction (urinary retention) after 6 hours in a child receiving chemotherapy.[6]

Diphenhydramine (0.5–1 mg/kg) has been used to treat these reactions.[21,24,25]

Gynecomastia related to metoclopramide use has been reported in pediatric patients.[26]

Drug interactions: Metoclopramide is associated with numerous drug interactions.[3] Consult appropriate resources for dosing recommendations before combining any drug with metoclopramide.

Other: Metoclopramide has been used for bedside transpyloric tube placement in pediatric ICU patients[27] and more recently to ease discomfort while placing nasogastric tubes in *adults*.[28]

Metoclopramide (0.05 mg/kg/dose given q 8 h) has been given to a small group of preterm infants (mean gestation 29 weeks) for approximately 3 weeks. No adverse effects were documented.[29]

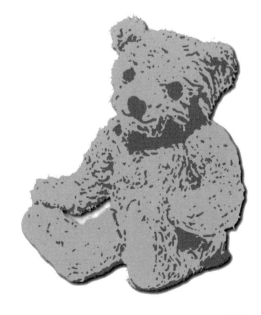

metroNIDAZOLE/metroNIDAZOLE HCl

Brand names	Flagyl IV RTU (metronidazole), Metronidazole Injection (metronidazole), Flagyl IV (metronidazole HCl)

Medication error potential

ISMP recommends the following tall man letters (not FDA approved): metroNIDAZOLE, metFORMIN.[1]

Look-alike, sound-alike drug names.

ISMP's *Confused Drug Names* lists confusion with metformin.[2]

USP reports confusion with fluconazole, mebendazole, meropenem, metformin, methocarbamol, methotrexate, methylprednisolone sodium succinate, metoclopramide, miconazole, omeprazole and potassium chloride. Confusion with metformin and metoclopramide has resulted in patient harm.[3]

Contraindications and warnings

US boxed warning: Known to be carcinogenic in mice and rats.[4] Avoid unnecessary use and reserve for indicated conditions.[4]

Contraindications: In patients with a prior history of hypersensitivity to metronidazole or other nitroimidazole derivatives.[4]

Other warnings: Convulsive seizures and peripheral neuropathy have been reported. The appearance of abnormal neurologic signs should be assessed and therapy discontinued as required. (See Rare adverse effects in Comments section.)

Infusion related cautions

None.

Dosage

Neonates: One report advocates a loading dose of 15 mg/kg.[4]

PNA	<1200 g	1200–2000 g	≥2000 g
<7 days	7.5 mg/kg q 24–48 h[5,7,8]*	7.5 mg/kg q 24 h[5,7,8]	15 mg/kg/day divided q 12 h[5-8]
≥7 days		15 mg/kg/day divided q 12 h[5,7,8]*	30 mg/kg/day divided q 12 h[5,7,8]

*Until 4 weeks of age.

Although doses of 22.5 mg/kg/day divided q 8 h have been given for 5 days without problems, the authors suggested that less frequent dosing would be appropriate in newborns.[5,6]

Infants and children: For mild-to-moderate infections, give 30–45 mg/kg/day divided q 6 h up to 4 g/day.[7,8,11,12] Not indicated for severe infections.[8]

***Clostridium difficile* infection:** 30 mg/kg/day divided q 6 h for 7–10 days.[8,13,14]

Surgical prophylaxis: 15 mg/kg over 30–60 minutes. Infusion should be completed 1 hour before surgery and followed by 7.5 mg/kg at 6 and 12 hours after the initial dose.[15]

Dosage adjustment in organ dysfunction

If CrCl is <10 mL/min, give 50% of the normal dose.[16] Decrease dose by 50% to 67% in patients with hepatic impairment.[16] Use a lower than recommended dose in patients with severe hepatic disease due to accumulation of metronidazole and its metabolites in the plasma.[4]

metroNIDAZOLE/metroNIDAZOLE HCl

Maximum dosage	4 g/day.[7]
Additives	14 mEq of sodium/500 mg of metronidazole.[17]
Suitable diluents	D5W, LR, or NS.[17]
Maximum concentration	5 mg/mL.[17]
Preparation and delivery	**Delivery system issues:** An interaction between aluminum hub needles and the initial reconstituted solution of Flagyl IV results in an orange, reddish-brown, or rust discoloration after ≥6 hours of contact.[14] **Compatibility:** See Appendix D for PN compatibility information.[18]
IV push	Not recommended.[17]
Intermittent infusion	≤8 mg/mL over 60 minutes.[17]
Continuous infusion	Not used.
Other routes of administration	None.
Comments	Seizures may occur with large cumulative doses and prolonged use. The cumulative dose is the most important factor in the pathogenesis of seizures.[19] In cases involving *adults* the cumulative dose has been >40 g. No correlation has been noted between this adverse effect and serum concentration of metronidazole.[20] Neuropathy has been reported when cumulative doses exceed 30 g.[21] It is usually reversible when the drug is discontinued.[22] Continuation of therapy, even at a lower dose, may potentiate symptoms.[21] Metronidazole is a nitroimidazole, and should be used cautiously in patients with evidence of or history of blood dyscrasia. Although a mild leukopenia has been observed, no persistent hematologic abnormalities have been seen in clinical studies.[4] **Monitoring:** Total and differential leukocyte counts before and after therapy. **Drug interactions:** Metronidazole inhibits alcohol dehydrogenase and other alcohol oxidizing enzymes to produce a disulfiram-type reaction (e.g., flushing, sweating, headache, and tachycardia) in patients who are concurrently given ethanol. Shown to potentiate the anticoagulant effect of warfarin and can result in an increase in prothrombin time.[4] Consult appropriate resources for dosing recommendations before combining any drug with metronidazole. **Laboratory interference:** Metronidazole may interfere with some assays to decrease values for AST, ALT, LDH, triglycerides, or glucose.[4]

Micafungin

Brand names	Mycamine

Medication error potential	None reported by ISMP or USP.[1-3]

Contraindications and warnings	**Contraindications:** Patients with known hypersensitivity to the drug or any of its components.[4]
	Warnings: Hypersensitivity reactions (see Infusion related cautions section), hematologic effects (acute intravascular hemolysis, hemoglobinuria, hemolytic anemia), abnormalities in liver function tests, hepatitis and hepatic failure, and renal dysfunction and acute renal failure have been reported.[4]

Infusion related cautions	Phlebitis and thrombophlebitis have been reported and occur more frequently with administration via a peripheral line.[4]
	Rapid infusions may result in histamine mediated reactions.[4] Isolated cases of serious hypersensitivity/anaphylaxis have also occurred.[4]

Dosage	Experience with micafungin in children, particularly neonates, is limited[5]; currently there is no established dose range for pediatric patients.

Treatment

Premature neonates (weight >1000 g) have received 0.75–3 mg/kg in a single-dose pharmacokinetic and safety study.[6] (See Pharmacokinetic considerations in Comments section.)

Infants and children: 1.5–12 mg/kg given once daily.[5,7-14] Larger doses may be necessary for children <8 years of age secondary to increased clearance.[5,15,16] (See Pharmacokinetic considerations in Comments section.)

Some papers dosed micafungin on patient weight as follows:

> **≤40 kg:** 1.5–2 mg/kg/day (up to 75 mg/day).[11,13,14]

> **>40 kg:** 75–100 mg/day.[11,14]

If infection or signs and symptoms persisted, dose has been increased every 1–7 days by 1.5 mg/kg (up to 75 mg) increments in patients ≤40 kg and by 75–100 mg increments in patients >40 kg.[11,14]

One study dosed micafungin based on patient weight and fungal species as follows[8]:

> **<40 kg:** 1 mg/kg/day (*Candida albicans*) or 2 mg/kg/day (nonalbicans or germ-tube negative).

> **≥40 kg:** 50 mg/day (*Candida albicans*) or 100 mg/day (nonalbicans or germ-tube negative).

The dose was increased by 50 mg (1 mg/kg for patients <40 kg) increments at 5 days if disease was stable or progressive.[8]

Prophylaxis: 1 mg/kg given once daily (studies in transplant patients).[17,18]

Dosage adjustment in organ dysfunction	No dosage adjustment necessary for renal dysfunction or moderate liver disease.[4,13,19-21] CVVH has little effect on micafungin kinetics; no dose adjustment or modification recommended.[18]

Micafungin

Maximum dosage	150 mg/day in *adults*.[4,5] One study reported the use of up to 200 mg/day in three patients.[8]
Additives	None.
Suitable diluents	D5W, NS.[4,22]
Maximum concentration	1.5 mg/mL.[4]
Preparation and delivery	NS recommended for reconstitution. D5W may also be used. Do not use diluents containing a bacteriostatic agent for reconstitution.[4,22] Further dilute reconstituted micafungin in a suitable diluent to a final concentration of 0.5–1.5 mg/mL.[4] Flush an existing line with NS prior to micafungin infusion.[4,22]
IV push	Not recommended.[4]
Intermittent infusion	0.5–1.5 mg/mL; infuse over 1 hour.[4]
Continuous infusion	No information available to support administration by this method.
Other routes of administration	No information available to support administration by other routes.
Comments	**Significant adverse effects:** Adverse effects most commonly occurring in one pediatric study were elevations in serum transaminases and alkaline phosphatase, hyperbilirubinemia, and nausea.[13] Arrhythmias and hypotension have been reported in *adults*.[4] **Drug interactions:** Micafungin is a poor substrate for the CYP3A4 isoenzyme and is associated with the potential for drug interactions. Consult appropriate resources for dosing recommendations before combining any drug with micafungin.[13] **Pharmacokinetic considerations:** One neonatal study compared three dosing regimens (0.75, 1.5, and 3 mg/kg/day) in two infant weight groups (500–1000 g, and >1000 g). Infants <1000 g only received 0.75 mg/kg per dose. The smaller infants had decreased serum concentrations and increased clearance when compared to the larger infants.[6]

Midazolam HCl

Brand names	Versed

Medication error potential

ISMP high-alert medication (moderate sedation agent, IV) that has an increased risk of causing significant patient harm if it is used in error.[1]

Look-alike, sound-alike drug names.

USP reports confusion with diazepam and lorazepam.[2] USP reports confusion for Versed with Valium, VePesid, and Vistaril.[2]

Contraindications and warnings

US boxed warning: Respiratory depression and arrest may occur, especially when used for sedation in noncritical care settings.[3] If not recognized promptly and treated effectively, death or hypoxic encephalopathy may occur.[3] Should only be used in hospital or ambulatory care settings that can continuously monitor respiratory and cardiac function. For deeply sedated pediatric patients, a dedicated individual, other than the practitioner performing the procedure, should monitor the patient throughout the procedures.

Should not be administered by rapid injection to neonates as severe hypotension and seizures have been reported, particularly when fentanyl is given concomitantly.[3] The use of the 1-mg/mL formulation or dilution of the 1- or 5-mg/mL formulation is recommended to facilitate slower injection.[3]

Contraindications: In patients with a known hypersensitivity to midazolam.[3] Although benzodiazepines are contraindicated in patients with acute narrow-angle glaucoma, they may be used in patients with open-angle glaucoma provided they are receiving appropriate therapy.[3]

Other warnings: Should not be used in patients with shock or coma, or in acute alcohol intoxication with depression of vital signs.[3] Use cautiously in patients with uncompensated acute illnesses, such as severe fluid or electrolyte disturbances.[3]

Infusion related cautions

Respiratory depression and arrest requiring mechanical ventilation may occur following excessive dosing, rapid administration,[3,4] or use with fentanyl.[3,5] Neonates may have profound and/or prolonged respiratory effects due to reduced and/or immature organ function.[3] Oxygen, resuscitative drugs, age- and size-appropriate equipment for bag/valve/mask ventilation and intubation, and skilled personnel for the maintenance of a patent airway and support of ventilation must be immediately availability.

Avoid intra-arterial injection or extravasation.[3]

Dosage

Flumazenil should be readily available for reversal. (See Other in Comments section and Flumazenil monograph.)

The dose should be calculated on ideal body weight in obese patients.[3] (See Appendix B.) Children <6 years of age may require larger doses (mg/kg) than older pediatric patients.[3]

Allow 3–5 minutes after dose to achieve peak central nervous system effect.[3]

Anesthesia induction: 0.15 mg/kg followed by up to three doses of 0.05 mg/kg at 2-minute intervals.[6] Time to induction was shorter with a dose of 0.3 mg/kg.[7] Doses of 0.6 mg/kg did not reliably induce anesthesia in children given atropine and meperidine.[8]

Procedural sedation: Midazolam is the preferred benzodiazepine because of its rapid onset and short duration.[9-12] It does not possess analgesic activity and must be combined with other agents (i.e., fentanyl) when analgesia is needed.[9]

Dosage *(cont.)*

0.05–0.4 mg/kg immediately before the procedure then q 2–5 min to effect.[11-19] Onset 2–5 minutes (IM 10–20 minutes) duration 30–60 minutes (IM 45–120 minutes)[9,10] up to 2 mg/dose[13,14] or 5 mg/dose[17,18] and a total of 10 mg.[13] Some recommend age dependent dosing: 0.05–0.1 mg/kg titrating up to 0.6 mg/kg (0.5–5 years) or 0.025–0.05 mg/kg titrating up to 0.4 mg/kg (6–12 years).[10,11]

Sedation with mechanical ventilation: 0.1–0.2 mg/kg over 2–5 minutes.[20-26] Do not administer a bolus dose to neonates.[21] Followed by 0.03–0.4 mg/kg/h.[20-25] Some recommend age dependent dosing in newborns with those <32 weeks gestation receiving 0.03 mg/kg/h and those >32 weeks receiving 0.06 mg/kg/h.[24]

Status epilepticus: A loading dose of 0.02–0.6 mg/kg[26-38] followed by a continuous infusion of 0.04–3 mg/kg/h.[26-38] Titrate by 0.06 mg/kg/h q 15 min.[30] The range of mean maintenance infusion was 0.14–3 mg/kg/h.[26-38] In a report of 306 pediatric patients the dose was <0.4 mg/kg/h in 81% of patients.[37] When weaning off midazolam, decrease dose by 0.06–0.12 mg/kg/h q 15 min.[30] Most patients regain full consciousness by an averaged 4 hours after discontinuation of midazolam.[27]

Tachyphylaxis may require progressively larger dose within the first 24–48 hours.[33]

Dosage adjustment in organ dysfunction

Patients with chronic renal failure and/or congestive heart failure eliminate midazolam more slowly, but no dosage adjustment required in renal dysfunction.[39] Adjust dosage in patients with hepatic dysfunction.[3]

Maximum dosage

Total doses >5 mg are not usually necessary for conscious sedation in *adults*.[3] For anesthesia induction, single doses of ≤0.6 mg/kg.[6,7] have been used not to exceed 5 mg/dose.[17,18] The largest dose given by continuous infusion was 3 mg/kg/h.[37]

Additives

0.14 mEq sodium/mL.[4] Some products may contain 1% benzyl alcohol.[4] (See Appendix C for specific information about benzyl alcohol's potential for toxicity.)

Suitable diluents

D5W, NS, D5NS.[4]

Maximum concentration

<5 mg/mL for IV push[3,4] and 1 mg/mL for IM administration.[3]

Preparation and delivery

Compatibility: For PN compatibility, please see Appendix D.[40]

IV push

1 or 5 mg/mL given over 20–30 seconds for anesthesia induction.[3,7] Rapid administration (<2 minutes) may cause severe hypotension in neonates, especially if concurrent fentanyl is given.[3] Seizures have also been reported in neonates following rapid administration.[3]

Intermittent infusion

Dilute to desired volume in suitable diluent and give over ≥2 minutes.[3]

Continuous infusion

Diluted to a concentration of 0.5 mg/mL with NS or D5W.[3]

Midazolam HCl

1 mg/mL.[3] IM doses of 0.15–0.5 mg/kg (maximum total dose 10 mg) have been administered safely in children requiring sedation or in patients in status epilepticus.[41,42] A 20% failure rate was noted following IM administration when midazolam was given prehospitalization.[42] Has been given by buccal administration.

Comments

Rare adverse effects: Paradoxical reactions, such as hyperactive, agitations, or aggressive behavior, have been reported with benzodiazepines, particularly in adolescent/pediatric or psychiatric patients.[3,4]

Involuntary epileptiform movements were reported in preterm infants <32-weeks-old given benzodiazepines.[43-47] Brief tonic-clonic seizures have occurred in patients with atypical absence (petit mal) status epileptics who receive a benzodiazepine.[3] Seizure activity and myoclonus have also been reported following administration of benzodiazepines, especially in very low birth weight neonates.[3,48-50] The movements generally began a few minutes after a bolus injection and continue for several hours.[49,50]

Severe hypotension has been observed in neonates receiving a continuous infusion of midazolam who then receive a rapid intravenous injection of fentanyl.[3]

Drug interactions: Midazolam is a substrate of CYP2B6 and 3A4 (major) and is a weak inhibitor of CYP2C8, 2C9, and 3A4.[4] Consult appropriate resources for dosing recommendations before combining any drug with midazolam.

Pharmacokinetic considerations: Pediatric patients generally require larger doses (mg/kg) than *adults.*[3] Those <6 years of age may require larger doses (mg/kg) than older pediatric patients.[3]

Pharmacodynamic considerations: Dosing in neonates is controversial since benzodiazepines may decrease blood pressure and cerebral blood flow velocity.[51] Midazolam should be used cautiously in this population.

Other: A withdrawal syndrome may begin 24 hours after cessation of prolonged continuous infusion (i.e., >5–10 days of continual use).[4,44,52-54] Other investigators have shown that cumulative doses >60 mg/kg are highly correlated with withdrawal syndromes.[55]

Some practitioners recommend weaning a patient from midazolam to oral lorazepam.[56]

Midazolam Rate	Equivalent Oral Dose of Lorazepam
1 mcg/kg/min = 1.44 mg/kg/day	0.3 mg/kg/day = 0.1 mg/kg q 8 h
2 mcg/kg/min = 2.88 mg/kg/day	0.6 mg/kg/day = 0.1–0.15 mg/kg q 6 h
3 mcg/kg/min = 4.32 mg/kg/day	0.9 mg/kg/day = 0.1–0.15 mg/kg q 4–6 h
4 mcg/kg/min = 5.76 mg/kg/day	0.3 mg/kg/day = 0.15 mg/kg q 4 h

Source: From Cyndi Reid, Pharm.D., Department of Pharmaceutical Services, Children's Hospital of Michigan, Detroit, MI.

Flumazenil, a specific benzodiazepine-receptor antagonist, is indicated for complete or partial reversal of benzodiazepine toxicity.[57] (See Flumazenil monograph.)

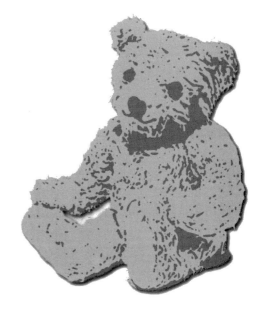

Milrinone Lactate

Brand names	Primacor

Medication error potential

ISMP high-alert medication (inotropic medication, IV) that has an increased risk of causing significant patient harm if it is used in error.[1]

Look-alike, sound-alike drug names.

USP reports confusion for Primacor with Natrecor.[2]

Contraindications and warnings

Contraindications: Milrinone is contraindicated in patients who are hypersensitive to it.[3]

Warnings: Regardless of route or method of delivery, milrinone has not been shown to be safe or effective when used longer than 48 hours in patients with heart failure.[3] (See Other in Comments section.) It should *not* be used in patients with severe obstructive aortic or pulmonic valvular disease[3] and may aggravate outflow tract obstruction in those with hypertrophic subaortic stenosis.[3] Use caution if vigorous diuretic therapy has been used or has been suspected of causing significant decreases in cardiac filling pressure.[3]

Infusion related cautions

Spontaneous bronchospasm has been reported.[3] IV site should be monitored and extravasation should be avoided.

Dosage

Important Correction Notice

...en established for pediatric patient patients.

Pediatric Injectable Drugs Ninth Edition (The Teddy Bear Book) – ISBN: 978-1-58528-2432
Order code: P2432

The publisher wishes to inform you of the following correction.

1. In the monograph for **Milrinone Lactate (pages 402–403)**

"Dosage" section – third paragraph should read:

A study in 29 premature neonates (<29 weeks) found that a loading dose of **0.75mcg/kg/min** over 3 hours,

Dosage adjustment in organ dysfunction

Adjust dosage in renal dysfunction (see below) as impaired milrinone clearance may result in significant hypotension.[3]

CrCl	Dose (mcg/kg/min)	CrCl	Dose (mcg/kg/min)
5	0.2	30	0.33
10	0.23	40	0.38
20	0.28	50	0.43

Milrinone Lactate

Maximum dosage	A loading dose of 100 mcg/kg[1,2] and a maintenance dose of 1.2 mcg/kg/min in infants and children.[16]
Additives	None.
Suitable diluents	D5W, NS, LR, ½NS.[18]
Maximum concentration	Loading dose may be given undiluted,[3] but may be diluted to allow for ease of administration. Normal dilution is 200 mcg/mL,[18] but 250 mcg/mL have been used for continuous infusion.[5,6,18] One study noted stability of a 400-mcg/mL solution in RL, D5W, ½NS, and NS.[19]
Preparation and delivery	**Stability:** Stable at 0.2 mg/mL for 72 hours at room temperature in normal light.[18]
	Compatibility: A precipitate will form when furosemide is injected into an IV line infusing milrinone.[3,18] See more specific references for other drug incompatibilities. See Appendix D for PN compatibility information.[20]
IV push	Although milrinone has been given over 30 seconds,[12] most references suggest longer infusion time.[3,18]
Intermittent infusion	Although milrinone has been given over 30 seconds to 5 minutes,[12] most references suggest that the loading dose should be given over 10–60 minutes.[11,18] One group has consistently reported infusing the loading dose over 3 hours.[12-14]
Continuous infusion	≤200 mcg/mL.[3,18]
Other routes of administration	Has been given by intraosseous administration.[11]
Comments	**Rare adverse effects:** Discontinue therapy if dose-related elevations in liver function test occur and clinical symptoms of hepatotoxicity are noted.[21,22]
	Hypokalemia and hypomagnesemia may occur.[21]
	Monitoring: Milrinone is a positive inotrope and vasodilator that has little chronotropic activity.[22] It does produce a slight shortening of AV node conduction time, indicating a potential for an increased ventricular response rate.[3] EKG should be monitored during infusion for supraventricular and ventricular arrhythmias.[3] Blood pressure and heart rate should be monitored during the infusion. If the patient develops excessive hypotension, the infusion should be decreased or stopped.[3] Fluid status should be monitored and diuretic and electrolyte therapy adjusted as needed. Monitor ALT and AST.
	Drug interactions: Consult appropriate resources before combining any drug with milrinone.
	Pharmacokinetic considerations: Half-life in very preterm infants was more than 10 hours, which is considerably longer than that reported for infants and children.[13]
	Other: In a multicenter trial of 1088 patients with Class III and IV heart failure, long-term *oral* therapy showed no improvement in symptoms and an increased risk of hospitalization and sudden death.[3] In this study, patients with Class IV symptoms appeared to be at particular risk of life-threatening cardiovascular reactions. There is no evidence that milrinone given by long-term continuous or intermittent infusion does not carry a similar risk.

Mivacurium

Brand names	Mivacron
Medication error potential	ISMP high-alert medication that has an increased risk of causing significant patient harm if it is used in error.[1]
Contraindications and warnings	**Contraindications:** Hypersensitivity to mivacurium or any of its components.[2] **Warnings:** Use carefully under the supervision of experienced clinicians; personnel should also be skilled in airway management, resuscitation and respiratory support.[2] Intubation and ventilatory support equipment, including oxygen therapy, should be readily available.[2] Also should have anticholinesterase inhibitors readily available when giving mivacurium.[2] Use with caution in patients with known or suspected homozygous atypical plasma cholinesterase gene.[2]
Infusion related cautions	Hypersensitivity reactions, hypotension, arrhythmias, and bronchospasm have been reported but appear to be rare.[2]
Dosage	*Respiratory function must be supported during use of this agent. Concurrent administration of a sedative is also necessary. Monitoring of neuromuscular transmission with a peripheral nerve stimulator is recommended during continuous infusion or with repeated dosing.*[2,3] Obese patients (≥30% of ideal body weight) should be dosed on ideal body weight.[2] (See Appendix B.) **Children 2–12 years of age:** 0.2 mg/kg repeated as needed to maintain pharmacological paralysis.[2-7] May follow initial dose by continuous infusion of 10–14 mcg/kg/min.[2-7]
Dosage adjustment in organ dysfunction	Standard doses may be used in patients with renal or hepatic dysfunction. Compared to healthy patients, the duration of neuromuscular blockade with mivacurium will be approximately one-and-a-half times longer in severe renal impairment and three times longer in end-stage liver disease.[2] Infusion rates should be decreased by 50% in patients with hepatic disease; no adjustment is necessary in patients with renal dysfunction.[2]
Maximum dosage	Infusion rates as large as 31 mcg/kg/min have been used.[2]
Additives	May contain benzyl alcohol.[2] See Appendix C for more specific information about potential adverse effects and/or benzyl alcohol toxicity in neonates.
Suitable diluents	D5W, D5NS, D5LR, LR, or NS.[2]
Maximum concentration	2 mg/mL for IV push and 0.5 mg/mL for continuous infusion.[2]
Preparation and delivery	Mivacurium is an acidic solution; do not administer with alkaline solutions.[2]
IV push	2 mg/mL over 5–15 seconds.[2]

Mivacurium

Intermittent infusion	Not administered by this method.
Continuous infusion	≤0.5 mg/mL.[2]
Other routes of administration	Not administered via other routes.
Comments	**Significant adverse effects:** Prolonged paralysis has been reported after mivacurium administration in pediatric and *adult* patients with reduced plasma cholinesterase activity.[2,8,9]
	Drug interactions: Concomitant administration of other drugs (e.g., aminoglycosides, clindamycin, inhalational anesthetics, ketamine, magnesium, quinidine, or succinylcholine) may prolong neuromuscular blockade.[2] Consult appropriate resources for additional information on drug interactions.

Morphine Sulfate

Brand names
Generics. Astramorph PF, Duramorph, Infumorph (preservative-free for microinfusion devices only)

Medication error potential
ISMP high-alert medication that has an increased risk of causing significant patient harm if it is used in error.[1]

Look-alike, sound-alike error potential.

ISMP reported that morphine was confused with hydromorphone.[2]

USP reported that morphine sulfate was confused with magnesium sulfate, methadone and OxyContin.[3] Patient harm resulted when morphine sulfate was confused with hydromorphone and meperidine.

Contraindications and warnings
US boxed warning: Because of the risk for severe adverse effects with the epidural or intrathecal routes of preservative-free morphine, patients must be observed in a fully equipped and staffed environment for at least 24 hours after the initial dose.[4]

Naloxone (opioid antagonist) injection and resuscitative equipment should be immediately available in case of life-threatening or intolerable side effects and whenever intrathecal or epidural preservative-free morphine therapy is being initiated.[4]

Contraindications: Those with known hypersensitivity to morphine should not receive morphine sulfate.[4,5] A manufacturer of generic morphine lists convulsive states (morphine stimulates the spinal cord), heart failure resulting from chronic lung disease, cardiac arrhythmias, and brain tumor as contraindications.[5] Those with acute bronchial asthma or upper airway obstruction should not receive morphine.[4,5]

Other warnings: Products containing preservatives (generics) are not for intrathecal or epidural use.[5]

Some products are for use with specific patient controlled analgesia pumps or auto-injectors.

Morphine sulfate is available in a variety of concentrations ranging from 0.5–50 mg/mL.[6] Choose products carefully.

Errors in programming patient controlled analgesia pumps, including the substitution of a more concentrated product than the pump was programmed to infuse, have resulted in deaths.[7]

The respiratory depressant effects of morphine and ability to increase intracranial pressure may be exaggerated in patients with head injury.[5]

Infusion related cautions
Confirm the choice of the correct morphine product and concentration on the vial prior to use.

Respiratory depression and arrest requiring mechanical ventilation may occur and is reversible with naloxone.[4] This is more likely to occur with rapid administration.[5]

Dosage
Dosing is titrated to effect and the lowest effective dose should be used. Chronic opioid use results in tolerance and an increased dose requirement. In these patients, a weaning protocol should be implemented when morphine is discontinued to avoid withdrawal symptoms.

Neonates (preservative-free morphine): 0.05 mg/kg IV, IM or SC q 4–6 h; maximum 0.1 mg/kg/dose or continuous infusion of 0.001–0.03 mg/kg/h.[8-15] Based on achieving a therapeutic morphine concentration of 15 ng/mL, an infusion of 0.0075 mg/kg/h would be appropriate at term birth and 0.0125 mg/kg/h at 1 month of age.[16,17] Of note, a decreased gestational age and postconceptional age are directly related to clearance.[11,13-15] Clearance is decreased in neonates who undergo cardiac surgery and dosing at 0.005 mg/kg/h has been recommended.[10] (See Comments section.)

Morphine Sulfate

Dosage *(cont.)*	**Infants/children:** 0.05–0.2 mg/kg but ≤15 mg q 2–4 h PRN[5,8,10-15,18] or continuous infusion of 0.005–0.03 mg/kg/h that may be preceded by a bolus.[8,17,19,20,21]
	
	Sickle cell disease with pain crisis: 0.15-mg/kg bolus followed by a continuous infusion of 0.03–0.15 mg/kg/h achieved adequate analgesia in hospitalized children.[22] Of note, a pharmacokinetic study found an eightfold variability in clearance in 18 children that resulted in a larger dose requirement (without increased side effects) in some patients.[23] This may be due to anemia-related changes in hepatic blood flow that accelerate renal or hepatic clearance.
	
	Severe pain: Larger doses may be needed in cancer, burn, or other patients with severe pain. In eight children with terminal malignancy, continuous infusions ranging from 0.03–0.15 provided adequate or complete pain relief.[24] However, doses from 0.76–2.6 mg/kg/h was needed in two of these.
	
	Epidural or intrathecal use of preservative-free morphine (under the direction of a physician experienced in this technique)[4,5]
	
	    Epidural: 0.03–0.05 mg preservative-free morphine/kg up to 0.1 mg/kg or 5 mg/day.[8]
	
	    Intrathecal (usually 1/10th the epidural dose): Forty-six children from 12–17 years old undergoing spinal fusion who received either 0.005 or 0.015 mg/kg (maximum dose 1 mg) preservative-free morphine intrathecally had decreased blood loss and postoperative need for opiates.[25]

Dosage adjustment in organ dysfunction	**CrCl 10–50 mL/min/1.73 m²:** 75% of the usual dose.[26] **CrCl ≤10 mL/min/1.73 m²:** 50% of the usual dose. Use with caution in severe liver disease.[4,5,8] During ECMO, dosage requirements are increased even though studies have shown that clearance is decreased because of binding to the polyvinyl chloride tubing and membrane oxygenator.[27,28]
Maximum dosage	0.1–0.2 mg/kg and ≤10 mg for IV use.[5] With repeated dosing, tolerance can develop resulting in increased dosage requirements. Epidural maximum dose is 5 mg in *adults*.[4,8] The intrathecal dose is usually 1/10 the epidural dose.[4]
Additives	Some morphine products contain chlorobutanol, phenol, sulfites, sodium phosphates, and/or formaldehyde sulfoxylate.[6] See Appendix C for specific information about adverse effects.
Suitable diluents	D5W, D10W, NS, ½NS, LR, R.[6]
Maximum concentration	Usually 1 mg/mL for continuous infusion[6]; however, concentrations may range from 0.5–5 mg/mL.[8]
Preparation and delivery	**Compatibility:** See Appendix D for PN compatibility information.

Morphine Sulfate

IV push	Over 4–5 minutes.[4,5,8]
Intermittent infusion	Over 15–30 minutes.[8]
Continuous infusion	May be given by continuous infusion.
Other routes of administration	May be given IM or SC using 0.5, 1, 2, 3, 4, or 5 mg/mL.[5] IM is preferred when repeat doses are needed since SC dosing causes local tissue irritation and pain.[5]
	Only preservative-free products are given via the epidural or intrathecal route.[4,5,8]
Comments	**Monitoring:** Patients should be monitored for adequacy of analgesia/sedation and signs and symptoms that would indicate toxicity such as decreased respiratory rate, oxygen saturation, and alertness.

Pharmacokinetics: A pharmacokinetic study in 17 preterm neonates (26–24 weeks of gestation) found a morphine clearance of 2.4 mL/min/kg, half-life of 8.75 hours, and volume of distribution of 1.82 L/kg.[29] Another study comparing preterm with term neonates found no statistically significant difference in half-life between the two groups (10.6 h ± 2.7 vs. 7.6 ± 2.6, respectively), clearance (2.23 mL/kg/min ± 0.95 vs. 2.03 ± 1.46), and volume of distribution (2.04 L/kg ± 1.01 vs. 2.07 ± 1.26).[30]

The age-related effects on morphine requirements and plasma concentrations of morphine and its metabolites were compared in postsurgical term infants from 0–4 weeks of age (n=57), from 4–26 weeks (n=55), 26–52 weeks (n=28), and 1–3 years (n=35). All received a 0.1-mg/kg bolus followed by a continuous infusion of 0.01 mg/kg/h or 0.03 mg/kg q 3 h. At 24 hours after surgery, neonates had higher morphine, morphine-3-glucuronide, and morphine-6-glucuronide concentrations than the 3 older age groups indicating a capacity for glucuronidation and a lower renal clearance.[31]

Drug interactions: Use morphine cautiously in patients receiving other CNS depressants as effects are additive.[5]

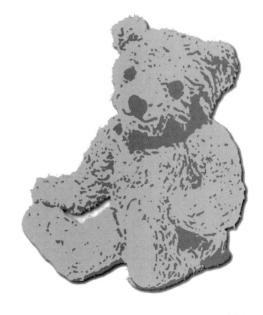

Multivitamins (Adult)

Brand names	MVI Adult, MVI Adult Unit Vial, MVI-12, Infuvite Adult
Medication error potential	None noted.
Contraindications and warnings	**Contraindications:** Known hypersensitivity to vitamins or excipients or pre-existing hypervitaminosis.[1,2]
Infusion related cautions	Rapid administration may result in dizziness, faintness, and tissue irritation.[1,2]

Dosage

Children ≥11 years and *adults*: 5 mL/day from vial 1 and 5 mL/day from vial 2 of MVI Adult (contains 150 mcg vitamin K) or Infuvite Adult (contains 150 mcg vitamin K) or 10 mL/day of mixed MVI–12 Unit Vial (does not contain vitamin K).[1,2]

Pediatric vitamin shortages[3]: The A.S.P.E.N. 2006 Pediatric Multivitamin Task Force recommended that when a shortage is recognized, the pediatric multivitamins should be reserved for infants <2.5 kg or <36 weeks gestation. Infants who are able to ingest 50% of their nutrient needs should be switched to oral vitamins. For those who must receive the parenteral product, the following doses of the *adult* parenteral multivitamins were recommended.

2.5 kg up to 11 years of age: Use half the *adult* dose (5 mL/day) and supplement vitamin K to a total dose of 200 mcg. (MVI Adult and Infuvite Adult contain 150 mcg of vitamin K; MVI–12 does not contain vitamin K.)

<2.5 kg or <36 weeks of gestation: If the Pediatric Multivitamin Product is unavailable, 1 mL/kg/day of an *adult* product. *Adult* multivitamins contain excipients that are known to be toxic in preterm infants. (See Additives section.)

Note: Vitamin K is not contained in MVI–12 but is included in the other products for use in *adults*.

Dosage adjustment in organ dysfunction

Hypervitaminosis A and D are potential complications in patients with renal failure.[1,2]

Maximum dosage

One-and-a-half to three times the usual daily dosage for 2 days for patients with multiple vitamin deficiencies or markedly increased requirements.[1,2,4] (See Comments section.)

Additives

The following excipients are included in the *adult* multivitamin products.[1-3] Infuvite Adult has been reformulated to contain less contaminant aluminum.

Product	Propylene glycol	Polysorbate 80	Polysorbate 20	Aluminum contaminant
MVI–Adult	3 g/10 mL	160 mg/10 mL	2.8 mg/10 mL	43–183 mcg/L
MVI–12	3 g/10 mL	160 mg/10 mL	2.8 mg/10 mL	43–78 mcg/L
Infuvite Adult	3 g/10 mL	140 mg/10 mL	none	70 mcg/L

See Appendix C for specific information about propylene glycol and polysorbate 80 potential adverse effects.

Multivitamins (Adult)

Suitable diluents	D5NS, D5W, D10W, D20W, LR, NS, PN solutions.[5]
Maximum concentration	Dilute dose in ≥500 mL of a compatible IV fluid.[1,2,5] Do not give undiluted.[1,2]
Preparation and delivery	**Stability:** Addition of these products to solutions containing bisulfites as antioxidants may result in thiamine inactivation.[6] **Photosensitivity:** Protect from light during storage.
IV push	Contraindicated.[6]
Intermittent infusion	Over a number of hours.[4] However, the contents of MVI–12 vials 1 and 2 (5 mL each) were diluted in 50 mL D5W and administered over 20 minutes without adverse effects in normal *adult* volunteers.[7]
Continuous infusion	May be infused continuously as in PN solutions.[1,2]
Other routes of administration	Not indicated.
Comments	**Laboratory interference:** Ascorbic acid in the urine may cause false negative urine glucose measurements.[1,2] **Monitoring:** For patients receiving larger doses than usual or who are on parenteral vitamins for 4–6 months, serum concentration measurement of vitamins A, C, D, and folic acid should be performed to ensure that concentrations are within the normal range.[1,2,8]

Multivitamins (Pediatric)

Brand names	MVI Pediatric, Infuvite Pediatric
Medication error potential	None noted.
Contraindications and warnings	**Contraindications:** Known hypersensitivity to vitamins or excipients or pre-existing hypervitaminosis.
Infusion related cautions	Rapid administration may result in dizziness, faintness, and tissue irritation.[1,2]
Dosage	Dosages listed are in terms of the reconstituted single dose 5-mL vial. **Neonates <1 kg:** 1.5 mL/day[1-3] or 2 mL/kg/day.[4] (See Comments section.) **Neonates and infants 1–3 kg:** 3.25 mL/day[1,2,3,5,6] *or* 2 mL/kg/day up to 5 mL/day.[4] **Infants and children ≥2.5 kg and <11 years:** 5 mL/day.[1,2,4-6]
Dosage adjustment in organ dysfunction	Hypervitaminosis A and D are potential complications in patients with renal failure.[1,2]
Maximum dosage	Usually 5 mL. However, larger doses may be indicated during certain diseases.[1,2]
Additives	The following excipients are included in the pediatric multivitamin products.[1,2,7] Infuvite Pediatric has been reformulated to contain less contaminant aluminum.

Product	Propylene glycol	Polysorbate 80	Polysorbate 20	Aluminum contaminant
MVI–Pediatric	None	50 mg/5 mL	0.8 mg/5 mL	42 mcg/L
Infuvite Pediatric	None	59 mg/5 mL	None	30 mcg/L

See Appendix C for specific information about potential adverse effects.

Suitable diluents	D5NS, D5W, D10W, D20W, LR, NS, PN solutions.[1,2]
Maximum concentration	Dilute dose in ≥100 mL of compatible IV fluid.[1,2] Do not give undiluted.[1,2]
Preparation and delivery	**Stability:** Addition of these products to solutions containing bisulfites as antioxidants may result in thiamine inactivation.[9] **Photosensitivity:** Protect from light during storage.[1,2] (See Comments section.)

Multivitamins (Pediatric)

IV push   Contraindicated.[1,2]

Intermittent infusion   Over a number of hours. Infants <6 months of age have received PN solutions (including micronutrients) cycled over 18 hours.[10]

Continuous infusion   May be infused continuously as in PN solutions.[1,2]

Other routes of administration   Not indicated.

Comments   Does not result in optimal vitamin dosing in low birth weight infants.[3,4,11-13] Doses of 1.5 mL/day did not maintain vitamin E levels in therapeutic range (1–3 mg/dL) in 56% of infants <1 kg.[3,11] Doses of 2 mL/kg in premature infants will not provide adequate vitamin A.[4]

The addition of sulfites to PN solutions results in thiamine inactivation. However, sulfites may slow the peroxidation of vitamins exposed to light. Whether to cover PN solutions and tubing to protect from light particularly in preterm neonates has been debated.[14,15]

Laboratory interference: Ascorbic acid in the urine may cause false negative urine glucose measurements.[1,2]

Muromonab-CD3

Brand names	Orthoclone OKT3
Medication error potential	None noted.

Contraindications and warnings

US boxed warning: Only physicians experienced in immunosuppressive therapy and management of solid organ transplant patients should use muromonab-CD3.[1]

Patients receiving muromonab-CD3 should be treated in facilities equipped and staffed for CPR and where the patient can be observed for an appropriate amount of time after infusion.

Anaphylactic and anaphylactoid reactions may occur following infusion of any dose. Serious, occasionally life-threatening or lethal, systemic, cardiovascular, and CNS reactions have been reported and include pulmonary edema (especially in patients with volume overload), shock cardiovascular collapse, cardiac or respiratory arrest, seizures, coma, cerebral edema, cerebral herniation, blindness and paralysis. Fluid status should be carefully monitored prior to and during treatment. Methylprednisolone pretreatment is recommended to minimize these symptoms known as the Cytokine-release syndrome.

Contraindications: Patients who have hypersensitivity to muromonab-CD3 or products of murine origin, are in uncompensated heart failure or fluid overload, have uncontrolled hypertension, have a history of seizures, are who are pregnant or breastfeeding.

Other warnings: Pediatric patients should be carefully evaluated for fluid retention and hypertension before initiating muromonab-CD3 due to the risk of cerebral edema and herniation.[1]

Infusion related cautions

See Contraindications and warnings section.

Dosage

Transplant (rejection) (several different dosing strategies have been used)

≤30 kg: 2.5 mg/day for 10–14 days.[1-6]
>30 kg: 5 mg/day for 10–14 days.[1-6]

<10 kg: 1.25 mg/day for 10 days.[7]
≥10–30 kg: 2.5 mg/day for 10 days.[7]
>30 kg: 5 mg/day for 10 days.[7]

<20 kg: 2.5 mg/day for 10–14 days.[8]
>20 kg: 5 mg/day for 10–14 days.[8]

1 mg/10 kg/day (≤5 mg) for 10–14 days.[9]

0.1–0.2 mg/kg/day (≤5 mg) for 7–14 days.[10-12]

CD3+ cell counts should be <25/mm³ and OKT3 serum concentration ≥800 ng/mL in children.[1,2]

Acute viral myocarditis: 5 children (15 months to 16 years of age) with left ventricular ejection fractions of 5% to 20% were treated with a variable combination of corticosteroids, cyclosporine, azathioprine, IVIG, and OKT3 dosed at 0.1 mg/kg/day for 10–14 days.[13]

Dosage adjustment in organ dysfunction

None noted.

Muromonab-CD3

Maximum dosage	15 mg.[1]
Additives	Contains polysorbate 80.[11] See Appendix C for specific information about polysorbate adverse effects.
Suitable diluents	None.
Maximum concentration	1 mg/mL.
Preparation and delivery	Do not shake solution.[1] Withdraw the solution from the ampule through a low protein-binding 0.2- or 0.22-micron filter. Discard this filter and attach a new needle prior to bolus injection.[1]
IV push	Over <1 minute.[1]
Intermittent infusion	Not indicated.[1]
Continuous infusion	Not indicated.
Other routes of administration	Not indicated.
Comments	**Monitoring:** Daily CD3 + T cells and OKT3 serum concentrations.[1,2,4-6,10,14,15]

Nafcillin Sodium

Brand names	Nafcil, Nallpen, Unipen

Medication error potential	USP reports confusion with ampicillin, ampicillin and sulbactam, oxacillin, piperacillin and tazobactam.[1]

Contraindications and warnings	**Warnings:** Individuals who have a Type I reaction to penicillin may have cross sensitivity to cephalosporins.[2] (See Appendix C for specific information.)

Infusion related cautions	If a decision is made to give this medication to a patient with known penicillin hypersensitivity, the patient should be closely observed for allergenicity.[2] (See Comments section.)
	Phlebitis was reported with a 15-minute infusion in a child.[3]
	Extravasation may cause tissue sloughing and necrosis.[4-6] (See Appendix E for management.)

Dosage	Serious anaphylactoid reactions may require immediate emergency treatment with epinephrine, oxygen, IV steroids, and airway management.

Neonates

PNA	<1200 g	≤2000 g	>2000 g
≤7 days	50 mg/kg/day divided q 12 h[7]*	50–100 mg/kg/day divided q 12 h[7,8]	75 mg/kg/day divided q 8 h[7,8]
>7 days	50–75 mg/kg/day divided q 12 h[7]*	50–75 mg/kg/day divided q 6–8 h[7,8]	100–140 mg/kg/day divided q 6 h[7,8]
≤4 weeks	50 mg/kg/day divided q 12 h[7]		

*Until 4 weeks of age.

Infants and children

Mild to moderate infections: 50–100 mg/kg/day divided q 6 h.[7,9-11]

Severe infections: (e.g., meningitis, osteomyelitis, pericarditis,) 100–200 mg/kg/day divided q 4–6 h.[7,9-11]

Endocarditis (oxacillin-susceptible): 200 mg/kg/day divided q 4–6 h for 6 weeks (native valve) with or without gentamicin.[12] If prosthetic valve related, add gentamicin (3 mg/kg/day divided q 8 h during the first 2 weeks of nafcillin) and oral rifampin (20 mg/kg/day divided q 8 h for 6 weeks or longer).[12]

Meningitis (staphylococcus aureus methicillin susceptible)

≤7 days and >2000 g: 100–150 mg/kg/day divided q 8–12 h.[2,12-15]

>7 days and >2000 g: 150–200 mg/kg/day divided q 6–8 h.[2,12-15]

Infants and children: See severe infections above.

Dosage adjustment in organ dysfunction	No adjustment in either renal[2,3] or hepatic failure[2]; however, the dosage should be adjusted in patients with combined renal and hepatic dysfunction.[2]

Nafcillin Sodium

Maximum dosage	200 mg/kg/day, not to exceed 6[2] to 12 g/day.[2] 18 g/day has been given to *adults* with severe infections.[16]
Additives	2.9 mEq sodium/g of nafcillin sodium.[2,17]
Suitable diluents	D5, D5R, D5LR, D5¼NS, D5½NS, D5NS, D10, D10NS, NS, R, LR.[17]
Maximum concentration	40 mg/mL.[17] Maximum concentration of 64 mg/mL (NS), 71 mg/mL (D5), 128 mg/mL (SW) for peripheral infusion in fluid-restricted patients.[17,18]
Preparation and delivery	**Delivery system issues:** The mixing of nafcillin with an aminoglycoside in vitro can result in substantial inactivation of the aminoglycoside.[9] (See Appendix C for more specific information.) **Compatibility:** See Appendix D for PN compatibility information.[17,24]
IV push	15–30 mL in ½NS, NS, or SW over 5–10 minutes through running IV.[2,18]
Intermittent infusion	2–40 mg/mL in D5W, NS, or R and infuse over 30–60 minutes.[18]
Continuous infusion	Although no information to support continuous infusion of nafcillin, other beta-lactam antibiotics have been given by this method.[17,25]
Other routes of administration	250 mg/mL in SW, BW, or NS by deep IM injection.[2,17]
Comments	**Rare adverse effects:** Has caused interstitial nephritis.[2]

Naloxone HCl

Brand names	Narcan

Medication error potential

ISMP's *Confused Drug Names* lists confusion for Narcan with Norcuron.[1]

USP reports confusion with nalbuphine and nalmefene and confusion between Narcan with Norcuron and Nubain.[2]

Contraindications and warnings

Contraindications: Hypersensitivity to naloxone or any component of the formulation.[3]

Warnings: An acute abstinence syndrome can be precipitated by abrupt and complete reversal of narcotic effects.[3] Naloxone should be administered cautiously to persons who are known or suspected to be physically dependent on opioids. This includes newborns of mothers who are physically dependent on opioids. (See Other in Comments section.)

Naloxone is not effective in (1) treating respiratory depression due to nonopioid drugs; (2) the management of acute toxicity caused by levopropoxyphene; and (3) reversal of respiratory depression by partial agonists (e.g., buprenorphine) or mixed agonist/antagonists (e.g., pentazocine). In the case of partial agonists or mixed agonist/antagonists reversal may be incomplete or may require larger doses due to the drugs prolonged duration, slow rate of binding, and slow dissociation from opioid receptor.[3]

Infusion related cautions

None.

Dosage

When used for acute opiate overdose, other resuscitative measures (e.g., maintenance of an adequate airway, artificial respiration, cardiac massage, vasopressor agents) should be readily available.

Neonatal opioid depression/asphyxia: Naloxone may be used to treat asphyxia in a neonate whose mother was given opiates during labor and delivery. Although it has been given to the mother shortly before delivery, the duration of action only lasts for the first 2 hours of the neonates life; hence, it is preferable to treat the neonate after delivery.[3] There is no role for naloxone in the resuscitation of a newborn with intrauterine asphyxia, which is unrelated to opioid use.

0.01 mg/kg (IV) administered into the umbilical vein and repeated q 2–3 min until clinical response; repeat q 1–2 h as needed.[3-5] Additional doses may be necessary at 1- to 2-hour intervals depending on the response of the neonate and the dosage and duration of action of the opiate administered to the mother. When the IV route cannot be used, the drug may be administered by IM or SC injection.

Opiate intoxication/dependency (known or suspected): *Smaller doses may be used to reverse respiratory depression associated with therapeutic opioid use.[6] Repeat doses may be necessary, because the duration of action of some narcotics may exceed that of naloxone. Monitor for at least 24 hours because relapse may occur as naloxone is metabolized.[3]*

> **<5 years or ≤ 20 kg (including neonates):** 0.1 mg/kg q 2–3 min as needed until opiate effects are reversed.[3,6-12] Repeat q 1–2 h if inadequate response or symptoms recur.[3]

> **≥5 years or >20 kg:** 2 mg/dose[3,8,10,13-15] with subsequent doses of 0.1 mg/kg q 1–2 min if no improvement occurs.[3,10,14,15] Repeat q 20–60 min if symptoms recur.[3]

Dosage *(cont.)*	When repeated doses are required, some suggest the use of continuous infusion (i.e., 2.5–160 mcg/kg/h).[16,17] After titrating clinical effectiveness, decrease by 25%.[15-17] Wean infusion in 50% increments over 6–12 hours, depending on the half-life of the opiate.[17]
	Postoperative opioid respiratory depression: Abrupt reversal of postoperative opioid depression may cause nausea, vomiting, sweating, trembling, tachycardia, hypertension, seizures, ventricular tachycardia and fibrillation, pulmonary edema, and cardiac arrest, which has resulted in death.[3]
	Dose is $\frac{1}{10}$ that used for opiate intoxication. 0.005–0.01 mg/kg q 2–3 min until clinical response is seen and then at 1- to 2-hour intervals as necessary.[3,4,18]
	Septic shock: Dose and dosage regimens have not been established. Although naloxone causes a sustained increase in the blood pressure of those with septic shock,[19-21] it does not appear to improve survival.[22] To date, there have not been any controlled trials in children. Three case reports have described success with 0.01–0.05 mg/kg/dose intermittently in infants and children with septic shock secondary to *Neisseria meningitides, Escherichia coli,* and group B streptococcus.[17,23,24] Intermittent doses have been followed by infusions of 0.13–0.45 mg/kg/h.[17]
Dosage adjustment in organ dysfunction	Although one reference notes no adjustment in renal dysfunction,[25] the manufacturer recommends use with caution in patients with renal or hepatic dysfunction.[3]
Maximum dosage	Not established.[3] 0.4 mg/kg in neonates[26] or 2 mg/dose in those >5 years or weighing >20 kg.[3,6,12,15] If no response is seen after 10-mg total dose, diagnosis of opioid toxicity is questionable.
	The following doses were given without evidence of toxicity: an 8-day-old received 0.45 mg/kg/h for 2 hours[17]; a total of 0.8 mg/kg was given in 27 hours to a 1-month-old[27]; a 0.16-mg/kg/h continuous infusion was given to infants for 5 days[16]; a 4½-year-old received 11 doses of 0.2 mg (2.2 mg) and a 2½-year-old was accidentally given 20 mg[3]; a 13-year-old required a cumulative dose of 0.65 mg/kg over 65.6 hours[28]; and a 17-year-old received 0.8 mg/h for 15.5 hours.[29]
Additives	Some products contain methylparabens or propylparabens.[3] (See Appendix C for specific information about parabens potential for toxicity.)
Suitable diluents	D5W or NS.[30]
Maximum concentration	1 mg/mL for IV push.[3,30] 0.4 mg/mL for continuous infusion.[3,30] Use of the 0.02-mg/mL concentration is no longer recommended, especially in neonates, because it requires unacceptably large fluid volumes. A solution of 0.8 mg/mL has been infused in an infant.[14]
Preparation and delivery	**Stability:** Diluted solutions should be used within 24 hours.[3]
	Compatibility: Do not mix with alkaline solutions or medications.[30]
	Photosensitivity: Should protect from excessive light.[30]
IV push	0.4 or 1 mg/mL undiluted over 30 seconds.[30]

Naloxone HCl

Intermittent infusion	Not given by this method.
Continuous infusion	2 mg in 500 mL (4 mcg/mL) in D5W or NS for continuous infusion.[3,30] A solution of 8 mcg/mL has been infused in an infant.[14]
Other routes of administration	SC, IM, and ET.[3,4,6] The American Academy of Pediatrics does not recommend IM or SC administration due to erratic absorption[10] but does suggest ET administration is acceptable.[10] Conversely, the American Heart Association notes that there is no evidence to support a specific ET dose.[6] When used, the ET dose is the same as that for opiate intoxication/dependency and should be followed by a 5 mL NS flush and five ventilations.[6] It can also be given intraosseously.[6]
Comments	**Rare adverse effects:** Two adolescents developed acute pulmonary edema postoperatively after receiving 0.1 mg and 0.5 mg (200 IV and 300 mg IM) of naloxone, respectively.[31] The pathogenesis of pulmonary edema is thought to be similar to neurogenic pulmonary edema.[3] In this condition, centrally mediated massive catecholamine response causes a dramatic shift of blood volume into the pulmonary vascular bed producing an increased hydrostatic pressures.
	Hypotension/hypertension, ventricular tachycardia/fibrillation, and cardiac arrest have occurred in patients given naloxone for reversal of postoperative opioid depression.[3] Naloxone should be used cautiously in patients with pre-existing cardiac disease and in those receiving medications known to cause cardiovascular effects.[3]
	Other: Signs and symptoms of withdrawal in those who are physically dependent on opioids may include, body aches, diarrhea, tachycardia, fever, runny nose, sneezing, piloerection, sweating, yawning, nausea or vomiting, nervousness, restlessness or irritability, shivering or trembling, abdominal cramps, weakness, and increased blood pressure.[3] Neonates may also display seizures, excessive crying, and hyperactive reflexes.[3]

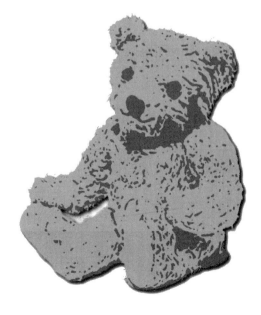

Nesiritide

Brand names	Natrecor

Medication error potential

ISMP high-alert medication that has an increased risk of causing significant patient harm if it is used in error.[1]

Look-alike, sound-alike error potential.

USP reports that nesiritide has been confused with Nipride; no patient harm resulted. USP reports that Natrecor has been confused with Primacor; no patient harm resulted. USP also reports that Natrecor has been confused with Norcuron; patient death resulted.[2]

Contraindications and warnings

Contraindications: Contraindicated in patients with hypersensitivity to the drug or any of its components. Should not be used in patients in cardiogenic shock or with systolic blood pressure <90 mm Hg.[3] Also avoid use in patients with known or suspected low cardiac filling pressures.[3]

Warnings: Be aware of the potential for allergic reactions, increased SCr, and hypotension.[3] (See Comments section.)

Infusion related cautions

Because hypotension is a dose-limiting adverse effect that may be prolonged, nesiritide should not be titrated at frequent intervals as is done with other medications that have a short half-life.[3] (See Comments section.)

Nesiritide is an *E. coli*–derived product; therefore, appropriate precautions should be taken during infusions in case of allergic reactions.[3]

Dosage

Per the manufacturer, safety and effectiveness in pediatric patients have not been established.[3]

Congestive heart failure: 1–2 mcg/kg IV bolus (see Comments section) followed by a continuous infusion of 0.01 mcg/kg/min.[4-10] Increases in continuous infusion rates by 0.005 mcg/kg/min are recommended at 2- to 3-hour intervals to a maximum of 0.03 mcg/kg/min.[4-10]

Infusions of up to 0.09 mcg/kg/min have been reported in children on ECMO.[11] Higher dosing requirements in patients on ECMO may be related to the drug's incompatibility with heparin.

Pulmonary hypertension: Limited success reported in children with pulmonary hypertension following postcardiac repair. Intermittent infusion up to 0.2 mcg/kg/min has been given directly into the pulmonary artery.[12]

Septic shock/trauma: Variable results reported in cases following infusions of 0.01–0.04 mcg/kg/min.[13-15]

Dosage adjustment in organ dysfunction

No dose adjustment is recommended for renal or hepatic insufficiency[5]; however, increases in serum creatinine have been reported during therapy.[3]

Maximum dosage

The maximum recommended dose by the manufacturer is 0.03 mcg/kg/min.[3] Reports of up to 0.09 mcg/kg/min in a pediatric ECMO patient treated for hypertension[11]; however, larger dosing requirements may be due to the drug's incompatibility with heparin in the ECMO circuit.

The manufacturer recommends the duration of infusion not exceed 72 hours[3]; however, it has been given for up to 45 days in a patient awaiting heart transplantation.[7]

Additives

None.

Suitable diluents	D5W, NS, D5½NS, D5¼NS.[3,16]
Maximum concentration	The maximum concentration for administration recommended by the manufacturer is 6 mcg/mL.[3,16]

Preparation and delivery

Preparation: Reconstitute nesiritide using 5 mL of suitable diluent; rock gently until solution is clear and colorless; add drug to 250-mL plastic infusion container to make a solution of 6 mcg/mL; invert several times to ensure adequate mixing.[3,16]

Compatibility: Although information on infusion compatibility is limited, known incompatibilities include heparin, bumetanide, enalaprilat, ethacrynic acid, furosemide, hydralazine, and insulin.[3]

Sodium metabisulfite is incompatible with nesiritide; thus, injectable drugs or solutions containing sodium metabisulfite as a preservative should not be co-infused with nesiritide.[3]

Delivery: Prime IV tubing with 5 mL of drug solution prior to initial bolus dose or initiation of the infusion.[3,16] Due to its incompatibility with heparin, infusion through a heparin-coated catheter is not recommended.[3,16]

IV push	Loading doses of 1–2 mcg/kg should be administered over 60 seconds.[3,16]
Intermittent infusion	Not recommended due to short half-life of agent.[3,17]
Continuous infusion	Recommended administration method.[3,16]
Other routes of administration	No information available to support administration by other routes.

Comments

Significant adverse effects: Concerns regarding increasing serum creatinine in *adults* given the recommended infusion rates prompted an FDA MedWatch to alert practitioners of its potential effects on renal function.[17] It is unclear whether increases in serum creatinine reflect hemodynamic effects or renal effects.[5,17] A recent report indicated the successful management of heart failure in a term infant with polycystic kidney disease without worsening of renal function.[18] Additionally, concerns for increased mortality rates in *adults* receiving nesiritide have prompted further investigation into its impact on survival of patients with congestive heart failure.[17] In hospitalized children with acute decompensated heart failure, continuous infusions of dopamine or nesiritide were associated with worsening renal failure.[19]

Hypotension is the dose-limiting adverse effect of nesiritide. Some pediatric intensivists recommend that the bolus dose be eliminated and that therapy begin with a continuous infusion at the recommended dose rate.[7,11] Others continue to recommend bolus dose.[6,9,10] When it occurs, hypotension may be prolonged (mean 2.2 hours); therefore, observation for a prolonged period of time may be necessary.[3] Dose reductions, discontinuation of therapy, and/or supportive measures may be required.[3]

Premature ventricular contractions have been reported in children with congestive heart failure.[6] Ventricular arrhythmias and bradycardia have been reported in *adults.*[3]

Other: An overdose of 36 mcg/kg was reported in a child with decompensated heart failure resulting in no hemodynamic change, renal function, and/or changes in inotropic and/or vasopressor support.[18] The patient later underwent successful heart transplantation and developed no untoward long-term effects.

Nesiritide has been found to improve hemodynamics in children with dilated cardiomyopathy.[20]

NiCARdipine

Brand names	Cardene

Medication error potential

Look-alike, sound-alike error potential.

ISMP and USP report that niCARdipine has been confused with NIFEdipine; no patient harm resulted.[1,2] USP also reports that niCARdipine has been confused with nimodipine and nitroprusside; patient harm resulted.[2]

USP reports that Cardene has been confused with Cardizem, Cordarone, and NIFEdipine; no patient harm resulted.[2]

Contraindications and warnings

Contraindications: Do not use in patients with hypersensitivity to nicardipine.[3] Contraindicated in patients with advanced aortic stenosis.[3]

Warnings: Use caution when administering nicardipine, particularly in combination with beta-blocker therapy, in patients with heart failure or significant left ventricular dysfunction.[3] (See Dosage adjustment in organ dysfunction section.) Also use caution when administering nicardipine to patients with pheochromocytoma.[3]

Avoid use in patients with space-occupying cerebral lesions due to increased intraocular pressure.[4]

Infusion related cautions

If administered via peripheral line, change sites q 12 h to avoid venous irritation/thrombophlebitis.[3,5]

Dosage

Hypertensive emergency/severe hypertension, hypertension on ECMO, during or postsurgery, and hypertension related to renal disease or postcoarctectomy

Neonates (preterm)[6,7]

Initial: 0.5 mcg/kg/min.

Maintenance: 0.5–2 mcg/kg/min; titrate q 15–30 min until target blood pressure achieved.

Has been given for up to 36–43 days.

Neonates (term) and infants

Initial: 0.5–1 mcg/kg/min.[8,9]

Maintenance: 1.5–3 mcg/kg/min[8,10]; titrate q 15–30 min until target blood pressure achieved.

Children 1–17 years

Initial: 1–5 mcg/kg/min[4,8,11-15]; some patients have received an initial dose of 10 mcg/kg/min.[11,13]

Maintenance: Typically 2–3 (range 1–6) mcg/kg/min; titrate q 15–30 min until target blood pressure achieved.[4,9,11-22]

In hypertensive emergencies, blood pressure should be frequently monitored to ensure that it does not decrease too quickly.[23,24] One group recommended that the blood pressure decrease by one third of the desired total blood pressure decrease within 6 hours, a further one-third decrease within the next 24–36 hours, with the final one-third decrease achieved over the next 48–72 hours.[17] Alternatively, a blood pressure decrease of <25% within minutes to 1 hour followed by further decreases over the next 2–6 hours if the patient is stable has been suggested.[23]

Dosage adjustment in organ dysfunction	No dose adjustment is recommended for renal impairment; however, conservative doses are recommended since patients with renal insufficiency may respond to lower doses or accumulate drug. [19,25] Since nicardipine is extensively metabolized by the liver, plasma concentrations will be elevated and half-life prolonged with hepatic failure; therefore, dose adjustment is warranted. [3,19] While one reference suggests that nicardipine may be used in children with cardiac disease, [26] the manufacturer recommends caution when administering nicardipine to patients with heart failure or significant left ventricular dysfunction due to a potential negative inotropic effect. [3]
Maximum dosage	**Initial:** 10 mcg/kg/min. [11,13] **Maintenance:** 6 mcg/kg/min. [21]
Additives	None.
Suitable diluents	D5W, D5NS, D5½NS, D5W with 40 mEq/L potassium, NS, ½NS. [5]
Maximum concentration	0.1 mg/mL per manufacturer. [3] A concentration of 3.6 mg/mL has been infused safely via a central line. [15]
Preparation and delivery	Nicardipine is not compatible with sodium bicarbonate or LR. [3,5]
IV push	Not recommended. [3,5]
Intermittent infusion	Not recommended. [3,5]
Continuous infusion	10 mL of nicardipine (25 mg) must be diluted before infusion by adding to 240 mL of suitable diluent to achieve a final concentration of 0.1 mg/mL. Titrate to desired effect. [3,5] More concentrated solutions (0.5 mg/mL) have been used in volume-restricted patients, [9,12,15] but thrombophlebitis has occurred. [12,15] A concentration of 3.6 mg/mL has been infused safely via a central line. [15]
Other routes of administration	No information available to support administration by other routes.
Comments	**Significant adverse effects:** May see tachycardia [11,16,17,19]; propranolol has been used to treat tachycardia. [11] One report describes the sudden drop in blood pressure in two of four severely asphyxiated term neonates; use nicardipine in asphyxiated patients with caution and under careful blood pressure monitoring. [27] **Drug interactions:** Nicardipine may have drug interactions with concomitant medications, including cyclosporine (increased cyclosporine concentrations), beta-blockers, cimetidine, and fentanyl. [3] Consult appropriate resources for dosing recommendations before combining any drug with nicardipine. **Other:** An accidental nicardipine overdose in a pregnant patient resulted in no serious maternal or neonatal consequence. [28]

Nitroglycerin

Brand names	Nitro-Bid I, Nitrostat I, Tridil, generic

Medication error potential

Look-alike, sound-alike error potential.

USP reports that nitroglycerin has been confused with Neo-Synephrine, nicotine, nitro-furantoin, nitroprusside and nystatin; no patient harm resulted. USP reports that Nitro-Bid IV has been confused Macrobid and Nitro-Dur; no patient harm resulted. USP reports that Tridil has been confused with Toradol; no patient harm resulted.[1]

Contraindications and warnings

Contraindications: Contraindicated in patients allergic to nitrates, and in patients with pericardial tamponade, restrictive cardiomyopathy, or constrictive pericarditis.[2]

Warnings: Many different IV preparations are available for nitroglycerin; attention should be paid to the dilution and dosage when switching from one product to another.[2]

Infusion related cautions

Severe hypotension and shock can occur with small doses.[2] Monitor blood pressure and heart rate closely.[2]

Dosage

Neonates, infants, and children: Begin infusion at 0.1–1 mcg/kg/min and increase by 0.5–1 mcg/kg/min q 3–5 min until desired clinical response,[3-6] usually ≤20 mcg/kg/min.[7]

The Pediatric Advanced Life Support (PALS) guidelines recommend 0.25–0.5 mcg/kg/min and increase 0.5–1 mcg/kg/min q 3–5 min as needed up to 1–5 mcg/kg/min (maximum 10 mcg/kg/min).[8]

Adolescents and *adults*: Begin infusion at 5 mcg/min and increase by 5 mcg/min q 3–5 min. If the desired response is not achieved at 20 mcg/min, increase by 10 mcg/min and later by 20 mcg/min until desired clinical response.[2] Responses are usually noted with infusion rates from 5–100 mcg/min.[3]

The PALS guidelines recommend 10–20 mcg/min and increase by 5–10 mcg/min q 5–10 min as needed (maximum 200 mcg/min).[8]

In hypersensitive emergencies, blood pressure should be frequently monitored to ensure that it does not decrease too quickly.[3] One group recommended that the blood pressure decrease by one third of the desired total blood pressure decrease within 6 hours, a further one-third decrease within the next 24–36 hours, with the final one-third decrease achieved over the next 48–72 hours.[9] A blood pressure decrease of <25% within minutes to 1 hour followed by further decreases over the next 2–6 hours if the patient is stable has been suggested.[3] (See Infusion related cautions section.)

Dosage adjustment in organ dysfunction

No dosage adjustment required.

Maximum dosage

60 mcg/kg/min was infused for ≤30 minutes to infants and children with congenital heart defects who had a low cardiac index postoperatively; however, the type of tubing used for the infusion was not stated.[5] (See Delivery system issues in Preparation and delivery section.) In *adults* with hypertension, doses up to 100 mcg/min have been used.[2,3] In *adults* with acute MI, the risk of hypotension increases with doses approaching 200 mcg/min.[2,3]

The Pediatric Advanced Life Support (PALS) guidelines state maximum doses of 10 mcg/kg/min in children and 200 mcg/min in adolescents.[8]

Nitroglycerin

Additives

One commercially available form of nitroglycerin injection contains 30% ethanol and 30% propylene glycol in water.[2] Another available form is in a solution of 50% dehydrated alcohol and 50% propylene glycol.[10] Nitroglycerin in dextrose solution also contains ethanol and propylene glycol.[11]

See Appendix C for more specific information about potential adverse effects of propylene glycol.

Suitable diluents

D5W or NS.[2,11]

Maximum concentration

400 mcg/mL.[2,11]

Preparation and delivery

Delivery system issues: Nitroglycerin readily absorbs too many plastics; therefore, glass infusion bottles and non-PVC administration sets are recommended. When standard polyvinyl chloride (PVC) IV tubing is used, significant drug is absorbed to the tubing.[2,3] Thus, the apparent doses required to achieve a desired clinical response are increased.[2,3] If PVC sets are used, larger doses are required.[2,3,11] Avoid filters, some of which absorb nitroglycerin.[2,3,11]

Compatibility: For PN compatibility information, please see Appendix D.

IV push

Not indicated.

Intermittent infusion

Not indicated.

Continuous infusion

Initial concentrations of 50–100 mcg/mL using an infusion control device are recommended; however, patient factors such as fluid requirements and duration of therapy may warrant use of more concentrated solutions.[2,3,11]

Other routes of administration

The PALS guidelines state nitroglycerin may also be given via intraosseous route.[8]

Other routes of administration are not indicated.

Comments

Significant adverse effects: Methemoglobinemia was associated with doses >7 mcg/kg/min in *adults*.[12,13] However, methemoglobinemia did not occur in 16 pediatric patients (3 days to 23.7 months) who received concomitant IV nitroglycerin (0.5–4 mcg/kg/min) and sodium nitroprusside (0.3–8.4 mcg/kg/min) for 0.5–7.6 days.[14]

Pharmacodynamic considerations: In *adults*, tolerance to hemodynamic effects of nitroglycerin is observed within 12–48 hours after beginning continuous infusion. If such tolerance occurs, intermittent therapy or a nitrate-free interval ≥8 hours after 12–48 hours of continuous infusion is recommended.[15]

Norepinephrine Bitartrate

Brand names	Levophed

Medication error potential

ISMP high-alert medication that has an increased risk of causing significant patient harm if it is used in error.[1]

Look-alike, sound-alike error potential.

USP reports that norepinephrine has been confused with epinephrine and nitroprusside; no patient harm resulted. USP reports that norepinephrine has been confused with Neo-Synephrine and phenylephrine; patient harm resulted.

USP reports that Levophed has been confused with Lopressor; no patient harm resulted.[2]

Contraindications and warnings

US boxed warning: Norepinephrine carries a boxed warning regarding the risk for extravasation and the appropriate use of the antidote, phentolamine mesylate, in cases of extravasation.[3] (See Infusion related cautions section.)

Contraindications: If used in hypotensive and volume depleted patients prior to volume replacement, peripheral and visceral vasoconstriction, decreased renal perfusion and urine output, decreased systemic flow, tissue hypoxia and lactic acidosis may occur.[3]

Do not use in patients with mesenteric or peripheral vascular thrombosis or in patients receiving cyclopropane and halothane anesthetics.[3]

Other warnings: Use with caution in patients on monoamine oxidase inhibitors or triptyline or imipramine antidepressants.[3] (See Comments section.)

Infusion related cautions

If possible, infuse via central,[4] large vein, particularly antecubital or femoral vein, using a plastic catheter, to decrease the risk of necrosis of overlying skin.[3]

Extravasation may cause local ischemia and tissue necrosis.[3-9] To prevent necrosis, the area should be infiltrated with 10–15 mL of a saline solution that contains 5–10 mg phentolamine mesylate.[3,4,8] Administer into and around the extravasation area using a fine hypodermic needle.[3] If the area is infiltrated with the antidote within 12 hours, reversal of the blanching should immediately occur.[3]

See Appendix E for additional information regarding extravasation treatment.

Dosage

Correct intravascular volume as fully as possible before starting norepinephrine.[3]

Avoid abrupt withdrawal by gradually reducing the dose.[3]

Infants and children: 0.05–0.1 mcg/kg/min titrated to the desired blood pressure up to usual maximum dose of 2 mcg/kg/min.[4,7,8,10]

Adolescents and *adults*: 4 mcg/min titrated to the desired blood pressure; the manufacturer states usual maintenance doses of 2–4 mcg/min,[3] while another reference states usual maintenance doses are 8–12 mcg/min.[11]

Dosage adjustment in organ dysfunction

No dosage adjustment required in renal dysfunction.

Maximum dosage

Large doses up to 68 mg/day have been used in *adults*.[3]

Additives

Contains sodium metabisulfite.[3,9] See Appendix C for more specific information about potential adverse effects of sulfites.

Norepinephrine Bitartrate

Suitable diluents	D5W, D5NS, or other D5S solution.[3,9] Dilution with dextrose-containing solutions protects against significant loss of potency from oxidation, thus use of NS alone for dilution is not recommended.[3,9]
Maximum concentration	16 mcg/mL.[11]
Preparation and delivery	**Preparation:** Standard concentration for infusion is 4 mcg/mL.[11] Norepinephrine is easily destroyed by oxidants and in alkaline solutions; therefore, solutions should be protected from light.[3] Do not infuse if solution is pinkish or darker than slightly yellow or if it contains a precipitate.[3] **Compatibility:** For PN compatibility information, please see Appendix D.
IV push	Not indicated.
Intermittent infusion	Not recommended.
Continuous infusion	4–16 mcg/mL infused into a large vein.[3,9,11]
Other routes of administration	Has been given via intraosseous route.[7,8,12]
Comments	Several drugs (e.g., tricyclic antidepressants, MAO inhibitors, etc.) may potentiate the pressor effects of norepinephrine.[3] Atropine may block the reflex bradycardia and enhance the pressor response caused by norepinephrine.[13] Consult appropriate resources before combining any drug with norepinephrine.

Octreotide Acetate

Brand names	SandoSTATIN, generic

Medication error potential

Do not confuse with Sandostatin LAR Depot, which should only be given via IM administration.[1]

Look-alike, sound-alike error potential.

ISMP and USP report that SandoSTATIN has been confused with SandIMMUNE; no patient harm resulted.[2,3] USP also reports that SandoSTATIN has been confused with sargramostim and simvastatin; no patient harm resulted.[3]

Contraindications and warnings

Contraindications: Hypersensitivity to octreotide or any of its components.[1]

Warnings: May inhibit gallbladder contraction and decrease bile secretion; gallstones, acute cholecystitis, ascending cholangitis, biliary obstruction, cholestatic hepatitis, and pancreatitis have been reported in patients receiving octreotide.[1]

Hypoglycemia or hyperglycemia, suppression of thyroid stimulating hormone and hypothyroidism, and cardiac conduction abnormalities have been reported in patients receiving octreotide. These effects may be seen more frequently in patients with acromegaly.[1]

Infusion related cautions

None known.

Dosage

Chylothorax/chyloperitoneum: 0.3–2 mcg/kg/h via continuous IV infusion initially; gradually increase dose until effect seen.[4-9]

10 mcg/kg/day in three divided SC doses; increase dose by 5–10 mcg/kg/day at 48- to 72-hour intervals until effect seen (typically up to 20–40 mcg/kg/day).[4,8,10-13]

A systematic review of 20 reports of octreotide for chylothorax recommended using higher doses (80–100 mcg/kg/day) earlier rather than starting with a low dose and titrating gradually upward.[14]

3.5 mcg/kg/h increased to 7 mcg/kg/h then to 12 mcg/kg/h has been used to decrease persistent pleural drainage in a 10-year-old after Fontan procedure.[15]

Diarrhea/increased gastrointestinal output: 13–200 mcg/day SC or IV in two divided doses.[16-21] Doses of 1.4–20 mcg/kg/day divided q 12 h have been used.[16,17,19-21] Begin at low end of dosage range and increase by 0.3 mcg/kg/dose every 3 days.[16] An alternative method is continuous infusion 1 mcg/kg/h.[22]

Fistula closure

Neonates: 1.4 mcg/kg/day SC divided BID, gradually increased up to 5 mcg/kg/day SC divided BID.[23]

Children: 50–300 mcg/day SC divided in two to three doses. Start at lower end of dosage range and increase gradually.[24,25]

Gastrointestinal bleeding: 1–2 mcg/kg bolus, followed by either 1 mcg/kg/h IV infusion or 3 mcg/kg/day IV divided q 8 h. Older children have received an *adult* dose of 50 mcg bolus over 5 minutes followed by 50 mcg/h. Continuous infusion can be increased q 8 h if no decrease in bleeding. Dose is tapered by 50% q 12 h when no active bleeding for 24 hours and can be stopped when dose is 25% of initial dose.[26-28] For chronic GI bleeding, 4–8 mcg/kg/day SC has been given with concurrent iron therapy.[29]

Hyperinsulinemia (congenital)/hypoglycemia of infancy: Initial doses of 2–10 mcg/kg/day in two to six doses SC.[30-37] Doses are titrated up to 40 mcg/kg/day based on glucose concentrations. Total daily dose may be given SC in divided doses or continuous infusion via a SC or IV infusion pump.[21,30,33]

Dosage *(cont.)*	**Pancreatitis/pancreatic tumors:** A 10-year-old child received 1.5 mcg/kg/h IV for pancreatic pseudocyst.[38] A 15-month-old infant received 2 mcg/kg SC q 6 h increased up to 20 mcg/kg for recurrent acute pancreatitis and ascites.[39] A 12-year-old received a maximum of 75 mcg/kg/dose SC in combination with chemotherapy for malignant pancreatic carcinoid tumor.[40]
	Sulfonylurea poisoning: In children, a single dose of 25 mcg can be given IV. Dose and duration vary depending on amount of sulfonylurea ingested and its half-life.[41-45] SC, IV, and continuous infusion are appropriate routes, and 2 mcg/kg/day SC divided q 12 h has also been cited as appropriate.[41] 2 mcg/kg followed by 2 mcg/kg/h has been used in a toddler with hypoglycemia unresponsive to dextrose infusion and glucagon.[46]
	Tall stature/excessive growth hormone (GH) secretion (use not established): 100–500 mcg two to three times daily up to 1500 mcg/day has been used but has not fully suppressed GH levels.[21,47]
	Children: 300–600 mcg/day in three divided doses.[21,47]
	Adolescents: 500–1500 mcg/day in two to three divided doses.[21]
	One study found 37.5 mcg (prepubertal) or 50 mcg (pubertal) given via SC injection 1 hour before bedtime to be effective in children.[48] Continuous SC infusion with the bulk of the total daily dose given overnight has been found to be superior to SC or depot injection therapy.[47]
Dosage adjustment in organ dysfunction	In patients with renal failure requiring dialysis, the dose may need to be adjusted secondary to increased half-life.[1]
Maximum dosage	No data for maximum dosage in children. (See Comments section.) In *adults*, the maximum dose is 1500 mcg/day divided q 8 h.[1] An infant has received as much as 2000 mcg/day.[18]
Additives	None.
Suitable diluents	D5W, NS.[1,49]
Maximum concentration	No information available.
Preparation and delivery	The manufacturer states that octreotide should not be added to PN because of the formation of glycosyl octreotide conjugate[1]; however, this is controversial.[49,50] For additional PN compatibility information, please see Appendix D.
IV push	In emergency situations, octreotide may be administered undiluted over 3 minutes.[1,49]
Intermittent infusion	Dilute with 50–200 mL and infuse over 15–30 minutes.[1,49]
Continuous infusion	Dilute and infuse over 24 hours.[1,49]

Octreotide Acetate

Other routes of administration	SC injection is the usual route of administration.[1,49] SC injection sites should be rotated.[1,49] IM administration with depot form only (Sandostatin LAR Depot).[1,49] Reconstitute with provided diluent and administer immediately after reconstitution into gluteal area at 4-week intervals.[1]
Comments	**Significant adverse effects:** A systematic review of somatostatin or octreotide in infants and young children reported side effects of cutaneous flush, nausea, loose stools, transient hypothyroidism, elevated liver function tests, strangulation ileus (with somatostatin) and transient abdominal distention, temporary hyperglycemia, and necrotizing enterocolitis (with octreotide).[4] Severe paradoxical hyperglycemia and bradycardia has been reported in an infant receiving 0.5 mcg/kg/day SC octreotide (divided four times daily) during surgery (pancreatectomy) for congenital hyperinsulinism.[51] A 6-month-old infant died of fulminant colitis after receiving somatostatin analogue in a dose of 18 mcg/kg/day.[52] Prior to the infant's death, the dose had been decreased to 3.5 mcg/kg/day. A 16-month-old with enterocutaneous fistula developed sudden abdominal pain and increased nasogastric drainage and died 8 hours after receiving a single dose of 100 mcg SC of somatostatin analogue.[1] Two reports in infants have associated the use of octreotide (one for postoperative chylothorax and the other for refractory hypoglycemia) to the development of necrotizing enterocolitis.[6,53] A neonate receiving 30 mcg/kg/day developed an increase in direct bilirubin and gamma glutamine transferase on day 7 of therapy. Ultrasound revealed ascites and biliary sludging. All symptoms resolved with termination of therapy.[10] Asymptomatic gallstones were found in an infant 1 year after being started on octreotide.[30] **Other:** Tachyphylaxis is a common occurrence, requiring larger doses to maintain similar effect, especially when used in patients with hyperinsulinism.[31,33,34] Octreotide has been used to improve GI symptoms (abdominal pain, nausea, vomiting) in a 12-year-old with bowel obstruction due to progression of adenocarcinoma despite surgery and chemotherapy.[54] May decrease B12 concentrations and alter dietary fat absorption.[1] Fat malabsorption documented by fecal fat testing was observed in one infant on prolonged octreotide therapy.[37]

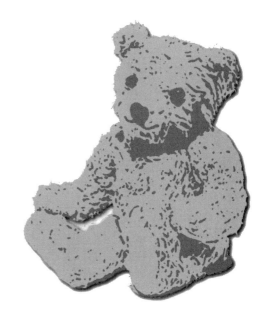

Ondansetron HCl

Brand names	Zofran

Medication error potential

Look-alike, sound-alike error potential.

USP reports that ondansetron has been confused with dolasetron, granisetron, and olanzapine.[1] No patient harm occurred. Zofran was confused with Reglan, Zantac, Zocor, Zoloft, Zometa, and Zosyn and no patient harm resulted. However, Zofran was confused with Zanaflex and patient harm did occur.

Contraindications and warnings

Contraindications: Patients with known hypersensitivity to the drug.[2]

Warnings: Hypersensitivity reactions may occur in patients with hypersensitivity to other 5-hydroxytryptamine 3 (5-HT3) antagonists.[2] An anaphylactoid reaction occurred in an 11-year-old girl.[3]

Infusion related cautions

Blood pressure changes and increased QTc interval have been reported during infusion in *adults*.[4]

Dosage

Prevention of chemotherapy-induced nausea and vomiting: 0.15 mg/kg over 15 minutes given 30 minutes before chemotherapy with two or three additional doses given 4 and 8 hours after the first dose.[2,5-10] A single dose of 0.6 mg/kg (≤32 mg/dose) was no more effective than 0.15 mg/kg (≤8 mg) q 4 h for four doses.[9] Similarly, no difference in efficacy was noted between 5 (≤8 mg) and 10 mg/m² (≤16 mg).[11] The inclusion of dexamethasone is recommended.[12]

In 26 children (18 months to 15 years) undergoing intrathecal chemotherapy who received 0.45 mg/kg given 30 minutes prior to treatment, vomiting was decreased compared to those who received 0.15 mg/kg.[11]

In *adults*, a dose of 32 mg is given 30 minutes before chemotherapy.[2,6]

Prevention of postoperative nausea and vomiting (PONV): ≥1 month old to ≤40 kg: 0.1 mg/kg.[2,14] >40 kg to 12 years of age: ≤4 mg.[2,14] Others report infusing 0.025–0.15 mg/kg immediately before induction of anesthesia or postoperatively in symptomatic patients.[15-23] One study noted that 0.075 mg/kg was as effective as 0.1–0.15 mg/kg.[21] Administration of a second dose in patients who fail to respond does not improve control.[2]

Emergency department treatment of acute gastroenteritis: 0.15 mg/kg, infused over 2 minutes in children 1 month to 22 years, reduced the need for hospital admission and decreased the number of vomiting episodes in the acute period of illness.[24]

Dosage adjustment in organ dysfunction

No dosage adjustment for renal or hepatic disease noted.[2]

Maximum dosage

0.45 mg/kg[13] up to 32 mg.[2,9] In *adults*, up to 150 mg/dose and up to 252 mg/day have been inadvertently given without adverse effects.[2]

Additives

Each mL of the 20-mL multidose vial contains 8.32 mg of methylparaben, and 0.15 mg of propylparaben.[2,25] See Appendix C for specific information about potential adverse effects.

Ondansetron HCl

Suitable diluents	D5W, D5 ½NS, D5NS, LR, NS, R.[2,25]
Maximum concentration	2 mg/mL (undiluted) for PONV prophylaxis.[2] Dilute for prevention of chemotherapy-induced nausea and vomiting.[2]
Preparation and delivery	**Stability:** Must be used within 24 hours of dilution.[2] **Compatibility:** See Appendix D for PN compatibility information.
IV push	In children <40 kg receiving 0.1 mg/kg and those >40 kg (including *adults*) receiving 4 mg for prevention of PONV, ondansetron may be infused over >30 seconds but over 2–5 minutes is preferable.[2]
Intermittent infusion	Infuse over 15 minutes for prevention of chemotherapy-induced nausea and vomiting.[2,7]
Continuous infusion	Although continuous infusion has been used in *adults*,[26] its use has not been reported for pediatric patients.
Other routes of administration	Can be given IM in *adults*.
Comments	**Pharmacokinetics:** Compared to those 4–12 months old, infants 1–4 months have decreased clearance resulting in a prolonged half-life.[2] Those <4 months old should be closely monitored.[2] Children and adolescents have increased clearance and shorter half-life than *adults*.[2] **Drug interactions:** Ondansetron is metabolized by the cytochrome P450 isozymes but neither induces or inhibits the isozymes. While ondansetron clearance is increased and concentrations are decreased by rifampin, carbamazepine, and rifampicin; no dosage adjustment for ondansetron is recommended.[2] **Adverse events:** Blurred vision has been noted. Transient blindness has been reported and resolves within a few minutes up to 48 hours.[2]

Oxacillin Sodium

Brand names	Bactocill, Prostaphlin

Medication error potential

Look-alike, sound-alike drug names.

USP reports confusion with ampicillin, cefazolin, nafcillin, and penicillin G potassium.[1]

Contraindications and warnings

Contraindications: Hypersensitivity to oxacillin or other penicillins or any component of the formulation.[2]

Warnings: Individuals who have a Type I reaction to penicillin may experience serious and occasionally fatal hypersensitivity (anaphylactic shock with collapse) reactions.[2] (See Appendix C for specific information.)

Prolonged use may cause superinfection and/or *Clostridium difficile*–associated diarrhea (CDAD), which has been reported and may range in severity from mild diarrhea to fatal colitis.[2] If CDAD is suspected or confirmed, appropriate fluid and electrolyte management, protein supplementation, antibiotic treatment of *C. difficile,* and surgical evaluation should be instituted as clinically indicated.[2]

Infusion related cautions

If a decision is made to give this medication to a patient with known penicillin hypersensitivity, the patient should be closely observed for allergenicity. Although rare, anaphylactoid reactions may require immediate emergency treatment with epinephrine, oxygen, IV steroids, antihistamines, pressor amines, and airway management.

Slowing the infusion (e.g., 60 minutes) may minimize vein irritation.[2]

Dosage

Neonates

PNA	≤1200 g	≤2000 g	>2000 g
≤7 days	50 mg/kg/day divided q 12 h[4,5]*	50–100 mg/kg/day divided q 12 h[4-6]	75–150 mg/kg/day divided q 8 h[4-6]
>7 days		75–150 mg/kg/day divided q 8 h[4-6]	100–200 mg/kg/day divided q 6 h[4-6]

*Until 4 weeks of age.

Infants and children

    Mild to moderate infections: 100–150 mg/kg/day divided q 6 h (up to 4 g/day).[4]

    Severe infections: 150–200 mg/kg/day divided q 4–6 h (up to 12 g/day).[4,5,7-10]

Dosage adjustment in organ dysfunction

Use the lower end of the dosage range if CrCl <10 mL/min.[2]

Maximum dosage

≤12 g/day for those with severe infections.[2,11] Although doses of 400 mg/kg/day have been given, they have been associated with hepatotoxicity.[12]

Additives

Contains 2.5–3.1 mEq sodium/g of oxacillin.[13]

Oxacillin Sodium

Suitable diluents	D5W, D10W, NS, ½NS, LR, SW, D5NS.[13] Specific references should be used as stability over time was variable in these diluents.[13]
Maximum concentration	100 mg/mL for IV push and ≤40 mg/mL for infusion.[2]
Preparation and delivery	**Delivery system issues:** The mixing of oxacillin with an aminoglycoside in vitro can result in substantial inactivation of the aminoglycoside.[2] (See Appendix C for more specific information.) **Compatibility:** See Appendix D for PN compatibility information.[14]
IV push	100 mg/mL over at least 10 minutes.[2,13]
Intermittent infusion	0.5–40 mg/mL administered over 15–30 minutes.[2,13] If given peripherally, consider infusing over 60 minutes at a maximum concentration of 20 mg/mL.[15]
Continuous infusion	Although the solution concentration and type of diluent were not specified, oxacillin has been given by this method.[2]
Other routes of administration	167 mg/mL in SW, NS, or ½NS may be given by deep IM injection in same doses as IV.[5,13]
Comments	**Rare adverse effects:** Hepatotoxicity, characterized by fever, nausea, and vomiting associated with abnormal liver function tests, mainly elevated AST levels, has been associated with the use of oxacillin.[16-18] Cholestatic hepatitis has been reported rarely. Neurotoxic (e.g., lethargy, confusion, twitching, multifocal myoclonus, localized or generalized epileptiform seizures) may occur with large doses, especially in patients with renal insufficiency.[2,19] **Monitoring:** AST (SGOT) and ALT (SGPT) values should be obtained periodically during therapy to monitor for possible liver function abnormalities.[2] **Laboratory interference:** Oxacillin may cause false-positive urinary glucose results when cupric sulfate solution-based tests (Clinitest, Benedict's solution, Fehling's solution) are used.[2] It is recommended that glucose tests (Diastix, TEST-TAPE, Clinistix) based on enzymatic glucose oxidase reactions be used.[2] **Drug interactions:** Concurrent use of tetracycline should be avoided as it may antagonize the bactericidal effect of penicillin.[2] Probenecid may decrease the tubular secretion of oxacillin and increase its concentration in the serum. Consult appropriate resources for dosing recommendations before combining any drug with oxacillin.

Palivizumab

Brand names	Synagis
Medication error potential	None noted.

Contraindications and warnings

Contraindications: Those with a previous hypersensitivity reaction to palivizumab.[1]

Warnings: Rare cases of acute hypersensitivity reactions or anaphylaxis have been reported after re-exposure to palivizumab.[1]

If milder hypersensitivity reactions occur with palivizumab, subsequent doses should be given with caution.

Infusion related cautions

Not given by IV infusion.

Dosage

Indications: Infants born at ≤35 weeks gestation or who have bronchopulmonary dysplasia (BPD) and infants who have stable hemodynamically significant (cyanotic or acyanotic) congenital heart disease (CHD).[1] Dosing should begin prior to the anticipated respiratory syncytial virus (RSV) season.[1]

15 mg/kg IM in the anterolateral aspect of the thigh repeated q 30 days during the RSV season for up to five doses (November through March).[1-8] Most infants and children who require palivizumab are treated as outpatients. However, it has been used in hospitalized preterm infants who met eligibility criteria during outbreaks[9,10] and during RSV season.[11]

In general, AAP recommends prophylaxis for[8]

Infants and children <24 months of age who have chronic lung disease (CLD) that required medical treatment 6 months before RSV season.

Infants with severe CLD and who continue to require medical treatment during their second RSV season.

Infants born ≤32 weeks gestation without CLD who are at the greatest risk from disease with two or more risk factors such as those in day care, with school-age siblings, who have exposure to environmental air pollution, with congenital abnormalities of the airway, or with severe neuromuscular disease.

Infants with CHD who require treatment for CHF, who have moderate to severe pulmonary hypertension, and who have cyanotic heart disease.

Dosage adjustment in organ dysfunction

None noted.

Maximum dosage

15 mg/kg monthly.[1]

Additives

Contains no preservatives.

Suitable diluents

Not given IV.

Maximum concentration

100 mg/mL for IM use.[1]

Preparation and delivery	Do not shake or agitate the vial.[1] 50- and 100-mg vials are single dose.[1] Do not re-enter the vial.
IV push	The manufacturer does not recommend IV infusion. However, palivizumab was infused over 2–5 minutes or 1–2 mL/min (10 mg/mL) in pharmacokinetic studies[12,13] and in infants with RSV infection who were mechanically ventilated.[14]
Intermittent infusion	Not indicated.
Continuous infusion	Not indicated.
Other routes of administration	IM is the usual route of administration. If the dosage volume exceeds 1 mL, the dose should be divided and given as separate injections.[1] Use of the combination of EMLA cream and 50/50 nitrous oxide/oxygen significantly decreased pain associated with injection than either used alone.[15]
Comments	Administration of palivizumab IV to patients in the acute phase of RSV illness did not improve clinical outcomes nor cause an exacerbation of the infection[13]; however, concentrations of virus in tracheal aspirates were reduced when administered at standard prophylactic doses.[14] Serum concentrations decreased by a mean of 58% following cardiopulmonary bypass in pediatric patients receiving open heart surgery, thus additional dosing after surgery may be required.[1] Lower doses (3–10 mg/kg) were associated with insufficient serum antibody concentrations.[6,12]

Pamidronate

Brand names	Aredia
Medication error potential	Look-alike, sound-alike error potential. USP reported the potential for confusion between pamidronate and papaverine.[1]
Contraindications and warnings	**Contraindications:** Hypersensitivity to pamidronate.[2] **Warnings:** Pamidronate should be infused slowly to avoid renal impairment.[2]
Infusion related cautions	Infusion site reactions are more likely to occur with larger doses.[2]
Dosage	**Osteogenesis imperfecta:** Regimens vary[3-6] but in general range from 1–1.5 mg/kg given every other month or q 3 mo.[7-9] Calcium and vitamin D supplements should be provided. Treatment may be continued for several years. Because of concerns over growth, one group discontinued treatment for 2 years and found that bone metabolism continued to be suppressed, improvements in bone mass continued, but children did not achieve normal bone growth.[10] **Osteoporosis/osteopenia:** 0.4–0.5 mg/kg over 2–4 hours for 3 days q 3–6 mo for up to 13 months in children with cerebral palsy.[11,12] Seventeen children on steroids for endocrine or renal disease who developed fractures were given 1 mg/kg q 2 mo for 1 or 2 years.[13] Patients were also prescribed calcium and vitamin D supplements.[12,13] **Hypercalcemia:** 0.5–1 mg/kg[14-18] or 35–50 mg/m^2[19] over 2–6 hours as a single dose or repeated for 1[19] or 2 more days.[18] One group repeated the initial 0.5-mg/kg dose on days 1–3 and then decreased the dose to 0.25 mg/kg on day 4 and 0.125 mg/kg on day 5.[20] **McCune Albright syndrome:** 0.5 mg/kg over 4 hours for 3 days each year, 1 mg/kg over 4 hours for 3 days q 6 mo, or 1 mg/kg for 3 days q 4 mo for up to 6 years,[21] or 1 mg/kg over 4 hours for 3 days q 6 mo for 2 years.[22]
Dosage adjustment in organ dysfunction	None recommended by manufacturer.[2] However, in those whose renal function deteriorates during treatment, the dose should be held until renal function returns to baseline.[2] One report described three children with renal failure or who were postrenal transplant with either fractures or hypercalcemia who were given one to three doses of 0.4–0.5 mg/kg without ill effects.[23]
Maximum dosage	1.5 mg/kg q 2 mo has been used in osteogenesis imperfecta.[9] 90 mg every 3–4 weeks in *adults* with metastatic bone disease.[2]
Additives	None.
Suitable diluents	D5W, ½NS, NS.[2]
Maximum concentration	0.36 mg/mL.[2]

Pamidronate

Preparation and delivery	Reconstitute 30 or 90 mg lyophilized powder in 10 mL SW. Dilute reconstitution in 250 mL to 1 L of D5W, ½ NS, NS.
	Compatibility: Incompatible with calcium containing fluids (including LR) and other parenteral drugs.[2]
IV push	Contraindicated.
Intermittent infusion	In *adults*, 30–90 mg over ≥2–4 hours. Longer infusion times decrease the risk for renal toxicity.[2]
Continuous infusion	90 mg infused over 24 hours in *adults*.[2]
Other routes of administration	Not indicated.[2]
Comments	**Monitoring:** Serum creatinine should be measured before each infusion.[2]
	Adverse effects: A transient, low-grade fever for 24–48 hours is common after the first infusion. The frequency of this reaction decreases with subsequent infusions.[2,7,8,13,14,21]
	Symptomatic and asymptomatic hypocalcemia has been reported.[2,3,17]
	Osteonecrosis of the jaw has been reported in *adult* cancer patients on chemotherapy who also receive pamidronate. It is recommended that while on pamidronate invasive dental procedures should be avoided.[2] Twenty-two children who underwent 38 dental procedures exhibited no evidence of jaw osteonecrosis.[24]

Pancuronium Bromide

Brand names Pavulon, generic

Medication error potential

ISMP high-alert medication that has an increased risk of causing significant patient harm if it is used in error.[1]

Look-alike, sound-alike error potential.

USP reports that pancuronium has been confused with vecuronium; no patient harm resulted.[2] USP also reports that pancuronium has been confused with Protonix; patient harm resulted.[2]

ISMP reports that Pavulon has been confused with Peptavlon.[3] USP reports that Pavulon has been confused with papaverine; no patient harm resulted.[2]

Contraindications and warnings

US boxed warning: Pancuronium should be administered only by adequately trained individuals familiar with the actions, characteristics and hazards of pancuronium.[4]

Contraindications: Hypersensitivity to pancuronium or any of its components.[4]

Other warnings: Use carefully under the supervision of experienced clinicians; personnel should also be skilled in airway management, resuscitation and respiratory support.[4] Intubation and ventilatory support equipment, including oxygen therapy, should be readily available.[4] Also should have anticholinesterase inhibitors readily available when giving pancuronium.[4]

Infusion related cautions

Cardiac dysrhythmias, tachycardia, and hypertension have been reported.[5-7]

Joint contractures have occurred in neonates.[8]

Anaphylaxis has occurred in *adults*.[9]

Dosage

Respiratory function must be supported during use of this agent. Concurrent administration of a sedative is also necessary. Monitoring of neuromuscular transmission with a peripheral nerve stimulator is recommended during continuous infusion or with repeated dosing.[4]

Endotracheal intubation and maintenance of neuromuscular blockade

> **Neonates:** Because neonates are particularly sensitive to nondepolarizing agents, a test dose of 0.02 mg/kg should be given to assess responsiveness.[1] 0.03–0.1 mg/kg repeated as necessary q 1–2 h to maintain muscle relaxation or 0.02–0.04 mg/kg/h as continuous infusion.[5,10-15]

> **Infants and children:** 0.08–0.15 mg/kg initially and then 0.02–0.2 mg/kg repeated as required or 0.03–0.1 mg/kg/h as continuous infusion.[4,6,16-18]

Dosage adjustment in organ dysfunction

Adjust dosage in patients with renal dysfunction.[19,20] If CrCl is 10–50 mL/min, give 50% of a normal dose; if CrCl is <10 mL/min, do not use.[19,20] Although clearance is decreased, volume of distribution is significantly increased in patients with liver dysfunction; hence, these patients may require larger doses.[4,21]

Maximum dosage

Cumulative dose of 0.3 mg/kg was given within several minutes to a newborn infant without adverse effects.[14] One study used up to 0.5 mg/kg as a single dose in neonates with hyaline membrane disease.[22] Large doses may increase frequency and severity of tachycardia.[23]

Additives

Benzyl alcohol: Multidose vials contain benzyl alcohol 0.9% as a preservative.[4] See Appendix C for more specific information about potential adverse effects and/or benzyl alcohol toxicity in neonates.

Pancuronium Bromide

Suitable diluents	D5W, D5NS, D5½NS, NS, LR.[4,24]
Maximum concentration	2 mg/mL for IV push or 0.8 mg/mL for continuous infusion.[4,23,24]
Preparation and delivery	No comments.
IV push	1 or 2 mg/mL given rapidly over seconds.[4,23,24]
Intermittent infusion	No information available to support administration by this method.
Continuous infusion	0.01–0.8 mg/mL.[23,25]
Other routes of administration	IM administration is not recommended.[4]
Comments	**Significant adverse effects:** Prolonged paralysis (mean duration of 9 weeks) has been reported following pancuronium infusion.[26-28] Factors that potentiate the duration of neuromuscular blockage include use of certain medications (see Drug interactions below), acidosis, hyponatremia, hypocalcemia, hypokalemia, and hypermagnesemia.[4,10,23] **Drug interactions:** Concomitant administration of corticosteroids with neuromuscular blockers has been shown to be a risk factor for prolonged paralysis.[29] Likewise, concomitant administration of pancuronium with certain antibiotics (e.g., aminoglycosides) and other drugs such as anesthetics, magnesium, and quinidine may also prolong neuromuscular blockade.[23] Consult appropriate resources for additional information on drug interactions.

Pantoprazole

Brand names	Protonix

Medication error potential

Look-alike, sound-alike error potential.

USP reports that Protonix has been confused with pancuronium; patient harm resulted.[1] USP also reports that pantoprazole has been confused with paroxetine, Pravachol, pravastatin, and propranolol and that pantoprazole has been confused with Paxil, Plavix, Pravachol, Primaxin, protamine sulfate, Proteinex, and Topamax; no patient harm resulted.[1]

ISMP reports that Protonix has been confused with Lotronex and protamine.[2]

Contraindications and warnings

Pantoprazole is contraindicated in patients with known hypersensitivity to the formulation.[3]

Infusion related cautions

Immediate hypersensitivity reactions, including anaphylaxis, may occur.[3]

Thrombophlebitis and injection site reactions have been reported.[3]

Dosage

Experience with IV pantoprazole in children, particularly neonates and infants, is limited; currently there is no established IV dose range for pediatric patients.

Initial pharmacokinetic studies of oral and IV pantoprazole in children 2–16 years of age have found similar pharmacokinetics to that observed in *adults*.[4-6] In *adults*, oral and IV dosage are similar in potency.

Doses used in pediatric IV pharmacokinetic studies[4-6]: 0.47–1.88 mg/kg/dose, maximum 80 mg/dose and 160 mg/day (children 2–16 years).

General dosing ranges from pediatric oral dosing studies

> **Gastroesophageal reflux/reflux esophagitis[7]:** 20 mg every day (0.5–1 mg/kg/day) for 28 days (children 6–13 years).

***Adult* dosing ranges (IV pantoprazole)**

> **Gastroesophageal reflux/reflux esophagitis[3]:** 40 mg every day for 7–10 days; oral formulation for maintenance.

> **Hypersecretory conditions[3]:** 80 mg q 12 h for up to 6 days; may increase frequency to q 8 h as needed to suppress acid production.

> **Peptic ulcer (use not established)[8-10]:** 80 mg bolus followed by continuous infusion of 8 mg/h for 3 days, followed by 40 mg q 12 h for 4–7 days.

> **Stress ulcer prophylaxis (use not established)[11]:** 80 mg q 8–12 h.

Dosage adjustment in organ dysfunction

No dosage adjustment recommended for renal or hepatic dysfunction.[3,12] Doses >40 mg/day have not been studied in patients with hepatic dysfunction.[3] Elimination half-life may be prolonged with hepatic dysfunction.[13]

Maximum dosage

80 mg/dose[5,6] and 160 mg/day[6] in children. 240 mg/day in *adults*.[3]

Additives

Edetate disodium (1 mg per 40-mg vial).[3,14] Edetate disodium is a chelator of metals, and the manufacturer recommends that zinc supplementation should be considered in patients receiving pantoprazole who are prone to zinc deficiency.[3]

Suitable diluents

Reconstitute to 4 mg/mL with NS. Further dilution may be done with D5W, LR, NS.[3,14]

Pantoprazole

Maximum concentration	4 mg/mL.[3,14]
Preparation and delivery	**Delivery:** Administer via a dedicated line or Y-site administration after flushing the line before and after with a suitable diluent.[3] **Compatibility:** Observe for any signs of precipitation when administering via Y-site.[3] Incompatible with midazolam, dobutamine, esmolol, norepinephrine, octreotide[13] and may be incompatible with zinc-containing solutions.[3]
IV push	May administer reconstituted 4-mg/mL solution over a minimum of at least 2 minutes.[3,14]
Intermittent infusion	Dilute to 0.4–0.8 mg/mL with suitable diluent and infuse over 15 minutes at a maximum rate of 7 mL/min.[3,14]
Continuous infusion	Not recommended.[3] In *adults*, a single 80-mg IV load followed by 8 mg/h has been used for 3 days.[8-10]
Other routes of administration	No information available to support administration by other routes.
Comments	**Significant adverse effects:** Administration of proton pump inhibitors has been associated with increased risk of developing gastroenteritis and pneumonia in children.[15] Adverse effects may include mild elevation of liver function tests.[3] Prolonged use (>3 years) may lead to impaired absorption of cyanocobalamin (vitamin B12) due to achlorhydria.[16] An *adult* patient developed generalized edema following the initiation of intermittent IV pantoprazole for the treatment of pyloric stenosis.[17] Peripheral edema has been more commonly reported in patients receiving proton pump inhibitors via continuous infusion of large volumes. **Drug interactions:** Pantoprazole is metabolized primarily by CYP2C19 and to a lesser extent by CYP3A4, CYP2D6, and CYP2C9. In vivo drug–drug interaction studies have found that pharmacokinetics are not significantly altered; therefore, there is no need for dosage reductions in general. Drug interaction potential is unknown in patients with hepatic dysfunction or in those receiving large doses.[3] Consult appropriate resources for dosing recommendations before combining any drug with pantoprazole. A known interaction exists between pantoprazole and clopidogrel. Since clopidogrel is metabolized to its active metabolite primarily via CYP2C19, and to a lesser extent, via CYP3A4 and CYP2C9, its use with pantoprazole may decrease the formation of the active metabolite and decrease antiplatelet effects.[18] **Pharmacokinetic considerations:** A randomized, open-label, multicenter trial in hospitalized patients 2–16 years of age found the pharmacokinetics of single oral and IV 0.8 or 1.6 mg/kg pantoprazole doses to be similar to 20, 40, or 80 mg doses in *adults*. The authors noted that plasma clearance in the children appears to be related to CYP2C19 genotype rather than age.[6] Another pharmacokinetic study (computer generated method) evaluated 19.9–140.6 mg/1.73 m^2/day IV pantoprazole in critically ill pediatric patients (10 days to 16.4 years of age) and found more rapid clearance in patients 6 months to 5 years compared to *adults*.[19] **Laboratory interference:** False-positive urine THC has been reported in patients taking proton pump inhibitors, including pantoprazole.[3]

Papaverine HCl

Brand names	Generic
Medication error potential	Look-alike, sound-alike error potential. USP reported that papaverine has the potential to be confused with pamidronate and was confused with Pavulon.[1]
Contraindications and warnings	**Contraindications:** Complete atrioventricular heart block.[2]
Infusion related cautions	May cause arrhythmias, apnea, or death if administered by rapid IV push.[3]
Dosage	**Prolong life of arterial catheters**[4,5]: 30 mg/250 mL heparinized (1 unit/mL) NS or ½NS. (See Comments section.) **Flush of femoral artery catheter after cardiac catheterization:** A single intra-arterial flush of 1.5 mg/kg papaverine or 1 unit heparin/0.25 mL NS was mixed to a volume of 4 mL and infused over 2 minutes in children (3–69 months; n = 56) after cardiac catheterization. Papaverine and heparin flush performed similar in terms of prevention of pulse loss.[6]
Dosage adjustment in organ dysfunction	No information available to support the need for dose adjustment.
Maximum dosage	Not established.
Additives	Multidose vials contain edentate disodium and chlorobutanol (preservative).[2]
Suitable diluents	NS, ½NS.[7]
Maximum concentration	30 mg/mL for vasospasm in *adults* (commercially available).
Preparation and delivery	**Compatibility:** Incompatible in LR.[2]
IV push	Over ≥2 minutes.[2,3]
Intermittent infusion	Diluted in NS and infused over at least 2 minutes.[2,3]
Continuous infusion	May be given continuously.[4,5]

Other routes of administration	IM.[2,3]

Comments	Studies evaluating the efficacy of papaverine in prolonging the life of arterial catheters are limited.

Peginterferon Alfa (alpha-2a, alpha-2b)

Brand names	PEGASYS (alpha-2a), PEG-Intron (alpha-2b)

Medication error potential

None noted.

Contraindications and warnings

US boxed warning: Alpha interferons cause or aggravate fatal or life-threatening neuropsychiatric, autoimmune, ischemic, and infectious disorders. Patients should be monitored closely, and periodic clinical and laboratory valuations should be performed. Treatment should be stopped in patients with persistently severe or worsening signs or symptoms of these conditions. In many cases, but not all, these disorders resolve after therapy is discontinued.[1,2]

Use with ribavirin[1,2]: Ribavirin is mutagenic and genotoxic and is potentially carcinogenic. It may cause birth defects and/or fetal death; therefore, pregnancy should be avoided during ribavirin therapy. Ribavirin causes hemolytic anemia.

Contraindications: Individuals with hypersensitivity to peginterferon alfa or any product components, autoimmune hepatitis, and decompensated liver disease.[1,2]

Infusion related cautions

Not intended for IV use.

Dosage

Interferon-pegylated alpha-2a (PEGASYS): BSA (m^2)/(1.73m^2) × 180 mcg SC once a week for 48 weeks has been used as monotherapy in 14 children from 2–8 years old with chronic hepatitis C.[3] In children who have hepatitis C and who survived cancer, 0.5 mcg/kg (with daily ribavirin) has been used.[4] In older children and *adults* with thalassemia major and chronic hepatitis C, 180 mcg SC once a week for 24 weeks was used with placebo (n = 12) or ribavirin (n = 8).[5] While poor patient recruitment ended the study early, investigators concluded that the combination was probably safe and effective and could be considered in patients with thalassemia and moderate transfusional iron overload.

Interferon-pegylated alpha-2b (PEG-Intron): 1–1.5 mcg/kg SC once a week (with daily ribavirin) has been used in children 2–17 years of age with chronic hepatitis C.[6-9] In *adults*, monotherapy dosing is different from combination (with daily ribavirin) therapy dosing. Both monotherapy and combination therapy are based on weight and concentration of product.[2]

Dosage adjustment in organ dysfunction

Peginterferon alpha-2a (PEGASYS)[1]

Hematologic

Absolute neutrophil count (ANC)

<750/mm³: Decrease dose to 135 mcg (25% decrease).

<500/mm³: Withhold treatment until ANC is 1000/mm³, resume treatment at 90 mcg/kg (50% usual dose).

Platelets

≥50,000/mm³: Continue treatment.

<50,000/mm³: Decrease dose to 90 mcg/kg (50% decrease).

<25,000/mm³: Withhold treatment.

Renal: Use with caution and observe for toxicity in those with CrCl <50 mL/min. In *adults* with end-stage renal disease and on hemodialysis, the dose should be decreased to 135 mcg (a 25% decrease in usual dose of 180 mcg).

Peginterferon Alfa (alpha-2a, alpha-2b)

Dosage adjustment in organ dysfunction (cont.)	**Hepatic:** For increases in ALT, the dose should be decreased. If the increases in ALT are accompanied by increases in bilirubin or are progressive despite a decreased dose, the drug should be discontinued.	

Peginterferon alpha-2b (PEG-Intron)[2]

Hematologic

Hemoglobin	<8.5 g/dL	Permanently discontinue
WBC	<1.5 × 10⁹/L	Reduce dose by 50%
	<1.0 × 10⁹/L	Permanently discontinue
Neutrophils	<0.75 × 10⁹/L	Reduce dose by 50%
	<0.5 × 10⁹/L	Permanently discontinue
Platelets	<80 × 10⁹/L	Reduce dose by 50%
	<50 × 10⁹/L	Permanently discontinue

Renal

CrCl 30–50 mL/min: Reduce dose by 25%.

CrCl 10–29 mL/min (including during hemodialysis): Reduce dose by 50%.

CrCl decreases during treatment: Discontinue.

Maximum dosage	**Peginterferon (PEGASYS):** 180 mcg daily for 1 week was given; no serious adverse effects were noted.[1] **Peginterferon alpha-2b (PEG-Intron):** 3.45 mcg/kg/week over a period of 12 weeks; this overdosage did not result in serious adverse effects.[2]
Additives	**Peginterferon alpha-2a (PEGASYS):** Vials and prefilled syringes contain polysorbate 80 and benzyl alcohol.[1] See Appendix C for specific information about potential benzyl alcohol toxicity in neonates. **Peginterferon alpha-2b (PEG-Intron):** Vials and syringes contain polysorbate 80.[2]
Suitable diluents	Not indicated.
Maximum concentration	**Interferon-pegylated alpha-2a (PEGASYS):** 180 mcg/mL.[1] **Interferon-pegylated alpha-2b (PEG-Intron):** 150 mcg/0.5 mL (also available as 50, 80, and 100 mcg/0.5 mL).[2]
Preparation and delivery	**Peginterferon alpha 2-a:** Single-use syringes or single-dose vials.[1] **Peginterferon alpha-2b (PEG-Intron REDIPEN and vials):** Single-use products, which do not contain preservatives. Once reconstituted, they should be used immediately or refrigerated and used within 24 hours.[2]
IV push	Not indicated.
Intermittent infusion	Not indicated.

Peginterferon Alfa (alpha-2a, alpha-2b)

Continuous infusion

Not indicated.

Other routes of administration

Given by SC injection. IM not indicated.

Comments

Monitoring: Routine monitoring should include CBC, chemistries (including liver function tests), TSH, and triglycerides.

Drug interactions: Interferon-pegylated alpha-2a (PEGASYS) increases theophylline area under the concentration curve by 25%. Theophylline serum concentrations should be monitored during treatment.[1]

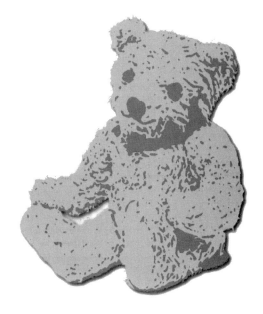

451

Penicillin G Potassium/Sodium

Brand names	Pfizerpen; various generics

Medication error potential

Look-alike, sound-alike drug names.

USP reports confusion with ampicillin, oxacillin, and penicillamine.[1]

Contraindications and warnings

Contraindications: A history of a hypersensitivity (anaphylactic) reaction to any penicillin.[2]

Warnings: Serious hypersensitivity and occasionally fatal anaphylactic reactions have been reported.[2] These are more likely in patients who are sensitive to multiple allergens (e.g., asthma) and in those with a history of Type I reaction to penicillin or cephalosporins.[2] (See Appendix C for specific information.)

Prolonged use may cause superinfection and/or *Clostridium difficile*–associated diarrhea (CDAD), which has been reported and may range in severity from mild diarrhea to fatal colitis.[2] If CDAD is suspected or confirmed, appropriate fluid and electrolyte management, protein supplementation, antibiotic treatment of *C. difficile,* and surgical evaluation should be instituted as clinically indicated.[2]

Infusion related cautions

If a decision is made to give this medication to a patient with known penicillin hypersensitivity, the patient should be closely observed for allergenicity. Although rare, anaphylactoid reactions may require immediate emergency treatment with epinephrine, oxygen, IV steroids, antihistamines, pressor amines, and airway management. Large-dose penicillin therapy (i.e., >10 million units) should be administered slowly due to potential adverse effects of electrolyte imbalance from the potassium content.[3] The total dose of potassium or sodium content should influence the rate of administration.[3] (See Additives section.) Avoid accidental intra-arterial administration; may cause thrombophlebitis.[3]

Dosage

Neonates

Congenital syphilis: If ≤7 days of age, give 100,000 units/kg/day divided q 12 h for 10 days.[3-6] If >7 days of age, give 100,000–150,000 units/kg/day divided q 8 h for 10 days.[3-6] If more than 1 day of therapy is missed, the entire therapy should be repeated.[4]

PNA	<1200 g	≤2000 g	>2000 g
≤7 days	50,000–100,000 units/kg/day divided q 12 h[5]	50,000–100,000 units/kg/day divided q 12 h[3,5,7]	75,000–150,000 units/kg/day divided q 8 h[3,5]
>7 days	50,000–100,000 units/kg/day divided q 12 h[5]*	75,000–225,000 units/kg/day divided q 8 h[3,5]	100,000–200,000 units/kg/day divided q 6 h[3,5]

*Until 4 weeks of age.

Meningitis: If ≤7 days of age and ≤2000 g, give 100,000 units/kg/day divided q 12 h[8]; if ≤7 days of age and >2000 g, give 150,000 units/kg/day divided q 8–12 h.[8,9] Smaller doses and prolonged intervals may be needed in very low birth weight infants. If ≥7 days of age, give 200,000 units/kg/day divided q 6–8 h.[9] For documented group B streptococci, give 250,000 to 450,000 units/kg/day divided q 8 h (if ≤7days of age) and 450,000–500,000 units/kg/day divided q 6 h (if >7 days of age).[5]

Penicillin G Potassium/Sodium

Dosage *(cont.)*	**Infants and children:** Give 100,000–200,000 units/kg/day divided q 6 h for mild-to-moderate infections,[5] and 250,000–400,000 units/kg/day divided q 4–6 h for severe infections.[5]

Bacterial endocarditis

Enterococcal endocarditis: 300,000 units/kg/day divided q 4–6 h for 4–6 weeks (plus gentamicin 3 mg/kg/day divided q 8 h for 2 weeks).[10]

Viridans group, streptococcal or S. bovis (penicillin sensitive): 200,000 units/kg/day divided q 4–6 h for 4 weeks if native valve and 300,000 units/kg/day divided q 4–6 h for 6 weeks if prosthetic valve (with or without gentamicin 3 mg/kg/day divided q 8 h for 2 weeks).[10]

Viridans group, streptococcal or S. bovis (relatively resistant): 300,000 units/kg/day divided q 4–6 h for 4 weeks for native valve and 6 weeks for prosthetic valve (plus gentamicin 3 mg/kg/day divided q 8 h for 2 weeks).[10]

Congenital syphilis: (>1 month after neonatal period) 200,000–300,000 units/kg/day divided q 4–6 h for 10 days.[3,4] If more than 1 day of therapy is missed, the entire course of therapy should be repeated.[4]

Meningitis: Initial empiric therapy should be vancomycin plus cefotaxime or ceftriaxone. If sensitive to penicillin, begin 250,000–400,000 units/kg/day (maximum 12 to 24 million units/day)[3,5,9] divided q 4 h (*Neisseria*) for 7 days[3] or 6 hours (*pneumococcus*) for 10 days.[3]

Dosage adjustment in organ dysfunction	If CrCl is 10–50 mL/min, administer 75% of normal dose; if CrCl is <10 mL/min, give 20% to 50% of normal dose.[11] Additional reduction in dose may be necessary in combined renal and hepatic dysfunction.[12]
Maximum dosage	500,000 units/kg/day,[5] not to exceed 24 million units/day[5] in those with normal renal function and 10 million units/day in end stage renal failure.[11]
Additives	Each million units of penicillin G potassium contain 1.7 mEq potassium and 0.3 mEq sodium, and each million units of penicillin G sodium contain 1.68 mEq sodium.[13]
Suitable diluents	**Penicillin G potassium:** D2.5W, D5W, D10W, NS, LR, ½NS, D5¼NS, D5½NS, D5NS, D5LR, dextran 6% in dextrose, and dextran 6.[13] **Penicillin G sodium:** Variable stability in D5W, NS.[13] See additional resource for more specific information.
Maximum concentration	1 million units/mL.[2] 146,000 units/mL in SW results in a maximum recommended osmolality for peripheral infusion in fluid-restricted patients.[14]
Preparation and delivery	**Delivery system issues:** The mixing of penicillin with an aminoglycoside in vitro can result in substantial inactivation of the aminoglycoside. (See Appendix C for more specific information.) **Stability:** Because of degradation or transformation penicillin G products form rapidly and may be responsible for sensitization, reconstituted solutions should be used immediately.[13] **Compatibility:** See Appendix D for PN compatibility information.[15]
IV push	Not recommended. Rapid administration of large doses my cause electrolyte imbalances due to the potassium content. Cardiac arrest occurred in an infant who erroneously received 500,000 units/kg (containing 1 mEq/kg of potassium) over 2 minutes.[16]

Penicillin G Potassium/Sodium

Intermittent infusion	Infuse over 15–30 minutes.[13] The electrolyte (potassium or sodium) content should be considered when determining the infusion rate. (See Additives section.)
Continuous infusion	Not generally administered by this method; however, large doses may be given by continuous infusion.[2] Sensitization, due to degradation or transformation of penicillin G products, may be increased with continuous infusions over 6–24 hours.[17,18]
Other routes of administration	≤100,000 units/mL cause little discomfort when given IM.[13]
Comments	**Rare adverse effects:** Neurotoxic (e.g., lethargy, confusion, twitching, multifocal myoclonus, localized or generalized epileptiform seizures) may occur with large doses, especially in patients with renal insufficiency.[2,19-22]

Laboratory interference: False-positive urinary glucose results when cupric sulfate solution-based tests (Clinitest, Benedict's solution, Fehling's solution) are used.[2] It is recommended that glucose tests (Diastix, TEST-TAPE, Clinistix) based on enzymatic glucose oxidase reactions be used. Positive direct Coombs' tests have been reported during treatment with penicillin.[2]

Other: Penicillin has been the drug of choice for *naturally* occurring anthrax; however, because of possible penicillin resistance or induction of resistance, the CDC does *not* recommend penicillin monotherapy to treat inhalational anthrax that occurs as the result of biologic warfare or bioterrorism.[23,24] Appropriate combination regimens include ciprofloxacin or doxycycline *and* one or two anti-infective agents that are predicted to be effective.

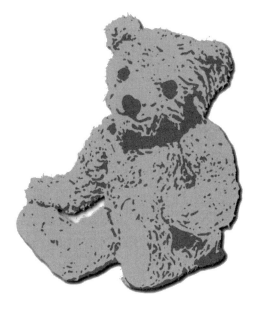

Pentamidine Isethionate

Brand names	Pentam 300
Medication error potential	None noted.

Contraindications and warnings

Contraindications: Patients with hypersensitivity to pentamidine isethionate.[1]

Warnings: Fatalities due to hypotension, cardiac dysrhythmias, hypoglycemia, and acute pancreatitis have been reported.[1-6]

Infusion related cautions

Severe hypotension, hypoglycemia, and cardiac arrhythmias have occurred following rapid administration.[1,3,4,7] Because of the risk of hypotension, the patient should be supine and have blood pressure monitored during IV infusion or IM injection.[1] After the dose is given, blood pressure should be monitored until stable.[1] Emergency equipment for resuscitation should be readily available.

In some cases extravasation has resulted in severe tissue damage requiring surgical debridement and grafting.[1,8] There is no known antidote for treatment of extravasation and management should be symptomatic.

Dosage

Pneumocystis jiroveci pneumonia (PCP)

Treatment (those who are intolerant of trimethoprim/sulfamethoxazole (TMP/SMX) or who do not respond to TMP/SMX): 4 mg/kg/day for 14–21 days.[1,2,9] If there is clinical improvement after 7–10 days, oral atovaquone or trimethoprim/dapsone can be used to complete the treatment.[9]

Prophylaxis: While IV pentamidine has been used, it is no longer recommended for PCP prophylaxis.[9] If TMP/SMX is not tolerated, aerosolized pentamidine via the Respirgard II nebulizer can be used in children (usually >5 years of age) who are able to use the device.[2,9] One study evaluated 4 mg/kg IV given monthly in pediatric oncology patients intolerant of TMP/SMX.[10] Breakthrough PCP was higher in infants than in older children leading investigators to suggest that other options need to be investigated in infants.[10]

Leishmaniasis

Cutaneous: 2–3 mg/kg/day or every other day for up to 7 doses.[11,12]

Visceral: Pentamidine 2 mg/kg IM every other day with daily allopurinol for 30 days was more effective than pentamidine 4 mg/kg every other day for 15 doses in antimony resistant disease in those 5–60 years old.[8]

Dosage adjustment in organ dysfunction

CrCl 10–30 mL/min: Usual dose q 36 h.[13]

CrCl <10 mL/min: Usual normal dose q 48 h.[13]

Neither the safety nor efficacy of dosage adjustments in renal or hepatic dysfunction is known.[1]

Maximum dosage	4 mg/kg.[1]
Additives	None.

Pentamidine Isethionate

Suitable diluents	D5W. Do not use NS to reconstitute because precipitation will occur.[1,14]
Maximum concentration	100 mg/mL for IM use. ~6 mg/mL for IV infusion.[1,11]
Preparation and delivery	**Preparation:** 3–5 mL SW is used to reconstitute the lyophilized powder (300 mg). Further dilution is required for IV infusion.[1,14] **Photosensitivity:** Protect from light during storage.[1]
IV push	Not indicated. Severe hypotension occurs with rapid infusion.[1]
Intermittent infusion	Over 60–120 minutes.[1]
Continuous infusion	Not indicated.
Other routes of administration	Deep IM in *adults*. To minimize local adverse effects, the Z-track injection technique should be used.[1] Nebulization.
Comments	Each 1.74 mg pentamidine isethionate is equivalent to 1 mg pentamidine.[1] **Adverse effects:** Renal toxicity is common following the use of parenteral pentamidine, and usually occurs after 2 weeks of therapy.[1,9] Maintaining adequate hydration and monitoring electrolytes and renal function can help minimize these effects. Nephrotoxicity is usually reversible with discontinuation of the drug.[1] Hypoglycemia and hyperglycemia can occur with parenteral or inhalational therapy and may persist for months after discontinuation. Monitor serum glucose concentrations before, during, and after treatment with pentamidine. Use with caution in patients predisposed to hypoglycemia or hyperglycemia.[1] **Monitoring:** Daily BUN, SCr, and blood glucose. Periodic assessment of CBC, liver function tests, serum calcium, and electrocardiograms is also recommended.[1] **Drug interactions:** Nephrotoxic effects may be additive with use of other drugs with known nephrotoxicity such as amphotericin and the aminoglycosides.[1] Close monitoring of renal function is recommended should it be necessary to combine these agents.

PENTobarbital Sodium

Brand names	Nembutal Sodium

Medication error potential	ISMP high-alert medication (moderate sedation agent IV and anesthetic) that has an increased risk of causing significant patient harm if it is used in error.[1] Look-alike, sound-alike drug names. ISMP recommends the following tall man letters (not FDA approved) to decrease confusion between PENTobarbital and PHENobarbital.[2] USP reports confusion with phenobarbital.[3]

Contraindications and warnings	**Contraindications:** In patients with known hypersensitivity to barbiturates and in patients with a history of manifest or latent porphyria.[4] **Warnings:** May be habit forming. Should be withdrawn gradually if large doses have been used for prolonged periods.[4] Rapid administration may cause respiratory depression, apnea, laryngospasm, or vasodilation with hypotension.[4] Paradoxical excitement may occur or important symptoms could be masked when given to patients with acute or chronic pain.[4]

Infusion related cautions	Respiratory depression and arrest requiring mechanical ventilation may occur. Monitor oxygen saturation. If hypotension occurs, the infusion rate should be decreased and/or the patient should be treated with IV fluids and/or vasopressors. Pentobarbital is an alkaline solution (pH = 9–10.5); therefore, extravasation may cause tissue necrosis.[4] Gangrene may occur following inadvertent intra-arterial injection.[4]

Dosage	**Procedural sedation:** 1–6 mg/kg over 30 seconds (≤50 mg/min).[8-10] If no response within 1 minute, give 1–2 mg/kg to desired effect.[9] Repeat up to a total dose of 7.5 mg/kg.[11] Patients chronically receiving barbiturates may require doses of 9 mg/kg.[11,12] **Sedation with mechanical ventilation:** A loading dose of 1–2 mg/kg followed by a continuous infusion of 1–2 mg/kg/h.[12-14] Reload and titrate infusion to desired effect. **Therapeutic coma (for persistently elevated ICP or refractory status epilepticus):** A loading dose of 15–35 mg/kg over 60–120 minutes[15-20] followed by 1.5–3.5 mg/kg/h.[15-20] Reload and titrate infusion to desired effect. If hypotension occurs, decrease infusion rate or treat with IV fluids and vasopressors.

Dosage adjustment in organ dysfunction	No dosage adjustment required in renal failure.[4,21] Use cautiously and decrease initial dose in hepatic dysfunction.[4]

Maximum dosage	**Sedation:** Total cumulative doses have ranged from 1.3–9.5 mg/kg,[6,7,21] with a mean of 4.4 mg/kg,[6] up to 100 mg/dose.[4,9] **Therapeutic coma:** Individualize therapy by titrating dosage based on EEG, ICP, cerebral perfusion pressure, and blood pressure.[15,22,23] Serum pentobarbital concentrations of 20–40 mg/L should produce an isoelectric EEG.[22]

Additives	Contains propylene glycol (40% v/v).[4] (See Appendix C for specific information about propylene glycol potential for toxicity.)

PENTobarbital Sodium

Suitable diluents	D2.5W, D5W, D10W, LR, ¼NS, ½NS, NS, D5LR, D5¼NS, D5½NS, dextran 6%-D5, dextran 6%-D5NS, and dextran 6%-RL.[4,24,25]
Maximum concentration	50 mg/mL for intermittent infusion.[24]
Preparation and delivery	**Stability:** Stored at room temperature (30°C). Brief exposure up to (40°C) does not adversely affect the product, but protect from freezing.[4] **Compatibility:** See Appendix D for PN compatibility information.[26]
IV push	Not recommended. Rapid infusion may cause hypotension and decreased myocardial contractility.[4,25]
Intermittent infusion	50 mg/mL given over 10–30 minutes,[4] not to exceed 50 mg/min.[4] In order to decrease hypotension, a loading dose should be given over 60–120 minutes.[4,19,21-23]
Continuous infusion	50 mg/mL.[24]
Other routes of administration	2–6 mg/kg (not to exceed 100 mg) as a single injection given deep into a large muscle.[4] The volume of the injection at any one site should not exceed 5 mL.[4]
Comments	**Rare adverse effects:** Administration of large doses of pentobarbital for more than 4 days may be associated with pulmonary edema, pneumonia, and ileus.[27] For these reasons, some practitioners suggest that tapering of pentobarbital should be attempted 12 hours after a burst-suppression pattern is obtained on EEG.[28] Anticonvulsant hypersensitivity syndrome is an acute, life-threatening, idiosyncratic reaction that has been reported in patients receiving phenytoin, phenobarbital, carbamazepine, primidone, and lamotrigine.[29-31] Symptoms generally develop within 1–12 weeks following initiation and include a classic triad of fever, rash, and lymphadenopathy.[29-31] Peripheral blood leucocytosis and eosinophilia and internal organ involvement may also be noted. Immediate discontinuation of the suspected anticonvulsant is essential for good outcome.[29-31] Cross-reactivity among the aromatic anticonvulsants has been noted; hence, these should not be used as alternative agents.[29-31] **Monitoring:** Large variability exists in patient response to initial and maintenance doses; hence, individualize dosage based on serum concentration and clinical response. Therapeutic serum concentrations are 1–5 mg/L (hypnotic) and 10–50 mg/L (coma).[25] **Drug interactions:** Pentobarbital is associated with numerous drug interactions[25]; consult appropriate resources for dosing recommendations before combining any drug with pentobarbital. **Pharmacodynamics:** Neonates may have an increased risk for complications from pentobarbital coma.[32] **Other:** One case report described pentobarbital desensitization in a 3-month-old with refractory status epilepticus who had a known allergy to phenobarbital.[33]

PHENobarbital Sodium

Brand names	Luminal Sodium

Medication error potential

ISMP high-alert medication that have an increased risk of causing significant patient harm if it is used in error.[1]

ISMP recommends the following tall man Letters to decrease confusion between PENTobarbital and PHENobarbital.[2]

Look-alike, sound-alike drug names.

USP reports confusion with pentobarbital, Phenergan, and phenytoin sodium. Confusion with phenytoin has resulted in patient harm and death[3]

Contraindications and warnings

Contraindications: In patients with known hypersensitivity to barbiturates or any component of the formulation.[4] Should not be used in patients with a history of manifest or latent porphyria, marked hepatic impairment, dyspnea or airway obstruction, nephritic patients (large doses) or in those with a history of sedative/hypnotic addiction.[4] Should not be given intra-arterially or subcutaneously.[4]

Warnings: May be habit forming.[4] Should be withdrawn gradually if large doses have been used for prolonged periods.[4] Rapid administration may cause respiratory depression, apnea, laryngospasm, or hypotension.[4] Paradoxical excitement may occur or important symptoms could be masked when given to patients with acute or chronic pain.[4] (See Rare adverse effects in Comments section for information on suicide).

Infusion related cautions

May cause respiratory depression or apnea if administered too rapidly or when combined with other sedatives.[4] Extravasation may cause tissue necrosis.[5] Inadvertent intra-arterial injection can cause spasms, severe pain, and other symptoms (e.g., discolored skin or white hand with cyanosed skin) along the involved artery, which can result in local reactions varying from transient pain to gangrene.[4,5]

Dosage

Hyperbilirubinemia: Studies evaluating the use to prevent or treat neonatal hyperbilirubinemia and decrease the need for phototherapy and exchange transfusion are mixed.[6-9] 5 mg/kg/day within 6 hours of life for 5 days reduced the duration of phototherapy[6]; however, 5 mg/kg/day for 3 days did not decrease the need for phototherapy or exchange transfusion.[7] 12 mg/kg as a single dose within hours of life significantly increased the rate of bilirubin disappearance, but the effect was not noted until day 7.[8] A dose of 20 mg/kg followed by 5 mg/kg/day for 1 week did not produce a clinically important difference when used with phototherapy.[9]

Neonatal abstinence syndrome: An opiate is the preferred initial therapy; however, addition of phenobarbital may decrease severity.[10,11] A loading dose of 20 mg/kg followed by 2–6 mg/kg/day.[12] If the severity score is <8, then a serum concentration of 20 mg/L is adequate and the dose should be maintained for 72 hours.[12] If the score is >8, give 10 mg/kg q 12 h until the syndrome is better or serum concentrations reach 70 mg/L.[12] Once the infant is stable for 72 hours, the dose should be decreased 15% per day.[12] When the severity score is <8 and serum concentration <15 mg/L, phenobarbital should be stopped.[12]

PHENobarbital Sodium

Dosage (cont.)

Prophylactic seizure therapy in severe perinatal asphyxia: There is little evidence from randomized controlled trials to support the use of any of the anticonvulsants.[13] 40 mg/kg/dose over 60 minutes given as soon as possible is associated with a 27% reduction in seizures and significant improvement in neurological outcome at 3 years of age.[14] Term infants with asphyxia had higher trough serum concentration than those without asphyxia[15] and require about half the maintenance dose of nonasphyxiated neonates.[16]

Seizures—nonstatus epilepticus

Neonates: Loading dose (see Seizures—status epilepticus below). Maintenance doses of 3.5–4.5 mg/kg/day if ≤35 weeks and 4–5 mg/kg/day if >35 weeks gestational age.[16] Dose >5 mg/kg/day are generally associated with toxicity.[17] Serum phenobarbital concentrations should be >40 mg/L before an additional anticonvulsant is used.[18]

Infants and children: Loading dose (see Seizures—status epilepticus below). Maintenance doses of ≤5 mg/kg/day.[19-21] If 1–5 years of age then 6–8 mg/kg/day, if 5–12 years of age then 4–6 mg/kg/day, and if 12 years of age give 1–3 mg/kg/day.[19] All doses may be given BID or once daily.[19-21]

Seizures—status epilepticus (persistent or recurrent)

Neonates: Some suggest that a benzodiazepine is the initial treatment of choice.[22] A loading dose of 8–10 mg/kg/day for 2 days,[23] 15–20 mg/kg,[17,24] or 30 mg/kg[25] has been suggested. Maintenance dose of ≤5 mg/kg/day divided BID or given once daily.[26]

Infants and children: Some suggest that this should only be used when maximum doses of benzodiazepine and hydantoin have failed.[25] Loading dose of 20 mg/kg[26-28] up to 1000 mg.[27] Some have advocated an additional 20 mg/kg/dose if no response within 15 minutes.[27]

Refractory status: May use a continuous infusion of a short-acting barbiturate (see Pentobarbital monograph). 10 mg/kg/dose q 30 min (maximum 120 mg/kg in 24 hours),[29] 5–10 mg/kg/dose to a total dose of 80 mg/kg.[30] (See Maximum dosage section.)

Maintenance dose: See Seizures—nonstatus epilepticus above.

Dosage adjustment in organ dysfunction

Adjust dosage using serum concentrations in patients with severe renal dysfunction.[31] If CrCl <10 mL/min, give 50% of normal dose q 24 h.[31] Larger dosages are necessary in children undergoing continuous cycling peritoneal dialysis[32] and in neonates on ECMO.[33,34]

Maximum dosage

<30[25]– 40[22,27] mg/kg as a loading dose. Up to 300 mg/dose[4,5] or 1 g/dose[23] for status epilepticus. Total doses of 70–120 mg/kg were given over 24 hours to children with refractory status epilepticus.[29,30] Because of interpatient variability in phenobarbital elimination, individualize dosage based on serum concentrations.

Additives

May contain benzyl alcohol and/or propylene glycol.[4] (See Appendix C for specific information about benzyl alcohol propylene glycol potential for toxicity.)

PHENobarbital Sodium

Suitable diluents	May be diluted with an equal volume of D2.5W, D5W, D10W, RI, LR, NS, ½NS, D-R, D-LR, D-saline combinations, dextran 6%-D5W, and dextran 6%-LR.[35]
Maximum concentration	130 mg/mL.[35]
Preparation and delivery	**Compatibility:** See Appendix D for PN compatibility information.[36] **Photosensitivity:** Protect from light.[5]
IV push	Not recommended.
Intermittent infusion	<30, 60, 65, or 130 mg/mL undiluted (available commercially)[4] and infuse over 3–5 minutes, not to exceed 30 mg/min[5] or 50–75 mg/min[4,26] or 1 mg/kg/min[5] to 2 mg/kg/min.[25,37] Large loading doses (e.g., 40 mg/kg) may be infused over 60 minutes.[14]
Continuous infusion	No information available.
Other routes of administration	May be given IM deep into muscle at a volume <5 mL.[4]
Comments	**Rare adverse effects** **Anticonvulsant hypersensitivity syndrome:** An acute, life-threatening, idiosyncratic reaction that has been reported in patients receiving phenytoin, phenobarbital, carbamazepine, primidone, and lamotrigine.[38-40] Symptoms generally develop within 1–12 weeks following initiation and include a classic triad of fever, rash, and lymphadenopathy.[38-40] Peripheral blood leucocytosis and eosinophilia and internal organ involvement may also be noted. Immediate discontinuation of the suspected anticonvulsant is essential for good outcome.[38-40] Cross-reactivity among the aromatic anticonvulsants has been noted; hence, these should not be used as alternative agents.[38-40] **Suicidal behavior/ideation:** The incidence of this adverse effect has been noted to be greater than placebo (0.43% vs 0.24% risk) in patients receiving 11 anticonvulsants (carbamazepine, divalproex sodium, felbamate, gabapentin, lamotrigine, levetiracetam, oxcarbazepine, pregabalin, tiagabine, topiramate, zonisamide) as either monotherapy or as adjuvant therapy for the treatment of epilepsy, psychiatric disorders, and other conditions.[41] The FDA will require that the product labeling of the entire class of antiepileptics include a warning concerning the risk of suicidality. **Monitoring:** Large variability exists in patient response to initial and maintenance dosages; individualize dosage based on serum concentration and clinical response. Therapeutic serum concentrations is 15–40 mg/L. Significantly higher serum concentrations are required if used for medically induced coma (>100 mg/L with no reflexes). **Drug interactions:** Phenobarbital is a substrate for CYP2C9, CYP2C19, and CYP2E1.[5] Because phenobarbital induces the CYP1A2; CYP2A6, CYP2C8, CYP2C9 and CYP3A4 and UGT, it is associated with numerous drug interactions[5]; consult appropriate resources for dosing recommendations before combining any drug with phenobarbital.

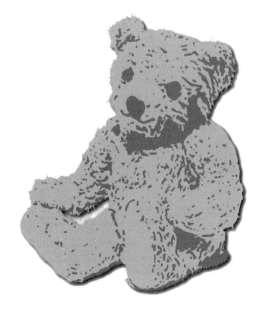

Phenytoin Sodium

Brand names	Dilantin, Phenytek

Medication error potential

Look-alike, sound-alike drug names.

USP reports confusion with Feldene, fluconazole, fosphenytoin, nystatin, phenazopyridine, phenobarbital, and phytonadione.[1] Dilantin has been confused with Diflucan, Dilaudid, Diltiazem, Neutrotin, and Nystatin.[1] Confusion with fosphenytoin and phenobarbital has resulted in patient harm and confusion with phenobarbital has resulted in death.[1]

Contraindications and warnings

Contraindications: Phenytoin is contraindicated in patients with a history of hypersensitivity to hydantoin products.[2] Parenteral phenytoin effects ventricular automaticity and is contraindicated in patients with sinus bradycardia, sino-atrial block, second and third degree A-V block, and Adams-Stokes syndrome.[2]

Warnings: Intravenous rate of administration should not exceed 50 mg/min in *adults* and 1–3 mg/kg/min in neonates.[2] Phenytoin should be used with caution in patients with hypotension and severe myocardial insufficiency.

The FDA is investigating the possibility of an increased risk of serious skin reactions (e.g., Stevens-Johnson syndrome and toxic epidermal necrolysis) in patients given phenytoin who have the human leukocyte antigen allele HLA-B*1502.[3] This allele occurs almost exclusively in individuals with ancestry across broad areas of Asia, including Han Chinese, Filipinos, Malaysians, South Asian Indians, and Thais.[3] Until the FDA evaluation is finalized, phenytoin should be avoided as an alternative for carbamazepine in patients who test positive for HLA-B*1502.[3] (See Monitoring in Comments section.)

A relationship between phenytoin and the development of localized or generalized lymphadenopathy including benign lymph node hyperplasia, pseudolymphoma, lymphoma and Hodgkin's disease has been noted.[2] Lymph node involvement may occur with or without symptoms and signs resembling anticonvulsant hypersensitivity syndrome. (See Comments section.)

Infusion related cautions

Rapid administration has resulted in hypotension, cardiovascular collapse, and CNS depression.[2]

Purple glove syndrome is the development of progressive distal limb edema, discoloration, and pain after peripheral administration of IV phenytoin.[4] Although this may occur from a reaction of the interstitial tissue to extravasation of phenytoin, it can occur in the absence of infiltration. It may result in extensive skin necrosis, limb ischemia, and compartmental syndrome, which may necessitate fasciotomies, skin grafting, or limb amputation. (See Appendix E for management.)

Because of the high risk of extravasation and local tissue irritation with peripheral administration of phenytoin, especially in neonates with peripheral scalp IV lines, fosphenytoin should be considered. (See Fosphenytoin monograph.)

Dosage

In obese patients with active seizures the loading doses should be calculated on adjusted body weight using the following equation[5] (see Appendix B):

Dosing weight (kg) = Ideal Body Weight (IBW) + 1.33 (measured weight − IBW)

Arrhythmias (Class 1B) (digoxin-induced tachyarrhythmias): 1.25 mg over 5 minutes. May repeat q 5 min titrated to a total of 15 mg/kg.[6]

Post-traumatic epilepsy (see status epilepticus for dosing): Although prophylactic phenytoin has been used for the prevention of epilepsy following head trauma, its use is controversial.[7,8] It should *not* be used for the prevention of late epilepsy.[9] Children with severe, acute neurotrauma have markedly altered protein binding and phenytoin metabolism and may require larger doses and more frequent dosing.[9,10] Free serum phenytoin concentration should be monitored.

Dosage *(cont.)*

Status epilepticus

Loading dose (assumes no previous phenytoin)

Neonates: 8–20 mg/kg[2,11-13] (may prefer to use phenobarbital or a benzodiazepine).

Infants and children: 10–20 mg/kg[14-16] not to exceed 1 g.[14]

Adolescents and *adults*: 10 to 15 mg/kg not to exceed 1 g.[2]

Maintenance dose

Neonates: 4–8 mg/kg/day divided q 12–24 h.[11,12] Some suggest smaller doses of 3–5 mg/kg/day.[13] Extremely difficult to obtain serum concentrations following conversion to oral therapy; therefore, consider an alternative anticonvulsant for oral dosing.[9,17]

Infants and children: For 4 weeks to <1 years, 4–8 mg/kg/day.[13] For 1–12 years, 8–10 mg/kg/day divided q 8 h.[13-15]

Adolescents and *adults*: If ≥12 years, 4–8 mg/kg/day divided q 8–12 h.[13] The manufacturer recommends 100 mg every 6–8 hours.[2]

Dosage adjustment in organ dysfunction

Dosage adjustment may be required in patients with hepatic[2] or renal dysfunction.[18,19]

Maximum dosage

20 mg/kg as a single dose,[20] not to exceed 1 g.[21,22] Doses as large as 25 mg/kg/day divided q 6 h were used to achieve total serum phenytoin concentrations within the "therapeutic range" in a neonate.[22] If large doses are used, free phenytoin concentrations should be monitored. Because of age-dependent variation in phenytoin elimination, individualize dosage based on total or free serum concentrations.

Additives

Undiluted injection contains 0.2 mEq sodium/mL of phenytoin.[23] Contains 40% propylene glycol. (See Appendix C for specific information about propylene glycol and potential for toxicity.)

Suitable diluents

Phenytoin is highly unstable in any IV solution; therefore, use only NS for dilution and do not mix with other medications.[23] An in-line 0.22–5 micron filter is recommended due to the high potential for precipitation of the solution.[23]

Maximum concentration

50 mg/mL (commercially available).[2]

Preparation and delivery

Stability: Use only a clear solution that is free from haziness or precipitant.[23] Although a faint yellow color may develop, this has no effect on potency.[23] Upon refrigeration or freezing, a precipitate might form; however, this will dissolve when allowed to stand at room temperature.[23] No evidence of DEHP leaching from PVC bag.[23]

Compatibility: See Appendix D for PN compatibility information.[24]

IV push

Not recommended.[2]

Intermittent infusion

≤50 mg/mL.[2] If necessary, dilute with NS[2,23] to a concentration <6 mg/mL[25] and infuse at a rate of 1–3 mg/kg/min in neonates, infants, and young children[2,20,22] or 50 mg/min in older children and *adults*.[2,20] Following administration, flush needle or catheter with NS.

Phenytoin Sodium

Continuous infusion

Not recommended.[2]

Other routes of administration

The manufacturer suggests that IM administration is acceptable, but does not recommend it for the treatment of status epilepticus.[2] Most practitioners would not administer phenytoin IM because of severe pain at the injection site, erratic absorption, possible precipitation of drug in tissue and severe damage due to infiltration.[26] Has been given intraosseously.[27]

Comments

Rare adverse effects

Anticonvulsant hypersensitivity syndrome: is an acute, life-threatening, idiosyncratic reaction that has been reported in patients receiving phenytoin, phenobarbital, carbamazepine, primidone, and lamotrigine.[28-30] Symptoms generally develop within 1–12 weeks following initiation and include a classic triad of fever, rash, and lymphadenopathy.[28-30] Peripheral blood leucocytosis and eosinophilia and internal organ involvement may also occur. Immediate discontinuation of the suspected anticonvulsant is essential for good outcome.[28-30] Cross-reactivity among the aromatic anticonvulsants has been noted; hence, these should not be used as alternative agents.[28-30]

Discontinuation of phenytoin abruptly may increase seizure frequency and/or precipitate status epilepticus. If an allergic or hypersensitivity reaction or if a life-threatening adverse event occurs, rapid substitution of an alternative anticonvulsant may be necessary. If phenytoin is discontinued due to development of a rash, an anticonvulsant *not* belonging to the hydantoin family and one structurally dissimilar should be used.[28-30]

Suicidal behavior/ideation: The risk of this adverse effect has been noted to be greater than placebo (0.43% vs 0.24% risk) in patients receiving 11 anticonvulsants (i.e., carbamazepine, divalproex sodium, felbamate, gabapentin, lamotrigine, levetiracetam, oxcarbazepine, pregabalin, tiagabine, topiramate, zonisamide) as either monotherapy or as adjuvant therapy for the treatment of epilepsy, psychiatric disorders, and other conditions.[31] The FDA will require that the product labeling of the entire class of antiepileptics include a warning concerning the risk of suicide.

Monitoring: Because large variability exists in patient response to dose, individualize dosage based on serum concentration and clinical response. Due to an increased fraction of unbound phenytoin in patients with renal or hepatic disease, or in those with hypoalbuminemia, the interpretation of total phenytoin plasma concentrations should be made with caution and unbound phenytoin concentrations may be more useful.[18] Free phenytoin serum concentrations should be measured in newborns, in patients with renal dysfunction, or in those who are hypoalbuminemic because of decreases in protein binding, increases in volume of distribution, and altered clearance.[10,18] Continuously monitor of blood pressure, respiratory function, heart rate, and ECG during IV loading doses and for approximately 10–20 minutes after the end of an infusion.[2] If the heart rate decreases by more than 10 beats/min the infusion rate should be decreased.[21]

The FDA does not recommend testing for the presence of *HLA-B*1502* prior to initiating phenytoin.[3]

Drug interactions: Because phenytoin induces the CYP2C19 and CYP3A families and UGT, it is associated with numerous drug interactions.[32] Phenytoin may also serve as a substrate and can be inhibited or induced by other drugs.[32] Consult appropriate resources for dosing recommendations before combining any drug with phenytoin.

Laboratory interference: Phenytoin may cause decreased serum levels of protein-bound iodine.[2] It may also produce lower than normal values for dexamethasone or metyrapone tests) and may cause increased serum levels of glucose, alkaline phosphatase and gamma glutamyl transpeptidase.[2]

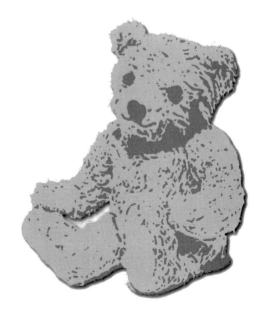

Physostigmine Salicylate

Brand names	Antilirium, generic

Medication error potential

Look-alike, sound-alike error potential.

USP reports that physostigmine has been confused with pyridostigmine; no patient harm resulted.[1]

Contraindications and warnings

Contraindicated in asthma, gangrene, diabetes, cardiovascular disease, and mechanical obstruction of the gastrointestinal or urogenital tract.[2] It should also not be used in patients receiving choline esters or depolarizing neuromuscular blocking agents (e.g., decamethonium, succinylcholine).[2]

Infusion related cautions

Bradycardia, asystole, convulsions, and hypersalivation have occurred following rapid injection.[2-4]

Physostigmine overdose may precipitate a cholinergic crisis.[2] Atropine sulfate injection should be available as an antagonist and antidote for physostigmine-associated life-threatening symptoms.[2,3] The dose of atropine should be 50% of the administered dose of physostigmine.[3]

Dosage

Anticholinergic toxicity

Pediatric patients: 0.02 mg/kg up to 0.5 mg/dose to reverse anticholinergic effects. If toxic effects persist, give 0.5 mg q 5–10 min up to 2 mg maximum dose.[2-8]

Adolescents and *adults*: 1–2 mg to reverse anticholinergic effects. If toxic effects persist, give 1 mg q 10–20 min up to 4 mg.[2-5,9]

Dosage adjustment in organ dysfunction

No information is available regarding dosage adjustment in organ dysfunction.

Maximum dosage

2 mg in pediatric patients[2-6] and 4 mg in adolescents or *adults*.[3]

No maximum cumulative dose established. A total of 22 mg was administered IV over 48 hours to a 22-year-old patient.[10]

Additives

Contains benzyl alcohol 2% as a preservative.[2] See Appendix C for more specific information about potential adverse effects and/or benzyl alcohol toxicity in neonates.

Contains sodium metabisulfite 0.1%.[2] Physostigmine should not be withheld from an individual with life-threatening anticholinergic toxicity who is sulfite sensitive.[4] Epinephrine should be available. See Appendix C for more specific information about potential adverse effects of sulfites.

Suitable diluents

D5W, NS.[11]

Maximum concentration

1 mg/mL.[2]

Physostigmine Salicylate

Preparation and delivery	Have atropine on hand.[2] (See Infusion related cautions section.)
IV push	Not recommended.[2] (See Infusion related cautions section.)
Intermittent infusion	1 mg/mL or dilute with 10-mL suitable diluent and infuse over 5–10 minutes, not to exceed 0.5 mg/min in children or 1 mg/min in *adults*.[2]
Continuous infusion	0.02 mg/mL in D5W has been given by continuous infusion to a 20-year-old.[12]
Other routes of administration	May be given IM at same doses as IV.[2]
Comments	**Significant adverse effects:** Two *adults* developed sinus bradycardia after receiving physostigmine for tricyclic overdose. Following 1 mg of atropine, both patients developed asystole.[13]
	Other: Although physostigmine has been used previously for tricyclic antidepressant toxicity in *adults* and children,[6,14] it now is recommended only for life-threatening symptoms unresponsive to other therapies.[15]
	The use of physostigmine in the central anticholinergic syndrome has been described in an infant and a child.[16,17]
	Physostigmine successfully treated post anesthesia emergence delirium (cognitive and psychomotor deficits, irritability, anxiety, apathy, and sleep disturbances, including nightmares) in a randomized, controlled trial in children 1–5 years of age. The dose of physostigmine was 0.03 mg/kg in NS given over 1 minute. Nausea and vomiting was increased in children receiving physostigmine. The authors suggested increasing the infusion to 5 minutes and giving dexamethasone to prevent theses symptoms.[18]

Piperacillin Sodium

Brand names	Pipracil

Medication error potential

Look-alike, sound-alike drug names.

USP reports confusion with ampicillin and ticarcillin.[1]

Contraindications and warnings

Contraindications: In those with a history of allergic reactions to any of the beta-lactams, including penicillins and/or cephalosporins.[2]

Warnings

Allergic reactions: Serious hypersensitivity and occasionally fatal anaphylactic reactions have been reported.[2] These are more likely in patients who are sensitive to multiple allergens (e.g., asthma) and in those with a history of penicillin, cephalosporins, or other beta-lactam hypersensitivity.[2]

Superinfection: Prolonged use may cause superinfection and/or *Clostridium difficile*–associated diarrhea (CDAD), which has been reported and may range in severity from mild diarrhea to fatal colitis.[2] If CDAD is suspected or confirmed, appropriate fluid and electrolyte management, protein supplementation, antibiotic treatment of *C. difficile,* and surgical evaluation should be instituted as clinically indicated.[2] Antibiotic use that is not directed against *C. difficile* may need to be discontinued.[2]

Infusion related cautions

Closely monitor patients with known penicillin hypersensitivity for allergenicity.[2] Anaphylactic reactions require immediate treatment with epinephrine. Oxygen, IV steroids, and airway management may be indicated.[2]

Thrombophlebitis has been reported in 4% to 13% of patients.[2]

Dosage

Neonates: 200 mg/kg/day divided q 12 h.[3] If <36 weeks gestational age, give 150 mg/kg/day divided q 12 h for 1 week and then 225 mg/kg/day divided q 8 h.[4] If >36 weeks gestational age, give 225 mg/kg/day divided q 8 h for 1 week and then 300 mg/kg/day divided q 6 h.[4]

Infants and children

Mild-to-moderate infections: 100–150 mg/kg/day divided q 6 h, up to 8 g/day.[5]

Severe infections: 200–300 mg/kg/day divided q 4–6 h, up to 24 g/day.[5-7]

Appendectomy (perforated): 200 mg/kg/day divided q 8 h.[8]

Cystic fibrosis: 300–600 mg/kg/day divided q 4–6 h.[9,10]

Febrile neutropenia: Administer 300 mg/kg/day divided q 8 h in conjunction with other antibiotics.[11,12]

Perioperative prophylaxis: In adolescents, give 2 g 30 minutes before the procedure.[13]

Dosage adjustment in organ dysfunction

If CrCl is 10–50 mL/min, give normal dose q 6–12 h; if CrCl is <10 mL/min, give q 12 h.[2,14,15]

Maximum dosage

500 mg/kg/day,[9] 600 mg/kg/day in patients with cystic fibrosis[9,10] not to exceed 18 g/day in children[5] and 24 g/day in *adults*.[2]

Additives

Contains 1.85 mEq sodium/g of piperacillin sodium.[2,16]

Piperacillin Sodium

Suitable diluents	D5NS, D5W, NS, LR, BW, or Dextran 6%NS.[2,16]
Maximum concentration	200 mg/mL for IV push,[2,16] 163 mg/mL for IV infusion,[17] and 400 mg/mL for IM administration.[2,16]
Preparation and delivery	**Delivery system issues:** The mixing of piperacillin with an aminoglycoside in vitro can result in substantial inactivation of the aminoglycoside.[18-22] (See Appendix C for more specific information.) **Stability:** Use immediately after reconstitution.[2] Unused portion that has been stored at room temperature (20°C to 25°C) for 24 hours or after 48 hours if refrigerated (2°C to 8°C) should be discarded.[2] **Compatibility:** See Appendix D for PN compatibility information.[23]
IV push	200 mg/mL infused over 3–5 minutes.[2,16]
Intermittent infusion	45–70 mg/mL over 20–60 minutes.[2,16]
Continuous infusion	Piperacillin/tazobactam and other beta-lactam antibiotics have been given by this method.[24-27]
Other routes of administration	May be given by IM administration using 400 mg/mL in SW, NS, bacteriostatic SW or NS, D5W or D5NS, or lidocaine HCl 0.5% to 1% (without epinephrine).[2,16] Should be injected deep into the upper-outer quadrant of the buttock. Maximum dose injected into one site should not exceed 2 g.[16]
Comments	**Rare adverse effects:** Piperacillin is more allergenic (e.g., fever, rash) in patients with cystic fibrosis.[28] Serum-like sickness and coagulopathy associated with fever, rash, and abnormal liver function tests occurred in two patients with cystic fibrosis.[29] Abnormal coagulation tests (e.g., clotting time, platelet aggregation, and prothrombin time) may occur, especially in patients with cystic fibrosis[2,29] or renal failure.[2] Piperacillin should be discontinued if bleeding occurs.[2] Tonic-clonic seizures have been reported in an 11-year-old child receiving IV piperacillin (3 g q 4 h) over 30 minutes.[30] **Monitoring:** Coagulation parameters should be monitored frequently during simultaneous administration of large doses of heparin, oral anticoagulants, or other drugs that may affect the blood coagulation system or the thrombocyte function.[2] **Drug interactions:** Piperacillin may decrease the clearance of methotrexate.[2,32] Antibiotics may diminish the therapeutic effect of Typhoid Vaccine, but only the live attenuated Ty21a strain is affected.[31] Perioperative use of piperacillin may prolong the neuromuscular blockade of vecuronium or other nondepolarizing muscle relaxants.[2,33] Probenecid may decrease the clearance of piperacillin.[2] Consult appropriate resources for dosing recommendations before combining any drug with piperacillin. **Laboratory interference:** A false-positive urinary glucose results when cupric sulfate solution-based tests (Clinitest, Benedict's solution, Fehling's solution) are used.[2] It is recommended that glucose tests (Diastix or TEST-TAPE) based on enzymatic glucose oxidase reactions be used.[2] Piperacillin/tazobactam may cause a false positive *Aspergillus* infection result when performed with the Bio-Rad Laboratories Platelia *Aspergillus* EIA test; hence, interpret reports cautiously and confirmed by other diagnostic measures.[2]

Piperacillin Sodium–Tazobactam Sodium

Brand names	Zosyn

Medication error potential

Look-alike, sound-alike drug names.

USP reports confusion between piperacillin and nafcillin.[1] Zosyn has been confused with cefazolin, Unasyn, Zofran and Zyvox.[1]

Contraindications and warnings

Contraindications: In those with a history of allergic reactions to any of the betalactams, including penicillins and/or cephalosporins.[2]

Warnings

Allergic reactions: Serious hypersensitivity and occasionally fatal anaphylactic reactions have been reported.[2] These are more likely in patients who are sensitive to multiple allergens (e.g., asthma) and in those with a history of penicillin, cephalosporins, or other beta-lactam hypersensitivity.[2]

Superinfection: Prolonged use may cause superinfection and/or *Clostridium difficile*-associated diarrhea (CDAD), which has been reported and may range in severity from mild diarrhea to fatal colitis.[2] If CDAD is suspected or confirmed, appropriate fluid and electrolyte management, protein supplementation, antibiotic treatment of *C. difficile,* and surgical evaluation should be instituted as clinically indicated.[2] Antibiotic use that is not directed against *C. difficile* may need to be discontinued.[2]

Infusion related cautions

If given to a patient with known penicillin hypersensitivity, closely observed for allergenicity.[2] Anaphylactic reactions require immediate treatment with epinephrine. Oxygen, IV steroids and airway management may be indicated.[2]

Thrombophlebitis has been reported in 4% to 13% of patients.[2]

Dosage

Tazobactam is a beta-lactamase inhibitor that extends the spectrum of piperacillin but has little antibacterial activity. Piperacillin/tazobactam is available in a ratio of 8:1 (piperacillin:tazobactam).[2] *Doses are based on piperacillin component*.[2]

Neonates: Safety in patients <2 months of age has not been established.[2] 100–300 mg/kg/day divided q 8–12 h.[3-5]

Infants and children: Inappropriate in mild-to-moderate infections.[6] For severe infections in those 2–9 months of age give 240 mg/kg/day divided q 8 h up to 18 g/day.[2,6] In those >9 months of age (up to 40 kg) give 300 mg/kg/day divided q 8 h up to 18 g/day.[2,6] Those weighing more than 40 kg should receive *adult* dose of 12 g/day divided q 6 h.[2] Based on a single-dose pharmacokinetic study, doses of 100 mg/kg q 8 h for bacteria whose MIC is 2 mg/L and q 6 h if the MIC is between 4 and 8 mg/L should be effective.[7]

Cystic fibrosis: 350–450 mg/kg/day divided q 6 h.[8,9]

Dosage adjustment in organ dysfunction

If CrCl is 30–50 mL/min, give 150–200 mg/kg/day divided q 6 h; if CrCl is 10–29 mL/min, give 150–200 mg/kg/day divided q 8 h; and if CrCl is <10 mL/min, give 150–200 mg/kg/day divided q 12 h.[10] No adjustment necessary in liver impairment.[11]

Maximum dosage

450 mg/kg/day[7,8] up to 18 g of piperacillin component daily.[5]

Additives

2.35 mEq of sodium/g of piperacillin.[12]

Piperacillin Sodium–Tazobactam Sodium

Suitable diluents	NS.[12]
Maximum concentration	200 mg/mL (piperacillin component); however, 20 mg/mL preferred.[12]
Preparation and delivery	**Delivery system issues:** The mixing of piperacillin with an aminoglycoside in vitro can result in substantial inactivation of the aminoglycoside.[13-17] (See Appendix C for more specific information.) **Stability:** Thaw frozen container at room temperature (20°C to 25°C) or under refrigeration (2°C to 8°C).[12] Do not force thaw by immersion in water baths and do not microwave.[12] **Compatibility:** See Appendix D for PN compatibility information.[18] Although amikacin and gentamicin are compatible in vitro for Y-site infusion, reformulated Zosyn contains EDTA, which is not compatible with tobramycin.[2]
IV push	Not administered by this method.
Intermittent infusion	Infuse over at least 30 minutes.[2]

Book Correction Notice for 'Pediatric Injectable Drugs, Ninth Edition'

BETHESDA, MD 07 July 2010-There is an important correction to the monograph for Piperacillin Sodium-Tazobactam Sodium in Pediatric Injectable Drugs, Ninth Edition (the Teddy Bear Book), published by ASHP.

On page 473, the Continuous Infusion section should read as follows:

Continuous infusions of 8-12 g piperacillin/24 h have been studied in adults

Please make this correction immediately in all copies of the ninth edition and communicate it to everyone who may use the book

should be discontinued if bleeding occurs.[~]

Tonic-clonic seizures have been reported in an 11-year-old child receiving IV piperacillin (3 g q 4 h) over 30 minutes.[24]

Monitoring: Coagulation parameters should frequently monitored during simultaneous administration of large doses of heparin, oral anticoagulants, or other drugs that may affect the blood coagulation system or the thrombocyte function.[2]

Drug interactions: Piperacillin may decrease the clearance of methotrexate.[2,25] Antibiotics may diminish the therapeutic effect of Typhoid Vaccine. Only the live attenuated Ty21a strain is affected.[26] Perioperative use of piperacillin may prolong the neuromuscular blockade of vecuronium or other nondepolarizing muscle relaxants.[2,27] Probenecid may decrease the clearance of piperacillin.[2] Consult appropriate resources for dosing recommendations before combining any drug with piperacillin–tazobactam.

Laboratory interference: A false-positive urinary glucose results when cupric sulfate solution-based tests (Clinitest, Benedict's solution, Fehling's solution) are used.[2] It is recommended that glucose tests (Diastix or TEST-TAPE) based on enzymatic glucose oxidase reactions be used.[2] Piperacillin–tazobactam may cause a false positive *Aspergillus* infection result when performed with the Bio-Rad Laboratories Platelia *Aspergillus* EIA test; hence, interpret reports cautiously and confirmed by other diagnostic measures.[2]

Potassium Chloride

Brand names	Various manufacturers

Medication error potential

ISMP high-alert medication that has an increased risk of causing significant patient harm if it is used in error.[1]

Look-alike, sound-alike error potential.

USP reports that potassium chloride was confused with metronidazole, potassium acetate, potassium bicarbonate, potassium citrate, potassium phosphates, and sodium chloride. No patient harm resulted.[2]

Contraindications and warnings

Administration of potassium chloride at excessive rates may result in fatal dysrhythmias.[3] The rate of potassium infusion should not exceed 0.5–1 mEq/kg/h and all sources should be considered.[4-8]

ECG monitoring should accompany infusions ≥0.5 mEq/kg/h.[8]

Infusion related cautions

Phlebitis occurs frequently with concentrations >40 mEq/L.[9,10]

Extravasation may cause tissue sloughing and necrosis.[11] See Appendix E for management of extravasation.

Dosage

Daily requirements[8]

Neonates >24 h of age: 2–6 mEq/kg/day.

Infants and children: 2–4 mEq/kg/day.

Hypokalemia: 0.5–1 mEq/kg given over ≥2 hours.[5,7]

During loop and thiazide diuretic therapy larger doses may be required.[6]

Dosage adjustment in organ dysfunction

Potassium is renally eliminated; therefore, extreme caution is required when dosing patients with renal insufficiency.[8-10]

In six 19–37 year old *adults* with sickle cell disease and normal glomerular filtration, urinary potassium excretion was significantly less than individuals without sickle cell disease during a 0.75 mEq/kg infusion over 2 hours.[12]

Maxim

Important Correction Notice

Pediatric Injectable Drugs Ninth Edition (The Teddy Bear Book)

The publisher wishes to inform you of the following corrections.

ns. Intermittent infu-

Serum potassium <2 mEq/L with ECG changes or muscle paralysis: 40 mEq/h up to 400 mEq/day.

Additives

Multidose vials contain methylparaben 0.05% and propylparaben 0.005%.[8-10] See Appendix C for specific information about potential paraben toxicity.

Contains contaminant aluminum.[10]

Suitable diluents

D–LR, D–R, D–S, D5LR, D5NS, D5W, D10W, D20W, LR, NS, ½NS, or R.[13]

Potassium Chloride

Maximum concentration	**Peripheral IV:** Generally, 40 mEq/L; however, concentrations 60–80 mEq/L may be required during severe hypokalemia.[9] Phlebitis is concentration related. **Central venous line:** ≤200 mEq/L.[8,9,14]
Preparation and delivery	Concentrated potassium solution addition to a maintenance fluid requires careful mixing including inversion, agitation, and kneading of the container to insure a uniform potassium concentration throughout the fluid. Inadequate mixing of with a diluent,[9,13] including the addition of potassium to a flexible container such as a Buretrol or Soluset, may result in inconsistent potassium concentrations in the solution and deliver potassium at a rate that may exceed recommendations. **Compatibility:** See Appendix D for PN compatibility information.
IV push	Contraindicated.[4,9,10]
Intermittent infusion	≤0.5–1 mEq/kg/h and all sources should be considered.[4-8] ECG monitoring should accompany infusion of individual doses >0.5 mEq/kg/h.[8]
Continuous infusion	Usual route of administration as a component of maintenance fluids.
Other routes of administration	Contraindicated.[9]
Comments	In *adults*, the addition of lidocaine (50 mg/65 mL of infusate) decreased the pain associated with infusion.[15]

In the monograph for **Potassium Chloride (pages 474-475)**

"Maximum Dosage " section – Second line should read:

"Intermittent infusions should not exceed 1 meq/kg/h"

Potassium Phosphates

Brand names	Various manufacturers
Medication error potential	ISMP high-alert medication that has an increased risk of causing significant patient harm if it is used in error.[1] Look-alike, sound-alike error potential. USP reports that potassium phosphates were confused with potassium chloride and sodium phosphates.[2] No patient harm occurred.
Contraindications and warnings	Administration of potassium at excessive rates may result in fatal dysrhythmias.[3-5] ECG monitoring should accompany potassium infusions ≥20 mEq/h in *adults*.[4]
Infusion related cautions	Phlebitis occurs frequently with potassium concentrations >40 mEq/L.[4] Extravasation may cause tissue sloughing and necrosis.[6] See Appendix E for management of extravasation. Potassium phosphates should not be administered through a Y-site with a calcium-containing solution.[7]

Dosage	Potassium phosphates are used to replace phosphate and not to replace potassium. The valence of phosphate changes with pH; therefore, the preferred units in which to express the amount of phosphate are mmol.[3,4,7]
	
	4.4 mEq of potassium = 3 mmol of phosphate.[3,4,7,8]
	
	Daily PN requirements (see Comments section)
	
	    Neonates and infants: 1–2 mol/kg/day.
	
	    Older infants and children: 0.5–1 mmol/kg/day.
	
	    Older children and adolescents: 15 mmol/L or per 1000 kilocalories.
	
	Diabetic ketoacidosis: If the phosphate concentration is low, one third to one half the potassium deficit can be replaced as phosphates.[10] These patients should be monitored for hypocalcemia and hypomagnesemia.[9,10]
	
	Hypophosphatemia in critically ill *adults* receiving 15 mmol potassium phosphate/L in PN[11]
	
	    Mild (serum phosphate concentration of 2.3–3 mg/dL): 0.16 mmol/kg over 4–6 hours.
	
	    Moderate (1.6–2.2 mg/dL): 0.32 mmol/kg over 4–6 hours.
	
	    Severe (<1.5 mg/dL): 0.64 mmol/kg over 8–12 hours.

Dosage adjustment in organ dysfunction	Potassium and phosphate ions are renally eliminated; therefore, extreme caution is required when dosing patients with renal insufficiency.[3,4,7]
Maximum dosage	Infants receiving PN may require daily doses of up to 2 mmol/kg for optimal bone growth.[12,13]
Additives	Contains contaminant aluminum.[3]

Potassium Phosphates

Suitable diluents	D–LR, D–R, D–S, D5LR, D5NS, D5W, D10W, LR, NS, ½NS, or R.[8]
Maximum concentration	**Peripheral IV:** 40 mEq potassium/L = 27 mmol phosphates/L.[4]
Preparation and delivery	Concentrated potassium solution addition to a maintenance fluid requires careful mixing including inversion, agitation, and kneading of the container to insure a uniform potassium concentration throughout the fluid. Inadequate mixing of with a diluent,[4] including the addition of potassium to a flexible container such as a Buretrol or Soluset, may result in inconsistent potassium concentrations in the solution and deliver potassium at a rate that may exceed recommendations. **Compatibility:** Compatibility with calcium is limited and depends on the calcium concentration, pH, and temperature of the final solution. See Appendix D for PN compatibility information. In compounding PN solutions, extreme care must be taken when calcium and phosphates are added to the same solution. Order of addition is critically important.[4]
IV push	Contraindicated.[3]
Intermittent infusion	In *adults* the dose has been diluted in 100 or 150 mL of NS or D5W and infused over 4–6 hours (mild/moderate hypophosphatemia) or over 8–12 hours (severe hypophosphatemia).[11] The final potassium concentration of the solution should be considered.
Continuous infusion	Usual route of administration as a component of maintenance fluids or PN.[7,8,11]
Other routes of administration	Contraindicated.[3]
Comments	Sodium phosphate is preferred as the phosphate source in pediatric PN because it contains less contaminant aluminum. Phosphate dosing is linked to calcium dosing. In neonates, the appropriate ratio is 2.5 mEq calcium:1 mmol of phosphates. The ratio gradually decreases to 1:1 as the infant approaches childhood.[12,13] Administration of large amounts of phosphate may cause hypocalcemia.[3,13]

Pralidoxime Chloride (2-PAM Chloride)

Brand names	Protopam Chloride

Medication error potential

Look-alike, sound-alike error potential.

None reported per USP and ISMP.[1,2]

Contraindications and warnings

Contraindications: Known hypersensitivity to the drug.[3]

Warnings: Should not be used for phosphorous, inorganic phosphate, or organophosphate poisoning not associated with anticholinesterase activity.[3] Also should not be used for carbamate class pesticide poisoning (may increase toxicity of carbaryl).[3]

Use with caution in patients with myasthenia gravis because drug may precipitate a myasthenic crisis.[3]

Infusion related cautions

Side effects (e.g., tachycardia, laryngospasm, and muscle rigidity) may be more common after rapid IV infusion of doses >30 mg/kg.[4,5] Weakness, blurred vision, dizziness, headache, nausea, and tachycardia have been noted with administration.[3,6]

Hypertension in *adults* has been related to dose and rate of administration.[6] If hypertension occurs, the rate of infusion should be reduced. IV administration of 5 mg of phentolamine may be used to reverse the hypertension.[6]

Dosage

Most effective if administered within 24–48 hours of exposure; however, patients presenting late (i.e., 2–6 days) may still benefit.[7,8]

Administered in combination with atropine.[3,6]

Chemical warfare: Dose and route are based on severity of symptoms and treatment setting.[6]

> **Outpatient setting, usually given IM as follows**[6]
>
> > **Mild-to-moderate symptoms:** 15 mg/kg.
> >
> > **Severe symptoms:** 25 mg/kg.
>
> **Emergency department, usually given as slow IV injection**[6]
>
> > **Mild-to-moderate or severe symptoms:** 15 mg/kg.

Organophosphate poisoning: For nicotinic (e.g., fasciculation, muscle weakness, paralysis, and decreased respiratory effort) and CNS symptoms.

> **Intermittent dosing:** 25–50 mg/kg, up to 2 g/dose, over 5–30 minutes; repeat dose after 1–2 hours and then q 6–12 h if cholinergic signs recur.[4,7-10]
>
> **Continuous infusion:** Loading dose of 25–50 mg/kg infused over 15–30 minutes followed by continuous infusion of 10–20 mg/kg/h for ≤60 hours while symptoms persist.[5,11] A loading dose of 50 mg/kg may be more appropriate in patients with severe organophosphate poisoning.[11]

Dosage adjustment in organ dysfunction

Should be used with caution and in reduced dosage in patients with renal dysfunction.[3,6]

Pralidoxime Chloride (2-PAM Chloride)

Maximum dosage	As much as 2 g/dose,[4] 12 g in 24 hours,[8] and 0.5 g/h by continuous infusion[6,12] have been used in *adults*, with the total dosage titrated according to cholinergic signs and clinical symptoms.
Additives	None.[3]
Suitable diluents	SW, NS. Diluents should be preservative-free due to larger volume required.[6]
Maximum concentration	50 mg/mL.[3,6]
Preparation and delivery	SW is used for reconstitution. NS is used for further dilution.[3,6]
IV push	20 mg/mL over at least 5 minutes in children.[6,7] In fluid-restricted patients, 50 mg/mL may be used.[6] Not to exceed 200 mg/min in *adults*.[3] (See Infusion related cautions section.)
Intermittent infusion	20 mg/mL over 15–30 minutes in *adults* and over 30 minutes in children.[6]
Continuous infusion	Although concentration and solution type were not provided, pralidoxime has been given by this method.[5,11]
Other routes of administration	May be given by IM or SC injection (300 mg/mL) when IV administration not possible. [3,6] May produce mild pain at the IM injection site.[3,6]
Comments	**Drug interactions:** Concomitant administration of pralidoxime may increase side effects of atropine.[3,6] **Other:** Morphine, theophylline, aminophylline, and succinylcholine are contraindicated in patients with anticholinesterase poisoning.[3,6] Pralidoxime has been given for up to 22 days following poisoning with highly lipophilic organophosphates.[8]

Procainamide HCl

Brand names	Pronestyl

Medication error potential	ISMP high-alert medication (antiarrhythmic agent) that has an increased risk of causing significant patient harm if it is used in error.[1]
	Look-alike, sound-alike drug names.
	USP reports confusion with probenecid.[2]
	The abbreviation PCA may be mistaken for "patient controlled analgesia" and should not be used.[3]

Contraindications and warnings	**US boxed warning:** Potentially fatal blood dyscrasias have occurred with normal doses. Long-term administration leads to the development of a positive antinuclear antibody (ANA) test in 50% of patients, which may result in a drug-induced lupus erythematosus-like syndrome in 20% to 30% of patients.[3]
	Contraindications: Complete heart block; second or third degree heart block without pacemaker; torsades de pointes (twisting of the points), an unusual ventricular tachycardia; pre-existing QT prolongation; myasthenia gravis or systemic lupus erythematosus.[3]

Infusion related cautions	To avoid the development of significant hypotension, limit the infusion rate to 20–30 mg/min.[3] Hypotension, atrioventricular block, cardiac dysrhythmias, and cardiac arrest may occur.[3]

Dosage	Monitor ECG. If QRS widens >50% or if the patient develops hypotension during the loading dose, the infusion should be discontinued and the maintenance dose held until signs of toxicity resolve.[4,5]
	Tachycardia: SVT unresponsive to vagal maneuvers and adenosine; VT unresponsive to synchronized cardioversion or adenosine.
	Loading dose: Two alternative regimens are recommended.
	2–5 mg/kg (max 100 mg) over 5 minutes and repeated q 5–10 min until the arrhythmia is controlled to a maximum of 15 mg/kg (500 mg) over 30 minutes.[3,4,6]
	or
	10–15 mg/kg over 30–60 minutes followed by maintenance infusion.
	Maintenance dose: 20–120 mcg/kg/min[3-7] to a maximum of 2 g in 24 hours[3] or 50–100 mg/kg/day divided q 4 h.[3]

Dosage adjustment in organ dysfunction	If CrCl is 10–50 mL/min, give normal dose q 6–12 h; if <10 mL/min, give q 8–24 h.[3]

Maximum dosage	2 g/day IV[3,4] and 4 g/day IM.[3,4]

Additives	Sodium bisulfate.[3] Some 100- and 500-mg/mL vials contain 0.9% benzyl alcohol.[3] (See Appendix C for specific information about sulfite hypersensitivity and benzyl alcohol's potential for toxicity.)

Procainamide HCl

Suitable diluents	D5W, NS, or SW.[8]
Maximum concentration	20–30 mg/mL for loading doses[3,8] or 4 mg/mL for intermittent infusions.[7,8]
Preparation and delivery	**Stability:** Variable stability has been reported in dextrose containing solutions with significant drug loss in as little as 4 hours, depending upon the pH adjustment of dextrose solution.[8]
IV push	20–30 mg/mL over 5–10 minutes at a maximum infusion rate of 20–30 mg/min (50 mg/min in *adults*).[3,4] Severe hypotension may occur with rapid administration.[5]
Intermittent infusion	2–4 mg/mL concentration solution over 25–30 minutes.[7,8]
Continuous infusion	2 or 4 mg/mL for continuous infusion preferably in NS or SW.[3,7,8]
Other routes of administration	Has been given IM and IO.[5]
Comments	**Monitoring:** Because large variability exists in patient response to initial and maintenance doses, individualize dosage based on serum concentration and clinical response. Reference range for procainamide is 4–10 mg/L and for combination of procainamide plus n-acetyl procainamide is 5–30 mg/L.[3,9] **Drug interactions:** Procainamide is primarily metabolized by CYP2D6.[3] Because it is associated with numerous pharmacokinetic and pharmacodynamic drug-drug interactions,[10] consult appropriate resources for dosing recommendations before combining any drug with procainamide.

Promethazine HCl

Brand names	Phenergan, Pentazine, Phenazine, Prorex, generic

Medication error potential

ISMP high-alert medication that has an increased risk of causing significant patient harm if it is used in error.[1]

Look-alike, sound-alike error potential.

USP reports that promethazine has been confused with perphenazine, phenazopyridine and prednisone; no patient harm resulted.[2] USP also reports that promethazine has been confused with Compazine and prochlorperazine; patient harm resulted.[2]

USP reports that Phenergan has been confused with Compazine, phenobarbital and phenylephrine; no patient harm resulted.[2]

Contraindications and warnings

US boxed warning: A black box warning was added to prescribing information in 2004 as follows[3]:

Promethazine contraindicated in pediatric patients <2 years of age because of the potential for fatal respiratory depression. Postmarketing cases of respiratory depression, including fatalities, have been reported with promethazine use in patients <2 years of age. A wide range of weight-based doses have resulted in respiratory depression in these patients.

Caution should be exercised when administering promethazine to pediatric patients >2 years of age. Use the lowest effective dose and avoid the use of concomitant therapy with respiratory depressants.

Contraindications: Contraindicated in patients <2 years of age, in comatose states, and in patients with a previous hypersensitivity to the drug.[3]

Other warnings: Promethazine use may result in CNS depression, respiratory depression, bone marrow depression, neuroleptic malignant syndrome, and lower seizure threshold.[3]

Infusion related cautions

Tissue irritation and damage can occur from promethazine injection regardless of the route of administration.[3] Extravasation may cause tissue necrosis.[3,4]

In an effort to increase awareness of the risk of severe tissue injury with IV promethazine administration, the Institute for Safe Medication Practices has recommended that institutions only stock the 25-mg/mL concentration, limit doses used, further dilute the 25-mg/mL concentration prior to administration, use large veins for administration, administer via a running IV at the furthest port from the patient, and administer slowly.[5]

Intra-arterial injection may result in gangrene of the affected extremity.[3,4]

Dosage

Antiemetic/sedation

> **Children >2 years of age:** 0.25–1 mg/kg (not to exceed 25 mg) q 4–6 h as needed.[6-8]

Dosage adjustment in organ dysfunction

No dosage adjustment required in *adult* patients with renal dysfunction. May cause excessive sedation in end stage renal disease.[9]

Maximum dosage

The dose should not exceed half of the suggested *adult* dose or up to 25 mg/dose in children or 50 mg/dose in adolescents.[3]

Additives

Each mL of solution (25 mg/mL and 50 mg/mL) contains 0.1 mg disodium edetate, 0.04 mg calcium chloride, 0.25 mg sodium metabisulfite, and 5 mg phenol.[10]

See Appendix C for more specific information about potential adverse effects of sulfites.

Promethazine HCl

Suitable diluents	NS, ½NS, D2.5W, D5W, D10W, LR, R, D–LR combinations, D–R combinations, D-saline combinations.[10]
Maximum concentration	25 mg/mL.[3,10]
Preparation and delivery	See Appendix D for PN compatibility information.
IV push	≤25 mg/mL; administer into tubing of a compatible infusion fluid at a rate <25 mg/min.[3,10]
Intermittent infusion	No information available to support administration by this method.
Continuous infusion	No information available to support administration by this method.
Other routes of administration	≤25 mg/mL via deep IM injection is the preferred route of administration.[3] SC injection is contraindicated.[3]
Comments	**Significant adverse effects:** All FDA-reported cases of serious adverse events (respiratory depression, apnea, cardiac arrest, dystonias, CNS effects, seizures, neuroleptic malignant syndrome) in children (0 to 16 years of age) were evaluated.[11] Respiratory depression occurred in 22 patients (1.5 months to 2 years of age) and seven of these patients died. A wide range of doses was represented (0.45–6.4 mg/kg). Nine patients received ≤1 mg/kg in addition to another drug with respiratory depressant effects.[11] Excessively large doses of antihistamines may cause hallucinations, convulsions, and sudden death in infants and children. Acutely ill children who are dehydrated may be more susceptible to dystonias. For these reasons, antiemetics are not recommended for the treatment of uncomplicated vomiting in children; their use should be limited to prolonged vomiting of unknown etiology.[3] **Laboratory interference:** An increase in blood glucose and false positive or false negative pregnancy tests (diagnostic tests utilizing HCG and anti-HCG) may occur with promethazine therapy.[3] **Other:** Meperidine, promethazine, and chlorpromazine have been used in combination (Demerol, Phenergan, Thorazine [DPT] cocktail) to sedate pediatric patients.[6,7,12-15] However, with the availability of safer and more effective agents,[13,16,17] this combination is no longer recommended.[15] Steroid-induced psychosis in a 32-month-old child with acute lymphocytic leukemia resolved with promethazine (0.5 mg/kg) therapy.[18]

Propofol

Brand names	Diprivan 1% and 2%, Propofol Injectable Emulsion 1% (generic)

Medication error potential

ISMP high-alert medication that has an increased risk of causing significant patient harm if it is used in error.[1]

ISMP's *Confused Drug Names* lists confusion for Diprivan and Ditropan.[2] USP reports confusion for Diprivan with Diflucan and Ditropan.[3] USP reports confusion with propranolol.[3]

Contraindications and warnings

Contraindications: Known hypersensitivity to DIPRIVAN Injectable Emulsion or its components (i.e., eggs, soybean) or when general anesthesia or sedation are contraindicated.[4]

Warnings: When used for general or monitored anesthesia should be administered only by persons trained in general anesthesia and who are not involved in the conduct of the surgical/diagnostic procedure.[4] For sedation of intubated, mechanically ventilated *adult* patients in the intensive care unit, should be administered only by persons skilled in the management of critically ill patients and trained in cardiovascular resuscitation and airway management.[4] Patients should be continuously monitored, and facilities for maintenance of a patent airway, artificial ventilation, and oxygen enrichment and circulatory resuscitation must be immediately available.

The Diprivan emulsion can support the growth of microorganisms as it is not an antimicrobially preserved product under USP standards.[4] Accordingly, strict aseptic technique must be adhered to. Do not use if contamination is suspected and discard unused portions as directed within the required time limits. Failure to use aseptic technique has been associated with microbial contamination of the product and with fever, infection/sepsis, and/or death.

Infusion related cautions

Transient pain during injection occurs frequently in pediatric patients (45%) when a small vein of the hand is used without lidocaine pretreatment.[4] With lidocaine (1 mL of a 1% solution; not to exceed 20 mg lidocaine per 200 mg propofol) pretreatment or when antecubital veins are used, the incidence of pain is <10% and well tolerated.[5]

Cardiorespiratory depression may occur during bolus dosing or after rapid increase in infusion rate.[4] Wait 3–5 minutes between dosage adjustments to assess patient response.[4]

Abrupt discontinuance of propofol may cause flushing of the hands and feet, agitation, tremors, hyperirritability, bradycardia, agitation, or jitteriness.[4]

Dosage

Anesthesia

Not recommended for the induction of anesthesia in patients <3 years of age and for the maintenance of anesthesia in patients <2 months of age.[4]

Induction doses (≥3 years of age): Mean dose 2.5 mg/kg (range: 1–4 mg/kg) given over 20–30 seconds until onset of induction.[4,6-14] Noncommunicative and nonverbal children (ASA III and IV) with cerebral palsy require less propofol than healthy children.[15]

Those older than 16 years should be given 40 mg (2–2.5 mg/kg) q 10 sec until onset of induction.[4] *Adults* >16 years who have neurosurgical diagnosis should receive smaller doses 20 mg (1–2 mg/kg) q 10 sec.[4]

Maintenance (≥2 months of age): If clinical signs of light anesthesia are not present following the first 30 minutes, the infusion rate should be decreased.[4]

Propofol

Dosage (cont.)	133–400 mcg/kg/min.[12,14,16] Younger children may require larger doses. During clinical trials mean doses were 125–300 mcg/kg/min (7.5–18 mg/kg/h).[4] Those >16 years received doses of 100–200 mcg/kg/min (6–12 mg/kg/h) or 40 mg (2–2.5 mg/kg) q 10 sec.[4]

Although rare, the propofol infusion syndrome has been reported following anesthesia. (See Rare adverse effects in Comments section.)

Epilepsy (refractory status epilepticus): Use in refractory status is based on non-randomized studies and case reports; hence, it should be used cautiously. Initial loading doses of 3 mg/kg followed by continuous infusion of 40–300 mcg/kg/min (2.4–18 mg/kg/h) for up to 48 hours have been used in patients from 9 months to 19 years.[17-21] (See Rare adverse effects in Comments section.)

Procedural sedation: 0.5–3 mg/kg initially followed by 50–200 mcg/kg/min (3–12 mg/kg/h)[22-24] with additional 1-mg/kg boluses as needed.[22,23] For the initial bolus, one group used 2.5 mg/kg in children and 3 mg/kg in infants.[23] As an alternative to continuous infusion, 0.2 to ≤1 mg/kg boluses for patient comfort have been used as needed.[22,25]

Sedation: The manufacturer stresses that propofol lacks approved labeling for sedation in critically ill, mechanically-ventilated pediatric patients.[4]

Given the current controversy regarding the propofol-related infusion syndrome (PRIS), the lowest effective dose should be used and the dose should not exceed 4 mg/kg/h.[26] The infusion rate should be increased by 5–10 mcg/kg/min (0.3–0.6 mg/kg/h) until the desired effect is achieved.[4] A minimum period of 5 minutes should be allowed for peak effect between titration events.[4] The patient should be switched to a benzodiazepine (i.e., midazolam or lorazepam) if adequate sedation cannot be achieved with dose of 4 mg/kg/h or if prolonged therapy (≥48 hours) is required.[26] While on propofol the patient should be monitored for clinical features and laboratory findings that have been attributed to the syndrome. Should symptoms occur propofol should be discontinued. (See Rare adverse effects in Comments section.)

Dosage adjustment in organ dysfunction	No adjustment in hepatic or renal dysfunction.[4,27]
Maximum dosage	Not established. (See Rare adverse effects in Comments section.)
Additives	The generic formulation contains sodium metabisulfite. (See Appendix C for specific information about sulfite hypersensitivity.) Each mL of Diprivan contains 100 mg soybean oil, 22.5 mg glycerol, 12 mg egg lecithin, and disodium edetate 0.005%. NaOH is used to adjust pH.[4,28] The generic contains 100 mg soybean oil, 22.5 mg glycerol, 12 mg egg yolk phospholipid, and 0.25 mg sodium metabisulfite. NaOH is used to adjust pH.[28] Patients who are allergic to eggs and/or soybean products should not be given propofol.[4] A 14-month-old patient with a history of egg and peanut allergies developed anaphylaxis after receiving propofol.[29]
Suitable diluents	D5W.
Maximum concentration	10 mg/mL[4] Should not be diluted to <2 mg/mL.[4]

Propofol

Preparation and delivery	**Delivery system issues:** To ensure proper delivery of propofol, in-line IV filters should be >5 microns.[4] Do not administer through the same IV catheter with blood or plasma. Tubing and any unused portions of propofol vials should be discarded after 12 hours.
	Stability: Store between 4°C to 22°C.[4] Do not freeze. If used directly from vial/prefilled syringe, use within 12 hours after vial has been spiked.[4] Several incidences of bacterial contamination have been reported following repackaging[30] or improper storage of propofol[31] and Intralipid.[32] If propofol is transferred to a syringe or other container, the transfer should be done as soon as the vial is opened and the product should be discarded and administration lines changed after 6 hours.[4] Shake well before use. Do not use if emulsion has separated.
	Compatibility: See Appendix D for PN compatibility information.
IV push	10 mg/mL[4] given over 20–30 seconds.[4,6-10] Has been given safely over 10 seconds.[6]
Intermittent infusion	Not routinely used.
Continuous infusion	2–10 mg/mL in D5W.[4] Do not dilute <2 mg/mL due to emulsion instability.[4]
Other routes of administration	IM not recommended.[4]
Comments	**Rare adverse effects:** PRIS is associated with a variety of symptoms, including progressive metabolic acidosis, lipemia, hypotension, MSOF, and rhabdomyolysis, which may culminate in cardiovascular collapse.[26] Several practitioners have successfully managed PRIS with venovenous hemodiafiltration and charcoal hemofiltration or ECMO.[26] Plasmapheresis was not beneficial.[26]
	Acute dystonia and seizures have also been reported in those with and without a history of epilepsy.[33-37] Subtherapeutic doses or withdrawal may contribute to this effect since increasing the dose can result in termination of the seizure activity.
	Acute pancreatitis has been reported.[38-40]
	A 9-month-old who received large doses of propofol for 5 days for status epilepticus developed first and secondary degree AV block, widened QRS, and ventricular tachycardia.[41]
	Monitoring: Arterial blood gases, potassium, CPK, AST and ALT, BUN, and creatinine. Serum triglyceride levels should be obtained prior to initiation of therapy and every 3–7 days thereafter, especially if receiving for >48 hours with doses exceeding 50 mcg/kg/min.[42] Collect blood from IV port opposite to the site of propofol infusion or temporarily suspend infusion and flush port prior to blood draw.
	Drug interactions: Propofol is a substrate of CYP2C9 and 2B6 (major) and a minor substrate for CYP1A2, 2A6, 2C19, 2D6, 2E1, and 3A4.[42] It inhibits CYP3A4 (major), CYP1A2 and 2C19 (moderate), and 2C9, 2D6, and (weak).[42] In pediatric patients, administration of fentanyl concomitantly with DIPRIVAN Injectable Emulsion may result in serious bradycardia.[4] Consult appropriate resources for dosing recommendations before combining any drug with propofol.
	Other: Diprivan contains EDTA an antimicrobial agent. Although rare, at large doses (2–3 g/day), EDTA may be toxic to the renal tubules.[4] In those predisposed to renal impairment, urinalysis and urine sediment should be assessed prior to initiation and on alternate days during therapy.[4] EDTA may bind zinc. Although this formulation has not been associated with decreased zinc levels or zinc deficiency-related adverse events, it should not be infused for longer than 5 days without providing a drug-free period.[4]

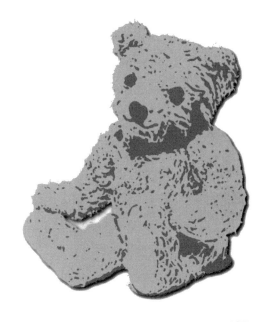

Propranolol HCl

Brand names	Inderal

Medication error potential

ISMP high-alert medication (adrenergic agonist) that has an increased risk of causing significant patient harm if it is used in error.[1]

Look-alike, sound-alike drug names.

Confusion has been reported between Inderal and Adderall,[2] Isordil, Isuprel, and Neoral.[3] Propranolol has been confused with nadolol, pantoprazole, Pravachol, pravastatin, prednisone, prochlorperazine, propantheline, and propofol.[3] Confusion with Imdur has resulted in patient harm.[3]

Contraindications and warnings

US boxed warning: Abrupt withdrawal in patients with coronary artery disease may exacerbate angina or precipitate myocardial infarction; hence, propranolol should be gradually discontinued over about 2 weeks.[4]

Contraindications: Propranolol is contraindicated in cardiogenic shock; sinus bradycardia and greater than first-degree block; and bronchial asthma.[4]

Other warnings: Use cautiously in patients with diabetes mellitus as propranolol may block hypoglycemia-induced tachycardia and blood pressure changes.[4] Acute elevations in blood pressure have been reported after insulin-induced hypoglycemia.[4] Beta-blockers may aggravate arterial insufficiency and should be used with caution in those with peripheral vascular disease.[4]

Patients with a history of anaphylactic reactions, may be more reactive to a repeated allergen challenge and may not respond to doses of epinephrine used to treat an allergic reaction.[4,5]

Infusion related cautions

Rapid administration may cause hypotension and cardiac standstill.[4-6]

Dosage

Significant differences exist between oral and IV dosing. Use caution when converting from one route of administration to another.

Arrhythmias: 0.01–0.25 mg/kg over 10 minutes[5,7-10] not to exceed 1 mg/min.[4,5] Repeat dose q 2 min.[7,8] (See Maximum dosage section.)

Burn patients: 0.5–1 mg/kg q 8 h for 5–10 days.[11,12] Used to decrease heart rate, cardiac work, and metabolic stress associated with severe burn.

Hypertensive emergency: Intravenous labetalol is the preferred beta-blocker.[13,14]

Infundibular spasm ("Tet" spell): Oxygen should be given before propranolol. 0.01–0.02 mg/kg over 10 minutes.[15-17] May repeat dose in 15 minutes.[16,17] Maximum initial dose 1 mg.[17]

Dosage adjustment in organ dysfunction

No adjustment in renal dysfunction.[18] Use cautiously in hepatic dysfunction and consider dosage reduction.[5]

Maximum dosage

0.2 mg/kg,[7,16] not to exceed 1 mg as initial dose for infants.[4,7,15] Although the AAP recommends a maximum initial dose in children of 10 mg,[7] the usual dose for *adults* is 1–3 mg.[4]

Additives

None.

Propranolol HCl

Suitable diluents	D5W, NS, D5NS, D5½NS, ½NS, LR.[18]
Maximum concentration	1 mg/mL.[18]
Preparation and delivery	**Compatibility:** Incompatible with bicarbonate.[19]
IV push	Not recommended.[4]
Intermittent infusion	1 mg/mL[19] administered over 10 minutes.[4,5,7] Not to exceed 1 mg/min.[4]
Continuous infusion	Not used.
Other routes of administration	None.
Comments	**Monitoring:** ECG and central venous pressure should be monitored during IV administration. Propranolol-induced bradycardia should be treated with atropine.[4] If no response to atropine, isoproterenol should be tried.[4,5]
	Drug interactions: Propranolol is primarily metabolized by CYP1A2, CYP2D6 and to a lesser extent by CYP2C18, and CYP2C19.[4] Mild inhibitor of CYP1A2 and CYP2D6.[4]
	Pharmacodynamic considerations: Caution should be exercised when administering propranolol with drugs that slow A-V nodal conduction (e.g., digitalis, lidocaine, and calcium channel blockers).[4,5]

Protamine Sulfate

Brand names	Generic

Medication error potential

Look-alike, sound-alike error potential.

ISMP reported that protamine sulfate was confused with Protonix.[1]

USP reported that protamine sulfate was confused with ProAmatine, protirelin, and Protonix.[2]

Contraindications and warnings

US boxed warning: Protamine sulfate can cause severe hypotension, cardiovascular collapse, noncardiogenic pulmonary edema, catastrophic pulmonary vasoconstriction, and pulmonary hypertension.[3] Appropriate facilities and supportive measures including resuscitative equipment and medications should be readily available in case of a severe reaction.[3]

Risk factors include high dose, overdose, rapid administration, repeated doses, previous administration of protamine, and current or previous use of protamine-containing drugs.[3] Allergy to fish, previous vasectomy, severe left ventricular dysfunction, and abnormal preoperative pulmonary hemodynamics may be risk factors. The risk to benefit should be considered in these patients.

Protamine sulfate should not be given when bleeding unrelated to heparin occurs.[3]

Infusion related cautions

See US boxed warning in Contraindications and warnings section.

In two case reports, doses of 3 and 4.5 mg/kg after cardiopulmonary bypass resulted in an anaphylactoid response in a 6- and a 2.5-year-old child, respectively.[4,5] Whether or not either child had any risk factors for this reaction was not clear.

Dosage

Heparin: 1 mg of protamine sulfate will neutralize about 100 USP heparin units.[3,6] Because heparin's half-life is short, over time less protamine is required. Only one half the dose of protamine should be used if IV heparin has been discontinued for 30 minutes.[1] (See Comments section.)

The following doses have been recommended for pediatric patients following IV injection of heparin[6]:

Time Since Last Heparin Dose Received	Protamine Dose (mg of protamine/100 units of heparin received)
<30 min	1 mg
30–60 min	0.5–0.75 mg
60–120 min	0.375–0.5 mg
>120 min	0.25–0.375 mg

If the heparin was administered by deep SC injection, 1–1.5 mg protamine/100 USP heparin units should be used. As an example, part of the dose (i.e., 25–50 mg) can be given over 10 minutes followed by an infusion of the remaining calculated dose over 8–16 hours.[7]

Low molecular weight heparin (LMWH): 1 mg protamine will neutralize about 1 mg enoxaparin or dalteparin.[7] If the aPTT remains increased 2–4 hours after the dose, a dose of 0.5 mg protamine/1 mg LMWH may be given.[7]

Protamine Sulfate

Dosage adjustment in organ dysfunction	None noted.
Maximum dosage	50 mg.[3,7]
Additives	Contains 9 mg NaCl/10 mg.[3]
Suitable diluents	D5W, NS.[3,8]
Maximum concentration	10 mg/mL.[3,6-8]
Preparation and delivery	**Compatibility:** A manufacturer states that protamine sulfate is incompatible with certain antibiotics, including several of the cephalosporins, and penicillins.[3]
IV push	Contraindicated. Rapid administration may result in hypotension, bradycardia, pulmonary hypertension, etc.[3,6,7]
Intermittent infusion	50 mg over 10 minutes,[3,6,7] and ≤5 mg/min.[3,6,7]
Continuous infusion	Not indicated.
Other routes of administration	Not indicated.
Comments	Note that the USP adopted new manufacturing controls for heparin. Beginning October 8, 2009, the reference standard for heparin products changed to the World Health Organization's International Standards (IS) unit dose definition.[9] This is about 10% less potent than the previous USP unit. Thus, the potency of heparin products is expected to decrease and this may lower the protamine dose required. **Adverse effects:** Following cardiopulmonary bypass (CPB), a 6-week-old infant experienced pulmonary hypertension and impending respiratory failure immediately after receiving protamine.[10] This infant was treated with high-frequency oscillation ventilation, inhaled nitric oxide (iNO), and prostacycline and recovered. Following CPB, a 3-year-old child developed pulmonary hypertension after protamine was given.[11] She failed to respond to conventional treatments and was started on iNO after which the pulmonary artery pressures decreased. She was subsequently weaned from iNO and mechanical ventilation and was discharged on postoperative day 4. One study in *adults* reported that when given prior to protamine, IV famotidine, but not diphenhydramine, prevented hypotension associated.[12] **Monitoring:** Coagulation studies including aPTT or ACT should help to guide therapy. Blood pressure should be monitored during infusion.[3,6,7]

Protein C Concentrate (Human)

Brand names	Ceprotin
Medication error potential	None reported by ISMP or USP.[1-3]
Contraindications and warnings	Protein C concentrate is made from human plasma. While the risk of transmission of infectious agents is low, the product may still transmit disease.[4] Consider vaccination for hepatitis A and B in patients receiving repeated doses of protein C concentrate.[4]
Infusion related cautions	The drug product may contain traces of mouse protein and/or heparin. If allergic/hypersensitivity symptoms occur, the infusion should be discontinued.[4]

Dosage

Dosage regimen (dose, frequency, duration) should be tailored to individual patient based on severity of protein C deficiency, age, patient's clinical condition, and protein C plasma concentrations.[4-6] The manufacturer reports that pediatric patients from 2 days of age to adolescence have been included in retrospective and prospective trials.[4] In general, dosing recommendations for pediatric patients and *adults* are as follows:

Acute episodes/short term prophylaxis[4-6]

> **Initial dose:** 100–120 International Units/kg.

> **Subsequent three doses:** 60–80 International Units/kg q 6 h.

> **Maintenance dose:** 45–60 International Units/kg q 6–12 h.

Long-term prophylaxis[4-6]: 45–60 International Units/kg q 12 h.

After the initial dose, subsequent doses should be adjusted to maintain peak protein C plasma activity of 100%. After the acute episode has subsided, continue same dose to maintain trough protein C plasma activity above 25%.[4-6]

Dosage adjustment in organ dysfunction	No information is known regarding dosage adjustment in organ dysfunction.[4]
Maximum dosage	In clinical trials, doses up to 600 International Units/kg/day (i.e., 150 International Units/kg q 6 h) for acute episodes/short-term prophylaxis and 291.7 International Units/kg/day for long-term prophylaxis have been used.[4]
Additives	Contains 8 mg/mL human albumin and 8.8 mg/mL sodium; thus, the total sodium content in the maximum daily dose is greater than 200 mg.[4] Monitor patients on a low sodium diet and/or with renal impairment closely.[4]
	Contains heparin; if heparin-induced thrombocytopenia is suspected, check platelets and discontinue therapy.[4]
Suitable diluents	SW.[4]
Maximum concentration	100 International Units/mL.[4]

Protein C Concentrate (Human)

Preparation and delivery	Product available in 500 International Units/vial and 1000 International Units/vial to be reconstituted with 5 mL and 10 mL SW, respectively (final concentration of 100 International Units/mL). Filter with filter needle provided prior to administration. Dose should be given within 3 hours of reconstitution.[4]
IV push	Not indicated.
Intermittent infusion	For patients ≥10 kg, infuse at 2 mL/min; for pediatric patients <10 kg, do not exceed an infusion rate of 0.2 mL/kg/min.[4]
Continuous infusion	No information available to support administration via continuous infusion.
Other routes of administration	Should only be administered via IV infusion.[4] No information available to support administration by other routes.
Comments	**Monitoring:** Protein C activity (using a chromogenic assay) should be measured to tailor dosage regimen.[4] (See Dosage section.) **Drug interactions:** Concomitant administration with thrombolytics or anticoagulants may increase the risk of bleeding.[4] **Pharmacokinetic considerations:** Protein C half-life may be decreased with acute thrombosis, purpura fulminans, and skin necrosis.[4] Pharmacokinetic parameters have been reported in a case report of two sisters who were both initiated on protein C concentrate therapy as infants for severe congenital protein C deficiency.[7] **Other:** Two infants with severe congenital protein C deficiency have received initial doses of 550 units (first infant) and 156 International Units/kg q 12 h (other infant) then 85–90 International Units/kg/dose given three times per week.[7]

Ranitidine

Brand names	Zantac, generic

Medication error potential

Look-alike, sound-alike error potential.

ISMP and USP report that Zantac has been confused with Xanax and Zyrtec.[1,2] USP reports that Zantac has been confused with Xanax, Zocor, and Zofran; no patient harm resulted.[2] USP also reports that Zantac has been confused with Zyrtec; patient harm resulted.[2]

USP reports that ranitidine has been confused with loratadine, nizatidine and rimantadine; no patient harm resulted.[2]

Contraindications and warnings

Known hypersensitivity to the drug.

Infusion related cautions

Bradycardia has been reported with rapid administration.[3]

Infusion of 50 mg over <5 minutes has resulted in transient hypotension in critically ill *adults*.[4]

Pain at the injection site (IV and IM administration) may occur. Burning and itching may also occur with IV administration.[3]

Dosage

Active GI bleeding, peptic ulcer disease, or hypersecretory conditions: 0.5–5 mg/kg/day given in divided doses or via continuous infusion.[5-7]

Prophylaxis against dexamethasone-associated ulceration in premature infants with bronchopulmonary dysplasia: 0.031–0.125 mg/kg/h during dexamethasone therapy.[8] An infusion of 0.0625 mg/kg/h was sufficient to increase and maintain gastric pH >4.[8]

Prophylaxis against stress ulceration

   Premature neonates: 0.5 mg/kg q 12 h.[9]

   Term neonates: Although one study recommended 1.5 mg/kg q 8 h,[9] another study reported that term neonates receiving 2 mg/kg/dose did not require dosing more frequently than q 12 h.[10] Ranitidine has also been given as a loading dose of 2 mg/kg over 10 minutes followed by 0.083 mg/kg/h.[10]

   ECMO: 2 mg/kg/dose q 12–24 h or as a continuous infusion.[3]

   Infants and children: Although doses of 1–6 mg/kg/day divided q 6–8 h have been used,[11-15] it has been suggested that critically ill infants and children require larger doses (i.e., >3 mg/kg/day) and more frequent dosing.[11,15-17] Alternatively, a loading dose of 0.15–0.6 mg/kg[5,6,15,18] over 15 minutes followed by a continuous infusion of 0.031–0.25 mg/kg/h has been used.[5,7,8,13-15,19-21]

Dosage adjustment in organ dysfunction

Adjust dosage in patients with severe renal dysfunction.[3,22]

CrCl 30–50 mL/min: 1 mg/kg q 12 h.[22]

CrCl 10–29 mL/min: 0.5 mg/kg q 12 h.[22]

CrCl <10 mL/min: 0.5 mg/kg q 24 h.[22]

Supplement doses above for hemodialysis and peritoneal dialysis (0.5 mg/kg q 24 h) and continuous renal replacement therapy (1 mg/kg q 12 h).[22]

Maximum dosage

200 mg/day in infants and children and 400 mg/day in *adults*.[3] 2.5 mg/kg/h and infusion rates of 220 mg/h have been used in *adults* with hypersecretory conditions.[3]

Ranitidine

Additives	Each mL of the premixed solution (50 mg/50 mL) contains 4.5 mg NaCl.[3]
Suitable diluents	D5W, D10W, LR, NS, or sodium bicarbonate 5%.[3]
Maximum concentration	2.5 mg/mL for IV and 25 mg/mL for IM administration.[3,23]
Preparation and delivery	Visually compatible with PN[23] and stable in PN and TNA solutions for 24 hours at room temperature.[24-26] See Appendix D for additional PN compatibility information.
IV push	Not recommended because of risk of bradycardia and hypotension.[4] Dilute to ≤2.5 mg/mL in D5W, D10W, LR, or NS and inject over at least 5 minutes,[3,23] not to exceed 4 mL/min (10 mg/min).[3,23]
Intermittent infusion	May give via intermittent infusion (≤0.5 mg/mL); infuse at 5–7 mL/min (15–20 minutes).[3,23]
Continuous infusion	May give via continuous infusion (<0.5 mg/mL).[3,23]
Other routes of administration	May give IM (25 mg/mL).[3,23]
Comments	**Significant adverse effects:** Bradycardia began 2 hours after ranitidine was infused in a neonate and gradually resolved within 24 hours of discontinuation.[27] No other cause of bradycardia could be determined.
	Ranitidine has produced a negative chronotropic effect in children receiving concomitant tolazoline.[28]
	Rare adverse effects: May precipitate acute porphyric attacks; do not use in patients with a history of acute porphyria.[3]
	Monitoring: Increases in ALT may occur when given at higher doses for 5 days or more; monitor ALT beginning at day 5 of therapy.[3]
	Drug interactions: Ranitidine inhibits a variety of CYP isoenzymes and is associated with numerous drug interactions.[3] Consult appropriate resources for dosing recommendations before combining any drug with ranitidine.
	Pharmacodynamic considerations: Several critically ill children have failed to respond to 6 mg/kg/day.[13,17] Tolerance developed in five of six infants who received continuous infusion ranitidine in PN solutions for 2–6 weeks.[19]
	Laboratory interference: May result in a false-positive urine protein test; testing with sulfosalicylic acid recommended.[3]
	Other: H2-blocker therapy has been associated with the incidence of necrotizing enterocolitis in very low birth weight infants.[29]

Rasburicase

Brand names	Elitek
Medication error potential	None known.

Contraindications and warnings

US boxed warning: May cause life-threatening anaphylaxis, hemolysis, methemoglobinemia.[1,2] Interference with uric acid assessment due to uric acid degradation may also occur.[1,2] (See Laboratory interference in Comments section.)

Contraindications: Patients with a known hypersensitivity to rasburicase or any components, past or known history of hemolytic reactions to drug or any components, and glucose-6-phosphatase dehydrogenase (G6PD) deficiencies.[1,2] (See Significant adverse effects in Comments section.)

Other warnings: Patients should receive concurrent hydration.[1]

Infusion related cautions

Hypersensitivity reactions have been reported.[3] (See Dosage section.)

Give concomitant IV hydration.[1]

Anaphylaxis may occur at any point during infusion. Immediately and permanently discontinue rasburicase should anaphylaxis occur.[1]

Dosage

Indicated for the initial management of plasma uric acid levels in pediatric patients who are expected to develop tumor lysis syndrome and subsequent elevations in uric acid as a result of their disease (lymphoma, leukemia, and solid tumor malignancies) and/or treatment regimen.[1]

Rasburicase may elicit an antibody response that may increase hypersensitivity reactions and decrease efficacy.[3] For this reason, the manufacturer recommends that it should be used for a single course of therapy only.[1] Rasburicase has been administered safely and effectively to pediatric and *adult* patients who had received prior therapy.[3,4]

Hyperuricemia: 0.15–0.2 mg/kg/day for up to 5–7 days.[1-9]

Chemotherapy should begin 4–24 hours after administration of rasburicase.[1]

Some trials have given 0.15–0.2 mg/kg q 12 h for the first 48–72 hours in patients at greatest risk of developing hyperuricemia.[3,4,6-9]

A single dose of 0.15 mg/kg was effective at decreasing uric acid levels in patients (18 months–72 years) with bulky tumor.[10]

A single 6-mg dose has been found to be effective in *adults*.[11]

Dosage adjustment in organ dysfunction	Not established.
Maximum dosage	0.2 mg/kg/dose or 0.4 mg/kg/day.[1]
Additives	None.
Suitable diluents	Reconstitute with diluents supplied.

Rasburicase

Maximum concentration	Not established. Desired dose of reconstituted rasburicase should be added to NS for a final total volume of 50 mL.[1]
Preparation and delivery	**Preparation:** Using aseptic technique and syringes of appropriate volume, remove the predetermined dose of rasburicase from the reconstituted vials and inject into an infusion bag containing the appropriate volume of NS to achieve a final total volume of 50 mL.[1] **Delivery:** Do not filter infusion. A separate line is preferred. Flushing the line with 15 mL of NS before and after administration is also acceptable.[1] Final solution for injection should be infused over 30 minutes.[1]
IV push	Not recommended.[1]
Intermittent infusion	Dilute rasburicase vials with 1 mL of provided diluent and add desired rasburicase dose to an infusion bag of NS for a final volume of 50 mL to be infused over 30 minutes.[1] Total dosing volumes of 10–50 mL have been given to infants.[7]
Continuous infusion	No information available to support administration by this method.
Other routes of administration	No information available to support administration by other routes.
Comments	**Significant adverse effects:** Patients with glucose-6-phosphate dehydrogenase deficiency (G6PD) are at increased risk of developing severe hemolysis. Rasburicase is contraindicated in G6PD since hydrogen peroxide is a major by-product in the conversion of uric acid to allantoin. High-risk G6PD populations should be screened prior to administration.[1] Methemoglobinemia and severe hypoxemia have occurred in two clinical trial patients. Immediately and permanently discontinue rasburicase and initiate supportive care.[1] Renal tubular damage was reported in a 7-year-old receiving rasburicase and alkalinization.[12] Renal damage has been related to alkalinization resulting in calcium phosphate precipitation.[3,12] Alkalinization should be avoided during rasburicase administration.[12] **Laboratory interference:** Rasburicase interferes with uric acid analysis. Collect blood in heparin-containing, prechilled tubes, which are immediately immersed in an ice bath. Analyze within 4 hours of collection.[1] **Monitoring:** CBC and plasma uric acid levels.[1,2]

Rifampin

Brand names

Rifadin IV

Medication error potential

Look-alike, sound-alike drug names.

ISMP's *Confused Drug Names* lists confusion between Rifadin and Rifater.[1]

USP reports confusion with ribavirin, rifabutin, and rifaximin.[2] Likewise, confusion between Rifadin and rifabutin and Rifamate.[2] Confusion with rifabutin has resulted in patient harm.[2]

Contraindications and warnings

Contraindications: Rifampin is contraindicated in patients with a history of hypersensitivity to any of the rifamycins.[3]

Warnings: May cause hepatic dysfunction.[3] Fatalities have occurred in patients with liver disease and in patients concurrently taking other hepatotoxic agents. Hyperbilirubinemia can also occur early in therapy.[3] An isolated, moderate rise in bilirubin and/or transaminases is not an indication for interrupting treatment. The decision should be predicated on the results of repeat tests and the patient's clinical condition. Discontinue if signs of hepatocellular damage are noted.[3] (See Monitoring in Comments section.)

Rifampin may induce delta amino levulinic acid synthetase and can exacerbate porphyria.[3]

Infusion related cautions

Extravasation may cause local irritation and inflammation.[3]

Dosage

Should not to be used for the treatment of meningococcal disease as rapid resistance may develop.[3]

Neonates: 10–20 mg/kg/day divided q 12 h.[4-6]

Infants and children: 10–20 mg/kg/day divided q 12 h or given as a single dose q 24 h.[6-8]

One study in children concluded that it may be more appropriate to shorten the dosing interval from 12 hours to 8 hours after 2 days of therapy to avoid prolonged periods of low plasma concentrations.[9]

Rifampin IV has been used synergistically in patients with persistent staphylococcal bacteremia unresponsive to vancomycin therapy and in patients with methicillin-resistant *Staphylococcus aureus* and methicillin-resistant coagulase-negative staphylococci.[10,11]

Biologic warfare or bioterrorism: The CDC and other experts recommend that treatment of inhalational anthrax spores due to biologic warfare or bioterrorism should be started on a multiple-drug parenteral regimen that includes ciprofloxacin or doxycycline and one or two additional anti-infective agents (e.g., chloramphenicol, clindamycin, rifampin, vancomycin, clarithromycin, imipenem, penicillin, or ampicillin).[12,13]

Prophylaxis of intraventricular shunt revision: 20 mg/kg as a single dose 1 hour prior to surgery.[14]

Dosage adjustment in organ dysfunction

No adjustment in renal[3,15] or hepatic dysfunction[3]; however, if CrCl is <10 mL/min, decrease dose by 50%.[3]

Maximum dosage

20 mg/kg/day[14,16] not to exceed 1200 mg/day in *adults*.[3,17]

Additives

None.

Rifampin

Suitable diluents	D5W, NS.[3,18]
Maximum concentration	≤6 mg/mL.[3,18]
Preparation and delivery	**Stability:** Infusion solution should be administered within 4 hours of preparation because rifampin may precipitate.[3]
IV push	Not recommended.[3]
Intermittent infusion	Over 30 minutes.[3,4,14]
Continuous infusion	Not used.
Other routes of administration	IM and SC not recommended.[3] Intraventricular administration (5 mg/dose) has been used in cases of central nervous system tuberculosis.[19]
Comments	**Rare adverse effects:** Thrombocytopenia has been reported.[3,20] It is generally associated with large dose intermittent therapy, but has also been reported after resumption of interrupted treatment.[3] Although it resolves if drug is stopped at the first appearance of purpura, cerebral hemorrhage and fatalities have been reported when rifampin is continued.[3]
	Elevations in BUN and serum uric acid have been reported.[3,21] Hemolysis, hemoglobinuria, hematuria, interstitial nephritis, acute tubular necrosis, and acute renal failure usually occur during intermittent therapy or when treatment is resumed following intentional or accidental interruption of a daily dosage regimen, and are reversible when rifampin is discontinued.
	Cutaneous reactions (e.g., of flushing and itching with or without a rash) are mild and self-limiting.[3] Although serious hypersensitivity associated cutaneous reactions have been reported (e.g., pruritus, urticaria, rash, pemphigoid reaction, erythema multiforme including Stevens-Johnson syndrome, toxic epidermal necrolysis, vasculitis, eosinophilia, sore mouth, sore tongue, and conjunctivitis), anaphylaxis is rare.[21]
	Monitoring: Monitor hepatic transaminases at baseline and then every 2 to 4 weeks during therapy.[3] The manufacturer notes that baseline tests are unnecessary in pediatric patients unless a complicating condition is known or suspected.[3]
	Drug interactions: Rifampin induces the CYP2C19 isozymes to cause numerous drug interactions. Consult appropriate resources before combining any drug with rifampin.[22]
	Laboratory interference: Rifampin may interfere with standard microbiological assays for serum folate and vitamin B12.[3] Cross-reactivity and false-positive urine screening tests for opiates have been reported.[3] Reduced biliary excretion of contrast media used for visualization of the gallbladder requires that tests be performed before the morning dose of rifampin.[3]
	Other: May discolor body secretions (e.g., sweat, urine, and tears).[3]

RiTUXimab

Brand names	Rituxan

Medication error potential

ISMP high-alert medication that has an increased risk of causing significant patient harm if it is used in error.[1]

Look-alike, sound-alike error potential.

ISMP and USP report that riTUXimab was confused with InFLIXimab; patient harm resulted.[2,3] USP also reports that riTUXimab was confused with Rituxan; patient death resulted.[3]

USP reports that Rituxan was confused with riTUXimab; no patient harm resulted.[3]

Contraindications and warnings

US boxed warning: Rituximab carries black box warnings for fatal infusion reactions (see Infusion related cautions section), tumor lysis syndrome (TLS), severe mucocutaneous reactions and progressive multifocal leukoencephalopathy (PML).

Tumor lysis syndrome (hyperkalemia, hypocalcemia, hyperuricemia, hyperphosphatemia, and acute renal failure) necessitating dialysis to prevent renal failure has been reported within 12–24 hours after the first rituximab infusion. Treatment should include supportive care with electrolyte correction and dialysis, as needed. Prophylaxis may be warranted in patients with a high tumor burden.

Severe mucocutaneous reactions with fatal outcomes have been reported 1–13 weeks after the initial rituximab dosage.[4]

Other warnings: May cause hepatitis B reactivation, increased risk of infection, life-threatening cardiac arrhythmias, renal toxicity, bowel obstruction, and bowel perforation.[4]

Infusion related cautions

Rituximab has been associated with the development of a fatal infusion reaction complex (hypoxia, pulmonary infiltrates, respiratory distress, myocardial infarction, ventricular fibrillation or cardiogenic shock). This complex most commonly occurs with the first dose.[4]

Severe infusion reactions (hypotension, hypoxia, bronchospasm, or angioedema) are most common with the first dose and generally occur within 30–120 minutes after beginning the infusion. Treatment should include interruption of the infusion and the use of supportive care measures, including oxygen, bronchodilators, and IV fluids. Often the infusion can be resumed with a 50% reduction in the infusion rate. Close monitoring in subsequent courses should occur.[4]

Other less serious hypersensitivity reactions are common and can be treated with a 50% reduction in infusion rate and acetaminophen and diphenhydramine. Bronchodilators and IV saline may also be used as needed.[4]

Premedication with acetaminophen and diphenhydramine is recommended to reduce the incidence of hypersensitivity reactions (e.g., fevers, chills, rigors).[4]

Dosage

Consult institutional protocols for complete dosing information.

Rituximab is part of combination therapy to treat newly diagnosed, relapsed, or refractory CD20 positive B-cell, non-Hodgkin's lymphoma or B-cell ALL, as well as other hematologic disorders.

CD20 positive B-cell, non-Hodgkin's lymphoma

Initial: 375 mg/m² once weekly for four to eight doses as monotherapy or in combination with CHOP (i.e., cyclophosphamide, doxorubicin, vincristine, and prednisone).[4-7]

Dosage *(cont.)*	**Retreatment:** 375 mg/m^2 once weekly for four doses or once weekly for four doses given q 6 mo for up to 2 years.[4,7]
	Refractory: 375 mg/m^2 on days 1 and 3 in combination with ifosfamide, mesna, carboplatin, and etoposide.[8]
	B-cell ALL: 375 mg/m^2 to conventional salvage therapy.[9]
	Relapsed or refractory low-grade, follicular, or transformed B-cell non-Hodgkin's lymphoma: 250 mg/m^2 administered 4 hours prior to Indium-111 ibritumomab; 7–9 days later, 250 mg/m^2 administered within 4 hours of Yttrium-90 ibritumomab.[4,10]
	Post-transplant lymphoproliferative disorder: 375 mg/m^2 once weekly for three to four doses.[11,12]
	Autoimmune hemolytic anemia: 375 mg/m^2 once weekly for three to six doses.[13,14]
Dosage adjustment in organ dysfunction	Not established.
Maximum dosage	Clinical trials have reported single dosages up to 500 mg/m^2.[4]
Additives	Contains 9 mg/mL NaCl.[4]
Suitable diluents	D5W or NS.[4]
Maximum concentration	4 mg/mL.[4]
Preparation and delivery	Do not mix or dilute with other drugs.[4]
IV push	Not recommended.[4]
Intermittent infusion	Dilute with suitable diluent to final concentration of 1–4 mg/mL and infuse at a beginning rate of 50 mg/h. If no hypersensitivity reactions occur, the rate may be escalated by 50 mg/h q 30 min to a maximum rate of 400 mg/h. In patients tolerating the first infusion, subsequent cycles may begin at a rate of 100 mg/h, escalating up to a maximum rate of 400 mg/h.[4]
Continuous infusion	No information available to support administration by this method.
Other routes of administration	No information available to support administration by other routes.

RiTUXimab

Significant adverse effects: Rituximab is associated with a minimal (<10%) risk of emesis.[15,16] Generally, prophylaxis for acute and delayed emesis is not needed. Patients may receive one time prophylaxis with a phenothiazine (e.g., prochlorperazine) or a butyrophenone (e.g., droperidol). Breakthrough medications should be offered, such as a phenothiazine (e.g., prochlorperazine), a butyrophenone (e.g., droperidol), a substituted benzamide (e.g., metoclopramide), or a benzodiazepine (e.g., lorazepam). Selection should be based on what the patient is currently receiving for acute antiemesis prophylaxis.[15,16]

Monitoring: CBC with platelets, cardiac and renal function, fluid balance, and vital signs.[4,17]

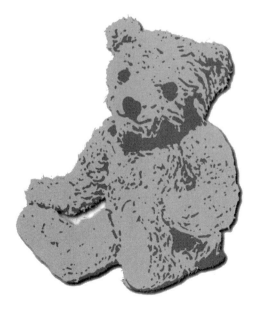

Rocuronium Bromide

Brand names	Zemuron

Medication error potential

ISMP high-alert medication that has an increased risk of causing significant patient harm if it is used in error.[1]

Look-alike, sound-alike error potential.

USP reports that rocuronium has been confused with Romazicon and vecuronium; no patient harm resulted.[2] USP also reports that Zemuron has been confused with vecuronium; patient death resulted.[2]

Contraindications and warnings

Contraindications: Hypersensitivity to rocuronium or any of its components.[3]

Warnings: Use carefully under the supervision of experienced clinicians; personnel should also be skilled in airway management, resuscitation, and respiratory support.[3] Intubation and ventilatory support equipment, including oxygen therapy, should be readily available.[3] Also should have anticholinesterase inhibitors readily available when giving rocuronium.[3]

Infusion related cautions

Hypersensitivity reactions, hypotension, arrhythmias, bronchospasm, and severe anaphylaxis (life-threatening in some cases) have been reported but appear to be rare.[3]

Dosage

Respiratory function must be supported during use of this agent. Concurrent administration of a sedative is also necessary. Monitoring of neuromuscular transmission with a peripheral nerve stimulator is recommended during continuous infusion or with repeated dosing.[3,4]

In obese patients, dose should be based on actual body weight, not ideal or lean body mass.[3]

When administered with inhalational anesthetics, such as halothane, isoflurane, or sevoflurane, the dose of rocuronium should be reduced by 20% to 50%.[5,6]

Infants: 0.5 mg/kg repeated q 20–30 min as needed to maintain pharmacological paralysis.[3,7]

Children: 0.6–0.8 mg/kg initially, followed by repeated doses of 0.075–0.125 mg/kg q 20–30 min as needed to maintain pharmacological paralysis.[3,7-10] May also give 10–12 mcg/kg/min as continuous infusion.[3,5,6,9,11]

Dosage adjustment in organ dysfunction

An increased initial dosage may be required for complete neuromuscular blockade in patients with hepatic impairment.[3] Duration of neuromuscular blockade in these patients may also be prolonged.[3] No dosage adjustment required in those with renal impairment.[3] In children with renal failure who were older than 1 year of age, a single bolus dose did not cause prolonged neuromuscular blockade but was associated with a slower onset of action than that noted in healthy children.[12]

Maximum dosage

Not established.

Additives

None.

Suitable diluents

D5W, D5NS, NS, LR.[3,13]

Maximum concentration

10 mg/mL for IV push; 5 mg/mL for infusion.[3]

Rocuronium Bromide

Preparation and delivery	Rocuronium is an acidic solution; do not administer with alkaline solutions.[3]
IV push	10 mg/mL over 5–10 seconds.[3]
Intermittent infusion	Not administered by this method.
Continuous infusion	0.5–1 mg/mL recommended.[3,14] The manufacturer provides information for continuous infusion with a 0.5-, 1-, and 5-mg/mL solution.[3]
Other routes of administration	Not recommended by manufacturer.[3] Although a single IM dose of 1 mg/kg in infants and 1.8 mg/kg in children has been used,[15] rocuronium should not be used as an alternative to IM succinylcholine when rapid intubation is necessary. The use of IM administration is not recommended since it does not consistently provide satisfactory tracheal intubating conditions.[15] When given in the deltoid muscle of infants and children, serum concentrations peak at 13 minutes, with about 80% of the dose absorbed systemically.[16]
Comments	**Significant adverse effects:** Prolonged neuromuscular blockade may occur. Factors that potentiate the duration of neuromuscular blockade include acidosis, hypokalemia, hypermagnesemia, neuromuscular disease, hepatic disease, and other medications.[3,7] (See Drug interactions below.) Patients with neurological diseases, such as myasthenia gravis, may exhibit increased sensitivity.[3] Decreased sensitivity to rocuronium may occur in patients with severe burns, muscle trauma, demyelinating lesions, neuropathy, or infection.[3] **Drug interactions:** Concomitant administration of other drugs (e.g., aminoglycosides, inhalational anesthetics, magnesium, succinylcholine, vancomycin) may prolong neuromuscular blockade.[3] Consult appropriate resources for additional information on drug interactions.

Ropivacaine HCl

Brand names	Naropin

Medication error potential

ISMP high-alert medication that has an increased risk of causing significant patient harm if it is used in error.[1]

Look-alike, sound-alike error potential.

USP reports that ropivacaine was confused with bupivacaine; no patient harm resulted.[2]

Contraindications and warnings

Contraindications: Ropivacaine is contraindicated in patients with known hypersensitivity to the drug or any amide anesthetic.[3]

Warnings: Ropivacaine should only be administered by persons specifically trained in the use of local anesthetics.[3]

The FDA notified healthcare professionals in November 2009 of the risk of chondrolysis following continuous intraarticular infusion of local anesthetics, including ropivacaine, via elastomeric infusion devices. The FDA has received 35 reports of chondrolysis, some were in previously healthy young *adults,* and most following shoulder surgery. The cases had received the local anesthetics for postoperative pain for periods of 48–72 hours. Chondrolysis symptoms (joint pain, stiffness, loss of motion) occurred as early as 2 (median 5) months following therapy with the local anesthetic.[4,5]

Infusion related cautions

Not for IV infusion or IM administration. Administer only by lumbar epidural injection or infusion, by thoracic epidural infusion, by injection for nerve block, and by infiltration.[3,4,6]

Accidental IV injection may result in cardiac arrhythmia or cardiac arrest, seizures, coma, and respiratory arrest.[3,4,7]

Oxygen, cardiopulmonary resuscitation and intubation equipment and medications and trained personnel in emergency management should be immediately available when using ropivacaine.[3]

Dosage

Dose varies with the anesthetic procedure, the area to be anesthetized, the vascularity of the tissues, the number of neuronal segments to be blocked, the depth and duration of anesthesia required, as well as individual response.

A test dose of epinephrine with or without lidocaine has been used to verify that the needle is not in the vascular space.[8,9] Once the catheter is placed, negative aspiration of blood or cerebrospinal fluid[3,10-13] and the absence of cardiovascular changes following a test dose indicates correct position of the catheter.[3,10,14] (See Significant adverse effects in Comments section.)

The manufacturer does not recommend the use of ropivacaine with or without epinephrine in children <12 years.[3]

Caudal/epidural block: Children 1.25–6.5 mg/kg.[4,8-12,14,15] or 1 mL/kg of 0.2% solution.[7]

Epidural continuous infusion

> **Children 4 months to 7 years:** A loading dose of 1 mg/kg followed by 0.2–0.4 mg/kg/h for 48 hours.[4,7,13,16] One group of investigators reported continuous infusion up to 96 hours without adverse events.[13]

Ropivacaine HCl

Dosage *(cont.)*	**Children from 7 to 12 years:** 24 children assigned to a patient-controlled infusion of a loading dose of 3.6 mg followed by a continuous infusion of 3.2 mg/h with dose titration up to 27.2 mg/h if needed required less drug than 24 children assigned to a standard treatment of a continuous infusion of 0.4 mg/kg/h (239 mg/48 h compared to 576 mg/48 h, respectively).[9] ***Adults:*** A loading dose of 10–14 mg (5–7 mL of 0.2% solution) followed by 12–28 mg/h (6–14 mL/h of 0.2% solution) for up to 72 hours.[3,4]
Dosage adjustment in organ dysfunction	Use with caution in patients with hepatic or cardiovascular disease.[3,4,7]
Maximum dosage	Not established.
Additives	None.
Suitable diluents	Not diluted.
Maximum concentration	1% (10 mg/mL).[3,4,6]
Preparation and delivery	Should not be mixed with alkaline solutions as precipitation is likely to occur.[3]
IV push	Do not administer IV.[3,4,7] (See Infusion related cautions section.)
Intermittent infusion	Do not administer IV.[2,3,11,14] (See Infusion related cautions section.) 1 mg/kg over 10 minutes has been administered via epidural catheter.[7]
Continuous infusion	Do not administer IV. (See Infusion related cautions section.) For epidural infusion only.[3,4,7,9,13,16] (See Dosage section.)
Other routes of administration	Do not administer IM.[3,4,6] (See Infusion related cautions section.)
Comments	**Significant adverse effects:** Systemic absorption of local anesthetics may result in toxic plasma concentrations, resulting in cardiovascular adverse effects, including decreased cardiac output, heart block, hypotension, bradycardia, ventricular arrhythmias, and cardiac arrest. Patients should be carefully monitored during injection. Use with caution in patients with underlying cardiovascular disease.[3,4,7] **Drug interactions:** Patients receiving class III antiarrhythmics (e.g., amiodarone) may be at increased risk for cardiac adverse effects.[3,4] Ropivacaine and its primary metabolite are metabolized via the CYP1A2 isoenzyme. Concomitant use of CYP1A2 inhibitors may be associated with the potential for serious drug interactions.[3] Consult appropriate resources for dosing recommendations before combining any drug with ropivacaine.

Sargramostim

Brand names	Leukine; yeast derived (*Saccharomyces cerevisiae*) recombinant human granulocyte-macrophage colony-stimulating factor (rhGM-CSF)
Medication error potential	Look-alike, sound-alike error potential. USP reported that sargramostim was confused with filgrastim and Sandostatin.[1]
Contraindications and warnings	**Contraindications:** Patients with ≥10% leukemic myeloid blasts in bone marrow or peripheral blood; patients with known hypersensitivity to GM-CSF, products derived from yeast, or any product component; 24 hours before or after chemotherapy or radiotherapy treatment.[2] **Warnings:** Allergic reactions have been reported. Should this occur, discontinue the infusion and institute appropriate therapy.[2]
Infusion related cautions	A first-dose response that includes respiratory distress, hypotension, tachycardia, and flushing is common with infusion of the first dose of a cycle and usually resolves with treatment.[2] This does not recur with subsequent doses in the cycle.[2]
Dosage	The products derived from *Escherichia coli* and Chinese hamster ovaries are not available in the US. Some of the studies cited evaluated these products, which may have different potencies, specific activities, and adverse effects.[1] **Neutropenia** **Postchemotherapy neutropenia:** 250–1000 mcg/m²/day IV over 2 hours for up to 14 days[2-4] or 5 mcg/kg/day IV (bacteria [*Escherichia coli*] derived) over 4 hours for up to 21 days.[5] Alternatively, 5 mcg/kg/day SC for up to 21 days following chemotherapy or irradiation.[6,7] (See Comments section.) **Bone marrow transplantation:** 250 mcg/m²/day IV over 2 hours beginning 2–4 hours after transplant and not earlier than 24 hours after chemotherapy or after radiation until absolute neutrophil count (ANC) >1500 cells/mm³ for 3 consecutive days.[2] Alternatively, 250 mcg/m²/day IV over 4 hours beginning after transplant for 21 days.[8] **Congenital neutropenia:** Five children (age 1, 2, 3, 9, and 19 years) were started on 3 mcg/kg/day IV over 30–60 minutes for 14 days that was increased to 10 mcg/kg/day if the ANC failed to increase and finally to 30 mcg/kg/day. Only one had an increase in ANC.[8] One patient received 10 mcg/kg/day as a continuous infusion for 4 weeks followed by SC dosing for another week without response.[9] **Associated with HIV or antiretroviral therapy:** 250 mcg/m²/day IV or SC for 2–4 weeks.[1] **Premature and term neonates (reconstitute lyophilized product in SW to avoid benzyl alcohol)** **Neutropenia and sepsis (≥28 weeks gestation):** 5 mcg/kg/day over 2 hours once daily for 5 days[10] or 4 mcg/kg/day over 2 hours q 12 h for up to 6 days or until neutropenia resolved.[11] **Neutropenia (≤31 weeks gestation):** 10 mcg/kg/day SC × 5 days.[12] **Aplastic anemia:** In nine children (0.7–19 years of age), induction phase continuous infusion doses of either 8 mcg/kg/day increased after 14 days to 16 mcg/kg/day for up to 14 more days if the hematologic response was inadequate or doses of 16 mcg/kg/day increased to 32 mcg/kg/day (Chinese hamster ovary cell derived).[13] After the induction phase, administration was changed to SC dosing.[13] Eighteen children received a standard immunosuppressive regimen for 5 days and then GM-CSF at 250 mcg/m²/day SC was started.[14]

Sargramostim

Dosage adjustment in organ dysfunction	None. Patients with renal or hepatic impairment should have renal function or liver function monitored weekly.[2]
Maximum dosage	32 mcg/kg[12] or 1500 mcg/m².[3]
Additives	The liquid product contains 1.1% benzyl alcohol, 40 mg/mL mannitol, 10 mg/mL sucrose, 1.2 mg/mL tromethamine.[2] After reconstitution with BW or SW, each mL of the lyophilized product contains 40 mg mannitol, 10 mg sucrose, and 1.2 mg/mL tromethamine.[2] BW contains benzyl alcohol. See Appendix C for information about potential benzyl alcohol toxicity in neonates.
Suitable diluents	NS.[2]
Maximum concentration	250 (reconstituted lyophilized powder) or 500 mcg/mL (liquid).[2]
Preparation and delivery	An in-line membrane filter should not be used when sargramostim is given IV.[2] **Stability:** The lyophilized product reconstituted with SW must be used within 6 hours of reconstitution because it contains no preservatives.[2] If the final concentration will be <10 mcg/mL, albumin should be added to the NS diluent to achieve a final albumin concentration of 0.1% prior to the addition of sargramostim to prevent adsorption to the drug delivery system.[2] **Compatibility:** See Appendix D for PN compatibility information.
IV push	Not indicated.[2]
Intermittent infusion	Usually infused over 2–4 hours[2-4] but has been given over 30 minutes.[9]
Continuous infusion	≥10 mcg/mL in NS.[2]
Other routes of administration	The liquid product (500 mcg/mL) can be given SC undiluted.[2] The lyophilized product is reconstituted to 250 mcg/mL and given SC without further dilution.[2] Not for IM administration.

Sargramostim

Comments

The use of colony-stimulating factor decreased febrile neutropenia, length of hospitalization, and number of infectious episodes but did not shorten the duration of neutropenia nor lessen treatment delays in children with ALL.[15]

Monitoring: A CBC with differential is recommended twice a week during therapy to evaluate for leukocytosis. If the ANC >20,000 cells/mm^3, or the platelet count >500,000 cells/mm^3, the dose should be decreased by 50% or held.[2]

Adverse effects: Children receiving multiple courses of SC GM-CSF have experienced acute toxicities at various times during their dosing including fever, tachycardia, hypotension and rash requiring discontinuation.[6]

Sargramostim has the potential to activate the coagulation system in pediatric patients receiving bone marrow or stem cell transplant.[16]

The severity of adverse reactions appears to be less with the yeast-derived product than those derived in Chinese hamster ovary cells or bacteria.[1]

Pericardial and pleural effusions, myalgias, and volume overload are dose-limiting side effects in *adults*.[2] Although adverse effects have been reported in children, they are usually mild[4,5] and unrelated to dose.[3] However, cardiopulmonary symptoms occurred in a child receiving continuous infusion of 24 mcg/kg/day[13] and a deep vein thrombosis occurred in a child being treated for myelosuppressive chemotherapy, who inadvertently received 1500 mcg/m^2/day for 7 days.[3]

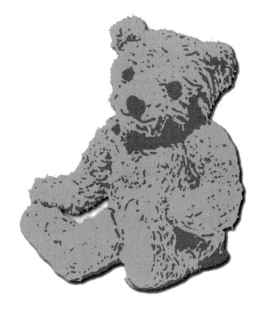

Sodium Bicarbonate

Brand names	Various manufacturers
	Available in concentrations of 0.5 mEq HCO₃/mL (4.2%), 0.6 mEq/mL (5%), 0.9 mEq/mL (7.5%), and 1 mEq/mL (8.4%)

Brand names Various manufacturers

Available in concentrations of 0.5 mEq HCO_3/mL (4.2%), 0.6 mEq/mL (5%), 0.9 mEq/mL (7.5%), and 1 mEq/mL (8.4%)

Medication error potential

Look-alike, sound-alike error potential.

USP reported that sodium bicarbonate was confused with sodium chloride and patient harm resulted.[1]

Contraindications and warnings

Contraindications: Ongoing chloride losses as in vomiting or gastrointestinal suction, those receiving diuretics known to cause a hypochloremic alkalosis.[2]

Infusion related cautions

Sodium bicarbonate should be infused slowly in neonates to decrease possible hypernatremia that may decrease CSF pressure and result in intracranial hemorrhage.[2-5]

Extravasation may cause local ischemia and tissue necrosis.[2,3,6] See Appendix E for management of extravasation of concentrated products.

Dosage

Cardiopulmonary resuscitation: Sodium bicarbonate should only be used after establishment of airway and adequate ventilation, administration of oxygen and medications (e.g., epinephrine and lidocaine), and restoration of effective circulation.[7,8] Routine use of sodium bicarbonate does not improve the outcome of cardiac arrest in children; however, there are certain times when its use can be considered.[7] The 4.2% solution (0.5 mEq/mL) should be used in neonates and infants.[3,8]

> **Prolonged cardiac arrest:** 1 mEq/kg.[7]
>
> **Cocaine-induced ventricular arrhythmia:** 1–2 mEq/kg.[7]
>
> **Tricyclic antidepressant, sodium channel blocker toxicity:** 1–2 mEq/kg until arterial pH is >7.45; then use continuous infusion to maintain alkalosis.[7,8]

Metabolic acidosis: Calculate the base deficit using the following equation[3]:

$$HCO_3 \text{ (mEq)} = 0.3 \times \text{weight (kg)} \times \text{base deficit (mEq/L)}$$

If laboratory measurements are not available: 1–2 mEq/kg.[3]

Adjunctive bicarbonate therapy is commonly used in children with severe DKA and a pH <6.9.[9] However, a retrospective study reported no difference in rate of metabolic recovery and complications between patients treated with or without bicarbonate, and hospitalization was prolonged in the bicarbonate group.[1]

Subsequent dosing should be based on current acid-base status.[2,3] Complete correction of the base deficit should occur over >24 hours because the compensatory response to changes in ventilation may be delayed.[2]

Urinary alkalinization (See Comments section.)

> **Poisonings (salicylate) in children**[11]**:** 25 mEq infused over 1 hour. Urine pH should be measured q 15–30 min and additional doses given until the urine pH is 7.5–8.5. Potassium concentrations should be measured hourly, the arterial pH should be ≤7.5.
>
> **Prevention of tumor lysis syndrome**[12]**:** D5¼NS with 50–100 mEq/L NaHCO₃ (no potassium) infused at 3–6 L/m²/day and titrated to a urinary pH of 7–7.5. Serum HCO₃ concentration should be kept ≤30 mEq/L.

Sodium Bicarbonate

Dosage adjustment in organ dysfunction	Use with caution in patients with renal insufficiency, congestive heart failure, or in those with edema and sodium retention.[2]
Maximum dosage	2 mEq/kg/dose,[2] 8 mEq/kg/day in infants,[2,5] 2–5 mEq/kg as intermittent infusions over 4–8 hours.[2,3]
Additives	Each gram of sodium bicarbonate contains 12 mEq sodium.[13] The 5% solution in 500-mL bottles also contains 0.9 mg/mL of edetate disodium.[2,13]
Suitable diluents	D5NS, D5W, D10W, D-LR, LR, R.[14]
Maximum concentration	**Neonates and infants:** 4.2% (0.5 mEq/mL).[2,3] **>2 years:** 8.4% (1 mEq/mL).[2]
Preparation and delivery	**Compatibility:** Bicarbonate inactivates norepinephrine and dobutamine.[2] Adequately flush the IV lines between administration of resuscitation drugs and sodium bicarbonate.[2,7] Incompatible with calcium containing fluids.[2] See Appendix D for PN compatibility information.
IV push	This method of administration is indicated in cardiac arrest.
Intermittent infusion	2–5 mEq/kg over 4–8 hours in older children.[2,3]
Continuous infusion	May be given continuously.
Other routes of administration	May be administered IO if unable to establish adequate IV access during cardiac arrest.[7]
Comments	Urinary alkalinization and forced diuresis has been used to prevent acute renal failure due to rhabdomyolysis. However, a retrospective review of 1771 *adults* with rhabdomyolysis due to trauma who received bicarbonate and mannitol forced diuresis found that renal failure was not decreased when compared to a group that did not receive this treatment.[14] **Monitoring:** Electrolytes, including potassium and calcium, should be monitored.[2,3] Measurement of arterial pH (blood gas) is indicated during resuscitation. Potassium concentration and pH are inversely related; therefore, increases in pH result in a decrease in potassium concentration. Blood calcium binding to albumin is enhanced with alkalosis resulting in decreased ionized calcium. Urinary pH should be measured during urinary alkalinization. **Adverse effects:** Rapid changes in serum sodium concentration should be avoided. Metabolic alkalosis is a complication that may result in hypokalemia, hypocalcemia, and impaired delivery of oxygen to the tissue.[5]

Sodium Chloride

Brand names

Various manufacturers

0.45% saline (½NS) = 77 mEq/L
0.9% saline (NS) = 154 mEq/L
3% saline = 513 mEq/L
5% saline = 855 mEq/L

Medication error potential

ISMP high-alert medication that has an increased risk of causing significant patient harm if it is used in error.[1]

USP reported that sodium chloride was confused with potassium chloride. Sodium chloride was confused with sodium bicarbonate and patient harm resulted.[2]

ISMP reported that use of hypotonic saline solutions post-operatively resulted in acute hyponatremia and death in two previously healthy children.[3]

Contraindications and warnings

A variety of sodium concentrations are available. The bulk packages are concentrated and are not intended for direct infusion.[4] Choose products carefully.

Infusion related cautions

During chronic hyponatremia, shifts of water and sodium occur to maintain normal cellular volume in the brain.[5,6] Too rapid correction of hyponatremia can result in osmotic demyelination syndrome (or central pontine; extrapontine myelinolysis).[5-10]

Similarly, during chronic hypernatremia the brain generates idiogenic osmoles to maintain cerebral intracellular osmolality.[5,6] Too rapid decreases in serum sodium water moves into the brain cells resulting in cerebral edema, seizures, and coma.

In general, the serum sodium should not be increased or decreased ≥10–12 mEq/day in these chronic conditions.[5,6]

Dosage

Hypotension/shock: 20 mL/kg of NS over 5–10 minutes that may be repeated. Up to 80 mL/kg may be required during the first hour; however, the child should continuously be assessed for fluid overload.[11,12]

Dehydration: 20 mL/kg of NS over 20 minutes that may be repeated to restore the intravascular volume.[6] In severe dehydration multiple boluses that are infused rapidly may be required to restore to prevent shock.[6] After intravascular volume is restored, correction of the fluid deficit (% dehydration × wt [kg]) should begin along with providing maintenance fluids.

Symptomatic hyponatremia: The initial goal of sodium replacement is symptom resolution and not correction of the serum sodium to normal. As an estimate, 1 mL/kg of 3% sodium chloride will raise the serum sodium by 1 mEq/L.[6] More aggressive replacement may be required in patients with severe symptoms such as seizures.[6] Following resolution of symptoms, the infusion should be adjusted to increase serum sodium concentration by no more than 10–12 mEq/L/day.[5,6] Frequent monitoring of serum sodium concentrations is essential. (See Comments section.)

Severe traumatic brain injury: 1.5% saline (268 mEq/L) infused to obtain a desired serum sodium concentration of 145–150 mEq/L[13] or 0.1–1 mL/kg/h 3% saline titrated to an intracranial pressure (ICP) of <20 mm Hg.[14-16]

Dosage adjustment in organ dysfunction

None required.

Sodium Chloride

Maximum dosage	None established.
Additives	Some products contain benzyl alcohol or parabens as a preservative.[17] See Appendix C for information about potential benzyl alcohol and parabens toxicity.
IV push	20 mL/kg given rapidly may be indicated in severe hypotension/shock.[5,6]
Intermittent infusion	20 mL/kg over 20 minutes to 1 hour in moderate dehydration.[5,6]
Continuous infusion	Usual method of administration.
Other routes of administration	IO.[11]
Maximum concentration	NS via a peripheral line (Osmolarity ~308 mOsm/L).[17] More concentrated saline infusions (i.e., 3% saline >1000 mOsm/L) may require infusion via central line.[17]
Comments	**Significant adverse effects:** Those who slowly develop hyponatremia may be relatively asymptomatic; however, those with a more rapid rate of decline of the sodium concentration may be symptomatic with mild hyponatremia. Symptoms associated with hyponatremia are primarily related to CNS effects and include symptoms of nausea, headache, lethargy, confusion, muscle aches, agitation, and seizures.[5,6] Too rapid correction of serum sodium (either hyper or hyponatremia) can result in cerebral edema with symptoms of seizures and coma. Too rapid decrease in serum sodium can be treated with 3% saline to acutely increase the serum sodium and reverse the cerebral edema.[5,6]

Sodium Nitroprusside

Brand names	Nitropress, generic

Medication error potential

ISMP high-alert medication that has an increased risk of causing significant patient harm if it is used in error.[1]

Look-alike, sound-alike error potential.

USP reported that nitroprusside was confused with norepinephrine and nitroglycerin.[2]

Nitroprusside confusion with nicardipine and Neo-Synephrine resulted in patient harm. USP reported that Nipride was confused with nesiritide.

Contraindications and warnings

US boxed warning[3]**:** The product must be diluted prior to infusion.

Precipitous decreases in blood pressure (BP) can occur. Patients must be continuously monitored with appropriate equipment and by trained personnel during infusion.

Cyanide ions can reach toxic levels during infusion. Failure to attain the desired response after maximum rate infusion for 10 minutes should result in termination of the infusion.

Contraindications[3]**:** Treatment of compensatory hypertension with primarily aortic coarctation or arteriovenous shunting, patients with known inadequate cerebral circulation or in moribund patients undergoing emergency surgery, patients with Leber's congenital optic atrophy or with tobacco amblyopia, or patients with acute CHF with reduced peripheral vascular resistance (high-output heart failure)

Infusion related cautions

Too rapid decrease in BP can result in serious and permanent neurological sequelae.[3-5] BP should be monitored continuously with an arterial line.[6,7] It has been recommended that the BP be gradually decreased ≤25% in the first 8 hours after presentation followed by gradual normalization of the BP over 26–48 hours.[8]

Nitroprusside should only be infused using a volumetric infusion device.[3]

Use with caution in those with increased intracranial pressure and those with compensatory hypertension, such as infants with arteriovenous shunt or coarctation of the aorta.[3,4]

Dosage

0.25–0.3 mcg/kg/min initially titrated by 0.25 mcg/kg/min q 5–10 min up to a maximum of 10 mcg/kg/min.[3-20] In neonates (n=58) infusion rates of 0.2–6 mcg/kg/min for 10 minutes to 126 hours[11] and in children infusion rates of 0.5–8 mcg/kg/min were reported.[5] Usual maintenance dose requirement is ≤3 mcg/kg/min in children and *adults*.[3] The infusion should be gradually tapered off to avoid potential rebound hypertension.[4]

Dosage adjustment in organ dysfunction

Use cautiously in severe renal or hepatic disease because the risk for thiocyanate toxicity is increased.[4] In anuric patients, the infusion should not exceed 1 mcg/kg/min to avoid accumulation of thiocyanate.[3]

Maximum dosage

8–10 mcg/kg/min.[3,4,6,9]

In *adults*, 400 mcg/kg/min was infused for short periods.[21]

Additives

Contains 0.335 mEq sodium/50 mg of sodium nitroprusside.[22,23]

Suitable diluents

D5W.[3,4,22]

Sodium Nitroprusside

Maximum concentration

200 mcg/mL.[3] 70 mcg/mL was used in children 8–17 years old.[13] In *adults*, a concentration of 800 mcg/mL was reported.[24]

Preparation and delivery

Preparation: The vial should be reconstituted with D5W or SW.[3] Do not use BW for reconstitution because the preservatives accelerate the rate of decomposition. The reconstituted product must be further diluted prior to infusion.

Delivery: Although it is not necessary to protect IV tubing, the bottle, burette, and/or syringe pump should be covered with an opaque protective covering.[3,4] Amber plastic coverings are ineffective.[22]

Photosensitivity: Protect from light.

Compatibility: See Appendix D for PN compatibility information.

IV push

Not indicated.

Intermittent infusion

Not indicated.

Continuous infusion

50–200 mcg/mL in D5W, LR, or NS.[3,21,22]

Other routes of administration

Not indicated.

Comments

Monitoring: Cyanide toxicity results in metabolic acidosis, air hunger, and confusion.[3] Most clinical laboratories do not have the capability to measure cyanide concentrations. And acidosis may not occur until 1 hour after cyanide concentrations are toxic.[3] During nitroprusside infusions (cumulative dose >10 mg/kg), hemoglobin can be sequestered as methemoglobin that is available as a laboratory measurement in most clinical laboratories. Methemoglobinemia (>10% of hemoglobin) results in signs of impaired oxygen delivery despite adequate cardiac output and arterial PaO_2.[3] Methylene blue is an antidote but should be used cautiously.[3]

Adverse effects: Cyanide toxicity (and the development of metabolic acidosis) usually occurs with prolonged use; however, it has been reported after as short a time as a few hours.[3,21,25,26] Those with decreased renal function may be at increased risk.[4,6] One study in children did not find an association between cumulative dose or duration of therapy and increased cyanide levels.[27]

In two pediatric studies including 52 and 63 children, the appearance of adverse events was not a reliable predictor of cyanide toxicity.[20,27] One group determined that the mean dose was most predictive of increased cyanide concentrations.[20]

Thiocyanate is a product of cyanide metabolism and a route for cyanide elimination.[3] Sodium thiosulfate has been administered with sodium nitroprusside at infusion rates of 5–10 times that of nitroprusside to accelerate the metabolism of cyanide; however, further study is needed before this can be recommended.[3]

Succinylcholine Chloride

Brand names	Anectine, Quelicin

Medication error potential

ISMP high-alert medication (neuromuscular blocking agent) that has an increased risk of causing significant patient harm if it is used in error.[1]

Contraindications and warnings

US boxed warning: Use of succinylcholine in children should be reserved for emergency intubation or instances where the airway must be immediately secured (e.g. laryngospasm, difficult airway, full stomach, or for intramuscular use when a suitable vein is inaccessible).[2]

Acute rhabdomyolysis with hyperkalemia, ventricular dysrhythmias, cardiac arrest, and death have been reported predominately in healthy children, but have also occurred in other age groups.[2] (See Rare adverse effects/Rhabdomyolysis in Comments section.)

Contraindications: Should not be given to individuals with a personal or familial history of malignant hyperthermia, skeletal muscle myopathies, and known hypersensitivity to the drug.[2] Because of severe hyperkalemia and possible cardiac arrest, should not be used in patients after the acute phase of injury following major burns, multiple trauma, extensive denervation of skeletal muscle, or upper motor neuron injury.[2] (See Rare adverse effects/Hyperkalemia in Comments section.)

Other warnings: Should be used only by those skilled in the management of artificial respiration and only when facilities are instantly available for tracheal intubation and ventilation, including the administration of oxygen under positive pressure and the elimination of carbon dioxide. Should be administered with extreme caution to patients suffering from electrolyte abnormalities and those who may have massive digitalis toxicity, because of the likelihood of serious cardiac arrhythmias or cardiac arrest due to hyperkalemia. (See Rare adverse effects/Hyperkalemia in Comments section.)

Should not be administered before unconsciousness has been induced.[2]

Succinylcholine is metabolized by plasma cholinesterase and should be used with caution, if at all, in patients known to be or suspected of being homozygous for the atypical plasma Cholinesterase gene.[2] (See Other in Comments section.)

Infusion related cautions

Rapid administration may cause bradyarrhythmias secondary to vagal stimulation.[2-5] Pretreatment with atropine may reduce this risk.[2,8,9] (See Dosage section.) Safety precautions must be maintained until full muscle tone has returned.[2]

Dosage

Bradycardia, which may progress to asystole, occurs more often following a second dose of succinylcholine.[2] Its incidence and severity is higher in children than *adults*. Pretreatment with atropine (0.01–0.02 mg/kg; minimum of 0.15 mg) should always be administered with or, preferably, before succinylcholine.[2]

Initial dose must be increased when nondepolarizing agent pretreatment is used because of the antagonism between succinylcholine and nondepolarizing neuromuscular-blocking agents.[6]

Dosing for rapid sequence intubation should be based on actual body weight.[7]

Test dose: Can evaluate sensitivity to succinylcholine, by cautiously administering 5–10 mg (1 mg/mL) by slow infusion.[2] (See Other in Comments section.)

Loading dose (for intubation or short surgical procedures): 1–2 mg/kg[3-5,8-10]; 1 mg/kg is recommended for older children and adolescents.[3,4,9-11]

Maintenance dose: 0.3–1 mg/kg q 5–10 min as needed.[3-5,8-10] Normal *adult* dosing is 0.04–0.07 mg/kg q 5–10 min as needed.[6] Monitoring neuromuscular transmission with a peripheral nerve stimulator is recommended with repeated dosing.[11]

Succinylcholine Chloride

Dosage adjustment in organ dysfunction	No adjustment in renal failure,[2] but use cautiously as succinylcholine can cause hyperkalemia.[2] Dose should be decreased in hepatic failure.[2]
Maximum dosage	2 mg/kg IV or 3–4 mg/kg IM.[2] Not to exceed 150 mg when given IM.[2]
Additives	May contain benzyl alcohol.[12] (See Appendix C for specific information about benzyl alcohol's potential for toxicity.)
Suitable diluents	D5W, D10W, LR, NS, ½NS, D5LR, D5NS, D5¼NS, D5½NS, dextran 6% in dextrose, dextran 6% in NS.[12]
Maximum concentration	100 mg/mL for IV push and 2 mg/mL for continuous infusion.[2,6]
Preparation and delivery	**Stability:** Stable for 45 days in polypropylene syringes (20 mg/mL) at room temperature. Stability diluted in D5W or NS (1–2 mg/mL) is 24 hours under refrigeration.[2]
IV push	100 mg/mL (available commercially) given over 10–30 seconds.[2] Flush needle or catheter with D5W or NS after administration.
Intermittent infusion	Not given.
Continuous infusion	Not recommended in infants and children.[2] It has been used successfully for neuromuscular relaxation in infants; however, tachyphylaxis and phase II nerve block have occurred during continuous infusion.[13] The risk of malignant hyperthermia also precludes continuous infusions in infants and children.[2]
Other routes of administration	3–4 mg/kg, not to exceed a total dose of 150 mg, by deep IM injection.[2]
Comments	**Rare adverse effects:** Numerous cases of sudden death have been attributed to succinylcholine. These generally are attributed to acute rhabdomyolysis with hyperkalemia and ventricular dysrhythmias; hyperkalemia; malignant hyperthermia; or a combination of all three. If a healthy patient develops unexplained sudden cardiac arrest soon after administration of succinylcholine, immediate treatment for hyperkalemia should be instituted.[2] One study reported the successful use of ECMO.[14] If indicated, treatment of malignant hyperthermia should also be instituted (see below).[2] **Rhabdomyolysis:** Succinylcholine has been reported to cause acute rhabdomyolysis and death in healthy children.[2,8,9,15,16] Many of these children were subsequently reported to have Duchenne's muscular dystrophy, but Duchenne's muscular dystrophy is not a contraindication to the use of succinylcholine.[2,17] Rhabdomyolysis may present with peaked T-waves and sudden cardiac arrest within minutes of administration. It appears to be most common in males ≤8 years old, but has also been reports in adolescents.[2] Routine resuscitative measures are generally unsuccessful.[2] However, extraordinary and prolonged resuscitative efforts have resulted in successful management in some cases.[2]

Succinylcholine Chloride

Comments (cont.)

Hyperkalemia: Hyperkalemia may occur, especially in patients who have trauma, severe burns, or neuromuscular disease.[2,18] The risk is dependent on the extent and location of the injury.[18,19] The precise time of onset and the duration of the risk period are not known, but hyperkalemia in these patients increases over time and usually peaks at 7 to 10 days after the injury.[18] If serum potassium is ≥5.5 mEq/L, succinylcholine should not be used.[2] Hyperkalemia occurs almost immediately after succinylcholine and peak in 5 minutes. Treat with calcium bicarbonate, glucose with insulin, and hyperventilation.[2] Should be used cautiously in patients with chronic abdominal infection, subarachnoid hemorrhage, or conditions causing degeneration of central and peripheral nervous systems.

Malignant hyperthermia: The risk of developing succinylcholine-associated acute malignant hyperthermia increases with the concomitant administration of volatile anesthetics.[2] It frequently presents as intractable spasm of the jaw muscles (masseter spasm), which may progress to generalized rigidity, increased oxygen demand, tachycardia, tachypnea, and profound hyperpyrexia.[20] Skin mottling, rising temperature, and coagulopathies may occur later. If sign or symptoms are present succinylcholine should be discontinued and correction of acidosis, support of circulation, assurance of adequate urinary output, and institution of measures to control rising temperature should be instituted. Intravenous dantrolene sodium is recommended as an adjunctive therapy.[20]

Succinylcholine-induced prolonged apnea secondary to neuromuscular blockade has occurred in neonates.[21]

Drug interactions: Aminoglycosides can cause neuromuscular blockade and potentiate the effects of neuromuscular blockers.[22] Because succinylcholine is associated with numerous drug interactions, consult appropriate resources for dosing recommendations before combining any drug with succinylcholine.

Pharmacodynamic considerations: Infants and children are more resistant than *adults* to the neuromuscular blockade produced by succinylcholine.[2-4]

Other: Plasma cholinesterase activity may be decreased or absent in the presence of genetic abnormalities of plasma cholinesterase (e.g., patients heterozygous or homozygous for atypical plasma cholinesterase gene), pregnancy, severe liver or kidney disease, malignant tumors, infections, burns, anemia, decompensated heart disease, peptic ulcer, or myxedema.[2] It may also be diminished by chronic administration of oral contraceptives, glucocorticoids, or certain monoamine oxidase inhibitors, and by irreversible inhibitors of plasma cholinesterase (e.g., organophosphate insecticides, echothiophate, and certain antineoplastic drugs).[2] Patients homozygous for atypical plasma cholinesterase gene (1 in 2500 patients) are extremely sensitive to the neuromuscular blocking effect of succinylcholine.[2] In these patients a test dose may be administered to evaluate sensitivity to succinylcholine.[2] Apnea or prolonged muscle paralysis should be treated with controlled respiration.

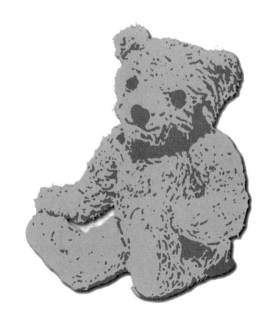

SUFentanil Citrate

Brand names	Sufenta
Medication error potential	ISMP high-alert medication that has an increased risk of causing significant patient harm if it is used in error.[1] Look-alike, sound-alike error potential. ISMP reports that SUFentanil has been confused with fentaNYL.[2] USP also reports that SUFentanil has been confused with alfentanil; no patient harm resulted.[3] USP reports that SUFentanil citrate has been confused with fentaNYL citrate; patient harm resulted.[3]
Contraindications and warnings	**Contraindications:** Sufentanil is contraindicated in patients with a hypersensitivity to the drug or know intolerance to opioid agonists.[4] **Warnings:** Alfentanil should only be administered by persons specifically trained in the use of IV anesthetics.[4]
Infusion related cautions	Significant bradycardia, muscle or chest wall rigidity (dose-related), and apnea may occur early in administration of sufentanil or following rapid administration. Pretreatment with atropine and a nondepolarizing neuromuscular blocking agent may aid in minimizing these adverse effects. Ventilation support is indicated.[4] An opioid antagonist, resuscitation and intubation equipment and oxygen should be readily available when using alfentanil.[4]

Dosage	Dosages vary depending on the desired degree of analgesia/anesthesia and adjunctive therapies (e.g., halothane, propofol). Repeat doses should be increased or decreased based on response to initial dose.[4]
	
	Use lean body weight when dosing patients whose weight is >20% of their ideal body weight.[4,5] (See Appendix B.)
	
	Infants and children (<2 years): 5–20 mcg/kg (0.5 mcg/kg dose when combined with halothane and nitric oxide)[4,6,7] followed by a continuous infusion of 1–2 mcg/kg/h.[4,8]
	
	Children (2–12 years): Initial 10–25 mcg/kg; maintenance 0.5–0.75 mcg/kg (max 25–50 mcg) as needed.[4]
	
	Children > 12 years and *adults*:
	
	    Analgesia (low dose): Initial 0.5–1 mcg/kg; maintenance 10–25 mcg as needed.[4,9]
	
	    Analgesia (moderate dose): Initial 2–8 mcg/kg; maintenance 10–50 mcg as needed.[4,9]
	
	    Anesthesia (high dose): Initial 8–30 mcg/kg; maintenance 10–50 mcg as needed.[4,9]

Dosage adjustment in organ dysfunction	No dosage adjustment required in patients with renal dysfunction.[10] Sufentanil should be administered with caution in patients with hepatic or renal impairment, since the drug undergoes metabolism mainly in the liver.[4]
Maximum dosage	Doses should be titrated to an appropriate level of anesthesia or pain control with manageable adverse effects.[4] In *adults* a maximum dose of 30 mcg/kg has been recommended for anesthesia and 8 mcg/kg for analgesia.[4] For procedures lasting >1 hour, the total sufentanil dose should not exceed 30 mcg/kg.[4,11] For all procedures, the total infusion dose should not exceed 1 mcg/kg/h of anticipated procedure time.[4,11]

SUFentanil Citrate

Additives None.

Suitable diluents D5W, NS.[12]

Maximum concentration 50 mcg/mL.[4,12]

Preparation and delivery No specific comments; see manufacturer labeling.

IV push 50 mcg/mL given over 2–5 minutes.[4,6,12,13]

Intermittent infusion Not given by this method.

Continuous infusion 12 mcg/mL.[4,7,8,12]

Other routes of administration Although sufentanil has been given by IM administration,[12] it is generally not administered via this route. It can be given by epidural injection.[12]

Comments **Significant adverse effects:** Caution should be used when administering sufentanil to patients with head trauma. It has been associated with increases in intracranial pressure in this population.[14]

Pharmacokinetic considerations: The elimination half-life is shorter in infants and children and longer in neonates compared to that of adolescents and *adults*.[4,15] Clearance can be further reduced by up to a third in neonates with cardiovascular disease.[4]

Tacrolimus

Brand names	Prograf

Medication error potential

Look-alike, sound-alike error potential.

USP reported that tacrolimus was confused with pimecrolimus, Sirolimus, tamsulosin, and tolterodine.[1]

Contraindications and warnings

US boxed warning[2]**:** Patients undergoing immunosuppressive therapies are at increased risk for infection and the development of lymphoma. Tacrolimus should only be prescribed by physicians with experience in immunosuppressive therapies. Patients receiving tacrolimus should be treated in facilities staffed and equipped with adequate laboratory and supportive medical resources. See the product literature for more complete information.

Contraindications: Patients with hypersensitivity to tacrolimus or who are allergic to polyoxyl 60 hydrogenated castor oil.[2]

Infusion related cautions

Anaphylaxis to the polyoxyl 60 hydrogenated castor oil vehicle has occurred.[2] Observe patient continuously for ≥30 minutes after start of infusion and frequently thereafter. Oxygen and an aqueous solution of epinephrine should be at the bedside during the infusion.[1,2]

Dosage

Tacrolimus should be started no earlier than 6 hours after transplantation. Patients should be changed to oral therapy as soon as possible. When converting from IV to oral dosing, the first oral dose should be given 8–12 hours after the infusion is stopped.[2]

Heart, liver, or kidney transplantation: 0.03–0.05 mg/kg/day by continuous infusion.[2] For kidney transplants, the dose may be delayed until renal function has recovered (SCr <4 mg/dL) and may be postponed >48 hours with postoperative oliguria.[2] Use lowest dose that attains the desired blood (preferred), serum, or plasma concentration.[1-6]

In children after heart transplant doses of 0.03–0.05 mg/kg/day as a continuous infusion were used if urine output was >1 mL/kg/h. These investigators recommended initial monitoring of blood concentrations 12 hours after the beginning of the infusion.[7]

Following liver transplant, doses have ranged from 0.03–0.15 mg/kg/day by continuous infusion.[3-6,8-10] One large, multicenter study in *adults* and children initially infused 0.075 mg/kg over 4 hours q 12 h but the dose was decreased to 0.05 mg/kg after an increase in renal toxicity was noted.[10]

In general, children require larger doses following liver transplant than *adults*.[2] In a pharmacokinetic study, children who received an intact child's liver had a greater than expected clearance of tacrolimus, while those who received a cut-down liver from an *adult* had lower clearance than expected.[11]

Graft-versus-host disease (GVHD) after bone marrow transplantation: 0.03 mg/kg/day as a continuous infusion plus mycophenolate mofetil or methotrexate beginning the day before transplantation has been used.[12,13] Another group treated an 18-year-old and a 9-year-old with steroid-resistant, severe, acute GVHD with 0.1 mg/kg/day as a continuous infusion, maintaining blood concentrations of 25–35 ng/mL.[14] (See Comments section.)

Dosage adjustment in organ dysfunction

Renal and hepatic insufficiency (Pugh ≤10): Initial doses should be the lowest in the recommended range and trough concentrations should be closely monitored.[2] In patients with oliguria therapy should be delayed 48 hours or longer after transplant.

Maximum dosage

Not established. 0.44 mg/kg/day has been given to *adults*.[10]

Additives

Contains polyoxyl 60 hydrogenated castor oil (HCO-60) and dehydrated alcohol.[2]

Suitable diluents	D5W, NS.[2]

Maximum concentration	0.02 mg/mL.[2]

Preparation and delivery	**Stability:** Tacrolimus absorbs to PVC; therefore, store in polyolefin containers or glass IV bottles. Infusion through PVC anesthesia extension tubing, PVC IV administration set tubing, or fat emulsion tubing does not result in decreased blood concentrations.[15,16] Surfactants in injectable products have been associated with leeching of the plasticizer DEHP when stored or administered in PVC containers. Only glass, polyethylene or non-DEHP plasticized administration, sets should be used for tacrolimus infusions.[17]
	Compatibility: See Appendix D for PN compatibility information.

IV push	Not indicated.

Intermittent infusion	Has been infused over 4 hours.[10]

Continuous infusion	Usually infused over 24 hours.[2-4,6,7,12-14]

Other routes of administration	Not indicated.

Comments	**Adverse effects:** The risk of lymphoproliferative disorders is greater in young children who are at risk for Epstein-Barr virus infection.[2]
	Reversible left ventricular wall thickening was noted in pediatric and *adult* patients who had trough concentrations >15 ng/mL.[18]
	Hypertension occurs frequently. Serum potassium should be monitored to be sure hyperkalemia has not developed.[2]
	Pharmacokinetics: To minimize toxicity, monitor whole blood, serum, or plasma concentrations.[2,4] Use the same matrix and assay type consistently for a given patient.[2] Whole blood is the preferred matrix and samples should be collected in EDTA tubes.[2] Trough concentrations should range from 5–20 ng/mL for whole blood.[2] Accuracy of whole blood measurements is diminished when microparticle enzyme immunoassay methods are used and concentrations are <9 ng/mL. Liquid chromatography—tandem mass spectrometry assays are associated with greater sensitivity and precision.[19]
	Drug interactions: Tacrolimus is a substrate of CYP3A4 and can be inhibited or induced by other drugs. Consult appropriate resources for dosing recommendations before combining any drug with tacrolimus.

Terbutaline Sulfate

Brand names	Brethine, generic
Medication error potential	Look-alike, sound-alike error potential.
	ISMP reported that Brethine was confused with Methergine.[1]
	USP reported that Brethine was confused with Methergine and thiethylperazine.[2]
Contraindications and warnings	**Contraindications:** Hypersensitivity to terbutaline or any product components.[3]
Infusion related cautions	The manufacturer does not recommend IV administration.[3] (See Comments section.)
Dosage	**Severe asthma exacerbations:** 0.01 mg/kg SC q 20 min for three doses then q 2–6 h as needed (in *adults* 0.25 mg q 20 min for three doses).[4] However, the *National Asthma Education and Prevention Program Expert Panel Report 3* states that there is no proven advantage of systemic terbutaline therapy over aerosol.[4]
	Status asthmaticus: Five adolescents received 0.25–0.3 mg SC q 12–15 min with a maximum of 10 mg in 24 hours.[5] In 11 children 7–33 months old who failed to respond to nebulizer treatments, a SC infusion of 0.2–0.3 mcg/kg/min was given over 20 minutes followed by 0.1 mcg/kg/min for an average of 6 days.[6]
	An IV loading dose of 2 mcg/kg over 5 minutes up to 10 mcg/kg over 30 minutes followed by 0.08–0.4 mcg/kg/min with increases of 0.1–0.2 mcg/kg/min q 30 min to desired response or toxicity has been reported.[7-9] Alternatively, an initial infusion of 0.5–1 mcg/kg/min increased by 0.1–0.2 mcg/kg/min q 2 h up to 5–10 mcg/kg/min according to respiratory symptoms.[10,11] Usual maximum infusion rates are ≤5 mcg/kg/min.[8-10]
	Chronic asthma: In eight children from 8–14 years old with chronic severe asthma, a continuous SC infusion of 2.5–5 mg/day increased to 10 mg/day as indicated (improvement in symptoms) and tolerated was used for ≥2 months.[12]
Dosage adjustment in organ dysfunction	None noted.[13]
Maximum dosage	10 mcg/kg as loading dose.[8,9] 10 mcg/kg/min for 6 hours was reported in an adolescent.[11]
Additives	Sodium chloride added for isotonicity.[3]
Suitable diluents	D5W, ½NS, NS.[14]
Maximum concentration	1 mg/mL (undiluted).[3,14] 0.05 mg/mL was used for SC infusion.[12]
Preparation and delivery	**Stability:** Sensitive to light and excessive heat.[14] Product should be stored in a controlled environment and protected from light and freezing.[14]
IV push	Over 5–10 minutes.[11,15,16]

Intermittent infusion	The length of the infusion is determined by the clinical effect. [7,16] In one study the infusion length ranged from 2–60 hours. [11]
Continuous infusion	May be infused continuously. [10,11,15,16]
Other routes of administration	Usually given SC. IM administration is not indicated.
Comments	**Adverse effects:** Increased heart rate, [6,7,10,11,16] increased systolic and decreased diastolic blood pressure, [7,11] tremor, [7,12] headache, [7,16] and decreased serum potassium [10] have been reported. An 11-year-old who received 10 mcg/kg/min for 6 hours had no evidence of arrhythmias, and creatine phosphokinase-MB (CPK-MB) cardiac isoenzymes were normal. [11] However, in that same study three children receiving a lower terbutaline dose (two were also receiving aminophylline) did have an elevated CPK-MB concentration. Two of 18 children developed ST segment depression following terbutaline and epinephrine. There was no correlation between CPK values and arrhythmias or ST changes.

The incidence of tremor and tachycardia may be increased in those receiving theophylline concomitantly. [7]

Bruising, tenderness, and site infection have been reported with continuous SC infusion. [12]

Pharmacokinetics: Although larger doses are used in children than in *adults*, there is no pharmacokinetic basis to support the need for larger doses. [15]

Drug interactions: Terbutaline may increase theophylline clearance. [17]

Thiopental Sodium

Brand names	Pentothal

Medication error potential

ISMP high-alert medication (anesthetic and moderate sedation) that has an increased risk of causing significant patient harm if it is used in error.[1]

Look-alike and sound-alike drug names.

USP reports confusion between thiopental and Nembutal and between Pentothal and Nembutal, which has resulted in patient harm.[2]

Contraindications and warnings

Contraindications: Hypersensitivity to thiopental, barbiturates, or any component of the formulation.[3] Absence of suitable veins for IV administration; should not be administered by intra-arterial injection.[3] Variegate porphyria (South African) or acute intermittent porphyria.[3]

Relative contraindications include severe cardiovascular disease, hypotension, or shock conditions in which the hypnotic effect may be prolonged or potentiated (e.g., excessive premedication, Addison's disease, hepatic or renal dysfunction, myxedema, increased BUN, severe anemia, asthma/status asthmaticus, and myasthenia gravis).

Warnings: May be habit forming.[3] Be prepared to provide respiratory support. Monitor oxygen saturation and keep oxygen available.[3]

Infusion related cautions

Respiratory depression, apnea, laryngospasm, and hypotension may occur if administered too rapidly.[3]

High alkaline pH (10.6) may cause tissue necrosis upon extravasation.[3] (See Appendix E for management of intra-arterial injection.)

Dosage

Anesthesia

Induction: Doses have ranged from 4 to 8.6 mg/kg over 10–60 minutes.[3-8] Although some have suggested that the induction doses of thiopental should be larger (relative to weight) in children (5–8 mg/kg)[10] and lower in neonates (3–4 mg/kg),[11] others have found no difference in dosing based on age.[12,13] If clinically indicated, 0.1 mg/kg/sec may be given until the face mask is tolerated.[9] Although rapid injection can cause hypotension and decreased cardiac output, 5 mg/kg have been given over 10 seconds when rapid induction was needed.[5]

Maintenance: 1 mg/kg as needed.[3]

Elevated intracranial pressure

Acute increases: 1.5–3.5 mg/kg, repeat as needed.[3,4]

Sustained elevations (medically induced coma)

Neonates: A loading dose of 10–30 mg/kg[14-16] followed by 2–4 mg/kg/h as a continuous infusion.[14,16] Two studies evaluated the effects of short-term[15] and prolonged coma with thiopental on outcome in neonates with asphyxia and reported no improvement; however, a greater complication rate (i.e., hypotension) was noted.[15,16]

Infants and children: A loading dose of 10–30 mg/kg.[14,18-20] Some investigators recommend administration of two loading doses: 20 mg/kg over 1 hour followed by 10 mg/kg over 6 hours.[15] The loading dose should be followed by a 1–2 mg/kg/h continuous infusion and should be titrated based on clinical response and/or serum thiopental concentration (20–40 mg/L).[14,17,20]

Dosage *(cont.)*	**Procedural sedation (for procedures <15 minutes):** Has been given rectally for this purpose[21]; however, other barbiturates are more frequently used. (See Pentobarbital monograph.)
	Status epilepticus
	Loading: 10–30 mg/kg.[22,23]
	Maintenance: 5–55 mg/kg/h.[22] Total doses of thiopental used to obtain and maintain burst suppression were 15–50 g over 48–120 hours and correlated with plasma thiopental levels of 25–40 mg/dL.[22] Most clinicians begin at 5 mg/kg/h and gradually increase by 1–2 mg/kg/h for 6–8 hours until all electrical brain activity is suppressed.[24,25]
Dosage adjustment in organ dysfunction	Because the hypnotic effect may be prolonged in renal or hepatic disease, use cautiously in these patients.[3,26] Adjust dose in renal dysfunction.[26,27] If CrCl is <10 mL/min, give 75% of normal dose.[24,28] May need to reduce dosage in hepatic failure/cirrhosis, but no specific recommendations.[27]
Maximum dosage	Not established.
Additives	4.9 mEq sodium/g of thiopental sodium.[3,29]
Suitable diluents	D2.5, D5W, NS, ½NS, D2.5NS, D2.5¼NS, D5¼NS, D5½NS, dextran 6% in D5W, and dextran 6% in NS.[3,29] SW should *not* be used for preparing solutions <2% thiopental since the resulting hypotonic solutions will cause hemolysis.[29]
Maximum concentration	50 mg/mL.[3]
Preparation and delivery	**Stability:** 3 days at room temperature (20°C to 25°C) and 7 days when refrigerated (2°C to 8°C).[3,29]
IV push	Over 20–30 seconds.[28] Twenty infants, age 12 months, received 5 mg/kg over 10 seconds for rapid anesthesia induction[9] and 10 mg was given over 2 minutes to neonates with resistant seizures without adverse effects.[23]
Intermittent infusion	20–50 mg/mL given over 10–60 minutes with rate titrated according to blood pressure.[14,16,19,28]
Continuous infusion	2–4 mg/mL in D5W or NS.[3,28]
Other routes of administration	IM administration not recommended due to tissue necrosis.[3,29]

Thiopental Sodium

Comments

Rare adverse effects: Renal failure may occur as a complication of barbiturate treatment. Monitor BUN and serum creatinine.[30]

Anticonvulsant hypersensitivity syndrome is an acute, life-threatening, idiosyncratic reaction that has been reported in patients receiving phenytoin, phenobarbital, carbamazepine, primidone, and lamotrigine.[30-32] Symptoms generally develop within 1–12 weeks following initiation and include a classic triad of fever, rash, and lymphadenopathy.[30-32] Peripheral blood leucocytosis and eosinophilia and internal organ involvement may also be noted. Immediate discontinuation of the suspected anticonvulsant is essential for good outcome.[30-32] Cross-reactivity among the aromatic anticonvulsants has been noted; hence, these should not be used as alternative agents.[30-32]

Monitoring: High-dose thiopental leads to a pronounced fall in serum potassium; therefore, measure diurnal urinary loss of potassium.[33] Therapeutic serum concentrations are 1–5 mg/L (hypnotic); 100 mg/L (coma); 7–130 mg/L (anesthesia).[28]

Drug interactions: Consult appropriate resources for dosing recommendations before combining any drug with thiopental.

Pharmacokinetic considerations: Recovery time after large or repeated doses may be more rapid for infants and children compared to *adults* because of a higher clearance.[34]

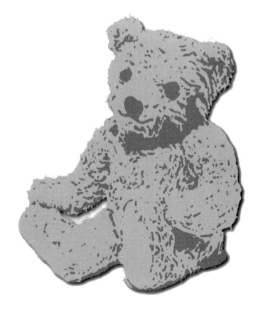

Ticarcillin Disodium–Clavulanate Potassium

Brand names	Timentin

Medication error potential

Look-alike, sound-alike drug names.

USP reports confusion with piperacillin.[1] Timentin may be confused with Tygacil and Ticar.[1]

Contraindications and warnings

Contraindications: in patients with a known hypersensitivity to ticarcillin, clavulanate or any of the penicillins.[2]

Warnings: Serious hypersensitivity and occasionally fatal anaphylactic reactions have been reported.[2] These are more likely in patients who are sensitive to multiple allergens (e.g., asthma) and in those with a history of Type I reaction to penicillin or cephalosporins.[2] (See Appendix C for specific information.)

Prolonged use may cause superinfection and/or *Clostridium difficile*–associated diarrhea (CDAD), which has been reported and may range in severity from mild diarrhea to fatal colitis.[2] If CDAD is suspected or confirmed, appropriate fluid and electrolyte management, protein supplementation, antibiotic treatment of *C. difficile,* and surgical evaluation should be instituted as clinically indicated.[2]

Infusion related cautions

If a decision is made to give this medication to a patient with known penicillin hypersensitivity, the patient should be closely observed for allergenicity. Although rare, anaphylactoid reactions may require immediate emergency treatment with epinephrine, oxygen, IV steroids, antihistamines, pressor amines, and airway management. Pain on injection and thrombophlebitis have been noted.[2]

Dosage

Dosage is based on ticarcillin component. Although clavulanate is a beta-lactamase inhibitor that extends the spectrum of ticarcillin, it has little antibacterial activity.[2]

In patients with meningeal seeding from a distant infection site or in whom meningitis is suspected or documented, or in patients who require prophylaxis against central nervous system infection, an alternate agent with demonstrated clinical efficacy in this setting should be used[2]

Neonates: Safety and efficacy has not been established in those <3 months of age.[2]

PNA	1200–2000 g	≥2000 g
<7 days	150 mg/kg/day divided q 12 h[3-7]	225 mg/kg/day divided q 8 h[3,4,7]
≥7 days	225 mg/kg/day divided q 8 h[3,4]*	300 mg/kg/day divided q 6 h[3-5]

*Until 4 weeks of age.

One study of 11 premature neonates weighing <2200 g suggested dose of 200 mg/kg/day divided q 6 h.[8]

Infants and children

Mild-to-moderate infections: 100–200 mg/kg/day divided q 6 h.[4]

Severe infections: 200–300 mg/kg/day divided q 4–6 h[4,9-14] or 9 g/m²/day divided q 6 h.[15-17]

Ticarcillin Disodium–Clavulanate Potassium

Dosage adjustment in organ dysfunction	Adjust dose in renal dysfunction.[2,18] If CrCl is between 10 and 50 mL/min, give a normal dose q 8 h; if CrCl is <10 mL/min, give a normal dose q 12 h.[18] Alternatively, the manufacturer recommends if CrCl 30–60 mL/min, give two-thirds normal dose q 4 h; if CrCl 10–30 mL/min, give two-thirds dose q 8 h; if CrCl <10 mL/min, give two-thirds dose q 12 h; and if CrCl <10 mL/min with hepatic insufficiency, give two-thirds dose q 24 h.[2]
Maximum dosage	300 mg/kg/day,[2,4] not to exceed 3 g/dose or 24 g/day, in those >12 years of age.[2,4]
Additives	Contains ~4.51 mEq of sodium and 0.15 mEq of potassium per g of ticarcillin.[2] The 3.1 g/100 mL frozen injection contains 0.187 mEq/mL of sodium and 0.005 mEq/mL of potassium.[19]
Suitable diluents	D5W, LR, SW, or NS.[19]
Maximum concentration	<100 mg/mL (ticarcillin).[2] 43 mg/mL in NS, 48 mg/mL in D5W, and 86 mg/mL in SW.[19]
Preparation and delivery	**Delivery system issues:** The mixing of ticarcillin with an aminoglycoside in vitro can result in substantial inactivation of the aminoglycoside. (See Appendix C for more specific information.) **Stability:** Store intact vials at <24°C.[2,19] Solutions in NS or LR are stable for 24 hours at room temperature, 7 days when refrigerated, or 30 days when frozen. Solution in D5W is stable for 24 hours at room temperature, 3 days when refrigerated, or 7 days when frozen. After freezing, thawed solution is stable for 8 hours at room temperature. Premixed solution: Store frozen at ≤−20°C. Thawed solution is stable for 24 hours at room temperature or 7 days under refrigeration. Do not refreeze. Darken solution indicates loss of potency of clavulanate.[2,19] **Compatibility:** See Appendix D for PN compatibility information.[20]
IV push	Not used.
Intermittent infusion	Over 30 minutes.[2,19]
Continuous infusion	Not used. One report in *adults*, but no concentration information provided.[21]
Other routes of administration	None.
Comments	**Rare adverse effects:** Neurotoxic (e.g., lethargy, confusion, twitching, multifocal myoclonus, localized or generalized epileptiform seizures) may occur with large doses, especially in patients with renal insufficiency.[2,22-26] Thrombocytopenia and bleeding disorders associated with abnormalities in clotting time, platelet aggregation, and prothrombin time have been reported.[2,27] These are more likely to occur in patients with renal impairment.[2] If bleeding manifestations appear, treatment should be discontinued and appropriate therapy instituted.

Ticarcillin Disodium–Clavulanate Potassium

Comments *(cont.)*

Elevation of serum transaminases, serum alkaline phosphatase, serum LDH, and serum bilirubin have been noted.[2] Hepatitis and cholestatic jaundice have also been reported.[2,28]

Laboratory interference: High urine concentrations may produce false-positive protein reactions (pseudoproteinuria) when testing is performed by sulfosalicylic acid and boiling test, acetic acid test, biuret reaction, and nitric acid test. The bromphenol blue reagent strip test (MULTI-STIX) appears reliable.[2] The presence of clavulanic acid may cause a nonspecific binding of IgG and albumin by red cell membranes leading to a false-positive Coombs' test.[2]

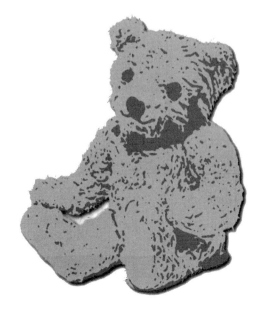

Tigecycline

Brand names	Tygacil

Medication error potential

Look-alike, sound-alike drug names.

USP reports confusion with Ticar and Timentin.[1]

Contraindications and warnings

Contraindications: In those with known hypersensitivity to tigecycline.[2]

Warnings: Tigecycline is a tetracycline derivative and should be administered cautiously in patients with hypersensitivity to tetracycline.[2] Life-threatening anaphylaxis/anaphylactoid reactions have occurred.

Use during tooth development (last half of pregnancy, infancy, and childhood to the age of 8 years) may cause permanent tooth discoloration (yellow-gray-brown).[2,3] This is more common during long-term use, but has been observed following repeated short-term courses.[2,3] Tetracycline drugs should not be used in this age group.

Elevation in transaminases, total bilirubin concentration, and prothrombin time have been noted and isolated cases of significant hepatic dysfunction/failure have occurred.[2] Patients who develop abnormal liver function tests should be monitored for worsening function and the risk to benefit of continuing therapy should be assessed.[2] (See Rare adverse effects in Comments section.)

Lower cure rates and higher mortality were seen when patients with ventilator-associated pneumonia were treated with tigecycline.[2]

Use caution when giving as monotherapy in those with complicated intra-abdominal infections secondary to clinically apparent intestinal perforation may develop sepsis/septic shock.[2] Although APACHE II scores were different from baseline, the relationship of this outcome to treatment cannot be established.[2]

Prolonged use may cause superinfection and/or *Clostridium difficile*–associated diarrhea (CDAD), which has been reported and may range in severity from mild diarrhea to fatal colitis.[2] If CDAD is suspected or confirmed, appropriate fluid and electrolyte management, protein supplementation, antibiotic treatment of *C. difficile,* and surgical evaluation should be instituted as clinically indicated.[2]

Infusion related cautions

Although rare, anaphylactoid reactions may require immediate emergency treatment with epinephrine, oxygen, IV steroids, antihistamines, pressor amines, and airway management.

Dosage

Safety and effectiveness in pediatric patients below the age of 18 years have not been established.[2]

If ≥12 years of age: 1.5 mg/kg as a single dose (maximum: 100 mg/dose) followed by 2 mg/kg/day (maximum: 50 mg/dose) divided q 12 h.[4]

Dosage adjustment in organ dysfunction

No dosage adjustment is necessary in renal impairment or mild to moderate hepatic impairment (Child Pugh A and Child Pugh B).[2] Patients with severe hepatic impairment (Child Pugh C) should be treated with caution. The initial dose should be 100 mg followed by a reduced maintenance dose of 25 mg q 12 h.[2]

Maximum dosage

100 mg initial dose and 50 mg/dose thereafter.[2]

Additives

None.

Suitable diluents

NS, D5W.[2]

Tigecycline

Maximum concentration	<1 mg/mL.[2]
Preparation and delivery	**Stability:** Reconstituted solution should be a red-orange color.[2]
IV push	Not used.
Intermittent infusion	30–60 minutes.[2]
Continuous infusion	Not used.
Other routes of administration	None.
Comments	**Rare adverse effects:** Tigecycline is structurally similar to tetracycline-class antibiotics and may have similar adverse effects including photosensitivity, pseudotumor cerebri, and anti-anabolic action (which has led to increased BUN, azotemia, acidosis, and hyperphosphatemia).[2] Hepatic toxicity frequently occurs in those receiving large dosages of tetracyclines (>2 g/day) or who have renal impairment or are pregnant.[2,5] Fatty degeneration of the liver and fatalities have occurred in pregnant women with concurrent acute pyelonephritis.[5] Pancreatitis is a known adverse effect of the tetracyclines and has also been reported with tigecycline.[2,6,7] **Monitoring:** Although tigecycline did not significantly alter the effects of warfarin on INR and did not affect the pharmacokinetic profile of tigecycline, the manufacturer recommends that prothrombin time or other suitable anticoagulation test should be monitored in those given warfarin.[2] Monitor patients periodically for abnormal liver function and observe for diarrhea.

Tissue Plasminogen Activator (t-PA)-Alteplase

Brand names	Activase, Cathflo Activase
Medication error potential	ISMP high-alert medication that has an increased risk of causing significant patient harm if it is used in error.[1] Look-alike, sound-alike error potential. ISMP reported that Activase was confused with TNKase.[2] USP reported that alteplase was confused with TNKase. Activase was confused with Retavase and TNKase.[3]
Contraindications and warnings	**Contraindications**[4]**:** Patients with acute myocardial infarction or pulmonary embolism when there is active internal bleeding, a history of a cerebrovascular accident, recent intracranial or intraspinal surgery or trauma, intracranial neoplasm, arteriovenous malformation or aneurysm, known bleeding diathesis, or severe uncontrolled hypertension. In acute ischemic stroke with evidence of intracranial hemorrhage; suspicion of subarachnoid hemorrhage; intracranial or intraspinal surgery, serious head trauma, or stroke within 3 months; history of intracranial hemorrhage; uncontrolled hypertension; seizure at stroke onset; active internal bleeding; intracranial neoplasm; arteriovenous malformation or aneurysm, known bleeding diathesis. **Warnings:** Bleeding is the most common complication.[4]
Infusion related cautions	Extravasation can cause ecchymosis and inflammation.[4,5] The infusion should be stopped and local treatment applied.
Dosage	**Recommendations for use of thrombolytics in pediatrics**[6]**:** • Neonates with a major vessel occluded and perfusion of limbs or vital organs that are being compromised—If thrombolytics are needed, plasminogen (fresh frozen plasma) should be given prior to infusion. • Children with deep vein thrombosis—Thrombolysis is not routinely recommended. If it is used and plasminogen deficiency is present, plasminogen should be supplemented. • Bilateral renal vein thrombosis with varying degrees of renal failure—Patients should first be anticoagulated with unfractionated heparin (UFH). Following thrombolytic therapy, patients should be anticoagulated with UFH or low molecular weight heparin (LMWH). • Those with blocked central venous lines (CVL)—Thrombolytic should be used to restore patency. A second dose may be stilled if the catheter remains blocked after the first instillation. • Children with limb-threatening or organ-threatening femoral artery thrombosis who fail initial UFH therapy. • Neonates with umbilical artery catheter related thrombosis with potentially life-, limb-, or organ-threatening symptoms—If thrombolysis is contraindicated, a surgical thrombectomy is recommended.

Tissue Plasminogen Activator (t-PA)-Alteplase

Dosage (cont.)

Thrombolytic therapy: 0.1–0.5 mg/kg over 10–20 minutes[7,8] followed by infusion of 0.04–0.6 mg/kg/h has been used.[10-16] Because of bleeding tendencies in 50% of patients, some suggest that initial doses of 0.1 mg/kg/h be increased gradually up to 0.5 mg/kg/h if clot dissolution does not occur at lower doses.[9] Another suggests 0.5 mg/kg/h for 1 hour followed by 0.25 mg/kg/h for 4–11 hours until clot lysis occurs; however, the incidence of bleeding was still approximately 50% with the lower infusion rate.[15] Continuous infusion for 8–11 days in neonates did not result in resolution of the thrombus and was associated with bleeding.[17,18]

In a 19-month-old child with pulmonary embolism, 0.1 mg/kg/h was infused for 11 hours via pulmonary artery.[19] One case report described the successful use of 2.5 mg given in repeated small boluses, intra-arterially for thrombolysis of middle cerebral artery occlusion.[20]

A 2-year-old with a superior vena cava thrombus was treated successfully with 0.03 mg/kg/h for 48 hours in combination with LMWH.[21] A 22-month-old with superior vena caval thrombosis received 1.5 mg/kg over 2 hours once daily for 2 days, after failing initial therapy with UFH.[22]

Three infants with brachial artery thrombosis and significant hand ischemia received UFH and intraarterial t-PA.[23]

Local instillation of low-dose (0.01–0.06 mg/kg/h) was effective in 12 of 17 children with acute thrombosis.[24]

CVL occlusion: Depending on catheter volume, 0.5–2 mg (1 mg/mL) for a dwell time of 20 minutes to 4 hours.[25-31] Some catheters may require more than one instillation.[25-28]

Glaucoma or cataract surgery complicated by hyphema and/or fibrin: Intracameral injection of 5–25 mg postoperatively.[32-34] An additional dose may be required.[32]

Myocardial infarction: A 7-year-old child with a thrombosed coronary aneurysm was given 5 mg IV push <1.5 hours after arrival, followed by 0.75 mg/kg over 0.5 hour, then 0.5 mg/kg over 1 hour and symptoms resolved.[35]

Occlusion of thoracentesis/peritoneal catheters: In a 16–month–old girl with parapneumonic effusion, 2 mg (2 mL) was infused via the catheter into the pleural space and the tube clamped for 4 hours. Drainage was re-established after one dose.[36] 2-mg/8 mL NS was infused via intraperitoneal catheter to aid in drainage of abdominal abscesses in a 4-week-old infant.[37]

Infective endocarditis: Seven high-risk infants overwhelming sepsis were treated with 0.2–0.3 mg/kg/h × 6 hours with the dose then increased to 0.5 mg/kg/h and continued until vegetations were no longer visible by echocardiogram.[38]

Dosage adjustment in organ dysfunction

None needed.

Maximum dosage

100 mg in *adults*.[4]

Additives

Contains arginine and polysorbate 80.[4,5,39] See Appendix C for information about polysorbate adverse effects.

Suitable diluents

D5W, NS.[4]

Maximum concentration

1 mg/mL.[4,39]

Tissue Plasminogen Activator (t-PA)-Alteplase

Preparation and delivery	Reconstitute with provided SW.[4] Swirl the vial to dissolve to avoid excessive foaming. Dilutions <0.5 mg/mL may result in precipitation.[40]
IV push	Not indicated.
Intermittent infusion	May be infused over several hours. Length of infusion depends on response.
Continuous infusion	Length of infusion depends on response.
Other routes of administration	Not indicated.
Comments	50 mg = 29 million International Units.[4]
	Significant adverse events: Bleeding is the most common adverse effect.[35] In children bleeding from venipuncture sites, extension of intraventricular hemorrhage, bruising, and other internal bleeding have been reported.[8,9,15]
	One investigator commented that higher bleeding rates may be associated with concomitant heparin infusions, larger doses, or use in patients with contraindications to antithrombolytic therapy, such as severe thrombocytopenia.[8]
	Two infants with fulminant meningococcemia made a full recovery after being given 0.5 mg/kg/h for 1–1.5 hours followed by 0.25 mg/kg/h for 1.5–4 hours.[41] Later these authors conducted a retrospective review of 62 infants with meningococcal purpura fulminans treated with a median dose of 0.3 mg/kg/h (range: 0.008–1.13 mg/kg/h) for a median duration of 9 hours (range of 1.2–83 hours), they found that 29 (47%) patients died, 17 (51%) of the 33 survivors had amputations, and five (8%) experienced intracranial hemorrhage.[42] Authors questioned the use of t-PA in patients with this disease.[42]

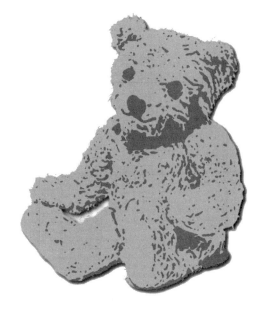

Tobramycin Sulfate

Brand names	Nebcin

Medication error potential

USP reports confusion with gentamicin.[1]

Contraindications and warnings

US boxed warning: Patients with impaired renal function and those receiving large doses or prolonged therapy have an increased risk for nephrotoxicity and ototoxicity (i.e., vestibular and auditory), both of which are generally irreversible.[2-4] The risk of toxicity can also be increased by prolonged elevations in serum concentrations, concurrent use of medications known to be nephro-, neuro-, or oto-toxic, dehydration, and advancing age.[2-4] (See Rare adverse effects and Monitoring in Comments section.)

Aminoglycosides can cause fetal harm when administered to a pregnant woman.[2]

Contraindications: Known hypersensitivity reaction to tobramycin or other aminoglycosides.[2]

Other warnings: Aminoglycosides can cause neuromuscular blockade and potentiate the effects of neuromuscular blockers.[2,5,6]

Infusion related cautions

None.

Dosage

In obese patients dosage should be based on the following equation[7]:

Dosing weight = IBW + 0.4 (TBW − IBW). (See Appendix B.)

Neonates

Loading dose: Although limited data are available, some practitioners advocate an initial 3–5 mg/kg dose in neonates.[8,9]

Maintenance dose: Estimated using age and weight[10,11] or gestational age.[12-14]

Based on age and weight

PNA	<1200 g	1200–2000 g	≥2000 g
<7 days	2.5 mg/kg q 18–24 h[10,11]	5 mg/kg/day divided 12 h[10-12]	5 mg/kg/day divided q 12 h[10-12]
≥7 days	2.5 mg/kg q 18–24 h[10,11]*	5–7.5 mg/kg/day divided q 8–12 h[10-12]	7.5 mg/kg/day divided q 8 h[10-12]

*Until 4 weeks of age.

Based on gestational age[12-14]

Gestational Age	Weight	Dose
≤26 weeks		2.5 mg/kg q 24 h[12]
27–34 weeks	AND ≥1.25 kg	2.5 mg/kg q 18 h[12-14]
	<1.25 kg	3 mg/kg q 24 h[13,14]
35–42 weeks		5 mg/kg/day divided q 12 h[12-14]

Tobramycin Sulfate

Dosage *(cont.)*	**Infants and children:** 7.5 mg/kg/day divided q 8 h.[10,12]
	Once-daily dosing: Several investigators have reported that once-daily dosing has comparable efficacy and perhaps less toxicity than classical 8–12 hours dosing.[15,16] A single dose of *aminoglycoside* has been given once daily (over 20–30 minutes) in critically ill infants and children with severe gram-negative infections,[17-19] bone marrow transplantation,[20] or in febrile neutropenic patients with cancer.[21-26] At this time, the use of once-daily dosing in infants and children is controversial.[27] The most recent edition of the *American Academy of Pediatrics Red Book: Report of the Committee on Infectious Diseases* continues to recommend 2.5 mg/kg/dose administered in multiple daily doses in all age groups and states that once daily dosing is investigational in children.[10]
	Cystic fibrosis: Patients require larger doses due to increased clearance and volume of distribution. Average dose is 10 mg/kg/day divided q 8 h[28,29]; however, doses have ranged from 7.5–20 mg/kg/day divided q 8 h.[28] Although several groups have investigated once-daily dosing in *adults*[30-32] and children,[29-34] this is not standard practice. Doses ranging from 7–20 mg/kg/day have been used.[28,29,31-38] No nephrotoxicity has been reported,[30,31] but one child given a 15 mg/kg dose over 5 minutes developed transient ototoxicity.[33]
Dosage adjustment in organ dysfunction	If CrCl is >50 mL/min, give a normal dose q 8–24 h; if CrCl is between 10–50 mL/min, give a normal dose q 24–48 h; if CrCl is <10 mL/min, give a normal dose q 48–72 h.[39]
Maximum dosage	Larger doses or shorter dosing intervals are sometimes required in patients with cystic fibrosis,[28-38] major thermal burns or dermal loss,[40] ascites, or in patients with febrile granulocytopenia.[21-26] Based on similarities between aminoglycosides, prolonged dosing interval may be required in those receiving ECMO.[41,42]
Additives	The premixed product contains 15.4 mEq of sodium/100 mL.[43] The 20 mg/2 mL and 80 mg/2 mL vials each contain 1.4 mg (0.06 mEq) of sodium.[2] Contains sodium bisulfite.[43] (See Appendix C for specific information about sulfite hypersensitivity.)
Suitable diluents	D5W, NS.[2,43]
Maximum concentration	5 mg/mL.[43] The volume must allow accurate measurement and delivery over 30 minutes.
Preparation and delivery	**Delivery system issues:** The mixing of tobramycin with an aminoglycoside in vitro can result in substantial inactivation of the aminoglycoside. (See Appendix C for more specific information.)
	Compatibility: See Appendix D for PN compatibility information.[44]
IV push	Not recommended. Aminoglycosides have been safely administered by rapid IV push (over 3–5 minutes)[45-47]; however, ototoxicity has been associated with elevated aminoglycoside peak serum concentrations following bolus administration in *adults*.[48]
Intermittent infusion	10 or 40 mg/mL or dilute in appropriate volume of D5W or NS to allow more accurate dosage measurement and infusion over 30–60 minutes.[43]
Continuous infusion	Not recommended. Toxicity occurs more frequently, and the value of this administration method compared to intermittent infusion has not been established.[48-50]

Tobramycin Sulfate

Other routes of administration

40 mg/mL may be given IM.[43] Solutions prepared from or commercially available in bulk packages, ADD-Vantage vials, and premixed solutions in NS should not be given IM.[2]

Comments

Rare adverse effects: Aminoglycosides accumulate in renal cortical tissue and may damage proximal tubule cells leading to oliguric renal failure. Risk of nephrotoxicity may be influenced by type of aminoglycoside, dose, duration (cumulative dose), frequency of therapy and elevated serum concentration.[2,6] It is also increased by advancing age, pre-existing renal or hepatic dysfunction, decrease renal perfusion, hypoalbuminemia, and dehydration.[2,4] Current administration of nephrotoxic medications may increase the risk of toxicity and should be avoided.[2]

Cochlear and/or vestibular ototoxicity has been associated with all aminoglycoside antibiotics.[4,5] Total AUC is a better indicator of ototoxic risk than either peak or trough serum concentration.[51,52] Use cautiously when giving with other drugs (e.g., macrolide antibiotics, loop diuretics, platinum-based chemotherapeutic agents) known to cause ototoxicity.

Aminoglycosides may potentiate the curare-like effects on the neuromuscular junction and should be used cautiously in patients with neuromuscular disorders since they may aggravate muscle weakness.[2,5,6] During or following tobramycin therapy, paresthesias, tetany, positive Chvostek and Trousseau signs and mental confusion have been described in patients with hypomagnesemia, hypocalcemia and hypokalemia.[2] Tetany and muscle weakness have been described in infants. Aminoglycosides may enhance the respiratory depressant effect of neuromuscular-blocking agents and may prolonged blockade.[2,53,54]

Monitoring: Because large variability exists in patient response to therapy, individualize dosage based on serum concentrations, clinical response, and renal function. Recommended peak and trough serum tobramycin concentration are 4–12 mg/L and <2 mg/L, respectively. Desired peak concentrations are dependent on the site of infection.

Although serum concentration monitoring has become routine practice in many institutions, not all patients require monitoring.[55,56] Monitoring is indicated if the patient is not clinically responding, is 3 months of age, has disease that requires large doses or high concentrations (CNS infections, endocarditis, pneumonia, ascites, burns), has decreased or unstable renal function, or will be treated more than 10 days.

Drug interactions: Consult appropriate resources before combining any drug with tobramycin.

Laboratory interference: Serum concentrations may be falsely elevated when blood samples are collected through central venous Silastic catheters.[57]

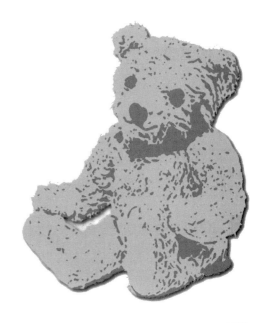

Topotecan HCl

Brand names	Hycamtin

Medication error potential

ISMP high-alert medication that has an increased risk of causing significant patient harm if it is used in error. [1]

Look-alike, sound-alike error potential.

USP reports that topotecan has been confused with irinotecan; no patient harm resulted. [2]

Contraindications and warnings

US boxed warning: Must be administered under the supervision of an experienced physician. Topotecan may cause severe bone marrow suppression, primarily neutropenia, and should not be administered to patients with baseline neutrophil counts less than 1,500 cells/mm^3. Monitor blood counts before and during therapy. [3] (See Monitoring in Comments section.)

Contraindications: Should not be used in patients with a history or known hypersensitivity to topotecan or any of the components. Should not be used in pregnant or breast-feeding patients or those with severe bone marrow suppression. [3]

Other warnings: May also cause thrombocytopenia and anemia. [3] (See Monitoring in Comments section.)

Infusion related cautions

Extravasation, causing mild reactions such as erythema and bruising, has been reported. [3,4] See Appendix E for additional information regarding extravasation treatment.

Dosage

Consult institutional protocol for complete dosing information.

Topotecan is a component of combination therapy or as single agent therapy to treat multiple pediatric solid tumors, including osteosarcoma, neuroblastoma, rhabdomyosarcoma, Ewing's sarcoma, retinoblastoma, ependymoma, as well as pediatric leukemia.

Combination therapy for solid tumors: 0.75 mg/m^2/day over 30 minutes for 5 days; repeat q 21 days. [5]

Single agent therapy for refractory solid tumors: 1.4–2.4 mg/m^2/day over 30 minutes for 5 days; repeat q 21 days. [6-8]

Pediatric solid tumors: 1 mg/m^2/day (range: 0.6–1.9 mg/m^2/day) for 3 days as a continuous infusion; repeat q 21 days [9,10] or over 30 minutes 5 days a week for 2 consecutive weeks; repeat q 24–28 days. [11]

Pediatric refractory acute leukemias: 2.4 mg/m^2/day over 30 minutes for 9 days; repeat q 21 days. [12,13]

Dosage adjustment in organ dysfunction

No dosage adjustment necessary in patients with hepatic dysfunction or mild renal impairment (CrCl 40–60 mL/min). [3] One reference recommends that patients with moderate renal failure (CrCl 20–39 mL/min) receive 50% of the standard dose. [14] Another reference recommends a 25% dose reduction for patients with CrCl <50 mL/min, a 50% reduction for CrCl of 10–50 mL/min, and a 75% reduction with CrCl <10 mL/min. [15]

Maximum dosage

Not established. One *adult* patient received a single dose of 35 mg/m^2 and developed reversible severe neutropenia. [3]

Additives

None.

Suitable diluents

Reconstitution with SW; further dilution with D5W or NS. [3,4]

Topotecan HCl

Maximum concentration	0.5 mg/mL.[14]
Preparation and delivery	Do not dilute in alkaline solutions.[4]
IV push	Not recommended.
Intermittent infusion	Dilute reconstituted drug (1 mg/mL) in 50–250 mL D5W or NS and infuse over 30 minutes.[3,4]
Continuous infusion	Has been administered via continuous infusion for up to 72 hours.[10]
Other routes of administration	No information available to support administration by other routes.
Comments	**Significant adverse effects:** Topotecan is associated with a low (10% to 30%) risk of emesis.[16] Patients should receive antiemetic therapy to prevent acute and delayed nausea and vomiting. The recommended therapy is a corticosteroid on every day chemotherapy is administered; alternatives are a phenothiazine (e.g., prochlorperazine) or a butyrophenone (e.g., droperidol).[16,17] Therapy for delayed nausea and vomiting is generally not needed. Breakthrough medications should also be offered, such as a phenothiazine (e.g., prochlorperazine), a butyrophenone (e.g., droperidol), a substituted benzamide (e.g., metoclopramide), or a benzodiazepine (e.g., lorazepam). Selection should be based on what the patient is currently receiving for acute emesis prophylaxis. **Monitoring:** Monitor CBC with platelets, renal function, and bilirubin.[3,14] Patients should have a baseline ANC >1500 cells/mm³ and a platelet count >100,000 cells/mm³ before drug administration.[3] The manufacturer recommends dose adjustments with severe neutropenia or thrombocytopenia.[3] (See Contraindications and warnings section.) **Drug interactions:** BCRP/ABCG2 inhibitors may increase serum concentrations of topotecan.[14] Consult appropriate resources for dosing recommendations before combining any drug with topotecan.

Tromethamine

Brand names	THAM
Medication error potential	None noted.

Contraindications and warnings

Contraindications: Uremia and anuria.[1,2] Also contraindicated in neonates with chronic respiratory acidosis and salicylate intoxication.

Warnings: Hypoglycemia can occur in preterm and term neonates.[1,2]

Infusion related cautions

Extravasations may result in tissue necrosis, severe inflammation, and sloughing.[1,3-5] Extravasations may be treated with procaine 1% added to hyaluronidase or with phentolamine infiltrated around the site.[3]

Infusion via low-lying umbilical catheters may result in hepatocellular necrosis.[1,2] (See Comments section.)

Rapid infusion may result in prolonged hypoglycemia.[1-3] Three of four *adults* given tromethamine to evaluate its effects on blood chemistries experienced decreases in blood glucose, which resulted in persistent symptoms for 24 hours in one *adult*.[6]

Too rapid administration may decrease the respiratory drive resulting in respiratory depression and apnea.[7]

Dosage

Doses (mL) are based on 0.3 M solution; 100 mL = 3.6 g, 30 mEq, 30 mmol.[1,2]

Neonates with acidosis associated with respiratory distress syndrome (RDS): 1 mL/kg for each pH unit <7.4.[1-3,8] One study reported using doses of 1.8–4.7 mmol/kg in six neonates (26–37 weeks of gestation).[9]

Infants and children: Dose (mL) = base deficit (mEq/L) × body weight (kg) × 1.1[1,2]

Dosage adjustment in organ dysfunction

Contraindicated in patients who are anuric or uremic.[1-3]

Maximum dosage

In neonates, the maximum dose is 5–7 mmol/kg/day.[4]

In *adults*, 35 g (291 mmol)/h[1] or 15 mmol/kg/day.[4,10]

Additives

Glacial acetic acid is added to decrease the pH to 8.6.[1-3] The buffering capacity is decreased about 10% with this addition.[1-3]

Suitable diluents

None noted.

Maximum concentration

Undiluted.[1,2]

Preparation and delivery

Vials do not contain preservatives and are intended for single use.[1]

Tromethamine

IV push	Not indicated.
Intermittent infusion	Over >1 hour.[1] In acute acidosis, 25% to 50% of the calculated deficit can be given over 5–10 minutes with the remainder infused over >1 hour.[4-5]
Continuous infusion	Not given continuously.
Other routes of administration	Not indicated.
Comments	**Significant adverse effects:** Postmortem evaluation of 67 neonates (24–38 weeks gestation) given 1.2 M tromethamine or sodium bicarbonate via umbilical vein reported hemorrhagic liver necrosis in 22 (32.8%).[11] Bladder necrosis has also been reported with tromethamine was infused via umbilical vein.[4] Of note, in these reports the tromethamine used was unbuffered and had a pH >10. Use of buffered tromethamine with a pH of ~8.6 does not seem to result in these adverse effects.[4] Irreversible ischemia of the hand was reported in an *adult* receiving unbuffered THAM 3.6% (pH 10.5) peripherally.[12] This product is not available in the US.

Valproate Sodium

Brand names	Depacon
Medication error potential	None.

Contraindications and warnings

US boxed warning

> **Hepatic failure:** Fatalities has occurred in patients receiving valproic acid and its derivatives.[1] Because of their increased risk for hepatotoxicity, valproate should be used cautiously in children <2 years of age, especially if they are receiving multiple anticonvulsants, have congenital metabolic disorders, severe seizures accompanied by mental retardation, or organic brain disease.[2-5]

> **Pancreatitis:** Life-threatening pancreatitis has been reported in both children and *adults* and has occurred shortly after initial use and after several years of use.[1,6-8] Some patients have developed hemorrhagic pancreatitis that progressed rapidly from onset of symptoms to death. If pancreatitis is diagnosed, valproate should be discontinued.

> **Teratogenicity:** Congenial malformations such as neural tube defects (e.g., spina bifida) have been reported.[1]

Contraindications: Should not be administered to patients with hepatic disease or significant hepatic dysfunction. It is contraindicated in patients with known hypersensitivity to the drug and should not be given to patients with known urea cycle disorders.[1]

Other warnings: Thrombocytopenia, hypothermia, and hyperammonemia may occur.[1] (See Rare adverse effects for information on suicide in Comments section.)

Infusion related cautions

Severe vein irritation and pain at the injection site may occur following administration of undiluted solution.[1]

Dosage

Intravenous use for >14 days has not been studied.[1] Convert to oral administration as soon as possible.

Headache: IV valproate has been safely and effectively used in *adults*[9-11] and adolescents.[12] Initial doses of 1000 mg were infused at 50 mg/min in 31 adolescents.[12] When response was not sufficient, a second 500 mg/dose was given.[12] In another study, patients were given a loading dose of 20–40 mg/kg followed by a continuous infusion of 1–1.5 mg/kg/h.[13]

Seizures (acute, nonstatus epilepticus)

> **Replacement therapy:** Individuals chronically receiving oral valproate may be converted to IV valproate using the same total daily dose (1:1 conversion); however, it should be administered q 6 h or by continuous infusion.[1]

> **Children (≥2 years) and adolescents:** 10–15 mg/kg administered q 6 h; for chronic therapy increase weekly by 5–10 mg/kg/day until seizures are controlled, therapeutic concentrations are reached, or the patient exhibits unacceptable toxicities.[1,14-19] Some have given a loading dose of 20–40 mg/kg followed by a continuous infusion of 1–1.5 mg/kg/h.[13] Maintenance dose in children ≥2 years: 30–60 mg/kg/day divided q 6 h.[13,16-22]

Valproate Sodium

Dosage *(cont.)*	**Seizures—generalize convulsive status epilepticus**
	Neonates and infants: Although IV valproate has been used safely in neonates to treat acute seizures and status epilepticus,[22,23] it should not be used unless all other options have failed. A single dose of 10–25 mg/kg was given and an apparent Vd of 0.245 L/kg and clearance of 25 mL/h/kg were estimated.[23] The elimination of valproate is significantly reduced in neonates and infants; therefore, doses may need to be administered less frequently than in older children. If used, it should be given with L-carnitine. (See Other in Comments section.)
	Children ≥2 years and adolescents: Loading dose of 13.4–40 mg/kg[13,24-28] or 500 mg.[24] The need for further loading doses should be guided by clinical response and serum concentrations. If the patient is on valproate monotherapy or other anticonvulsants that do not induce the cytochrome P450 system, begin with 1 mg/kg/h; if the patient is on one or more inducers (e.g., phenobarbital, phenytoin, rifampin), begin with 2 mg/kg/h; if the patient is receiving inducers and is in pentobarbital coma, begin with 4–6 mg/kg/h.[22] One group recommends beginning at 5 mg/kg/h; once the patient is seizure free for 6 hours the dose should be reduced by 1 mg/kg/h q 2 h.[28]
	Seizures—nonconvulsive status epilepticus
	Children ≥2 years and adolescents: A loading dose of 13.4–25 mg/kg[21,27] followed by 4 mg/kg q 6 h.[27]
	Seizures—prophylaxis for post-traumatic epilepsy: Because a clinical study in *adults* with head trauma showed a higher mortality rate than that observed for phenytoin, IV valproate is not recommended for seizure prophylaxis following head trauma.[1,29]
Dosage adjustment in organ dysfunction	No dosage adjustment necessary in renal dysfunction.[1,30] However, renal failure may cause a disproportionate increase in free-to-total valproate ratios, causing total serum concentrations to be misleading.[1,31] Should not be administered to patients with hepatic disease or significant hepatic dysfunction.[1]
Maximum dosage	Has not been established. A loading dose of 40 mg/kg[23] and a continuous infusion of 6 mg/kg/h have been used in children.[20] A dose of 240 mg/h has been given to a 67-year-old *adult*.[32] Children receiving one or more medications known to increase the metabolism of valproate may require doses up to 100 mg/kg/day, while children in pentobarbital coma may require larger doses (150 mg/kg/day).[22,33]
Additives	None.
Suitable diluents	The parenteral injection has been used undiluted; however, severe vein irritation occurred.[1] Administer in a 1:1 or 2:1 dilution in at least 50 mL of D5W, NS, or LR.[1]
Maximum concentration	25–50 mg/mL.[1]
Preparation and delivery	**Stability:** When stored in glass or polyvinyl chloride bags at room temperature (15°C to 30°C) the product is stable for at least 24 hours.[1] Any unused portion of a vial should be discarded.[1]
IV push	Although not recommended by the manufacturer,[1] some have given as a bolus without adverse effects: loading dose of 20–40 mg/kg over 1–5 minutes[28]; one report gave 7.5–41.5 mg/kg at a rate of 1.5–11 mg/kg/min[34]; and 10 mg/kg/min and doses of up to 30 mg/kg.[35] (See Rare adverse effects in Comments section.)

Valproate Sodium

Intermittent infusion	60 minutes (but not more than 20 mg/min)[1,13] 1–6 mg/kg/min.[23,24] Others have given ≤15 minutes (8.2–15.4 mg/kg).[36] (See Rare adverse effects in Comments section.)
Continuous infusion	2–4 mg/mL in D5W or NS at a rate of 1–6 mg/kg/h.[1,22]
Other routes of administration	None.
Comments	

Rare adverse effects

Hypotension and arrhythmia: The manufacturer's recommendation to infusion over 60 minutes is predicated on concerns about hemodynamic instability. An 11-year-old girl who received 30 mg/kg (480 mg) over 20 minutes (0.5 mg/kg/h) developed significant, but reversible, hypotension 12 minutes into the infusion.[36] Another 11-year-old girl developed hypotension 20 minutes after receiving 30 mg/kg (960 mg) over 60 minutes.[24] Others have noted that 11 mg/kg/min[12] and 1.5–11 mg/kg/min[26,24,37-39] did not produce hypotension, bradycardia, or arrhythmias. In one clinical safety study, about 90 patients with epilepsy were given a single infusions of (up to 15 mg/kg and mean dose of 1184 mg) over 5–10 minutes (1.5–3.0 mg/kg/min).[1] Patients generally tolerated the more rapid infusions.[1]

Thrombocytopenia: About 25% of those given 50 mg/kg/day developed thrombocytopenia (platelet counts $<75 \times 10^9$/L).[1,40,41] The likelihood increases when total serum valproate concentrations exceed 100 mg/L.

Hyperammonemia: Despite normal liver function tests, hyperammonemic encephalopathy accompanied by unexplained acute alterations in level of consciousness and/or cognitive function with lethargy or vomiting have been reported.[1] An ammonia level should be measured and valproate should be stopped if the level is elevated. Concomitant administration of topiramate and valproic acid has been associated with hyperammonemia with or without encephalopathy in patients who have tolerated either drug alone.[1,42]

Hypothermia (unintentional drop to <35°C): Has occurred in patients receiving valproate and those given concomitant topiramate with valproate.[1,43,44] It has been noted in patients with and without hyperammonemia.[1]

Suicidal behavior/ideation: The incidence of this adverse effect has been noted to be greater than placebo (0.43% vs 0.24% risk) in patients receiving 11 anticonvulsants (carbamazepine, divalproex sodium, felbamate, gabapentin, lamotrigine, levetiracetam, oxcarbazepine, pregabalin, tiagabine, topiramate, zonisamide) as either monotherapy or as adjuvant therapy for the treatment of epilepsy, psychiatric disorders, and other conditions.[45] The FDA will require that the product labeling of the entire class of antiepileptics include a warning concerning the risk of suicidality.

Monitoring: Although dosing is often guided by total serum valproate concentrations (50–150 mg/L), the relationship between serum concentration and clinical response is not well documented. The variability in serum concentrations may be attributed to the nonlinear, concentration-dependent protein binding of valproate, which affects it clearance.[45] Patients planning surgery should have platelet count and coagulation parameters monitored before surgery.[1]

Pharmacokinetics: Infants ≤2 months of age have a decreased ability to eliminate valproate compared to older children and *adults.* This is attributed to a combination of immature development of glucuronosyltransferase and other hepatic enzyme and an increased volume of distribution due to decreased plasma protein binding.[46] Pediatric patients (i.e., between 3 months and 10 years) have 50% higher clearances expressed on weight (i.e., mL/min/kg) than do *adults.*[18,19] Over the age of 10 years, children have pharmacokinetic parameters that approximate those of *adults.*[18,19]

Comments *(cont.)*

Drug interactions: Because valproate inhibits CYP2C9, epoxide hydroxylase, and beta-oxidation, it is associated with numerous drug interactions.[47] Valproate can also serve as a substrate and can be inhibited or induced by other drugs. Consult appropriate resources for dosing recommendations before combining any drug with valproate.

Other: Some have advocated that the concomitant administration of L-carnitine may improve survival of those with severe valproate-induced hepatotoxicity. L-carnitine may enhance beta-oxidation of valproate, thereby limiting cytosolic omega-oxidation and the production of toxic metabolites that have been implicated in liver toxicity and ammonia accumulation.[48]

Vancomycin HCl

Brand names	Lyphocin, Vancocin, Vancoled

Medication error potential

Look-alike, sound-alike drug names.

USP reports confusion with clindamycin, gentamicin, tobramycin, valacyclovir, vecuronium, and Vibramycin.[1] Confusion with vecuronium has resulted in patient harm.[1]

Contraindications and warnings

Contraindications: Documented hypersensitivity to vancomycin or any of its components.[2] Solutions containing dextrose may be contraindicated in patients with known allergy to corn or corn products.[2] If possible, avoid in patients with previous severe hearing loss.[3]

Warnings: Rapid administration may cause exaggerated hypotension, including shock, and, rarely, cardiac arrest.[2] (See Infusion related cautions section; see Rare adverse effects in Comments section.)

Transient or permanent hearing loss has been reported in those given excessive doses of vancomycin, who have underlying hearing loss, or received therapy with other ototoxic agents.[2] (See Rare adverse effects in Comments section.)

Use cautiously in renal insufficiency.[2] (See Dosage adjustment in organ dysfunction section.)

Prolonged use may cause superinfection and/or *Clostridium difficile*–associated diarrhea (CDAD), which has been reported and may range in severity from mild diarrhea to fatal colitis.[2] If CDAD is suspected or confirmed, appropriate fluid and electrolyte management, protein supplementation, antibiotic treatment of *C. difficile,* and surgical evaluation should be instituted as clinically indicated.[2]

Infusion related cautions

Administration over <60 minutes may cause red man syndrome.[2] (See Rare adverse effects in Comments section.) Concomitant administration with anesthetic agents has resulted in erythema histamine-like flushing and anaphylaxis.[2]

Thrombophlebitis can be minimized by using dilute solutions (e.g., 2.5–5 mg/mL) and rotating injection sites.[2] Extravasation should be avoided.[2] (See Appendix E for information regarding infiltration.)

Dosage

Dose obese individuals using actual or total body weight.[2,4,5] Shorter dosing intervals may be needed to maintain trough serum vancomycin concentration above 5 mg/L.[4,5]

Neonates

Some advocate a loading dose of 15–20-mg/kg.[6]

Although a variety of neonatal dosing recommendations have been published,[7-9] the following continue to be the most common and are based on gestational age and weight or postconceptional age.

Based on weight and gestational age[10-15]

PNA	<1200 g	1200–2000 g	≥2000 g
<7 days	15 mg/kg q 24 h*	20–30 mg/kg/day divided q 12–18 h	30–45 mg/kg/day divided q 8–12 h
≥7 days		30–45 mg/kg/day divided q 8–12 h*	40–60 mg/kg/day divided q 6–8 h

*Until 4 weeks of age.

554

Dosage *(cont.)*

Based on postconceptional age[16]

Postconceptional Age	Dose
≤26 weeks	15 mg/kg q 24 h
27–34 weeks	15 mg/kg q 18 h
35–42 weeks	30 mg/kg/day divided q 12 h
≥43 weeks	45 mg/kg/day divided q 8 h

Infants and children

Mild-to-moderate infections: 40 mg/kg/day divided q 6–8 h up to 2 g/day.[10,16]

Severe infections (including meningitis): 60 mg/kg/day divided q 6 h up to 4 g/day.[10,17] In *adults* give loading dose of 25–30 mg/kg over at least 60 minutes followed by 45–60 mg/kg/day divided q 8–12 h.[18]

Each dose should be administered no faster than 10 mg/min or over a period of at least 60 minutes, whichever is longer.[2]

Bacterial endocarditis (prophylaxis)

Genitourinary and gastrointestinal procedures: Prophylactic antibiotics solely to prevent endocarditis is not recommended.[19] Patients with underlying cardiac conditions associated with the highest risk of adverse outcome (see Other in Comments section), have *established* GI or GU tract infection, those receiving antibiotics to prevent wound infection or sepsis associated with a GI or GU procedure, and have an organism suspected to be resistant to methicillin may receive a single dose of vancomycin 30–60 minutes before a procedure.[19]

Infected skin, skin structure, or musculoskeletal: Prophylactic antibiotics solely to prevent endocarditis is not recommended.[19] Patients with underlying cardiac conditions associated with the highest risk of adverse outcome (see Other in Comments section), who have an organism suspected to be resistant to methicillin, and who cannot tolerate a beta-lactam antibiotic may receive a single dose of vancomycin 30–60 minutes before a procedure.[19]

Respiratory tract procedures: Prophylactic antibiotics solely to prevent endocarditis is not recommended.[19] Patients with underlying cardiac conditions associated with the highest risk of adverse outcome (see Other in Comments section), and who have *established* respiratory tract infection, require an invasive procedure (e.g., incision or biopsy of the respiratory mucosa; abscess drainage) and have an organism suspected to be resistant to methicillin may receive a single dose of vancomycin 30–60 minutes before a procedure.[19]

Bacterial endocarditis (treatment)

Culture positive (native valve or prosthetic valve)

Strains susceptible to penicillin, gentamicin, and vancomycin: Patients unable to tolerate penicillin or ceftriaxone may receive 40 mg/kg/day divided q 8–12 h plus gentamicin (3 mg/kg/day divided q 8 h) for 6 weeks.[20] If resistant to gentamicin, give streptomycin 20–30 mg/kg/day divided q 12 h.[20]

Enterococcal resistant to penicillin, and susceptible to gentamicin, and vancomycin: If beta-lactamase-producing and patient is unable to tolerate ampicillin-sulbactam, give receive 40 mg/kg/day divided q 8–12 h plus gentamicin (3 mg/kg/day divided q 8 h) for 6 weeks.[20] If intrinsic penicillin resistance, give 40 mg/kg/day divided q 8–12 h plus gentamicin (3 mg/kg/day divided q 8 h) for 6 weeks.[20]

Vancomycin HCl

Dosage *(cont.)*	**Staphylococci resistant to oxacillin:** Those without prosthetic material should receive 40 mg/kg/day divided q 8–12 h for 6 weeks.[20] Patients *with* prosthetic material should receive 40 mg/kg/day divided q 8–12 h for ≥6 weeks plus rifampin (20 mg/kg/day divided q 8 h for ≥6 weeks) and gentamicin (3 mg/kg/day divided q 8 h for 2 weeks).[20]
	Viridans Group Streptococci and *Streptococcus bovis*: Regardless of penicillin sensitivity, patients unable to tolerate penicillin or ceftriaxone may receive 40 mg/kg/day divided q 8–12 h for 6 weeks.[20]
	Culture negative (including *Bartonella*)
	Native valve: Should not be used in native value diseases unless the patient cannot tolerate penicillin.[20] 40 mg/kg/day divided q 8–12 h plus ampicillin-sulbactam (300 mg/kg/day divided q 4–6 h, gentamicin (3 mg/kg/day divided q 8 h) and ciprofloxacin 20–30 mg/kg/day divided q 12 h for 4–6 weeks.[20]
	Prosthetic valve/material: If 1 year since prosthetic valve placement, give 40 mg/kg/day divided q 8–12 h plus gentamicin (3 mg/kg/day divided q 8 h), cefepime (150 mg/kg/day divided q 8 h), and rifampin (20 mg/kg/day divided q 8 h). With the exception of rifampin (2 weeks) antibiotics should be given for weeks.[20]
	Biologic warfare or bioterrorism: The CDC and other experts recommend that treatment of inhalational anthrax spores due to biologic warfare or bioterrorism should be started on a multiple-drug parenteral regimen that includes ciprofloxacin or doxycycline and one or two additional anti-infective agents (i.e., chloramphenicol, clindamycin, rifampin, vancomycin, clarithromycin, imipenem, penicillin, or ampicillin).[21,22]
	Central venous catheter infection: 25 mg/L of vancomycin added to parenteral nutrition solution as a continuous infusion[23-25] or as a flush/lock.[26,27] Although this dose has been used for prophylaxis to decrease catheter-related coagulase-negative staphylococcal sepsis, the Centers for Disease Control and Prevention discourage this practice.[24]
	Ventricular shunt infection: *ISMP high-alert medication that has an increased risk of causing significant patient harm if it is used in error.*[1] This warning is related to intrathecal administration only.
	60 mg/kg/day divided q 6 h by intravenous administration. 5–20 mg/dose (50 mg/mL diluted with preservative free NS to a final concentration of 1–5 mg/mL) directly into the ventricle (if the shunt is not externalized) or via the externalized shunt, which is then clamped for 1 hour after administration.[28-31]
Dosage adjustment in organ dysfunction	Adjust dosage in renal dysfunction.[32] If CrCl is 30–50 mL/min, give a normal dose q 12 h; if 10–29 mL/min, give normal dose q 18–24 h; and if CrCl is <10 mL/min, adjust dosage based on serum concentrations.[32]

Patients on ECMO have an increased circulating volume and transiently altered renal function; therefore, a suggested dose is 20 mg/kg q 24 h.[33] Patients with malignancy may have increased clearance and require larger doses (i.e., mean dose of 71.5 mg/kg/day).[34,35] Although serum vancomycin concentration should not be routinely monitored, trough concentration may be helpful in patients who are not clinically responding. |
Maximum dosage	60 or 80 mg/kg/day[10,17,18] not to exceed *adult* dose of 4 g/day.[2]
Additives	None.
Suitable diluents	NS, LR, D5W, D10W, D5NS, Sodium Bicarbonate 3.75%, Dextran 6% + NS.[36,37]
Maximum concentration	<5 mg/mL.[37]

Vancomycin HCl

Preparation and delivery

Delivery system issues: The potential for toxic effects from chemicals that may leach from the plastic containers into the single-dose, premixed intravenous preparation has not been determined.[38]

Stability: Solutions prepared in D5W or NS are stable for 14 days when refrigerated or 24 hours at room temperature.[2] Frozen premixed solutions are stable for 90 days from the date of shipping when stored at ~20C. Thawed solutions are stable for 72 hours at room temperature and 30 days when refrigerated.

Compatibility: See Appendix D for PN compatibility information.[39]

IV push

Not recommended.[2]

Intermittent infusion

Over ≥ 60 minutes or ≤10 mg/min in *adults.*[2] Has been given safely in 30 minutes,[13,15,40,41] but the likelihood of adverse effects in significant. (See Infusion related cautions section; see Rare adverse effects in Comments section.)

Continuous infusion

Vancomycin has a slow bactericidal activity, a low MIC against most organisms, and exhibits time-dependent killing. Some have proposed that administration by continuous infusion would maximize the time that vancomycin serum concentrations exceed the MIC for the suspected organism and thereby enhance efficacy, prevent bacterial regrowth, and perhaps decrease toxicity.[42-48] Data for the administration of vancomycin by continuous infusion are extremely limited and have focused on *adults*[42-46] and neonates.[47,48]

Other routes of administration

IM administration is not recommended because it may cause local tissue necrosis and has erratic absorption.[2] Has been given by inhalation[49,50] and intraventricular routes[28-31] for the treatment of methicillin-resistant *Staphylococcus aureus*. No information available to support administration by other routes. Chemical peritonitis (abdominal pain, fever, and changes in dialysate fluid) has been reported following intraperitoneal delivery of vancomycin during continuous ambulatory peritoneal dialysis.[2] Discontinuation of intraperitoneal vancomycin has shown to reverse the chemical peritonitis.

Comments

Rare adverse effects: Rapid IV administration may result in red man syndrome.[2] This syndrome may be accompanied by flushing and/or a maculopapular rash or erythematous rash on the face, neck, chest, and upper extremities. Severe hypotension and cardiac arrest have occurred in *adults* and children after rapid administration.[51,52] Symptoms usually begin minutes after start of the infusion. Symptoms usually resolve spontaneously after discontinuation of the infusion. Lengthen the infusion time to 2 hours and/or pretreatment with an antihistamine diphenhydramine HCl 1 mg/kg IV) or H-2 antagonist (cimetidine 4 mg/kg/IV) may prevent the syndrome.[53,54]

Although extremely rare, nephrotoxicity may occur in patients with underlying kidney dysfunction, those receiving large doses, or in patients receiving concurrent nephrotoxicity medications.[2] When vancomycin was discontinued, azotemia resolves in most patients.[2] Although most of these have occurred in patients who were given aminoglycosides concomitantly, the literature does not support the contention that the combination is more nephrotoxic in the pediatric population.[55-58]

Vancomycin-associated hearing loss has been reported in patients with kidney dysfunction, preexisting hearing loss, and/or those receiving other ototoxic agents.[2] Vertigo, dizziness, and tinnitus have been reported rarely.

Vancomycin HCl

Comments

Monitoring: Studies have shown,[59,60] and the American Academy of Pediatrics[10] recommends, that routine monitoring of serum vancomycin concentrations is unnecessary.

Drug interactions: Combination with other nephrotoxic or neurotoxic drugs requires close monitoring. Consult appropriate resources for dosing recommendations before combining any drug with vancomycin.

Laboratory interference: Some fluorescence immunoassay and radioimmunoassay for vancomycin may overestimate serum vancomycin concentrations in patients with renal failure.[61] This occurs due to accumulation of vancomycin crystalline degradation products (CDP-1). Some assay do not suffer from this problem[62]; hence practitioners should check with their clinical laboratory.

Other: Cardiac conditions associated with the highest risk of adverse outcome from endocarditis for which prophylaxis with dental procedures is reasonable: (1) prosthetic cardiac valve or prosthetic material used for cardiac valve repair; (2) previous IE; (3) congenital heart disease (CHD)* in a person with a) unrepaired cyanotic CHD, including palliative shunts and conduits, b) completely repaired congenital heart defect with prosthetic material or device, whether placed by surgery or by catheter intervention, during the first 6 months after the procedure,† c) repaired CHD with residual defects at the site or adjacent to the site of a prosthetic patch or prosthetic device (which inhibit endothelialization); and (4) cardiac transplantation recipients who develop cardiac valvulopathy.[19]

---

*Except for the conditions listed above, antibiotic prophylaxis is no longer recommended for any other form of CHD.

†Prophylaxis is reasonable because endothelialization of prosthetic material occurs within 6 months after the procedure.

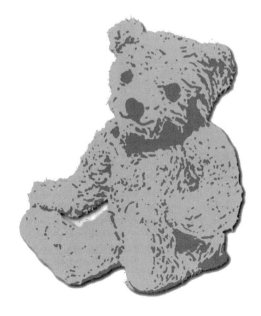

Vasopressin

Brand names	Pitressin
Medication error potential	Look-alike, sound-alike error potential. USP reported that vasopressin was confused with desmopressin and oxytocin. Pitressin was confused with pitocin.[1]
Contraindications and warnings	**Contraindications:** Hypersensitivity to vasopressin or any of its components.[2]
Infusion related cautions	Extravasation of IV infusion may result in tissue necrosis.[3] (See Appendix E for extravasation management.)

Dosage	**Central diabetes insipidus:** Initially 0.0005 unit/kg/h doubling the dose q 30 min until urine osmolality is twice that of plasma and urine output is <2 mL/kg/h.[3] The dosage required rarely exceeds 0.01 unit/kg/h.[4] A 3-day-old and a 3-year-old were started on 0.003 unit/kg/h.[5] Polyuria resolved and the drug was weaned over several days.[5]
	
	Shock refractory to standard therapy (vasopressors): Starting doses range from 0.0002–0.0006 unit/kg/min increased to 0.002–0.005 titrated to a response in blood pressure.[6-8] Blood pressure stabilized in an older 14-year-old who received 0.04 unit/min.[8]
	
	In *adults* with septic shock, continuous low-dose infusion of 0.01 and 0.04 unit/min (not titrated) in conjunction with other pressors is supported.[9] The Surviving Sepsis Campaign guidelines warn against the use of >0.04 unit/min because it has been associated with myocardial ischemia and cardiac arrest.[10]
	
	Gastrointestinal bleeding (other therapies have decreased the use of vasopressin for this indication)
	
	    Age-based[11]
	
	        0.1 unit/min as a continuous infusion; increased by 0.05 unit/min each hour up to a maximum of
	
	        <5 years: 0.2 unit/min.
	
	        5–12 years: 0.3 unit/min.
	
	        >12 years: 0.4 unit/min.
	
	    Weight-based[12]
	
	        An initial infusion of 0.3 unit/kg (up to 20 units) infused over 20 minutes may be used prior to a continuous infusion of 0.2–0.4 unit/1.73 m²/min. The infusion is maintained for 12 hours after bleeding stops and then tapered to off over the next 24–36 hours.[12]
	
	        In 17 children an average of 7.2 years old, 0.1–0.2 unit/min was titrated to control bleeding.[13] Maximum dosage was 0.004–0.04 unit/kg/min. The low dose group (<0.01 unit/kg/min) and high dose (≥0.01 unit/kg/min) were not different in controlling bleeding; however, significantly more complications (electrolyte disturbances, fluid overload, hypertension, cardiac dysrhythmias) occurred with the larger dose.
	
	Cardiac arrest: A four-patient case series found evidence that vasopressin administration may be beneficial during prolonged pediatric cardiac arrest.[14] However, there is not enough evidence for the PALS guidelines for resuscitation to recommend for or against its use.[15]

Vasopressin

Dosage adjustment in organ dysfunction	No dosage adjustment required in renal dysfunction.[16]
Maximum dosage	Generally the dose is titrated to effect. **Diabetes insipidus:** 0.01 unit/kg/h. **Gastrointestinal bleeding:** ≥0.01 unit/kg/min has been used but resulted in significantly more adverse effects.
Additives	9 mg NaCl/mL and chlorobutanol as a preservative.[2]
Suitable diluents	D5W, NS.[3]
Maximum concentration	1 unit/mL.[17]
Preparation and delivery	Undiluted for SC or IM use.[2,17] Diluted to 0.1–1 unit/mL in D5W or NS for continuous infusion.[17]
IV push	Not indicated.[3]
Intermittent infusion	Not indicated.
Continuous infusion	May be administered by continuous infusion.[2,3]
Other routes of administration	IM or SC.[2,17]
Comments	**Monitoring:** Fluid status and electrolytes should be monitored.[3] **Drug interactions:** The antidiuretic effects of vasopressin may be potentiated when used with carbamazepine, chlorpropamide, clofibrate, urea, fludrocortisone, and tricyclic antidepressants. Conversely concomitant use of demeclocycline, norepinephrine, lithium, and heparin may antagonize the effects of vasopressin.[2]

Vecuronium Bromide

Brand names	Norcuron, generic

Medication error potential

ISMP high-alert medication that has an increased risk of causing significant patient harm if it is used in error.[1]

Look-alike, sound-alike error potential.

USP reports that vecuronium has been confused with pancuronium and rocuronium; no patient harm resulted.[2] USP reports that vecuronium has been confused with vancomycin; patient harm resulted.[2] USP also reports that vecuronium has been confused with Zemuron; patient death resulted.[2]

ISMP and USP report that Norcuron has been confused with Narcan; no patient harm resulted.[2,3] USP also reports that Norcuron has been confused with Natrecor; patient death resulted.[2]

Contraindications and warnings

US boxed warning: Vecuronium should be administered only by adequately trained individuals familiar with the actions, characteristics, and hazards of vecuronium.[4]

Contraindications: Hypersensitivity to vecuronium or any of its components.[4]

Other warnings: Use carefully under the supervision of experienced clinicians; personnel should also be skilled in airway management, resuscitation, and respiratory support.[4] Intubation and ventilatory support equipment, including oxygen therapy, should be readily available.[4] Also should have anticholinesterase inhibitors readily available when giving vecuronium.[4]

Infusion related cautions

Flushing, erythema, pruritus, urticaria, bronchospasm, and hypotension are uncommon but may occur.[5,6]

Dosage

Respiratory function must be supported during use of this agent. Concurrent administration of a sedative is also necessary. Monitoring of neuromuscular transmission with a peripheral nerve stimulator is recommended during continuous infusion or with repeated dosing.[4,7]

Because vecuronium does not cause histamine release, it is considered the neuromuscular blocking agent of choice in patients with allergies and/or asthma.[8]

0.08–0.1 mg/kg as required to maintain desired neuromuscular blockade[8-13] followed by a continuous infusion of 0.06–0.1 mg/kg/h titrated up to 0.17 mg/kg/h based on individual response.[8-13] One paper suggests 0.06–0.09 mg/kg/h for infants and 0.09–0.15 mg/kg/h for children.[8]

Dosage adjustment in organ dysfunction

To avoid prolonged neuromuscular blockade, give smaller initial doses to anephric patients.[4] Patients with cirrhosis and cholestasis may experience prolonged recovery times.[4]

Maximum dosage

A single, 0.4 mg/kg dose has been used safely in children 2–9 years old with normal renal and hepatic function.[12] The largest reported continuous infusion rate was 0.27 mg/kg/h for 21 hours.[11]

In a study of 11 infants and children, the mean infusion rate was 0.14 mg/kg/h (range 0.1–0.27 mg/kg/h).[11] One neonate required 0.18 mg/kg/h.[11]

Vecuronium Bromide

Additives

Multidose vials contain benzyl alcohol 0.9% as a preservative.[4,14] See Appendix C for more specific information about potential adverse effects and/or benzyl alcohol toxicity in neonates.

Suitable diluents

D5W, D5NS, NS, LR.[4,14]

Maximum concentration

1 mg/mL.[4,14]

Preparation and delivery

In neonates, use SW for reconstitution to avoid the administration of benzyl alcohol.[14]

Vecuronium should not be mixed or administered with alkaline solutions.[14]

For PN compatibility information, please see Appendix D.

IV push

1 mg/mL administered rapidly over seconds.[4,14]

Intermittent infusion

Not administered by this method.

Continuous infusion

0.1–0.2 mg/mL preferred.[4,10,11,14] Another reference states that up to 1 mg/mL may be given via continuous infusion.[15]

Other routes of administration

Should not be given IM.[4,14] No information available to support administration by other routes.

Comments

Significant adverse effects: Prolonged paralysis has been reported in several patients after long-term infusion of vecuronium.[16-18] Acute quadriplegic myopathy resulted when a 17-month-old infant was intubated for 24 days and treated with vecuronium and high-dose methylprednisolone.[19]

Sinus node exit block occurred in a 14-year-old after administration of 0.08 mg/kg.[20]

Drug interactions: Concomitant administration of corticosteroids[21,22] and certain antibiotics (e.g., aminoglycosides and polymyxin B)[23,24] with neuromuscular blockers has been shown to be a risk factor for prolonged paralysis.

Reduce vecuronium dose to 0.04–0.06 mg/kg in patients receiving succinylcholine, enflurane, or isoflurane.[4] Concomitant use with atracurium in an equipotent dose is more potent than either agent alone.[13]

Other: Disruption of the blood brain barrier in critical illness may cause penetration of vecuronium into the CNS, resulting in dilated, nonreactive pupils. Three such cases were reported in a pediatric oncology unit.[25]

Verapamil HCl

Brand names	Generic

Medication error potential

ISMP high-alert medication that has an increased risk of causing significant patient harm if it is used in error.[1]

Contraindications and warnings

Contraindications[2]: Severe hypotension or cardiogenic shock, second- or third-degree atrioventricular (AV) block (unless patient has a pacemaker), sick sinus syndrome (unless patient has a pacemaker), severe CHF, treatment with beta-blockers (should be administered hours apart), atrial flutter or atrial fibrillation with an accessory bypass tract (Wolff-Parkinson-White syndrome,[3,4] ventricular tachycardia, and known hypersensitivity to verapamil.

The initial use should be in facilities with appropriate monitoring and resuscitation facilities including direct-current cardioversion availability.[2,5]

Continuous ECG monitoring should be performed during infusion.[5,6]

Infusion related cautions

Hypotension, bradycardia, tachycardia, asystole, and arrhythmias may occur, particularly in patients with sinus node dysfunction or impaired AV conduction.[7]

Calcium chloride 10 mg/kg should be at the bedside in the event of hypotension.[5]

Dosage

PALS guidelines state that verapamil should not be used in infants during CPR because it may cause refractory hypotension and cardiac arrest.[8]

Tachyarrhythmias

Neonates and infants: While verapamil has been used in this age group, severe hemodynamic side effects including death have been reported.[9-12] Doses of 0.1–0.2 mg/kg (usually 0.75–2 mg) with continuous ECG monitoring have been used.[2,5,13-17] If necessary, the dose can be repeated 30 minutes after the initial dose.[5,13]

Children 1–15 years: Initially, 0.1–0.3 mg/kg[2,6,7,13-15,17] (usually 2–5 mg).[2] If necessary, the dose (≤10 mg) can be repeated one time 30 minutes after the initial dose.[2]

Dosage adjustment in organ dysfunction

Use with caution and monitor (ECG, blood pressure) for signs of toxicity in patients with renal insufficiency.[5]

In patients with liver disease, the dose should be halved.[18]

Maximum dosage

Neonates and infants: 0.2 mg/kg and ≤2 mg/dose.[2]

1–15 years: 0.3 mg/kg and ≤10 mg/dose.[2]

An 18-year-old with anticholinergic-induced torsades de pointes and prolonged QT interval unresponsive to standard therapies was successfully treated with three 5-mg (0.1 mg/kg) doses of verapamil followed by an infusion of 5 mcg/kg/min.[19]

Additives

Contains 8.5 mg sodium chloride/mL.[2,20]

Suitable diluents

D5W, D5½NS, D5NS, D5LR, D5R, ½NS, NS, LR, R.[20]

Verapamil HCl

Maximum concentration	2.5 mg/mL (undiluted).[2]
Preparation and delivery	**Photosensitivity:** Protect from light during storage.[2]
IV push	Over ≥2–3 minutes.[2,20]
Intermittent infusion	Not indicated.
Continuous infusion	Has been infused continuously in *adults*.[21-23]
Other routes of administration	Not indicated.
Comments	**Adverse effects:** Apnea, cardiovascular collapse, and respiratory arrest have been reported in pediatric patients, particularly those <1 year of age.[9-12] Brief myoclonic seizures developed in an 18-month-old patient following intravenous verapamil.[24] A 15-year-old with Duchenne's muscular dystrophy was given seven 5-mg doses of verapamil over 20 hours and had resolution of the tachyarrhythmia.[25] However, 4 hours after the last dose, severe bradycardia and hypotension occurred and the child was not able to be resuscitated. The death was not felt to be related to the verapamil because of the length of time since the last dose and the short half-life of verapamil. A 17-year-old with Duchenne's muscular dystrophy developed irreversible respiratory failure felt to be related to verapamil.[26] **Drug interactions:** Verapamil is a substrate for CYP3A4 and moderately inhibits CPY3A4 and, thus, is subject to a number of drug interactions. Appropriate references should be consulted prior to combining any drug with verapamil.

VinBLAStine Sulfate

Brand names	Velban, generic

Medication error potential

ISMP high-alert medication that has an increased risk of causing significant patient harm if it is used in error.[1]

Look-alike, sound-alike error potential.

ISMP and USP report that vinBLAStine has been confused with vinCRIStine; no patient harm resulted.[2,3]

Contraindications and warnings

US boxed warning: Should only be administered by individuals with experience in the administration of vinblastine. Vinblastine may cause extravasation. (See Infusion related cautions section.) Vinblastine is fatal if given intrathecally.[4]

Contraindications: Vinblastine should not be administered to patients with significant granulocytopenia or in the presence of a bacterial infection.[4] (See Significant adverse effects in Comments section.)

Other warnings: May cause serious stomatitis, neurological toxicity, leukopenia, and dyspnea.[4] (See Significant adverse effects in Comments section.)

Infusion related cautions

Vinblastine is only administered IV. Intrathecal administration of vinblastine is fatal.[4,5]

Extravasation of vinblastine can cause considerable local tissue irritation.[4,6] The infusion should be stopped if the patient complains of discomfort. Because of extravasation and infiltration risk, small veins in the dorsum of the hand or foot and scalp veins should be avoided if at all possible. Local injection of hyaluronidase and application of moderate heat to the area may lessen pain and potential damage.[4] See Appendix E for additional information regarding extravasation treatment.

Dosage

Consult institutional protocol for complete dosing information.

Vinblastine is used alone and in combination with a variety of antineoplastic agents for the treatment of Hodgkin's lymphoma, non-Hodgkin's lymphoma, histiocytic lymphoma, testicular cancer, Kaposi's sarcoma, histiocytosis X, and others. While it can be used as monotherapy, it is often part of a multidrug regimen, and the timing of doses for all drugs is critical to achieve the optimal outcome.

Vinblastine is usually dosed once a week; however, there are specific protocols that vary. Some regimens that have been used in children are listed below:

Histiocytosis X: 6.5 mg/m^2 weekly for 24 weeks.[7]

Hodgkin's disease (combined with other agents): 6 mg/m^2 on protocol day 7.[8]

Testicular cancer (combined with other agents): 3 mg/m^2 on two separate days[9] or on protocol days 22 and 23 or days 1 and 2.[10]

In *adults*, the initial dose is usually 3.7 mg/m^2 and this is increased by 1.8 mg/m^2 weekly until the WBC is 3000/m^2 or a maximum dose of 18.5 mg/m^2 is reached. Once the dose that suppresses the WBC to <3000/m^2 is reached, the maintenance dose should be decreased by one step (1.8 mg/m^2). Usual weekly range of doses in *adults* is 5.5–7.4 mg/m^2.[11]

Dosage adjustment in organ dysfunction

No dose reduction is needed in patients with renal dysfunction.[12] Vinblastine doses should be reduced in patients with hepatic insufficiency.[13] The manufacturer recommends a 50% dose reduction in patients with a direct serum bilirubin >3 mg/dL.[4]

Maximum dosage

Maximum weekly dose should not exceed 18.5 mg/m^2 in *adults*.[4] Refer to treatment protocols for maximum-dose guidelines.

VinBLAStine Sulfate

Additives

May contain benzyl alcohol 0.9%.[5] (See Preparation and delivery section.) See Appendix C for more specific information about potential adverse effects and/or benzyl alcohol toxicity in neonates.

Suitable diluents

D5W, LR, NS.[4,5]

Maximum concentration

1 mg/mL.[4,5]

Preparation and delivery

Reconstitute with NS or bacteriostatic NS (with benzyl alcohol). Also available as a 1-mg/mL solution (preserved with benzyl alcohol).[5]

Preparation: Vinblastine must be dispensed with a sticker affixed directly to the container that states "Fatal if given intrathecally. For IV use only."[4,5] Vinblastine must also be dispensed in overwrap which bears the statement "Do not remove covering until the moment of injection. Fatal if given intrathecally. For IV use only."[4,5]

IV push

1 mg/mL administered via an intact, free-flowing IV needle or catheter over 1 minute.[5]

Intermittent infusion

Although vinblastine has been administered by this method, it is not recommended because of the risk of infiltration.[5]

Continuous infusion

Not recommended.[5]

Other routes of administration

Contraindicated.[4,5]

Comments

Significant adverse effects: Vinblastine is associated with severe hematologic effects, primarily leukopenia (granulocytopenia), and rarely anemia and thrombocytopenia. The hematologic effects appear to be dose-related. Vinblastine should not be given if the WBC is <4000/m^3.[4]

Neurotoxicity has been observed following vinblastine administration, but this adverse effect is much less common than with vincristine.[14]

Dyspnea has not been observed with vinblastine alone,[15] but there have been numerous case reports of an acute, temporally related, respiratory distress syndrome that occurs within 1–5 hours following the combination of vinblastine and mitomycin C. Some of these acute reactions have been fatal.[15-21] The incidence of this toxic pulmonary reaction has been estimated to be as high as 3% to 6%.[17]

Vinblastine is associated with a minimal (<10%) risk of emesis.[22,23] Generally, prophylaxis for acute and delayed emesis is not needed. Patients may receive one-time prophylaxis with a phenothiazine (e.g., prochlorperazine) or a butyrophenone (e.g., droperidol). Breakthrough medications may be offered, such as a phenothiazine (e.g., prochlorperazine), a butyrophenone (e.g., droperidol), a substituted benzamide (e.g., metoclopramide), or a benzodiazepine (e.g., lorazepam). Selection should be based on what the patient is currently receiving for acute antiemesis prophylaxis.

Monitoring: CBC with differential, serum uric acid, and hepatic function.[4,5]

Drug interactions: Vinblastine is major substrate for CYP3A4 and a minor substrate for CYP2D6; there is a potential for drug interactions.[4,5] Consult appropriate resources for dosing recommendations before combining any drug with vinblastine.

VinCRIStine Sulfate

Brand names	Vincasar PFS, Oncovin, generic
Medication error potential	ISMP high-alert medication that has an increased risk of causing significant patient harm if it is used in error.[1] Look-alike, sound-alike error potential. ISMP and USP report that vinCRIStine has been confused with vinBLAStine; no patient harm resulted.[2,3] USP also reports that vinCRIStine has been confused with vinorelbine; no patient harm resulted.[3]
Contraindications and warnings	**US boxed warning:** Should only be administered by individuals with experience in the administration of vincristine. Vincristine may cause extravasation. (See Infusion related cautions section.) Vincristine is fatal if given intrathecally.[4] **Contraindications:** Vincristine should not be administered to patients with demyelinating forms of Charcot-Marie-Tooth syndrome.[4] **Other warnings:** Vincristine has been associated with serious constipation, neurotoxicity, respiratory effects, and urinary tract disturbances.[4] (See Significant adverse effects in Comments section.)
Infusion related cautions	Vincristine is only administered IV.[4,5] IT administration of vincristine is fatal.[4-7] Because extravasation may cause tissue sloughing and necrosis, the infusion should be stopped if the patient complains of discomfort.[8,9] Because of extravasation and infiltration risk, small veins in the dorsum of the hand or foot and scalp veins should be avoided if at all possible. Local injection of hyaluronidase and application of moderate heat to the area may lessen pain and potential damage.[4] See Appendix E for additional information regarding extravasation treatment.
Dosage	Please consult institutional protocol for complete dosing information. Vincristine is used as a component of combination therapy to treat childhood acute lymphocytic (lymphoblastic) leukemia, Hodgkin's disease, non-Hodgkin's lymphoma, neuroblastoma, rhabdomyosarcoma, Wilms' Tumor, Kaposi's sarcoma, brain tumors, small cell lung cancer, and other neoplastic diseases. One protocol for high-risk acute lymphoblastic leukemia included vincristine on induction days 8, 15, 22, and 29; during block 1 of therapy on days 1 and 8; and as part of reinduction on days 8, 15, 22, and 29.[10] A protocol for treating Hodgkin's disease included doses of vincristine on day 0 (with the complete schedule of chemotherapies repeated q 28 days) or on day 42 of a 63-day multiple chemotherapy regimen.[11] Usual doses given no more frequently than weekly[8,12,13]: **<10 kg or BSA <1 m²:** 0.05 mg/kg (up to 2 mg). **≥10 kg:** 1.5–2 mg/m² (up to 2 mg). ***Adults:*** 1.4 mg/m² (up to 2 mg). In infants, vincristine clearance is more closely related to body weight than BSA.[14]
Dosage adjustment in organ dysfunction	Dose should be reduced in patients with hepatic insufficiency.[15] A 50% reduction in dose is recommended if direct serum bilirubin is >3 mg/dL.[8] No dose reduction is needed in patients with renal dysfunction.[16]

VinCRIStine Sulfate

Maximum dosage	Most, but not all, clinical trials and treatment protocols have maximum-dose guidelines of 2 mg in order to minimize neurotoxicity.[12,13,17] However, some clinicians have questioned the appropriateness of the 2-mg maximum vincristine dose.[18] Refer to treatment protocols for maximum-dose guidelines.
Additives	None.
Suitable diluents	D5W, NS.[4,5]
Maximum concentration	1 mg/mL.[5]
Preparation and delivery	Vincristine must be dispensed with a sticker affixed directly to the container which states "Fatal if given intrathecally. For IV use only." Vincristine must also be dispensed in overwrap which bears the statement "Do not remove covering until the moment of injection. Fatal if given intrathecally. For IV use only."[4,5]
IV push	1 mg/mL administered via an intact, free-flowing IV needle or catheter over 1 minute.[5]
Intermittent infusion	May dilute with suitable diluent and infuse over 4–8 hours.[5]
Continuous infusion	May dilute with suitable diluent and infuse continuously.[5]
Other routes of administration	Not recommended; for IV infusion only.[4,5]
Comments	**Significant adverse effects:** The dose-limiting effect of vincristine is neurotoxicity.[4,8] Severe vincristine-associated neurotoxicity has been observed with concurrent administration of drugs that inhibit hepatic cytochrome P450 isoenzymes.[19] (See Drug interactions below.)
	Vincristine is associated with a minimal (<10%) risk of emesis.[20,21] Generally, prophylaxis for acute and delayed emesis is not needed. Patients may receive one time prophylaxis with a phenothiazine (e.g., prochlorperazine) or a butyrophenone (e.g., droperidol). Breakthrough medications should be offered, such as a phenothiazine (e.g., prochlorperazine), a butyrophenone (e.g., droperidol), a substituted benzamide (e.g., metoclopramide), or a benzodiazepine (e.g., lorazepam). Selection should be based on what the patient is currently receiving for acute antiemetic prophylaxis.
	Monitoring: CBC with differential, uric acid levels, serum electrolytes, hepatic function, and neurologic examination.[4,8]
	Drug interactions: Vincristine is a major substrate for CYP3A4. Concomitant use with drugs that inhibit the CYP3A4 isoenzyme (e.g., azole antifungals, cyclosporine, and macrolide antibiotics) may result in severe neurotoxicity.[19] Consult appropriate resources for dosing recommendations before combining any drug with vincristine.
	Other: Vincristine should not be given to patients receiving radiation through ports that include the liver due to risk of potentially fatal hepatitis.[22]
	In overdose, treatment includes fluid restriction due to likelihood of syndrome of inappropriate antidiuretic hormone (SIADH), prophylactic phenobarbital, enemas to prevent ileus, daily hemoglobin and hematocrit to evaluate need for transfusion, and monitoring the cardiovascular system. Some have suggested that leucovorin calcium 100 mg IV q 3 h for 24 hours and then q 6 h for at least 48 hours may be of value.[8]

Vitamin A

Brand names	Aquasol A Parenteral (water-miscible vitamin A palmitate)
Medication error potential	Look-alike, sound-alike error potential. USP reported that Aquasol A was confused with Aquasol E.[1]
Contraindications and warnings	**Contraindications:** Hypersensitivity to any product components.[2]
Infusion related cautions	Not intended for IV use.

Dosage

Vitamin A deficiency[2]

> **Infants:** 7500–15,000 units/day IM for 10 days.

> **1–8 years of age:** 17,500–35,000 units/day IM for 10 days.

Decrease morbidity from bronchopulmonary dysplasia in preterm infants: 2000 units (n = 20) or placebo (n = 20) IM was given to infants with increased risk for bronchopulmonary dysplasia (BPD) on day 1 of life and then every other day for 28 days. Vitamin A status was improved and morbidity associated with BPD was decreased.[3] In a follow-up multicenter study, either 5000 units (n = 405) or placebo (n = 402) was given IM three times weekly for 4 weeks in premature infants as small as 770 ± 135 g. Compared to controls, the treated infants had improved vitamin A serum concentrations and the risk of chronic lung disease decreased (62% vs. 55%, respectively).[4] A follow-up study evaluating the long-term outcome when these infants were 18 to 22 months of age found no evidence that hospitalizations or pulmonary problems were different between the vitamin A group and controls.[5]

One group recommended 2000 units IM on day of life 1 and every other day until enteral feedings are established.[6] Once 75% of enteral feedings is attained, the route is changed to enteral and the dose increased to 4000 units given until discharge from the neonatal intensive care unit. Should the patient be placed NPO, the IM dose and route are resumed. Vitamin A and retinol binding protein concentrations should be measured weekly. (See Comments section.)

Dosage adjustment in organ dysfunction	Elevated serum retinol concentrations accompanied by clinical toxicity have been reported in one *adult* and two children with renal failure who were on PN.[7]
Maximum dosage	15,000 units in children,[2] 5000 units in neonates.[3]
Additives	Contains 12% polysorbate 80 and 0.5% chlorobutanol.[2] See Appendix C for specific information about potential polysorbate adverse effects.
Suitable diluents	Not applicable.
Maximum concentration	50,000 USP units (15 mg retinol)/mL (undiluted).[2]
Preparation and delivery	**Photosensitivity:** Protect from light.[2]

IV push	Not for IV use.[2]
Intermittent infusion	Not for IV use.[2]
Continuous infusion	Not for IV use.[2]
Other routes of administration	For IM administration only.[2]
Comments	The target serum concentration range is 30–60 mcg/dL. Concentrations >100 mcg/dL are potentially toxic.[6] In particular, measuring serum concentrations is recommended in patients receiving glucocorticoids because steroids increase plasma concentrations of vitamin A.[8] This confounds the assessment of adequacy of vitamin A intake.

Vitamin K$_1$–Phytonadione

Brand names	AquaMEPHYTON; various manufacturers
Medication error potential	Look-alike, sound-alike error potential. USP reported that vitamin K was confused with Urocit-K and that phytonadione was confused with coumadin and phenytoin sodium.[1]
Contraindications and warnings	**US boxed warning:** Severe reactions including fatalities have occurred during and after IV administration even when the product is diluted and infusion has been slow. Severe reactions have been noted following IM administration. Usually these resemble anaphylaxis or hypersensitivity type reactions. Restrict IV and IM use to situations when the SC route is not feasible.[2] **Contraindications:** Hypersensitivity to phytonadione or any of its components.[2]
Infusion related cautions	See US boxed warning in Contraindications and warnings section.[2]

Dosage	**Neonatal hemorrhagic disease**
	
	    Prophylaxis: Usually given within 1 hour of birth.[2,3]
	
	        ≤1500 g: 0.5 mg IM.[2-7]
	
	        >1500 g: 1 mg IM.[2-7]
	
	    Treatment: Usually 1 mg; however, larger doses may be needed if the mother was receiving anticoagulant therapy.[2,4,8-11]
	
	Prothrombin deficiency (malabsorption syndromes, broad spectrum antibiotics, etc.)
	
	    Infants: 2 mg.[12]
	
	    Older children: 5–10 mg.[12]
	
	Reversal of over-warfarinization in children: 30 mcg/kg IV (0.35–1 mg) was used in seven children (age not reported).[13]

Dosage adjustment in organ dysfunction	None noted. Those with liver dysfunction may require larger than usual doses[2] or more than one dose. Measurement of the INR and/or PT may be used to guide dosing.[12]
Maximum dosage	5 mg in children.[13] In *adults* with anticoagulant-induced hypoprothrombinemia, doses are usually 2.5–10 mg; however, doses up to 50 mg may be needed.[2] It is prudent to limit the dose to the lowest effective amount so the patient can resume anticoagulation at the appropriate level.[14] Failure to respond may indicate that the underlying disease may be unresponsive to vitamin K.
Additives	Contains benzyl alcohol.[2] See Appendix C for specific information about potential benzyl alcohol toxicity.

Vitamin K$_1$–Phytonadione

Suitable diluents	D5W, D10W, D-R combinations, D-LR combinations, ½NS, NS, LR, R.[2,15]
Maximum concentration	10 mg/mL (undiluted).[2]
Preparation and delivery	**Compatibility:** See Appendix D for PN compatibility information. **Photosensitivity:** Protect from light during storage.[2]
IV push	Over >1 mg/min in *adults*.[2,13] IV administration should be restricted due to the potential for severe adverse reactions.[2]
Intermittent infusion	Over 15–30 minutes.[13]
Continuous infusion	Specified dose can be added to PN solutions.[16]
Other routes of administration	SC is the referred route of administration.[2]
Comments	**Monitoring:** Improvement in hemostasis will not be seen until 1–2 hours after administration.[2,13] Some recommend measurement of INR 4–6 hours after the dose in those at high risk of bleeding or 12 hours after the dose in less severe cases of over-warfarinization.[13] Hyperbilirubinemia and severe hemolytic anemia have occurred in neonates receiving larger doses.[2] Two neonates who received IV phytonadione for prophylaxis developed late-onset hemorrhagic disease.[17]

Voriconazole

Brand names	Vfend

Medication error potential	Look-alike, sound-alike error potential. USP reports that Vfend has been confused with Venofer; no patient harm resulted.[1]

Contraindications and warnings	**Contraindications:** Concomitant administration with astemizole, cisapride, pimozide, quinidine, or terfenadine is contraindicated due to the increased risk of QT prolongation and torsades de pointes. Also contraindicated with concomitant use of sirolimus, rifampin, carbamazepine, long-acting barbiturates, ritonavir, rifabutin, ergot alkaloids, and St. John's Wort.[2] (See Drug interactions in Comments section.) Voriconazole is contraindicated in patients with a hypersensitivity to the drug or any of its components.[2] **Warnings:** Visual adverse effects are commonly reported with voriconazole therapy.[2] The effect of voriconazole on visual function is not known if therapy is prolonged beyond 28 days.[2] Visual function should be monitored in patients receiving voriconazole beyond 28 days.[2] Prolonged therapy should be used with caution in infants and children who are unable to vocalize visual effects.[2,3] Voriconazole has been associated with uncommon cases of hepatotoxicity, including liver failure and death. Liver function should be monitored before and during therapy. Cessation of therapy should be considered in patients with clinical signs and symptoms of liver disease.[2] Voriconazole can be teratogenic when given to pregnant women.[2] Contains hydroxypropyl-beta-cyclodextrin.[2] (See Dosage adjustment in organ dysfunction and Additives sections.)

Infusion related cautions	Anaphylactic-type reactions, typically presenting upon initiation of the infusion, have occurred uncommonly.[2]

Dosage	The most commonly reported dosage regimen in pediatric patients is a loading dose of 6 mg/kg q 12h for two doses followed by a maintenance dose of 4 mg/kg q 12 h.[4]
	
	Other published doses are summarized below:
	
	Neonates and infants: Experience with voriconazole in neonates and infants is limited.[5] One report of two cases of VLBW infants receiving 3 mg/kg IV q 12 h for two doses, then 2 mg/kg IV q 12 h documented serum concentrations below that seen in *adults*; therapy was successful in both infants.[6]
	
	Two reports in infants (one preterm) utilized initial dosing of 6 mg/kg IV q 12 h.[7,8] The dose in the preterm infant was increased to 6 mg/kg IV q 8 h to obtain serum concentrations similar to that seen in *adults*.[7]
	
	A 3-month-old received 6 mg/kg IV q 12 h for two doses, then 4 mg/kg IV q 12 h.[9]
	
	One reference suggests a dosing regimen of 8 mg/kg IV q 12 h for two doses, then 6 mg/kg IV q 12 h.[10]
	
	Children[3,5,10-14]
	
	    Loading dose: 6–8 mg/kg IV q 12 h for two doses.
	
	    Maintenance dose: 4–7 mg/kg IV q 12 h.
	
	Children have required larger doses than *adults* to maintain similar concentrations.[3,13,14]

Voriconazole

Dosage adjustment in organ dysfunction	**Hepatic impairment:** Patients with mild-to-moderate hepatic cirrhosis (Child-Pugh Class A or B) should receive a standard loading dose and 50% of maintenance dose.[2] Dosing has not been evaluated in patients with severe hepatic cirrhosis (Child-Pugh Class C) or chronic hepatitis B or C.[2] **Renal impairment:** Oral voriconazole is preferred in patients with CrCl <50 mL/min due to accumulation of the vehicle, sulfobutyl ether beta-cyclodextrin sodium (SBECD).[2,15] Peritoneal dialysis or hemodialysis does not remove a sufficient amount of voriconazole to warrant dose adjustment.[2,15,16]
Maximum dosage	No specific maximum dosage has been defined. A critically ill 3-year-old with neuroblastoma has received 5 mg/kg q 12 h increased every 2 days to 13 mg/kg q 12 h then up to 21 mg/kg q 12 h in conjunction with therapeutic drug monitoring.[17]
Additives	Each 200-mg vial contains 160 mg/mL sulfobutyl ether beta-cyclodextrin sodium or SBECD.[2,18] (See Dosage adjustment in organ dysfunction section.)
Suitable diluents	D5W, D5NS, D5½NS, D5W + 20 mEq/L potassium chloride, NS, ½NS, LR, D5LR.[2,18]
Maximum concentration	5 mg/mL.[2,18]
Preparation and delivery	Dilute reconstituted product to a final concentration of 0.5–5 mg/mL with appropriate diluent.[2,18] Do not administer through the same catheter or admix with other drugs, blood products, or PN.[2,18]
IV push	Not recommended.[2]
Intermittent infusion	Infuse over 1–2 hours at a maximum rate of 3 mg/kg/h.[2,18]
Continuous infusion	No information available to support administration by this method.
Other routes of administration	No information available to support administration by other routes.
Comments	**Significant adverse effects:** The most commonly reported adverse effects in children are dose-dependent visual disturbances and increases in transaminases and bilirubin, and photosensitivity.[4] Therapy has been associated with prolongation of QT interval.[2] Serum electrolytes (potassium, magnesium, calcium) should be within range before starting therapy to reduce risk of arrhythmias.[2] Stevens-Johnson syndrome has been reported rarely.[2]

Voriconazole

Drug interactions: Voriconazole is a major substrate for CYP2C9 and CYP2C19 and a minor substrate for CYP3A4; it is a weak inhibitor of CYP2C9 and CYP2C19 and a moderate inhibitor of CYP3A4.[19] Voriconazole is associated with numerous serious drug interactions.[2] Consult appropriate resources for dosing recommendations before combining any drug with fluconazole.

Patients on concomitant phenytoin therapy may require an increase in voriconazole maintenance dosing to 5 mg/kg.[12]

Pharmacokinetic considerations: Voriconazole metabolism may be variable among patients due to disease state, concomitant drug therapy and genetic polymorphisms.[2,4] Therapeutic drug monitoring is recommended to ensure optimal therapy, particularly in critically ill patients and patients receiving concomitant therapy that may affect voriconazole concentrations.[20,21] While efficacy has been correlated with trough concentrations greater than 2.05 mg/L, neurologic effects have been associated with trough concentrations above 5.5 mg/L; thus, it is prudent to adjust therapy to maintain a trough concentration between 2 and 5.5 mg/L.[4] Pediatric patients have required increased doses to achieve therapeutic drug concentrations.[17,22]

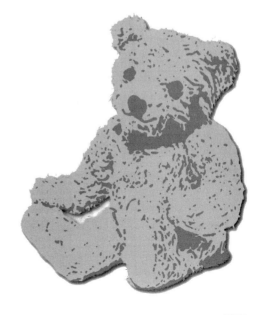

Zidovudine

Brand names	Retrovir (formerly called Azidothymidine, AZT)

Medication error potential

Look-alike, sound-alike error potential.

USP reports that zidovudine has been confused with lamivudine; no patient harm resulted.[1]

ISMP and USP report that Retrovir has been confused with ritonavir; patient harm resulted.[1,2] USP reports that Retrovir has been confused with acyclovir and Epivir; no patient harm resulted. USP also reports that Retrovir has been confused with Norvir; patient harm resulted.[1]

Contraindications and warnings

US boxed warning: Zidovudine has been associated with hematologic toxicity (neutropenia and anemia), and myopathy. Nucleoside analogues have been associated with lactic acidosis and severe hepatomegaly with steatosis.[3]

Contraindications: Life-threatening allergic reactions to any components of the medication.[3]

Other warnings: Combivir and Trizivir contain zidovudine, and thus should not be given concomitantly with zidovudine. Patients receiving interferon alpha with or without ribavirin concomitantly with zidovudine should be monitored closely.[3]

Infusion related cautions

May cause pain or irritation at injection site.[3]

Dosage

HIV-infected children should receive aggressive antiretroviral therapy with at least three drugs. Refer to www.aidsinfo.nih.gov or 1-800-TRIALS-A for the most up-to-date information regarding HIV treatment protocols in children.[4,5]

Initiation of zidovudine postexposure prophylaxis therapy in the infant should begin as soon as possible after delivery and preferably within 6–12 hours. Therapy initiating after 48 hours is not likely to be effective.[6]

For conversion from IV to oral dosing, the oral dose is one-third greater than the IV dose.[7,8] According to the manufacturer, in *adults* the IV dosage regimen equivalent to 100 mg q 4 h PO is approximately 1 mg/kg q 4 h IV.[3]

Antiretroviral therapy[4-14]

Premature neonates[4]

<30 weeks GA: 1.5 mg/kg IV q 12 h, then 1.5 mg/kg IV q 8 h at 4 weeks of age.

≥30 weeks GA: 1.5 mg/kg IV q 12 h, then 1.5 mg/kg IV q 8 h at 2 weeks of age.

Term neonates and infants <6 weeks of age[4]**:** 1.5 mg/kg IV q 6 h.

Infants and children (6 weeks to 12 years of age)[5]**:** 120 mg/m^2 IV q 6 h or 20-mg/m^2/h continuous infusion.

Continuous infusion of 0.5–1.4 mg/kg/h (360–1000 mg/m^2/day) has been beneficial in children as young as 6 months with symptomatic HIV infection, especially those with encephalopathy.[11,13,14]

Prevention of perinatal transmission[4,6]**:** Maternal zidovudine 100 mg five times a day beginning at 14–34 weeks gestation and continued through pregnancy. During labor, 2 mg/kg zidovudine IV over 1 hour followed by continuous infusion of 1 mg/kg/h until delivery. Begin treatment in newborn as soon as possible after delivery (see recommended doses above), preferably within 6–12 hours, and continue for the first 6 weeks of life. Continuation of therapy determined by virologic test results.

Zidovudine

Dosage adjustment in organ dysfunction

Adjust dosage in patients with severe renal dysfunction.[3,5,15] If CrCl is <10 mL/min, give 50% of a normal dose.[15] May also be necessary to adjust dose or interrupt therapy in patients with significant anemia and/or neutropenia.[3,7,10,11,14] Insufficient data suggest a reduction in dose may be needed in patients with liver disease; these patients should be monitored for hematologic toxicity.[3]

Maximum dosage

640 mg/m^2/day for intermittent infusion.[7,12] 1.8 mg/kg/h (1300 mg/m^2/day) for continuous infusion.[13,14]

Additives

None.[3]

Suitable diluents

D5W.[3,16]

Maximum concentration

4 mg/mL.[3,16]

Preparation and delivery

Stability: Once diluted, the solution is stable for 24 hours at room temperature and 48 hours if refrigerated at 2°C to 8°C. Because it contains no preservatives, the manufacturer suggests administering the solution within 8 hours if stored at room temperature or within 24 hours if refrigerated at 2°C to 8°C as an additional precaution.[3]

Compatibility: For PN compatibility information, please see Appendix D.

IV push

Not recommended.[3,16]

Intermittent infusion

≤4 mg/mL in D5W infused over 60 minutes.[3,16]

Continuous infusion

Although concentration and solution type were not specified, has been given by this method.[11,13,14,16]

Other routes of administration

IM administration not recommended by manufacturer. No information available to support administration by other methods.[3,16]

Comments

Significant adverse effects: Anemia necessitating treatment with partial volume exchange transfusion was reported in a 36-week-gestation infant born via emergent c-section (secondary to decreased fetal movement) to an HIV-positive woman receiving zidovudine, lamivudine, and nevirapine who developed macrocytic anemia at 29 weeks gestation (treated with packed red blood cell transfusion).[17]

Severe lactic acidosis has been reported in a neonate receiving zidovudine; symptoms resolved following zidovudine discontinuation.[18]

Drug interactions: Because zidovudine is associated with numerous drug interactions,[3] consult appropriate resources for dosing recommendations before combining any drug with zidovudine.

Zoledronic Acid

Brand names	Zometa, Reclast
Medication error potential	Look-alike, sound-alike error potential. USP reports potential for confusion between Zometa and Zofran and Zoladex.[1]
Contraindications and warnings	**Contraindications:** Previous hypersensitivity to zoledronic acid; uncorrected hypocalcemia.[2,3]
Infusion related cautions	None noted.
Dosage	**Bone disease:** 0.0125–0.05 mg/kg over 30 minutes.[4-7] Depending on the dose, the infusion may be repeated in 6 weeks or 3 months. The incidence of hypocalcemia is decreased with the lower dose.[4] There are no reports of zoledronic acid use to treat hypercalcemia in children.
Dosage adjustment in organ dysfunction	Do not use in patients with CrCl <35 mL/min.[2,3]
Maximum dosage	4[2] or 5[3] mg.
Additives	None.
Suitable diluents	D5W, NS.[2,4]
Maximum concentration	0.04 mg/mL.[2] 0.05 mg/mL (ready to infuse solution).[2]
Preparation and delivery	**Compatibility:** Incompatible with calcium containing fluids (including LR) and other parenteral drugs.[2]
IV push	Not indicated.
Intermittent infusion	Over ≥15 minutes.[2,3]
Continuous infusion	Not indicated.
Other routes of administration	Not indicated.

Zoledronic Acid

Comments

Monitoring: Serum creatinine should be measured before each infusion.[2]

Adverse effects: A transient, low-grade fever, arthralgia, hypocalcemia, and headache within 3 days of infusion is common. The frequency of this reaction decreases with subsequent infusions.[2,3] Bone pain has also been reported frequently.[4,6]

Osteonecrosis of the jaw has been reported in *adult* cancer patients on chemotherapy who also receive zoledronate. It is recommended that while on zoledronate invasive dental procedures should be avoided.[3] A report in children receiving pamidronate or zoledronate found no evidence of jaw osteonecrosis in 22 patients who underwent 38 dental procedures.[7]

Drug interactions: Aminoglycoside and loop diuretics may increase the risk for hypocalcemia.[2,3] Use nephrotoxic drugs with caution.[2,3]

Appendix A

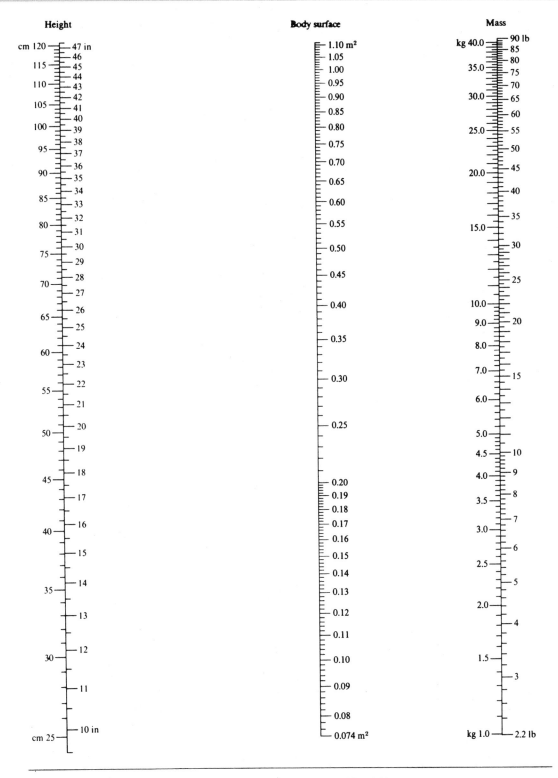

Height   Body surface   Mass

From the formula of DuBois and DuBois, *Arch. intern. Med.*, **17**, 863 (1916): $S = M^{0.425} \times H^{0.725} \times 71.84$, or $\log S = \log M \times 0.425 + \log H \times 0.725 + 1.8564$ (S: body surface in cm², M: mass in kg, H: height in cm).

Reproduced with permission, from Geigy scientific tables, volume 1. 8th ed. Lentner C, ed. Basel, Switzerland: CIBA-GEIGY Limited; 1993:226.

Appendix B

Nomogram for Estimating Ideal Body Mass in Children

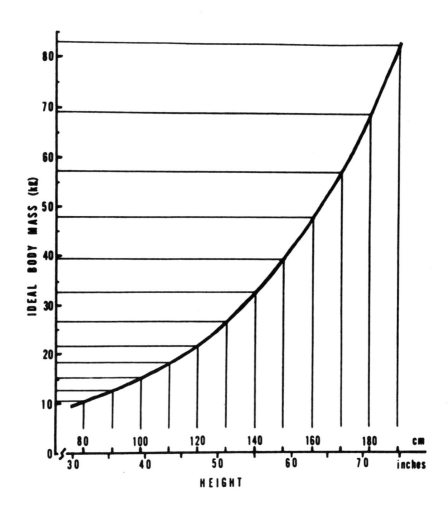

$$IBM \text{ (kg)} = 2.396 \ e^{0.01863(\text{height in cm})}$$

Appendix C

Additives and Antibiotic Considerations

Additives

Benzyl alcohol: Benzyl alcohol in small doses as a preservative in drugs is considered safe in newborns.[1] However, a 3-week-old, very low birth weight (710 g) infant experienced a profound oxygen desaturation that required resuscitation after the third and fourth doses of clindamycin that was subsequently related to the benzyl alcohol preservative.[2] Administration of saline flushes containing benzyl alcohol (bacteriostatic water for injection) was associated with a fatal gasping syndrome, intraventricular hemorrhage, metabolic acidosis, and increased mortality in preterm infants.[3] This should not be used in neonates. Hypersensitivity reactions to benzyl alcohol in parenteral products have been reported in *adults*.[4,5]

Paraben: Paraben preservatives may cause hypersensitivity reactions that are more common with cutaneous exposure.[6] However, one case of pruritus and bronchospasm following infusion of hydrocortisone that contained a paraben has been reported.[7]

Propylene glycol: Propylene glycol is added to parenteral drugs as a solubilizer. Rapid infusion of medications that contain propylene glycol has resulted in respiratory depression and cardiac dysrhythmias.[8] Its half-life is three times longer in neonates than in *adults*[1] and has caused hyperosmolality[9] and refractory seizures[10] in preterm neonates receiving 3 g/day.

Sulfites: Sulfites may cause hypersensitivity reactions that are more common in *adults* with asthma. Most reactions are mild but can include anaphylactic symptoms and life-threatening or less severe asthma episodes.[1, 11,12] Epinephrine may be required in severe cases, and if the sulfite-free product is not available, the sulfite-preserved epinephrine should be used.[1]

Antibiotic considerations

Type I reaction to penicillin: Certain infections (i.e., syphilis) require penicillin for cure. It is recommended that a desensitization protocol for penicillin-allergic individuals should be performed in a hospital setting. This can usually be completed in about 4 hours, at which time the first dose of penicillin can be given.[13]

Patients with a history of type I reaction to penicillin should not receive beta-lactam antibiotics. From 5% to 15% of patients allergic to penicillin will also be allergic to cephalosporins.[14]

Inactivation aminoglycoside/penicillin: The beta-lactam ring of penicillins can link with an amino sugar of the aminoglycoside and inactivate the aminoglycoside.[15-17] To avoid this potential interaction, administer penicillins 1 hour before or after an aminoglycoside, adequately flush the infusion line between each infusion, or infuse them through separate lines. In vivo inactivation that is dose dependent can also occur particularly in patients with renal failure.[17-19] In patients with end-stage renal failure, gentamicin half-life was decreased by 22–31 hours after carbenicillin or ticarcillin was added to the drug regimen.[18]

Aminoglycosides/neuromuscular blockade: Aminoglycosides may cause neuromuscular blockade and this effect is pronounced in patients with renal insufficiency, neuromuscular disease, and hypocalcemia.[17,20]

The effects of nondepolarizing neuromuscular blockers may be prolonged during aminoglycoside use.[20]

Cephalosporins and bleeding: The N-methyl-thiotetrazole (NMTT) side chain may inhibit vitamin K dependent clotting factors resulting in a prolonged PTT time.[17] The coagulopathy is more pronounced in patients with renal insufficiency.[17] The non-NMTT side chain antibiotics have also been associated with bleeding in patients with renal insufficiency.

The NMTT side chain causes a disulfiram-like reaction (e.g., flushing sweating, headache, and tachycardia) when combined with alcohol.

Appendix C

References

1. American Academy of Pediatrics Committee on Drugs. "Inactive" ingredients in pharmaceutical products: update. *Pediatrics.* 1997;99:268-278.
2. Hall CM, Milligan DWA, Berrington J. Probable adverse reaction to a pharmaceutical excipient. *Arch Dis Child Fetal Neonatal Ed.* 2004;89:F184.
3. Hiller JL, Benda GI, Rahatzad M, et al. Benzyl alcohol toxicity: impact on mortality and intraventricular hemorrhage among very low birth weight infants. *Pediatrics.* 1986;77:500-506.
4. Grant JA, Bilodeau PA, Guernsey BG, et al. Unsuspected benzyl alcohol hypersensitivity. *N Engl J Med.* 1982;306:108.
5. Wilson JP, Solimando DA, Edwards MS. Parenteral benzyl alcohol-induced hypersensitivity reaction. *Drug Intell Clin Pharm.* 1986;20:689-691.
6. Soni MG, Taylor SL, Greenberg NA, et al. Evaluation of the health aspects of methyl paraben: a review of the published literature. *Food Chem Toxicol.* 2002;40:1335-1373.
7. Nagel JE, Fuscaldo JT, Firemen P. Paraben allergy. *JAMA.* 1977;237:1594-1595.
8. Louis S, Kutt H, McDowell F. The cardiocirculatory changes caused by intravenous Dilantin and its solvent. *Am Heart J.* 1967;74:523-529.
9. Glasgow AM, Boeckx RL, Miller MK, et al. Hyper-osmolality in small infants due to propylene glycol. *Pediatrics.* 1983;72:353-355.
10. MacDonald MG, Getson PR, Glasgow AM, et al. Propylene glycol: increased incidence of seizures in low birth weight infants. *Pediatrics.* 1987;79:622-625.
11. Smolinske SC. Review of parenteral sulfite reactions. *J Toxicol Clin Toxicol.* 1992;30:597-606.
12. Lester MR. Sulfite sensitivity: significance in human health. *J Am Col Nutr.* 1995;14:229-232.
13. CDC. Sexually transmitted diseases treatment guidelines, 2006. *MMWR.* 2006;55(No. RR11):1-94.
14. Anderson JA. Cross-sensitivity to cepalosporins in patients allergic to penicillin. *Pediatr Infect Dis.* 1986;5:557-561.
15. McLaughlin JE, Reeves DS. Clinical and laboratory evidence for inactivation of gentamicin by carbenicillin. *Lancet.* 1971;1:261-264.
16. Riff LJ, Jackson GG. Laboratory and clinical conditions for gentamicin inactivation by carbenicillin. *Arch Intern Med.* 1972;130:887-891.
17. Manian FA, Stone WJ, Alford RH. Adverse antibiotic effects associated with renal insufficiency. *Rev Infect Dis.* 1990;12:236-249.
18. Davies M, Morgan JR, Anand C. Interactions of carbenicillin and ticarcillin with gentamicin. *Antimicrob Agents Chemother.* 1975;7:431-434.
19. Weibert R, Keane W, Shapiro F. Carbenicillin inactivation of aminoglycosides in patients with severe renal failure. *Trans Amer Soc Artif Int Organs.* 1976;22:439-443.
20. Snavely SR, Hodges GR. The neurotoxicity of antibacterial agents. *Ann Intern Med.* 1984;101;92-104.

Appendix D

Y-Site Compatibility of Medications with Parenteral Nutrition

Christine A. Robinson, Pharm.D. and Jaclyn E. Lee, Pharm.D.

Many pediatric conditions such as abdominal wall defects of the newborn and short bowel syndrome warrant the use of parenteral nutrition. Obtaining and maintaining venous access in pediatric patients complicates the administration of this form of nutrition. Many patients require multiple treatment modalities to be administered intravenously including, medications, fluids, blood products, and nutrition. Clinicians must optimize available access to ensure appropriate and timely administration of all products prior to establishing additional access. This may require simultaneous administration of medications and parenteral nutrition; therefore, compatibility considerations become essential. It is important to recognize that compatibility only reflects the physical interactions such as formation of a precipitate and does not necessarily address stability or pharmacologic activity of the products. Published data may report both compatibility and stability; however, most evaluate compatibility alone. Currently there are multiple resources to use when answering the question of compatibility with parenteral nutrition. We strove to evaluate and present the available published data as a comprehensive and practical reference. We sought out primary literature regarding Y-site compatibility of multiple drugs commonly used in pediatric patients with three different parenteral nutrition formulas, 3-in-1, 2-in-1, and lipids alone. When conflicting results were encountered, the clinical strength was considered. When published data was not accessible, Lawrence Trissel's *Handbook on Injectable Drugs*[1] was used. Below please find each of the classifications utilized in this reference:

C Compatibility has been demonstrated. When Y-site compatibility was not available, medications compatible in solution for 24 hours were assumed to be Y-site compatible. Medications compatible with 3-in-1 admixtures were assumed to be compatible with lipids alone.[1]

I Incompatibility has been demonstrated

— Compatibility data not available

C/I Conflicting compatibility has been demonstrated and strength of the evidence supports compatible

I/C Conflicting compatibility has been demonstrated and strength of the evidence supports incompatible

Medication	Admixture Type			Comments	References	
	2-in-1	**Lipids**	**3-in-1**		**C**	**I**
Acetazolamide	I	—	—	White precipitate forms immediately		2
Acyclovir	I	I	I	White precipitate forms immediately		2,3,4
Amikacin	C	C/I	C/I	Visual breaking of emulsion within 1 h in select formulations	2,3,4,5,6,7	8
Aminophylline	C/I	C	C		3,4,9,10	2
Amphotericin B	I	I	I	Yellow precipitate formed immediately		3,4
Ampicillin sodium	C/I	C	C		3,4,11	2,5,7,12
Ampicillin sodium–sulbactam sodium	C	C	C		3,4	
Atracurium besylate	C	—	—		13	
Aztreonam	C	C	C		3,4	
Bumetanide	C	C	C		3,4	
Caffeine	C	—	—		14	
Cefazolin sodium	C/I	C	C	Incompatible at a dextrose concentration of 25%	3,4,5,14	3
Cefepime	C	—	—		15	
Cefoperazone sodium	C	C	C		3,4,5	
Cefotaxime sodium	C	C	C		2,3,4,5	
Cefotetan disodium	C	C	C		3,4	

Appendix D

Cefoxitin sodium	C	C	C		3,4,5,11	
Ceftazidime	C	C	C		2,3,4,16	
Ceftriaxone sodium	C	C	C		3,4,13	
Cefuroxime sodium	C	C	C		3,4	
Chloramphenicol sodium succinate	C	C	—		1,5	
Chlorpromazine HCl	C	C	C		3,4	
Cimetidine HCl	C	C	C		3,4,17	
Ciprofloxacin lactate	I	C	C	Amber discoloration in 1 to 4 h	4	3
Cisplatin	I	C	C	Amber discoloration in 1 to 4 h	4	3
Clindamycin phosphate	C	C	C		4,5,11	
Co-trimoxazole	C	C	C		3,4	
Cyclophosphamide	C	C	C		3,4	
Cyclosporine	C/I	C/I	C/I	For 2:1, found to be compatible with Dextrose 5%/Amino Acid 4.25%, but not compatible with Dextrose 25%/Amino Acid 3.5%	3,4,18	3,4
Dexamethasone sodium phosphate	C	C	C		2,3,4	
Digoxin	C	C	C		3,4,19	
Diphenhydramine HCl	C	C	C		3,4	
Dobutamine HCl	C	C	C		2,3,4,6	
Dopamine HCl	C	C/I	C/I		2,3,4,19	4
Doxycycline hyclate	C	I	I	Emulsion disruption occurs immediately	3,5	4
Droperidol	C	I	I	Emulsion disruption occurs in 1 to 4 h	3	4
Enalaprilat	C	C	C		3,4	
Epinephrine HCl	C	—	—		13	
Epoetin alfa	C	—	—		20	
Erythromycin lactobionate	C	C	C		5,11,13	
Famotidine	C	C	C		3,4,17,21,22, 23,24,25	
Fentanyl citrate	C	C	C		2,3,4,26	
Fluconazole	C	C	C		3,4,27	
Foscarnet	C	—	—		28	
Furosemide	C/I	C	C	Small amount of precipitate formed in 4 h in select formulations	2,4,13,19	3
Ganciclovir sodium	I/C	I	I	Concentrations of ≥10 mg/mL resulted in precipitation within 0–30 min	29,30	3,4,29
Gentamicin sulfate	C	C	C		2,3,4,5,6,7, 8,11,12,13	
Granisetron HCl	C	C	C		3,4	
Haloperidol lactate	C	I	I	Emulsion disruption occurs immediately	3,13	4
Heparin sodium	C	I	I	Emulsion disruption occurs immediately with heparin 100 units/mL	3,13	4

Hydrochloric acid	C	—	—		31	
Hydrocortisone sodium/phosphate/succinate	C	C	C		3,4,13	
Ifosfamide	C	C	C		3,4	
Imipenem–cilastatin sodium	C	C	C		3,4	
Immune globulin	—/C	—	—	Only supportive of Gammagard® 2.5%; not recommended to infuse with other drugs or solutions	32	
Indomethacin sodium trihydrate	I	—	—			33
Insulin, regular human	C	C	C		3,4,13	
Iron dextran	C/I	—	I/C	For 2:1, found to be compatible in solution at amino acid concentrations of 2% or greater	34,35,36	35,37
Isoproterenol HCl	C	C	C	For 2:1, compatible with dextrose 25%/amino acids 4.25% (electrolytes were not added)	19,38	
Kanamycin sulfate	C	C	C		11,12,38,39	
Lidocaine HCl	C	C	C	For 2:1, compatible with dextrose 25%/amino acids 4.25% (electrolytes were not added)	19,38	
Linezolid	C	—	—	Compatible with dextrose 20%/amino acids 4.9%; electrolytes were not added	40	
Lorazepam	C	I	I	Partial emulsion disruption occurs in 1 h	3	4
Magnesium sulfate	C	C	C		3,4	
Mannitol	C	C	C		3,4	
Meperidine HCl	C	C	C		3,4,41	
Meropenem	—	C	C		4	
Methotrexate	I	C	C	For 2:1, hazy precipitate formed in 0 to 1 h	4	3
Methyldopate HCl	C	C/I	C/I	For 2:1, compatible with dextrose 25%/amino acids 4.25% (electrolytes were not added); cracked the lipid emulsion in select formulations	19,38	20
Methylprednisolone sodium succinate	C	C	C		3,4	
Metoclopramide HCl	I/C	C	C	Substantial loss of natural turbidity occurred immediately in select formulations	1,4	3
Metronidazole HCl	C	C	C		2,3,4,13	
Midazolam HCl	I/C	I	I	White precipitate forms immediately in select formulations	42	3,4,13
Milrinone lactate	C	—	—		43,44	
Morphine sulfate	C	C/I	C/I	For 3:1, morphine 1 mg/mL compatible, but 15 mg/mL was not compatible; emulsion disruption occurs immediately in select formulations	3,4,13,41	4

Appendix D

Nafcillin sodium	C	C	C		3,4,5,7	
Nitroglycerin	C	C	C		3,4	
Norepinephrine bitartrate	C	C	C		3,19	
Octreotide acetate	C	C	C		3,4	
Ondansetron HCl	C	I	I	Emulsion disruption occurs immediately	3	4
Oxacillin sodium	C	C	C		5,7,11	
Penicillin G potassium	C	C	C		2,5,7,11,13	
Penicillin G sodium	C	—	—		5,7	
Pentobarbital sodium	C	I	I	Emulsion disruption occurs immediately	3	4
Phenobarbital sodium	C	I	I	Emulsion disruption occurs immediately	3	4
Phenytoin sodium	I	I	—	Heavy white precipitate forms immediately; incompatible with dextrose		1,13
Piperacillin sodium	C	C	C		3,4,5,7	
Piperacillin sodium–tazobactam sodium	C	C	C		3,4	
Potassium chloride	C	C	C		3,4	
Potassium phosphate	I	I	I	Emulsion disruption occurs immediately; increased turbidity occurs immediately		3,4
Promethazine HCl	C/I	C	C	Amber discoloration in 4 h in select formulations	3,4	3
Propofol	C	—	—	Propofol injection contains approximately 10 g fat/100 mL	45	
Ranitidine HCl	C	C	C		2,3,4,13,17	
Sargramostim	C	—	—		46	
Sodium bicarbonate	I/C	C	C	Small amount of precipitate formed in 1 h in select formulations	3,5	3
Sodium nitroprusside	C	C	C		3,4	
Tacrolimus	C	C	C		3,4	
Ticarcillin disodium	C	C	C		3,4,5,7,11	
Ticarcillin disodium–clavulanate potassium	C	C	C		3,4,13	
Tobramycin sulfate	C	C	C		2,3,4,5,6,7,8,11	
Vancomycin HCl	C	C	C		2,3,4,5,6,13	
Vecuronium bromide	C	—	—		13	
Vitamin K$_1$–phytonadione	C	C	—		12,47	
Zidovudine	C	C	C		2,3,4	

Source: Adapted with permission from Robinson CA, Lee JE. Y-Site compatibility of medications with parenteral nutrition. *J Pediatr Pharmacol Ther.* 2007;12.

Appendix E

Extravasation Treatment (early treatment is recommended to minimize injury)

Medication	Cold/Warm Packs × 15–20 Min Several Times a Day	Antidote	Regimen
Aminophylline Calcium salts Dextrose >10% Nafcillin Oxacillin Phenytoin Potassium salts Sodium bicarbonate (8.4%) Sodium chloride (>0.9%) Tetracycline Vancomycin	Cold	Hyaluronidase	Add 1 mL NS to the lyophylized hyaluronidase vial resulting in a 150 units/mL reconstituted solution. Infuse five separate 0.2 mL SC or intradermal injections around the edge of the affected area. The needle (25 or 27 gauge) should be changed with each injection. (Some pediatric institutions dilute further by adding 0.1 mL of the 150 units/mL reconstituted dose to 1 mL NS resulting in a 15 units/mL product.)
Dobutamine Dopamine Epinephrine Norepinephrine Vasopressin	None	Phentolamine	Add 5 mg phentolamine to 9 mL NS. Inject a small amount of the dilution around the area. (Some suggest a dilution of 1 mg/mL and infusing five separate 0.1–0.2 mL injections around the affected area. The needle should be changed with each injection.) Blanching should reverse immediately. This can be repeated if necessary.
Vinblastine Vincristine	Warm	Hyaluronidase	Add 1 mL NS to the lyophylized hyaluronidase vial resulting in a 150 units/mL reconstituted solution. Infuse five separate 0.2 mL SC or intradermal injections around the edge of the affected area. The needle (25 or 27 gauge) should be changed with each injection. (Some pediatric institutions dilute further by adding 0.1 mL of the 150 units/mL reconstituted dose to 1 mL NS resulting in a 15 units/mL product.)
Cisplatin	Cold	Sodium thiosulfate	Use of antidote is based on infiltration size and cisplatin concentration. Infiltrates <20 mL and <0.5 mg/mL cisplatin concentration: no treatment other than cool packs. In *adults*: Infiltrates >20 mL and cisplatin concentration >0.5 mg/mL use sodium thiosulfate, add 4 mL of 10% sodium thiosulfate (1/6 molar) to 6 mL SWI and inject 3–5 mL.
Dactinomycin	Cold	None	
Irinotecan Topotecan	Cold		

Sources: Bey D, El-Chaar GM, Bierman F, et al. The use of phentolamine in the prevention of dopamine-induced tissue extravasation. *J Crit Care.* 1998;13:13-20; Camp-Sorrell D. Developing extravasation protocols and monitoring outcomes. *J Intraven Nurs.* 1998;21:232-239; Zenk KE, Dungy CI, Greene GR. Nafcillin extravasation injury: use of hyaluronidase as an antidote. *Am J Dis Child.* 1981;135:1113-1114; and Extravasation Treatment. Lexi-Comp® Online with AHFS® (database). Bethesda, MD: American Society of Health-System Pharmacists; Updated June 10, 2009.

References

Abatacept

1. Available at: http://www.usp.org/hqi/similarProducts/choosy.html. Accessed February 27, 2009.
2. Orencia [prescribing information]. Princeton, NJ: Bristol-Myers Squibb; April 2008.
3. Ruperto N, Lovell DJ, Quartier P, et al. Abatacept in children with juvenile idiopathic arthritis: a randomized, double-blind, placebo controlled withdrawal trial. *Lancet.* 2008;372:383-391.
4. Angeles-Han S, Flynn T, Lehman T. Abatacept for refractory juvenile idiopathic arthritis-associated uveitis—a case report (letter). *J Rheumatol.* 2008;35:1897-1898.

Acetazolamide

1. Available at: http://ismp.org/Tools/highalertmedications.pdf. Accessed June 19, 2009.
2. Available at: http://ismp.org/Tools/confuseddrugnames.pdf. Accessed June 19, 2009.
3. Thomson Healthcare Inc. USP DI® drug information for the health care professional. Available at: http://www.thomsonhc.com. MICROMEDEX® Healthcare Series [database online]. Accessed June 19, 2009.
4. Acetazolamide. Lexi-Comp® Online with AHFS® (database). Hudson, OH: Lexi-Comp Inc; updated March 19, 2009.
5. Acetazolamide [package insert]. Bedford, OH: Ben Venue Laboratories Inc; December 2002.
6. Guignard JP. Diuresis. In: Yaffe SJ, Aranda JV, eds. *Neonatal and Pediatric Pharmacology.* 3rd ed. Philadelphia, PA: Lippincott Williams & Wilkins; 2005:595-611.
7. Manzi SF, Arnold A, Patterson A. Pediatric drug formulary. In: Yaffe SJ, Aranda JV, eds. *Neonatal and Pediatric Pharmacology.* 3rd ed. Philadelphia, PA: Lippincott Williams & Wilkins; 2005:890.
8. Shirkey JC, ed. *Pediatric Therapy.* 4th ed. St. Louis, MO: Mosby; 1972.
9. International PHVD Drug Trial Group. International randomized controlled trial of acetazolamide and furosemide in posthemorrhagic ventricular dilatation in infancy. *Lancet.* 1998;352:433-440.
10. Kennedy CR, Ayers S, Campbell MJ, et al. Randomized, controlled trial of acetazolamide and furosemide in posthemorrhagic ventricular dilation in infancy: follow-up at 1 year. *Pediatrics.* 2001;108:597-607.
11. Libenson MH, Kaye EM, Rosman NP, et al., Acetazolamide and Furosemide for Posthemorrhagic Hydrocephalus of the Newborn. *Pediatr Neurol,* 1999, 20:185-191.
12. Lieh-Lai M, Sarnaik AP. Therapeutic applications in pediatric intensive care. In: Yaffe SJ, Aranda JV, eds. *Neonatal and Pediatric Pharmacology.* 3rd ed. Philadelphia, PA: Lippincott Williams & Wilkins; 2005:261-277.
13. Aronoff GR, Berns JS, Brier ME, et al. Drug prescribing in renal failure. 4th ed. Available at: http://www.kdp-baptist.louisville.edu/renalbook/. Accessed June 19, 2009.
14. Trissel LA, ed. *Handbook on Injectable Drugs.* 15th ed. Bethesda, MD: American Society of Health-System Pharmacists; 2009.
15. Robinson CA, Sawyer JE. Y-site compatibility of medications with parenteral nutrition. *J Pediatr Pharmacol Ther.* 2009;14:49-57.

Acetylcysteine (NAC)

1. Available at: http://www.ismp.org/tools/confuseddrugnames.pdf Accessed June 19, 2009.
2. Available at: http://www.usp.org/hqi/similarProducts/choosy.html. Accessed June 19, 2009.
3. Acetadote [package insert]. Nashville, TN: Cumberland Pharmaceuticals Inc; April 2009.
4. Tolar J, Orchard PJ, Bjoraker KJ, et al. N-acetyl-cysteine improves outcome of advanced cerebral adrenoleukodystrophy. *Bone Marrow Transplant.* 2007;39:211-215.
5. Tepel M, van der Giet M, Schwarzfeld C, et al. Prevention of radiographic-contrast-agent-induced reductions in renal function by acetylcysteine. *N Engl J Med.* 2000;343:180-184.
6. Safirstein R, Andrade L, Vieira JM. Acetylcysteine and nephrotoxic effects of radiographic contrast agents—a new use for an old drug. *N Engl J Med.* 2000;343:210-212.
7. Marenzi G, Assanelli E, Marana I, et al. N-Acetylcysteine and contrast-induced nephropathy in primary angioplasty. *N Engl J Med.* 2006;354:2773-2782.
8. Ahola T, Lapatto R, Raivio KO, et al. N-acetylcysteine does not prevent bronchopulmonary dysplasia in immature infants: a randomized controlled trial. *J Pediatr.* 2003;143:713-719.
9. Mager DR, Marcon M, Wales P, et al. Use of N-acetyl cysteine for the treatment of parenteral nutrition-induced liver disease in children receiving home parenteral nutrition. *J Pediatr Gastroenterol and Nutr.* 2008;46:220-223.
10. Aronoff GR, Berns JS, Brier ME, et al. Drug prescribing in renal failure. 4th ed. Available at: http://www.kdp-baptist.louisville.edu/renalbook/. Accessed August 28, 2009.
11. Ahola T, Fellman V, Laaksonen R, et al. Pharmacokinetics of intravenous N-acetylcysteine in pre-term newborn infants. *Eur J Clin Pharmacol.* 1999;55:645-550.
12. Available at: http://online.lexi.com/crlsql/servlet/crlonline. Accessed June 19, 2009.
13. Horowitz RS, Dart RC, Jarvie DR, et al. Placental transfer of N-acetylcysteine following human maternal acetaminophen toxicity. *J Toxicol Clin Toxicol.* 1997;35:447-451.

Acyclovir Sodium

1. Available at: http://www.usp.org/hqi/similarProducts/choosy.html. Accessed August 24, 2009.
2. Available at: http://ismp.org/Tools/confuseddrugnames.pdf. Accessed August 24, 2009.
3. Acyclovir [package insert]. Bedford, OH: Bedford Laboratories; June 2005.
4. Brigden D, Rosling AE, Woods NC. Renal function after acyclovir intravenous injection. *Am J Med.* 1982;73:182-185.
5. Robbins MS, Stromquist C, Tan LH. Acyclovir pH—possible cause of extravasation tissue injury. *Ann Pharmacother.* 1993;27:238.
6. Bacigalupo A, Frassoni F, Van Lint MT. Acyclovir for the treatment of severe aplastic anemia. *N Engl J Med.* 1984;310:1606-1607.
7. Yeager AS. Use of acyclovir in premature and term neonates. *Am J Med.* 1982;73:205-209.
8. Meyers JD, Reed EC, Shepp DH, et al. Acyclovir for prevention of cytomegalovirus infection and disease after allogeneic marrow transplantation. *N Engl J Med.* 1988;318:70-75.
9. Mitchell CD, Gentry SR, Boen JR, et al. Acyclovir therapy for mucocutaneous herpes simplex infections in immunocompromised patients. *Lancet.* 1981;1:1389-1392.
10. O'Meara A, Hillary IB. Acyclovir in the management of herpes virus infections in immunosuppressed children. *Ir J Med Sci.* 1981;150:73-77.
11. Gould JM, Chessells JM, Marshall WC, et al. Acyclovir in herpes virus infections in children: experience in an open study with particular reference to safety. *J Infect.* 1982;5:283-289.
12. Balfour HH. Intravenous acyclovir therapy for varicella in immunocompromised children. *J Pediatr.* 1984;104:134-136.
13. Balfour HH, Bean B, Laskin OL, et al. Acyclovir halts progression of herpes zoster in immunocompromised patients. *N Engl J Med.* 1983;308:1448-1453.
14. Prober CG, Kirk LE, Keeney RE. Acyclovir therapy of chickenpox in immunosuppressed children. A collaborative study. *J Pediatr.* 1982;101:622-625.

15. American Academy of Pediatrics. Pickering LK, Baker CJ, Kimberlin DW, et al., eds. *2009 Red Book: Report of the Committee on Infectious Diseases.* 28th ed. Elk Grove Village, IL: American Academy of Pediatrics; 2009.
16. Kimberlin DW, Lin CY, Jacobs RF, et al. Safety and efficacy of high-dose intravenous acyclovir in the management of neonatal herpes simplex virus infections. *Pediatrics.* 2001;108:230-238.
17. Balfour HH Jr. Antiviral drugs. *N Engl J Med.* 1999;340:1255-1268.
18. Carcao MD, Lau RC, Gupta A, et al. Sequential use of intravenous and oral acyclovir in the therapy of varicella in immunocompromised children. *Pediatr Infect Dis J.* 1998;17:626-631.
19. Kashtan CE, Cook M, Chavers BM, et al. Outcome of chickenpox in 66 pediatric renal transplant recipients. *J Pediatr.* 1997;131:874-877.
20. Prentice HG, Gluckman E, Powles RL, et al. Impact of long-term acyclovir on cytomegalovirus infection and survival after allogeneic bone marrow transplantation. *Lancet.* 1994;343:749-753.
21. Laskin OL, Longstreth JA, Whelton A, et al. Acyclovir kinetics in end-stage renal disease. *Clin Pharmacol Ther.* 1982;31:594-601.
22. Englund JA, Fletcher CV, Balfour HH. Acyclovir therapy in neonates. *J Pediatr.* 1991;119:129-135.
23. Aronoff GR, Berns JS, Brier ME, et al. Drug prescribing in renal failure. 4th ed. Available at: http://www.kdp-baptist.louisville.edu/renalbook/. Accessed October 15, 2009.
24. Baker KL, Baker DS, Morgan DL. Largest dose of acyclovir inadvertently administered to a neonate. *Pediatr Infect Dis J.* 2003;22:842.
25. Trissel LA, ed. *Handbook on Injectable Drugs.* 15th ed. Bethesda, MD: American Society of Health-System Pharmacists; 2009.
26. Rosenberry KR, Bryan CK, Sohn CA. Acyclovir: evaluation of a new antiviral agent. *Clin Pharm.* 1982;1:399-406.
27. Van der Meer JW, Versteeg J. Acyclovir in severe herpes virus infections. *Am J Med.* 1982;73:271-274.
28. Buck ML, Vittone SB, Zaglul HF. Vesicular eruptions following acyclovir administration. *Ann Pharmacother.* 1993;27:1458-1459.
29. Feder HM, Goyal RK, Krause PJ. Acyclovir-induced neutropenia in an infant with herpes simplex encephalitis: case report. *Clin Infect Dis.* 1995;20:1557-1559.
30. Vachvanichsanong P, Patamasucon P, Malagon M. Acute renal failure in a child associated with acyclovir. *Pediatr Nephrol.* 1995;9:346-347.
31. Zeng L, Nath CE, Blair EYL, et al. Population pharmacokinetics of acyclovir in children and young people with malignancy after administration of intravenous acyclovir or oral valacyclovir. *Antimicrob Agents Chemother.* 2009;53:2918-2927.
32. DiCarlo A, Amon E, Gardner M, et al. Eczema herpeticum in pregnancy and neonatal herpes infection. *Obestrics Gynecology.* 2008;112:455-457.
33. Yamada K, Yamamoto Y, Uchiyama A, et al. Successful treatment of neonatal herpes simplex-type 1 infection complicated by hemophagocytic lymphohistiocytosis and acute liver failure. *Tohoku J Exp Med.* 2008;214:1-5.

Adalimumab

1. Humira [package insert]. North Chicago, IL: Abbott Laboratories; December 2002.
2. Adalibumab. Lexi-Comp® Online with AHFS® (database). Bethesda, MD: American Society of Health-System Pharmacists; updated March 19, 2009.
3. Lovell DJ, Ruperto N, Goodman S, et al. Adalimumab with or without methotrexate in juvenile rheumatoid arthritis. *N Engl J Med.* 2008;359:810-820.
4. Vazques-Cobian LB, Flynn T, Lehman TJA. Adalimumab therapy for childhood uveitis. *J Pediatr.* 2006;149:572-575.
5. Foeldvari I, Nlelson S, Kummerl-Deschner J, et al. Tumor necrosis factor-α blocker in treatment of juvenile idiopathic arthritis-associated uveitis refractory to second-line agents: results of a multinational survey. *J Rheumatol.* 2007;34:1146-1150.
6. Beister S, Deueter C, Doycheva D, et al. Adalimumab in the therapy of uveitis in childhood. *Br J Ophthamol.* 2007;91:319-324.
7. Costamagna P, Furst K, Tully K, et al. Tuberculosis associated with blocking agents against tumor necrosis factor-alpha—California, 2002–2003. *MMWR Morb Mortal Wkly Rep.* 2004;53(30):683-686.

Adenosine

1. Available at: http://ismp.org/Tools/highalertmedications.pdf. Accessed August 29, 2009. Available at: http://www.usp.org/hqi/similarProducts/choosy.html. August 29, 2009.
2. Adenosine [package insert]. Bedford, OH: Bedford Laboratories; January 2006.
3. American Heart Association. Guidelines 2005 for cardiopulmonary resuscitation and emergency cardiovascular care. Part 12: pediatric advanced life support. *Circulation.* 2005;112:167-187.
4. Delacrétaz E. Clinical practice: supraventricular tachycardia. *N Engl J Med.* 2006, 354:1039-1051.
5. DeGroff CG, Silka MJ. Bronchospasm after intravenous administration of adenosine in a patient with asthma. *J Pediatr.* 1994;125:822-823.
6. Burkhart KK. Respiratory failure following adenosine administration. *Am J Emer Med.* 1993;11:249-250.
7. Aggarwal A, Farber NE, Warltier DC. Intraoperative bronchospasm caused by adenosine. *Anesthesiology.* 1993;79:1132-1135.
8. Konduri GG, Garcia DC, Kazzi NJ, et al. Adenosine infusion improves oxygenation in term infants with respiratory failure. *Pediatrics.* 1996;97:295-300.
9. Praghu AS, Singh TP, Morrow WR, et al. Safety and efficacy of intravenous adenosine for pharmacologic stress testing in children with aortic valve disease or Kawasaki disease. *Am J Cardiol.* 1999;83:284-286.
10. Paul T, Pfammatter JP. Adenosine: An effective and safe antiarrhythmic drug in pediatrics. *Pediatr Cardiol.* 1997;18:118-126.
11. Rossi AF, Steinburg LG, Kipel G, et al. Use of adenosine in the management of perioperative arrhythmias in the pediatric cardiac intensive care unit. *Crit Care Med.* 1992;20:1107-1111.
12. Ralston MA, Knilans TK, Hannon DW, et al. Use of adenosine for diagnosis and treatment of tachyarrhythmias in pediatric patients. *J Pediatr.* 1994;24:139-143.
13. Luedtke SA, Kuhn RJ, McCaffrey FM. Pharmacologic management of supraventricular tachycardias in children. Part 1: Wolff-Parkinson-White and atrioventricular nodal reentry. *Ann Pharmacother.* 1997;31:1227-1242.
14. Losek JD, Endom E, Dietrich A, et al. Adenosine and pediatric supraventricular tachycardia in the emergency department: multicenter study and review. *Ann Emer Med.* 1999;33:85-191.
15. Kugler JD, Danford DA. Management of infants, children, and adolescents with paroxysmal supraventricular tachycardia. *J Pediatr.* 1996;129:324-338.
16. Dixon J, Foster K, Wyllie J, et al. Guidelines and adenosine dosing in supraventricular tachycardia. *Arch Dis Child.* 2005;90:1190-1191.
17. Rosenthal E. Pitfalls in the use of adenosine. *Arch Dis Child.* 2005;91:451.
18. Aronoff GR, Berns JS, Brier ME, et al. Drug prescribing in renal failure. 4th ed. Available at: http://www.kdp-baptist.louisville.edu/renalbook/. Accessed August 30, 2009.
19. Berul CI. Higher adenosine dosage required for supra-ventricular tachycardia in infants treated with theophylline. *Clin Pediatr.* 1993;32:167-168.
20. Fitzsimmons CL, Withington DE. Use of andeosine in multiple doses for supraventricular tachycardia in an infant. *Pediatr Cardiol.* 1997;18:432-433.
21. Trissel LA, ed. *Handbook on Injectable Drugs.* 15th ed. Bethesda, MD: American Society of Health-System Pharmacists; 2009.
22. Till J, Shinebourne EA, Rigby ML, et al. Efficacy and safety of adenosine in the treatment of supraventricular tachycardia in infants and children. *Br Heart J.* 1989;62:204-211.
23. Watt AH, Bernard MS, Webster J, et al. Intravenous adenosine in the treatment of supraventricular tachycardia: a dose-ranging study and interaction with dipyridamole. *Br J Clin Pharmacol.* 1986;21:227-230.

References

Albumin (Normal Human Serum)

1. Albumin. Lexi-Comp® Online with AHFS® (database). Bethesda, MD: American Society of Health-System Pharmacists; updated May 26, 2009.
2. Stafford CT, Lobel SA, Fruge BC, et al. Anaphylaxis to human serum albumin. *Ann Allergy*. 1988;61:85-88.
3. Goldberg RN, Chung D, Goldman SL, et al. The association of rapid volume expansion and intraventricular hemorrhage in the preterm infant. *J Pediatr*. 1980;96:1060-1063.
4. Lambert HJ, Baylis PH, Coulthard MG. Central-peripheral temperature difference, blood pressure, and arginine vasopressin in preterm neonates undergoing volume expansion. *Arch Dis Child Fetal Neonatal Ed*. 1998;78:F43-F45.
5. Ruelas-Orozco G, Varga-Origel A. Assessment of therapy for arterial hypotension in critically ill preterm infants. *Am J Perinatol*. 2000;17:95-99.
6. Lay KS, Bancalari E, Malkus H, et al. Acute effects of albumin infusion on blood volume and renal function in premature infants with respiratory distress syndrome. *J Pediatr*. 1980;97:619-623.
7. Greissman A, Silver P, Nimkoff L, et al. Albumin bolus administration versus continuous infusion in critically ill hypoalbuminemic pediatric patients. *Intensive Care Med*. 1996;22:495-499.
8. Hardin TC, Page CP, Schwesinger WH. Rapid replacement of serum albumin in patients receiving total parenteral nutrition. *Surg Gynecol Obstet*. 1986;163:359-362.
9. Cochran EB, Hogue SL. Prediction of serum albumin concentration after albumin supplementation in pediatric patients receiving parenteral nutrition. *Clin Pharm*. 1991;10:704-706.
10. Weiss RA, Schoeneman M, Greifer I. Treatment of severe nephrotic edema with albumin and furosemide. *NY State J Med*. 1984;84:384-386.
11. Haws RM, Baum M. Efficacy of albumin and diuretic therapy in children with nephrotic syndrome. *Pediatrics*. 1993;91:1142-1146.
12. Roth KS, Amaker BG, Chan JCM. Nephrotic syndrome: pathogenesis and management. *Pediatr Rev*. 2002;23:237-247.
13. Trissel LA. *Handbook on Injectable Drugs*. 15th ed. Bethesda, MD: American Society of Health-System Pharmacists; 2009.
14. Hemolysis associated with 25% human albumin diluted with sterile water—United States, 1994–1998. *MMWR*. 1999;48:157-159.
15. Pierce LR, Gaines A, Barricchio F, et al. Hemolysis and renal failure associated with use of sterile water for injection to dilute 25% human albumin solution. *Am J Health-Syst Pharm*. 1998;55:1057, 1062, 1070.
16. Snyder RL. Filter clogging caused by albumin in I.V. nutrient solution. *Am J Hosp Pharm*. 1993;50:63-64.
17. Feldman F, Bergman G. Filter clogging caused by albumin in I.V. nutrient solution (response). *Am J Hosp Pharm*. 1993;50:64.

Alfentanil

1. Available at: http://ismp.org/Tools/highalertmedications.pdf. ISMP 2008. Accessed August 24, 2009.
2. Available at: http://www.usp.org/hqi/similarProducts/choosy.html. Accessed August, 24, 2009.
3. Alfenta [package insert]. Decatur, IL: Taylor Pharmaceuticals; June 2005.
4. Pokela ML, Ryhanen PT, Koivisto ME, et al. Alfentanil-induced rigidity in newborn infants. *Anesth Analg*. 1992;75:252-257.
5. Alfentanil. Lexi-Comp Online with AHFS (database). Hudson, OH: Lexi-Comp Inc; updated August 13, 2009.
6. Klemola U, Mennander S, Saarnivaara L. Tracheal intubation without the use of muscle relaxants: remifentanil or alfentanil in combination with propofol. *Acta Anaesthesthiol Scand*. 2000;44:465-469.
7. Marlow N, Weindling AM, Van Peer A, et al. Alfentanil pharmacokinetics in preterm infants. *Arch Dis Child*. 1990;65;349-351.
8. Killian A, Davis PJ, Stiller RL, et al. Influence of gestational age on pharmacokinetics of alfentanil in neonates. *Dev Pharmacol Ther*. 1990;15:82-85.
9. Leoni F, Benni F, Iacobucci T, et al. Pain control with low-dose alfentanil in children undergoing minor abdominal and genitor-urinary surgery. *Eur J Anaesth*. 2004;21:738-742.
10. Meistelman C, Saint-Maurice C, LePaul M, et al. A comparison of alfentanil pharmacokinetics in children and adults. *Anesthesiology*. 1987;66:13-16.
11. Davis PJ, Lerman J, Suresh S, et al. A randomized multicenter study of remifentanil compared with alfentanil, isoflurane, or propofol in anesthetized pediatric patients undergoing elective strabismus surgery. *Anesth Analg*. 1997;84:982-989.
12. Mulroy JJ, Davis PJ, Rymer DB, et al. Safety and efficacy of alfentanil and halothane in paediatric surgical patients. *Can J Anesth*. 1991;38 (4 pt 1):445-449.
13. den Hollander JM, Hennis PJ, Burm AG, et al. Alfentanil in infants and children with congenital heart defects. *J Cardiothorac Anesth*. 1988;2:1-7.
14. Aronoff GR, Berns JS, Brier ME, et al. Drug prescribing in renal failure. 4th ed. Available at: http://www.kdp-baptist.louisville.edu/renalbook/. Accessed November 17, 2009.
15. Trissel LA, ed. *Handbook on Injectable Drugs*. 15th ed. Bethesda, MD: American Society of Health-System Pharmacists; 2009.
16. Keene DL, Roberts D, Splinter WM, et al. Alfentanil mediated activation of epileptiform activity in the electrocorticogram during resection of epileptogenic foci. *Can J Neurol Sci*. 1997;24:37-39.
17. Cascino GD, So EL, Sharbrough FW, et al. Alfentanil-induced epileptiform activity in patients with partial epilepsy. *J Clin Neurophysiol*. 1993;10:520-525.

Allopurinol Sodium

1. Available at: http://www.usp.org/hqi/similarProducts/choosy.html. Accessed March 4, 2009.
2. Aloprim [product information]. Lake Forest, IL: Biioniche Pharma USA LLC; April 2008.
3. Allopurinol. Lexi-Comp® Online with AHFS® (database). Bethesda, MD: American Society of Health-System Pharmacists; updated May 26, 2009.
4. Donnenberg A, Holton CP, Mayer CM, et al. Evaluation of intravenous allopurinol (NSC-1390) in pediatric neoplasia. *Cancer Chemother Rep*. 1974;58:737-739.
5. Brown CH, Stashick E, Carbone PP. Clinical efficacy and lack of toxicity of allopurinol (NSC-1390) given intravenously. *Cancer Chemother Rep*. 1970;54:125-129.
6. Smalley RV, Guaspari A, Haase-Statz S, et al. Allopurinol: intravenous use for prevention and treatment of hyperuricemia. *J Clin Oncol*. 2000;18:1758-1763.
7. Van Bel F, Shadid M, Moison RM, et al. Effect of allopurinol on postasphyxial free radical formation, cerebral hemodynamic, and electrical brain activity. *Pediatrics*. 1998;101:185-193.
8. Marro PJ, Baumgart S, Delivoria-Papadopoulos M, et al. Purine metabolism and inhibition of xanthine oxidase in severely hypoxic neonates going onto extracorporeal membrane oxygenation. *Pediatr Res*. 1997;41:513-521.
9. McGaurn SP, Davis LE, Krawczeniuk MM, et al. The pharmacokinetics of injectable allopurinol in newborns with the hypoplastic left heart syndrome. *Pediatrics*. 1994;94:820-823.
10. Clancy RR, McGaurn SA, Goin JE, et al. Allopurinol neurocardiac protection trial in infants undergoing heart surgery using deep hypothermic circulatory arrest. *Pediatrics*. 2001;108:61-70.
11. Trissel LA, ed. *Handbook on Injectable Drugs*. 13th ed. Bethesda, MD: American Society of Health-System Pharmacists; 2005.
12. Breithaupt H, Tittel M. Kinetics of allopurinol after single intravenous and oral doses. *Eur J Clin Pharmacol*. 1982;22:77-84.
13. Appelbaum SJ, Mayersohn M, Dorr RT, et al. Allopurinol kinetics and bioavailability. *Cancer Chemother Pharmacol*. 1982;8:93-98.
14. Lin YW, Okazaki S, Hamahata K, et al. Acute pure red cell aplasia associated with allopurinol therapy. *Am J Hematol*. 1999;61:209-211.

References

Alprostadil

1. Prostin VR [package insert]. Bedford, OH: Bedford Laboratories; January 2005.
2. Peled N, Dagan O, Babyn P, et al. Gastric-outlet obstruction induced by prostaglandin therapy in neonates. *N Engl J Med*. 1992;327:505-510.
3. Merkus JFM, Cromme-Dijkhuis AH, Robben SGF, et al. Prostaglandin E1 and gastric outlet obstruction in infants. *Lancet*. 1993;342:747.
4. Ernst JA, Williams JM, Glick MR, et al. Osmolality of substances used in the intensive care nursery. *Pediatrics*. 1983;72:347-352.
5. Schlegel PG, Haber HP, Beck J, et al. Hepatic veno-occlusive disease in pediatric stem cell recipients: successful treatment with continuous infusion of prostaglandin E1 and low-dose heparin. *Ann Hematol*. 1998;76:37-41.
6. Neutze JM, Starling MB, Elliott RB, et al. Palliation of cyanotic congenital heart disease in infancy with E-type prostaglandins. *Circulation*. 1977;55:238-241.
7. Lewis AB, Takahashi M, Lurie PR. Administration of prostaglandin E1 in neonates with critical congenital cardiac defects. *J Pediatr*. 1978;93:481-485.
8. Eades, S. Pharmacotherapy of congenital heart disease. *J Pediatri Pharmacol Ther*. 2004;9:160-178.
9. Benson LN, Olley PM, Patel RG, et al. Role of prostaglandin E1 infusion in the management of transposition of the great arteries. *Am J Cardiol*. 1979;44:691-696.
10. Lang P, Freed MD, Bierman FZ, et al. Use of prostaglandin E1 in infants with d-transposition of the great arteries and intact ventricular septum. *Am J Cardiol*. 1979;44:76-81.
11. Freed MD, Heymann MA, Lewis AB, et al. Prostaglandin E1 in infants with ductus arteriosus-dependent congenital heart disease. *Circulation*. 1981;64:809-905.
12. Heymann MA, Clyman RI. Evaluation of alprostadil (prostaglandin E1) in the management of congenital heart disease in infancy. *Pharmacotherapy*. 1982;2:148-155.
13. Von Planta M, Fasnacht M, Holm C, et al. Atypical Kawasaki disease with peripheral gangrene and myocardial infarction: therapeutic implications. *Eur J Pediatr*. 1995;154:830-834.
14. Kwan CM, Chang WC, Chen JH, et al. The effect of intravenous infusion of prostaglandin E1 on cutaneous microcirculation in black foot disease. *J Formos Med Assoc*. 1993;92:603-608.
15. Bauer J, Dapper F, Demirakea S, et al. Perioperative management of pulmonary hypertension after heart transplantation in childhood. *J Heart Lung Transplant*. 1997;16:1238-1247.
16. Radovancevic B, Vrtovec B, Thomas CD, et al. Nitric oxide versus prostaglandin E1 for reduction of pulmonary hypertension in heart transplant candidates. *J Heart Lung Transplant*. 2005;24:690-695.
17. Zimmerman AA, Howard TK, Huddleston BC. Combined lung and liver transplantation in a girl with cystic fibrosis. *Can J Anesth*. 1999;46:571-575.
18. Giostra E, Chen H, Deng H, et al. Prophylactic administration of prostaglandin E1 in liver transplantation: results of a pilot trial. *Transplant Proc*. 1997;29:2381-2384.
19. Tancharoen S, Jones RM, Angus PW, et al. Prostaglandin E1 therapy in orthotopic liver transplantation recipients: indications and outcome. *Transplant Proc*. 1992;24:2248-2249.
20. Mollison LC, Angus PW, Jones RM. Prostaglandin E1 for the treatment of primary non-function of the donor organ in liver transplantation. *Med J Aust*. 1991;155:51-53.
21. Gaber AO, Thistlethwaite JR Jr, Busse-Henry S, et al. Improved results of preservation of hepatic grafts preflushed with albumin and prostaglandins. *Transplant Proc*. 1988;20:992-993.
22. Host A, Halken S, Kamper J, et al. Prostaglandin E1 treatment in ductus dependent congenital cardiac malformation: a review of 34 neonates. *Dan Med Bull*. 1988:35:81-84.
23. Trissel LA, ed. *Handbook on Injectable Drugs*. 15th ed. Bethesda, MD: American Society of Health-System Pharmacists; 2009.
24. Carter EL, Garzon MC. Neonatal urticaria due to prostaglandin E1. *Pediatr Dermatol*. 2000;17:58-61.
25. Rao J, Campbell ME, Krol A. The harlequin color change and association with prostaglandin E1. *Pediatr Dermatol*. 2005;21:573-576.
26. Raboi CA, Smith W. Brown fat necrosis in the setting of congenital heart disease and prostaglandin E1 use: a case report. *Pediatr Radiol*. 1999;29:61-63.
27. Vanhaesebrouck S, Allegaert K, Vanhole C, et al. Pseudo-Bartter syndrome in a neonate on prostaglandin infusion. *Eur J Pediatr*. 2003;162:569-571.
28. Arav-Boger R, Baggett HC, Spevak PJ, et al. Leukocytosis caused by prostaglandin E1 in neonates. *J Pediatr*. 2001;138:263-265.
29. Kaufman MB, El-Chaar GM. Bone and tissue changes following prostaglandin therapy in neonates. *Ann Pharmacother*. 1996;20:269-274.
30. NadrooAm, Shringari S, Garg M, et al. Prostaglandin induced cortical hyperostosis in neonates with cyanotic heart disease. *J Perinat Med*. 2000;28:447-452.
31. Velaphi S, Cilliers A, Beckh-Arnold E, et al. Corticol hyperostosis in an infant on prolonged prostaglandin infusion: case report and literature review. *J Perinatol*. 2004;24:263-265.
32. Jureidine S, Chase NA, Alpert BS, et al. Soft-tissue swelling in two neonates during prostaglandin E1 therapy. *Pediatr Cardiol*. 1986;7:157-160.

Amikacin Sulfate

1. Available at: http://ismp.org/Tools/confuseddrugnames.pdf. Accessed November 15, 2009.
2. Available at: http://www.usp.org/hqi/similarProducts/choosy.html. Accessed November 15, 2009.
3. Amikacin [package insert]. Irvine, CA: Sicor Pharmaceuticals; November 2003.
4. Pannu N, Nadim MK. An overview of drug-induced acute kidney injury. *Crit Care Med*. 2008;36(4 Suppl):S216-S223.
5. Guthrie OW. Aminoglycoside induced ototoxicity. *Toxicology*. 2008;249:91-96.
6. Snavely SR, Hodges GR. The neurotoxicity of antibacterial agents. *Ann Intern Med*. 1984;101:92-104.
7. Paradelis AG. Aminoglycoside antibiotics and neuromuscular blockade. *J Antimicrob Chemother*. 1979;5:737-738.
8. Schwartz SN, Pazin GJ, Lyon JA, et al. A controlled investigation of the pharmacokinetics of gentamicin and tobramycin in obese subjects. *J Infect Dis*. 1978;138:499-505.
9. Bauer LA, Blouin RA, Griffen WO, et al. Amikacin pharmacokinetics in morbidly obese patients. *Am J Hosp Pharm*. 1980;37:519-522.
10. Isemann BT, Kotagal UR, Mashni SM, et al. Optimal gentamicin therapy in preterm neonates includes loading doses and early monitoring. *Ther Drug Monit*. 1996;18:549-555.
11. Semchuk W, Shevchuk YM, Sankaran K, et al. Prospective, randomized, controlled evaluation of a gentamicin loading dose in neonates. *Biol Neonate*. 1995; 67:13-20.
12. Gal P, Ransom JL, Weaver RL. Gentamicin in neonates: the need for loading doses. Am J Perinatol. 1990;7:254-257.
13. Berger A, Kretzer V, Gludovatz P, et al. Evaluation of an amikacin loading dose for nosocomial infections in very low birthweight infants. *Acta Paediatr*. 2004;93:356-360.
14. American Academy of Pediatrics. Pickering LK, Baker CJ, Kimberlin DW, et al., eds. *2009 Red Book: Report of the Committee on Infectious Diseases*. 28th ed. Elk Grove Village, IL: American Academy of Pediatrics; 2009.
15. Prober CG, Yeager AS, Arvin AM. The effect of chronologic age on the serum concentrations of amikacin in sick term and premature infants. *J Pediatr*. 1981;98:636-640.
16. Nelson JD, Bradley JS, eds. *Nelson's Pocket Book of Pediatric Antimicrobial Therapy*. 17th ed. Chicago, IL: American Academy of Pediatrics; 2009.

References

17. Sherwin CM, Svahn S, Van Der Linden A, et al. Individualised dosing of amikacin in neonates: a pharmacokinetic/pharmacodynamic analysis. *Eur J Clin Pharmacol.* 2009;65:705-713.
18. Yow M. An overview of pediatric experience with amikacin. *Am J Med.* 1977;62:954-958.
19. Marik PE, Lipman J, Kobilski S, et al. A prospective randomized study comparing once- versus twice-daily amikacin dosing in critically ill adult and paediatric patients. *J Antimicrob Chemother.* 1991;28:753-764.
20. Myers MG, Roberts RJ, Mirhij NJ. Effects of gestational age, birth weight, and hypoxemia on pharmacokinetics of amikacin in serum of infants. *Antimicrob Agents Chemother.* 1977;11:1027-1032.
21. Sanderman H, Colding H, Hendel J, et al. Kinetics and dose calculations of amikacin in the newborn. *Clin Pharmacol Ther.* 1976;20:59-66.
22. Vogelstein B, Kowarski AA, Lietman PS. The pharmacokinetics of amikacin in children. *J Pediatr.* 1977;91:333-339.
23. Amikacin. In: Kucer A, Crowe SM, Grayson ML, et al., eds. *The Use of Antibiotics: A Clinical Review of Antibacterial, Antifungal and Antiviral Drugs.* 5th ed. Boston, MA: Butterworth Heinemann; 1997;504-521.
24. Contopoulos-Ioannidis DG, Giotis ND, Baliatsa DV, et al. Extended-interval aminoglycoside administration for children: a meta-analysis. *Pediatrics.* 2004;114:e111-e118.
25. Kraus DM, Pai MP, Rodvold KA. Efficacy and tolerability of extended-interval aminoglycoside administration in pediatric patients. *Paediatr Drugs.* 2002;4:469-484.
26. Kotze A, Bartel PR, Sommers DK. Once versus twice daily amikacin in neonates: prospective study on toxicity. *J Paediatr Child Health.* 1999;35:283-286.
27. Marik PE, Lipman J, Kobilski S, et al. A prospective randomized study comparing once- versus twice-daily amikacin dosing in critically ill adult and paediatric patients. *J Antimicrob Chemother.* 1991;28:753-764.
28. Kafetzis DA, Sianidou L, Vlachos E, et al. Clinical and pharmacokinetic study of a single daily dose of amikacin in paediatric patients with severe gram-negative infections. *J Antimicrob Chemother.* 1991;27:105-112.
29. Trujillo H, Robledo J, Robledo C, et al. Single dose amikacin in paediatric patients with severe gram-negative infections. *J Antimicrob Chemother.* 1991;27:141-147.
30. Viscoli C, Dudley M, Ferrea G, et al. Serum concentration and safety of a single daily dose of amikacin in children undergoing bone marrow transplantation. *J Antimicrob Chemother.* 1991;27:113-120.
31. Bouffet E, Fuhrmann C, Frappaz D, et al. Once daily antibiotic regimen in paediatric oncology. *Arch Dis Child.* 1994;70:484-487.
32. International Antimicrobial Therapy Cooperative Group of the European Organization for Research and Treatment of Cancer. Efficacy and toxicity of single daily doses of amikacin and ceftriaxone versus multiple daily doses of amikacin and ceftazidime for infection in patients with cancer and granulocytopenia. *Ann Intern Med.* 1993;119:584-593.
33. Krivoy N, Postovsky S, Elhasid R, et al. Pharmacokinetic analysis of amikacin twice and single daily dosage in immunocompromised pediatric patients. *Infection.* 1998;26:396-398.
34. Hamidah A, Rizal AM, Nordiah AJ et al. Piperacillin-tazobactam plus amikacin as an initial empirical therapy of febrile neutropenia in paediatric cancer patients. *Singapore Med J.* 2008; 49:26-30.
35. Gauthier M, Chevalier I, Sterescu A, et al. Treatment of urinary tract infections among febrile young children with daily intravenous antibiotic therapy at a day treatment center. *Pedaitrics.* 2002;114:e469-e476.
36. Chicella M. Once-daily aminoglycoside dosing in pediatrics. What is its role? *J Pediatr Pharm Pract.* 2000:5;98-103.
37. Aronoff GR, Berns JS, Brier ME, et al. Drug prescribing in renal failure. 4th ed. Available at: http://www.kdp-baptist.louisville.edu/renalbook/. Accessed November 15, 2009.
38. Pea F, Viale P, Furlanut M. Antimicrobial therapy in critically ill patients: a review of pathophysiological conditions responsible for altered disposition and pharmacokinetic variability. *Clin Pharmacokinet.* 2005;44:1009-1034.
39. Kelly HB, Menendez R, Fan L, et al. Pharmacokinetics of tobramycin in cystic fibrosis. *J Pediatr.* 1982;100:318-321.
40. Loirat P, Rohan J, Baillet A, et al. Increased glomerular filtration rate in patients with major burns and its effect on the pharmacokinetics of tobramycin. *N Engl J Med.* 1978;299:915-919.
41. Kopcha RG, Fant WK, Warden GD. Increased dosing requirements for amikacin in burned children. *J Antimicrob Chemother.* 1999;28:747-752.
42. Buck ML. Pharmacokinetic changes during extracorporeal membrane oxygenation. *Clin Pharmacokinet.* 2003;42:403-417.
43. Trissel LA, ed. *Handbook on Injectable Drugs.* 15th ed. Bethesda, MD: American Society of Health-System Pharmacists; 2009.
44. Robinson CA, Sawyer JE. Y-site compatibility of medications with parenteral nutrition. *J Pediatr Pharmacol Ther.* 2009;14:49-57.
45. Pagliaro LA, Pagliaro AM, eds. *Problems in Pediatric Drug Therapy.* 2nd ed. Hamilton, IL: Drug Intelligence Publications Inc; 1987.
46. Gillett AP, Falk RH, Andrews J, et al. Rapid intravenous injection of tobramycin: suggested dosage schedule and concentrations in serum. *J Infect Dis.* 1976;134:S110-S113.
47. Dobbs SM, Mawer GE. Intravenous injection of gentamicin and tobramycin without impairment of hearing. *J Infect Dis.* 1976;134 (suppl):S114-S117.
48. Mendelson J, Portnoy J, Dick V, et al. Safety of the bolus administration of gentamicin. *Antimicrob Agents Chemother.*1976;9:633-638.
49. Bodey GP, Chang HY, Rodriguez V, et al. Feasibility of administering aminoglycoside antibiotics by continuous intravenous infusion. *Antimicrob Agents Chemother.* 1975;8:328-333.
50. Powell SH, Thompson WL, Luthe MA, et al. Once daily vs. continuous aminoglycoside dosing: efficacy and toxicity in animal and clinical studies of gentamicin, netilmicin and tobramycin. *J Infect Dis.* 1983;147:918-932.
51. Giacoia GP, Schentag JJ. Pharmacokinetics and nephrotoxicity of continuous intravenous infusion of gentamicin in low birth weight infants. *J Pediatr.* 1986;109:715-719.
52. Beaubien AR, Desjardins S, Ormsby E, et al. Incidence of amikacin ototoxicity: a sigmoid function of total drug exposure independent of plasma levels. *Am J Otolaryngol.* 1989;10:234-243.
53. Beaubien AR, Ormsby E, Bayne A, et al. Evidence that amikacin ototoxicity is related to total perilymph area under the concentration-time curve regardless of concentration. *Antimicrob Agents Chemother.* 1991;35:1070-1074.
54. Brownsberger RJ, Morrelli HF. Neuromuscular blockade due to gentamicin sulfate.*West J Med.* 1988;148:215.
55. Warner WA, Sanders E. Neuromuscular blockade associated with gentamicin therapy. *JAMA.* 1971;215:1153-1154.
56. Massey KL, Hendeles L, Neims A. Identification of children for whom routine monitoring of aminoglycoside serum concentrations is not cost effective. *J Pediatr.* 1986;109:897-901.
57. Logsdon BA, Phelps SJ. Routine monitoring of gentamicin serum concentrations in pediatric patients with normal renal function is unnecessary. *Ann Pharmacother.* 1997;31:1514-1518.
58. Franson TR, Ritch PS, Quebbeman EJ. Aminoglycoside serum concentration sampling via central venous catheters: a potential source of clinical error. *JPEN J Parenter Enteral Nutr.* 1987;11:77-79.

Aminocaproic Acid

1. Available at: http://www.usp.org/hqi/similarProducts/choosy.html. Accessed April 1, 2009.
2. Amicar injection [package insert]. Newport, KY: Xanodyne Pharmaceuticals Inc; June 2007.
3. Aminocaproic acid. Lexi-Comp® Online with AHFS® (database). Bethesda, MD: American Society of Health-System Pharmacists; updated May 26, 2009.
4. Florentino-Pineda I, Thompson GH, et al. The effect of Amicar on perioperative blood loss in idiopathic scoliosis: the results of a prospective, randomized double-blind study. *Spine.* 2004;29:233-238.

5. Downard CD, Betit P, Chang RW, et al. Impact of Amicar on hemorrhagic complications of ECMO: a ten-year review. *J Pediatr Surg.* 2003;38:1212-1216.
6. Wilson JM, Bower LK, Fackler JC, et al. Aminocaproic acid decreases the incidence of intracranial hemorrhage and other hemorrhagic complications of ECMO. *J Pediatr Surg.* 1993;28:536-541.
7. Horwitz JR, Cofer BR, Warner BW, et al. A multicenter trial of 6-aminocaproic acid (Amicar) in the prevention of bleeding in infants on ECMO. *J Pediatr Surg.* 1998;33:1610-1613.
8. Williams GD, Bratton SI, Riley EC, et al. Efficacy of epsilon-aminocaproic acid in children undergoing cardiac surgery. *J Cardiothorac Vasc Anesth.* 1999;13:304-308.
9. Florentino-Pineda I, Blakemore LC, Thompson GH, et al. The effect of epsilon-aminocaproic acid on perioperative blood loss in patients with idiopathic scoliosis undergoing posterior spinal fusion: a preliminary prospective study. *Spine.* 2001;26:1147-1151.
10. Chauhan S, Kumar BA, Rao BH, et al. Efficacy of aprotinin, epsilon aminocaproic acid, or combination in cyanotic heart disease. *Ann Thorac Surg.* 2000;70:1308-1312.
11. Chauhan S, Das SN, Bisoi A, et al. Comparison of epsilon aminocaproic acid and tranexamic acid in pediatric cardiac surgery. *J Cartiothorac Vasc Anesth.* 2004;18:141-143.
12. Ghosh K, Shetty S, Jijina F, Mohanty D. Role of epsilon amino caproic acid in the management of haemophilic patients with inhibitors. *Haemophilia.* 2004;10:58-62.
13. Grizelj R, Vukovic J, Filipovic-Grcic B, Saric D, Luetic T. Successful use of recombinant activated FVII and aminocaproic acid in four neonates with life-threatening hemorrhage. *Blood Coagul Fibrinolysis.* 2006;17:413-415.
14. Brant-Zawadzski PB, Fenton SJ, Nichol PF, et al. The split abdominal wall muscle flap repair for large congenital diaphragmatic hernias on extracorporeal membrane oxygenation. *J Pediatr Surg.* 2007;42:1047-1051.
15. Winter SS, Chaffee S, Kahler SG, et al. e-Aminocaproic acid-associated myopathy in a child. *J Pediatr Hematol Oncol.* 1995;17:53-55.
16. Trissel LA. *Handbook on Injectable Drugs.* 15th ed. Bethesda, MD: American Society of Health-System Pharmacists; 2009.
17. Ririe DG, James RL, O'Brien JJ, et al. The pharmacokinetics of epsilon-aminocaproic acid in children undergoing surgical repair of congenital heart defects. *Anesth Analg.* 2002;94:44-49.

Aminophylline

1. Available at: http://www.usp.org/hqi/similarProducts/choosy.html. Accessed October 10, 2009.
2. Aminophylline [package insert]. Lake Forest, IL: Hospira Inc; June 2004.
3. Aminophylline. Lexi-Comp® Online with AHFS® (database). Hudson, OH: Lexi-Comp Inc; updated July 17, 2009.
4. Bada HS, Khanna NN, Somani SM, et al. Interconversion of theophylline and caffeine in newborn infants. *J Pediatr.* 1979;94:993-995.
5. Aranda JV, Sitar DS, Parsons WD, et al. Pharmacokinetic aspects of theophylline in premature newborns. *N Engl J Med.* 1976;295:413-416.
6. Tserng KY, Takieddine FN, King KC. Developmental aspects of theophylline metabolism in premature infants. *Clin Pharmacol Ther.* 1983;33:522-528.
7. Al-Omran A, Al-Alaiyan S. Theophylline concentration following equal doses of intravenous aminophylline and oral theophylline in preterm infants. *Amer J Perinatol.* 1997;14:147-149.
8. Muttitt SC, Tierney AJ, Finer NN. The dose response of theophylline in the treatment of apnea of prematurity. *J Pediatr.* 1988;112:115-121.
9. Bairam A, Boutroy M-J, Badonnel Y, et al. Theophylline versus caffeine: comparative effects in treatment of idiopathic apnea in the preterm infant. *J Pediatr.* 1987;110:636-639.
10. Tserng K-Y, King KC, Takieddine FN. Theophylline metabolism in premature infants. *Clin Pharmacol Ther.* 1981;29:594-600.
11. Latini R, Assael BM, Bonati M, et al. Kinetics and efficacy of theophylline in the treatment of apnea of prematurity in the premature newborn. *Eur J Clin Pharmacol.* 1978;13:203-207.
12. Muttitt SC, Tierney AJ, Finer NN. The dose response of theophylline in the treatment of apnea of prematurity. *J Pediatr.* 1988;112:115-121.
13. Ritschel WA, Kearns GL, eds. *Handbook of Basic Pharmacokinetics.* 5th ed. Washington, DC: American Pharmacists Association; 1999.
14. Zainudin BM, Ismail O, Yusoff K. Effect of adding aminophylline infusion to nebulized salbutamol in severe acute asthma. *Thorax.* 1994;49:267-269.
15. Rodrigo C, Rodrigo G. Lack of therapeutic benefit and increase of the toxicity from aminophylline given in addition to high doses of salbutamol delivered by metered-dose inhaler with a spacer. *Chest.* 1994;106:1071-1076.
16. Murphy DG, McDermott MF, Rydman RJ, et al. Aminophylline in the treatment of acute asthma when 2-adrenergics and steroids are provided. *Arch Intern Med.* 1993;153:1784-1788.
17. Self TH, Abou-Shala N, Burns R, et al. Inhaled albuterol and oral prednisone therapy in hospitalized adult asthmatics. *Chest.* 1990;98:1317-1321.
18. Strauss RE, Wertheim DL, Bonagura VR, et al. Aminophylline therapy does not improve outcome and increases adverse effects in children hospitalized with acute asthmatic exacerbation. *Pediatrics.* 1994;93:205-210.
19. Needleman JP, Kaifer MC, Nold JT, et al. Theophylline does not shorten hospital stay for children admitted for asthma. *Arch Pediatr Adolesc Med.* 1995;149:206-209.
20. Carter E, Cruz M, Chesrown S, et al. Efficacy of intravenously administered theophylline in children hospitalized with severe asthma. *J Pediatr.* 1993;122:470-476.
21. DiGiulio GA, Kercsmar CM, Krug SE, et al. Hospital treatment of asthma: lack of benefit from theophylline given in addition to nebulized albuterol and intravenously administered corticosteroids. *J Pediatr.* 1993;122:464-469.
22. Huang D, O'Brien RG, Harman E, et al. Does aminophylline benefit adults admitted to the hospital for acute exacerbation of asthma? *Ann Intern Med.* 1993;119:1155-1160.
23. Mitra A, Bassler D, Goodman K, et al. Intravenous aminophylline for acute severe asthma in children over two years receiving inhaled bronchodilators. *Cochrane Database Syst Rev.* 2001;(4):CD001276.
24. Self TH, Redmond AM, Nguyen WT. Reassessment of theophylline use for severe asthma exacerbation: is it justified in critically ill hospitalized patients? *J Asthma.* 2002;39:677-686.
25. Zahorska-Markiewicz B, Waluga M, Zieliński M, et al. Pharmacokinetics of theophylline in obesity. *Int J Clin Pharmacol Ther.* 1996;34:393-395.
26. Visram N, Friesen EG, Jamali F. Theophylline loading dose in obese patients. *Clin Pharm.* 1987;6:188-189.
27. Gal P, Jusko WJ, Yurchak AM, et al. Theophylline disposition in obesity. *Clin Pharmacol Ther.* 1978;23:438-444.
28. Hendeles L, Weinberger M. Guidelines for avoiding theophylline overdose. *N Engl J Med.* 1979;300:1217.
29. Hendeles L, Weinberger M. Theophylline: a state of the art review. *Pharmacotherapy.* 1983;3:2-44.
30. Hogue SL, Phelps SJ. Evaluation of three theophylline dosing equations for use in infants up to one year of age. *J Pediatr.* 1993;123:651-656.
31. Bonati M, Latini R, Marra G, et al. Theophylline metabolism during the first month of life and development. *Pediatr Res.* 1981;15:304-308.
32. Gilman JT, Gal P, Levine RS, et al. Factors influencing theophylline disposition in 179 newborns. *Ther Drug Monit.* 1986;8:4-10.
33. Gal P, Boer HR, Toback J, et al. Effect of asphyxia on theophylline clearance in newborns. *South Med J.* 1982;75:836-838.
34. Trissel LA, ed. *Handbook on Injectable Drugs.* 15th ed. Bethesda, MD: American Society of Health-System Pharmacists; 2009.
35. Robinson CA, Sawyer JE. Y-site compatibility of medications with parenteral nutrition. *J Pediatr Pharmacol Ther.* 2009;14:49-57.
36. Sessler CN. Theophylline toxicity: clinical features of 116 consecutive cases. *Am J Med.* 1990;88:567-576.
37. Shannon M. Life-threatening events after theophylline overdose: a 10-year prospective analysis. *Arch Intern Med.* 1999;159:989-994.
38. Shannon M, Lovejoy FH Jr. Effect of acute versus chronic intoxication on clinical features of theophylline poisoning in children. *J Pediatr.* 1992;121:125-130.

References

39. Blake KV, Massey KL, Hendeles L, et al. Relative efficacy of phenytoin and phenobarbital for the prevention of theophylline-induced seizures in mice. *Ann Emerg Med*. 1988;17:1024-1028.
40. Goldberg MJ, Spector R, Miller G. Phenobarbital improves survival in theophylline-intoxicated rabbits. *J Toxicol Clin Toxicol*. 1986;24:203-211.
41. Self TH, Heilker GM, Alloway RR, et al. Reassessing the therapeutic range for theophylline on laboratory report forms: the importance of 5-15 micrograms/ml. *Pharmacotherapy*. 1993;13:590-594.
42. Weinberger MM, Hendeles L. Reassessing the therapeutic range for theophylline: another perspective. *Pharmacotherapy*.1993;13:598-601.

Amphotericin B

1. Available at: http://ismp.org/Tools/confuseddrugnames.pdf. Accessed August 25, 2009.
2. Available at: http://www.usp.org/hqi/similarProducts/choosy.html. Accessed August 25, 2009.
3. Fungizone [package insert]. Princeton, NJ: Bristol-Myers Squibb Company; June 2009.
4. Grasela TH, Goodwin SD, Walawander MK, et al. Prospective surveillance of intravenous amphotericin B use patterns. *Pharmacotherapy*. 1990;10:341-348.
5. Murray H. Allergic reactions to amphotericin B. *N Engl J Med*. 1974;290:693.
6. Wilson R, Feldman S. Toxicity of amphotericin B in children with cancer. *Am J Dis Child*. 1979;133:731-734.
7. American Academy of Pediatrics. Antifungal drugs for systemic fungal infections. In: Pickering LK, Baker CJ, Kimberlin DW, et al., eds. *2009 Red Book: Report of the Committee on Infectious Diseases*. 28th ed. Elk Grove Village, IL: American Academy of Pediatrics; 2009:765-776.
8. Maddux MS, Barriere SL. A review of complications of amphotericin-B therapy: recommendations for prevention and management. *Drug Intell Clin Pharm*. 1980;14:177-181.
9. Labadie EL, Hamilton RH. Survival improvement in coccidioidal meningitis by high-dose intrathecal amphotericin B. *Arch Intern Med*. 1986;146:2013-2018.
10. Tyler EM, Salamone FR, Brown AE. Management and prevention of amphotericin B-induced side effects. *Hosp Pharm*. 1988;23:254-259.
11. Medoff G, Kobayashi GS. Strategies in the treatment of systemic fungal infections. *N Engl J Med*. 1980;302:145-155.
12. Trissel LA, ed. *Handbook on Injectable Drugs*. 15th ed. Bethesda, MD: American Society of Health-System Pharmacists; 2009.
13. Moreau P, Milpied N, Fayette N, et al. Reduced renal toxicity and improved clinical tolerance of amphotericin B in neutropenic patients. *J Antimicrob Chemother*. 1992;30:535-541.
14. Chavanet PY, Garry I, Charlier N, et al. Trial of glucose versus fat emulsion in preparation of amphotericin for use in HIV infected patients with candidiasis. *Br Med J*. 1992;305:921-925.
15. Arbuthnot R, Dullea A, Rippel S. Controlling thrombophlebitis from amphotericin B. *Am J Hosp Pharm*. 1978;35:129.
16. Googe JH, Walterspiel JN. Arrhythmia caused by amphotericin B in a neonate. *Pediatr Infect Dis J*. 1988;7:73.
17. Bennett JE. Chemotherapy of systemic mycoses (first of two parts). *N Engl J Med*. 1974;290:30-32.
18. Butler WT, Bennett JE, Hill GJ. Electrocardiographic and electrolyte abnormalities caused by amphotericin B in dog and man. *Proc Soc Exp Biol Med*. 1964;116:857-863.
19. Fields BT, Bates JH, Abernathy RS. Effect of rapid intravenous infusion on serum concentrations of amphotericin B. *Appl Microbiol*. 1971;22:615-617.
20. Barreuther AD, Dodge RR, Blondeaux AM. Administration of amphotericin B. *Drug Intell Clin Pharm*. 1977;11:368-369.
21. Tarala RA, Smith JD. Cryptococcosis treated by rapid infusion of amphotericin B. *Br Med J*. 1980;281:28.
22. Pappas PG, Rex JH, Sobel JD, et al. Guidelines for treatment of candidiasis. *Clin Infect Dis*. 2004;38:161-189.
23. Chapman RL. Candida infections in the neonate. *Curr Opin Pediatr*. 2003;15:97-102.
24. Fernandez M, Moylett EH, Noyola DE, et al. Candidal meningitis in neonates: a 10-year review. *Clin Infect Dis*. 2000;31:458-463.
25. Driessen M, Ellis JB, Cooper PA, et al. Fluconazole vs. amphotericin B for the treatment of neonatal fungal septicemia: a prospective randomized trial. *Pediatr Infect Dis J*. 1996;15:1107-1112.
26. Van Den Anker JN, Van Popele NML, Sauer PJJ. Antifungal agents in neonatal systemic candidiasis. *Antimicrob Agents Chemother*. 1995;39:1391-1397.
27. Donowitz LG, Hendley JO. Short-course amphotericin B therapy for candidemia in pediatric patients. *Pediatrics*. 1995;95:888-891.
28. Baley JE, Meyers C, Kliegman RM, et al. Pharmacokinetics, outcome of treatment, and toxic effects of amphotericin B and 5-fluorocytosine in neonates. *J Pediatr*. 1990;116:791-797.
29. Sanchez PJ, Siegel JD, Fishbein J. Candida endocarditis: successful medical management in three preterm infants and review of the literature. *Pediatr Infect Dis J*. 1991;10:239-243.
30. Zenker PN, Rosenberg EM, Van Dyke RB, et al. Successful medical treatment of presumed Candida endocarditis in critically ill infants. *J Pediatr*. 1991;119:472-477.
31. Butler KM, Rench MA, Baker CJ. Amphotericin B as a single agent in the treatment of systemic candidiasis in neonates. *Pediatr Infect Dis J*. 1990;9:51-56.
32. Sanchez PJ, Cooper BH. Candida lusitaniae: sepsis and meningitis in a neonate. *Pediatr Infect Dis J*. 1987;6:758-759.
33. Turner RB, Donowitz LG, Hendley JO. Consequences of candidemia for pediatric patients. *Am J Dis Child*. 1985;139:178-180.
34. Smego RA, Devoe PW, Sampson HA, et al. Candida meningitis in two children with severe combined immunodeficiency. *J Pediatr*. 1984;104:902-904.
35. Chesney PJ, Teets KC, Mulvihill JJ, et al. Successful treatment of Candida meningitis with amphotericin B and 5-fluorocytosine in combination. *J Pediatr*. 1976;89:1017-1019.
36. Adler S, Randall J, Plotkin SA. Candidal osteomyelitis and arthritis in a neonate. *Am J Dis Child*. 1972;123:595-596.
37. Turner DJ, Wadlington WB. Blastomycosis in childhood: treatment with amphotericin B and a review of the literature. *J Pediatr*. 1969;75:708-717.
38. Cherry JD, Lloyd CA, Quilty JF, et al. Amphotericin B therapy in children. *J Pediatr*. 1969;75:1063-1069.
39. Hill HR, Mitchell TG, Masten JM, et al. Recovery from disseminated candidiasis in a premature neonate. *Pediatrics*. 1974;53:748-752.
40. Fosson AR, Wheeler WE. Short-term amphotericin B treatment of severe childhood histoplasmosis. *J Pediatr*. 1975;86:32-36.
41. Keller MA, Sellers BB, Melish ME, et al. Systemic candidiasis in infants: a case presentation and literature review. *Am J Dis Child*. 1977;131:1260-1263.
42. Ward RM, Sattler FR, Dalton AS. Assessment of antifungal therapy in an 800-gram infant with candidal arthritis and osteomyelitis. *Pediatrics*. 1983;72:234-238.
43. Faix RG. Systemic candida infections in infants in intensive care nurseries: high incidence of central nervous system involvement. *J Pediatr*. 1984;105:616-622.
44. Loke HL, Verber I, Szymonowicz W, et al. Systemic candidiasis and pneumonia in preterm infants. *Aust Paediatr J*. 1988;24:138-142.
45. Leibovitz E, Iuster-Reicher A, Amitai M, et al. Systemic candidal infections associated with use of peripheral venous catheters in neonates: a 9-year experience. *Clin Infect Dis*. 1992;14:485-491.
46. Starke JR, Mason EO, Kramer WG, et al. Pharmacokinetics of amphotericin B in infants and children. *J Infect Dis*. 1987;155:766-774.
47. Koren G, Lau A, Klein J, et al. Pharmacokinetics and adverse effects of amphotericin B in infants and children. *J Pediatr*. 1988;113:559-563.
48. Johnson DE, Thompson TR, Green TP, et al. Systemic candidiasis in very low-birth-weight infants (<1,500 grams). *Pediatrics*. 1984;73:138-143.
49. Baley JE, Kliegman RM, Fanaroff AA. Disseminated fungal infections in very low-birth-weight infants: therapeutic toxicity. *Pediatrics*. 1984;73:153-157.
50. Glick C, Graves GR, Feldman S. Neonatal fungemia and amphotericin B. *South Med J*. 1993;86:1368-1371.

References

51. Aronoff GR, Berns JS, Brier ME, et al. Drug prescribing in renal failure. 4th ed. Available at: http://www.kdp-baptist.louisville.edu/renalbook/. Accessed October 27, 2009.
52. Weber ML, Abela A, de Repentigny L, et al. Myeloperoxidase deficiency with extensive candidal osteomyelitis of the base of the skull. *Pediatrics.* 1987;80:876-879.
53. Butler WT, Bennett JE, Alling DW, et al. Nephrotoxicity of amphotericin B: early and late effects in 81 patients. *Ann Intern Med.* 1964;61: 175-187.
54. Graybill JR. Is there a correlation between serum antifungal drug concentration and clinical outcome? *J Infect.* 1994;28(S1):17-24.
55. Cleary JD, Hayman J, Sherwood J, et al. Amphotericin B overdose in pediatric patients with associated cardiac arrest. *Ann Pharmacother.* 1993;27:715-718.
56. Amphotericin B Conventional. Lexi-Comp Online with AHFS (database). Hudson, OH: Lexi-Comp Inc; updated October 5, 2009.
57. Utz JP, Bennett JE, Brandriss MW, et al. Amphotericin B toxicity. General side effects. *Ann Intern Med.* 1964;61:340-343.
58. Lee MD, Hess MM, Boucher BA, et al. Stability of amphotericin in 5% dextrose injection stores at 4 or 25ºC for 120 hours. *Am J Hosp Pharm.* 1994;51:394-396.
59. Wiest DB, Maish WA, Garner SS, et al. Stability of amphotericin B in four concentrations of dextrose injection. *Am J Hosp Pharm.* 1991;48:2430-2433.
60. Holler B, Omar SA, Farid MD, et al. Effects of fluid and electrolyte management on amphotericin B-induced nephrotoxicity among extremely low birth weight infants. *Pediatrics.* 2004;113:e608-e616.
61. Christenson JC, Shalit I, Welch DF, et al. Synergistic action of amphotericin B and rifampin against *Rhizopus* species. *Antimicrob Agents Chemother.* 1987;31:1775-1778.

Amphotericin B Cholesteryl Sulfate Complex

1. Available at: http://ismp.org/Tools/highalertmedications.pdf. ISMP 2008. Accessed August 25, 2009.
2. Amphotec [package insert]. Cranberry Township, PA: Three Rivers Pharmaceuticals LLC; July 2005.
3. American Academy of Pediatrics. Pickering LK, Baker CJ, Kimberlin DW, et al., eds. *2009 Red Book: Report of the Committee on Infectious Diseases.* 28th ed. Elk Grove Village, IL: American Academy of Pediatrics; 2009.
4. Janknegt R, de Marie S, Bakker-Woudenberg I, et al. Liposomal and lipid complex formulations of amphotericin B: clinical pharmacokinetics. *Clin Pharmacokinet.* 1992;23:279-291.
5. Henry N, Hoeker JL, Rhodes KH. Antimicrobial therapy for infants and children: guidelines for the inpatient and outpatient practice of pediatric infectious disease. *Mayo Clinic Proceed.* 2000;75:86-97.
6. Quilitz R. The use of lipid formulations of amphotericin B in cancer patients. *Cancer Control.* 1998;5:439-449.
7. Sandler ES, Mustafa MM, Tkaczewski I, et al. Use of amphotericin B colloidal dispersion in children. *J Pediatr Hematol Oncol.* 2000;22:242-246.
8. Bowden R, Chandrasekar P, White MH, et al. A double-blind, randomized, controlled trial of amphotericin B colloidal dispersion versus amphotericin B for treatment of invasive aspergillosis in immunocompromised patients. *Clin Infect Dis.* 2002;35:359-366.
9. Linder N, Klinger G, Shalit I, et al. Treatment of candidaemia in premature infants: comparison of three amphotericin B preparations. *J Antimicrob Chemother.* 2003;52:663-667.
10. Trissel LA, ed. *Handbook on Injectable Drugs.* 15th ed. Bethesda, MD: American Society of Health-System Pharmacists; 2009.
11. White MH, Bowden RA, Sandler ES, et al. Randomized, double-blind, clinical trial of amphotericin B colloidal dispersion vs amphotericin B in the empiric treatment of fever and neutropenia. *Clin Infect Dis.* 1998;27:296-302.

Amphotericin B Lipid Complex

1. Available at: http://ismp.org/Tools/highalertmedications.pdf. ISMP 2008. Accessed August 25, 2009.
2. Available at: http://www.usp.org/hqi/similarProducts/choosy.html. Accessed August 25, 2009.
3. Available at: http://ismp.org/Tools/confuseddrugnames.pdf. Accessed August 25, 2009.
4. Abelcet [package insert]. Bridgewater, NJ: Enzon Pharmaceuticals Inc.
5. Wingard JR, White MH, Anaissie E. A randomized, double blind comparative trial evaluating the safety of liposomal amphotericin B versus amphotericin B lipid complex in the empirical treatment of febrile neutropenia. *CID.* 2000;31:1155-1163.
6. Rowles DM, Fraser SL. Amphotericin B Lipid complex (ABLC)-associated hypertension: case report and review of the literature. *Clin Infect Dis.* 1999;29:1564-1565.
7. American Academy of Pediatrics. Antifungal drugs for systemic fungal infections. In: Pickering LK, Baker CJ, Kimberlin DW, et al., eds. *2009 Red Book: Report of the Committee on Infectious Diseases.* 28th ed. Elk Grove Village, IL: American Academy of Pediatrics; 2009:765-776.
8. Wurthwein G, Groll AH, Hempel G, et al. Population pharmacokinetics of amphotericin B lipid complex in neonates. *Antimicrob Agent Chemother.* 2005;5092-5098.
9. Janknegt R, de Marie S, Bakker-Woudenberg I, et al. Liposomal and lipid complex formulations of amphotericin B: clinical pharmacokinetics. *Clin Pharmacokinet.* 1992;23:279-291.
10. Wiley JM, Seibel NL, Walsh TJ. Efficacy and safety of amphotericin B lipid complex in 548 children and adolescents with invasive fungal infections. *Pediatr Infect Dis J.* 2005;24:167-174.
11. Herbrecht R, Auvrignon A, Andres E, et al. Efficacy of amphotericin B lipid complex in the treatment of invasive fungal infections in immunosuppressed paediatric patients. *Eur J Clin Microbiol Infect Dis.* 2001;20:77-82.
12. Adler-Shohet F, Waskin H, Lieberman JM. Amphotericin B lipid complex for neonatal invasive candidiasis. *Arch Dis Child Fetal Neonatal Ed.* 2001;84:131-133.
13. Aronoff GR, Berns JS, Brier ME, et al. Drug prescribing in renal failure. 4th ed. Available at: http://www.kdp-baptist.louisville.edu/renalbook/. Accessed October 27, 2009.
14. Alexander BD, Wingard JR. Study of renal safety in amphotericin B lipid complex-treated patients. *Clin Infect Dis.* 2005;40:S414-S421.
15. Hooshmand-Rad R, Reed MD, Chu A, et al. Retrospective study of the renal effects of amphotericin B lipid complex when used at higher-than recommended dosages and longer durations compared with lower dosages and shorter durations in patients with systemic fungal infections. *Clin Ther.* 2004;26:1652-1662.
16. Trissel LA, ed. *Handbook on Injectable Drugs.* 15th ed. Bethesda, MD: American Society of Health-System Pharmacists; 2009.

Amphotericin B Liposomal

1. Available at: http://ismp.org/Tools/highalertmedications.pdf. ISMP 2008. Accessed August 25, 2009.
2. Available at: http://www.usp.org/hqi/similarProducts/choosy.html. Accessed August 25, 2009.
3. Available at: http://ismp.org/Tools/confuseddrugnames.pdf. Accessed August 25, 2009.
4. Ambisome [package insert], San Dimas, CA: Gilead Sciences Inc; October 2008.
5. Roden MM, Nelson LD, Knudsen TA, et al. Triad of acute infusion-related reactions associated with liposomal amphotericin B: analysis of clinical and epidemiological characteristics. *Clin Infect Dis.* 2003;36:1213-1220.

References

6. Johnson MD, Drew RH, Perfect JR. Chest discomfort associated with liposomal amphotericin B: report of three cases and review of the literature. *Pharmacotherapy.* 1998;18:1053-1061.
7. Walsh TJ, Finberg RW, Arndt C, et al. Liposomal amphotericin B for empirical therapy in patients with persistent fever and neutropenia. National Institute of Allergy and Infectious Diseases Mycoses Study Group. *N Engl J Med.* 1999;340:764-771.
8. Wingard JR, White MH, Anaissie E. A randomized, double blind comparative trial evaluating the safety of liposomal amphotericin B versus amphotericin B lipid complex in the empirical treatment of febrile neutropenia. *CID.* 2000;31:1155-1163.
9. Pasic S, Flannagan L, Cant AJ. Liposomal amphotericin (AmBisome) is safe in bone marrow transplantation for primary immunodeficiency. *Bone Marrow Transplant.* 1997;19:1229-1232.
10. Tollemar J, Hockerstedt K, Ericzon BG, et al. Liposomal amphotericin B prevents invasive fungal infections in liver transplant recipients. A randomized, placebo-controlled study. *Transplantation.* 1995;59:45-50.
11. Noskin G, Gurwith M, Bowden R. Treatment of invasive fungal infections with amphotericin B colloidal dispersion in bone marrow transplant recipients. *Bone Marrow Transplant.* 1999;23:697-703.
12. Ringden O, Andstrom EE, Remberger M, et al. Prophylaxis and therapy using liposomal amphotericin B (AmBisome) for invasive fungal infections in children undergoing organ or allogenic bone-marrow transplantation. *Pediatr Transplant.* 1997;1:124-129.
13. Mehta P, Vinks A, Filipovich A, et al. High-dose weekly AmBisome antifungal prophylaxis in pediatric patients undergoing hematopoietic stem cell transplantation: a pharmacokinetic study. *Biol Blood Marrow Transplant.* 2006;12:235-240.
14. American Academy of Pediatrics. Antifungal drugs for systemic fungal infections. In: Pickering LK, Baker CJ, Kimberlin DW, et al., eds. *2009 Red Book: Report of the Committee on Infectious Diseases.* 28th ed. Elk Grove Village, IL: American Academy of Pediatrics; 2009:765-776.
15. Scarcella A, Pasquariello MB, Giugliano B, et al. Liposomal amphotericin B treatment for neonatal fungal infections. *Pediatr Inf Dis J.* 1998;146-148.
16. Weitkamp JH, Poets CF, Sievers R, et al. Candida infection in very low birth-weight infants: outcome and nephrotoxicity of treatment with liposomal amphotericin B (AmBisome). *Infection.* 1998;26:11-15.
17. Dornbusch HJ, Urban CE, Pinter H, et al. Treatment of invasive pulmonary aspergillosis in severely neutropenic children with malignant disorders using liposomal amphotericin B (AmBisome), granulocyte colony-stimulating factor, and surgery: report of five cases. *Pediatr Hemat Oncol.* 1995;12:577-586.
18. Seaman J, Boer C, Wilkinson R, et al. Liposomal amphotericin B (AmBisome) in the treatment of complicated kala-azar under field conditions. *Clin Infect Dis.* 1995;21:188-193.
19. Ng TT, Denning DW. Liposomal amphotericin B (AmBisome) therapy in invasive fungal infections. Evaluation of United Kingdom compassionate use data. *Arch Intern Med.* 1995;155:1093-1098.
20. Linder N, Klinger G, Shalit I, et al. Treatment of candidaemia in premature infants: comparison of three amphotericin preparations. *J Antimicrob Chemother.* 2003;52:663-667.
21. Juster-Reicher A, Flidel-Rimon O, Amitay M, et al. High-dose liposomal amphotericin B in the therapy of systemic candidiasis in neonates. *Eur J Clin Microbiol Infect Dis.* 2003;22:603-607.
22. Juster-Reicher A, Leibovitz E, Linder N, et al. Liposomal amphotericin B (AmBisome) in the treatment of neonatal candidiasis in very low birth weight infants. *Infection.* 2000;28:223-226.
23. Santos RP, Sanchez PJ, Mejias A, et al. Successful medical treatment of cutaneous aspergillosis in a premature infant using liposomal amphotericin B, voriconazole and micafungin. *Pediatr Infect Dis J.* 2007;26:364-366.
24. Karatza AA, Dimitriou G, Marangos M, et al. Successful resolution of cardiac mycetomas by combined liposomal amphotericin B with fluconazole treatment in premature neonates. *Eur J Pediatr.* 2008;267:1021-1023.
25. Jeon GW, Koo SH, Lee JH, et al. A comparison of AmBisome to Amphotericin B for treatment of systemic candidiasis in very low birth weight infants. *Yonsei Med J.* 2007;48:619-626.
26. Walsh TJ, Goodman JL, Pappas P, et al. Safety, tolerance, and pharmacokinetics of high-dose liposomal amphotericin B (AmBisome) in patients infected with Aspergillus species and other filamentous fungi: Maximum tolerated dose study. *Antimicrob Agent Chemother.* 2001;45:3487-3496.
27. Davidson RN, di Martino L, Gradoni L, et al. Short-course treatment of visceral leishmaniasis with liposomal amphotericin B (AmBisome). *Clin Infect Dis.* 1996;22:938-943.
28. Minodier P, Retornaz K, Horelt A, et al. Liposomal amphotericin B in the treatment of visceral leishmaniasis in immunocompetent patients. *Fundam Clin Pharm.* 2003;17:183-188.
29. Syriopoulou V, Daikos GL, Theodoridou M, et al. Two doses of a lipid formulation of amphotericin B for the treatment of Mediterranean visceral leishmaniasis. *Clin Infect Dis.* 2003;36:560-566.
30. Trissel LA, ed. *Handbook on Injectable Drugs.* 15th ed. Bethesda, MD: American Society of Health-System Pharmacists; 2009.
31. Sutherland SM, Hong DK, Balagtas J, et al. Liposomal amphotericin B associated with severe hyperphosphatemia. *Pediatr Infect Dis J.* 2008;27:77-79.
32. Jain A, Butani L. Severe hyperphosphatemia resulting from high-dose liposomal amphotericin in a child with leukemia. *J Pediatr Hematol Oncol.* 2003;25:324-326.
33. Buckler BS, Sams RN, Goei VL, et al. Treatment of central venous catheter fungal infection using liposomal amphotericin-B lock therapy. *Pediatr Infect Dis J.* 2008;27:762-764.

Ampicillin Sodium

1. Available at: http://www.usp.org/hqi/similarProducts/choosy.html. Accessed October 1, 2009.
2. Ampicillin [package insert]. Schaumburg, IL: American Pharmaceutical Partners; February 2007.
3. Prober CG, Stevenson DK, Benitz WE. The use of antibiotics in neonates weighing less than 1200 grams. *Pediatr Infect Dis J.* 1990;9:111-121.
4. American Academy of Pediatrics. Pickering LK, Baker CJ, Kimberlin DW, et al., eds. *2009 Red Book: Report of the Committee on Infectious Diseases.* 28th ed. Elk Grove Village, IL: American Academy of Pediatrics; 2009:746, 753.
5. Nelson JD, Bradley JS, eds. *Nelson's Pocket Book of Pediatric Antimicrobial Therapy.* 17th ed. Chicago, IL: American Academy of Pediatrics; 2009.
6. Wilson W, Taubert K, Gewitz M, et al. Prevention of infective endocarditis. Guidelines from the American Heart Association Rheumatic Fever, Endocarditis, and Kawasaki Disease Committee, Council on Cardiovascular Disease in the Young, and the Councils on Clinical Cardiology, Council on Cardiovascular Surgery and Anesthesia and the Quality of Care and Outcomes Research Interdisciplinary Working Group. *Circulation.* 2007;116:1736-1754.
7. Baddour LM, Wilson WR, Bayer AS, et al. Infective endocarditis: diagnosis, antimicrobial therapy, and management of complications: a statement for healthcare professionals from the Committee on Rheumatic Fever, Endocarditis, and Kawasaki Disease, Council on Cardiovascular Disease in the Young, and the Councils on Clinical Cardiology, Stroke, and Cardiovascular Surgery and Anesthesia, American Heart Association: endorsed by the Infectious Diseases Society of America. *Circulation.* 2005;111:e394-e434.
8. Feigin RD, McCracken GH, Klein JO. Diagnosis and management of meningitis. *Pediatr Infect Dis J.* 1992;11:785-814.
9. Tunkel AR, Hartman BJ, Kaplan SL, et al. Practice guidelines for the management of bacterial meningitis. *Clin Infect Dis.* 2004;39:1267-84.
10. Klein JO, Feigin RD, McCracken GH. Report of American Academy of Pediatrics task force on diagnosis and management of meningitis. *Pediatrics.* 1986;78(suppl):959-982.
11. American Academy of Pediatrics. Committee on Infectious Diseases. Treatment of bacterial meningitis. *Pediatrics.* 1988;6:904-907.
12. Fleming PC, Murray JDM, Fujiwara MW, et al. Ampicillin in the treatment of bacterial meningitis. *Antimicrob Agents Chemother.* 1966;47-52.

13. Odio CM, Faingezicht I, Salas JL, et al. Cefotaxime vs. conventional therapy for the treatment of bacterial meningitis of infants and children. *Pediatr Infect Dis J.* 1986;5:402-407.
14. Jadavji T, Biggar WD, Gold R, et al. Sequelae of acute bacterial meningitis in children treated for seven days. *Pediatrics.* 1986;78:21-25.
15. Aronoff GR, Berns JS, Brier ME, et al. Drug prescribing in renal failure. 4th ed. Available at: http://www.kdp-baptist.louisville.edu/renalbook/. Accessed Octover 10, 2009.
16. American Academy of Pediatrics Committee on Infectious Diseases. Ampicillin-resistant strains of Hemophilus influenza type B. *Pediatrics.* 1975;55:145-146.
17. Ampicillin. Lexi-Comp® Online with AHFS® (database). Bethesda, MD: American Society of Health-System Pharmacists; updated September 2009.
18. Trissel LA, ed. *Handbook on Injectable Drugs.* 15th ed. Bethesda, MD: American Society of Health-System Pharmacists; 2009.
19. Pagliaro LA, Pagliaro AM, eds. *Problems in Pediatric Drug Therapy.* 2nd ed. Hamilton, IL: Drug Intelligence Publications Inc; 1987.
20. Robinson CA, Sawyer JE. Y-site compatibility of medications with parenteral nutrition. *J Pediatr Pharmacol Ther.* 2009;14:49-57.
21. Shaffer CL, Davey AM, Ransom JL, et al. Ampicillin-induced neurotoxicity in very-low-birth-weight neonates. *Ann Pharmacother.* 1998;32:482-484.
22. Barrons RW, Murray KM, Richey RM. Populations at risk for penicillin-induced seizures. *Ann Pharmacother.* 1992;26:26-29.
23. Manian FA, Stone WJ, Alford RH. Adverse antibiotic effects associated with renal insufficiency. *Rev Infect Dis.* 1990;12:236-249.
24. Kagan, BM. Ampicillin rash. *West J Med.* 1977;126:333-335.

Ampicillin Sodium–Sulbactam Sodium

1. Available at: http://www.usp.org/hqi/similarProducts/choosy.html. Accessed June 19, 2006.
2. Ampicillin sodium and sulbactam sodium [package insert]. Deerfield, IL: Baxter Healthcare Corporation; MLT-01107/2.0.
3. American Academy of Pediatrics. Pickering LK, Baker CJ, Kimberlin DW, et al., eds. *2009 Red Book: Report of the Committee on Infectious Diseases.* 28th ed. Elk Grove Village, IL: American Academy of Pediatrics; 2009:746, 753.
4. Bassetti D, Solbiati M, Ravelli A, et al. Clinical evaluation of sulbactam plus ampicillin in the treatment of general pediatric infections. *APMIS.* 1989;5:41-44.
5. Kanra G, Secmeer G, Akalin E, et al. Sulbactam/ampicillin in the treatment of pediatric infections. *Diagn Microbiol Infect Dis.* 1989;12:185S-187S.
6. Azimi PH, Barson WJ, Janner D, et al. Efficacy and safety of ampicillin/sulbactam and cefuroxime in the treatment of serious skin and skin structure infections in pediatric patients. *Pediatr Infect Dis J.* 1999;18:609-613.
7. Wald E, Reilly JS, Bluestone CD, et al. Sulbactam/ampicillin in the treatment of acute epiglottitis in children. *Rev Infect Dis.* 1986;8:6617-6619.
8. Bluestone CD. Role of sulbactam/ampicillin and sultamicillin in the treatment of bacterial infections of the upper respiratory tract of children. *APMIS.* 1989;5:35-40.
9. Collins MD, Dajani AS, Kim KS, et al. Comparison of ampicillin/sulbactam plus aminoglycoside vs. ampicillin plus clindamycin plus aminoglycosides in the treatment of intra-abdominal infections in children. *Pediatr Infect Dis J.* 1998;17:S15-S18.
10. Kulhanjian J, Dunphy MG, Hamstra S, et al. Randomized comparative study of ampicillin/sulbactam vs. ceftriaxone for treatment of soft tissue and skeletal infections in children. *Pediatr Infect Dis J.* 1989;8:605-610.
11. Meier H, Springsklee M, Wildfeuer A. Penetration of ampicillin and sulbactam into human costal cartilage. *Infection.* 1994;22:152-155.
12. Aronoff SC, Scoles PV, Makley JT, et al. Efficacy and safety of sequential treatment with parenteral sulbactam/ampicillin and oral sultamicillin for skeletal infections in children. *Rev Infect Dis.* 1986;8:S639-S643.
13. Syriopoulou V, Bitsi M, Theodoridis C, et al. Clinical efficacy of sulbactam/ampicillin in pediatric infections caused by ampicillin-resistant or penicillin-resistant organisms. *Rev Infect Dis.* 1986;8:S630-S633.
14. Baddour LM, Wilson WR, Bayer AS, et al. Infective endocarditis: diagnosis, antimicrobial therapy, and management of complications: a statement for healthcare professionals from the Committee on Rheumatic Fever, Endocarditis, and Kawasaki Disease, Council on Cardiovascular Disease in the Young, and the Councils on Clinical Cardiology, Stroke, and Cardiovascular Surgery and Anesthesia, American Heart Association: endorsed by the Infectious Diseases Society of America. *Circulation.* 2005;111:e394-e434.
15. Unasyn. Lexi-Comp® Online with AHFS® (database). Bethesda, MD: American Society of Health-System Pharmacists; updated September 2009.
16. Foulds G, McBride TJ, Knirsch AK, et al. Penetration of sulbactam and ampicillin into cerebrospinal fluid of infants and young children with meningitis. *Antimicrob Agents Chemother.* 1987;31:1703-1705.
17. Tunkel A, Hartman BJ et al. Practice guidelines for the management of bacterial meningitis. *Clin Infect Dis.* 2004;39:1267-1284.
18. Foster MC, Morris DL, Legan C, et al. Perioperative prophylaxis with sulbactam and ampicillin compared with metronidazole and cefotaxime in the prevention of wound infection in children undergoing appendectomy. *J Pediatr Surg.* 1987;22:869-872.
19. Aronoff GR, Berns JS, Brier ME, et al. Drug prescribing in renal failure. 4th ed. Available at: http://www.kdp-baptist.louisville.edu/renalbook/. Accessed October 1, 2009.
20. Trissel LA, ed. *Handbook on Injectable Drugs.* 15th ed. Bethesda, MD: American Society of Health-System Pharmacists; 2009.
21. Robinson CA, Sawyer JE. Y-site compatibility of medications with parenteral nutrition. *J Pediatr Pharmacol Ther.* 2009;14:49-57.
22. Shaffer CL, Davey AM, Ransom JL, et al. Ampicillin-induced neurotoxicity in very-low-birth-weight neonates. *Ann Pharmacother.* 1998;32:482-484.
23. Barrons RW, Murray KM, Richey RM. Populations at risk for penicillin-induced seizures. *Ann Pharmacother.* 1992;26:26-29.
24. Kagan, BM. Ampicillin rash. *West J Med.* 1977;126:333-335.

Anidulafungin

1. Available at: http://ismp.org/Tools/highalertmedications.pdf. Accessed August 24, 2009.
2. Available at: http://ismp.org/Tools/confuseddrugnames.pdf. Accessed August 24, 2009.
3. Available at: http://www.usp.org/hqi/similarProducts/choosy.html. Accessed August 24, 2009.
4. Eraxis [package insert]. New York, NY: Pfizer Inc; June 2009.
5. Benjamin DK, Driscoll T, Seibel NL, et al. Safety and pharmacokinetics of intravenous anidulafungin in children with neutropenia at high risk for invasive fungal infections. *Antimicrob Agents Chemother.* 2006;50:632-638.
6. American Academy of Pediatrics. Antifungal drugs for systemic fungal infections. In: Pickering LK, Baker CJ, Kimberlin DW, et al., eds. *2009 Red Book: Report of the Committee on Infectious Diseases.* 28th ed. Elk Grove Village, IL: American Academy of Pediatrics; 2009:765-776.
7. Pannaraj PS, Walsh TJ, Baker CJ. Advances in antifungal therapy. *Pediatr Infect Dis J.* 2005;24:921-922.
8. Steinbach WJ, Benjamin DK. New Antifungal agents under development in children and neonates. *Curr Opin Infect Dis.* 2005;18:484-489.
9. Trissel LA, ed. *Handbook on Injectable Drugs.* 15th ed. Bethesda, MD: American Society of Health-System Pharmacists; 2009.

Argatroban

1. Available at: http://ismp.org/Tools/highalertmedications.pdf. ISMP 2008.
2. Available at: http://ismp.org/Tools/confuseddrugnames.pdf. Updated April 1, 2005.
3. Available at: http://www.usp.org/hqi/similarProducts/choosy.html. Accessed March 3, 2009.

References

4. Argatroban [prescribing information]. Research Triangle Park, NC: GlaxoSmithKline; May 2008.
5. Argatroban. Lexi-Comp® Online with AHFS® (database). Bethesda, MD: American Society of Health-System Pharmacists; updated March 19, 2009.
6. Hursting MJ, Dubb J, Verme-Gibboney CN. Argatroban anticoagulation in pediatric patients: a literature analysis. *J Pediatr Hematol Oncol.* 2006;28:4-10.
7. John TE, Hallisey RK. Argatroban and lepirudin requirements in a 6-year old. *Pharmacotherapy.* 2005;25:1383-1388.
8. Dyke PC 2nd, Russo P, Mureebe L, et al. Argatroban for anticoagulation during cardiopulmonary bypass in an infant. *Paediatr Anaesth.* 2005;15:328-333.
9. Tcheng WY, Wong WY. Successful use of argatroban in pediatric patients requiring anticoagulant alternatives to heparin. *Blood.* 2004;104:107b-108b. Abstract.
10. Trissel LA. *Handbook on Injectable Drugs.* 15th ed. Bethesda, MD: American Society of Health-System Pharmacists; 2009.
11. Monagle P, Chalmers E, Chan A, et al. Antithrombotic therapy in neonates and children. *Chest.* 2008;133:887S-968S.

Arginine HCl

1. Arginine. Lexi-Comp® Online with AHFS® (database). Bethesda, MD: American Society of Health-System Pharmacists; updated March 19, 2009.
2. Tiwary CM, Rosenbloom AI, Julius RL. Anaphylactic reactions to arginine infusion. *N Engl J Med.* 1973;288:218. Letter.
3. Resnick DJ, Softness B, Murphy AR et al. Case report of an anaphylactoid reaction to arginine. *Ann Allergy Asthma Immunol.* 2002;88:67-68.
4. Keller A, Donaubauer J, Kratzsch J, et al. Administration of arginine plus growth hormone releasing hormone to evaluate growth hormone (GH) secretory status in children with GH deficiency. *J Pediatr Endocrinol Metabol.* 2007;20:1307-1314.
5. Root AW, Saenz-Rodriguez C, Bongiovanni AM, et al. The effect of arginine infusion on plasma growth hormone and insulin in children. *J Pediatr.* 1969;74:187-197.
6. Nelin LD, Hoffman GM. L-arginine infusion lowers blood pressure in children. *J Pediatr.* 2001;139:747-749.
7. Summar MS. Current strategies for the management of neonatal urea cycle disorders. *J Pediatr.* 2001;138:S30-S39.
8. Batshaw ML, MacArthur RB, Tuchman M. Alternative pathway therapy for urea cycle disorders: twenty years later. *J Pediatr.* 2001;138:S46-S55.
9. Enns GM, Berry SA, Berry GT, et al. Survival after treatment with phenylacetate and benzoate for urea-cycle disorders. *N Engl J Med.* 2007;356:2282-2292.
10. Martin WF, Matzke GR. Treating severe metabolic alkalosis. *Clin Pharm.* 1982;1:42-48.
11. McCaffrey MJ, Bose CL, Reiter PD, et al. Effect of L-Arginine infusion on infants with persistent pulmonary hypertension of the newborn. *Biol Neonate.* 1995;67:240-243.
12. Mehta S, Stewart DJ, Langleben D et al. Short-term pulmonary vasodilation with L-arginine in pulmonary hypertension. *Circulation.* 1995;92:1539-1545.
13. Schulze-Nick I, Penny DJ, Rigby ML, et al. L-arginine and substance P reverse the pulmonary endothelial dysfunction caused by congenital heart surgery. *Circulation.* 1999;100:749-755.
14. Bushinsky DA, Gennari FJ. Life-threatening hyperkalemia induced by arginine. *Ann Intern Med.* 1978;89:632-634.
15. Hertz P, Richardson JA. Arginine-induced hyperkalemia in renal failure patients. *Arch Intern Med.* 1972;130:778-780.
16. Lee B. Management of urea cycle disorders. Available at: www.uptodate.com. Accessed March 4, 2009.
17. Bowlby HA, Elanjian SI. Necrosis caused by extravasation of arginine hydrochloride. *Ann Pharmacother.* 1992;26:263-264.
18. Salameh Y, Shoufani A. Full-thickness skin necrosis after arginine extravasation—a case report and review of literature. *J Pediatr Surg.* 2004;39:E9-E11.
19. Gerard JM, Luisiri A. A fatal overdose of arginine hydrochloride. *Clin Toxicol.* 1997;35:621-625.

Asparaginase

1. Available at: http://ismp.org/Tools/highalertmedications.pdf. ISMP 2008. Accessed October 25, 2009.
2. Available at: http://www.usp.org/hqi/similarProducts/choosy.html. Accessed October 25, 2009.
3. Elspar [package insert]. Deerfield, IL: Ovation Pharmaceuticals; May 2007.
4. Asparaginase. Lexi-Comp® Online with AHFS® (database). Bethesda, MD: American Society of Health-System Pharmacists; updated May 26, 2009.
5. Asparaginase. Lexi-Comp® Online with AHFS® (database). Hudson, OH: Lexi-Comp Inc; updated October 22, 2009.
6. Kung FH, Nythan WL, Cuttner J, et al. Vincristine, prednisone, and L-asparaginase in the induction of remission in children with acute lymphoblastic leukemia following relapse. *Cancer.* 1979;41(2):428-434.
7. Jones B, Holland JF, Glidewell O. Optimal use of asparaginase in acute lymphocytic leukemia. *Med Pediatr Oncol.* 1979;3(4):387-400.
8. Ertel IJ, Nesbit ME, Hammond D, et al. Effective dose of L-asparaginase for induction of remission in previously treated children with acute lymphoblastic leukemia: a report from Children's Cancer Study Group. *Cancer Res.* 1979;39(10):3893-3896.
9. Ortega JA, Nesbit ME, Donaldson MH, et al. L-asparaginase, vincristine, and prednisone for induction of first remission in acute lymphocytic leukemia. *Cancer Res.* 1977;37(2):535-540.
10. Pession A, Valsecchi MG, Masera G, et al. Long-term results of a randomized trial on extended use of high dose L-asparaginase for standard risk childhood acute lymphoblastic leukemia. *J Clin Oncol.* 2005;23(28):7161-7167.
11. Haskell CM, Canellos GP, Leventhal BG, et al. L-asparaginase: therapeutic and toxic effects in patients with neoplastic disease. *N Engl J Med.* 1969;281(19):1028-1034.
12. Trissel LA, ed. *Handbook on Injectable Drugs.* 15th ed. Bethesda, MD: American Society of Health-System Pharmacists; 2009.
13. Rodriguez T, Baumgarten E, Fengler R, et al. Long-term infusion of L-asparaginase—an alternative to intramuscular injection? *Klin Pediatr.* 1995;207(4):207-210.
14. Nesbit M, Chard R, Evans A. Evaluation of intramuscular versus intravenous administration of L-asparaginase in childhood leukemia. *Am J Pediatr Hematol Oncol.* 1979;1(1):9-13.
15. Tan C, Oettgen H. Clinical experience with L-asparaginase administered intrathecally. *Proc Am Assoc Cancer Res.* 1969;10:92 (abstract 365).
16. Dorr RT, Fritz WL. *Cancer Chemotherapy Handbook.* New York, NY: Elsevier; 1980:230-239.
17. Yang L, Panetta JC, Cai X, et al. Asparaginase may influence dexamethasone pharmacokinetics in acute lymphoblastic leukemia. *J Clin Oncol.* 2008;26:1932-1939.

Asparaginase–pegylated (Pegaspargase)

1. Available at: http://ismp.org/Tools/highalertmedications.pdf. ISMP 2008. Accessed August 24, 2009.
2. Available at: http://www.usp.org/hqi/similarProducts/choosy.html. Accessed August 24, 2009.
3. Oncaspar [package insert]. Bridgewater, NJ: Enzon Pharmaceuticals Inc; July 2006.
4. Solimando DA, ed. *Lexi-Comp's Drug Information Handbook for Oncology.* 4th ed. Hudson, OH: Lexi-Comp; 2004:651-654.

5. Pegaspargase. Lexi-Comp® Online with AHFS® (database). Bethesda, MD: American Society of Health-System Pharmacists; updated December 2008.
6. Pegaspargase. Lexi-Comp Online with AHFS (database). Hudson, OH: Lexi-Comp Inc; updated October 22, 2009.
7. Avramis AI, Sencer S, Periclou, et al. A randomized comparison of native *Escherichia coli* asparaginase and polyethylene glycol conjugated asparaginase for treatment of children with newly diagnosed standard-risk acute lymphoblastic leukemia: a Children's Cancer Group study. *Blood.* 2002;99:1986-1994.
8. Abshire TC, Pollock BH, Billett AL, et al. Weekly polyethylene glycol conjugated L-asparaginase compared with biweekly dosing produces superior induction remission rates in childhood relapsed acute lymphoblastic leukemia: a pediatric oncology group study. *Blood.* 2000;96:1709-1715.
9. Hawkins DS, Park JR, Thomson BG, et al. Asparaginase pharmacokinetics after intensive polyethylene glycol-conjugated L-asparaginase therapy for children with relapsed acute lymphoblastic leukemia. *Clin Cancer Res.* 2004;10:5335-5341.

Atenolol

1. Available at: http://ismp.org/Tools/highalertmedications.pdf. June 19, 2009.
2. Available at: http://ismp.org/Tools/confuseddrugnames.pdf. June 19, 2009.
3. AstraZeneca Pharmaceuticals. Tenormin® (atenolol) IV injection prescribing information. Wilmington, DE; 2005 Feb.
4. The American Heart Association. Guidelines 2005 for cardiopulmonary resuscitation and emergency cardiovascular care. *Circulation.* 2005; 112(Suppl I): IV1-211.
5. National High Blood Pressure Education Program Working Group on High Blood Pressure in Children and Adolescents. The fourth report on the diagnosis, evaluation, and treatment of high blood pressure in children and adolescents. *Pediatrics.* 2004 Aug;114(2 suppl 4th Report):555-576.
6. Kay JD, Sinaiko AR, Daniels SR. Pediatric hypertension. *Am Heart J.* 2001;142:422-432.
7. Buck ML, Wiest D, Gillette PC, et al. Pharmacokinetics and pharmacodynamics of atenolol in children. *Clin Pharmacol Ther.* 1989;46:629-633.
8. Aronoff GR, Berns JS, Brier ME, et al. Drug prescribing in renal failure. 4th ed. Available at: http://www.kdp-baptist. louisville.edu/renalbook/. Accessed June 18, 2009.
9. Atenolol. Lexi-Comp® Online with AHFS® (database). Bethesda, MD: American Society of Health-System Pharmacists; updated February 2008.
10. Ramsdale DR, Faragher EB, Bennett DH, et al. Ischemic pain relief in patients with acute myocardial infarction by intravenous atenolol. *Am Heart J.* 1982;103:459-467.
11. Trissel LA, ed. *Handbook on Injectable Drugs.* 17th ed. Bethesda, MD: American Society of Health-System Pharmacists; 2009.

Atracurium Besylate

1. Available at: http://ismp.org/Tools/highalertmedications.pdf. ISMP 2008. Accessed August 24, 2009.
2. Atracurium besylate [package insert]. Bedford, OH: Bedford Laboratories; May 2004.
3. Martin LD, Bratton SL, O'Rourke PP. Clinical uses and controversies of neuromuscular blocking agents in infants and children. *Crit Care Med.* 1999;27:1358-1368.
4. Goudsouzian NG, Young ET, Moss J, et al. Histamine release during the administration of atracurium or vecuronium in children. *Br J Anaesth.* 1986;58:1229-1233.
5. Basta SJ, Savarese JJ, Ali HH, et al. Histamine-releasing potencies of atracurium, dimethyltubocurarine and tubocurarine. *Br J Anaesth.* 1983; 55:105S-106S.
6. McHutchon A, Lawler PG. Bradycardia following atracurium. *Anaesthesia.* 1983;38:597-598.
7. Carter ML. Bradycardia after the use of atracurium. *BMJ.* 1983;287:247-248.
8. Rowlee SC. Monitoring neuromuscular blockade in the intensive care unit: the peripheral nerve stimulator. *Heart Lung.* 1999;28:352-362.
9. Atracurium besylate injection. Lexi-Comp Online with AHFS (database). Bethesda, MD: American Society of Health-System Pharmacists; updated January 2009.
10. Meakin G, Shaw EA, Baker RD, et al. Comparison of atracurium-induced neuromuscular blockade in neonates, infants and children. *Br J Anaesth.* 1988;60:171-175.
11. Piotrowski A. Comparison of atracurium and pancuronium in mechanically ventilated neonates. *Intensive Care Med.* 1993;19:401-405.
12. Meretoja OA, Wirtavori K. Influence of age on the dose-response relationship of atracurium in paediatric patients. *Acta Anaesthesiol Scand.* 1988;32:614-618.
13. Nightingale DA, Bush GH. Atracurium in paediatric anaesthesia. *Br J Anaesth.* 1983;55:115S.
14. Brandom BW, Rudd GD, Cook DR. Clinical pharmacology of atracurium in paediatric patients. *Br J Anaesth.* 1983;55:117S-121S.
15. Brandom BW, Woelfel SK, Cook DR, et al. Clinical pharmacology of atracurium in infants. *Anesth Analg.* 1984;63:309-312.
16. Goudsouzian NG, Liu LM, Cote CJ, et al. Safety and efficacy of atracurium in adolescents and children anesthetized with halothane. *Anesthesiology.* 1983;59:459-462.
17. Goudsouzian NG, Liu LM, Gionfriddo M, et al. Neuromuscular effects of atracurium in infants and children. *Anesthesiology.* 1985;62:75-79.
18. Brandom BW, Stiller RL, Cook DR, et al. Pharmacokinetics of atracurium in anaesthetized infants and children. *Br J Anaesth.* 1986;58:1210-1213.
19. Eagar BM, Flynn P, Hughes R. Infusion of atracurium for long surgical procedures. *Br J Anaesth.* 1984;56:447-452.
20. Wait CM, Goat VA. Atracurium infusion during paediatric craniofacial surgery. *Anaesthesia.* 1989;44:567-570.
21. Brandom BW, Cook DR, Woelfel SK, et al. Atracurium infusion requirements in children during halothane, isoflurane, and narcotic anesthesia. *Anesth Analg.* 1985;64:471-476.
22. Playfor SD, Thomas DA, Choonara I. Duration of action of atracurium when given by infusion to critically ill children. *Paediatr Anaesth.* 2000;10:77-81.
23. Kushimo OT, Darowski MJ, Hollis S, et al. Dose requirements of atracurium in paediatric intensive care patients. *Br J Anaesth.* 1991;67:781-783.
24. Ridley SA, Hatch DJ. Post-tetanic count and profound neuromuscular blockade with atracurium infusion in paediatric patients. *Br J Anaesth.* 1988;60:3135.
25. Aronoff GR, Berns JS, Brier ME, et al. Drug prescribing in renal failure. 4th ed. Available at: http://www.kdp-baptist.louisville.edu/renalbook/. Accessed November 13, 2009.
26. Simpson DA, Green DW. Use of atracurium during major abdominal surgery in infants with hepatic dysfunction from biliary atresia. *Br J Anaesth.* 1986;58:1214-1217.
27. Kalli I, Metetoja OA. Infusion of atracurium in neonates, infants, and children. *Br J Anaesth.* 1988;60:651-654.
28. Branney SW, Haenel JB, Moore FA, et al. Prolonged paralysis with atracurium infusion: a case report. *Crit Care Med.* 1994;22:1699-1701.
29. Trissel LA, ed. *Handbook on Injectable Drugs.* 15th ed. Bethesda, MD: American Society of Health-System Pharmacists; 2009.
30. Watling SM, Dasta JF. Prolonged paralysis in intensive care unit patients after the use of neuromuscular blocking agents: a review of the literature. *Crit Care Med.* 1994;22:884-893.
31. Grigore AM, Brusco L, Kuroda M, et al. Laudanosine and atracurium in a patient receiving long-term atracurium infusion. *Crit Care Med.* 1998;26:180-183.
32. Fahey MR, Rupp SM, Canfell C, et al. Effect of renal failure on laudansoine excretion in man. *Br J Anaesth.* 1985;576:1049-1051.
33. Brandom BW, Woelfel SK, Cook DR, et al. Relative potency of atracurium in children during halothane, isoflurane, or thiopental–fentanyl anesthesia. *Anesthesiology.* 1983;59:A442.

References

Atropine Sulfate

1. Atropine. Lexi-Comp® Online with AHFS® (database). Hudson, OH: Lexi-Comp Inc; updated July 17, 2009.
2. AtroPen [package insert]. Columbia, MD: Meridian Medical Technologies Inc. NDA 17-106/S0928. Available at: http://129.128.185.122/drugbank2/drugs/DB00572/fda_labels/63. Accessed July 28, 2009.
3. 2005 American Heart Association guidelines for cardiopulmonary resuscitation and emergency cardiovascular care. Part 12: Pediatric advanced life support. *Circulation.* 2005;112(24 suppl):IV-167–IV-187.
4. Roberts KD, Leone TA, Edwards WH, et al. Premedications for nonemergent neonatal intubations: a randomized, controlled trial comparing atropine and fentanyl to atropine, fentanyl, and mivacurium. *Pediatrics.* 2006;118:1583-1591.
5. American Academy of Pediatrics Committee on Drugs. Emergency drug doses for infants and children. *Pediatrics.* 1998;101(1):e1-e11.
6. Gaviotaki A, Smith RM. Use of atropine in pediatric anesthesia. *Int Anesthesiol Clin.* 1962;1:97-113.
7. Bachman L, Freeman A. The cardiac rate and rhythm in infants during anesthesia induction with cyclopropane. Atropine versus scopolamine as preanesthetic medication. *J Pediatr.* 1961;59:922-927.
8. Wark HJ, Overton JH, Marian P. The safety of atropine premedication in children with Down's syndrome. *Anaesthesia.* 1983;38:871-874.
9. Hofley MA, Hofley PM, Keom TP, et al. A placebo-controlled trial using intravenous atropine as an adjunct to conscious sedation in pediatric esophagogastroduodenoscopy. *Gastrointest Endosc.* 1995;42:457-460.
10. The International Liaison Committee on Resuscitation (ILCOR) Consensus on Science with Treatment Recommendations for Pediatric and Neonatal Patients: Neonatal Resuscitation. *Pediatrics.* 2006;117:e978-e988.
11. Thomson Healthcare Inc. POISINDEX® Managements. Available at: http://www.thomsonhc.com-MICROMEDEX® Healthcare Series [database on the Internet]. Accessed April 7, 2009.
12. Rotenberg JS, Newmark J. Nerve agent attacks on children: diagnosis and management. *Pediatrics.* 2003;112;648-658.
13. Zwiener RJ, Ginsburg CM. Organophosphate and carbamate poisoning in infants and children. *Pediatrics.* 1988;81:121-125.
14. Sungur M, Guven M. Intensive care management of organophosphate insecticide poisoning. *Crit Care.* 2001;5:211-215.
15. Trissel LA, ed. *Handbook on Injectable Drugs.* 15th ed. Bethesda, MD: American Society of Health-System Pharmacists; 2009.
16. LeBlanc FN, Benson BE, Gilig AD. A severe organophosphate poisoning requiring the use of an atropine drip. *J Toxicol Clin Toxicol.* 1986;24:69-76.
17. Sullivan KJ, Berman LS, Koska J, et al. Intramuscular atropine sulfate in children: comparison of injection sites. *Anesth Analg.* 1997;84:54-58.
18. Chhabra A, Mishra S, Kumar A, et al. Atropine-induced lens extrusion in an open eye surgery. *Pediatr Anesthesia.* 2006;16:59-62.

Azithromycin

1. Available at: http://www.usp.org/hqi/similarProducts/choosy.html. Accessed June 10, 2009.
2. Zithromax® (azithromycin) for injection for IV infusion only [prescribing information]. New York, NY: Pfizer Labs; October 2003.
3. Plouffe J, Schwartz DB, Kolokathis A, et al. Clinical efficacy of intravenous followed by oral azithromycin monotherapy in hospitalized patients with community-acquired pneumonia. *Antimicrob Agents Chemother.* 2000;44:1796-1802.
4. Vergis EN, Indorf A, File TM, et al. Azithromycin vs. cefuroxime plus erythromycin for empirical treatment of community-acquired pneumonia in hospitalized patients: a prospective, randomized, multicenter trial. *Arch Intern Med.* 2000;160:1294-1300.
5. Bartlett JG, Dowell SF, Mandell LA, et al. Practice guidelines for the management of community-acquired pneumonia in adults. *Clin Infect Dis.* 2000;31:347-382.
6. American Academy of Pediatrics. Pickering LK, Baker CJ, Kimberlin DW, et al., eds. *2009 Red Book: Report of the Committee on Infectious Diseases.* 28th ed. Elk Grove Village, IL: American Academy of Pediatrics; 2009.
7. Workowski KA, Berman SM; Centers for Disease Control and Prevention. Pelvic inflammatory disease. Sexually transmitted diseases treatment guidelines 2006 [published errata in *MMWR Morb Mortal Wkly Rep.* 2006;55:997]. *MMWR Morb Mortal Wkly Rep.* 2006;55(RR-11):56-61.
8. Aronoff GR, Berns JS, Brier ME, et al. Drug prescribing in renal failure. 4th ed. Available at: http://www.kdp-baptist.louisville.edu/renalbook/. Accessed August 28, 2009.
9. Jacobs RF, Maples HD, Aranda JV, et al. Pharmacokinetics of intravenously administered azithromycin in pediatric patients. *Pediatr Infect Dis J.* 2005;24:34-39.
10. Luke DR, Foulds G, Cohen SF, et al. Safety, toleration, and pharmacokinetics of intravenous azithromycin. *Antimicrob Agents Chemother.* 1996;40:2577-2581.
11. Trissel LA, ed. *Handbook on Injectable Drugs.* 15th ed. Bethesda, MD: American Society of Health-System Pharmacists; 2009.
12. Bizjak ED, Haug MT, Schilz RJ, et al. Intravenous azithromycin-induced ototoxicity. *Pharmacotherapy.* 1999;19:245-248.
13. Azithromycin. Lexi-Comp® Online with AHFS® (database). Bethesda, MD: American Society of Health-System Pharmacists; updated August 13, 2009.
14. Owens RC Jr, Nolin TD. Antimicrobial-associated QT interval prolongation: pointes of interest. *Clin Infect Dis.* 2006;43:1603-1611.

Aztreonam

1. Available at: http://www.usp.org/hqi/similarProducts/choosy.html. Accessed October 30, 2009.
2. Azactam [package insert]. Princeton, NJ: Bristol-Myers Squibb Co; January 2004.
3. Joint Task Force on Practice Parameters; American Academy of Allergy, Asthma and Immunology; American College of Allergy, Asthma and Immunology; Joint Council of Allergy, Asthma and Immunology. The diagnosis and management of anaphylaxis: an updated practice parameter. *J Allergy Clin Immunol.* 2005;115:S483-S523.
4. Adkinson NF Jr, Swabb EA, Sugerman AA. Immunology of the monobactam aztreonam. *Antimicrob Agents Chemother.* 1984;25:93-97.
5. Saxon A, Hassner A, Swabb EA, et al. Lack of cross-reactivity between aztreonam, a monobactam antibiotic, and penicillin in penicillin-allergic subjects. *J Infect Dis.* 1984;149:16-22.
6. Afrumin J, Gallagher JC Allergic cross-sensitivity between penicillin, carbapenem, and monobactam antibiotics: what are the chances? *Ann Pharmacother.* 2009;43:304-315.
7. de la Fuente PR, Armentia MA, Sanchez PP, et al. Urticaria caused by sensitization to aztreonam. *Allergy.* 1993;8:634-636.
8. American Academy of Pediatrics. Pickering LK, Baker CJ, Kimberlin DW, et al. *2009 Red Book: Report of the Committee on Infectious Diseases.* 28th ed. Elk Grove Village, IL: American Academy of Pediatrics; 2009.
9. Nelson JD, Bradley JS, eds. *Nelson's Pocket Book of Pediatric Antimicrobial Therapy.* 17th ed. Chicago, IL: American Academy of Pediatrics; 2009.
10. Stutman HR. Clinical experience with aztreonam for treatment of infections in children. *Rev Infect Dis.* 1991;13:S582-S585.
11. Bosso JA, Black PG. The use of aztreonam in pediatric patients: a review. *Pharmacotherapy.* 1991;11:20-25.
12. Stutman HR, Chartrand SA, Tolentino T, et al. Aztreonam therapy for serious gram-negative infections in children. *Am J Dis Child.* 1986;140:1147-1151.
13. Kline MW, Kaplan SL, Mason EO. Aztreonam therapy of gram-negative infections predominantly of the urinary tract in children. *Curr Ther Res.* 1986;39:625-631.

References

14. Bosso JA, Black PG, Matsen JM. Efficacy of aztreonam in pulmonary exacerbations of cystic fibrosis. *Pediatr Infect Dis J.* 1987;6:393-397.
15. Bosso JA, Black PG. Controlled trial of aztreonam vs. tobramycin and azlocillin for acute pulmonary exacerbations of cystic fibrosis. *Pediatr Infect Dis J.* 1988;7:171-176.
16. Aronoff GR, Berns JS, Brier ME, et al. Drug prescribing in renal failure. 4th ed. Available at: http://www.kdp-baptist.louisville.edu/renalbook/. Accessed Otocber 30, 2009.
17. Trissel LA, ed. *Handbook on Injectable Drugs.* 15th ed. Bethesda, MD: American Society of Health-System Pharmacists; 2009.
18. Aztreonam. Lexi-Comp® Online with AHFS® (database). Bethesda, MD: American Society of Health-System Pharmacists; updated September 16, 2009.
19. Robinson CA, Sawyer JE. Y-site compatibility of medications with parenteral nutrition. *J Pediatr Pharmacol Ther.* 2009;14:49-57.
20. McCoy KS, Quittner AL, Oermann CM, et al. Inhaled aztreonam lysine for chronic airway *Pseudomonas aeruginosa* in cystic fibrosis. *Am J Respir Crit Care Med.* 2008;178:921-928.
21. Retsch-Bogart GZ, Quittner AL, Gibson RL, et al. Efficacy and safety of inhaled aztreonam lysine for airway *Pseudomonas* in cystic fibrosis. *Chest.* 2009;135:1223-1232.

Baclofen

1. Available at: http://www.ismp.org/tools/confuseddrugnames.pdf. Accessed June 10, 2009.
2. Available at: http://www.usp.org/hqi/similarProducts/choosy.html. Accessed June 10, 2009.
3. Lioresal Intrathecal [package insert]. Minneapolis, MN: Medtronics; March 2002.
4. Bardutzky J, Tronnier V, Schwab S, et al. Intrathecal baclofen for stiff-person syndrome: life-threatening intermittent catheter leakage. *Neurology.* 2003;60:1976-1978.
5. Dickerman RD, Schneider SJ. Recurrent intrathecal baclofen pump catheter leakage: a surgical observation with recommendations. *J Pediatr Surg.* 2002;37:E17-E19.
6. Al-Khodairy AT, Vuagnat H, Uebelhart D. Symptoms of recurrent intrathecal baclofen withdrawal resulting from drug delivery failure: a case report. *Am J Phys Med Rehabil.* 1999;78:272-277.
7. Disabato J, Ritchie A. Intrathecal baclofen for the treatment of spasticity of cerebral origin. *JSPN.* 2003;8:31-34.
8. Campbell WM, Ferrel A, McLaughlin JF, et al. Long-term safety and efficacy of continuous intrathecal baclofen. *Dev Med Child Neurol.* 2002;44:660-665.
9. Buonaguro V, Scelsa B, Curci D, et al. Epilepsy and intrathecal baclofen therapy in children with cerebral palsy. *Pediatr Neurol.* 2005;33:110-113.
10. Stokic DS, Yablon SA, Hayes A. Comparison of clinical and neurophysiologic responses to intrathecal baclofen bolus administration in moderate-to-severe spasticity after acquired brain injury. *Arch Phys Med Rehabil.* 2005;86:1801-1806.
11. Stempien L, Tsai T. Intrathecal baclofen pump use for spasticity. *Am J Phys Med Rehabil.* 2000;79:536-541
12. Ward LA. Spasticity in kids: an intrathecal option. *RN.* 2001;64:39-41.
13. Van Schaeybroeck P, Nuttin B, Lagae L, et al. Intrathecal baclofen for intractable cerebral spasticity: a prospective, placebo-controlled, double-blind study. *Neurosurgery.* 2000;46:603-612.
14. Bjornson KF, McLaughlin JF, Loeser JD, et al. Oral motor, communication, and nutritional status of children during intrathecal baclofen therapy: a descriptive pilot study. *Arch Phys Med Rehabil.* 2003;84:500-506.
15. Armstrong RW, Steinbok P, Cochrane DD, et al. Intrathecally administered baclofen for treatment of children with spasticity of cerebral origin. *J Neurosurg.* 1997;87:409-414.
16. Pohl M, Rockstroh G, Rückriem S, et al. Time course of the effect of a bolus dose of intrathecal baclofen on severe cerebral spasticity. *J Neurol.* 2003;250:1195-2000.
17. Baclofen. Lexi-Comp® Online with AHFS® (database). Bethesda, MD: American Society of Health-System Pharmacists; updated March 13, 2009.
18. Dressnandt J, Knostanzer A, Weinzierl FX, et al. Intrathecal baclofen in tetanus: four cases and a review of reported cases. *Intensive Care Med.* 1997;23:896-902.
19. Engrand N, Guerot E, Alexis R, et al. The efficacy of intrathecal baclofen in severe tetanus. *Anesthesiology.* 1999;90:1773-1776.
20. Coffey RJ, Edgar TS, Francisco GE, et al. Abrupt withdrawal from intrathecal baclofen: recognition and management of a potentially life-threatening syndrome. *Arch Phys Med Rehabil.* 2002;83:735-741.
21. Kao LW, Amin Y, Kirk MA, et al. Intrathecal baclofen withdrawal mimicking sepsis. *J Emerg Med.* 2003;24:423-427.
22. Samson-Fang L, Gooch J, Norlin C. Intrathecal baclofen withdrawal simulating neuroleptic malignant syndrome in a child with cerebral palsy. *Dev Med Child Neurol.* 2000;42:561-565.
23. Douglas AF, Weiner HL, Schwartz DR. Prolonged intrathecal baclofen withdrawal syndrome. *J Neurosurg.* 2005;102:1133-1136.
24. Green LB, Nelson VS. Death after acute withdrawal of intrathecal baclofen: case report and literature review. *Arch Phys Med Rehabil.* 1999;80:1600-1604.
25. Colachis SC, Rea GL. Monitoring of creatinine kinase during weaning of intrathecal baclofen and with symptoms of early withdrawal. *Am J Phys Med Rehabil.* 2003;82:489-492.
26. Hansen CR, Gooch JL, Such-Neibar T. Prolonged, severe intracheal baclofen withdrawal syndrome: a case report. *Arch Phys Med Rehabil.* 2007;88:1468-1471.
27. Cruikshank M, Eunson P. Intravenous diazepam infusion in the management of planned intrathecal bacolfen withdrawal. *Dev Med Child Neurol.* 2007;49:626-628.
28. Khorasani A, Peruzzi WT. Dantrolene treatment for abrupt intrathecal baclofen withdrawal. *Anesth Analg.* 1995;80:1054-1056.
29. Meythaler JM, Roper JF, Brunner RC. Cyproheptadine for intrathecal baclofen withdrawal. *Arch Phys Med Rehabil.* 2003;84:638-642.
30. Greenberg MI, Hendrickson RG. Baclofen withdrawal following removal of an intrathecal baclofen pump despite oral baclofen replacement. *J Toxicol Clin Toxicol.* 2003;41:83-85.
31. Vaidyanathan S, Soni BM, Oo T, et al. Bladder stones—red herring for resurgence of spasticity in a spinal cord injury patient with implantation of Medtronic Synchromed pump for intrathecal delivery of baclofen—a case report. *BMC Urology.* 2003;3:1-7.
32. Albright AL, Ferson S, Carlos S. Occult hydrocephalus in children with cerebral palsy. *Neurosurgery.* 2005;56:93-97.
33. Schuele SU, Kellinghaus C, Shook SJ, et al. Incidence of seizures in patients with multiple sclerosis treated with intrathecal baclofen. *Neurology.* 2005;64:1086-1087.
34. Schuele SU, Ahrens CL, Kellinghaus C, et al. Incidence of seizures in patients with multiple sclerosis treated with intrathecal baclofen. *Neurology.* 2005;66:784-785.
35. Segal LS, Wallach DM, Kanev PM. Potential complications of posterior spine fusion and instrumentation in patients with cerebral palsy treated with intrathecal baclofen infusion. *Spine.* 2005;30:E219-E224.
36. Sansone JM, Mann D, Noonan K, et al. Rapid progression of scoliosis following insertion of intrathecal baclofen pump. *J Pediatr Orthop.* 2006;26:125-128.

Bumetanide

1. Available at: http://www.usp.org/hqi/similarProducts/choosy.html. Accessed April 13, 2009.
2. Bumetanide injection, USP [package insert]. Bedford, OH: Bedford Laboratories; June 2005.
3. Bumetanide. Lexi-Comp® Online with AHFS® (database). Bethesda, MD: American Society of Health-System Pharmacists; updated May 26, 2009.

References

4. Turmen T, Thom P, Louridas AT, et al. Protein binding and bilirubin displacing properties of bumetanide and furosemide. *J Clin Pharmacol.* 1982;22:551-556.
5. Wells TG. The pharmacology and therapeutics of diuretics in the pediatric patient. *Pediatr Clin North Am.* 1990;37:463-504.
6. Sullivan JE, Witte MK, Yamashita TS, et al. Dose-ranging evaluation of bumetanide pharmacodynamics in critically ill infants. *Clin Pharmacol Ther.* 1996;60:424-434.
7. Ward OC, Lam LK. Bumetanide in heart failure in infancy. *Arch Dis Child.* 1977;52:877-882.
8. Shankaran S, Ilagan N, Liang KC, et al. Bumetanide pharmacokinetics in preterm neonates. *Pediatr Res.* 1989;25:72A. Abstract.
9. Gale R, Armon Y, Aranda JV. Pharmacodynamic profile of bumetanide in newborn infants. *Pediatr Res.* 1988;23:257A. Abstract.
10. Wells TG, Fasules JW, Taylor BJ, et al. Pharmacokinetics and pharmacodynamics of bumetanide in neonates treated with extracorporeal membrane oxygenation. *J Pediatr.* 1992;121:974-980.
11. Lopez-Samblas AM, Adams JA, Goldberg RN, et al. The pharmacokinetics of bumetanide in the newborn infant. *Biol Neonate.* 1997;72:265-272.
12. Marshall JD, Wells TG, Letzig L, et al. Pharmacokinetics and pharmacodynamics of bumetanide in critically ill pediatric patients. *J Clin Pharmacol.* 1998;38:994-1002.
13. Sullivan JE, Witte MK, Yamashita TS, et al. Analysis of the variability in the pharmacokinetics and pharmacodynamics of bumetanide in critically ill infants. *Clin Pharmacol Ther.* 1996;60:414-423.
14. Sullivan JE, Witte MK, Yamashita TS, et al. Pharmacokinetics of bumetanide in critically ill infants. *Clin Pharmacol Ther.* 1996;60:405-413.
15. Trissel LA. Handbook on Injectable Drugs. 15th ed. Bethesda, MD: American Society of Health-System Pharmacists; 2009.
16. Rudy DW, Voelker JR, Greene PK, et al. Loop diuretics for chronic renal insufficiency: a continuous infusion is more efficacious than bolus therapy. *Ann Intern Med.* 1991;115:360-366.
17. Howard PA, Dunn MI. Severe musculoskeletal symptoms during continuous infusion of bumetanide. *Chest.* 1997;111:359-364.

Bupivacaine

1. Available at: http://ismp.org/Tools/highalertmedications.pdf. ISMP 2008. Accessed August 24, 2009.
2. Available at: http://www.usp.org/hqi/similarProducts/choosy.html. Accessed August 24, 2009.
3. Bupivacaine hydrochloride [package insert]. Lake Forest, IL: Hospira; January 2007.
4. Bupivacaine. Lexi-Comp Online with AHFS (database). Hudson, OH: Lexi-Comp; updated November 16, 2009.
5. Available at: http://www.fda.gov/Drugs/DrugSafety/PostmarketDrugSafetyInformationforPatientsandProviders/ucm190302.htm. Accessed November 20, 2009.
6. Trissel LA, ed. *Handbook on Injectable Drugs.* 15th ed. Bethesda, MD: American Society of Health-System Pharmacists; 2009.
7. Hansen TG, Henneberg SW, Walther-Larsen S, et al. Caudal bupivacaine supplemented with caudal or intravenous clonidine in children undergoing hypospadias repair: a double-blind study. *Br J Anaesth.* 2004;92:223-227.
8. Bozkurt P, Arslan I, Bakan M, et al. Free plasma levels of bupivacaine and ropivacaine when used for caudal block in children. *Eur J Anaesth.* 2005;22:634-643.
9. Brindley N, Taylor R, Brown S. Reduction of incarcerated inguinal hernia in infants using caudal epidural anaesthesia. *Pediatr Surg Int.* 2005;21:715-717.
10. Hansen TG, Morton NS, Cullen PM, et al. Plasma concentrations and pharmacokinetics of bupivacaine with and without adrenaline following caudal anaesthesia in infants. *Acta Anaesthesiol Scand.* 2001;45:42-47.
11. Khalil S, Campos C, Farag AM, et al. Caudal block in children: ropivacaine compared with bupivacaine. *Anesthesiology.* 1999;91:1279-1284.
12. Meunier JF, Goujard E, Dubousset AM, et al. Pharmacokinetics of bupivacaine after continuous epidural infusion in infants with and without biliary atresia. *Anesthesiology.* 2001;95:87-95.
13. Larsson BA, Lonnqvist PA, Olsson GL. Plasma concentrations of bupivacaine in neonates after continuous epidural infusion. *Anesth Analg.* 1997;84:501-505.
14. Kumar P, Rudra A, Pan AK, et al. Caudal additives in pediatrics: a comparison among midazolam, ketamine, and neostigmine coadministered with bupivacaine. *Br J Anaesth.* 2005;101:69-73.
15. Shlizerman L, Ashkenazi D. Peripheral facial nerve paralysis after peritonsillar infiltration of bupivacaine: a case report. *Am J Otolaryngol.* 2005;26:406-407.

Caffeine Citrate

1. Caffeine citrate [package insert]. Detroit, MI: Caraco Pharmaceutical Laboratories Ltd; November 2009.
2. Schmidt B, Roberts RS, Davis P, et al. Caffeine therapy for apnea of prematurity. *N Engl J Med.* 2006;354:2112-2121.
3. Erenberg A, Leff RD, Haack DG. Caffeine citrate for the treatment of apnea of Prematurity: a double-blind, placebo-controlled study. *Pharmacotherapy.* 2000;20:644-652.
4. Bauer J, Maier K, Linderkamp O, et al. Effect of caffeine on oxygen consumption and metabolic rate in very low birth weight infants with idiopathic apnea. *Pediatrics.* 2001;107:660-663.
5. Thomson AH, Kerr S, Wright S. Population pharmacokinetics of caffeine in neonates and young infants. *Ther Drug Monit.* 1996;18:245-253.
6. Lee TC, Charles C, Steer P et al. Population pharmacokinetics of intravenous caffeine in neonates with apnea of prematurity. *Clin Pharmacol Ther.* 1997;61:628-640.
7. Steer P, Flenady V, Shearman A, et al. High dose caffeine citrate for extubation of preterm infants: a randomized controlled trial. *Arch Dis Child Fetal Neonatal Ed.* 2004;89:F499-F503.
8. Caffeine. Lexi-Comp® Online with AHFS® (database). Hudson, OH: Lexi-Comp Inc; updated October 9, 2009.
9. Trissel LA, ed. *Handbook on Injectable Drugs.* 15th ed. Bethesda, MD: American Society of Health-System Pharmacists; 2009.
10. Robinson CA, Sawyer JE. Y-site compatibility of medications with parenteral nutrition. *J Pediatr Pharmacol Ther.* 2009;14:49-57.
11. Schmidt B, Roberts RS, Davis P, et al. Long-term effects of caffeine therapy for apnea of prematurity. *N Engl J Med.* 2007;357:1893-1902.
12. Natarajan G, Botica ML, Thomas R, Aranda JV. Therapeutic drug monitoring for caffeine in preterm neonates: an unnecessary exercise? *Pediatrics.* 2007;119:936-940.
13. Charles BG, Townsend SR, Steer PA, et al. Caffeine citrate treatment for extremely premature infants with apnea: population pharmacokinetics, absolute bioavailability, and implications for therapeutic drug monitoring. *Ther Drug Monit.* 2008;30:709-716.

Calcitriol

1. Available at: http://www.usp.org/hqi/similar Products/choosy.html. Accessed June 30, 2009.
2. Calcijex [prescribing information]. North Chicago, IL: Abbott Laboratories; July 2007.
3. Calcitriol. Lexi-Comp® Online with AHFS® (database). Bethesda, MD: American Society of Health-System Pharmacists; updated May 26, 2009.
4. Greenbaum LA, Grenda R, Qiu P, et al. Intravenous calcitriol for treatment of hyperparathyroidism in children on hemodialysis. *Pediatr Nephrol.* 2005;20:622-630.

5. Salusky IB, Kuizon BD, Belin TR, et al. Intermittent calcitriol therapy in secondary hyperparathyroidism: a comparison between oral and intraperitoneal administration. *Kid Internat.* 1998;54:907-914.
6. Bellazzini MA, Howes DS. Pediatric hypocalcemic seizures: a case of rickets. *J Emerg Med.* 2005;28:161-164.
7. Venkataraman PS, Tsang RC, Steichen JJ, et al. Early neonatal hypocalcemia in extremely preterm infants. High incidence, early onset, and refractoriness to supraphysiologic doses of calcitriol. *Am J Dis Child.* 1986;140:1004-1008.
8. Salusky IB, Goodman WG, Horst R, et al. Pharmacokinetics of calcitriol in continuous ambulatory and cycling peritoneal dialysis patients. *Am J Kidney Dis.* 1990;16:126-132.
9. Trissel LA, ed. *Handbook on Injectable Drugs.* 15th ed. Bethesda, MD: American Society of Health-System Pharmacists; 2009.
10. Pecosky DA, Parasrampuria J, Luk CL, et al. Stability and sorption of calcitriol in plastic tuberculin syringes. *Am J Hosp Pharm.* 1992;49:1463-1466.
11. Mouser JF, Cochran EB, McKay CP, et al. Relationship between 1, 25 dihydroxyvitamin D (calcitriol) plasma concentrations and parathyroid hormone suppression in pediatric hemodialysis patients. *Pharmacotherapy.* 1994;14:366. Abstract.

Calcium Chloride

1. Available at: http://www.usp.org/hqi/similarProducts/choosy.htmo. Accessed July 1, 2009.
2. Calcium chloride injection, USP 10%. Shirley, NJ: American Regent Laboratories Inc; February 2000.
3. Rocephin [prescribing information]. Nutley, NJ: Roche Laboratories Inc; March 2009.
4. Calcium chloride. Lexi-Comp® Online with AHFS® (database). Hudson, OH: Lexi-Comp Inc; updated May 7, 2009.
5. Calcium supplements. Lexi-Comp® Online with AHFS® (database). Hudson, OH: Lexi-Comp Inc; updated June 22, 2009.
6. Upton J, Mulliken JB, Murray JE. Major intravenous extravasation injuries. *Am J Surg.* 1979;137:497-506.
7. Heckler FR, McCraw JB. Calcium-related cutaneous necrosis. *Surg Forum.* 1976;27:553-555.
8. Yosowitz P, Ekland DA, Shaw RC, et al. Peripheral intravenous infiltration necrosis. *Ann Surg.* 1975;182:553-556.
9. MacCara ME. Extravasation: a hazard of intravenous therapy. *Drug Intell Clin Pharm.* 1983;17:713-717.
10. Broner CW, Stidham GL, Westerkirchner DF, et al. A prospective randomized, double-blind comparison of calcium chloride and calcium gluconate therapies for hypocalcemia in critically ill children. *J Pediatr.* 1990;117:986-989.
11. Cote CJ, Drop LJ, Hoaglin DC, et al. Ionized hypocalcemia after fresh frozen plasma administration to thermally injured children: effects of infusion rate, duration, and treatment with calcium chloride. *Anesth Analg.* 1988;67:152-160.
12. 2005 American Heart Association guidelines for cardiopulmonary resuscitation and emergency cardiovascular care: Part 12: pediatric advanced life support. *Circulation.* 2005;112(24)(suppl1):IV167-IV187.
13. Trissel LA. *Handbook on Injectable Drugs.* 15th ed. Bethesda, MD: American Society of Health-System Pharmacists; 2009.

Calcium Gluconate

1. Available at: http://www.usp.org/hqi/similarProducts/choosy.htmo. Accessed July 1, 2009.
2. Calcium gluconate injection, USP 10%. Schaumburg, IL. APP Pharmaceuticals, LLC. December 2007.
3. Rocephin [prescribing information]. Nutley, NJ: Roche Laboratories Inc; March 2009.
4. Calcium gluconate. Lexi-Comp® Online with AHFS® (database). Hudson, OH: Lexi-Comp Inc; updated May 7, 2009.
5. Calcium supplements. Lexi-Comp® Online with AHFS® (database). Hudson, OH: Lexi-Comp Inc; updated June 22, 2009.
6. Upton J, Mulliken JB, Murray JE. Major intravenous extravasation injuries. *Am J Surg.* 1979;137:497-506.
7. Heckler FR, McCraw JB. Calcium-related cutaneous necrosis. *Surg Forum.* 1976;27:553-555.
8. Lee FA, Gwinn JL. Roentgen patterns of extravasation of calcium gluconate in the tissues of the neonate. *J Pediatr.* 1975;86:598-601.
9. Weiss Y, Ackerman C, Shmilovitz L. Localized necrosis of scalp in neonates due to calcium gluconate infusions: a cautionary note. *Pediatrics.* 1975;56:1084-1086.
10. MacCara ME. Extravasation: a hazard of intravenous therapy. *Drug Intell Clin Pharm.* 1983;17:713-717.
11. Book LS, Herbst JJ, Stewart D. Hazards of calcium gluconate therapy in the newborn infant: intra-arterial injection producing intestinal necrosis in rabbit ileum. *J Pediatr.* 1978;92:793-797.
12. Bifano E, Kavey R, Pergolizzi J, et al. The cardiopulmonary effects of calcium infusion in infants with persistent pulmonary hypertension of the newborn. *Pediatr Res.* 1989;25:262-265.
13. Venkataraman PS, Wilson DA, Sheldon RE, et al. Effect of hypocalcemia on cardiac function in very-low-birth-weight preterm neonates: studies of blood ionized calcium, echocardiography, and cardiac effect of intravenous calcium therapy. *Pediatrics.* 1985;76:543-550.
14. Brown DR, Steranka BH, Taylor FH. Treatment of early onset neonatal hypocalcemia. *Am J Dis Child.* 1981;135:24-28.
15. Mizrahi A, London RD, Gribetz D. Neonatal hypocalcemia—its causes and treatment. *N Engl J Med.* 1968; 278:1163-1165.
16. Scott SM, Ladenson JH, Aguanna JJ, et al. Effect of calcium therapy in the sick premature infant with early neonatal hypocalcemia. *J Pediatr.* 1984;104:747-751.
17. Tsang RC, Steichen JJ, Chan GM. Neonatal hypocalcemia. Mechanism of occurrence and management. *Crit Care Med.* 1977;5:56-61.
18. Trissel LA. *Handbook on Injectable Drugs.* 15th ed. Bethesda, MD: American Society of Health-System Pharmacists; 2009.
19. Millard TP, Harris AJ, MacDonald DM. Calcinosis cutis following intravenous infusion of calcium gluconate. *Br J Derm.* 1999;140:184-186.
20. Broner CW, Stidham GL, Westerkirchner DF, et al. A prospective randomized, double-blind comparison of calcium chloride and calcium gluconate therapies for hypocalcemia in critically ill children. *J Pediatr.* 1990;117:986-989.
21. Cote CJ, Drop LJ, Hoaglin DC, et al. Ionized hypocalcemia after fresh frozen plasma administration to thermally injured children: effects of infusion rate, duration, and treatment with calcium chloride. *Anesth Analg.* 1988;67:152-160.
22. Frey OR, Maier L. Polyethylene vials of calcium gluconate reduce aluminum contamination of TPN. *Ann Pharmacother.* 2000;34:811-812.

Caspofungin

1. Available at: http://ismp.org/Tools/confuseddrugnames.pdf. Accessed August 24, 2009.
2. Available at: http://www.usp.org/hqi/similarProducts/choosy.html. Accessed August 24, 2009.
3. Caspofungin Acetate [package insert]. Whitehouse Station, NJ: Merck & Co Inc; July 2008.
4. Castagnola E, Machetti M, Cappelli B. Caspofungin associated with liposomal amphotericin B or voriconazole for treatment of refractory fungal pneumonia in children with acute leukaemia or undergoing allogeneic bone marrow transplant. *Clin Microbiol Infect.* 2004;10:255-257.
5. Smith PB, Steinbach WJ, Cotten CM, et al. Caspofungin for the treatment of azole resistant candidemia in a premature infant. *J Perinatol.* 2007;27:127-129.
6. Natarajan G, Lulic-Botica M, Rongkavilit C, et al. Experience with caspofungin in the treatment of persistent fungemia in neonates. *J Perinatol.* 2005;25:770-777.
7. Mrowczynski W, Wojtalik M. Caspofungin for Candida endocarditis. *Pediatr Infect Dis J.* 2004;23:376.
8. Hesseling M, Weindling M, Neal T. First reported use of caspofungin in an extremely low-birth-weight neonate. *J Matern Fetal Neonatal Med.* 2003;14:212.

References

9. Odio CM, Araya R, Pinto LE, et al. Caspofungin therapy of neonates with invasive candidiasis. *Pediatr Infect Dis J.* 2004;23(12):1093-1097.
10. Manzar S, Kamat M, Pyati S. Caspofungin for refractory candidemia in neonates. *Pediatr Infect Dis J.* 2006;25(3):282-283.
11. Pannaraj PS, Walsh TJ, Baker CJ. Advances in antifungal therapy. *Pediatr Infect Dis J.* 2005;24:921-922.
12. Yalaz M, Akisu M, Hilmioglu S, et al. Successful caspofungin treatment of multidrug resistant *Candida parapsilosis* septicaemia in an extremely low birth weight neonate. *Mycoses.* 2006;49:242-245.
13. American Academy of Pediatrics. Antifungal drugs for systemic fungal infections. In: Pickering LK, Baker CJ, Kimberlin DW, et al., eds. *2009 Red Book: Report of the Committee on Infectious Diseases.* 28th ed. Elk Grove Village, IL: American Academy of Pediatrics; 2009:765-776.
14. Neely M, Jafri HS, Seibel N, et al. Pharmacokinetics and safety of caspofungin in older infants and toddlers. *Antimicrob Agents Chemother.* 2009;53(4):1450-1456.
15. Walsh T, Adamson P, Seibel N, et al. Pharmacokinetics, safety, and tolerability of caspofungin in children and adolescents. *Antimicrob Agents Chemother.* 2005;49:4536-4545.
16. Groll AH, Attarbaschi A, Schuster FR, et al. Treatment with caspofungin in immunocompromised paediatric patients: a multicentre survey. *J Antimicrob Chemother.* 2006;57:527-535.
17. Cesaro S, Toffolutti T, Messina C, et al. Safety and efficacy of caspofungin and liposomal amphotericin B, followed by voriconazole in young patients affected by refractory invasive mycosis. *Eur J Haematol.* 2004;73:50-55.
18. Pancham S, Hemmaway C, New H, et al. Caspofungin for invasive fungal infections: Combination treatment with liposomal amphotericin B in children undergoing hemopoietic stem cell transplantation. *Pediatr Transplantation.* 2005;9:254-257.
19. Pacetti SA, Gelone SP. Caspofungin acetate for treatment of invasive fungal infections. *Ann Pharmacother.* 2003;37(1):90-98.
20. Bliss JM, Wellington M, Gigliotti F. Antifungal pharmacotherapy for neonatal candidiasis. *Semin Perinatol.* 2003;27:365-374.
21. Kontny U, Walsh TJ, Rossler J, et al. Successful treatment of refractory chronic disseminated candidiasis after prolonged administration of caspofungin in a child with acute myeloid leukemia. *Pediatr Blood Cancer.* 2007;49:360-362.
22. Trissel LA, ed. *Handbook on Injectable Drugs.* 15th ed. Bethesda, MD: American Society of Health-System Pharmacists; 2009.
23. Fallon RM, Girotto JE. A review of clinical experience with newer antifungals in children. *J Pediatr Pharmacol Ther.* 2008;13:124-140.
24. Elanjikal Z, Sorensen J, Schmidt H, et al. Combination therapy with caspofungin and liposomal amphotericin B for invasive aspergillosis. *Pediatr Infect Dis J.* 2003;22:653-656.

CeFAZolin Sodium

1. Available at: http://www.ismp.org/tools/tallmanletters.pdf. Accessed June 14, 2009.
2. Available at: http://www.usp.org/hqi/similarProducts/choosy.html. Accessed June 14, 2009.
3. Cefazolin [package insert]. Bedford, OH: Bedford Laboratories; January 2005.
4. Prober CG, Stevenson DK, Benitz WE. The use of antibiotics in neonates weighing less than 1200 grams. *Pediatr Infect Dis J.* 1990;9:111-121.
5. Nelson JD, Bradley JS, eds. *Nelson's Pocket Book of Pediatric Antimicrobial Therapy.* 17th ed. Chicago, IL: American Academy of Pediatrics; 2009.
6. Pickering LK, O'Connor DM, Anderson D, et al. Comparative evaluation of cefazolin and cephalothin in children. *J Pediatr.* 1974;85:842-847.
7. Pickering LK, O'Connor DM, Anderson D, et al. Clinical and pharmacologic evaluation of cefazolin in children. *J Infect Dis.* 1973;128:S407-S414.
8. American Academy of Pediatrics. Pickering LK, Baker CJ, Kimberlin DW, et al., eds. *2009 Red Book: Report of the Committee on Infectious Diseases.* 28th ed. Elk Grove Village, IL: American Academy of Pediatrics; 2009.
9. Rhodes KH, Henry NK. Antibiotic therapy for severe infections in infants and children. *Mayo Clin Proc.* 1992;67:59-68.
10. Wilson W, Taubert K, Gewitz m, et al. Prevention of infective endocarditis. Guidelines from the American Heart Association Rheumatic Fever, Endocarditis, and Kawasaki Disease Committee, Council on Cardiovascular Disease in the Young, and the Councils on Clinical Cardiology, Council on Cardiovascular Surgery and Anesthesia and the Quality of Care and Outcomes Research Interdisciplinary Working Group. *Circulation.* 2007;115:1736-1754; correction *Circulation.* 2007;116:e376-e377.
11. Baddour LM, Wilson WR, Bayer AS, et al. Infective endocarditis: diagnosis, antimicrobial therapy, and management of complications: a statement for healthcare professionals from the Committee on Rheumatic Fever, Endocarditis, and Kawasaki Disease, Council on Cardiovascular Disease in the Young, and the Councils on Clinical Cardiology, Stroke, and Cardiovascular Surgery and Anesthesia, American Heart Association: endorsed by the Infectious Diseases Society of America. *Circulation.* 2005;111:e394-e434.
12. Hiner LB, Baluarte HJ, Polinsky MS, et al. Cefazolin in children with renal insufficiency. *J Pediatr.* 1980;96:335-339.
13. Trissel LA, ed. *Handbook on Injectable Drugs.* 15th ed. Bethesda, MD: American Society of Health-System Pharmacists; 2009.
14. Robinson DC, Cookson TL. Concentration guidelines for parenteral antibiotics in fluid-restricted patients. *Drug Intell Clin Pharm.* 1987;21:985-989.
15. McLaughlin JE, Reeves DS. Clinical and laboratory evidence for inactivation of gentamicin by carbenicillin. *Lancet.* 1971;1:261-264.
16. Riff LJ, Jackson GG. Laboratory and clinical conditions for gentamicin inactivation by carbenicillin. *Arch Intern Med.* 1972;130:887-891.
17. Manian FA, Stone WJ, Alford RH. Adverse antibiotic effects associated with renal insufficiency. *Rev Infect Dis.* 1990;12:236-249.
18. Davies M, Morgan JR, Anand C. Interactions of carbenicillin and ticarcillin with gentamicin. *Antimicrob Agents Chemother.* 1975;7:431-434.
19. Weibert R, Keane W, Shapiro F. Carbenicillin inactivation of aminoglycosides in patients with severe renal failure. *Trans Amer Soc Artif Int Organs.* 1976;22:439-443.
20. Robinson CA, Sawyer JE. Y-site compatibility of medications with parenteral nutrition. *J Pediatr Pharmacol Ther.* 2009;14:49-57.
21. Craig WA, Ebert SC. Continuous infusion of beta-lactam antibiotics. *Antimicrob Agents Chemother.* 1992;36:2577-2583.
22. Bell MJ, Stockwell DC, Luban NLC, et al. Ceftriaxone-induced hemolytic anemia and hepatitis in an adolescent with hemoglobin SC disease. *Pediatr Crit Care Med.* 2005;6:363-366.
23. Torun D, Sezer S, Kayaselcuk F, et al. Acute Interstitial Nephritis Due to Cefoperazone. *Ann Pharmacother.* 2004;38:1446-1448.

Cefepime

1. Available at: http://www.usp.org/hqi/similarProducts/choosy.html. Accessed July 27, 2009.
2. Cefepime [package insert]. Deerfield, IL: Baxter Healthcare Inc.
3. Capparelli E, Hochwald C, Rasmussen M, et al. Population pharmacokinetics of cefepime in the neonate. *Antimicrob Agents Chemother.* 2005;49:2760-2766.
4. American Academy of Pediatrics. Pickering LK, Baker CJ, Kimberlin DW, et al., eds. *2009 Red Book: Report of the Committee on Infectious Diseases.* 28th ed. Elk Grove Village, IL: American Academy of Pediatrics; 2009.
5. Shahid SK. Efficacy and safety of cefepime in laste-onset ventilator-associated pneumonia in infants: pilot randomized and controlled study. *Ann Tropical Med Parasitol.* 2008;1:63-71.
6. Baddour LM, Wilson WR, Bayer AS, et al. Infective endocarditis: diagnosis, antimicrobial therapy, and management of complications: a statement for healthcare professionals from the Committee on Rheumatic Fever, Endocarditis, and Kawasaki Disease, Council on Cardiovascular Disease in the Young, and the Councils on Clinical Cardiology, Stroke, and Cardiovascular Surgery and Anesthesia, American Heart Association: endorsed by the Infectious Diseases Society of America. *Circulation.* 2005;111:e394-e434.
7. Hamelin BA, Moore N, Knupp CA, et al. Cefepime pharmacokinetics in cystic fibrosis. *Pharmacotherapy.* 1993;465-470.

References

8. Arguedas AG, Stutman HR, Zaleska M, et al. Pharmacokinetics and clinical response in patients with cystic fibrosis. *Am J Dis Child.* 1992;146;797-802.
9. Chastagner P, Plouvier E, Eyer D, et al. Efficacy of cefepime and amikacin in the empiric treatment of febrile neutropenic children with cancer. *Med Ped Oncol.* 2000;34:306-308.
10. Mustafa MM, Carlson L, Tkaczewski I, et al. Comparative study of cefepime versus ceftazidime in the empiric treatment of pediatric cancer patients with fever and neutropenia. *Pediatr Infect Dis J.* 2001;20:362-369.
11. Borbolla JR, Lopez-Hernandez MA, Gonzalez-Avante M, et al. Comparison of cefepime versus ceftriaxone-amikacin as empirical regimens for the treatment of febrile neutropenia in acute leukemia patients. *Chemotherapy.* 2001;47:381-384.
12. Hamidah A, Lim YS, Zulkifli SA, et al. Cefepime plus amikacin as an initial empirical therapy of febrile neutropenia in paediatric cancer patients. *Singapore Med J.* 2007;48:615-619.
13. Saez-Llorens X, Castano E, Garcia R, et al. Prospective randomized comparison of cefepime and cefotaxime for treatment of bacterial meningitis in infants and children. *Antimicrob Agents Chemother.* 1995;39:937-940.
14. Saez-Llorens X, O'Ryan M. Cefepime in the empiric treatment of meningitis in children. *Pediatr Infect Dis J.* 2001;20:356-361.
15. Schaad, UB, Eskola J, Kafetzis D, et al. Cefepime vs. ceftazidime treatment of pyelonephritis: a European randomized, controlled study of 300 pediatric cases. *Pediatr Infect Dis J.* 1998;17:639-644.
16. Reed MD, Yamashita TS, Knupp CK, et al. Pharmacokinetics of intravenously or intramuscularly administered cefepime in infants and children. *Antimicrob Agents Chemother.* 1997;41:1783-1787.
17. Henry N, Hoeker JL, Rhodes KH. Antimicrobial therapy for infants and children: guidelines for the inpatient and outpatient practice of pediatric infectious disease. *Mayo Clinic Proceed.* 2000;5:86-97.
18. Bradley JS, Arrieta A. Empiric use of cefepime in the treatment of lower respiratory tract infections in children. *Pediatr Infect Dis.* 2001;20:343-349.
19. Arrieta AC, Bradley JS. Empiric use of cefepime in the treatment of serious urinary tract infections in children. *Pediatr Infect Dis J.* 2001;20:350-355.
20. Aronoff GR, Berns JS, Brier ME, et al. Drug prescribing in renal failure. 4th ed. Available at: http://www.kdp-baptist.louisville.edu/renalbook/. Accessed September 23, 2009.
21. Sampol E, Jacquet A, Viggiano M, et al. Plama, urine, and skin pharmacokinetics of cefepime in burn patients. *J Antimicrob Chemother.* 2000;46:315-317.
22. Trissel LA, ed. *Handbook on Injectable Drugs.* 15th ed. Bethesda, MD: American Society of Health-System Pharmacists; 2009.
23. Garrelts JC, Wagner DJ. The pharmacokinetics, safety, and tolerance of cefepime administered as an intravenous bolus or a rapid infusion. *Ann Pharmacother.* 1999;33:1258-1261.
24. Burgess DS, Hastings RW, Hardin TC. Pharmacokinetic and pharmacodynamics of cefepime administration by intermittent and continuous infusion. *Clin Ther.* 2000;22:66-75.

Cefotaxime Sodium

1. Available at: http://www.usp.org/hqi/similarProducts/choosy.html. Accessed September 24, 2009.
2. Claforan [package insert]. Bridgewater, NJ: Sanofi-Aventis US LLC; September 2008.
3. Prober CG, Stevenson DK, Benitz WE. The use of antibiotics in neonates weighing less than 1200 grams. *Pediatr Infect Dis J.* 1990;9:111-121.
4. American Academy of Pediatrics. Pickering LK, Baker CJ, Kimberlin DW, et al., eds. *2009 Red Book: Report of the Committee on Infectious Diseases.* 28th ed. Elk Grove Village, IL: American Academy of Pediatrics; 2009.
5. McCracken GH, Threlkeld NE, Thomas ML. Pharmacokinetics of cefotaxime in newborn infants. *Antimicrob Agents Chemother.* 1982;21:683-684.
6. Kearns GL, Jacobs RF, Thomas BR, et al. Cefotaxime and desacetylcefotaxime pharmacokinetics in very low birth weight neonates. *J Pediatr.* 1989;114:461-467.
7. Gouyon JB, Pechinot A, Safran C, et al. Pharmacokinetics of cefotaxime in preterm infants. *Dev Pharmacol Ther.* 1990;14:29-34.
8. Kafetzis DA, Brater DC, Kanarios J, et al. Clinical pharmacology of cefotaxime in pediatric patients. *Antimicrob Agents Chemother.* 1981;20:487-490.
9. Kearns GL, Young RA, Jacobs RF. Cefotaxime dosage in infants and children: pharmacokinetic and clinical rationale for an extended dosage interval. *Clin Pharmacokinet.* 1992;22:284-297.
10. Tunkel AR, Hartman BJ, Kaplan SL, et al. Practice guidelines for the management of bacterial meningitis. *Clin Infect Dis.* 2004;39:1267-1284.
11. Kaplan SL, Patrick CC. Cefotaxime and aminoglycoside treatment of meningitis caused by gram-negative enteric organisms. *Pediatr Infect Dis J.* 1990;9:810-814.
12. Trang JM, Jacobs RF, Kearns GL, et al. Cefotaxime and desacetylcefotaxime pharmacokinetics in infants and children with meningitis. *Antimicrob Agents Chemother.* 1985;28:791-795.
13. Odio CM, Faingezicht I, Salas JL, et al. Cefotaxime vs. conventional therapy for the treatment of bacterial meningitis of infants and children. *Pediatr Infect Dis J.* 1986;5:402-407.
14. Fillastre JP, Leroy A, Humbert G, et al. Pharmacokinetics of cefotaxime in subjects with normal and impaired renal function. *J Antimicrob Chemother.* 1980;6(suppl A):103-111.
15. Aronoff GR, Berns JS, Brier ME, et al. Drug prescribing in renal failure. 4th ed. Available at: http://www.kdp-baptist.louisville.edu/renalbook/. Accessed September 19, 2009.
16. Trissel LA, ed. *Handbook on Injectable Drugs.* 15th ed. Bethesda, MD: American Society of Health-System Pharmacists; 2009.
17. Robinson DC, Cookson TL, Frisafe JA. Concentration guidelines for parenteral antibiotics in fluid-restricted patients. *Drug Intell Clin Pharm.* 1987;21:985-989.
18. Robinson CA, Sawyer JE. Y-site compatibility of medications with parenteral nutrition. *J Pediatr Pharmacol Ther.* 2009;14:49-57.
19. Zhanel GG. Cephalosporin-induced nephrotoxicity: does it exist? *DICP.* 1990;24:262-265.
20. Williams KJ, Bax RP, Brown H, et al. Antibiotic treatment and associated prolonged prothrombin time. *J Clin Pathol.* 1991;44:738-741.
21. Grill MF, Maganti R. Cephalosporin-induced neurotoxicity: clinical manifestations, potential pathogenic mechanisms, and the role of electroencephalographic monitoring. *Ann Pharmacother.* 2008;42:1843-1850.
22. Cefotaxime. Lexi-Comp® Online with AHFS® (database). Hudson, OH: Lexi-Comp Inc; updated August 13, 2009.

Cefotetan Disodium

1. Available at: http://www.usp.org/hqi/similarProducts/choosy.html. Accessed September 13, 2009.
2. Cefotan [package insert]. Wilmington, DE: AstraZeneca Pharmaceuticals LP; January 2004.
3. Johnson ST, Fueger JT, Gottschall JL. One center's experience: the serology and drugs associated with drug-induced immune hemolytic anemia—a new paradigm. *Transfusion.* 2007;47:697-702.
4. American Academy of Pediatrics. Pickering LK, Baker CJ, Kimberlin DW, et al., eds. *2009 Red Book: Report of the Committee on Infectious Diseases.* 28th ed. Elk Grove Village, IL: American Academy of Pediatrics; 2009.
5. Hemsell DL, Little BB, Faro S, et al. Comparison of three regimens recommended by the Centers for Disease Control and Prevention for the treatment of women hospitalized with acute pelvic inflammatory disease. *Clin Infect Dis.* 1994;19:720-727.

References

6. Available at: http://www.cdc.gov/std/treatment/2006/GonUpdateApril2007.pdf Accessed September 13, 2009.
7. Aronoff GR, Berns JS, Brier ME, et al. Drug prescribing in renal failure. 4th ed. Available at: http://www.kdp-baptist.louisville.edu/renalbook/. Accessed September 3, 2009.
8. Trissel LA, ed. *Handbook on Injectable Drugs.* 15th ed. Bethesda, MD: American Society of Health-System Pharmacists; 2009.
9. McLaughlin JE, Reeves DS. Clinical and laboratory evidence for inactivation of gentamicin by carbenicillin. *Lancet.* 1971;1:261-264.
10. Riff LJ, Jackson GG. Laboratory and clinical conditions for gentamicin inactivation by carbenicillin. *Arch Intern Med.* 1972;130:887-891.
11. Manian FA, Stone WJ, Alford RH. Adverse antibiotic effects associated with renal insufficiency. *Rev Infect Dis.* 1990;12:236-249.
12. Davies M, Morgan JR, Anand C. Interactions of carbenicillin and ticarcillin with gentamicin. *Antimicrob Agents Chemother.* 1975;7:431-434.
13. Weibert R, Keane W, Shapiro F. Carbenicillin inactivation of aminoglycosides in patients with severe renal failure. *Trans Amer Soc Artif Int Organs.* 1976;22:439-443.
14. Robinson CA, Sawyer JE. Y-site compatibility of medications with parenteral nutrition. *J Pediatr Pharmacol Ther.* 2009;14:49-57.
15. Craig WA, Ebert SC. Continuous infusion of beta-lactam antibiotics. *Antimicrob Agents Chemother.* 1992;36:2577-2583.
16. Williams KJ, Bax RP, Brown H, et al. Antibiotic treatment and associated prolonged prothrombin time. *J Clin Pathol.* 1991;44:738-741.
17. Cefotetan. Lexi-Comp® Online with AHFS® (database). Hudson, OH: Lexi-Comp Inc; updated August 13, 2009.

Cefoxitin Sodium

1. Available at: http://www.usp.org/hqi/similarProducts/choosy.html. Accessed June 19, 2009.
2. Cefoxitin sodium [package insert]. Deerfield, IL: Merck & Co Inc; October 2006.
3. Regazzi MB, Chirico G, Cristiani D, et al. Cefoxitin in newborn infants. A clinical and pharmacokinetic study. *Eur J Clin Pharmacol.* 1983;25:507-509.
4. Farmer K. Use of cefoxitin in the newborn. *N Z Med J.* 1982;95:398.
5. Yogev R, Delaplane D, Wiringa K. Cefoxitin in a neonate. *Pediatr Infect Dis.* 1983;2:342-343.
6. American Academy of Pediatrics. Pickering LK, Baker CJ, Kimberlin DW, et al., eds. *2009 Red Book: Report of the Committee on Infectious Diseases.* 28th ed. Elk Grove Village, IL: American Academy of Pediatrics; 2009.
7. The Lexi-Comp® Online with AHFS® database is comprised of material copyrighted independently by Lexi-Comp and the American Society of Health-System Pharmacists (ASHP); updated August 12, 2009.
8. Gnehm HE, Seger RA, Boyle CM. The efficacy and tolerance of cefoxitin in the treatment of paediatric infections. *Curr Med Res Opin.* 1982;8:44-50.
9. Jacobson JA, Santos JI, Palmer WM. Clinical and bacteriological evaluation of cefoxitin in children. *Antimicrob Agents Chemother.* 1979;16:183-185.
10. Feldman WE, Moffitt S, Sprow N. Clinical and pharmacokinetic evaluation of parenteral cefoxitin in infants and children. *Antimicrob Agents Chemother.* 1980;17:669-674.
11. Available at: http://www.cdc.gov/std/treatment/2006/GonUpdateApril2007.pdf. Accessed August 29, 2009.
12. Gutierrez C, Vila J, Garcia-Sala C, et al. Study of appendicitis in children treated with four different antibiotic regimens. *J Pediatr Surg.* 1987;22:865-868.
13. Aronoff GR, Berns JS, Brier ME, et al. Drug prescribing in renal failure. 4th ed. Available at: http://www.kdp-baptist.louisville.edu/renalbook/. Accessed August 28, 2009.
14. Trissel LA, ed. *Handbook on Injectable Drugs.* 15th ed. Bethesda, MD: American Society of Health-System Pharmacists; 2009.
15. Robinson DC, Cookson TL, Frisafe JA. Concentration guidelines for parenteral antibiotics in fluid-restricted patients. *Drug Intell Clin Pharm.* 1987;21:985-989.
16. McLaughlin JE, Reeves DS. Clinical and laboratory evidence for inactivation of gentamicin by carbenicillin. *Lancet.* 1971;1(7693):261-264.
17. Riff LJ, Jackson GG. Laboratory and clinical conditions for gentamicin inactivation by carbenicillin. *Arch Intern Med.* 1972;130:887-891.
18. Manian FA, Stone WJ, Alford RH. Adverse antibiotic effects associated with renal insufficiency. *Rev Infect Dis.* 1990;12:236-249.
19. Davies M, Morgan JR, Anand C. Interactions of carbenicillin and ticarcillin with gentamicin. *Antimicrob Agents Chemother.* 1975;7:431-434.
20. Weibert R, Keane W, Shapiro F. Carbenicillin inactivation of aminoglycosides in patients with severe renal failure. *Trans Amer Soc Artif Int Organs.* 1976;22:439-443.
21. Robinson CA, Sawyer JE. Y-site compatibility of medications with parenteral nutrition. *J Pediatr Pharmacol Ther.* 2009;14:49-57.
22. Craig WA, Ebert SC. Continuous infusion of beta-lactam antibiotics. *Antimicrob Agents Chemother.* 1992;36:2577-2583.
23. El-Bitar MK, Boustany RM. Common causes of uncommon seizures. *Pediatr Neurol.* 2009;41:83-87.
24. Grill MF, Maganti R. Cephalosporin-induced neurotoxicity: clinical manifestations, potential pathogenic mechanisms, and the role of electroencephalographic monitoring. *Ann Pharmacother.* 2008;42:1843-1850.
25. Strauss AA. Di(2-ethylhexyl)phthalate (DEHP). *J Pediat Pharmacol Ther.* 2004;89-95.

Ceftazidime

1. Available at: http://www.usp.org/hqi/similarProducts/choosy.html. Accessed September 24, 2009.
2. Ceftazidime [package insert]. Research Triangle Park, NC: GlaxoSmithKline; January 2007.
3. American Academy of Pediatrics. Pickering LK, Baker CJ, Kimberlin DW, et al., eds. *2009 Red Book: Report of the Committee on Infectious Diseases.* 28th ed. Elk Grove Village, IL: American Academy of Pediatrics; 2009.
4. Nelson JD, Bradley JS, eds. *Nelson's Pocket Book of Pediatric Antimicrobial Therapy.* 17th ed. Chicago, IL: American Academy of Pediatrics; 2009.
5. Mulhall A, de Louvois J. The pharmacokinetics and safety of ceftazidime in the neonate. *J Antimicrob Chemother.* 1985;15:97-103.
6. Tessin L, Trollfors B, Thiringer K, et al. Concentrations of ceftazidime, tobramycin, and ampicillin on the cerebrospinal fluid of newborn infants. *Eur J Pediatr.* 1989;148:679-681.
7. Tessin L, Thiringer K, Trollfors B, et al. Comparison of serum concentrations of ceftazidime and tobramycin in newborn infants. *Eur J Pediatr.* 1988;147:405-407.
8. McCracken GH, Threlkeld N, Thomas ML. The pharmacokinetics of ceftazidime in newborn infants. *Antimicrob Agents Chemother.* 1984;26:583-584.
9. Assael BM, Boccazi A, Caccamo ML, et al. Clinical pharmacology of ceftazidime in paediatrics. *J Antimicrob Chemother.* 1983;12(suppl A):341-346.
10. Prinsloo JG, Delport SD, Moncrieff J, et al. A preliminary pharmacokinetic study of ceftazidime in premature, newborn and small infants. *J Antimicrob Chemother.* 1983;12(suppl A):361-364.
11. Mulhall A, de Louvois J. The pharmacokinetics and safety of ceftazidime in the neonate. *J Antimicrob Chemother.* 1985;15:97-103.
12. van den Anker JN, Schoemaker RC, van der Heijden BJ. Once-daily versus twice-daily administration of ceftazidime in the premature infant. *Antimicrob Chemother.* 1995;39:2048-2050.
13. van den Anker JN, Schoemaker RC, Hop WC, et al. Ceftazidime pharmacokinetics in preterm infants: effect of renal function and gestational age. *Clin Pharmacol Ther.* 1995;58:650-659.
14. Rodriguez WJ, Khan WN, Gold B, et al. Ceftazidime in the treatment of meningitis in infants and children over one month of age. *Am J Med.* 1985;79(suppl 2A):52-55.
15. Hatch D, Overturf GD, Kovacs A, et al. Treatment of bacterial meningitis with ceftazidime. *Pediatr Infect Dis.* 1986;5:416-420.

16. Rodriguez WJ, Puig JR, Khan W, et al. Ceftazidime vs. standard therapy for pediatric meningitis: therapeutic, pharmacologic and epidemiologic observations. *Pediatr Infect Dis J.* 1986;5:408-415.
17. Viscoli C, Moroni C, Boni L, et al. Ceftazidime plus amikacin versus ceftazidime plus vancomycin as empiric therapy in febrile neutropenic children with cancer. *Rev Infect Dis.* 1991;13:397-404.
18. Granowetter L, Wells H, Lange BJ. Ceftazidime with or without vancomycin vs. cephalothin, carbenicillin and gentamicin as the initial therapy of the febrile neutropenic pediatric cancer patient. *Pediatr Infect Dis.* 1988;7:165-170.
19. Jacobs RF, Vats TS, Pappa KA, et al. Ceftazidime versus ceftazidime plus tobramycin in febrile neutropenic children. *Infection.* 1993;21:223-228.
20. Tunkel AR, Hartman BJ, Kaplan SL, et al. Practice guidelines for the management of bacterial meningitis. *Clin Infect Dis.* 2004;39:1267-1284.
21. Cullen RT, McCrae WM, Govan J, et al. Ceftazidime in cystic fibrosis: clinical, microbiological and immunological studies. *J Antimicrob Chemother.* 1983;12(suppl A):369-375.
22. Schadd UB, Wedgwood-Krucko J, Suter S, et al. Efficacy of inhaled amikacin as adjunct to intravenous combination therapy (ceftazidime and amikacin) in cystic fibrosis. *J Pediatr.* 1987;111:599-605.
23. Gold R, Carpenter S, Heurter H, et al. Randomized trial of ceftazidime versus placebo in the management of acute respiratory exacerbations in patients with cystic fibrosis. *J Pediatr.* 1987;111:907-913.
24. DeBoeck K, Breysem L. Treatment of pseudomonas aeruginosa lung infection in cystic fibrosis with high or conventional doses of ceftazidime. *J Antimicrob Chemother.* 1998;41:407-409.
25. Munzenberger PJ, Man-Ching J, Holliday SJ. Relationship of ceftazidime pharmacokinetics indices with therapeutic outcomes in patients with cystic fibrosis. *Pediatr Infect Dis J.* 1993;12:997-1001.
26. Latzin P, Fehling M, Bauernfeind A, et al. Efficacy and safety of intravenous meropenem and tobramycin versus ceftazidime and tobramycin in cystic fibrosis. *J Cystic Fibrosis.* 2008;7:142-146.
27. Bosso JA, Bonapace CR, Flume PA, et al. A pilot study of the efficacy of constant infusion ceftazidime in the treatment of endobronchial infections in adults with cystic fibrosis. *Pharmacotherapy.* 1999;19:620-626.
28. Chuang YY, Hung IJ, Yang CP, et al. Cefepime versus ceftazidime as empiric monotherapy for fever and neutropenia in children with cancer. *Pediatr Infect Dis J.* 2002;21:203-209.
29. Ohkawa M, Nakashima T, Shoda R, et al. Pharmacokinetics of ceftazidime in patients with renal insufficiency and in those undergoing hemodialysis. *Chemotherapy.* 1985;31:410-416.
30. Welage LS, Schultz RW, Schentag JJ. Pharmacokinetics of ceftazidime in patients with renal insufficiency. *Antimicrob Agents Chemother.* 1984;25:201-204.
31. Ackerman BH, Ross J, Tofte RW, et al. Effect of decreased renal function on the pharmacokinetics of ceftazidime. *Antimicrob Agents Chemother.* 1984;25:785-786.
32. Aronoff GR, Berns JS, Brier ME, et al. Drug prescribing in renal failure. 4th ed. Available at: http://www.kdp-baptist.louisville.edu/renalbook/. Accessed September 24, 2009.
33. Yost RL, Ramphal R. Ceftazidime review. *Drug Intell Clin Pharm.* 1985;19:509-513.
34. Scully BE, Neu HC. Clinical efficacy of ceftazidime: treatment of serious infection due to multiresistant Pseudomonas and other gram-negative bacteria. *Arch Intern Med.* 1984;144:57-62.
35. Trissel LA, ed. *Handbook on Injectable Drugs.* 15th ed. Bethesda, MD: American Society of Health-System Pharmacists; 2009.
36. Robinson DC, Cookson TL, Frisafe JA. Concentration guidelines for parenteral antibiotics in fluid-restricted patients. *Drug Intell Clin Pharm.* 1987;21:985-989.
37. Robinson CA, Sawyer JE. Y-site compatibility of medications with parenteral nutrition. *J Pediatr Pharmacol Ther.* 2009;14:49-57.
38. Dalle JH, Gnansounou M, Husson MO, et al. Continuous infusion of ceftazidime in the empiric treatment of febrile neutropenic children with cancer. *J Pediatr Hem Onc.* 2002;24:714-716.
39. Zhanel GG. Cephalosporin-induced nephrotoxicity: does it exist? *DICP.* 1990;24:262-265.
40. Williams KJ, Bax RP, Brown H, et al. Antibiotic treatment and associated prolonged prothrombin time. *J Clin Pathol.* 1991;44:738-741.
41. Grill MF, Maganti R. Cephalosporin-induced neurotoxicity: clinical manifestations, potential pathogenic mechanisms, and the role of electroencephalographic monitoring. *Ann Pharmacother.* 2008;42:1843-1850.
42. van den Anker JN, Hop WC, Schoemaker RC, et al. Ceftazidime pharmacokinetics in preterm infants: effect of postnatal age and postnatal exposure to indomethacin. *Br J Clin Pharmacol.* 1995;40:439-443.

CefTRIAXone Sodium

1. Available at: http://www.ismp.org/Tools/tallmanletters.pdf. Accessed September 19, 2009.
2. Available at: http://www.usp.org/hqi/similarProducts/choosy.htm. Accessed September 19, 2009.
3. Ceftriaxone [package insert]. Deerfield, IL: Baxter Healthcare Corp; September 2008.
4. Available at: http://www.accessdata.fda.gov/scripts/cdrh/cfdocs/psn/transcript.cfm?show=88#4/. Accessed September 19, 2009.
5. American Academy of Pediatrics. Pickering LK, Baker CJ, Kimberlin DW, et al., eds. *2009 Red Book: Report of the Committee on Infectious Diseases.* 28th ed. Elk Grove Village, IL: American Academy of Pediatrics; 2009.
6. McCracken GH, Siegel JD, Threlkeld N, et al. Ceftriaxone pharmacokinetics in newborn infants. *Antimicrob Agents Chemother.* 1983;23:341-343.
7. Nelson JD, Bradley JS, eds. *Nelson's Pocket Book of Pediatric Antimicrobial Therapy.* 17th ed. Chicago, IL: American Academy of Pediatrics; 2009.
8. Higham M, Cunningham FM, Teele DW. Ceftriaxone administered once or twice a day for treatment of bacterial infections of childhood. *Pediatr Infect Dis.* 1985;4:22-26.
9. Chadwick EG, Connor EM, Shulman ST, et al. Efficacy of ceftriaxone in treatment of serious childhood infections. *J Pediatr.* 1983;103:141-145.
10. Tunkel AR, Hartman BJ, Kaplan SL, et al. Practice guidelines for the management of bacterial meningitis. *Clin Infect Dis.* 2004;39:1267-1284.
11. Congeni BL, Bradley J, Hammerschlag MR. Safety and efficacy of once daily ceftriaxone for the treatment of bacterial meningitis. *Pediatr Infect Dis.* 1986;5:293-297.
12. Lebel MH, Hoyt MJ, McCracken GH. Comparative efficacy of ceftriaxone and cefuroxime for treatment of bacterial meningitis. *J Pediatr.* 1989;114:1049-1054.
13. Kavaliotis J, Manios SG, Kansouzidou A, et al. Treatment of childhood bacterial meningitis with ceftriaxone once daily: open, prospective randomized, comparative study of short-course versus standard-length therapy. *Chemotherapy.* 1989;35:296-303.
14. Frenkel LD. Multicenter Ceftriaxone Pediatric Study Group. Once-daily administration of ceftriaxone for the treatment of selected serious bacterial infections in children. *Pediatrics.* 1988;82:486-491.
15. Peltola H, Anttila M, Renkonen O, et al. Randomized comparison of chloramphenicol, ampicillin, cefotaxime, and ceftriaxone for childhood bacterial meningitis. *Lancet.* 1989;1:1281-1287.
16. Grubbauer HM, Dornbusch HJ, Dittrich P, et al. Ceftriaxone monotherapy for bacterial meningitis in children. *Chemotherapy.* 1990;36:441-447.
17. Tuncer AM, Gur I, Ertem U, et al. Once daily ceftriaxone for meningococcemia and meningococcal meningitis. *Pediatr Infect Dis.* 1988;7:711-713.
18. Del Rio MA, Chrane D, Shelton S, et al. Ceftriaxone versus ampicillin and chloramphenicol for treatment of bacterial meningitis in children. *Lancet.* 1983;1:1241-1244.
19. Steele RW, Eyre LB, Bradsher RW, et al. Pharmacokinetics of ceftriaxone in pediatric patients with meningitis. *Antimicrob Agents Chemother.* 1983;23:191-194.

References

20. Steele RW, Bradsher RW. Comparison of ceftriaxone with standard therapy for bacterial meningitis. *J Pediatr.* 1983;103:138-140.
21. Chonmaitree T, Congeni BL, Munoz J, et al. Twice daily ceftriaxone therapy for serious bacterial infections in children. *J Antimicrob Chemother.* 1984;13:511-516.
22. Prado V, Cohen J, Banfi A, et al. Ceftriaxone in the treatment of bacterial meningitis in children. *Chemotherapy.* 1986;32:383-390.
23. Craig JC, Abbott GD, Mogridge NB. Ceftriaxone for pediatric bacterial meningitis: a report of 62 children and a review of the literature. *NZ Med J.* 1992;105:441-444.
24. Gavalda J, Len O, Miró JM, et al. Brief communication: treatment of *enterococcus faecalis* endocarditis with ampicillin plus ceftriaxone. *Ann Intern Med.* 2007;146:574-579.
25. Workowski KA, Berman SM. Sexually transmitted diseases treatment guidelines, 2008. *Morbid Mortal Weekly.* 2006;55:RR-11.
26. Green SM, Rothrock SG. Single-dose intramuscular ceftriaxone for acute otitis media in children. *Pediatrics.* 1993;91:23-30.
27. Chamberlain JM, Boenning DA, Waisman Y, et al. Single-dose ceftriaxone versus 10 days of cefaclor for otitis media. *Clin Pediatr.* 1994;33:642-646.
28. Barnett ED, Teele DW, Klein JO, et al. Comparison of ceftriaxone and trimethoprim-sulfamethoxazole for acute otitis media. Greater Boston Otitis Media Study Group. *Pediatrics.* 1997;99:23-28.
29. Aronoff GR, Berns JS, Brier ME, et al. Drug prescribing in renal failure. 4th ed. Available at: http://www.kdp-baptist.louisville.edu/renalbook/. Accessed September 25, 2009.
30. Patel IH, Sugihara JG, Weinfeld RE, et al. Ceftriaxone pharmacokinetics in patients with various degrees of renal impairment. *Antimicrob Agents Chemother.* 1984;5:438-442.
31. Trissel LA, ed. *Handbook on Injectable Drugs.* 15th ed. Bethesda, MD: American Society of Health-System Pharmacists; 2009.
32. Robinson CA, Sawyer JE. Y-site compatibility of medications with parenteral nutrition. *J Pediatr Pharmacol Ther.* 2009;14:49-57.
33. Baumgartner JD, Glauser MP. Single daily dose treatment of severe refractory infections with ceftriaxone. *Arch Intern Med.* 1983;143:1868-1873.
34. Grubbauer HM, Dornbusch HJ, Dittrich P, et al. Ceftriaxone monotherapy for bacterial meningitis in children. *Chemotherapy.* 1990;36:441-447.
35. Lossos IS, Lossos A. Hazards of rapid administration of ceftriaxone. *Ann Pharmacother.* 1994;28:807. Letter.
36. Craig JC, Abbott GD, Mogridge NB. Ceftriaxone for pediatric bacterial meningitis: a report of 62 children and a review of the literature. *NZ Med J.* 1992;105:441-444.
37. Zhanel GG. Cephalosporin-induced nephrotoxicity: does it exist? *DICP.* 1990;24:262-265.
38. Bonnet JP, Abid L, Dabhar A, et al. Early biliary pseudolithiasis during ceftriaxone therapy for acute pyelonephritis in children: a prospective study in 34 children. *Eur J Pediatr Surg.* 2000;10:368-371.
39. Prince JS, Senac MO Jr. Ceftriaxone-associated nephrolithiasis and biliary pseudolithiasis in a child. *Pediatr Radiol.* 2003;33:648-651. Epub 2003 Jun 26.
40. Mattis LE, Saavedra JM, Shan H, et al. Life-threatening ceftriaxone-induced immune hemolytic anemia in a child with Crohn's disease. *Clin Pediatr.* 2004;43:175-178.
41. Williams KJ, Bax RP, Brown H, et al. Antibiotic treatment and associated prolonged prothrombin time. *J Clin Pathol.* 1991;44:738-741.
42. Grill MF, Maganti R. Cephalosporin-induced neurotoxicity: clinical manifestations, potential pathogenic mechanisms, and the role of electroencephalographic monitoring. *Ann Pharmacother.* 2008;42:1843-1850.

Cefuroxime Sodium

1. Available at: http://www.usp.org/hqi/similarProducts/choosy.html. Accessed September 25, 2009.
2. Cefuroxime [package insert]. Research Triangle Park, NC: GlaxoSmithKline; February 2007.
3. Nelson JD, Bradley JS, eds. *Nelson's Pocket Book of Pediatric Antimicrobial Therapy.* 17th ed. Chicago, IL: American Academy of Pediatrics; 2009.
4. Renlund M, Petty O. Pharmacokinetics and clinical efficacy of cefuroxime in the newborn period. *Proc R Soc Med.* 1977;70(suppl 9):179-182.
5. Wilkinson PJ, Belohradsky BH, Marget W. A clinical study of cefuroxime in neonates. *Proc R Soc Med.* 1977; 70(suppl 9):183-185.
6. American Academy of Pediatrics. Pickering LK, Baker CJ, Kimberlin DW, et al., eds. *2009 Red Book: Report of the Committee on Infectious Diseases.* 28th ed. Elk Grove Village, IL: American Academy of Pediatrics; 2009.
7. Nelson JD. Cefuroxime: a cephalosporin with unique applicability to pediatric practice. *Pediatr Infect Dis.* 1983;2:394-396.
8. Barson WJ, Miller MA, Marcon MJ, et al. Cefuroxime therapy for bacteremic soft-tissue infections in children. *Am J Dis Child.* 1985;139:1141-1144.
9. Nelson JD, Kusmiesz H, Shelton S. Cefuroxime therapy for pneumonia in infants and children. *Pediatr Infect Dis.* 1982;1:159-163.
10. Nelson JD, Bucholz RW, Kusmiesz H, et al. Benefits and risks of sequential parenteral-oral cephalosporin therapy for suppurative bone and joint infections. *J Pediatr Orthop.* 1982;2:255-262.
11. Azimi PH, Barson WJ, Janner D, et al. Efficacy and safety of ampicillin/sulbactam and cefuroxime in the treatment of serious skin and skin structure infections in pediatric patients. *Pediatr Infect Dis J.* 1999;18:609-613.
12. Lebel MH, Hoyt MJ, Waagner DC, et al. Magnetic resonance imaging and dexamethasone therapy for bacterial meningitis. *Am J Dis Child.* 1989;143:301-306.
13. Lebel MH, Hoyt MJ, McCracken GH. Comparative efficacy of ceftriaxone and cefuroxime for treatment of bacterial meningitis. *J Pediatr.* 1989;114:1049-1054.
14. Trissel LA, ed. *Handbook on Injectable Drugs.* 15th ed. Bethesda, MD: American Society of Health-System Pharmacists; 2009.
15. Robinson DC, Cookson TL, Frisafe JA. Concentration guidelines for parenteral antibiotics in fluid-restricted patients. *Drug Intell Clin Pharm.* 1987;21:985-989.
16. Robinson CA, Sawyer JE. Y-site compatibility of medications with parenteral nutrition. *J Pediatr Pharmacol Ther.* 2009;14:49-57.
17. Schaad UB, Suter S, Gianella-Borradori A, et al. A comparison of ceftriaxone and cefuroxime for the treatment of bacterial meningitis in children. *N Engl J Med.* 1990;322:141-147.
18. Zhanel GG. Cephalosporin-induced nephrotoxicity: does it exist? *DICP.* 1990;24:262-265.
19. Grill MF, Maganti R. Cephalosporin-induced neurotoxicity: clinical manifestations, potential pathogenic mechanisms, and the role of electroencephalographic monitoring. *Ann Pharmacother.* 2008;42:1843-1850.
20. Williams KJ, Bax RP, Brown H, et al. Antibiotic treatment and associated prolonged prothrombin time. *J Clin Pathol.* 1991;44:738-741.

Chloramphenicol Sodium Succinate

1. Chloramphenicol [package insert] Bristol, TN: Monarch Pharmaceuticals; April 2007.
2. American Academy of Pediatrics. Pickering LK, Baker CJ, Kimberlin DW, et al., eds. *2009 Red Book: Report of the Committee on Infectious Diseases.* 28th ed. Elk Grove Village, IL: American Academy of Pediatrics; 2009.
3. Mulhall A, Berry DJ, de Louvois J. Chloramphenicol in paediatrics: current prescribing practice and the need to monitor. *Eur J Pediatr.* 1988;147:574-578.
4. Rajchgot P, Prober CG, Soldin S, et al. Initiation of chloramphenicol therapy in the newborn infant. *J Pediatr.* 1982;101:1018-1021.
5. Feder HM. Chloramphenicol: what we have learned in the last decade. *South Med J.* 1986;79:1129-1134.
6. Prober CG, Stevenson DK, Benitz WE. The use of antibiotics in neonates weighing less than 1200 grams. *Pediatr Infect Dis J.* 1990;9:111-121.

References

7. Glazer JP, Danish MA, Plotkin SA, et al. Disposition of chloramphenicol in low birth weight infants. *Pediatrics*. 1980;66:573-578.
8. Meissner HC, Smith AL. The current status of chloramphenicol. *Pediatrics*. 1979;64:348-356.
9. Laferriere CI, Marks MI. Chloramphenicol: properties and clinical use. *Pediatr Infect Dis*. 1982;1:257-264.
10. Bartlett JG. Chloramphenicol. *Med Clin North Am*. 1982;66:91-102.
11. Smith AL, Weber A. Pharmacology of chloramphenicol. *Pediatr Clin North Am*. 1983;30:209-236.
12. Friedman CA, Lovejoy FC, Smith AL. Chloramphenicol disposition in infants and children. *J Pediatr*. 1979;95:1071-1077.
13. Sack CM, Koup JR, Smith AL. Chloramphenicol pharmacokinetics in infants and young children. *Pediatrics*. 1980;66:579-584.
14. Kauffman RE, Thirumoorthi MC, Buckley JA, et al. Relative bioavailability of intravenous chloramphenicol succinate and oral chloramphenicol palmitate in infants and children. *J Pediatr*. 1981;99:963-967.
15. Burckhart GJ, Barrett FF, Straughn AB, et al. Chloramphenicol clearance in infants. *J Clin Pharmacol*. 1982;22:49-52.
16. Rodriguez WJ, Puig JR, Khan W, et al. Ceftazidime vs. standard therapy for pediatric meningitis: therapeutic, pharmacologic and epidemiologic observations. *Pediatr Infect Dis J*. 1986;5:408-415.
17. Nahata MC. Serum concentrations and adverse effects of chloramphenicol in pediatric patients. *Chemotherapy*. 1987;33:322-327.
18. Craig JC, Abbott GD, Mogridge NB. Ceftriaxone for pediatric bacterial meningitis: a report of 62 children and a review of the literature. *NZ Med J*. 1992;105:441-444.
19. Mato SP, Robinson S, Begue RE. Vancomycin-resistant enterococcus faecium meningitis successfully treated with chloramphenicol. *Pediatr Infect Dis J*. 1999;18:483-484.
20. Marks WA, Stutman HR, Marks MI, et al. Cefuroxime versus ampicillin plus chloramphenicol in childhood bacterial meningitis: a multicenter randomized controlled trial. *J Pediatr*. 1986;109:123-130.
21. Odio CM, Faingezicht I, Salas JL, et al. Cefotaxime vs. conventional therapy for the treatment of bacterial meningitis of infants and children. *Pediatr Infect Dis J*. 1986;5:402-407.
22. Brasfield JH, Record KE, Griffen WO, et al. Chloramphenicol and chloramphenicol succinate concentrations in patients with renal impairment. *Clin Pharm*. 1983;2:355-358.
23. Phelps SJ, Tsiu W, Barrett FF, et al. Chloramphenicol-induced cardiovascular collapse in an anephric patient. *Pediatr Infect Dis J*. 1987;6:285-288.
24. American Society of Health-System Pharmacists. American Hospital Formulary System. Available at: http://ahfsfirst.firstdatabank.com/AHFSfirst/NSAHFSFirstSearchmain.asp. Accessed August 11, 2006.
25. Weiss CF, Glazko AJ, Weston JK. Chloramphenicol in the newborn infant: a physiologic explanation of its toxicity when given in excessive doses. *N Engl J Med*. 1960;262:787-794.
26. Trissel LA, ed. *Handbook on Injectable Drugs*. 15th ed. Bethesda, MD: American Society of Health-System Pharmacists; 2009.
27. Robinson CA, Sawyer JE. Y-site compatibility of medications with parenteral nutrition. *J Pediatr Pharmacol Ther*. 2009;14:49-57.
28. Rapp RP, Wermeling DP, Piecoro JJ Jr. Guidelines for the administration of commonly used intravenous drugs—1984 update. *Drug Intell Clin Pharm*. 1984;18:217-232.
29. Weber MW, Gatchalian SR, Ogunlesi O, et al. Chloramphenicol pharmacokinetics in infants less than three months of age in the Philippines and the Gambia. *Pediatr Infect Dis J*. 1999;18:896-901.
30. Scapellato PG, Ormazabal C, Scapellato JL, et al. Meningitis due to vancomycin-resistant *enterococcus faecium* successfully treated with combined intravenous and intraventricular chloramphenicol. *J Clin Microbiol*. 2005;43:3578-3579.
31. Brown RT. Chloramphenicol toxicity in an adolescent. *J Adolesc Health Care*. 1982;3:53-55.
32. Biancaniello T, Meyer RA, Kaplan S. Chloramphenicol and cardiotoxicity. *J Pediatr*. 1981;98:828-830.
33. Krasinski K, Perkin R, Rutledge J. Gray baby syndrome revisited. *Clin Pediatr*. 1982;21:571-572.
34. Wilkinson JD, Pollack MM, Costello J. Chloramphenicol toxicity: hemodynamic and oxygen utilization effects. *Pediatr Infect Dis J*. 1985;4:69-72.
35. Craft AW, Brocklebank JT, Hey EN, et al. The grey toddler: chloramphenicol toxicity. *Arch Dis Child*. 1974;49:235-237.
36. Evans LS, Kleiman MB. Acidosis as a presenting feature of chloramphenicol toxicity. *J Pediatr*. 1986;108:475-477.
37. Chlorampenicol. Lexi-Comp® Online with AHFS® (database). Hudson, OH: Lexi-Comp Inc; August 13, 2009.
38. Koup JR, Gibaldi M, McNamara P, et al. Interaction of chloramphenicol with phenytoin and phenobarbital. *Clin Pharmacol Ther*. 1978;24:571-575.
39. Bui LL, Huang DD. Possible interaction between cyclosporin and chloramphenicol. *Ann Pharmacother*. 1999;33:252-253.
40. Schulman SL, Shaw LM, Jabs K, et al. Interaction between tacrolimus and chloramphenicol in a renal transplant recipient. *Transplantation*. 1998;65:1397-1398.

ChlorproMAZINE HCl

1. Available at: http://ismp.org/Tools/confuseddrugnames.pdf. Accessed August 26, 2009.
2. Available at: http://www.usp.org/hqi/similarProducts/choosy.html. Accessed August 24, 2009.
3. Available at: http://www.fda.gov/Drugs/DrugSafety/PostmarketDrugSafetyInformationforPatientsandProviders/ucm124830.htm. Accessed September, 15 2009.
4. Chlorpromazine hydrochloride [package insert]. Deerfield, IL: Baxter Healthcare Corporation; MLT-19/1.0.
5. Riemenschneider TA, Nielsen HC, Ruttenberg HD, et al. Disturbances of the transitional circulation: spectrum of pulmonary hypertension and myocardial dysfunction. *J Pediatr*. 1976;89:622-625.
6. Nordeng H, Lindemann R, Perminov KV, et al. Neonatal withdrawal syndrome after *in utero* exposure to selective serotonin reuptake inhibitors. *Acta Paediatr*. 2001;90:288-291.
7. Infants of drug-dependent mothers. In: Kagan BM, Gellis SS, eds. *Current Pediatric Therapy Eleven*. Philadelphia, PA: WB Saunders Company; 1984:653.
8. Larsson LE, Ekstrom-Jodal B, Hjalmarson O. The effect of chlorpromazine in severe hypoxia in newborn infants. *Acta Paediatr Scand*. 1982;71:399-402.
9. Chlorpromazine hydrochloride. Lexi-Comp Online with AHFS (database). Bethesda, MD: American Society of Health-System Pharmacists; 2009. Accessed September 15, 2009.
10. Marshall G, Kerr S, Vowels M, et al. Antiemetic therapy for chemotherapy-induced vomiting: metoclopramide, benztropine, dexamethasone, and lorazepam regimens compared with chlorpromazine alone. *J Pediatr*. 1989;115:156-160.
11. Mehta P, Gross S, Graham-Pole J, et al. Methylprednisolone for chemotherapy-induced emesis: a double-blind randomized trial in children. *J Pediatr*. 1986;108:774-776.
12. Graham-Pole J, Weare J, Engle S, et al. Antiemetics in children receiving cancer chemotherapy: a double-blind prospective randomized study comparing metoclopramide with chlorpromazine. *J Clin Oncol*. 1986;4:1110-1113.
13. Relling RV, Mulhern RK, Fairclough D, et al. Chlorpromazine with and without lorazepam as antiemetic therapy in children receiving uniform chemotherapy. *J Pediatr*. 1993;12:811-816.
14. Chlorpromazine. Lexi-Comp Online with AHFS (database). Hudson, OH: Lexi-Comp Inc. Accessed September 13, 2009.
15. Miscellaneous drugs. In: Roberts RJ, ed. *Drug Therapy in Infants: Pharmacologic Principles and Clinical Experience*. Philadelphia, PA: WB Saunders Company; 1984:296-308.
16. Ruckman RN, Keane JF, Freed MD, et al. Sedation for cardiac catheterization: a controlled study. *Pediatr Cardiol*. 1980;1:263-268.

References

17. Aronoff GR, Berns JS, Brier ME, et al. Drug prescribing in renal failure. 4th ed. Available at: http://www.kdp-baptist.louisville.edu/renalbook/. Accessed August 17, 2009.
18. Trissel LA, ed. *Handbook on Injectable Drugs*. 15th ed. Bethesda, MD: American Society of Health-System Pharmacists; 2009.
19. Abajo FJ, Montero D, Madurga M, et al. Acute and clinically relevant drug induced liver injury: a population based case-control study. *Br J Clin Pharmacol.* 2004;58:71-80.
20. Fixler DE, Carrell T, Browne R, et al. Oxygen consumption in infants and children during cardiac catheterization under different sedation regimens. *Circulation.* 1974;50:788-794.
21. Nahata MC, Clotz MA, Krogg EA. Adverse effects of meperidine, promethazine, and chlorpromazine for sedation in pediatric patients. *Clin Pediatr.* 1985;24:558-560.
22. Nahata MC. Sedation in pediatric patients undergoing diagnostic procedures. *Drug Intell Clin Pharm.* 1988;22:711-715.
23. Cook BA, Bass JW, Nomizu S, et al. Sedation of children for technical procedures: current standards of practice. *Clin Pediatr.* 1992;31:137-142.
24. American Academy of Pediatrics. Committee on Drugs. Reappraisal of lytic cocktail/demerol, phenergan, and thorazine (DPT) for the sedation of children. *Pediatrics.* 1995;95:598-602.
25. Snodgrass WR, Dodge WF. Lytic/DPT cocktail: time for rational and safer alternatives. *Pediatr Clin North Am.* 1989;36:1285-1291.
26. Brown ET, Corbett SW, Green SM. Iatrogenic cardiopulmonary arrest during pediatric sedation with meperidine, promethazine, and chlorpromazine. *Pediatr Emerg Care.* 2001;17:351-353.
27. Kelly AM, Ardagh M, Curry C, et al. Intravenous chlorpromazine versus intramuscular sumatriptan for acute migraine. *J Accid Emerg Med.* 1997;14:209-211.
28. Nakano T, Kado H, Shiokawa Y, et al. The low resistance strategy for the perioperative management of the Norwood procedure. *Ann Thorac Surg.* 2004;77:908-912.
29. Isbister CK, Balit CR, Kilham HA. Antipsychotic poisoning in young children. *Drug Safety.* 2005;28:1029-1044.

Cimetidine

1. Available at: http://www.usp.org/hqi/similarProducts/choosy.html. Accessed August 24, 2009.
2. Cimetidine [package insert]. Lake Forest, IL: Hospira Inc; August 2006.
3. Jefferys DB, Vale JA. Cimetidine and bradycardia. *Lancet.* 1978;1:828. Letter.
4. Mahon WA, Kolton M. Hypotension after intravenous cimetidine. *Lancet.* 1978;1:828. Letter.
5. Smith CL, Bardgett DM, Hunter JM. Haemodynamic effects of the IV administration of cimetidine or ranitidine in the critically ill patient. A double-blind prospective study. *Br J Anaesth.* 1987;59:1397-1402.
6. Shaw RG, Mashford ML, Desmond PV. Cardiac arrest after intravenous injection of cimetidine. *Med J Aust.* 1980;2:629-630.
7. Aranda JV, Outerbridge EW, Schentag JJ. Pharmacodynamics and kinetics of cimetidine in a premature newborn. *Am J Dis Child.* 1983;137:1207.
8. Ziemniak JA, Wynn RJ, Aranda JV, et al. The pharmacokinetic and metabolism cimetidine in neonate. *Dev Pharmacol Ther.* 1984;7:30-38.
9. Chhattriwalla Y, Colon AR, Scanion JW. The use of cimetidine in the newborn. *Pediatrics.* 1980;65:301-302.
10. Vandenplas Y, Sacre L. Cimetidine influence on gastric emptying time in neonates. *Drug Intell Clin Pharm.* 1986;20:232-233.
11. Lloyd CW, Martin WJ, Taylor BD. The pharmacokinetics of cimetidine and metabolites in a neonate. *Drug Intell Clin Pharm.* 1985;19:203-205.
12. Vandenplas Y, Sacre L. The use of cimetidine in newborns. *Am J Perinatol.* 1987;4:131-133.
13. Agarwal AK, Saili A, Pandey KK, et al. Role of cimetidine in prevention and treatment of stress-induced gastric bleeding in neonates. *Indian Pediatr.* 1990;27:465-469.
14. Lacroix J, Infante-Rivard C, Gauthier M, et al. Upper gastrointestinal tract bleeding acquired in a pediatric intensive care unit: prophylaxis trial with cimetidine. *J Pediatr.* 1986;108:1015-1018.
15. Chin TWF, MacLeod SM, Fenje P, et al. Pharmacokinetics of cimetidine in critically ill children. *Pediatr Pharmacol.* 1982;2:285-292.
16. Somogyi A, Becker M, Gugler R. Cimetidine pharmacokinetics and dosage requirements in children. *Eur J Pediatr.* 1985;144:72-76.
17. Lloyd CW, Martin WJ, Taylor BD, et al. Pharmacokinetics and pharmacodynamics of cimetidine and metabolites in critically ill children. *J Pediatr.* 1985;107:295-300.
18. Martyn JAJ. Cimetidine and/or antacid for the control of gastric acidity in pediatric burn patients. *Crit Care Med.* 1985;13:1-3.
19. Kelly DA. Do H$_2$ receptor antagonists have a therapeutic role in childhood? *J Pediatr Gastroenterol Nutr.* 1994;19:270-276.
20. Crill CM, Hak EB. Upper gastrointestinal bleeding in critically ill pediatric patients. *Pharmacotherapy.* 1999;19:162-180.
21. Ostro MJ, Russell JA, Soldin SJ, et al. Control of gastric pH with cimetidine: boluses versus primed infusions. *Gastroenterology.* 1985;89:532-537.
22. Frank W, Karlstadt R, Rockhold F, et al. Comparison between continuous and intermittent infusion regimens of cimetidine in ulcer patients. *Clin Pharmacol Ther.* 1989;46:234-239.
23. Martin LF, Booth FV, Karlstadt RG, et al. Continuous intravenous cimetidine decreases stress-related upper gastrointestinal hemorrhage without promoting pneumonia. *Crit Care Med.* 1993;21:19-30.
24. Larsson R, Erlanson P, Bodemar G, et al. The pharmacokinetics of cimetidine and its sulphoxide metabolite in patients with normal and impaired renal function. *Br J Clin Pharmacol.* 1982;13:163-170.
25. Priebe HJ, Skillman JJ, Bushnell LS, et al. Antacid versus cimetidine in preventing acute gastrointestinal bleeding. *N Engl J Med.* 1980;302:426-430.
26. Trissel LA, ed. *Handbook on Injectable Drugs*. 15th ed. Bethesda, MD: American Society of Health-System Pharmacists; 2009.
27. Hatton J, Leur M, Hirsch J, et al. Histamine receptor antagonists and lipid stability in total nutrient admixtures. *J Parenter Enteral Nutr.* 1994;18:308-312.
28. Baptista RJ, Palombo JD, Tahan SR, et al. Stability of cimetidine hydrochloride in a total nutrient admixture. *Am J Hosp Pharm.* 1985;42:2208-2210.
29. Morgan DJ, Uccellini DA, Raymond K, et al. The influence of duration of intravenous infusion of an acute dose on plasma concentrations of cimetidine. *Eur J Clin Pharmacol.* 1983;25:29-34.
30. Thompson J, Lilly J. Cimetidine-induced cerebral toxicity in children. *Lancet.* 1979;1:725.
31. Bale JF, Roberts C, Book LS. Cimetidine-induced cerebral toxicity in children. *Lancet.* 1979;1:725-726.
32. Kuint J, Linder N, Reichman B. Hypoxemia associated with cimetidine therapy in a newborn infant. *Am J Perinatol.* 1996;13:301-303.
33. Martyn JA, Greenblatt DJ, Hagen J, et al. Alteration by burn injury of the pharmacokinetics and pharmacodynamics of cimetidine in children. *Eur J Clin Pharmacol.* 1989;36:361-367.
34. Ziemniak JA, Assael BM, Padoan R, et al. The bioavailability and pharmacokinetics of cimetidine and its metabolites in juvenile cystic fibrosis patients: age related differences as compared to adults. *Eur J Clin Pharmacol.* 1984;26:183-189.
35. Guillet R, Stoll BJ, Cotton CM, et al. Association of H2-blocker therapy and higher incidence of necrotizing enterocolitis in very low birth weight infants. *Pediatrics.* 2006;117:e137-e142.

Ciprofloxacin Lactate

1. Available at: http://www.usp.org/hqi/similarProducts/choosy.html. Accessed August 27, 2009.
2. Ciprofloxacin lactate [package insert] Irvine, CA: Teva Parenteral Medicines Inc; December 2007.

References

3. Davis H, McGoodwin E, Reed TG. Anaphylactoid reactions reported after treatment with ciprofloxacin. *Ann Intern Med.* 1989;111:1041-1043.
4. Deamer RL, Prichard JG, Loman GJ. Hypersensitivity and anaphylactoid reactions to ciprofloxacin. *DICP Ann Pharmacother.* 1992;26:1081-1084.
5. Arcieri GM. Safety of intravenous ciprofloxacin: a review. *Am J Med.* 1989;87(suppl 5A):92-97.
6. American Academy of Pediatrics. Pickering LK, Baker CJ, Kimberlin DW, et al., eds. *2009 Red Book: Report of the Committee on Infectious Diseases.* 28th ed. Elk Grove Village, IL: American Academy of Pediatrics; 2009.
7. Lumbiganon P, Pengsaa K, Sookpranee T, et al. Ciprofloxacin in neonates and its possible adverse effect on teeth. *Pediatr Infect Dis J.* 1991;10:619-620.
8. Wessalowski R, Thomas L, Kivit J, et al. Multiple brain abscesses caused by Salmonella enteritidis in a neonate: successful treatment with ciprofloxacin. *Pediatr Infect Dis J.* 1993;12:683-688.
9. Van den Oever HL, Versteegh FG, Thewessen EA, et al. Ciprofloxacin in preterm neonates: case report and review of the literature. *Eur J Pediat.* 1998;157:843-845.
10. Krcmery V, Filka J, Uher J, et al. Ciprofloxacin in treatment of nosocomial meningitis in neonates and in infants: report of 12 cases and review. *Diagn Microbiol Infect Dis.* 1999;35:75-80.
11. Drossou-Agakidou V, Roilides E, Papakyriakidou-Koliouska P, et al. Use of ciprofloxacin in neonatal sepsis: lack of adverse events up to one year. *Pediatr Infect Dis J.* 2004;23:346-349.
12. Lipman J, Gous AG, Mathivha LR, et al. Ciprofloxacin pharmacokinetic profiles in paediatric sepsis: how much ciprofloxacin is enough? *Intensive Care Med.* 2002;28:493-500.
13. Goepp JG, Lee CK, Anderson T, et al. Use of ciprofloxacin in an infant with ventriculitis. *J Pediatr.* 1992;121:303-305.
14. Inglesby TV, O'Toole T, Henderson DA, et al., for the Working Group on Civilian Biodefense. Anthrax as a biological weapon 2002: updated recommendations for management. *JAMA.* 2002;287:2236-2252.
15. Centers for Disease Control and Prevention. Update: Investigation of bioterrorism-related anthrax and interim guidelines for exposure management and antimicrobial therapy, October 2001. *MMWR Morb Mortal Wkly Rep.* 2001;50:909-919.
16. Heggers JP, Villarreal C, Edgar P, et al. Ciprofloxacin as a therapeutic modality in pediatric burn wound infections. *Arch Surg.* 1998;133:1247-1250.
17. Church DA, Kanga JF, Kuhn RJ, et al. Sequential ciprofloxacin therapy in pediatric cystic fibrosis: comparative study vs. ceftazidime/tobramycin in the treatment of acute pulmonary exacerbations. *Pediatr Infect Dis J.* 1997;16:97-105.
18. Schaefer HG, Stass H, Wedgwood J, et al. Pharmacokinetics of ciprofloxacin in pediatric cystic fibrosis patients. *Antimicrob Agents Chemother.* 1996;40:29-34.
19. Rubio TT, Miles MV, Lettieri JT, et al. Pharmacokinetic disposition of sequential intravenous/oral ciprofloxacin in pediatric cystic fibrosis patients with acute pulmonary exacerbation. *Pediatr Infect Dis J.* 1997;16:112-117.
20. Dutta P, Rasaily R, Saha R, et al. Ciprofloxacin for treatment of severe typhoid fever in children. *Antimicrob Agents Chemother.* 1993;37:1197-1199.
21. Thomsen LL, Paerregaard A. Treatment with ciprofloxacin in children with typhoid fever. *Scand J Infect Dis.* 1998;30:355-357.
22. Aronoff GR, Berns JS, Brier ME, et al. Drug prescribing in renal failure. 4th ed. Available at: http://www.kdp-baptist.louisville.edu/renalbook/. Accessed November 15, 2009.
23. Gasser TC, Ebert SC, Graversen PH, et al. Ciprofloxacin pharmacokinetics in patients with normal and impaired renal function. *Antimicrob Agents Chemother.* 1987;31:709-712.
24. Gasser TC, Ebert SC, Graversen PH, et al. Pharmacokinetic study of patients with impaired renal function. *Am J Med.* 1987;82:139-141.
25. Esposito S, Miniero M, Barba D, et al. Pharmacokinetics of ciprofloxacin in impaired liver function. *Int J Clin Pharm Res.* 1989;9:37-41.
26. Chysky V, Kapila K, Hullman R, et al. Safety of ciprofloxacin in children: worldwide clinical experience based on compassionate use. Emphasis on joint evaluation. *Infection.* 1991;19:289-296.
27. Hussey G, Kibel M, Parker N, et al. Ciprofloxacin treatment of multiply drug-resistant extrapulmonary tuberculosis in a child. *Pediatr Infect Dis J.* 1992;11:408-409.
28. Trissel LA, ed. *Handbook on Injectable Drugs.* 15th ed. Bethesda, MD: American Society of Health-System Pharmacists; 2009.
29. Robinson CA, Sawyer JE. Y-site compatibility of medications with parenteral nutrition. *J Pediatr Pharmacol Ther.* 2009;14:49-57.
30. Schaad UB, Stoupis C, Wedgewood J, et al. Clinical, radiologic and magnetic resonance monitoring for skeletal toxicity in pediatric patients with cystic fibrosis receiving a three-month course of ciprofloxacin. *Pediatr Infect Dis J.* 1991;10:723-729.
31. Orenstein DM, Pattishall EN, Noyes BE, et al. Safety of ciprofloxacin in children with cystic fibrosis. *Clin Pediatr.* 1993;32:504-506.
32. Schaad UB, Sander E, Wedgewood J, et al. Morphologic studies for skeletal toxicity after prolonged ciprofloxacin therapy in two juvenile cystic fibrosis patients. *Pediatr Infect Dis J.* 1992;11:1047-1049.
33. Schaad UB, Wedgewood J. Lack of quinolone-induced arthropathy in children. *J Antimicrob Chemother.* 1992;30:414-416.
34. Hampel B, Hullmann R, Schmidt H. Ciprofloxacin in pediatrics: worldwide clinical experience based on compassionate use-safety report. *Pediatr Infect Dis J.* 1997;16:127-129.
35. Jick S. Ciprofloxacin safety in a pediatric population. *Pediatr Infect Dis J.* 1997;16:130-134.
36. Camp KA, Miyagi SL, Schroeder DJ. Potential quinolone-induced cartilage toxicity in children. *Ann Pharmacother.* 1994;28:336-338.
37. Erdem G, Staat MA, Connelly BL, et al. Anaphylactic reaction to ciprofloxacin in a toddler: successful desensitization. *Pediatr Infect Dis J.* 1999;18:563-564.
38. Lantner RR. Ciprofloxacin desensitization in a patient with cystic fibrosis. *J Allergy Clin Immunol.* 1995;96:1001-1002.
39. Atasoy H, Erdem G, Ceyhan M, et al. Hypertension associated with ciprofloxacin use in an infant. *Ann Pharmacother.* 1995;29:1049.
40. Darwish T. Ciprofloxacin-induced seizures in a healthy patient. *N Z Med J.* 2008;121:104-105.
41. Agbaht K, Bitik B, Piskinpasa S, et al. Ciprofloxacin-associated seizures in a patient with underlying thyrotoxicosis: case report and literature review. *Int J Clin Pharmacol Ther.* 2009;47:303-310.
42. Kushner JM, Peckman HJ, Snyder CR. Seizures associated with fluoroquinolones. *Ann Pharmacother.* 2001;35:1194-1198.
43. Tattevin P, Messiaen T, Pras V, et al. Confusion and general seizures following ciprofloxacin administration. *Nephrol Dial Transplant.* 1998;13:2712-2713.

Cisatracurium Besylate

1. Available at: http://ismp.org/Tools/highalertmedications.pdf. ISMP 2008. Accessed November 15, 2009.
2. Nimbex [package insert]. Lake Forest, IL: Hospira Inc.
3. Legros CB, Oreliaguet GA, Mayer M, et al. Severe anaphylactic reaction to cisatracurium in a child. *Anesth Analg.* 2001;92:648-649.
4. Rowlee SC. Monitoring neuromuscular blockade in the intensive care unit: the peripheral nerve stimulator. *Heart Lung.* 1999;28:352-362.
5. Martin LD, Bratton SL, O'Rourke PP. Clinical uses and controversies of neuromuscular blocking agents in infants and children. *Crit Care Med.* 1999;27:1358-1368.
6. de Ruiter J, Crawford MW. Dose-response relationship and infusion requirements of cisatracurium besylate in infants and children during nitrous oxide-narcotic anesthesia. *Anesthesiology.* 2001;94:790-792.
7. Reich DL, Hollinger I, Harrington DJ, et al. Comparison of cisatracurium and vecuronium by infusion in neonates and small infants after congenital heart surgery. *Anesthesiology.* 2004;101:1122-1127.
8. Burmester M, Mok Q. Randomised controlled trial comparing cisatracurium and vecuronium infusions in a paediatric intensive care unit. *Intensive Care Med.* 2005;31:686-692.

References

9. Aronoff GR, Berns JS, Brier ME, et al. Drug prescribing in renal failure. 4th ed. Available at: http://www.kdp-baptist.louisville.edu/renalbook/. Accessed November 13, 2009.
10. Trissel LA, ed. *Handbook on Injectable Drugs*. 15th ed. Bethesda, MD: American Society of Health-System Pharmacists; 2009.
11. Davis NA, Rodgers JE, Gonzalez ER, et al. Prolonged weakness after cisatracurium infusion: a case report. *Crit Care Med*. 1998;26:1290-1292.
12. Watling SM, Dasta JF. Prolonged paralysis in intensive care unit patients after the use of neuromuscular blocking agents: a review of the literature. *Crit Care Med*. 1994;22:884-893.
13. Panacek EA, Sherman B. Hydrocortisone and pancuronium bromide: acute myopathy during status asthmaticus. *Crit Care Med*. 1988;16:732.
14. Cooper MK, Bateman ST. Cisatracurium in "weakening doses" assist in weaning from sedation and withdrawal following extended use of inhaled isoflurane. *Pediatr Crit Care Med*. 2007;8:58-60.

CISplatin

1. Available at: http://ismp.org/Tools/highalertmedications.pdf. ISMP 2008. Accessed August 24, 2009.
2. Available at: http://ismp.org/Tools/confuseddrugnames.pdf. Accessed August 24, 2009.
3. Available at http://www.usp.org/hqi/similarProducts/choosy.html. Accessed August 24, 2009.
4. Platinol [package insert]. Princeton, NJ: Bristol-Myers Squibb; March 2006.
5. Cisplatin. Lexi-Comp® Online with AHFS® (database). Bethesda, MD: American Society of Health-System Pharmacists; updated January 2009.
6. MacCara ME. Extravasation: a hazard of intravenous therapy. *Drug Intell Clin Pharm*. 1983;17:713-717.
7. Kushner B, Helson L. Coordinated use of sequentially escalated cyclophosphamide and cell-cycle-specific chemotherapy (N4SE Protocol) for advanced neuroblastoma: experience with 100 patients. *J Clin Oncol*. 1987;5:1746-1751.
8. West DC, Shamberger RC, Macklis RM, et al. Stage III neuroblastoma over 1 year of age at diagnosis: improved survival with intensive multimodality therapy including multiple alkylating agents. *J Clin Oncol*. 1993;11:84-90.
9. McWilliams NB, Hayes FA, Green AA, et al. Cyclophosphamide/doxorubicin vs. cisplatin/teniposide in the treatment of children older than 12 months of age with disseminated neuroblastoma: a pediatric oncology group randomized phase II study. *Med Ped Onc*. 1995;24:176-180.
10. Gasparini M, Tondini C, Rottoli L, et al. Continuous cisplatin infusion in combination with vincristine and high-dose methotrexate for advanced osteogenic sarcoma. *Am J Clin Oncol*. 1987;10:152-155.
11. Uchida A, Myoui A, Araki N, et al. Neoadjuvant chemotherapy for pediatric osteosarcoma patients. *Cancer*. 1997;79:411-415.
12. Harris MB, Gieser P, Goorin AM, et al. Treatment of metastatic osteosarcoma at diagnosis: a pediatric oncology group study. *J Clin Onc*. 1998;16:3641-3648.
13. Walker RW, Allen, JC. Cisplatin in the treatment of recurrent childhood primary brain tumors. *J Clin Oncol*. 1988;6:62-66.
14. Nitsche R, Starling K, et al. Cis-diamminedichloroplatinum (NSC-119875) in childhood malignancies. A southwest oncology group study. *Med Ped Onc*. 1978;4:127-132.
15. Kamalakar P, Freeman A, Higby DJ, et al. Clinical response and toxicity with cis-dichlorodiammineplatinum(II) in children. *Cancer Treat Rep*. 1977; 61:835-839.
16. Aronoff GR, Berns JS, Brier ME, et al. Drug prescribing in renal failure. 4th ed. Available at: http://www.kdp-baptist.louisville.edu/renalbook/. Accessed November 14, 2009.
17. Cisplatin. Lexi-Comp Online with AHFS (database). Hudson, OH: Lexi-Comp Inc; updated October 22, 2009.
18. Trissel LA, ed. *Handbook on Injectable Drugs*. 15th ed. Bethesda, MD: American Society of Health-System Pharmacists; 2009.
19. Gutierrez ML, Crooke ST. Pediatric cancer chemotherapy: an updated review I. Cis-diamminedichloroplatinum II (cisplatin), VM-26 (teniposide), VP-16 (etoposide), mitomycin C. *Cancer Treat Rev*. 1979;6:153-164.
20. Jaffe N, Keifer R III, Robertson R, et al. Renal toxicity with cumulative doses of cis-diamminedichloroplatinum II in pediatric patients with osteosarcoma. *Cancer*. 1987;59:1577-1581.
21. Marin AC, Rierson B. Peripheral neuropathy secondary to cis-Dichlorodiammino-platinum (II) (Platinol). Treatment for advanced ovarian cancer. *Ariz Med*. 1979;36:898-899.
22. Mollman JE. Cisplatin neurotoxicity. *N Engl J Med*. 1990;2:126-127.
23. Greenspan A, Treat J. Peripheral neuropathy and low dose cisplatin. *Am J Clin Onc*. 1988;11:660-662.
24. Blachley JD, Hill JB. Renal and electrolyte disturbances associated with cisplatin. *Ann Intern Med*. 1981;95:628-632.
25. Piel IJ, Meyer D, Perlia CP, et al. Effects of cis-diamminedichloroplatinum (NSC-119875) on hearing function in man. *Cancer Chemother Rep*. 1974;58:871.
26. Moroso MJ, Blair R. A review of cis-platinum ototoxicity. *J Otolaryngol*. 1983;12:365-369.
27. Reddel RR, Kefford RF, Grant JM, et al. Ototoxicity in patients receiving cisplatin: importance of dose and method of drug administration. *Cancer Treat Rep*. 1982;66:19.
28. National Comprehensive Cancer Network (NCCN) Antiemesis Panel Members. NCCN Clinical Practice Guidelines in Oncology. Antiemesis, v.1.2006. Available at www.nccn.org. Accessed March 29, 2006.
29. Roila F, Feyer P, Maranzamo E, et al. Antiemetics in children receiving chemotherapy. *Support Care Cancer*. 2005;13:129-131.

Clindamycin Phosphate

1. Available at: http://www.usp.org/hqi/similarProducts/choosy.html. Accessed October 18, 2009.
2. Clindamycin Phosphate [package insert]. Schaumburg, IL: American Pharmaceutical Partners; November 2007.
3. American Academy of Pediatrics. Pickering LK, Baker CJ, Kimberlin DW, et al., eds. *2009 Red Book: Report of the Committee on Infectious Diseases*. 28th ed. Elk Grove Village, IL: American Academy of Pediatrics; 2009.
4. Nelson JD, Bradley JS, eds. *Nelson's Pocket Book of Pediatric Antimicrobial Therapy*. 17th ed. Chicago, IL: American Academy of Pediatrics; 2009.
5. Koren G, Zarfin Y, Maresky D, et al. Pharmacokinetics of intravenous clindamycin in newborn infants. *Pediatr Pharmacol*. 1986;5:287-292.
6. Bell M, Shackelford P, Smith R, et al. Pharmacokinetics of clindamycin phosphate in the first year of life. *J Pediatr*. 1984;105:482-486.
7. Faix RG, Polley TZ, Grasela TH. A randomized controlled trial of parenteral clindamycin in neonatal necrotizing enterocolitis. *J Pediatr*. 1988;112:271-277.
8. Jacobson SJ, Griffiths K, Diamond S, et al. A randomized controlled trial of penicillin vs. clindamycin for the treatment of aspiration pneumonia in children. *Arch Pediatr Adolesc Med* 1997;151:701-704.
9. Peltola H, Paakkonen M, Kallio P, et al.; Osteomyelitis-Septic Arthritis (OM-SA) Study Group. Prospective, randomized trial of 10 days versus 30 days of antimicrobial treatment, including a short-term course of parenteral therapy, for childhood septic arthritis. *CID*. 2009;48:1201-1210.
10. Lin JJ, Wu CT, Hsia SH, Chiu CH. Bullous impetigo: a rare presentation in fulminant streptococcal toxic shock syndrome. *Pediatric Emergency Care*. 2007;23:318-320.
11. Wilson W, Taubert K, Gewitz m, et al. Prevention of infective endocarditis. Guidelines from the American Heart Association Rheumatic Fever, Endocarditis, and Kawasaki Disease Committee, Council on Cardiovascular Disease in the Young, and the Councils on Clinical Cardiology, Council on Cardiovascular Surgery and Anesthesia and the Quality of Care and Outcomes Research Interdisciplinary Working Group. *Circulation*. 2007;115:1736-1754; correction *Circulation*. 2007;116:1736-1754.

12. Inglesby TV, O'Toole T, Henderson DA, et al.; Working Group on Civilian Biodefense. Anthrax as a biological weapon 2002: updated recommendations for management. *JAMA.* 2002;287:2236-2252.
13. Centers for Disease Control and Prevention. Update: investigation of bioterrorism0related anthrax and interim guidelines for exposure management and antimicrobial therapy, October 2001. *MMWR Morb Mortal Wkly Rep.* 2001;50:909-919.
14. Ciftci AO, Tanyel FC, Buyukpamukcu N, et al. Comparative trial of four antibiotics combinations for perforated appendicitis in children. *Eur J Surg.* 1997;163:591-596.
15. Bratzler DW, Houck PM, et al. Antimicrobial prophylaxis for surgery: an advisory statement from the Nation Surgical Infection Prevention Project. *Clin Infect Dis.* 2004;38:1706-1715.
16. Aronoff GR, Berns JS, Brier ME, et al. Drug prescribing in renal failure. 4th ed. Available at: http://www.kdp-baptist.louisville.edu/renalbook/. Accessed October 1, 2009.
17. Trissel LA, ed. *Handbook on Injectable Drugs.* 15th ed. Bethesda, MD: American Society of Health-System Pharmacists; 2009.
18. Strauss AA. Di(2-ethylhexyl)phthalate (DEHP). *J Pediat Pharmacol Ther.* 2004;89-95.
19. Robinson CA, Sawyer JE. Y-site compatibility of medications with parenteral nutrition. *J Pediatr Pharmacol Ther.* 2009;14:49-57.
20. Aucoin P, Beckner RR, Gantz NM. Clindamycin-induced cardiac arrest. *South Med J.* 1983;75:768.
21. Fulghum DD, Catalano PM. Stevens-Johnson syndrome from clindamycin: a case report. *JAMA.* 1973;223:318-319.
22. Chiou CS, Lin SP, Chang WG, et al. Clindamycin-induced Anaphylactic Shock During General Anesthesia. *J Chin Med Assoc.* 2006;69:549-561.
23. Beavers-May T, Jacobs RF. Clinical and laboratory issues in community-acquired MRSA. J Pediatr Pharmacol Ther. 2004;9:82-88.
24. Thomas RJ. Neurotoxicity of antibacterial therapy. *South Med J.* 1994;87:869-874.
25. Al Ahdal O, Bevan DR. Clindamycin-induced neuromuscular blockade. *Can J Anaesth.* 1995;42:614-617.
26. Annear DI. Interaction between erythromycin and lincomycin. *J Med Microbiol.* 1978;194-198.

Co-Trimoxazole (Trimethoprim–Sulfamethoxazole)

1. Available at: http://www.usp.org/hqi/similarProducts/choosy.html. Accessed October 30, 2009.
2. Sulfamethoxazole and trimethoprim injection [package insert]. Irvine, CA: Sicor Pharmaceuticals Inc; September 2008.
3. Sulfamethoxazole and Trimethoprim. Lexi-Comp® Online with AHFS®. Hudson, OH: Lexi-Comp Inc; updated August 13, 2009.
4. American Academy of Pediatrics. Pickering LK, Baker CJ, Kimberlin DW, et al., eds. *2009 Red Book: Report of the Committee on Infectious Diseases.* 28th ed. Elk Grove Village, IL: American Academy of Pediatrics; 2009.
5. Tunkel AR, Hartman BJ, Kaplan SL, et al. Practice guidelines for the management of bacterial meningitis. *Clin Infect Dis.* 2004;39:1267-1284.
6. Armstrong RW, Slater B. Listeria monocytogenes meningitis treated with trimethoprim–sulfamethoxazole. *Pediatr Infect Dis.* 1986;5:712-713.
7. Ferlauto JJ, Wells DH. Flavobacterium meningosepticum in the neonatal period. *South Med J.* 1981;74:757-759.
8. Murphy TF, Fernald GW. Trimethoprim–sulfamethoxazole therapy for relapses of Salmonella meningitis. *Pediatr Infect Dis.* 1983;2:465-468.
9. Tamer MA, Bray JD. Trimethoprim–sulfamethoxazole treatment of multiantibiotic-resistant staphylococcal endocarditis and meningitis. *Clin Pediatr.* 1982;21:125-126.
10. Hughes WT, Feldman S, Chaudhary SC, et al. Comparison of pentamidine isethionate and trimethoprim–sulfamethoxazole in the treatment of Pneumocystis carinii pneumonia. *J Pediatr.* 1978;92:285-291.
11. Sattler FR, Remington JS. Intravenous trimethoprim–sulfamethoxazole therapy for Pneumocystis carinii pneumonia. *Am J Med.* 1981;70:1215-1221.
12. Wharton JM, Coleman DL, Wofsy CB, et al. Trimethoprim–sulfamethoxazole or pentamidine for Pneumocystis carinii pneumonia in the acquired immunodeficiency syndrome: a prospective randomized trial. *Ann Intern Med.* 1986;105:37-44.
13. Small CB, Harris CA, Friedland GH, et al. The treatment of Pneumocystis carinii pneumonia in the acquired immunodeficiency syndrome. *Arch Intern Med.* 1985;145:837-840.
14. Hughes WT. Trimethoprim–sulfamethoxazole therapy for Pneumocystis carinii pneumonitis in children. *Rev Infect Dis.* 1982;4:602-607.
15. Lipson A, Marshall WC, Hayward AR. Treatment of Pneumocystis carinii pneumonia in children. *Arch Dis Child.* 1977; 52:314-319.
16. Larter WE, John TJ, Sieber OF, et al. Trimethoprim–sulfamethoxazole treatment of Pneumocystis carinii pneumonitis. *J Pediatr.* 1978;92:826-828.
17. Siegel SE, Wolff LJ, Baehner RL, et al. Treatment of Pneumocystis carinii pneumonitis. A comparative trial of sulfamethoxazole–trimethoprim vs. pentamidine in pediatric patients with cancer: report from the children's cancer study group. *Am J Dis Child.* 1984;138:1051-1054.
18. Aronoff GR, Berns JS, Brier ME, et al. Drug prescribing in renal failure. 4th ed. Available at: http://www.kdp-baptist.louisville.edu/renalbook/. Accessed October 30, 2009.
19. Hoppu K, Koskimies O, Tuomisto J. Trimethoprim pharmacokinetics in children with renal insufficiency. *Clin Pharmacol Ther.* 1987;42:181-186.
20. Siber GR, Gorham CC, Ericson JF, et al. Pharmacokinetics of intravenous trimethoprim–sulfamethoxazole in children and adults with normal and impaired renal function. *Rev Infect Dis.* 1982;4:566-578.
21. Welling PG, Craig WA, Amidon GL, et al. Pharmacokinetics of trimethoprim and sulfamethoxazole in normal subjects and in patients with renal failure. *J Infect Dis.* 1973;128(suppl):S556-S566.
22. Trissel LA, ed. *Handbook on Injectable Drugs.* 15th ed. Bethesda, MD: American Society of Health-System Pharmacists; 2009.
23. Baumgartner TG, Russell WL. Intravenous trimethoprim–sulfamethoxazole administration alert. *Am J IV Ther Clin Nutr.* 1983;10:14-15.
24. Robinson CA, Sawyer JE. Y-site compatibility of medications with parenteral nutrition. *J Pediatr Pharmacol Ther.* 2009;14:49-57.
25. Koh MJ, Tay YK. An update on Stevens-Johnson syndrome and toxic epidermal necrolysis in children. *Curr Opin Pediatr.* 2009;21:505-510.
26. Zaman F, Ye G, Abreo KD, et al. Successful orthotopic liver transplantation after trimethoprim-sulfamethoxazole associated fulminant liver failure. *Clin Transplant.* 2003;17:461-464.
27. Abusin S, Johnson S. Sulfamethoxazole/Trimethoprim induced liver failure: a case report. *Cases J.* 2008;1:44-47.
28. Perazella MA. Trimethoprim-induced hyperkalaemia: clinical data, mechanism, prevention and management. *Drug Saf.* 2000;22:227-236.

Coagulation Factor VIIa (Recombinant) (rFVIIa)

1. NovoSeven®RT (Coagulation Factor VIIa recombinant) [prescribing information]. Princeton, NJ: Novo Nordisk Inc; May 9, 2008.
2. O'Connell KA, Wood JJ, Wise RP, et al. Thromboembolic adverse events after use of recombinant human coagulation factor VIIa. *JAMA.* 2006;295:293-298.
3. Schulman S. Continuous infusion of recombinant factor VIIa in hemophilic patients with inhibitors: safety, monitoring, and cost effectiveness. *Semin Thromb Hemost.* 2000;26:421-424.
4. Pruthi RK, Mathew P, Valentino LA, et al. Haemostatic efficacy and safety of bolus and continuous infusion of recombinant factor VIIa are comparable in haemophilia patients with inhibitors undergoing major surgery. *Thromb Haemost.* 2007;98:726-732.
5. Schulman S. Safety, efficacy, and lessons from continuous infusion with rFVIIa. *Haemophilia.* 1998;4:564-567.
6. Pirrello R, Siragusa S, Giambona C, et al. Bleeding prophylaxis in a child with cleft palate and factor VII deficiency: a case report. *Cleft Palate Craniofac J.* 2006;43:108-111.
7. Pychynska-Pokorska M, Moll JJ, Krajewski W, et al. The use of recombinant factor VIIa in uncontrolled postoperative bleeding in children undergoing cardiac surgery with cardiopulmonary bypass. *Pediatr Crit Care Med.* 2004;5:246-250.
8. Tobias JD, Berkenbosch JW, Russo P. Recombinant factor FIIa to treat bleeding after cardiac surgery in an infant. *Pediatr Crit Care Med.* 2003;4:49-51.
9. Malherbe S, Tsui BCH, Stobart K, et al. Argatroban as an anticoagulant in cardiopulmonary bypass in an infant and attempted reversal with recombinant activated factor VII. *Anesthesiol.* 2004;100:443-445.

References

10. Ekert H, Brizard C, Eyers R, et al. Elective administratin in infants of low-dose recombinant activated factor VII (rFVIIa) in cardiopulmonary bypass surgery for congenital heart disease does not shorten time to chest closure or reduce blood loss and the need for transfusions: a randomized, double-blind, parallet group, placebo-controlled study of rFVIIa and standard haemostatic replacement therapy versus standard haemostatic replacement therapy. *Blood Coagul Fibrinolysis.* 2006;17:389-398.
11. Dominguez TE, Mitchell M, Friess SH, et al. Use of recombinant factor VIIa for refractory hemorrhage during extracorporeal membrane oxygenation. *Pediatr Crit Care Med.* 2005;6:348-351.
12. Wittenstein B, Ravn H, Goldman A. Recombinant factor VII for severe bleeding during extracorporeal membrane oxygenation following open heart surgery. *Pediatr Crit Care Med.* 2005;6:473-476.
13. Velik-Salchner C, Sergi C, Fries D, et al. Use of recombinant factor FVIIa (Novoseven®) in combination with other coagulation products led to a thrombotic occlusion of the truncus brachiocephalicus in a neonate supported by extracorporeal membrane oxygenation. *Anesth Analg.* 2005;101:920-929.
14. Tofil NM, Winkler MK, Watts RG, et al. The use of recombinant factor VIIa in a patient with Noonan syndrome and life-threatening bleeding. *Pediatr Crit Care Med.* 2005;6:352-354.
15. Kurekci AE, Atay AA, Okutan V, et al. Recombinant activated factor VII for severe gastrointestinal bleeding after chemotherapy in an infant with acute megakaryoblastic leukemia. *Blood Coagul Fibrinolysis.* 2005;16:145-147.
16. Brown JB, Emerick KM, Brown DL, et al. Recombinant factor VIIa improves coagulopathy caused by liver failure. *J Pediatr Gastroenterol Nutr.* 2003;37:268-272.
17. Pettersson M, Fischler B, Petrini P, et al. Recombinant FVIIa in children with liver disease. *Thrombosis Res.* 2005;116:185-197.
18. Atkison PR, Jardine L, Williams S, et al. Use of recombinant factor VIIa in pediatric patients with liver failure and severe coagulopathy. *Transplant Proc.* 2005;37:1091-1093.
19. Barro C, Brobleski I, Piolat C, et al. Successful use of recombinant factor VIIa for severe surgical liver bleeding in a 5 month old baby. *Haemophilia.* 2004;10:183-185.
20. Kalicinski P, Kaminski A, Drewniak T, et al. Quick correction of hemostasis in two patients with fulminant liver failure undergoing liver transplantation by recombinant activated factor VII. *Transplant Proc.* 1999;31:378-379.
21. Markiewicz M, Kalicinski P, Kaminski A, et al. Acute coagulopathy after reperfusion of the liver graft in children correction with recombinant activated factor VII. *Transplant Proc.* 2003;35:2318-2319.
22. Pavese P, Bonodona A, Beaubien J, et al. FVIIa corrects the coagulopathy of fulminant hepatic failure but may be associated with thrombosis: a report of four cases. *Can J Anesth.* 2005;52:26-29.
23. Ozelo MC, Svirin P, Larina L. Use of recombinant factor VIIa in the management of severe bleeding episodes in patients with Bernard-Soulier syndrome. *Ann Hematol.* 2005;84:816-822.
24. Poon MC, Demers C, Jobin F, et al. Recombinant factor VIIa is effective for bleeding and surgery in patients with glanzmann thromboasthenia. *Blood.* 1999;94:3951-3953.
25. Almeida AM, Khair K, Hann I, et al. The use of recombinant factor VIIa in children with inherited platelet function disorders. *Br J Hematol.* 2003;121:477-481.
26. Veldman A, Josef J, Fischer D, et al. A prospective pilot study of prophylactic treatment of preterm neonates with recombinant activated factor VII during the first 72 hours of life. *Pediatr Crit Care Med.* 2006;7:34-39.
27. Duncan A, Benson L, Critz A, et al. Neonatal coagulopathy treatment with rFVIIa. *Pediatr Res.* 2001;49:290A.
28. Filan PM, Mills JF, Clarnette TD, et al. Spontaneous liver hemorrhage during laparotomy for necrotizing enterocolitis: a potential role for recombinant factor VIIa. *J Pediatr.* 2005;147:857-859.
29. Olomu N, Kulkarni R, Manco-Johnson M. Treatment of severe pulmonary hemorrhage with activated recombinant factor VII (rFIIa) in very low birth weight infants. *J Perinatol.* 2002;22:672-674.
30. Cetin H, Yalaz M, Akisu M, et al. The use of recombinant activated factor VII in the treatment of massive pulmonary hemorrhage in a preterm infant. *Blood Coagul Fibrinolysis.* 2006;17:213-216.
31. Erhardtsen E. Pharmacokinetics of recombinant activated factor VII (rFVIIa). *Semin Thromb Hemost.* 2000;26:385-391.

Conivaptan

1. Available at: http://ismp.org/Tools/highalertmedications.pdf. Accessed November 13, 2009.
2. Available at: http://ismp.org/Tools/confuseddrugnames.pdf. Accessed November 13, 2009.
3. Available at: http://www.usp.org/hqi/similarProducts/choosy.html. Accessed November 13, 2009.
4. Conivaptan hydrochloride injection [package insert]. Deerfield, IL: Astellas Pharma US Inc; October 2008.
5. Hline SS, Phuong-Truc TP, Phuong-Thu TP, et al. Conivaptan: a step forward in the treatment of hyponatremia? *Therapeutics and Clinical Risk Management.* 2008:4(2);315-326.
6. Chagan L. Conivaptan HCl for injection (Vaprisol): a vasopressin antagonist for the management of euvolemic hyponatremia. *P&T.* 2007;32(3):140-149.
7. Conivaptan Hydrochloride. Lexi-Comp® Online with AHFS® (Adult). Hudson, OH: Lexi-Comp Inc; updated November 17, 2009.
8. Conivaptan Hydrochloride. Lexi-Comp® Online with AHFS® (Adult and Pediatric). Bethesda, MD: American Society of Health-System Pharmacists; updated January 2009.
9. Rianthavorn P, Cain JP, Turman MA. Use of conivaptan to allow aggressive hydration to prevent tumor lysis syndrome in a pediatric patient with large-cell lymphoma and SIADH. *Pediatr Nephrol.* 2008;23:1367-1370.

Cyclophosphamide

1. Available at: http://ismp.org/Tools/highalertmedications.pdf. ISMP 2008. Accessed August 26, 2009.
2. Available at: http://www.usp.org/hqi/similarProducts/choosy.html. Accessed August 26, 2009.
3. Cytoxan [package insert]. Deerfield, IL: Baxter Healthcare Corp; September 2005.
4. Cyclophosphamide. Lexi-Comp® Online with AHFS® (database). Bethesda, MD: American Society of Health-System Pharmacists; updated January 2009.
5. Cyclophosphamide. Lexi-Comp Online with AHFS (database). Hudson, OH: Lexi-Comp; updated October 22, 2009.
6. Spunt SL, Smith LM, Ruymann FB, et al. Cyclophosphamide dose intensification during induction therapy for intermediate-risk pediatric rhabdomyosarcoma is feasible but does not improve outcome: a report from the soft tissue sarcoma committee of the children's oncology group. *Clin Cancer Res.* 2004;10(18 Pt 1):6072-6079.
7. Lehman TJ, Onel K. Intermittent intravenous cyclophosphamide arrests progression of the renal chronicity index in childhood systemic lupus erythematosus. *J Pediatr.* 2000;136(2):243-247.
8. Yee CS, Gordon C, Dostal C, et al. EULAR randomised controlled trial of pulse cyclophosphamide and methylprednisolone versus continuous cyclophosphamide and prednisolone followed by azathioprine and prednisolone in lupus nephritis. *Ann Rheum Dis.* 2004;63(5):525-529.
9. Cassileth PA, Harrington DP, Appelbaum FR, et al. Chemotherapy compared with autologous or allogeneic bone marrow transplantation in the management of acute myeloid leukemia in first remission. *N Engl J Med.* 1998;339(23):1649-1656.

References

10. Aronoff GR, Berns JS, Brier ME, et al. Drug prescribing in renal failure. 4th ed. Available at: http://www.kdp-baptist.louisville.edu/renalbook/. Accessed November 25, 2009.
11. Trissel LA, ed. *Handbook on Injectable Drugs*. 15th ed. Bethesda, MD: American Society of Health-System Pharmacists; 2009.
12. National Comprehensive Cancer Network (NCCN) Antiemesis Panel Members. NCCN Clinical Practice Guidelines in Oncology. Antiemesis, v.1.2006. Available at: www.nccn.org. Accessed October 3, 2009.
13. Roila F, Feyer P, Maranzamo E, et al. Antiemetics in children receiving chemotherapy. *Support Care Cancer.* 2005;13(2):129-131.

CycloSPORINE

1. Available at: http://www.usp.org/hqi/similarProducts/choosy.html. Accessed July 7, 2009.
2. Sandimmune [prescribing information]. East Hanover, NJ. Novartis Pharmaceuticals Corp; June 2008.
3. Theis JG, Liau-Chu M, Chan HS, et al. Anaphylactoid reactions in children receiving high-dose intravenous cyclosporine for reversal of tumor resistance: the causative role of improper dissolution of cremophor EL. *J Clin Oncol.* 1995;13:2508-2516.
4. Bisogno G, Cowie F, Boddy A, et al. High-dose cyclosporin with etoposide- toxicity and pharmacokinetic interaction in children with solid tumours. *Br J Cancer.* 1998;77:2304-2309.
5. Margarit C, Ibanez VM, Potau N, et al. Cyclosporine in pediatric liver transplantation: is there a therapeutic blood level that abrogates rejection? *Transplant Proc.* 1988;20(suppl 3):369-374.
6. Burckart G, Starzl T, Williams L, et al. Cyclosporine monitoring and pharmacokinetics in pediatric liver transplant patients. *Transplant Proc.* 1985;17:1172-1175.
7. Wonigeit K, Brolsch C, Neuhaus P, et al. Special aspects of immunosuppression with cyclosporine in liver transplantation. *Transplant Proc.* 1983;15:2586-2591.
8. Yee GC, Lennon TP, Gmur DJ, et al. Age-dependent cyclosporine: pharmacokinetics in marrow transplant recipients. *Clin Pharmacol Ther.* 1986;40:438-443.
9. Clardy CW, Schroeder TJ, Myre SA, et al. Clinical variability of cyclosporine pharmacokinetics in adult and pediatric patients after renal, cardiac, hepatic, and bone-marrow transplants. *Clin Chem.* 1988;34:2012-2015.
10. Burckart GJ, Venkataramanan R, Ptachcinski RJ, et al. Cyclosporine absorption following orthotopic liver transplantation. *J Clin Pharmacol.* 1986;26:647-651.
11. Tzakis AG, Reyes J, Todo S, et al. FK506 versus cyclosporine in pediatric liver transplantation. *Transplant Proc.* 1991;23:3010-3015.
12. McDiarmid SV, Busuttil RW, Ascher NL, et al. FK506 (Tacrolimus) compared with cyclosporine for primary immunosuppression after pediatric liver transplantation. *Transplantation.* 1995;59:530-536.
13. Chiavarelli M, Boucek MM, Nehlsen-Cannarella SL, et al. Neonatal cardiac transplantation. *Arch Surg.* 1992;127:1072-1076.
14. Kahan BD, Conley S, Portman R, et al. Parent-to-child transplantation with cyclosporine immunosuppression. *J Pediatr.* 1987;111:1012-1016.
15. Conley SB, al-Urzi A, So S, et al. Prevention of rejection and graft loss with an aggressive quadruple immunosuppressive therapy regimen in children and adolescents. *Transplantation.* 1994;57:540-544.
16. Houtenbos I, Bracho F, Davenport V, et al. Autologous bone marrow transplantation for childhood acute lymphoblastic leukemia: a novel combined approach consisting of ex vivo marrow purging, modulation of multi-drug resistance, induction of autograft vs. leukemia effect, and post-transplant immuno- and chemotherapy (PTIC). *Bone Marrow Transplant.* 2001;27:145-153.
17. Alvarez F, Atkinson PR, Grant DR, et al. NOF-11: A one-year pediatric randomized double-blind comparison of neoral versus sandimmune in orthotopic liver transplantation. *Transplantation.* 2000;69:87-92.
18. Benfield MR, Tejani A, Harmon WE, et al. A randomized multicenter trial of OKT3 mAbs induction compared with intravenous cyclosporine in pediatric renal transplantation. *Pediatr Transplant.* 2005;9:282-292.
19. Salomon R, Gagnadoux M, Niaudet P. Intravenous cyclosporine therapy in recurrent nephrotic syndrome after renal transplantation in children. *Transplantation.* 2003;75:810-814.
20. Schwinghammer TL, Bloom EJ, Rosenfield CS, et al. High-dose cyclosporine and corticosteroids for prophylaxis of acute and chronic graft-versus-host disease. *Bone Marrow Transplant.* 1995;16:147-154.
21. Koga Y, Nagatoshi Y, Kawano Y, et al. Methotrexate *vs* Cyclosporin A as a single agent for graft-versus-host-disease prophylaxis in pediatric patients with hematological malignancies undergoing allogeneic bone marrow transplantation from HLA-identical siblings: a single-center analysis in Japan. *Bone Marrow Transplant.* 2003;32:171-176.
22. Ross M, Schmidt GM, Niland JC, et al. Cyclosporine, methotrexate, and prednisone compared with cyclosporine and prednisone for prevention of acute graft-vs.-host disease: effect on chronic gravt-vs.-host disease and long-term survival. *Biol Blood Marrow Transplant.* 1999;5:285-291.
23. Locatelli F, Zecca M, Rondelli R, et al. Graft versus host disease prophylaxis with low-dose cyclosporine-A reduces the risk of relapse in children with acute leukemia given HLA identical sibling bone marrow transplantation: results of a randomized trial. *Blood.* 2000;95:1572-1579.
24. Chao NJ, Snyder DS, Jain M, et al. Equivalence of 2 effective graft-versus-host disease prophylaxis regimens: results of a prospective double-blind randomized trial. *Biol Blood Marrow Transplant.* 2000;6:254-261.
25. Locatelli F, Bruno B, Zecca M, et al. Cyclosporin A and short-term methotrexate versus cyclosporine A as graft versus host disease prophylaxis in patients with severe aplastic anemia given allogeneic bone marrow transplantation from an HLA-identical sibling: results of a GITMO/EBMT randomized trial. *Blood.* 2000;96:1690-1697.
26. Dahl GV, Lacayo NJ, Brophy N, et al. Mitoxantrone, etoposide, and cyclosporine therapy in pediatric patients with recurrent or refractory acute myeloid leukemia. *J Clin Oncol.* 2000;18:1867-1875.
27. Santos JV, Baudat JA, Casellas FJ, et al. Intravenous cyclosporine for steroid-refractory attacks of Crohn's Disease. *J Clin Gastroenterol.* 1995;20:207-210.
28. Santos J, Baudat S, Casellas FJ, et al. Efficacy of intravenous cyclosporine for steroid refractory attacks of ulcerative colitis. *J Clin Gastroenterol.* 1995;20:285-289.
29. Gurudu SR, Griffel LH, Gialanella RJ, et al. Cyclosporine therapy in inflammatory bowel disease. *J Clin Gastroenterol.* 1999;29:151-154.
30. Carbonnel F, Boruchowicz A, Duclos B, et al. Intravenous cyclosporine in attacks of ulcerative colitis. *Dig Diseases and Sciences.* 1996;41:2471-2476.
31. Egan LJ, Sandborn WJ, Tremaine WJ. Clinical outcome following treatment of refractory inflammatory and fistulizing Crohn's Disease with intravenous cyclosporine. *Am J Gastroenterol.* 1998;93:442-447.
32. Cohen RD, Stein R, Hanauer SB. Intravenous cyclosporin in ulcerative colitis: a five-year experience. *Am J Gastroenterol.* 1999;94:1587-1592.
33. Bernstein EF, Whitington PF. Successful treatment of atypical sprue in an infant with cyclosporine. *Gastroenterology.* 1988;95:199-204.
34. Trissel LA. *Handbook on Injectable Drugs*. 15th ed. Bethesda, MD: American Society of Health-System Pharmacists; 2009.
35. Ptachcinski RJ, Logue LW, Burckart GJ, et al. Stability and availability of cyclosporine in 5% dextrose injection or 0.9% sodium chloride injection. *Am J Hosp Pharm.* 1986;43:94-97.
36. Kahan BD. Cyclosporine. *N Engl J Med.* 1989;321:1725-1738.
37. Venkataramanan R, Burckart GJ, Ptachcinski RJ, et al. Leaching of diethylhexyl phthalate from polyvinyl chloride bags into intravenous cyclosporine solution. *Am J Hosp Pharm.* 1986;43:2800-2802.
38. Gotardo MA, Monteiro M. Migration of diethylhexyl phthalate from PVC bags into intravenous cyclosporine solutions. *J Pharm Biomed Anal.* 2005;38:709-713.

References

39. Friedman LS, Dienstag JL, Nelson PW, et al. Anaphylactic reaction and cardiopulmonary arrest following intravenous cyclosporine. *Am J Med.* 1985;78:343-345.
40. Howrie DL, Ptachcinski RJ, Griffith BP, et al. Anaphylactoid reactions associated with parenteral cyclosporine use: possible role of Cremophor EL. *Drug Intell Clin Pharm.* 1985;19:425-427.
41. Chapuis B, Helg C, Jeannet M, et al. Anaphylactic reaction to intravenous cyclosporine. *N Engl J Med.* 1985;312:1259. Letter.
42. Napoli KL, Kahan BD. Nonselective measurement of cyclosporine for therapeutic drug monitoring by fluorescence polarization immunoassay with a rabbit polyclonal antibody: I. Evaluation of the serum methodology and comparison with a sheep polyclonal antibody in an ^{3}H tracer-mediated radioimmunoassay. *Transplant Proc.* 1990;22:1175-1181.
43. Napoli KL, Kahan BD. Nonselective measurement of cyclosporine for therapeutic drug monitoring by fluorescence polarization immunoassay with a sheep polyclonal antibody: II. Evaluation of the whole blood methodology and comparison with an ^{3}H tracer-mediated radioimmunoassay with a sheep polyclonal antibody. *Transplant Proc.* 1990;22:1181-1185.
44. Bertault-Peres P, Berland Y, Mucke MK, et al. A novel technique for plasma CSA determination-application to drug monitoring during transplantation. *Transplant Proc.* 1989;21:904-905.
45. Strologo LD, Campagnano P, Federici G, et al. Cyclosporine A monitoring in children: abbreviated area under curve formulas and C2 level. *Pediatr Nephrol.* 1999;13:95-97.
46. Weber LT, Armstrong VW, Shipkova M, et al. Cyclosporin A absorption profiles in pediatric renal transplant recipients predict the risk of acute rejection. *Ther Drug Monit.* 2004;26:415-424.
47. Bowers LD, Canafax DM. Cyclosporine: experience with therapeutic monitoring. *Ther Drug Monit.* 1984;6:142-147.
48. Rodriguez E, Delucchi MA, Cano F. Comparison of cyclosporine concentrations 2 hours post-dose determined using 3 different methods and trough level in pediatric renal transplantation. *Transplant Proc.* 2005;37:3354-3357.
49. Senner AM, Johnston K, McLachlan AJ. A comparison of peripheral and centrally collected cyclosporine A blood levels in pediatric patients undergoing stem cell transplant. *Oncol Nurs Forum.* 2005;32:73-77.
50. Leson CL, Bryson SM, Giesbrecht EE, et al. Therapeutic monitoring of cyclosporine following pediatric bone marrow transplantation: problems with sampling from silicone central venous lines. *DICP Ann Pharmacother.* 1989;23:300-303.
51. Duffner U, Bergstraesser E, Sauter S, et al. Spuriously raised cyclosporin concentrations drawn through polyurethane central venous catheter. *Lancet.* 1998;352:1442.

Cytomegalovirus Immunoglobulin

1. Available at: http://ismp.org/Tools/confuseddrugnames.pdf.
2. Available at: http://www.usp.org/hqi/similarProducts/choosy.html. Accessed October 26, 2009.
3. Available at: http://www.formularyproductions.com/blackbox/. Accessed October 26, 2009.
4. CytoGam [package insert]. King of Prussia, PA: CSL Behring; July 2008.
5. Gungor T, Funk M, Linde R, et al. Combined therapy in human immunodeficiency virus infected children: a four year experience. *Eur J Pediatr.* 1993;152:650-654.
6. Snydman DR, Werner BG, Meissner HC, et al. Use of cytomegalovirus immunoglobulin in multiply transfused premature neonates. *Pediatr Infect Dis J.* 1995;14:34-40.
7. Bowden RA, Fisher LD, Rogers K, et al. Cytomegalovirus (CMV)-specific intravenous immunoglobulin for the prevention of primary CMV infection and disease after marrow transplant. *J Infect Dis.* 1991;164:483-487.
8. Falagas ME, Syndman DR, Ruthazer R, et al. Cytomegalovirus immune globulin (CMVIG) prophylaxis is associated with increased survival after orthotopic liver transplantation. *Clin Transplant.* 1997;11:432-437.
9. Tzakis AG. Cytomegalovirus prophylaxis with ganciclovir and cytomegalovirus immune globulin in liver and intestinal transplantation. *Transpl Infect Dis.* 2001;3:35-39.
10. Fontana I, Verrina E, Timitilli A, et al. Cytomegalovirus infection in pediatric kidney transplantation. *Transplant Proc.* 1994;26:18-19.
11. Snydman DR, Werner BG, Heinze-Lacey B, et al. Use of cytomegalovirus immune globulin to prevent cytomegalovirus disease in renal-transplant recipients. *N Engl J Med.* 1987;317:1049-1054.
12. Murray JC, Bernini JC, Bijou HL, et al. Infantile cytomegalovirus-associated autoimmune hemolytic anemia. *J Pediatr Hematol Oncol.* 2001;23:318-320.

DACTINomycin

1. Available at: http://ismp.org/Tools/highalertmedications.pdf. ISMP 2008. Accessed October 25, 2009.
2. Available at: http://ismp.org/Tools/confuseddrugnames.pdf. Accessed October 25, 2009.
3. Available at: http://www.usp.org/hqi/similarProducts/choosy.html. Accessed October 25, 2009.
4. Cosmegen [package insert]. Whitestation, NJ: Merck & Co; March 2009.
5. Dactinomycin. Lexi-Comp® Online with AHFS® (database). Bethesda, MD: American Society of Health-System Pharmacists; updated April 2007.
6. Green DM, Norkool P, Breslow NE, et al. Severe hepatic toxicity after treatment with vincristine and dactinomycin using single-dose or divided-dose schedules: a report from the National Wilms' Tumor Study. *J Clin Oncol.* 1990; 8(9):1525-1530.
7. de Carmargo B, Franco EL. A randomized clinical trial of single-dose versus fractionated-dose dactinomycin in the treatment of Wilms' tumor. Results after extended follow-up. Brazilian Wilms' Tumor Study Group. *Cancer.* 1994;73(12):3081-3086.
8. D'Angio GJ, Breslow N, Beckwith JB, et al. Treatment of Wilms' tumor. Results of the Third National Wilms' Tumor Study. *Cancer.* 1989;64(2):349-360.
9. Craft AW, Cotterill SJ, Bullimore JA, et al. Long-term results from the first UKCCSG Ewing's Tumour Study (ET-1). United Kingdom Children's Cancer Study Group (UKCCSG) and the medical research council bone sarcoma working party. *Eur J Cancer.* 1997;33(7):1061-1069.
10. Meany HJ, Seibel NL, Sun J, et al. Phase 2 trial of recombinant tumor necrosis factor-alpha in combination with dactinomycin in children with recurrent Wilms tumor. *J Immunother.* 2008;31:679-683.
11. Vugrin D, Herr HW, Whitmore WF, et al. VAB-6 combination chemotherapy in disseminated cancer of the testis. *Ann Intern Med.* 1981;95(1):59-61.
12. Osathanondh R, Goldstein DP, Pastorfide GB, et al. Actinomycin D as the primary agent for gestational trophoblastic disease. *Cancer.* 36(3):863-866.
13. Newlands ES, Bagshawe KD, Begent RH, et al. Results with the EMA/CO (etoposide, methotrexate, actinomycin D, cyclophosphamide, vincristine) regimen in high risk gestational trophoblastic tumours, 1979 to 1989. *Br J Obstet Gynaecol.* 1991;98(6):550-557.
14. Trissel LA, ed. Handbook on Injectable Drugs. 15th ed. Bethesda, MD: American Society of Health-System Pharmacists; 2009.
15. Arndt C, Hawkins D, Anderson JR, et al. Age is a risk factor for chemotherapy-induced hepatopathy with vincristine, dactinomycin, and cyclophosphamide. *J Clin Oncol.* 2004;22(10):1894-1901.
16. National Comprehensive Cancer Network (NCCN) Antiemesis Panel Members. NCCN Clinical Practice Guidelines in Oncology. Antiemesis, v.1.2006. Available at www.nccn.org. Last accessed March 29, 2006.
17. Roila F, Feyer P, Maranzamo E, et al. Antiemetics in children receiving chemotherapy. *Supportive Care Cancer.* 2005;13:129-131.

References

Darbepoetin

1. Available at: http://www.usp.org/hqi/similarProducts/choosy.html. Accessed August 26, 2009.
2. Aranesp [package insert]. Thousand Oaks, CA: Amgen Inc; April 2009.
3. Pirker R, Vansteenkiste J, Gateley J, et al. A phase III, double-blind, placebo-controlled, randomized study of novel erythropoiesis stimulating protein (NESP) in patients undergoing platinum-treatment for lung cancer. *Eur J Cancer.* 2001;37 (suppl 6)abstract:254.
4. Smith RE Jr, Tchekmedyian NS, Chan D, et al. A dose- and schedule-finding study of darbepoetin alpha for the treatment of chronic anaemia of cancer. *Cancer.* 2003;88:1851-1858
5. Glaspy J, Jadeja J, Justice G, et al. Darbepoetin alfa given every 1 or 2 weeks alleviates anaemia associated with cancer chemotherapy. *Br J Cancer.* 2002;87:268-276.
6. Kotasek D, Steger G, Faught W, et al. Darbepoetin alfa administered every 3 weeks alleviates anaemia in patients with solid tumours receiving chemotherapy; results of a double-blind, placebo-controlled, randomised study. *Eur J Cancer.* 2003;39:2026-2034.
7. Blumer J, Berg S, Adamson PC, et al. Pharmacokinetic evaluation of darbepoetin alfa for the treatment of pediatric patients with chemotherapy-induced anemia. *Pediatr Blood Cancer.* 2007;49:687-693.
8. Lerner G, Kale AS, Warady BA, et al. Pharmacokinetics of darbepoetin alfa in pediatric patients with chronic kidney disease. *Pediatr Nephrol.* 2002;17:933-937.
9. Geary DF, Keating LE, Vigneux A, et al. Darbepoetin alfa (Aranesp™) in children with chronic renal failure. *Kidney International.* 2005;68:1759-1765.
10. De Palo T, Giordano M, Palumbo F, et al. Clinical experience with darbepoietin alfa (NESP) in children undergoing hemodialysis. *Pediatr Nephrol.* 2004;19:337-340.
11. Durkan AM, Keating LE, Vigneux A, et al. The use of darbepoetin in infants with chronic renal impairment. *Pediatr Nephrol.* 2006;21:694-697.
12. Joy MS. Darbepoetin alfa: a novel erythropoiesis-stimulating protein. *Ann Pharmacother.* 2002;36:1183-1192.
13. Warady BA, Arar MY, Lerner G, et al. Darbepoetin alfa for the treatment of anemia in pediatric patients with chronic kidney disease. *Pediatr Nephrol.* 2006;21:1144-1152.
14. André JL, Deschênes G, Boudailliez B, et al. Darbepoetin, effective treatment of anaemia in paediatric patients with chronic renal failure. *Pediatr Nephrol.* 2007;22:708-714.
15. Rijk Y, Raaijmakers R, van de Kar N, Schröder C. Intraperitoneal treatment with darbepoetin for children on peritoneal dialysis. *Pediatr Nephrol.* 2007;22:436-440.
16. Ohls RK, Dai A. The effect of Aranesp on the growth of fetal and neonatal erythroid progenitors. *Blood.* 2003;102:18b (abstract).
17. Warwood TL, Ohls RK, Wiedmeier SE, et al. Single-dose darbepoetin administration to anemic preterm neonates. *J Perinatol.* 2005;25:725-730.
18. Warwood TL, Ohls RK, Lambert DK, et al. Intravenous administration of darbepoetin to NICU patients. *J Perinatol.* 2006;26:296-300.
19. Kuo DJ, Bruckner AL, Jeng MR. Darbepoetin alfa and ferric gluconate ameliorate the anemia associated with recessive dystrophic epidermolysis bullosa. *Pediatr Dermatol.* 2006;23:580-585.

Deferoxamine Mesylate

1. Available at: http://www.usp.org/hqi/similarProducts/choosy.html. Accessed August 26, 2009.
2. Desferal [package insert]. East Hanover, NJ: Novartis Pharmaceuticals Corp; November 2007.
3. Mills KC, Cury SC. Acute iron poisoning. *Emerg Med Clin North Am.* 1994;12:397-413.
4. Bentur Y, McGuigan M, Koren G. Deferoxamine (desferrioxamine). New toxicities for an old drug. *Drug Safety.* 1991;6:37-46.
5. Miller KB, Rosenwasser LJ, Bessette JM, et al. Rapid desensitization for desferrioxamine anaphylactic reaction. *Lancet.* 1981;1:1059.
6. Cohen AR, Mizanin J, Schwartz E. Rapid removal of excessive iron with daily, high-dose intravenous chelation therapy. *Pediatrics.* 1989;115:151-155.
7. Peck MG, Rogers JF, Rivenbark JF. Use of high doses of deferoxamine (Desferal) in an adult patient with acute iron overdosage. *J Toxicol Clin Toxicol.* 1982;19:865-869.
8. Banner W Jr, Tong TG. Iron poisoning. *Pediatr Clin North Am.* 1986;33:393-409.
9. Deferoxamine. Lexi-Comp Online with AHFS (database). Bethesda, MD: American Society of Health-System Pharmacists; 2009. Accessed October 3, 2009.
10. Gallant T, Mizanin J, Schwartz E, et al. Serial studies of auditory neurotoxicity in patients receiving deferoxamine therapy. *Am J Med.* 1987;83:1085-1090.
11. Graziano JH, Markensen A, Miller DR, et al. Chelation therapy in ß-thalassemia major. I. Intravenous and subcutaneous deferoxamine. *J Pediatr.* 1978;92:648-652.
12. Porter JB, Jaswon MS, Huehns ER, et al. Desferrioxamine ototoxicity: evaluation of risk factors in thalassemic patients and guidelines for safe dosage. *Br J Haematol.* 1989;73:403-409.
13. National Kidney Foundation. K/DOQI clinical practice guidelines for bone metabolism and disease in chronic kidney disease. *Am J Kidney Dis.* 2003;42:S1-S201.
14. Aronoff GR, Berns JS, Brier ME, et al. Drug prescribing in renal failure. 4th ed. Available at: http://www.kdp-baptist.louisville.edu/renalbook/. Accessed October 3, 2009.
15. Propper RD, Shurin SB, Nathan DG. Reassessment of the use of desferrioxamine B in iron overload. *N Engl J Med.* 1976;294:1421-1143.
16. Cohen AR, Martin M, Mizanin J, et al. Vision and hearing during deferoxamine therapy. *J Pediatr.* 1990;117:326-330.
17. Scanderberg AC, Izzi GC, Butturini A, et al. Pulmonary syndrome and intravenous high-dose desferrioxamine. *Lancet.* 1990;336:1511.
18. Davies SC, Hungerford JL, Arden GB, et al. Ocular toxicity of high-dose intravenous desferrioxamine. *Lancet.* 1983;23:181-184.
19. Bentur Y, Koren G, Tesoro A, et al. Comparison of deferoxamine pharmacokinetics between asymptomatic thalassemic children and those exhibiting severe neurotoxicity. *Clin Pharmacol Ther.* 1990;47:478-482.
20. Carlsson M, Cortes D, Jepsen S, Kanstrup T. Severe iron intoxication treated with exchange transfusion. *Arch Dis Child.* 2007;93:321-322.
21. Trissel LA, ed. *Handbook on Injectable Drugs.* 15th ed. Bethesda, MD: American Society of Health-System Pharmacists; 2009.
22. Dickerhoff R. Acute aphasia and loss of vision with deferoxamine overdose. *Am J Pediatr Hematol Oncol.* 1987;9:287-288.
23. Freedman MH, Grisaru D, Olivieri N, et al. Pulmonary syndrome in patients with thalassemia major receiving intravenous deferoxamine infusions. *Am J Dis Child.* 1990;144:565-569.
24. Adamson IY, Sienko A, Tenenbein M. Pulmonary toxicity of deferoxamine in iron poisoned mice. *Toxicol Appl Pharm.* 1993;120:13-19.
25. Tenenbein M, Kowalski S, Sienko A, et al. Pulmonary toxic effects of continuous desferrioxamine administration in acute poisoning. *Lancet.* 1992;339:699-701.
26. Chan KW, Bond M, Fernandez W. Desferrioxamine in acute iron poisoning. *Lancet.* 1992;339:1601-1602.
27. Anderson KJ, Rivers RPA. Desferrioxamine in acute iron poisoning. *Lancet.* 1992;339:1602.
28. Macarol V, Yawalkar SH. Desferrioxamine in acute iron poisoning. *Lancet.* 1992;339:1601.
29. Shannon M. Desferrioxamine in acute iron poisoning. *Lancet.* 1992;339:1601.
30. Cheney K, Gumbiner C, Blaine B, et al. Survival after a severe iron poisoning treated with intermittent infusions of deferoxamine. *Clin Toxicol.* 1995;33:61-66.
31. Koren G, Bentur Y, Strong D, et al. Acute changes in renal function associated with deferoxamine therapy. *Am J Dis Child.* 1989;143:1077-1080.
32. Eisen TF, Lacouture PG, Woolf A. Visual detection of ferrioxamine color changes in urine. *Vet Hum Toxicol.* 1988;30:369-370.
33. Valentine K, Mastropietro C, Sarnaik AP. Infantile iron poisoning: challenges in diagnosis and management. *Pedaitr Crit Care Med.* 2009;10:e31-e33.

References

Dexamethasone Sodium Phosphate

1. Available at: http://www.usp.org/hqi/similarProducts/choosy.html. Accessed August 9, 2009.
2. Dexamethasone sodium phosphate injection, USP. Schaumburg, IL: American Pharmaceutical Partners Inc; March 2004.
3. Chamberlin P, Meyer WJ. Management of pituitary-adrenal suppression secondary to corticosteroid therapy. *Pediatrics.* 1981;67:245-251.
4. Gross SJ, Anbar RD, Mettelman BB. Follow-up at 15 years of preterm infants from a controlled trial of moderately early dexamethasone for the prevention of chronic lung disease. *Pediatrics.* 115;681-687.
5. LeFlore JL, Salhab WA, Broyles RS, et al. Association of antenatal and postnatal dexamethasone exposure with outcomes in extremely low birth weight neonates. *Pediatrics.* 2002;110:275-279.
6. Durand M, Sardesai S, McEvoy C. Effects of early dexamethasone therapy on pulmonary mechanics and chronic lung disease in very low birth weight infants: a randomized, controlled trial. *Pediatrics.* 1995;95:584-590.
7. The Vermont Oxford Network Steroid Study Group. Early postnatal dexamethasone therapy for the prevention of chronic lung disease. *Pediatrics.* 2001;108:741-748.
8. American Academy of Pediatrics, Canadian Paediatric Society: Postnatal corticosteroids to treat or prevent chronic lung disease in preterm infants. *Pediatrics.* 2002;109:330-338.
9. Tellez DW, Galvis AG, Storgion SA, et al. Dexamethasone in the prevention of postextubation stridor in children. *J Pediatr.* 1991;118:289-294.
10. Couser RJ, Ferrara B, Falde B, et al. Effectiveness of dexamethasone in preventing extubation failure in preterm infants at increased risk for airway edema. *J Pediatr.* 1992;121:591-596.
11. Doyle LW, Davis PG, Morley CJ, et al. Low-dose dexamethasone facilitates extubation among chronically ventilator dependent infants: a multicenter, international, randomized, controlled. *Pediatrics.* 2006;117:75-83.
12. Anene O, Meert KL, Uy H, et al. Dexamethasone for the prevention of post-extubation airway obstruction: a prospective, randomized, double-blind, placebo-controlled trial. *Crit Care Med.* 1996;24:1666-1669.
13. Alvarez O, Freeman A, Bedros A, et al. Randomized double-blind crossover ondansetron-dexamethasone versus ondansetron-placebo study for the treatment of chemotherapy-induced nausea and vomiting in pediatric patients with malignancies. *J Pediatr Hematol Oncol.* 1995;17:145-150.
14. Holdsworth MT, Raisch DW, Frost J. Acute and delayed nausea and emesis control in pediatric oncology patients. *Cancer.* 2006;106:931-940.
15. Kris MG, Hesketh PJ, Somerfield MR, et al. American Society of Clinical Oncology Guideline for antiemetics in ocology: update 2006. *J Clin Oncology.* 2006;24:2932-2947.
16. Madan R, Bhatia A, Chakithandy S, et al. Prophylactic dexamethasone for postoperative nausea and vomiting in pediatric strabismus surgery: a dose ranging and safety evaluation study. *Anesth Analg.* 2005;100:1622-1666.
17. Subramaniam B, Madan R, Sadhasivam S, et al. Dexamethasone is a cost-effective alternative to ondansetron in preventing PONV after paediatric strabismus repair. *Br J Anaesthesia.* 2001;86:84-89.
18. Fazel MR, Yegane-Moghaddam A, Forghani, et al. The effect of dexamethasone on postoperative vomiting and oral intake after adenotonsillectomy. *Int J Pediatr Otorhinolaryngol.* 2007;71:1235-1238.
19. Elhakim M, Ali NM, Rashed I, et al. Dexamethasone reduces postoperative vomiting and pain after pediatric tonsillectomy. *Can J Anesth.* 2003;50:392-397.
20. Hanasono MM, Lalakea L, Mikulec AA, et al. Perioperative steroids in tonsillectomy using electrocautery and sharp dissection techniques. *Arch Otolaryngol Head Neck Surg.* 2004;130:917-921.
21. Super DM, Cartelli NA, Brooks LJ, et al. A prospective randomized double-blind study to evaluate the effect of dexamethasone in acute laryngotracheitis. *J Pediatr.* 1989;115:323-329.
22. Fitzgerald DA, Kilham HA. Croup: assessment and evidence-based management. *Med J Austral.* 2003;179:372-377.
23. Rittichier KK, Ledwith CA. Outpatient treatment of moderate croup with dexamethasone: intramuscular versus oral dosing. *Pediatrics.* 2000;106:1344-1348.
24. Klassen T. Croup: a current perspective. *Pediatr Clin North Am.* 1999;46:1167-1178.
25. Chub-Uppakarn S, Sangsupawanich P. A randomized comparison of dexamethasone 0.25 mg/kg versus 0.6 mg/kg for the treatment of moderate to severe croup. *Int J Pediatr Otorhinolaryngol.* 2007;71:473-477.
26. Arditi M, Mason EO, Bradley JS, et al. Three-year multicenter surveillance of pneumococcal meningitis in children: clinical characteristics, and outcome related to penicillin susceptibility and dexamethasone use. *Pediatrics.* 1998;102:1087-1097.
27. Molyneux EM, Walsh AL, Forsyth H, et al. Dexamethasone treatment in childhood bacterial meningitis in Malawi: a randomized controlled trial. *Lancet.* 2002;360:211-218.
28. Tunkel AR, Hartman BJ, Kaplan SL, et al. Practice guidelines for the management of bacterial meningitis. *Clin Infect Dis.* 2004;39:1267-1284.
29. Mongelluzzo J, Mohamad Z, Ten Have TR, Shah SS. Corticosteroids and mortality in children with bacterial meningitis. *JAMA.* 2008;299:2048-2055.
30. National Asthma Education and Prevention Program Expert Panel Report 3: Guidelines for the diagnosis and management of asthma. National Institutes of Health Publication No. 07-4051, Bethesda, MD. August 2007.
31. Ghajar J, Hariri RJ. Management of pediatric head injury. *Pediatr Clin North Am.* 1992;39:1093-1125.
32. Trissel LA. *Handbook on Injectable Drugs.* 13th ed. Bethesda, MD: American Society of Health-System Pharmacists; 2005.
33. Dexamethasone, dexamethasone acetate, dexamethasone sodium phosphate. Lexi-Comp® Online with AHFS® (database). Bethesda, MD: American Society of Health-System Pharmacists; updated May 26, 2009.
34. Atkinson WL, Pickering LK, Schwartz B, et al. General recommendations on immunization. Recommendations of the Advisory Committee on Immunization Practices (ACIP) and the American Academy of Family Physicians (AAFP). *MMWR Recomm Rep.* 2002;51(RR-2):1-35.
35. Stark AR, Carlo WA, Tyson JE, et al. Adverse effects of early dexamethasone treatment in extremely-low-birth-weight infants. *N Engl J Med.* 2001;344:95-101.
36. Kaempf JW, Campbell B, Sklar RS, et al. Implementing potentially better practices to improve neonatal outcomes after reducing postnatal dexamethasone use in infants born between 501 and 1250 grams. *Pediatrics.* 2003;111:e534-e541.

Dexmedetomidine HCl

1. Available at: http://www.usp.org/hqi/similarProducts/choosy.html. Accessed August 8, 2009.
2. Precedex [prescribing information]. Lake Forest, IL: Hospira; October 2008.
3. Berkenbosch JW, Wankum PC, Tobias JD. Prospective evaluation of dexmedetomidine for noninvasive procedural sedation in children. *Pediatr Crit Care Med.* 2005;6:435-439.
4. Koroglu A, Demirbilek S, Teksan H, et al. Sedative, haemodynamic and respiratory effects of dexmedetomidine in children undergoing magnetic resonance imaging examination: preliminary results. *Br J Anaesth.* 2005;94:821-824.
5. Heard C, Burrows F, Johnson K, et al. A comparison of dexmedetomidine-midazolam with propofol for maintenance of anesthesia in children undergoing magnetic resonance imaging. *Anesth Analg.* 2008;107:1832-1839.
6. Tobias JD, Berkenbosch JW. Sedation during mechanical ventilation in infants and children: dexmedetomidine versus midazolam. *S Med J.* 2004;97:451-455.
7. Buck ML, Willson DF. Use of dexmedetomidine in the pediatric intensive care unit. *Pharmacother.* 2008;1:51-57.
8. Chrysostomou C, Di Filippo S, Manrique AM, et al. Use of dexmedetomidine in children after cardiac and thoracic surgery. *Pediatr Crit Care Med.* 2006;7:126-131.

9. Finkel JC, Johnson YJ, Quezado ZMN. The use of dexmedetomidine to facilitate acute discontinuation of opioids after cardiac transplantation in children. *Crit Care Med.* 2005;33:2110-2112.
10. Trissel LA. *Handbook on Injectable Drugs.* 15th ed. Bethesda, MD: American Society of Health-System Pharmacists; 2009.
11. Saadawy I, Boker A, Elshahawy MA, et al. Effect of dexmedetomidine on the characteristics of bupivacaine in a caudal block in pediatrics. *Acta Anaesthesiol Scand.* 2009;53:251-256.
12. Yuen VM, Hui TW, Irwin MG, Yuen MK. A comparison of intranasal dexmedetomidine and oral midazolam for premedication in pediatric anesthesia: a double-blind randomized controlled trial. *Anesth Analg.* 2008;106:1715-1721.
13. Berkenbosch JW, Tobias JD. Development of bradycardia during sedation with dexmedetomidine in an infant concurrently receiving digoxin. *Pediatr Crit Care Med.* 2004;4:203-205.
14. Hammer GB, Drove DR, Cao H, et al. The effects of dexmedetomidine on cardiac electrophysiology in children. *Anesth Analg.* 2008;106:79-83.
15. Ludwig K, Sorrell M, Liu P. Severe rash associated with dexmedetomidine use during mechanical ventilation. *Pharmacother.* 2009;29:479-481.
16. Petroz GC, Sikich N, James M, et al. A Phase I, Two-center study of the pharmacokinetics and pharmacodynamics of dexmedetomidine in children. *Anesthesiol.* 2006;105:1098-1110.
17. Diaz SM, Rodarte A, Foley J, Capparelli EV. Pharmacokinetics of dexmedetomidine in postsurgical pediatric intensive care unit patients: Preliminary study. *Pediatr Crit Care Med.* 2007;8:419-424.
18. Potts AL, Warman GR, Anderson BJ. Dexmedetomidine disposition in children: a population analysis. *Pediatr Anesthesia.* 2008;18:722-730.

Dextrose

1. Available at: http://ismp.org/Tools/highalertmedications.pdf. Accessed March 3, 2009.
2. 20%, 30%, 40%, 50% and 70% Dextrose Injection, USP [package insert]. Lake Forest, IL: Hospira; September 2005.
3. Frankel L, Stevenson DK. Metabolic emergencies of the newborn: hypoxemia and hypoglycemia. *Compr Ther.* 1987;13:14-19.
4. Dextrose. Lexi-Comp® Online with AHFS® (database). Hudson, OH: Lexi-Comp Inc; updated June 12, 2009.
5. Polk DH. Disorders of carbohydrate metabolism. In: Tauesch HW, Ballard RA, eds. *Avery's Diseases of the Newborn.* 7th ed. Philadelphia, PA: WB Saunders Company; 1998:1235-1241.
6. Sperling MA. Hypoglycemia. In: Behrman RE, Kliegman RM, Jenson HB, eds. *Nelson Textbook of Pediatrics.* 17th ed. Philadelphia, PA: WB Saunders Company; 2004:505-508.
7. Pryds O, Christensen NJ, Friis-Hansen B. Increased cerebral blood flow and plasma epinephrine in hypoglycemic, preterm neonates. *Pediatrics.* 1990;85:172-176.
8. LaFranchi S. Hypoglycemia of infancy and childhood. *Pediatr Clin North Am.* 1987;34:961-982.
9. Lilien LD, Grajwer LA, Pildes RS. Treatment of neonatal hypoglycemia with continuous intravenous glucose infusion. *J Pediatr.* 1977;91:779-782.
10. Lilien LD, Pildes RS, Srinivasan G, et al. Treatment of neonatal hypoglycemia with minibolus and intravenous glucose infusion. *J Pediatr.* 1980;97:295-298.
11. Mehta A. Prevention and management of neonatal hypoglycemia. *Arch Dis Child.* 1994;70:F54-F65.
12. American Heart Association guidelines for cardiopulmonary resuscitation and emergency cardiovascular care. *Circulation.* 2005;112:167-187.
13. Lui K, Thungappa U, Nair A, et al. Treatment with hypertonic dextrose and insulin in severe hyperkalemia of immature infants. *Acta Paediatr.* 1992;81:213-216.
14. Collins JE, Leonard JV. Hyperinsulinism in asphyxiated and small-for-dates infants with hypoglycemia. *Lancet.* 1984;2:311-313.
15. Okada A, Imura K. Parenteral nutrition in neonates. In: Rombeau JL, Caldwell MD, eds. *Clinical Nutrition: Parenteral Nutrition.* 2nd ed. Philadelphia, PA: WB Saunders Company; 1993:756-769.

Diazepam

1. Available at: http://ismp.org/Tools/highalertmedications.pdf. Accessed October 9, 2009.
2. Available at: http://www.usp.org/hqi/similarProducts/choosy.html. Accessed October 7, 2009.
3. Diazepam [package insert]. Deerfield, IL: Baxter Healthcare; MLT-01161/1.
4. Upton J, Mulliken JB, Murray JE. Major intravenous extravasation injuries. *Am J Surg.* 1979;137:497-506.
5. Sillers BR. Irritant properties of diazepam. *Br Dent J.* 1968;124:295.
6. Shankar V, Deshpande JK. Procedural sedation in the pediatric patient. *Anesthesiol Clin N Am.* 2005;23:635-654, viii.
7. Flood RG, Krauss B. Procedural sedation and analgesia for children in the emergency department. *Emerg Med Clin North Am.* 2003;21:121-139.
8. Krauss B, Green S. Procedural sedation and analgesia in children. *Lancet.* 2006;367:766-780.
9. Bavdekar SB, Mahajan MD, Chandu KV. Analgesia and sedation in paediatric intensive care unit. *J Postgrad Med.* 1999;45:95-102.
10. Wheless JW, Clarke DF, Carpenter D. Treatment of pediatric epilepsy: expert opinion, 2005. *J Child Neurol.* 2005;20(suppl 1):1-57.
11. Maytal J, Novak GP, King KC. Lorazepam in the treatment of refractory neonatal seizures. *J Child Neurol.* 1991;6:319-323.
12. Zupanc ML. Neonatal seizures. *Pediatr Clin N Amer.* 2004;51:961-978.
13. Chamberlain JM, Altieri MA, Futterman C, et al. A prospective randomized study comparing intramuscular midazolam with intravenous diazepam for the treatment of seizures in children. *Pediatr Emerg Care.* 1997;13:92-94.
14. Giang DW, McBride MC. Lorazepam versus diazepam for the treatment of status epilepticus. *Pediatr Neurol.* 1988;4:358-361.
15. American Academy of Pediatrics Committee on Drugs. Emergency drug doses for infants and children. *Pediatrics.* 1998;101:e1-e11.
16. Camfield PR. Treatment of status epilepticus in children. *Can Med Assoc J.* 1983;128:671-672.
17. Eriksson K, Kalviainen R. Pharmacologic management of convulsive status epilepticus in childhood. *Expert Rev Neurotherapeutics.* 2005;5:777-783.
18. Hegenbarth MA; American Academy of Pediatrics Committee on Drugs. Preparing for pediatric emergencies: drugs to consider. *Pediatrics.* 2008;121:433-443.
19. Khoo BH, Lee EL, Lam KL. Neonatal tetanus treated with high dosage diazepam. *Arch Dis Child.* 1978;53:737-739.
20. Tekur U, Gupta A, Tayal G, et al. Blood concentrations of diazepam and its metabolites in children and neonates with tetanus. *J Pediatr.* 1983;102:145-147.
21. Aronoff GR, Berns JS, Brier ME, et al. Drug prescribing in renal failure. 4th ed. Available at: http://www.kdp-baptist.louisville.edu/renalbook/. Accessed August 28, 2009.
22. Neale BW, Mesler EL, Young M, et al. Proylene glycol-induced lactic acidosis in a patient with normal renal function: a proposed mechanism and monitoring recommendations. *Ann Pharmacother.* 2005;39:1732-1736.
23. Yaucher NE, Fish JT, Smith HW, et al. Propylene glycol-associated renal toxicity from lorazepam infusion. *Pharmacotherapy.* 2003;23:1094-1099.
24. Smith BT, Masotti RE. Intravenous diazepam in the treatment of prolonged seizure activity in neonates and infants. *Dev Med Child Neurol.* 1971;13:630-634.
25. Thong YH, Abramson DC. Continuous infusion of diazepam in infants with severe recurrent convulsions. *Med Ann DC.* 1974;43:63-65.
26. Lopez-Herce J, Bonet C, Meana A, et al. Benzyl alcohol poisoning following diazepam intravenous infusion. *Ann Pharmacother.* 1995;29:632.
27. Trissel LA, ed. *Handbook on Injectable Drugs.* 15th ed. Bethesda, MD: American Society of Health-System Pharmacists; 2009.
28. Delgado-Escueta AV, Wasterlain C, Treiman DM, et al. Current concepts in neurology. Management of status epilepticus. *N Engl J Med.* 1982;306:1337-1340.
29. Bell HE, Bertino JS. Constant diazepam infusion in the treatment of continuous seizure activity. *Drug Intell Clin Pharm.* 1984;18:965-970.

References

30. Cronin CM. Neurotoxicity of lorazepam in a premature infant. *Pediatrics.* 1992;89:1129.
31. Reiter PD, Stiles AD. Lorazepam toxicity in a premature infant. *Ann Pharmacother.* 1993;27:727-729.
32. Chess PR, D'Angio CT. Clonic movement following lorazepam administration in full-term infants. *Arch Pediatr Adolesc Med.* 1998;152:98-99.
33. Diazepam. Lexi-Comp® Online with AHFS® (database). Bethesda, MD: American Society of Health-System Pharmacists; updated September 8, 2009.
34. Straaten HL, Rademaker CM, de Vries LS. Comparison of the effect of midazolam or vecuronium on blood pressure and cerebral blood flow velocity in premature newborns. *Dev Pharmacol Ther.* 1992;19:191-195.
35. Tobias JD. Sedation analgesia in paediatric intensive care units. *Pediatr Drugs.*1999;1:109-126.
36. Hoffman EJ, Warren EW. Flumazenil: a benzodiazepine antagonist. *Clin Pharm.* 1993;12:614-656.
37. Flumazenil Injection USP [package insert]. Bedford, OH: Bedford Laboratories; December 2007.

Digoxin

1. Available at: http://ismp.org/Tools/highalertmedications.pdf. Accessed September 13, 2009.
2. Available at: http://www.usp.org/hqi/similarProducts/choosy.html. Accessed September 13, 2009.
3. Available at: http://ismp.org/Tools/confuseddrugnames.pdf. Accessed September 13, 2009.
4. Lanoxin injection pediatric [prescribing information]. Research Triangle Park, NC: GlaxoSmithKline; July 2002.
5. Berman W, Whitman V, Marks KH, et al. Inadvertent overadministration of digoxin to low-birth-weight infants. *J Pediatr.* 1978;92:1024-1025.
6. Bhambhani V, Beri RS, Puliyel JM. Inadvertent overdosing of neonates as a result of the dead space of the syringe hub and needle. *Arch Dis Child Fetal Neonatal Ed.* 2005;90:F444-F446.
7. Halkin H, Radomsky M, Blieden L, et al. Steady state serum digoxin concentrations in relation to digitalis toxicity in neonates and infants. *Pediatrics.* 1978;61:184-188.
8. Bendayan R, McKenzie MW. Digoxin pharmacokinetics and dosage requirements in pediatric patients. *Clin Pharm.* 1983;2:224-235.
9. Pinsky WW, Jacobsen JR, Gillette PC, et al. Dosage of digoxin in premature infants. *J Pediatr.* 1979;96:639-642.
10. Park MK. Use of digoxin in infants and children, with specific emphasis on dosage. *J Pediatr.* 1986;108:871-877.
11. Lang D, von Bernuth G. Serum concentrations and serum half-life of digoxin in premature and mature newborns. *Pediatrics.* 1977;59:902-906.
12. Berman W, Dubynsky O, Whitman V, et al. Digoxin therapy in low-birth-weight infants with patent ductus arteriosus. *J Pediatr.* 1978;93:652-655.
13. Gortner L, Hellenbrecht D. Estimation of digoxin dosage in VLBW infants using serum creatinine concentrations. *Acta Paediatr Scand.* 1986;75:433-438.
14. Johnson GL, Desai NS, Pauly TH, et al. Complications associated with digoxin therapy in low-birth weight infants. *Pediatrics.* 1982;69:463-465.
15. Nyberg L, Wettrell G. Pharmacokinetics and dosage of digoxin in neonates and infants. *Eur J Clin Pharmacol.* 1980;18:69-74.
16. Rutkowski MM, Cohen SN, Doyle EF. Drug therapy of heart disease in pediatric patients II. The treatment of congestive heart failure in infants and children with digitalis preparations. *Am Heart J.* 1973;86:270-275.
17. Hastreiter AR, van der Horst RL, Voda C, et al. Maintenance digoxin dosage and steady-state plasma concentration in infants and children. *J Pediatr.* 1985;107:140-146.
18. Bakir M, Bilgic A. Single daily dose of digoxin for maintenance therapy of infants and children with cardiac disease: is it reliable? *Pediatr Cardiol.* 1994;15:229-232.
19. Aronoff GR, Berns JS, Brier ME, et al. Drug prescribing in renal failure. 4th ed. Available at: http://www.kdp-baptist.louisville.edu/renalbook/. Accessed September 13, 2009.
20. American Academy of Pediatrics. Committee on Drugs. Emergency drug doses for infants and children. *Pediatrics.* 1988;81:462-465.
21. Trissel LA, ed. *Handbook on Injectable Drugs.* 15th ed. Bethesda, MD: American Society of Health-System Pharmacists; 2009.
22. Robinson CA, Sawyer JE. Y-site compatibility of medications with parenteral nutrition. *J Pediatr Pharmacol Ther.* 2009;14:49-57.
23. Fenner KS, Troutman MD, Kempshall S, et al. Drug-Drug interactions mediated through p-glycoprotein: clinical relevance and *in vitro–in vivo* correlation using digoxin as a probe drug. *Clin Pharm and Ther.* 2009:85:173-181.
24. Phelps SJ, Kamper CA, Bottorff MB, et al. Effect of age and serum creatinine on endogenous digoxin-like substances in infants and children. *J Pediatr.* 1987;110:136-139.
25. Pudek MR, Seccombe DW, Whitfield MF, et al. Digoxin-like immunoreactivity in premature and full-term infants not receiving digoxin therapy. *N Engl J Med.* 1983;308:904-905.
26. Valdes R, Graves SW, Brown BA, et al. Endogenous substance in newborn infants causing false positive digoxin measurements. *J Pediatr.* 1983;102:947-950.
27. Ebara H, Suzuki S, Nagashima K, et al. Digoxin-like immunoreactive substances in urine and serum from preterm and term infants: relationship to renal excretion of sodium. *J Pediatr.* 1986;108:760-762.
28. Graves SW, Brown B, Valdes R. An endogenous digoxin-like substance in patients with renal impairment. *Ann Intern Med.* 1983;99:604-608.
29. Greenway DC, Nanji AA. Falsely increased results of digoxin sera from patients with liver disease: ten immunoassay kits compared. *Clin Chem.* 1985;31:1078-1079.
30. Digoxin. Lexi-Comp® Online with AHFS® (database). Hudson, OH: Lexi-Comp Inc; updated August 4, 2009.
31. Digibind [prescribing information]. Research Triangle Park, NC: GlaxoSmithKline; September 2003.
32. Martiny SS, Phelps SJ, Massey KL. Treatment of severe digitalis intoxication with digoxin-specific antibody fragments: a clinical review. *Crit Care Med.* 1988;16:629-635.

Digoxin Immune Fab

1. Available at: http://www.usp.org/hqi/similarProducts/choosy.html. Accessed September 13, 2009.
2. Digibind [prescribing information]. Research Triangle Park, NC: GlaxoSmithKline; September 2003.
3. Allen NM, Dunham GD. Treatment of digitalis intoxication with emphasis on the clinical use of digoxin FAB. *DICP Ann Pharmacother.* 1990;24:991-998.
4. Martiny SS, Phelps SJ, Massey KL. Treatment of severe digitalis intoxication with digoxin-specific antibody fragments: a clinical review. *Crit Care Med.* 1988;16:629-635.
5. Zucker AR, Lacina SJ, DasGupta DS, et al. Fab fragments of digoxin-specific antibodies used to reverse ventricular fibrillation induced by digoxin ingestion in a child. *Pediatrics.* 1982;70:468-471.
6. Murphy DJ, Bremner WF, Haber E, et al. Massive digoxin poisoning treated with Fab fragments of digoxin-specific antibodies. *Pediatrics.* 1982;70:472-473.
7. Presti S, Friedman D, Saslow J, et al. Digoxin toxicity in a premature infant: treatment with Fab fragments of digoxin-specific antibodies. *Pediatr Cardiol.* 1985;6:91-94.
8. Hursting MF, Raisys VA, Opheim KE, et al. Determination of free digoxin concentrations in serum for monitoring Fab treatment of digoxin overdose. *Clin Chem.*1987;33:1652-1655.

9. Kaufman J, Leikin J, Kendzierski D, et al. Use of digoxin Fab immune fragments in a seven-day-old infant. *Pediatr Emerg Care*. 1990;6:118-121.
10. American Academy of Pediatrics Committee on Drugs. Emergency drug doses for infants and children. *Pediatrics*. 1998;101:e1-e11.
11. Digoxin Immune Fab. Lexi-Comp® Online with AHFS® (database). Hudson, OH: Lexi-Comp Inc; updated July 17, 2009.
12. Woolf AD, Wenger T, Smith TW, et al. The use of digoxin-specific Fab fragments for severe digitalis intoxication in children. *N Engl J Med*. 1992;326:1739-1744.
13. Fazio A. Fab fragments in the treatment of digoxin overdose: pediatric considerations. *South Med J*. 1987;80:1553-1556.
14. Wenger TL, Butler VP Jr, Haber E, et al. Treatment of 63 severely digoxin-specific Fab patients with digoxin-specific antibody fragments. *J Am Coll Cardiol*. 1985;5:118A-123A.
15. Lemon M, Andrews DJ, Binks AM, et al. Concentrations of free serum digoxin after treatment with antibody fragments. *Br Med J*. 1987;295:1520-1521.
16. Ujhelyi MR, Green PJ, Cummings DM, et al. Determination of free serum digoxin concentrations in digoxin toxic patients after administration of digoxin Fab antibodies. *Ther Drug Monitor*. 1992;14:147-154.
17. Ujhelyi MR, Colucci RD, Cummings DM, et al. Monitoring serum digoxin concentrations during digoxin immune Fab therapy. *DICP Ann Pharmacother*. 1991;25:1047-1049.
18. Ujhelyi MR, Robert S, Cummings DM, et al. Influence of digoxin immune Fab therapy and renal dysfunction on the disposition of total and free digoxin. *Ann Intern Med*. 1993;119:273-277.
19. Ocal IT, Green TR. Serum digoxin in the presence of digibind: determination of digoxin by the Abbott AxSYM and Baxter Stratus II immunoassays by direct analysis without pretreatment of serum samples. *Clin Chem*. 1998;44:1947-1950.

Dihydroergotamine Mesylate

1. Available at: http://ismp.org/Tools/confuseddrugnames.pdf. Accessed August 30, 2009.
2. Available at: http://www.usp.org/hqi/similarProducts/choosy.html. Accessed August 30, 2009.
3. D.H.E. 45—dihydroergotamine mesylate [package insert]. Costa Mesa, CA: Valeant Pharmaceuticals; 2002.
4. Padon A, Ostadian M, Wright C, et al. Dihydroergotamine-associated intestinal ischemia in a child with cyclic vomiting syndrome. *J Pediatr Gastroenterol Nutr*. 2006;42:573-575.
5. Ford RG, Ford KT. Continuous intravenous dihydroergotamine in the treatment of intractable headache. *Headache*. 1997;37:129-136.
6. Winner P, Dalessio D, Mathew N, et al. Concomitant administration of antiemetics is not necessary with intramuscular dihydroergotamine. Concomitant administration of antiemetics is not necessary with intramuscular dihydroergotamine. *Am J Emerg Med*. 1994;12:138-141.

Diltiazem HCl

1. Available at: http://www.usp.org/hqi/similarProducts/choosy.html. Accessed August 1, 2009.
2. Diltiazem hydrochloride injection [package insert]. Bedford, OH: Bedford Laboratories; May 2005.
3. Pass RH, Libermam L, Al-Fayadd HM, et al. Continuous intravenous diltiazem infusion for short-term ventricular rate control in children. *Am J Cardiol*. 2000; 86:559-562.
4. Porter CJ, Garson A, Gillette PC. Verapamil: an effective calcium blocking agent for pediatric patients. *Pediatrics*. 1983;71:748-755.
5. Flynn JT, Pasko DA. Calcium channel blockers: pharmacology and place in therapy of pediatric hypertension. *Pediatr Nephrol*. 2000;15:302-316.
6. Islam S, Masiakos P, Schnitzer JJ, et al. Diltiazem reduces pulmonary arterial pressures in recurrent pulmonary hypertension associated with pulmonary hypoplasia. *J Pediatr Surg*. 1999;34:712-714.
7. Houde C, Bohn DJ, Freedom RM, et al. Profile of paediatric patients with pulmonary hypertension judged by responsiveness to vasodilators. *Br Heart J*. 1993;70:461-468.

DiphenhydrAMINE HCl

1. Available at: http://ismp.org/Tools/confuseddrugnames.pdf. Accessed August 26, 2009.
2. Available at: http://www.usp.org/hqi/similarProducts/choosy.html. Accessed August 26, 2009.
3. Benadryl [package insert]. New York, NY: Parke Davis, Division of Pfizer Inc; May 2006.
4. Hegenbarth MA; American Academy of Pediatrics Committee on Drugs. Preparing for pediatric emergencies: drug to consider. *Pediatrics*. 2008;121:433-443.
5. Gupta JM, Lovejoy FH Jr. Acute phenothiazine toxicity in childhood: a five-year survey. *Pediatrics*. 1967;39:771-774.
6. American Academy of Pediatrics. Committee on Drugs. Anaphylaxis. *Pediatrics*. 1973;51:136-140.
7. Cohen GH, Casta A, Sapire DW, et al. Decorticate posture following cardiac cocktail. *Pediatr Cardiol*. 1982;2:251-253.
8. Knight ME, Roberts RJ. Phenothiazine and butyrophenone intoxication in children. *Pediatr Clin North Am*. 1986;33:298-309.
9. Relling RV, Mulhern RK, Fairclough D, et al. Chlorpromazine with and without lorazepam as antiemetic therapy in children receiving uniform chemotherapy. *J Pediatr*. 1993;12:811-816.
10. Aronoff GR, Berns JS, Brier ME, et al. Drug prescribing in renal failure. 4th ed. Available at: http://www.kdp-baptist.louisville.edu/renalbook/. Accessed September 12, 2009.
11. Rapp RP, Wermeling DP, Piecoro JJ Jr. Guidelines for the administration of commonly used intravenous drugs—1984 update. *Drug Intell Clin Pharm*. 1984;18:217-232.
12. Trissel LA, ed. *Handbook on Injectable Drugs*. 15th ed. Bethesda, MD: American Society of Health-System Pharmacists; 2009.
13. Hestand HE, Teske DW. Diphenhydramine hydrochloride intoxication. *J Pediatr*. 1977;90:1017-1018.
14. Simons FER. Diphenhydramine in infants. *Arch Pediatr Adolesc Med*. 2007;161:105.
15. Santiago-Palma J, Fischberg D, Kornick C, et al. Diphenhydramine as an analgesic adjuvant in refractory cancer pain. *J Pain Symptom Manage*. 2001;22:699-703.

DOBUTamine HCl

1. Available at: http://ismp.org/Tools/highalertmedications.pdf. ISMP 2008. Accessed October 24, 2009.
2. Available at: http://ismp.org/Tools/confuseddrugnames.pdf. Accessed October 24, 2009.
3. Available at: http://www.usp.org/hqi/similarProducts/choosy.html. Accessed October 24, 2009.
4. Dobutamine hydrochloride injection [package insert]. Bedford, OH: Bedford Laboratories Inc; June 2007.
5. Dobutamine hydrochloride. Lexi-Comp Online with AHFS (database). Bethesda, MD: American Society of Health-System Pharmacists; updated May 26, 2009.
6. American Academy of Pediatrics and American Heart Association. *Pediatric Advanced Life Support*. (Provider manual.) Dallas, TX: American Heart Association; 2006.

References

7. Bohn DJ, Poirier CS, Edmonds JF, et al. Hemodynamic effects of dobutamine after cardiopulmonary bypass in children. *Crit Care Med.* 1980;8:367-371.
8. Hegenbarth MA; American Academy of Pediatrics Committee on Drugs. Preparing for pediatric emergencies: drugs to consider. *Pediatrics.* 2008;121:433-443.
9. Driscoll DJ, Gillette PC, Duff DF, et al. The hemodynamic effect of dobutamine in children. *Am J Cardiol.* 1979;43:581-585.
10. Jose JB, Niguidula F, Botros S, et al. Hemodynamic effects of dobutamine in children. *Anesthesiology.* 1981;55:A61.
11. Schranz D, Stopfkuchen H, Jungst BK, et al. Hemodynamic effects of dobutamine in children with cardiovascular failure. *Eur J Pediatr.* 1982;139:4-7.
12. Perkin RM, Levin DL, Webb R, et al. Dobutamine: a hemodynamic evaluation in children with shock. *J Pediatr.* 1982;100:977-983.
13. Martinez AM, Padbury JF, Thio S. Dobutamine pharmacokinetics and cardiovascular responses in critically ill neonates. *Pediatr* 1992;89:47-51.
14. Greenough A, Emery EF. Randomized trial comparing dopamine and dobutamine in preterm infants. *Eur J Pediatr.* 1993;152:925-927.
15. Roze JC, Tohier C, Maingueneau C, et al. Response to dobutamine and dopamine in the hypotensive very preterm infant. *Arch Dis Child.* 1993;69:59-63.
16. Berg RA, Donnerstein RL, Padbury JF, et al. Dobutamine infusions in stable, critically ill children: pharmacokinetics and hemodynamic actions. *Crit Care Med.* 1993;21:678-686.
17. Klarr JM, Faix RG, Pryce CJE, et al. Randomized, blind trial of dopamine versus dobutamine for treatment of hypotension in preterm infants with respiratory distress syndrome. *J Pediatr.* 1994;125:117-122.
18. Hentschel R, Hensel D, Brune T, et al. Impact on blood pressure and intestinal perfusion of dobutamine or dopamine in hypotensive preterm infants. *Biol Neonate.* 1995;68:318-324.
19. Ruelas-Orozco G, Vargas-Origel A. Assessment of therapy for arterial hypotension in critically ill preterm infants. *Am J Perinatol.* 2000;17:95-99.
20. Committee on Drugs. Drugs for pediatric emergencies. *Pediatrics.* 1998;101:e13.
21. American Heart Association guidelines for cardiopulmonary resuscitation and emergency Cardiovascular care. Part 12: pediatric advanced life support. *Circulation.* 2005;112(suppl 1):167-187.
22. Banner W, Vernon DD, Minton SD, et al. Nonlinear dobutamine pharmacokinetics in a pediatric population. *Crit Care Med.* 1991;19:871-873.
23. Berg RA, Padbury JF, Donnerstein RL, et al. Dobutamine pharmacokinetics and pharmacodynamics in normal children and adolescents. *J Pharmacol Experiment Ther.* 1993;265:1232-1238.
24. Aronoff GR, Berns JS, Brier ME, et al. Drug prescribing in renal failure. 4th ed. Available at: http://www.kdp-baptist.louisville.edu/renalbook/. Accessed August 17, 2009.
25. Trissel LA, ed. *Handbook on Injectable Drugs.* 15th ed. Bethesda, MD: American Society of Health-System Pharmacists; 2009.
26. Allen EM, Van Boerum DH, Olsen AF, et al. Difference between the measured and ordered dose of catecholamine infusion. *Ann Pharmacother.* 1995;29:1095-1100.
27. Rich DS. New JCAHO medication management standards for 2004. *Am J Health-Syst Pharm.* 2004;61:1349-1358.
28. Buck ML, Wiggins BS, Sesler JM. Intraosseous Drug Administration in Children and Adults During Cardiopulmonary Resuscitation. *Ann Pharmacother.* 2007;41:1679-1686.
29. Unverferth DV, Blanford M, Kates RE, et al. Tolerance to dobutamine after a 72-hour continuous infusion. *Am J Med.* 1980;69:262-266.

Dolasetron Mesylate

1. Available at: http://www.usp.org/hqi/similarProducts/choosy.html. Accessed July 23, 2009.
2. Available at: http://ismp.org/Tools/confuseddrugnames.pdf. updated April 1, 2005.
3. Anzemet injection [prescribing information]. Bridgewater, NJ: Sanofi-Aventis US LLC; June 2006.
4. Coppes MJ, Lau R, Ingram LC, et al. Open-label comparison of the antiemetic efficacy of single intravenous doses of dolasetron mesylate in pediatric cancer patients receiving moderately to highly emetogenic chemotherapy. *Med Pediatr Onco.* 1999;33:99-105.
5. ASHP Therapeutic guidelines on the pharmacologic management of nausea and vomiting in adult and pediatric patients receiving chemotherapy or radiation therapy or undergoing surgery. *Am J Health Syst Pharm.* 1999;56:729-764.
6. Kris MG, Hesketh PJ, Somerfield MR, et al. American Society of Clinical Oncology Guideline for antiemetics in ocology: update 2006. *J Clin Oncology.* 2006;24:2932-2947.
7. Wagner D, Pandit U, Voepel-Lewis T, et al. Dolasetron for the prevention of postoperative vomiting in children undergoing strabismus surgery. *Paediatr Anaesth.* 2003;13:522-526.
8. Sukhani R, Pappas AL, Lurie J, Ondansetron and dolasetron provide equivalent postoperative vomiting control after ambulatory tonsillectomy in dexamethasone-pretreated children. *Anesth Analg.* 2002;95:1230-1235.
9. Trissel LA. *Handbook on Injectable Drugs.* 15th ed. Bethesda, MD: American Society of Health-System Pharmacists; 2009.

DOPamine HCl

1. Available at: http://ismp.org/Tools/highalertmedications.pdf. ISMP 2008. Accessed October 24, 2009.
2. Available at: http://ismp.org/Tools/confuseddrugnames.pdf. Accessed October 24, 2009.
3. Available at: http://www.usp.org/hqi/similarProducts/choosy.html. Accessed October 24, 2009.
4. Dopamine hydrochloride injection USP [package insert]. Lake Forest, IL: Hospira, Inc; October 2004.
5. Gaze NR. Tissue necrosis caused by commonly used intravenous infusions. *Lancet.* 1978;2:417-419.
6. American Academy of Pediatrics and American Heart Association. *Pediatric Advanced Life Support.* (Provider manual.) Dallas, TX: American Heart Association; 2006.
7. Stier PA, Bogner MP, Webster K, et al. Use of subcutaneous terbutaline to reverse peripheral ischemia. *Am J Emerg Med.* 1999;17:91-94.
8. Maggi JC, Angelats J, Scott JP. Gangrene in a neonate following dopamine therapy. *J Pediatr.* 1982;100:323-325.
9. Koerber RK, Haven GT, Cohen SM, et al. Peripheral gangrene associated with dopamine infusion in a child. *Clin Pediatr.* 1984;23:106-107.
10. Goenka S, Mehta AV, Powers PJ. An unusual peripheral vascular response to dopamine in a neonate. *Tenn Med.* 1999;92:375-376.
11. Zenk KE, Noerr B, Ward R. Severe sequelae from umbilical arterial catheter administration of dopamine. *Neonatal Network.* 1994;13:89-91.
12. American Heart Association Guidelines for Cardiopulmonary Resuscitation and Emergency Cardiovascular Care. Part 12: Pediatric Advanced Life Support. *Circulation.* 2005;112(suppl 1):167-187.
13. Han YY, Carcillo JA, Dragotta MA. Early reversal of pediatric-neonatal septic shock by community physicians is associated with improved outcome. *Pediatrics.* 2003;112:793-799.
14. Hegenbarth MA; American Academy of Pediatrics Committee on Drugs. Preparing for pediatric emergencies: drugs to consider. *Pediatrics.* 2008;121:433-443.
15. Driscoll DJ, Gillette PC, McNamara DG. The use of dopamine in children. *J Pediatr.* 1978;92:309-314.
16. Bhatt-Mehta V, Nahata MC, McClead RE, et al. Dopamine pharmacokinetics in critically ill newborn infants. *Eur J Clin Pharmacol.* 1991;40:593-597.
17. Greenough A, Emery EF. Randomized trial comparing dopamine and dobutamine in preterm infants. *Eur J Pediatr.* 1993;152:925-927.

18. Hentschel R, Hensel D, Brune R, et al. Impact on blood pressure and intestinal perfusion of dobutamine or dopamine in hypotensive preterm infants. *Biol Neonate*. 1995;68:318-324.
19. Lang P, Williams RG, Norwood WI, et al. The hemodynamic effects of dopamine in infants after corrective cardiac surgery. *J Pediatr*. 1980;96:630-634.
20. DiSessa TG, Leitner M, Ti CC, et al. The cardiovascular effects of dopamine in the severely asphyxiated neonate. *J Pediatr*. 1981;99:772-776.
21. Fiddler GI, Chatrath R, Williams GJ, et al. Dopamine infusion for the treatment of myocardial dysfunction associated with a persistent transitional circulation. *Arch Dis Child*. 1980;55:194-198.
22. Seri I, Rudas G, Bors Z, et al. Effects of low-dose dopamine infusion on cardiovascular and renal functions, cerebral blood flow, and plasma catecholamine levels in sick preterm neonates. *Pediatr Res*. 1993;34:742-749.
23. Klarr JM, Faix RG, Pryce C, et al. Randomized, blind trial of dopamine versus dobutamine for treatment of hypotension in preterm infants with RDS. *J Pediatr*. 1994;125:117-122.
24. Roze JC, Tohier C, Maingueneau, et al. Response to dobutamine and dopamine in the hypotensive very preterm infant. *Arch Dis Child*. 1993;69:59-63.
25. Dopamine hydrochloride. Lexi-Comp Online with AHFS (database). Bethesda, MD: American Society of Health-System Pharmacists; updated May 26, 2009.
26. Rennie JM. Cerebral blood flow velocity variability after cardiovascular support in premature babies. *Arch Dis Child*. 1989;64:897-901.
27. Ruelas-Orozco G, Vargas-Origel A. Assessment of therapy for arterial hypotension in critically ill preterm infants. *Am J Perinatol*. 2000;17:95-99.
28. Valverde E, Pellicer A, Madero R, et al. Dopamine versus epinephrine for cardiovascular support in low birth weight infants: analysis of systemic effects and neonatal clinical outcomes. *Pediatrics*. 2006;117:e1213-e1222.
29. Holmes CL, Walley KR. Bad medicine: low-dose dopamine in the ICU. *Chest*. 2003;123(4):1266-1275.
30. Seri I. Cardiovascular, renal, and endocrine actions of dopamine in neonates and children. *J Pediatr*. 1995;126:333-344.
31. Guller B, Fields AI, Coleman MG, et al. Changes in cardiac rhythm in children treated with dopamine. *Crit Care Med*. 1978;6:151-154.
32. Zaritsky A, Lotze A, Stull R, et al. Steady-state dopamine clearance in critically ill infants and children. *Crit Care Med*. 1988;16:217-220.
33. Trissel LA, ed. *Handbook on Injectable Drugs*. 15th ed. Bethesda, MD: American Society of Health-System Pharmacists; 2009.
34. Dopamine hydrochloride. Lexi-Comp Online with AHFS (database). Hudson, OH: Lexi-Comp Inc; updated August 13, 2009.
35. Allen EM, Van Boerum DH, Olsen AF, et al. Difference between the measured and ordered dose of catecholamine infusion. *Ann Pharmacother*. 1995;29:1095-1100.
36. Rich DS. New JCAHO medication management standards for 2004. *Am J Health-Syst Pharm*. 2004;61:1349-1358.
37. Buck ML, Wiggins BS, Sesler JM. Intraosseous drug administration in children and adults during cardiopulmonary resuscitation. *Ann Pharmacother*. 2007;41:1679-1686.
38. Driscoll DJ, Gillette PC, Duff DF, et al. The hemodynamic effect of dopamine in children. *J Thorac Cardiovasc Surg*. 1979;78:765-768.
39. Booker PD, Evans C, Franks R. Comparison of haemodynamic effects of dopamine and dobutamine in young children undergoing cardiac surgery. *Br J Anaesth*. 1995;74:419-423.
40. Hoffman TM, Bush DM, Wernovsky G, et al. Postoperative junctional ectopic tachycardia in children: incidence, risk factors, and treatment. *Ann Thorac Surg*. 2002;74:1607-1611.
41. Padbury JF, Agata Y, Baylen BG, et al. Dopamine pharmacokinetics in critically ill newborn infants. *J Pediatr*. 1986;110:293-298.
42. Banner W, Vernon DD, Dean JM, et al. Nonlinear dopamine pharmacokinetics in a pediatric population. *J Pharmacol Exp Ther*. 1989;249:131-133.
43. Notternan DA, Greenwald BM, Moran F, et al. Dopamine clearance in critically ill infants and children: effect of age and organ system dysfunction. *Clin Pharmacol Ther*. 1990;48:138-147.

Doxapram HCl

1. Doxapram hydrochloride injection USP [package insert]. Bedford, OH: Bedford Laboratories; March 2007.
2. Barrington KJ, Finer NN, Peters KL, et al. Physiologic effects of doxapram in idiopathic apnea of prematurity. *J Pediatr*. 1986;108:125-129.
3. Ruggins NR. Pathophysiology of apnoea in preterm infants. *Arch Dis Child*. 1991;66:70-73.
4. Peliowski A, Finer NN. A blinded, randomized, placebo-controlled trial to compare theophylline and doxapram for the treatment of apnea of prematurity. *J Pediatr*. 1990;116:648-653.
5. Kumita H, Mizuno S, Shinohara M, et al. Low-dose doxapram therapy in premature infants and its CSF and serum concentrations. *Acta Paediatr Scand*. 1991;80:786-791.
6. Eyal F, Alpan G, Sagi E, et al. Aminophylline versus doxapram in idiopathic apnea of prematurity: a double-blind controlled study. *Pediatrics*. 1985;75:709-713.
7. Barrington KJ, Finer NN, Torok-Both G, et al. Dose-response relationship of doxapram in the therapy of refractory idiopathic apnea of prematurity. *Pediatrics*. 1987;80:22-27.
8. Eyal FG, Sagi EF, Alpan G, et al. Aminophylline versus doxapram in weaning premature infants from mechanical ventilation: preliminary report. *Crit Care Med*. 1985;13:124-125.
9. Barrington KJ, Muttitt, SC. Randomized, controlled, blinded trial of doxapram for extubation of the very low birthweight infant. Acta Paediatr. 1998;87:191-194.
10. Henderson-Smart DJ, Davis PG. Prophylactic doxapram for the prevention of morbidity and mortality in preterm infants undergoing endotracheal extubation. *Cochrane Database Syst Rev*. 2000;(3):CD001966.
11. Trissel LA. *Handbook on Injectable Drugs*. 15th ed. Bethesda, MD: American Society of Health-System Pharmacists; 2009.
12. Sreenam C, Etches PC, Demianczuk N, et al. Isolated mental developmental delay in very low birth weight infants: association with prolonged doxapram therapy for apnea. *J Pediatr*. 2001;139:832-837.
13. Dani C, Bertini G, Pezzati M, et al. Brain hemodynamic effects of doxapram in preterm infants. *Biol Neonate*. 2006;98:69-74.
14. Maillard C, Boutroy MJ, Fresson J et al. QT interval lengthening in premature infants treated with doxapram. *Clin Pharmacol Ther*. 2001;70:540-545.

Doxycycline Hyclate

1. Available at: http://www.usp.org/hqi/similarProducts/choosy.html. Accessed August 29, 2009.
2. Doxycycline hyclate [package insert]. Bedford, OH: Bedford Laboratories; September 2004.
3. Smith M, Ubkel JH, Fenton SJ, DeVincenzo JP. The use of tetracyclines in pediatric patients. *J Pediatr Pharmacol Ther*. 2001;66:71.
4. Doxycycline. Lexi-Comp® Online with AHFS® (database). Bethesda, MD: American Society of Health-System Pharmacists; updated August 13, 2009.
5. American Academy of Pediatrics. Pickering LK, Baker CJ, Kimberlin DW, et al., eds. *2009 Red Book: Report of the Committee on Infectious Diseases*. 28th ed. Elk Grove Village, IL: American Academy of Pediatrics; 2009.
6. Holloway WJ. Preliminary report on intravenous doxycycline. *Del Med J*. 1971;43:394-397.
7. Hackett E, Axelrod M. Intravenous doxycycline (Vibramycin I.V.): a clinical evaluation. *Curr Ther Res*. 1972;14:626-637.
8. Heaney D, Eknoyan G. Minocycline and doxycycline kinetics in chronic renal failure. *Clin Pharmacol Ther*. 1978;24:233-239.
9. Aronoff GR, Berns JS, Brier ME, et al. Drug prescribing in renal failure. 4th ed. Available at: http://www.kdp-baptist.louisville.edu/renalbook/. Accessed August 28, 2009.

References

10. Whelton A. Tetracyclines in renal insufficiency: resolution of a therapeutic dilemma. *Bull NY Acad Med.* 1978;54:223-237.
11. Whelton A, von Wittenau MS, Twomey TM, et al. Doxycycline pharmacokinetics in the absence of renal function. *Kidney International.* 1974;5:365-371.
12. Trissel LA, ed. *Handbook on Injectable Drugs.* 15th ed. Bethesda, MD: American Society of Health-System Pharmacists; 2009.
13. Robinson CA, Sawyer JE. Y-site compatibility of medications with parenteral nutrition. *J Pediatr Pharmacol Ther.* 2009;14:49-57.
14. Akcam M, Artan R, Akcam FY, et al. Nail discoloration induced by doxycycline. *Pediatr Infect Dis J.* 2005;9:845-846.

Droperidol

1. Available at: http://www.usp.org/hqi/similarProducts/choosy.html. Accessed August 26, 2009.
2. Inapsine [package insert]. Decatur, IL: Taylor Pharmaceuticals; April 2006.
3. Lin DM, Furst ST, Rodarte A. A double-blinded comparison of metoclopramide and droperidol for prevention of emesis following strabismus surgery. *Anesthesiol.* 1992;76:357-361.
4. Watcha MF, Simeon RM, White PF, et al. Effect of propofol on the incidence of postoperative vomiting after strabismus surgery in pediatric outpatients. *Anesthesiology.* 1992;75:204-209.
5. Larsson S, Jonmarker C. Postoperative emesis after pediatric strabismus surgery: the effect of dixyrazine compared to droperidol. *Anaesthesiol Scand.* 1990;34:227-230.
6. Abramowitz MD, Oh TH, Epstein BS, et al. The antiemetic effect of droperidol following outpatient strabismus surgery in children. *Anesthesiology.* 1983;59:579-583.
7. Lerman J, Eustis S, Smith DR. Effect of droperidol pretreatment on postanesthetic vomiting in children undergoing strabismus surgery. *Anesthesiology.* 1986;65:322-325.
8. Christensen S, Farrow-Gillespie A, Lerman J. Incidence of emesis and postanesthetic recovery after strabismus surgery in children: a comparison of droperidol and lidocaine. *Anesthesiology.* 1989;70:251-254.
9. ASHP Commission on Therapeutics. ASHP therapeutic guidelines on the pharmacologic management of nausea and vomiting in adult and pediatric patients receiving chemotherapy or radiation therapy or undergoing surgery. *Am J Health-Syst Pharm.* 1999;56:729-764.
10. Blanc VF. Antiemetic prophylaxis with promethazine or droperidol in paediatric outpatient strabismus surgery. *Can J Anaesth.* 1991;38:54-60.
11. Trissel LA, ed. *Handbook on Injectable Drugs.* 15th ed. Bethesda, MD: American Society of Health-System Pharmacists; 2009.
12. Park CK, Choi HY, In YO, et al. Acute dystonia by droperidol during intravenous patient-controlled analgesia in young patients. *J Korean Med Sci.* 2002;17:715-717.

Edetate Calcium Disodium

1. Available at: http://ismp.org/Tools/confuseddrugnames.pdf. Accessed August 24, 2009.
2. Available at: http://www.usp.org/hqi/similarProducts/choosy.html. Accessed August 24, 2009.
3. Available at: http://www.fda.gov/Drugs/DrugSafety/PublicHealthAdvisories/ucm051138.html. Accessed October 2, 2009.
4. Baxter AJ, Krenzelok EP. Pediatric fatality secondary to EDTA chelation. *Clin Toxicol.* 2008;46:1083-1084.
5. Preventing lead poisoning in young children. Washington, DC: Centers for Disease Control, US Department of Health and Human Services; October 1991.
6. Centers for Disease Control and Prevention (CDC). Deaths associated with hypocalcemia from chelation therapy—Texas, Pennsylvania, and Oregon, 2003–2005. *MMWR Morb Mortal Wkly Rep.* 2006;55:204-207.
7. Calcium disodium versenate [package insert]. Northridge, CA: 3M Pharmaceuticals; July 2004.
8. Piomelli S, Rosen JF, Chisolm JJ, et al. Management of childhood lead poisoning. *J Pediatr.* 1984;105:523-532.
9. Available at: http://formularyproductions.com/blackbox/. Accessed October 2, 2009.
10. American Academy of Pediatrics. Committee on Drugs. Treatment guidelines for lead exposure in children. *Pediatrics.* 1995;96:155-160.
11. Trissel LA. *Handbook on Injectable Drugs.* 15th ed. Bethesda, MD: American Society of Health-System Pharmacists; 2009.
12. Markowitz ME, Rosen JF. Need for the lead mobilization test in children with lead poisoning. *J Pediatr.* 1991;119:305-310.
13. Markowitz ME, Rosen JF. Assessment of lead stores in children: validation of an 8-hour $CaNa_2EDTA$ provocative test. *J Pediatr.* 1984;104:337-341.
14. Iniguez JL, Leverger G, Dollfus C, et al. Lead mobilization test in children with lead poisonings: validation of a 5-hours edetate calcium disodium provocation test. *Arch Pediatr Adolesc Med.* 1995;149:338-340.
15. Kassner J, Shannon M, Graef J. Role of forced diuresis on urinary lead excretion after the ethylenediaminetetraacetic acid mobilization test. *J Pediatr.* 1990;117:914-916.
16. Garrettson LK. Lead poisoning. In: Haddad LM, Winchester JF, eds. *Clinical Management of Poisoning and Drug Overdose.* Philadelphia, PA: WB Saunders Company; 1983:652-655.
17. Moel DI, Kumar K. Reversible nephrotoxic reactions to a combined 2,3-dimercapto-1-propanol and calcium disodium ethylenediaminetetraacetic acid regimen in asymptomatic children with elevated blood levels. *Pediatrics.* 1982;70:259-262.
18. Chisolm JJ. The use of chelating agents in the treatment of acute and chronic lead intoxication in childhood. *J Pediatr.* 1968;73:1-38.
19. Edetate calcium disodium. Lexi-Comp Online with AHFS (database). Bethesda, MD: American Society of Health-System Pharmacists; updated August 2009.
20. Cory-Slechta DA, Weiss B, Cox C. Mobilization of lead over the course of calcium disodium ethylenediamine tetraacetate chelation therapy. *J Pharmacol Exp Ther.* 1987;243:804-813.
21. Mycyk MB, Leikin JB. Combined exchange transfusion and chelation therapy for neonatal lead poisoning. *Ann Pharmacother.* 2004;38:821-824.
22. Horowitz BZ, Mirkin DB. Lead poisoning and chelation in a mother-neonate pair. *J Toxicol Clin Toxicol.* 2001;39:727-731.

Edrophonium Chloride

1. Available at: http://www.usp.org/hqi/similarProducts/choosy.html. Accessed August 26, 2009.
2. Enlon [package insert]. Deerfield, IL: Baxter Healthcare Corporation.
3. Edrophonium. Lexi-Comp Online with AHFS (database). Bethesda, MD: American Society of Health-System Pharmacists; updated May 26, 2009.
4. Leih-Lai m, Sarnaik AP. Therapeutic applications in pediatric intensive care. In: Yaffe SJ, Aranda JV, eds. *Neonatal and Pediatric Pharmacology.* 3rd ed. Philadelphia, PA: Lippincott Williams & Wilkins; 2005:264.
5. Fisher DM, Cronnelly R, Sharma M, et al. Clinical pharmacology of edrophonium in infants and children. *Anesthesiology.* 1984;61:428-433.
6. Gwinnutt CL, Walker RW, Meakin G. Antagonism of intense atracurium-induced neuromuscular block in children. *Br J Anaesth.* 1991;67;13-16.
7. Kirkegaard-Nielsen H, Meretoja OA, Wirtavuori K. Reversal of atracurium-induced neuromuscular block in paediatric patients. *Acta Anaesthesiol Scand.* 1995;39:906-911.
8. Abdulatif M, El-Sanabary M. Edrophonium antagonism of cisatracurium-induced neuromuscular block: dose requirements in children and adults. *Anaesth Intensive Care.* 2001;29:364-370.

References

9. Suzuki T, Lien CA, Belmont MR, et al. Edrophonium effectively antagonizes neuromuscular block at the laryngeal adductors induced by rapacuronium, rocuronium and cisatracurium, but not mivacurium. *Can J Anaesth.* 2003;50:879-885.
10. Trissel LA, ed. *Handbook on Injectable Drugs.* 15th ed. Bethesda, MD: American Society of Health-System Pharmacists; 2009.

Enalaprilat

1. Available at: http://ismp.org/Tools/confuseddrugnames.pdf. Accessed August 30, 2009.
2. Available at: http://www.usp.org/hqi/similarProducts/choosy.html. Accessed August 30, 2009.
3. Enalaprilat injection [package insert]. Bedford, OH: Ben Venue Laboratories; June 2005.
4. Marcadis ML, Kraus DM, Hatzopoulos FK, et al. Use of enalaprilat for neonatal hypertension. *J Pediatr.* 1991;119:505. Letter.
5. Wells TG, Bunchman TE, Kearns GL. Treatment of neonatal hypertension with enalaprilat. *J Pediatr.* 1990;117:664-667.
6. Manzi SF, Arnold A, Patterson A. Pediatric drug formulary. In: Yaffe SJ, Aranda JV, eds. *Neonatal and Pediatric Pharmacology.* 3rd ed. Philadelphia, PA: Lippincott Williams & Wilkins; 2005:901.
7. Mason T, Polak MJ, Pyles L, et al. Treatment of neonatal renovascular hypertension with intravenous enalapril. *Am J Perinatol.* 1993;9:254-257.
8. National High Blood Pressure Education Program Working Group on High Blood Pressure in Children and Adolescents. The fourth report on the diagnosis, evaluation, and treatment of high blood pressure in children and adolescents. *Pediatrics.* 2004;114(2 suppl 4th report):555-576.
9. Miller K. Pharmacological management of hypertension in paediatric patients. *Drugs.* 1994;46:868-887.
10. Webster MWI, Neutze JM, Calder AL. Acute hemodynamic effects of converting enzyme inhibition in children with intracardiac shunts. *Pediatr Cardiol.* 1992;13:129-135.
11. Sluysmans L, Styns-Cailteux M, Tremouroux-Wattiez M, et al. Intravenous enalaprilat and oral enalapril in congestive heart failure secondary to ventricular septal defect in infancy. *Am J Cardiol.* 1992;70:959-961.
12. Rheuban KS, Carpenter MA, Ayers CA, et al. Acute hemodynamic effects of converting enzyme inhibition in infants with congestive heart failure. *J Pediatr.* 1990;117:668-670.
13. Wells TG, Ilyas M. Antihypertensive agents. In: Yaffe SJ, Aranda JV, eds. *Neonatal and Pediatric Pharmacology.* 3rd ed. Philadelphia, PA: Lippincott Williams & Wilkins; 2005:683.
14. Aronoff GR, Berns JS, Brier ME, et al. Drug prescribing in renal failure. 4th ed. Available at: http://www.kdp-baptist.louisville.edu/renalbook/. Accessed August 30, 2009.
15. Trissel LA, ed. *Handbook on Injectable Drugs.* 15th ed. Bethesda, MD: American Society of Health-System Pharmacists; 2009.

Enoxaparin Sodium

1. Available at: http://ismp.org/Tools/highalertmedications.pdf. ISMP 2008.
2. Available at: http://www.usp.org/hqi/similarProducts/choosy.html. Accessed August 25, 2009.
3. Lovenox [package insert]. Bridgewater, NJ: Sanofi-Aventis US LLC; July 2008.
4. Monagle P, Chan A, Massicotte P, et al. Antithrombotic therapy in children. American College of Chest Physicians evidence-based clinical practice guidelines (8th ed.). *Chest.* 2008;133 (Suppl):887S-968S.
5. Merkel N, Gunther G, Schobess R. Long-term treatment of thrombosis with enoxaparin in pediatric and adolescent patients. *Acta Haematol.* 2006;115:230-236.
6. Michaels LA, Gurian M, Hegyi T, et al. Low molecular weight heparin in the treatment of venous and arterial thromboses in the premature infant. *Pediatrics.* 2004;114:703-707.
7. Dix D, Andrew M, Marzinotto V, et al. The use of low molecular weight heparin in pediatric patients: a prospective cohort study. *J Pediatr.* 2000;136:439-445.
8. Massicotte P, Adams M, Marzinotto V, et al. Low-molecular-weight heparin in pediatric patients with thrombotic disease: a dose finding study. *J Pediatr.* 1996;128:313-318.
9. Burak CR, Bowen MD, Barron TF. The use of enoxaparin in children with acute, nonhemorrhagic ischemic stroke. *Pediatr Neurol.* 2003;29:295-298.
10. Streif W, Goebel G, Chan AK, et al. Use of low molecular mass heparin (enoxaparin) in newborn infants: a prospective cohort study of 62 patients. *Arch Dis Child Fetal Neonatal Ed.* 2003;88:F365-F370.
11. Ho SH, Wu JK, Hamilton DP, et al. An assessment of published pediatric dosage guidelines for enoxaparin: a retrospective review. *J Pediatr Hematol Oncol.* 2004;26:561-566.
12. Malowany JI, Knoppert DC, Chan AKC, Pepelasis D, Lee DSC. Enoxaparin use in the neonatal intensive care unit: experience over 8 years. *Pharmacother.* 2007;27:1263-1271.
13. Malowany JI, Monagel P, Knoppert DC, et al. Enoxaparin for neonatal thrombosis: a call for a higher dose for neonates. *Thromb Res.* 2008;122:826-830.
14. Massicotte MP, Adams M, Leaker M, et al. A nomogram to establish therapeutic levels of the low molecular weight heparin (LMWH), clivarine in children requiring treatment for venous thromboembolism (VTE) [abstract]. *Thromb Haemost.* 1997;(suppl):282-283.
15. Michelson AD, Bovill E, Monagle P, et al. Antithrombotic therapy in children. *Chest.* 1998;114:748S-769S.
16. Clary SE, van Orden H, Journeycake JM. Experience with intravenous enoxaparin in critically ill infants and children. *Pediatr Crit Care Med.* 2008;9:647-649.
17. Dager WE, Gosselin RC, King JH, et al. Anti-Xa stability of diluted enoxaparin for use in pediatrics. *Ann Pharmacother.* 2004;38:569-573.
18. Dunaway KK, Gal P, Ransom JL. Use of enoxaparin in a preterm infant. *Ann Pharmacother.* 2000;34:1410-1413.
19. Dager WE, White RH. Low-molecular weight heparin-induced thrombocytopenia in a child. *Ann Pharmacother.* 2004;38:247-250.

EPINEPHrine HCl

1. Available at: http://ismp.org/Tools/highalertmedications.pdf. Accessed August 26, 2009.
2. Available at: http://ismp.org/Tools/confuseddrugnames.pdf. Accessed August 26, 2009.
3. Available at: http://www.usp.org/hqi/similarProducts/choosy.html. Accessed August 26, 2009.
4. Epinephrine. Lexi-Comp Online with AHFS (database). Hudson, OH: Lexi-Comp Inc; updated September 11, 2009.
5. Epinephrine. Lexi-Comp Online with AHFS (database). Bethesda, MD: American Society of Health-System Pharmacists; updated May 26, 2009.
6. Horak A, Raine R, Opie LH, et al. Severe myocardial ischemia induced by intravenous adrenaline. *Br Med J.* 1983;286:519.
7. Sullivan TJ. Cardiac disorders in penicillin-induced anaphylaxis. Association with intravenous epinephrine therapy. *JAMA.* 1982;248:2161-2162.
8. Levine DH, Levkoff AH, Pappu LD, et al. Renal failure and other serious sequelae of epinephrine toxicity in neonates. *South Med J.* 1985;78:874-877.
9. American Academy of Pediatrics and American Heart Association. *Pediatric Advanced Life Support. Provider Manual.* Dallas, TX: American Heart Association; 2006.
10. Gaze NR. Tissue necrosis caused by commonly used intravenous infusions. *Lancet.* 1978;2:417-419.
11. MacCara ME. Extravasation: a hazard of intravenous therapy. Drug Intell Clin Pharm 1983;17:713-717.

References

12. Hegenbarth MA; American Academy of Pediatrics Committee on Drugs. Preparing for pediatric emergencies: drugs to consider. *Pediatrics.* 2008;121:433-443.
13. Stier PA, Bogner MP, Webster K, et al. Use of subcutaneous terbutaline to reverse peripheral ischemia. *Am J Emerg Med.* 1999;17:91-94.
14. American Academy of Pediatrics. Pickering LK, Baker CJ, Kimberlin DW, et al., eds. *2009 Red Book: Report of the Committee on Infectious Diseases.* 28th ed. Elk Grove Village, IL: American Academy of Pediatrics; 2009.
15. Available at: http://www.nhlbi.nih.gov/guidelines/asthma/asthsumm.htm. Accessed October 18, 2009.
16. Berg RA, Otto CW, Kern KB, et al. High-dose epinephrine results in greater early mortality after resuscitation from prolonged cardiac arrest in pigs: a prospective, randomized study. *Crit Care Med.* 1994;22:282-290.
17. Perondi M, Reis A, Paiva E, et al. A comparison of high-dose and standard-dose epinephrine in children with cardiac arrest. *N Engl J Med.* 2004;350:1722-1730.
18. Berg RA, Otto CW, Kern KB, et al. A randomized, blinded trial of high-dose epinephrine versus standard-dose epinephrine in a swine model of pediatric asphyxial cardiac arrest. *Crit Care Med.* 1996;24:1695-1700.
19. Tang W, Weil MH, Sun S, et al. Epinephrine increases the severity of postresuscitation myocardial dysfunction. *Circulation.* 1995;92:3089-3093.
20. Rivers EP, Wortsman J, Rad MY et al. The effect of the total cumulative epinephrine dose administered during human CPR on hemodynamic, oxygen transport, and utilization variables in the postresuscitation period. *Chest.* 1994;106:1499-1507.
21. American Heart Association. 2005 guidelines for cardiopulmonary resuscitation and emergency cardiovascular care. Part 13: Neonatal Resuscitation Guidelines. *Pediatrics.* 2006;117:e989-e1004.
22. Goetting MG, Paradis NA. High dose epinephrine in refractory pediatric cardiac arrest. *Crit Care Med.* 1989;17:1258-1262.
23. Goetting MG, Paradis NA. High dose epinephrine improves outcome from pediatric cardiac arrest. *Ann Emerg Med.* 1991;20:22-26.
24. Dieckmann RA, Vardis R. High-dose epinephrine in pediatric out-of-hospital cardiopulmonary arrest. *Pediatrics.* 1995;95:901-913.
25. Trissel LA, ed. Handbook on Injectable Drugs. 15th ed. Bethesda, MD: American Society of Health-System Pharmacists; 2009.
26. Allen EM, Van Boerum DH, Olsen AF, et al. Difference between the measured and ordered dose of catecholamine infusion. *Ann Pharmacother.* 1995;29:1095-1100.
27. Barach EM, Nowak RM, Lee TG, et al. Epinephrine for treatment of anaphylactic shock. *JAMA.* 1984;251:2118-2122.
28. Zaritsky A, Chernow B. Use of catecholamines in pediatrics. *J Pediatr.* 1984;105:341-350.
29. Rich DS. New JCAHO medication management standards for 2004. *Am J Health-Syst Pharm.* 2004;61:1349-1358.
30. Kuracheck SC, Rockoff MA. Inadvertent intravenous administration of racemic epinephrine. *JAMA.* 1985;253:1441-1442.

Epoetin Alfa

1. Available at: http://www.usp.org/hqi/similarProducts/choosy.html. Accessed August 26, 2009.
2. Epogen [package insert]. Thousand Oaks, CA: Amgen Inc; February 2009.
3. Trissel LA, ed. *Handbook on Injectable Drugs.* 15th ed. Bethesda, MD: American Society of Health-System Pharmacists; 2009.
4. Rigden SPA, Montini G, Morris M, et al. Recombinant human erythropoietin therapy in children maintained on hemodialysis. *Pediatr Nephrol.* 1990;4:618-622.
5. Montini G, Zacchello G, Baraldi E, et al. Benefits and risks of anemia correction with recombinant human erythropoietin in children maintained on hemodialysis. *J Pediatr.* 1990;117:556-560.
6. Bianchetti MG, Hammerli I, Roduit C, et al. Epoetin alfa in anemic children or adolescents on regular dialysis. *Eur J Pediatr.* 1991;150:509-512.
7. Campos A, Garin EH. Therapy of renal anemia in children and adolescents with recombinant human erythropoietin (rHuEPO). *Clin Pediatr.* 1992;31:94-99.
8. Tenbrock K, Muller-Berghaus J, Michalk D, et al. Intravenous iron treatment of renal anemia in children on hemodialysis. *Pediatr Nephrol.* 1999;13:580-582.
9. Mak RH. Effect of recombinant human erythropoietin on insulin, amino acid, and lipid metabolism in uremia. *J Pediatr.* 1996;129:97-104.
10. Offner G, Hoyer PF, Latta K, et al. One year's experience with recombinant erythropoietin in children undergoing continuous ambulatory or cycling peritoneal dialysis. *Pediatr Nephrol.* 1990;4:498-500.
11. Caselli D, Maccabruni A, Zuccotti GV, et al. Recombinant erythropoietin for treatment of anaemia in HIV-infected children. *AIDS.* 1996;10:929-931.
12. Razzouk BI, Hord JD, Hockenberry M, et al. Double-blind, placebo-controlled study of quality of life, hematologic endpoints, and safety of weekly epoetin alfa in children with cancer receiving myelosuppressive chemotherapy. *J Clin Oncol.* 2006;24:3583-3589.
13. Freeman BB 3rd, Hinds P, Iacono LC, et al. Pharmacokinetics and pharmacodynamics of intravenous epoetin alfa in children with cancer. *Pediatr Blood Cancer.* 2006;47:572-579.
14. Zoubek A, Kronberger M. Early epoetin alfa treatment in children with solid tumors. *Med Pediatr Oncol.* 2002;39:459-462.
15. Abdelrazik N, Fouda M. Once weekly recombinant human erythropoietin treatment for cancer-induced anemia in children with acute lymphoblastic leukemia receiving maintenance chemotherapy: a randomized case-controlled study. *Hematology.* 2007;12:533-541.
16. Shannon KM, Mentzer WC, Abels RI, et al. Recombinant human erythropoietin in the anemia of prematurity: results of a placebo-controlled pilot study. *J Pediatr.* 1991;118:949-955.
17. Carnielli V, Montini G, Da Riol R, et al. Effect of high doses of human recombinant erythropoietin on the need for transfusions in preterm infants. *J Pediatr.* 1992;121:98-102.
18. Wandstrat TL, Maxwell SR. Erythropoietin to treat anemia or prematurity. *Ann Pharmacother.* 1997;31:645-646.
19. Carnielli VP, da Riol R, Montini G. Iron supplementation enhances response to high doses of recombinant human erythropoietin in preterm infants. *Arch Dis Child Fetal Neonatal Ed.* 1998;79:F44-F48.
20. Ohls RK, Harcum J, Schibler KR, et al. The effect of erythropoietin on the transfusion requirements of preterm infants weighing 750 grams or less: a randomized, double-blind, placebo-controlled study. *J Pediatr.* 1997;131:661-665.
21. Klipp M, Holzwarth AU, Poeschl JM, et al. Effects of erythropoietin on erythrocyte deformability in non-transfused preterm infants. *Acta Paediatr.* 2007;96:253-256.
22. Ohls RK, Veerman MW, Christensen RD. Pharmacokinetics and effectiveness of recombinant erythropoietin administered to preterm infants by continuous infusion in total parenteral nutrition solution. *J Pediatr.* 1996;128:518-523.
23. Maier RF, Obladen M, Muller-Hansen I et al. Early treatment with erythropoietin beta ameliorates anemia and reduces transfusion requirements in infants with birth weights below 1000g. *J Pediatr.* 2002;141:8-15.
24. Reiter PD, Rosenberg AA, Valuck R, et al. Effect of short-term erythropoietin therapy in anemic premature infants. *J Perinatol.* 2005;25:125-129.
25. Donato H, Vain N, Rendo P, et al. Effect of early versus late administration of human recombinant erythropoietin on transfusion requirements in premature infants: results of a randomized, placebo-controlled, multicenter trial. *Pediatrics.* 2000;5:1066-1072.
26. Fridge JL, Vichinsky EP. Correction of the anemia of epidermolysis bullosa with intravenous iron and erythropoietin. *J Pediatr.* 1998;132:871-873.
27. National Kidney Foundation. KDOQI Clinical Practice Guidelines and Clinical Practice Recommendations for Anemia in Chronic Kidney Disease. *Am J Kidney Dis.* 2006;47 (suppl 3):S1-S146.
28. Shimpo H, Mizumoto T, Kouji O, et al. Erythropoietin in pediatric cardiac surgery. *Chest.* 1997;111:1565-1570.
29. Chikada M, Furuse A, Kotsuka Y, et al. Open-heart surgery in Jehovah's Witness patients. *Cardiovascular Surg.* 1996;4:311-314.
30. Krajewski K, Ashley RK, Pung N, Wald, et al. Successful blood conservation during craniosynostotic correction with dual therapy using procrit and cell saver. *J Craniofac Surg.* 2008;19:101-105.
31. Gumy-Pause F, Ozsahin H, Mermillod B, et al. Stepping up versus standard doses of erythropoietin in preterm infants. *Pediatr Hematol Onc.* 2005;22:667-678.

32. Huynh-Delerme C, Penaud JF, Lacombe C. Stability and biological activity of epoietin beta in parenteral nutrition solutions. *Biol Neonate.* 2002;81:158-162.
33. Ohls RK, Christensen RD. Stability of human recombinant epoetin alfa in commonly used neonatal intravenous solutions. *Ann Pharmacother.* 1996;5:466-468.
34. Delanty N, Vaughan C, Frucht S, et al. Erythropoietin-associated hypertensive posterior leukoencephalopathy. *Neurology.* 1997;49:686-689.
35. Latini G, Rosati G. Transient neutropenia may be a risk of treating preterm neonates with high doses of recombinant erythropoietin. *Eur J Pediatr.* 1998;157:443-444.
36. Snanoudj R, Beaudreuil S, Arzouk N. Recovery from pure red cell aplasia caused by anti-erythropoietin antibodies after kidney transplantation. *Am J Transplant.* 2004;4:274-277.
37. Brandt JR, Avner ED, Hickman RO, et al. Safety and efficacy of erythropoietin in children with chronic renal failure. *Pediatr Nephrol.* 1999;13:143-147.

Ertapenem

1. Available at: http://www.ismp.org/tools/tallmanletters.pdf. Accessed September 1, 2009.
2. Available at: http://ismp.org/Tools/confuseddrugnames.pdf. Accessed September 1, 2009.
3. Available at: http://www.usp.org/hqi/similarProducts/choosy.html. Accessed September 1, 2009.
4. Ertapenem [package insert]. Clermont-Ferrand Cedex, France: Merck Sharp & Dohme-Chibret; August 2009.
5. Yellin AE, Johnson J, Higareda I, et al. Ertapenem or ticarcillin/clavulanate for the treatment of intra-abdominal infections or acute pelvic infections in pediatric patients. *Amer J Surg.* 2007;194:367-374.
6. Arguedas A, Cespedes J, Botet FA, et al. Safety and efficacy in a double-blind study of ertapenem vs. ceftriaxone in pediatric patients with complicated urinary tract infections, community acquired pneumonia, or skin and soft tissue infections. *Int J Antimicro Agents.* 2009;33:163-167.
7. Keating GM, Perry CM. Ertapenem: a review of its use in the treatment of bacterial infections. *Drugs.* 2005;65:2151-2178.
8. Trissel LA, ed. *Handbook on Injectable Drugs.* 15th ed. Bethesda, MD: American Society of Health-System Pharmacists; 2009.
9. Legua P, Lema J, Moll J. Safety and local tolerability of intramuscularly administered ertapenem diluted in lidocaine: a prospective, randomized, double-blind study versus intramuscular ceftriaxone. *Clin Ther.* 2002;24:434-444.
10. Norrby SR. Neurotoxicity of the carbapenem antibacterials. *Drug Safety.* 1996;15:87-90.
11. Norrby SR. Carbapenems in serious infections: a risk-benefit assessment. *Drug Safety.* 2000;22:191-194.
12. Calandra G, Lydick E, Carrigan J, et al. Factors predisposing to seizures in seriously ill infected patients receiving antibiotics: experience with imipenem/cilastatin. *Am J Med.* 1988;84:911-918.
13. Lunde JL, Nelson RE, Storandt HF. Acute seizures in a patient receiving divalproex sodium after starting ertapenem therapy. *Pharmacotherapy.* 2007;27:1202-1205.

Erythromycin Gluceptate/Lactobionate

1. Available at: http://www.usp.org/hqi/similarProducts/choosy.html. Accessed September 23, 2009.
2. Erythrocin lactobionate IV [package insert]. Lake Forrest, IL: Hospira Inc; 2004.
3. Eichenwald HF. Adverse reactions to erythromycin. *Pediatr Infect Dis.* 1986;5:147-150.
4. Baier RJ, Loggins J, Kruger TE. Failure of erythromycin to eliminate airway colonization with ureaplasma urealyticum in very low birth weight infants. *BMC Pediatrics.* 2003;3:10-15.
5. Nogami K, Nishikubo T, Minowa H, et al. Intravenous low-dose erythromycin administration for infants with feeding intolerance. *Pediatr Int.* 2001;43:605-610.
6. Waites KB, Sims PJ, Crouse DT, et al. Serum concentrations of erythromycin after intravenous infusion in preterm neonates treated for Ureaplasma urealyticum infection. *Pediatr Infect Dis J.* 1994;13:840-841.
7. Mabanta CG, Pryhuber GS, Weinberg GA, Phelps DL. Erythromycin for the prevention of chronic lung disease in intubated preterm infants at risk for, or colonized or infected with Ureaplasma urealyticum. *Cochrane Database Syst Rev.* 2003;4:CD003744
8. American Academy of Pediatrics. Pickering LK, Baker CJ, Kimberlin DW, et al., eds. *2009 Red Book: Report of the Committee on Infectious Diseases.* 28th ed. Elk Grove Village, IL: American Academy of Pediatrics; 2009.
9. Available at: http://www.cdc.gov/std/treatment/2006/GonUpdateApril2007.pdf Accessed September 13, 2009.
10. Patole S, Rao S, Doherty D. Erythromycin as a prokinetic agent in preterm neonates: a systematic review. *Arch Dis Child Fetal Neonatal Ed.* 2005;90:F301-F306.
11. Stenson BJ, Middlemist L, Lyon AJ. Influence of erythromycin on establishment of feeding in preterm infants: observations from a randomised controlled trial. *Arch Dis Child Fetal Neonatal Ed.* 1998;79:F212-F214.
12. Cucchiara S, Minella R, Scoppa A, et al. Antroduodenal motor effects of intravenous erythromycin in children with abnormalities of gastrointestinal motility. *J Pediatr Gastrointest Nutr.* 1997;24:411-418.
13. Di Lorenzo C, Lucanto C, Flores AF, et al. Effect of sequential erythromycin and octreotide on antroduodenal manometry. *J Pediatr Gastrointest Nutr.* 1999;29:293-296.
14. Su BH, Lin HC. Erythromycin for treatment of feeding intolerance in preterm infants. *J Pediatr.* 2007;150:e30-e31.
15. Ng E, Shah V. Erthromycin for feeding intolerance in preterm infants. *Cochrane Database Syst Rev.* 2008;3:CD001815.
16. Aronoff GR, Berns JS, Brier ME, et al. Drug prescribing in renal failure. 4th ed. Available at: http://www.kdp-baptist.louisville.edu/renalbook/. Accessed August 28, 2009.
17. Barre J, Mallat A, Rosenbaum J, et al. Pharmacokinetics of erythromycin in patients with severe cirrhosis. Respective influence of decreased serum binding and impaired liver metabolic capacity. *Br J Clin Pharmacol.* 1987;23:753-757.
18. Trissel LA, ed. *Handbook on Injectable Drugs.* 15th ed. Bethesda, MD: American Society of Health-System Pharmacists; 2009.
19. Nelson JD, Bradley JS, eds. *Nelson's Pocket Book of Pediatric Antimicrobial Therapy.* 17th ed. Chicago, IL: American Academy of Pediatrics; 2009.
20. Robinson CA, Sawyer JE. Y-site compatibility of medications with parenteral nutrition. *J Pediatr Pharmacol Ther.* 2009;14:49-57.
21. Haydon RC, Thelin JW, Davis WE. Erythromycin ototoxicity: analysis and conclusions based on 22 case reports. *Otolaryngol Head Neck Surg.* 1984;92:678-684.
22. Kroboth PD, McNeil MA, Kreeer A, et al. Hearing loss and erythromycin pharmacokinetics in a patient receiving hemodialysis. *Arch Intern Med.* 1983;143:1263-1265.
23. Schweitzer VG. Ototoxic effect of erythromycin therapy. *Arch Otolaryngol.* 1984;110:258-260.
24. Owens RC Jr, Nolin TD. Antimicrobial-associated QT interval prolongation: pointes of interest. *Clin Infect Dis.* 2006;43:1603-1611.
25. Schweitzer VG. Ototoxic effect of erythromycin therapy. *Arch Otolaryngol.* 1984;110:258-260.
26. McComb JM, Campbell NP, Cleland J. Recurrent ventricular tachycardia associated with QT prolongation after mitral valve replacement and its association with intravenous administration of erythromycin. *Am J Cardiol.* 1984;54:922-923.
27. Farrar HC, Walsh-Sukys MC, Kyllonen K, et al. Cardiac toxicity associated with erythromycin lactobionate: two case reports and a review of the literature. *Pediatric Infect Dis J.* 1993;12:688-691.
28. Sims PJ, Waites KB, Crouse DT. Erythromycin lactobionate toxicity in preterm neonates. *Pediatr Infect Dis J.* 1994;13:164-165.
29. Farrar HC, Walsh-Sukys MC, Kyllonen K, et al. Erythromycin lactobionate toxicity in preterm neonates (reply). *Pediatr Infect Dis J.* 1994;13:166-167.
30. Dan M, Feigll D. Erythromycin associated hypotension. *Pediatr Infect Dis J.* 1993;12:692.

References

Esmolol HCl

1. Available at: http://ismp.org/Tools/highalertmedications.pdf. Accessed October 4, 2009.
2. Available at: http://www.usp.org/hqi/similarProducts/choosy.html. Accessed October 4, 2009.
3. Esmolol [package insert]. Deerfield, IL: Baxter Healthcare Corp; August 2005.
4. Trippel DI, Wiest DB, Gillette PC. Cardiovascular and antiarrhythmic effects of esmolol in children. *J Pediatr.* 1991;119:142-147.
5. Cuneo BF, Zales VR, Blahunka PC, et al. Pharmaco-dynamics and pharmacokinetics of esmolol, a short-acting beta-blocking agent, in children. *Pediatr Cardiol.* 1994;15:296-301.
6. Luyt D, Dance M, Litmanovitch M, et al. Esmolol in the treatment of severe tachycardia in neonatal tetanus. *Anaesth Intensive Care.* 1994;22:303-304.
7. Wiest DB, Trippel DL, Gillette PC, et al. Pharmacokinetics of esmolol in children. *Clin Pharmacol Ther.* 1991;49:6186-6123.
8. Temple ME, Nahata MC. Treatment of pediatric hypertension. *Pharmacotherapy.* 2000;20:140-150.
9. Wells TG, Ilyas M. Antihypertensive agents. In: Yaffe SJ, Aranda JV, eds. *Neonatal and Pediatric Pharmacology.* 3rd ed. Philadelphia, PA: Lippincott Williams & Wilkins; 2005:683.
10. National High Blood Pressure Education Program Working Group on High Blood Pressure in Children and Adolescents. The fourth report on the diagnosis, evaluation, and treatment of high blood pressure in children and adolescents. *Pediatrics.* 2004;114(2 suppl 4th Report):555-576.
11. Tabutt S, Nicolson SC, Adamson PC, et al. The safety, efficacy, and pharmacokinetics of esmolol for blood pressure control immediately after repair of coarctation of the aorta in infants and children: a multicenter, double-blind, randomized trial. *J Thorac Cardiovasc Surg.* 2008;136:321-328.
12. Smerling A, Gersony WM. Esmolol for severe hypertension following repair of aortic coarctation. *Crit Care Med.* 1990;18:1288-1290.
13. Aronoff GR, Berns JS, Brier ME, et al. Drug prescribing in renal failure. 4th ed. Available at: http://www.kdp-baptist.louisville.edu/renalbook/. Accessed October 5, 2009.
14. Trissel LA, ed. *Handbook on Injectable Drugs.* 15th ed. Bethesda, MD: American Society of Health-System Pharmacists; 2009.
15. Leih-Lai M, Sarnaik AP. Therapeutic applications in pediatric intensive care. In: Yaffe SJ, Aranda JV, eds. *Neonatal and Pediatric Pharmacology.* 3rd ed. Philadelphia, PA: Lippincott Williams & Wilkins; 2005:262.
16. Esmolol. Lexi-Comp® Online with AHFS® (database). Hudson, OH: Lexi-Comp Inc; updated August 13, 2009.

Esomeprazole

1. Available at: http://www.usp.org/hqi/similarProducts/choosy.html. Accessed October 27, 2009.
2. Nexium® IV [package insert]. Wilmington, DE: AstraZeneca; December 2008.
3. Available at: http://clinicaltrials.gov/ct2/show/NCT00474019. Accessed October 27, 2009.
4. Omari T, Davidson G, Bondarov P, et al. Pharmacokinetics and acid-suppressive effects of esomeprazole in infants 1–24 months old with symptoms of gastroesophageal reflux disease. *J Pediatr Gastroenterol Nutr.* 2007;45:530-537.
5. Zhao J, Li J, Hamer-Maansson JE, et al. Pharmacokinetic properties of esomeprazole in children aged 1 to 11 yars with symptoms of gastroesophageal reflux disease: a randomized, open-label study. *Clin Ther.* 2006;28:1868-1876.
6. Gilger MA, Tolia V, Vandenplas Y, et al. Safety and tolerability of esomeprazole in children with gastroesophageal reflux disease. *J Pediatr Gastroenterol Nutr.* 2008;46:524-533.
7. Li J, Zhai J, Hamer-Maansson, et al. Pharmacokinetics properties of esomeprazole in adolescent patients aged 12 to 17 years with symptoms of gastroesophageal reflux disease: a randomized, open-label study. *Clin Ther.* 2006;28:419-427.
8. Gold BD, Gunasekaran T, Tolia V, et al. Safety and symptom improvement with esomeprazole in adolescents with gastroesophageal reflux disease. *J Pediatr Gastroenterol Nutr.* 2007;45:520-529.
9. Kupiec TC, Aloumanis V, Ben M, et al. Physical and chemical stability of esomeprazole sodium solutions. *Ann Pharmacother.* 2008;42:1247-1251.
10. Baldassarre E, Sagaon MM, Ferrarini A, et al. Severe systemic adverse reaction to proton pump inhibitors in an infant. *Pediatr Pulmonol.* 2007;42:563-564.
11. Canani RB, Cirillo P, Roggero P, et al. Therapy with gastric acidity inhibitors increases the risk of acute gastroenteritis and community-acquired pneumonia in children. *Pediatrics.* 2006;117:817-820.
12. Hirschowitz BI, Worthington J, Mohnen J. Vitamin B12 deficiency in hypersecretors during long-term acid suppression with proton pump inhibitors. *Aliment Pharmacol Ther.* 2008;27:1110-1121.
13. Last EJ, Sheehan AH. Review of recent evidence: potential interaction between clopidogrel and proton pump inhibitors. *Am J Health-Syst Pharm.* 2009;66:e11-e16.

Etanercept

1. Available at: http://ismp.org/Tools/confuseddrugnames.pdf. Updated April 1, 2005.
2. Enbrel [prescribing information]. Thousand Oaks, CA: Immunex Corp; December 2008.
3. Available at: http://www.fda.gov/Drugs/DrugSafety/PostmarketDrugSafetyInformationforPatientsandProviders/DrugSafetyInformationforHeathcareProfessionals/ucm174474.htm. Accessed August 23, 2009.
4. Etanercept. Lexi-Comp® Online with AHFS® (database). Bethesda, MD: American Society of Health-System Pharmacists; updated March 19, 2009.
5. Lovell DJ, Reiff A, Jones OY, et al. Long-term safety and efficacy of etanercept in children with polyarticular-course juvenile rheumatoid arthritis. *Arthritis Rheum.* 2006;54:1987-1994.
6. Lovell DJ, Reiff A, Ilowite NT, et al. Safety and efficacy of up to eight years of continuous etanercept therapy in patients with juvenile rheumatoid arthritis. *Arthritis Rheum.* 2008;58:1496-1504.
7. Paller AM, Siegfried EC, Langley RG, et al. Etanercept treatment for children and adolescents with plaque psoriasis. *N Engl J Med.* 2008;358:241-251.
8. Papoutsaki M, Costanzo A, Mazzotta A, et al. Etanercept for the treatment of severe childhood psoriasis. *Br J Dermatol.* 2006;154:177-204.
9. Safa G, Loppin M, Bousser AM, et al. Etanercept in a 7-year-old boy with severe and recalcitrant psoriasis. *J Am Acad Dermatol.* 2007;56:S19-S20.
10. Reiff A, Takei S, Sadeghi, et al. Etanercept therapy in children with treatment-resistant uveitis. *Arthritis Rheum.* 2001;44:1411-1415.
11. Smith JR, Levinson RD, Holland GN, et al. Differential efficacy of tumor necrosis factor inhibition in the management of inflammatory eye disease and associated rheumatic disease. *Arthritis Care Res.* 2001;45:252-257.
12. Tynjala P, Lindahl P, Honkanen V, et al. Infliximab and etanercept in the treatment of chronic uveitis associated with refractory juvenile idiopathic arthritis. *Ann Rheum Dis.* 2007;66:548-550.
13. Foeldvari I, Nielsen S, Kummerle-Deschner J, et al. Tumor necrosis factor-a blocker in treatment of juvenile idiopathic arthritis-associated uveitis refractory to second-line agents: results of a multinational survey. *J Rheumatol.* 2007;34:1146-1150.
14. Costamagna A, Furst K, Tully K, et al. Tuberculosis associated with blocking agents against tumor necrosis factor-alpha—California, 2002–2003. *MMWR Morb Mortal Wkly Rep.* 2004;53:683-686.
15. Vojvodich PF, Hansen JB, Andersson U, et al. Etanercept treatment improves longitudinal growth in prepubertal children with juvenile idiopathic arthritis. *J Rheumatol.* 2007;34:2481-2485.

References

Ethacrynate Sodium

1. Ethacrynic acid. Lexi-Comp® Online with AHFS® (database). Bethesda, MD: American Society of Health-System Pharmacists; updated March 19, 2009.
2. Intravenous Sodium Edecrin [package insert]. Greenville, NC: DSM Pharmaceuticals Inc; October 2007.
3. VanDerLinde LP, Campbell RK, Jackson E. Guidelines for the intravenous administration of drugs. *Drug Intell Clin Pharm*. 1977;11:30-55.
4. Loggie JMH, Kleinman LI, Maanen EFV. Renal function and diuretic therapy in infants and children. Part III. *J Pediatr*. 1975;86:825-832.
5. Friedman WF, George BL. New concepts and drugs in the treatment of congestive heart failure. *Pediatr Clin North Am*. 1984;31:1197-1227.
6. Whitman V, Stern RC, Bellet P, et al. Studies on cor pulmonale in cystic fibrosis: I. Effects of diuresis. *Pediatrics*. 1975;55:83-85.
7. Sparrow AW, Friedberg DZ, Nadas AS. The use of ethacrynic acid in infants and children with congestive heart failure. *Pediatrics*. 1968;42:291-302.
8. Chemtob S, Doray JL, Laudignon N, et al. Alternating sequential dosing with furosemide and ethacrynic acid in drug tolerance in the newborn. *Am J Dis Child*. 1989;143:850-854.
9. Scalais E, Papageorgiou A, Aranda JV. Effects of ethacrynic acid in the newborn infant. *J Pediatr*. 1984;104:947-950.
10. Serratto M. Diagnosis and management of heart failure in infants and children. *Comprehensive Ther*. 1992;18:11-19.
11. Trissel LA, ed. *Handbook on Injectable Drugs*. 15th ed. Bethesda, MD: American Society of Health-System Pharmacists; 2009.
12. Raymond G, Day P, Rabb M. Sodium content of commonly administered intravenous drugs. *Hosp Pharm*. 1982;17:560-561.
13. Robertson CMT, Tyebkhan JM, Peliowski A, et al. Ototoxic drugs and sensorineural hearing loss following severe neonatal respiratory failure. *Acta Paediatrica*. 2006;95:214-223.
14. Kjellstrand CM. Ethacrynic acid in acute tubular necrosis: indications and effect on the natural course. *Nephron*. 1972;9:337-348.
15. Slone D, Jick H, Lewis GP, et al. Intravenously given ethacrynic acid and gastrointestinal bleeding. *JAMA*. 1969;209:1668-1671.

Etomidate

1. Available at: http://ismp.org/Tools/highalertmedications.pdf. Accessed October 9, 2009.
2. Available at: http://www.usp.org/hqi/similarProducts/choosy.html. Accessed October 9, 2009.
3. Etomidate [package insert]. Lake Forest, IL: Hospira Inc; May 2004.
4. Kienstra AJ, Ward MA, Sasan F, et al. Etomidate versus pentobarbital for sedation of children for head and neck CT imaging. *Pediatr Emerg Care*. 2004;20:499-506.
5. Deitch S, Davis DP, Schatteman J, et al. The use of etomidate for prehospital rapid-sequence intubation. *Prehosp Emerg Care*. 2003;7:380-383.
6. Guldner G, Schultz J, Sexton P, et al. Etomidate for rapid-sequence intubation in young children: hemodynamic effects and adverse events. *Acad Emerg Med*. 2003;10:134-139.
7. Di Liddo L, D'Angelo A, Nguyen B, et al. Etomidate versus midazolam for procedural sedation in pediatric outpatients: a randomized controlled trial. *Ann Emerg Med*. 2006;48:433-440.
8. Bozeman WP, Young S. Etomidate as a sole agent for endotracheal intubation in the prehospital air medical setting. *Air Med J*. 2002;21:2-35.
9. Editomate. Lexi-Comp® Online with AHFS® (database). Hudson, OH: Lexi-Comp Inc; updated August 13, 2009.
10. Cotton BA, Guillamondegui OD, Fleming SB, et al. Increased risk of adrenal insufficiency following etomidate exposure in critically injured patients. *Arch Surg*. 2008;143:62-67.
11. Levy ML, Aranda M, Zelman V, et al. Propylene glycol toxicity following continuous etomidate infusion for the control of refractory cerebral edema. *Neurosurgery*. 1995;37:363-371.
12. Schulte HM, Benker G, Reinwein D, et al: Infusion of low dose etomidate: Correction of hypercortisolaemia in patients with Cushing's syndrome and dose-related relationship in normal subjects. *J Clin Endocrinol Metab*. 1990;70:1426-1430.
13. Drake WM, Perry LA, Hinds CJ, et al: Emergency and prolonged use of intravenous etomidate to control hypercortisolemia in a patient with Cushing's syndrome and peritonitis. *J Clin Endocrinol Metab*. 1998;83:3542-3544.
14. Greening JE, Brain CE, Perry LA, et al: Efficient short-term control of hypercortisolaemia by low dose etomidate in severe paediatric Cushing's disease. *Horm Res*. 2005;64:140-143.
15. Allolio B, Schulte HM, Kaulen D, et al: Nonhypnotic low-dose etomidate for rapid correction of hypercortisolaemia in Cushing's syndrome. *Klin Wochenschr*. 1988;66:361-364.
16. Mettauer N, Brierley J. A novel use of etomidate for intentional adrenal suppression to control severe hypercortisolemia in childhood. *Pediatr Crit Care Med*. 2009;10:418-419.
17. Aronoff GR, Berns JS, Brier ME, et al. Drug prescribing in renal failure. 4th ed. Available at: http://www.kdp-baptist.louisville.edu/renalbook/. Accessed September 10, 2009.
18. den Brinker M, Hokken-Koelega AC, Hazelzet JA, et al. One single dose of etomidate negatively influences adrenocortical performance for at least 24h in children with meningococcal sepsis. *Intensive Care Med*. 2008;34:163-168.
19. Ledingham IM, Watt I. Influence of sedation on mortality in critically ill multiple trauma patients. *Lancet*. 1983;1:1270.
20. Greenberg M, Hilty C. Myoclonus after prolonged infusion of etomidate treated with dantrolene. *J Clin Anesth*. 2003;15:489-490.
21. Van Keulen SG, Burton JH. Myoclonus associated with etomidate for ED procedural sedation and analgesia. *Am J Emerg Med*. 2003;21:556-558.

Etoposide

1. Available at: http://ismp.org/Tools/highalertmedications.pdf. ISMP 2008. Accessed August 24, 2009.
2. Etoposide [package insert]. Bedford, OH: Bedford Laboratories; February 2006.
3. Etoposide. Lexi-Comp® Online with AHFS® (database). Bethesda, MD: American Society of Health-System Pharmacists; updated January 2009.
4. Etoposide. Lexi-Comp® Online with AHFS® (database). Hudson, OH: Lexi-Comp Inc; updated October 22, 2009.
5. Dahl GV, Lacayo NJ, Brophy N, et al. Mitoxantrone, etoposide, and cyclosporine therapy in pediatric patients with recurrent or refractory acute myeloid leukemia. *J Clin Oncol*. 2000;18(9):1867-1875.
6. Wells RJ, Adams MT, Alonzo TA, et al. Mitoxantrone and cytarabine induction, high-dose cytarabine, and etoposide intensification for pediatric patients with relapsed or refractory acute myeloid leukemia: Children's Cancer Group Study 2951. *J Clin Oncol*. 2003;21(15):2940-2947.
7. Massimo M, Gandola L, Luksch R, et al. Sequential chemotherapy, high-dose thiotepa, circulating progenitor cell rescue and radiotherapy childhood high-grade glioma. *Neuro-Oncol*. 2005;7(1):41-48.
8. Coze C, Hartmann O, Michon J, et al. NB87 induction protocol for stage 4 neuroblastoma in children over 1 year of age: a report from the French Society of Pediatric Oncology. *J Clin Oncol*. 1997;15(12):3433-3440.
9. Rodriguez-Galindo C, Daw NC, Kaste SC, et al. Treatment of refractory osteosarcoma with fractionated cyclophosphamide and etoposide. *J Pediatr Hematol Oncol*. 2002;24(4):250-255.
10. Le Deley MC, Guinebretiere JM, Gentet JC, et al. SFOP OS94: a randomised trial comparing preoperative high-dose methotrexate plus doxorubicin to high-dose methotrexate plus etoposide and ifosfamide in osteosarcoma patients. Eur J Cancer 2007;43:752-761.
11. Ayas M, Al-Seraihi A, Al-Mahr M, et al. The outcome of children with acute myeloid leukemia (AML) post-allogeneic stem cell transplantation (SCT) is not improved by the addition of etoposide to the conditioning regimen. *Pediatr Blood Cancer*. 2006;47(7):926-930. Epub ahead of print.

References

12. Sandler ES, Hagg R, Coppes MJ, et al. Hematopoietic stem cell transplantation (HSCT) with a conditioning regimen of busulfan, cyclophosphamide, and etoposide for children with acute myelogenous leukemia (AML): a phase I study of the Pediatric Blood and Marrow Transplant Consortium. *Med Pediatr Oncol*. 2000;35(4):403-409.
13. Aronoff GR, Berns JS, Brier ME, et al. Drug prescribing in renal failure. 4th ed. Available at: http://www.kdp-baptist.louisville.edu/renalbook/. Accessed October 23, 2009.
14. Solimando DA, ed. *Lexi-Comp's Drug Information Handbook for Oncology*. 4th ed. Hudson, OH: Lexi-Comp; 2004:313-319.
15. Trissel LA, ed. *Handbook on Injectable Drugs*. 15th ed. Bethesda, MD: American Society of Health-System Pharmacists; 2009.
16. Damon LE, Johnston LJ, Ries CA, et al. Treatment of acute leukemia with idarubicin, etoposide, and cytarabine (IDEA). A randomized study of etoposide schedule. *Cancer Chemother Pharmacol*. 2004;53(6):468-474.
17. National Comprehensive Cancer Network (NCCN) Antiemesis Panel Members. NCCN Clinical Practice Guidelines in Oncology. Antiemesis, v.1.2006. Available at: www.nccn.org. Accessed October 5, 2009.
18. Roila F, Feyer P, Maranzamo E, et al. Antiemetics in children receiving chemotherapy. *Support Care Cancer*. 2005;13:129-131.

Famotidine

1. Available at: http://www.usp.org/hqi/similarProducts/choosy.html. Accessed August 26, 2009.
2. Pepcid [package insert]. Whitehouse Station, NJ: Merck & Co Inc; October, 2006.
3. James LP, Marotti T, Stowe CD, et al. Pharmacokinetics and pharmacodynamics of famotidine in infants. *J Clin Pharmacol*. 1998;38:1089-1095.
4. Behrens R, Hofbeck M, Singer H, et al. Frequency of stress lesions of the upper gastrointestinal tract in paediatric patients after cardiac surgery: effects of prophylaxis. *Br Heart J*. 1994;72:186-189.
5. Kraus G, Krishna DR, Chmerlarsch D, et al. Famotidine. Pharmacokinetic properties and suppression of acid secretion in paediatric patients following cardiac surgery. *Clin Pharmacokinet*. 1990;18:77-81.
6. Treem WR, Davis PM, Hyams JS. Suppression of gastric acid secretion by intravenous administration of famotidine in children. *J Pediatr*. 1991;118:812-816.
7. James LP, Kearns GL. Pharmacokinetics and pharmacodynamics of famotidine in paediatric patients. *Clin Pharmacokinet*. 1996;31:103-110. Review.
8. James LP, Marshall JD, Heulitt MJ, et al. Pharmacokinetics and pharmacodynamics of famotidine in children. *J Clin Pharmacol*. 1996;36:48-54.
9. Santeiro ML, Riggs CD, Weibley RE. Famotidine pharmacodynamics and dosing requirements in critically ill children. *Pharmacotherapy*. 1997;17:1103, A175.
10. Jahr JS, Burckart G, Smith SS, et al. Effects of famotidine on gastric pH and residual volume in pediatric injury. *Acta Anaesthesiol Scand*. 1991;35:457-460.
11. Nagita A, Manago M, Aoki S, et al. Pharmacokinetics and pharmacodynamics of famotidine in children with gastroduodenal ulcers. *Ther Drug Monit*. 1994;16:444-449.
12. Maples HD, James LP, Stowe CD, et al. Famotidine Disposition in Children and Adolescents with Chronic Renal Insufficiency. *J Clin Pharmacol* 2003;43:7-14.
13. Aronoff GR, Berns JS, Brier ME, et al. Drug prescribing in renal failure. 4th ed. Available at: http://www.kdp-baptist.louisville.edu/renalbook/. Accessed September 12, 2009.
14. Trissel LA, ed. *Handbook on Injectable Drugs*. 15th ed. Bethesda, MD: American Society of Health-System Pharmacists; 2009.
15. DiStefano JE, Mitrano FP, Baptista RJ, et al. Long-term stability of famotidine 20 mg/L in a total parenteral nutrient solution. *Am J Hosp Pharm*. 1989;46:2333-2335.
16. Montoro JB, Pou L, Salvador P, et al. Stability of famotidine 20 and 40 mg/L in total nutrient admixtures. *Am J Hosp Pharm*. 1989;46:2329-2332.
17. Watanabe Y, Tsumura H, Sasaki H, et al. The effects of intermittent and continuous intravenous infusion of famotidine on gastric acidity in patients with peptic ulcers. *Clin Ther*. 1990;12:534-546.
18. Kirch W, Halabi A, Linde M, et al. Negative effects of famotidine on cardiac performance assessed by noninvasive hemodynamic measurements. *Gastroenterology*. 1989;96:1388-1392.
19. Guillet R, Stoll BJ, Cotton CM, et al. Association of H2-blocker therapy and higher incidence of necrotizing enterocolitis in very low birth weight infants. *Pediatrics*. 2006;117:e137-e142.

Fenoldopam

1. Corlopam [package insert]. Lake Forest, IL: Hospira Inc; March 2005.
2. Verghese ST, Hammer GB, Lavandosky G, et al. A multicenter, randomized study to determine the pharmacokinetics and pharmacodynamics of fenoldopam mesylate in pediatric patients. *Am J Ther*. 1999;6:283-288.
3. Tobias JD. Fenoldopam for controlled hypotension during spinal fusion in children and adolescents. *Paediatr Anaesthesia*. 2000;10:261-266.
4. Costello JM, Thiagarajan RR, Dionne RE, et al. Initial experience with fenoldopam after cardiac surgery in neonates with an insufficient response to conventional diuretics. *Pediatr Crit Care Med*. 2006;7:28-33.
5. Ricci Z, Stazi GV, Di Chiara L, et al. Fenoldopam in newborn patients undergoing cardiopulmonary bypass:controlled clinical trial. *Interact Cardiovasc Thorac Surg*. 2008;7:1049-1053.
6. US Department of Health and Human Services, National Institutes of Health, National Heart, Lung, and Blood Institute. *Diagnosis, Evaluation, and Treatment of High Blood Pressure in Children and Adolescents, 4th report*. NIH Publication 05-5267. Bethesda, MD: NIH; revised May 2005.
7. Knoderer CA, Leiser JD, Nailescu C, et al. Fenoldopam for acute kidney injury in children. *Pediatr Nephrol*. 2008;23:495-498.
8. Trissel LA, ed. *Handbook on Injectable Drugs*. 15th ed. Bethesda, MD: American Society of Health-System Pharmacists; 2009.
9. Lechner BL, Pascual JF, Roscelli JD. Failure of fenoldopam to control severe hypertension secondary to renal graft rejection in a pediatric patient. *Mil Med*. 2005;170:130-132.

FentaNYL Citrate

1. Available at: http://ismp.org/Tools/confuseddrugnames.pdf. Updated April 1, 2005.
2. Available at: http://www.usp.org/hqi/similarProducts/choosy.html. Accessed August 13, 2009.
3. Fentanyl citrate injection [prescribing information]. Lake Forest, IL: Hospira; March 2008.
4. Robinson S, Gregory G. Fentanyl-air-oxygen anesthesia for ligation of patent ductus arteriosus in preterm infants. *Anesth Analg*. 1981;60:331-334.
5. Comstock MK, Carter JG, Moyers JR, et al. Rigidity and hypercarbia on fentanyl–oxygen induction. *Anesthesiology*. 1979;51:328.
6. Jarvis AP, Arancibia CU. A case of difficult neonatal ventilation. *Anesth Analg*. 1987;66:196-199.
7. Collins C, Koren G, Crean P, et al. Fentanyl pharmacokinetics and hemodynamic effects in preterm infants during ligation of patient ductus arteriosus. *Anesth Analg*. 1985;64:1078-1080.
8. Koehntop DE, Rodman JH, Brundage DM, et al. Pharmacokinetics of fentanyl in neonates. *Anesth Analg*. 1986;65:227-232.
9. Wells S, Williamson M, Hooker D. Fentanyl-induced chest wall rigidity in a neonate: a case report. *Heart Lung*. 1994;23:196-198.

References

10. Anand KJ, Sippell WG, Aynsley-Green A. Randomized trial of fentanyl anesthesia in preterm babies undergoing surgery: effects on the stress response. *Lancet.* 1987;243-248.
11. Friesen R, Henry D. Cardiovascular changes in preterm neonates receiving isofluorane, halothane, fentanyl, and ketamine. *Anesthesiology.* 1986;64:238-242.
12. Hickey PR, Hansen DD, Wessel DL, et al. Pulmonary and systemic hemodynamic responses to fentanyl in infants. *Anesth Analg.* 1985;64:483-486.
13. Yaster M. The dose response of fentanyl in neonatal anesthesia. *Anesthesiology.* 1987;66:433.
14. Koren G, Goresky G, Crean P, et al. Pediatric fentanyl dosing based on pharmacokinetics during cardiac surgery. *Anesth Analg.* 1984;63:577-582.
15. Fentanyl. Lexi-Comp® Online with AHFS® (database). Hudson, OH: Lexi-Comp Inc; updated August 13, 2009.
16. Roth B, Schlunder C, Houben F, et al. Analgesia and sedation in neonatal intensive care using fentanyl by continuous infusion. *Dev Pharmacol Ther.* 1991;17:121-127.
17. Leuschen MP, Willwitt LD, Hoie EB, et al. Plasma fentanyl levels in infants undergoing extracorporeal membrane oxygenation. *J Thorac Cardiovasc Surg.* 1993;105:885-891.
18. Arnold JH, Truog RD, Scavone JM, et al. Changes in the pharmacodynamic response to fentanyl in neonates during continuous infusion. *J Pediatr.* 1991;119:639-643.
19. Koren G, Maurice L. Pediatric uses of opioids. *Pediatr Clin North Am.* 1989;36:1141-1157.
20. Tobias JD. Sedation and analgesia in paediatric intensive care units. *Paediatric Drugs.* 1999;1:109-126.
21. Lago P, Benini F, Zacchello F. Randomized controlled trial of low dose fentanyl infusion in preterm infants with hyaline membrane disease. *Arch Dis Child Fetal Neonatal Ed.* 1998;79:F194-F197.
22. Buck ML. Pharmacokinetic changes during extracorporeal membrane oxygenation. Implications for drug therapy of neonates. *Clin Pharmacokinet.* 2003;42:403-417.
23. Hansen DD, Hickey PR. Anesthesia for hypoplastic left heart syndrome: use of high-dose fentanyl in 30 neonates. *Anesth Analg.* 1986;65:127-132.
24. Trissel LA. *Handbook on Injectable Drugs.* 15th ed. Bethesda, MD: American Society of Health-System Pharmacists; 2009.
25. Tobias JD. Subcutaneous administration of fentanyl and midazolam to prevent withdrawal after prolonged sedation in children. *Crit Care Med.* 1999;27:2262-2265.
26. Billmire DA, Neale HW, Gregory R. Use of IV fentanyl in the outpatient treatment of pediatric facial trauma. *J Trauma.* 1985;25:1079-1080.
27. Lane JC, Tennison MB, Lawless ST, et al. Movement disorder after withdrawal of fentanyl infusion. *J Pediatr.* 1991;119:649-651.
28. Katz R, Kelly HW, Hsi A. Prospective study on the occurrence of withdrawal in critically ill children who receive fentanyl by continuous infusion. *Crit Care Med.* 1994;22:763-767.
29. Bragonier R, Bartle D, Langton-Hewer S. Acute dystonia in a 14-yr-old following propofol and fentanyl anaesthesia. *Br J Anaesth.* 2000;84:828-829.
30. Aouad MT, Kanzi GE, Siddik-Sayyid SM, et al. Preoperative caudal block prevents emergence agitation in children following sevoflurane anesthesia. *Acta Anaesthesiol Scand.* 2005;49:300-304.
31. Demirbilek S, Togal T, Cicek M, et al. Effects of fentanyl on the incidence of emergence agitation in children receiving desflurane or sevoflurane anaesthesia. *Eur J Anaesthesiol.* 2004;21:538-542.

Ferric Gluconate

1. Ferrlecit (sodium ferric gluconate complex in sucrose injection) [product information]. Corona CA: Watson Pharma Inc; September 2006.
2. Ferric gluconate. Lexi-Comp® Online with AHFS® (database). Hudson, OH: Lexi-Comp Inc; updated August 13, 2009.
3. Fishbane S, Kowalski EA. The comparative safety of intravenous iron dextran, iron saccharate, and sodium ferric gluconate. *Seminars in Dialysis.* 2000;13:381-384.
4. Chertow GM, Mason PD, Vaage-Nilsen O, et al. On the relative safety of parenteral iron formulations. *Nephrol Dial Transplant.* 2004;19:1571-1575.
5. Baile GR, Clark JA, Lane CE, et al. Hypersensitivity reactions and deaths associated with intravenous iron preparations. *Nephrol Dial Transplant.* 2005;20:1443-1449.
6. Fishbane S. Safety in iron management. *Am J Kid Disease.* 2003;41:S18-S36.
7. Micheal B, Coyne DW, Fishbane S, et al. Sodium ferric gluconate complex in haemodialysis patients: adverse reactions compared to placebo and iron dextran. *Kidney International.* 2002;61:1830-1839.
8. Saadeh C, Srkalovic G. Acute hypersensitivity reaction to ferric gluconate in a premedicated patient. *Ann Pharmacother.* 2005;39:2124-2127.
9. NDOQI clinical practice guidelines and clinical practice recommendations for anemia in chronic kidney disease. *Am J Kid Dis.* 2006:47(suppl 3):S1-S145.
10. Tenbrok K, Muller-Berghaus J, Michalk D, et al. Intravenous iron treatment of renal anemia in children on hemodialysis. *Pediatr Nephrol.* 1999;13:580-582.
11. Yorgin PD, Belson A, Sarwal M, et al. Sodium ferric gluconate therapy in renal transplant and renal failure patients. *Pediatr Nephrol.* 2000;15:171-175.
12. Gillespie RS, Symons JM. Sodium ferric gluconate for post-transplant anemia in pediatric and young adult renal transplant recipients. *Pediatr Transplantation.* 2005;9:43-46.
13. Warady BA, Zobrist RH, Wu J, et al. Sodium ferric gluconate complex therapy in anemic children on hemodialysis. *Pediatr Nephrol.* 2005;20:1320-1327.
14. Warady BA, Seligman PA, Dahl N. Single-dosage pharmacokinetics of sodium ferric gluconate complex in iron-deficient pediatric hemodialysis patients. *Clin J Am Soc Nephrol.* 2007;2:1140-1146.

Filgrastim

1. Available at: http://www.usp.org/hqi/similarProducts/choosy.html. Accessed August 14, 2009.
2. Available at: http://ismp.org/Tools/confuseddrugnames.pdf. Updated April 1, 2005.
3. Filgrastim [prescribing information]. Thousand Oaks, CA: Amgen Manufacturing Limited; September 9, 2007.
4. Kojima S, Fukada M, Miyajima Y, et al. Treatment of aplastic anemia in children with recombinant human granulocyte colony-stimulating factor. *Blood.* 1991;77:937-941.
5. Kojima S, Hibi S, Kosaka Y, et al. Immunosuppressive therapy using antithymocyte globulin, cyclosporine, and danazol with or without human granulocyte colony-stimulating factor in children with acquired aplastic anemia. *Blood.* 2000;96:2049-2054.
6. Little MA, Morland B, Chisholm J, et al. A randomized study of prophylactic G-CSF following MRC UKALL XI intensification regimen in childhood ALL and T-NHL. *Med Pediatr Oncol.* 2002;38:98-103.
7. Alonzo TA, Kobrinsky NL, Aledo A, et al. Impact of granulocyte colony-stimulating factor use during induction for acute myelogenous leukemia in children: a report from the Children's Cancer Group. *J Pediatr Hematol Oncol.* 2002;24:627-635.
8. Furman WL, Crist WM. Biology and clinical applications of hemopoietins in pediatric practice. *Pediatrics.* 1992;90:716-728.
9. Riikonen P, Rahiala J, Salonvarra M, et al. Prophylactic administration of granulocyte colony-stimulating factor (filgrastim) after conventional chemotherapy in children with cancer. *Stem Cells.* 1995;13:289-294.
10. Hawkins DS, Felgenhauer J, Park J, et al. Peripheral blood stem cell support reduces the toxicity of intensive chemotherapy for children and adolescents with metastatic sarcomas. *Cancer.* 2002;95:1354-1365.

References

11. Welte K, Zeidler C, Reiter A, et al. Differential effects of granulocyte-macrophage colony-stimulating factor and granulocyte colony-stimulating factor in children with severe congenital neutropenia. *Blood.* 1990;75:1056-1063.
12. Bonilla MA, Gillio AP, Ruggeiro M, et al. Effects of recombinant human granulocyte colony-stimulating factor on neutropenia in patients with congenital agranulocytosis. *N Engl J Med.* 1989;320:1574-1580.
13. Gillan ER, Christensen RD, Suen Y, et al. A randomized, placebo-controlled trial of recombinant human granulocyte colony-stimulating factor administration in newborn infants with presumed sepsis: significant induction of peripheral and bone marrow neutrophilia. *Blood.* 1994;84:1427-1433.
14. Makhlouf RA, Doron MW, Bose CL, et al. Administration of granulocyte colony-stimulating factor to neutropenic low birth weight infants of mothers with pre-eclampsia. *J Pediatr.* 1995;126:454-456.
15. Kucukoduk S, Sezer T, Yildiran A, et al. Randomized, double-blinded, placebo-controlled trial of early administration of recombinant human granulocyte colony-stimulating factor to non-neutropenic preterm newborns between 33 and 36 weeks with presumed sepsis. *Scand J Infect Dis.* 2002;34:893-897.
16. Ahmad A, Laborada G, Bussel J, et al. Comparison of recombinant granulocyte colony-stimulating factor, recombinant human granulocyte-macrophage colony-stimulating factor and placebo for treatment of septic preterm infants. *Pediatr Infect Dis J.* 2002;21:1061-1065.
17. Schroten H, Roesler J, Breidenbach T, et al. Granulocyte and granulocyte-macrophage colony-stimulating factors for treatment of neutropenia in glycogen storage disease type Ib. *J Pediatr.* 1991;119:748-754.
18. Calderwood S, Kilpatrick L, Douglas SD, et al. Recombinant human granulocyte colony-stimulating factor therapy for patients with neutropenia and/or neutrophil dysfunction secondary to glycogen storage disease type 1b. *Blood.* 2001;97:376-382.
19. de la Rubia J, Arbona C, de Arriba F, et al. Analysis of factors associated with low peripheral blood progenitor cell collection in normal donors. *Transfusion.* 2002;42:4-9.
20. Madero L, Gonzalez-Vicent M, Molina J, et al. Use of concurrent G-CSF + GM-CSF vs G-CSF alone for mobilization of peripheral blood stem cells in children with malignant disease. *Bone Marrow Transplant.* 2000;26:365-369.
21. Perez-Duenas B, Alcorta I, Estella J, et al. Safety and efficacy of high-dose G-CSF (24 mcg/kg) alone for PBSC mobilization in children. *Bone Marrow Transplant.* 2002;30:987-988.
22. Trissel LA. *Handbook on Injectable Drugs.* 15th ed. Bethesda, MD: American Society of Health-System Pharmacists; 2009.
23. Sasse EC, Sasse AD, Brandalise ST, et al. Colony-stimulating factors for prevention of myelosuppressive therapy-induced febrile neutropenia in children with acute lymphoblastic leukemia. *Cochrane Database Syst Rev.* 2005;(3):CD004139.

Fluconazole

1. Available at: http://www.usp.org/hqi/similarProducts/choosy.html. Accessed August 27, 2009.
2. Available at: http://ismp.org/Tools/confuseddrugnames.pdf. Accessed August 27, 2009.
3. Diflucan [prescribing information]. New York, NY: Pfizer Inc; May 2008.
4. Saxen H, Hoppu K, Pohjavuori M. Pharmacokinetics of fluconazole in very low birth weight infants during the first two weeks of life. *Clin Pharmacol Ther.* 1993;54:269-277.
5. Brammer KW, Coates PE. Pharmacokinetics of fluconazole in pediatric patients. *Eur J Clin Microbiol Infect Dis.* 1994;13:325-329.
6. Viscoli C, Castagnola E, Corsini M, et al. Fluconazole therapy in an underweight infant. *Eur J Clin Microbiol Infect Dis.* 1989;8:925-926.
7. Wiest DB, Flower SL, Garner SS, et al. Fluconazole in neonatal disseminated candidiasis. *Arch Dis Child.* 1991;66:1002.
8. Bergman KA, Meis JF, Horrevorts AM, et al. Acute renal failure in a neonate due to pelviureteric candidal bezoars successfully treated with long-term systemic fluconazole. *Acta Pediatr.* 1992;81:709-711.
9. Huttova M, Hartmanova I, Kralinsky K, et al. Candida fungemia in neonates treated with fluconazole: report of forty cases, including eight with meningitis. *Pediatr Infect Dis J.* 1998;17:1012-1015.
10. Novelli V, Holzel H. Safety and tolerability of fluconazole in children. *Antimicrob Agents Chemother.* 1999;43:1955-1960.
11. Driessen M, Ellis JB, Cooper PA, et al. Fluconazole vs. amphotericin B for the treatment of neonatal fungal septicemia: a prospective randomized trial. *Pediatr Infect Dis J.* 1996;15:1107-1112.
12. Wainer S, Cooper PA, Gouws H, et al. Prospective study of fluconazole therapy in systemic neonatal fungal infection. *Pediatr Infect Dis J.* 1997;16:763-767.
13. Bliss JM, Wellington M, Gigliotti F. Antifungal pharmacotherapy for neonatal candidiasis. *Semin Perinatol.* 2003;27:365-374.
14. Kaufman D, Boyle R, Hazen KC, et al. Fluconazole prophylaxis against fungal colonization and infection in preterm infants. *N Engl J Med.* 2001;345:1660-1666.
15. Kicklighter SD, Springer SC, Cox T, et al. Fluconazole for prophylaxis against candidal rectal colonization in the very low birth weight infant. *Pediatrics.* 2001;107:293-298.
16. Manzoni P, Stolfi I, Pugni L, et al. A multicenter, randomized trial of prophylactic fluconazole in preterm neonates. N Engl J Med 2007;356:2483-95.
17. Clerihew L, Austin N, McGuire W. Systemic antifungal prophylaxis for very low birthweight infants: a systematic review. *Arch Dis Child Fetal Neonatal Ed.* 2008;93:F198-F200.
18. American Academy of Pediatrics. Antifungal drugs for systemic fungal infections. In: Pickering LK, Baker CJ, Kimberlin DW, et al., eds. *2009 Red Book: Report of the Committee on Infectious Diseases.* 28th ed. Elk Grove Village, IL: American Academy of Pediatrics; 2009:765-776.
19. Viscoli C, Castagnola E, Fioredda F, et al. Fluconazole in the treatment of candidiasis in immunocompromised children. *Antimicrob Agents Chemother.* 1991;35:365-367.
20. Lee JW, Seibel NL, Amantea M, et al. Safety and pharmacokinetics of fluconazole in children with neoplastic diseases. *J Pediatr.* 1992;120:987-993.
21. Santeiro ML, Riggs D, Weibley RE. Fluconazole therapy in a child with candida tropicalis fungemia. *Ann Pharmacother.* 1992;26:840. Letter.
22. Simon G, Simon G, Erdos M, et al. Invasive Cryptococcus laurentii disease in a nine-year-old boy with X-linked Hyper-immunoglobulin M syndrome. *Pediatr Infect Dis J.* 2005;24:935-937.
23. Humphrey MJ, Jevons S, Tarbit MH. Pharmacokinetic evaluation of UK-49858, a metabolically stable triazole antifungal agent, in animals and humans. *Antimicrob Agents Chemother.* 1985;28:648-653.
24. Dudley MN. Clinical pharmacology of fluconazole. *Pharmacotherapy.* 1990;10(suppl):141-145.
25. Aronoff GR, Berns JS, Brier ME, et al. Drug prescribing in renal failure. 4th ed. Available at: http://www.kdp-baptist.louisville.edu/renalbook/. Accessed November 9, 2009.
26. Nicolau DP, Crowe H, Nightingale CH, et al. Effect of continuous arteriovenous hemodiafiltration on the pharmacokinetics of fluconazole. *Pharmacotherapy.* 1994;14:502-505.
27. Bafeltowska JJ, Buszman E. Pharmacokinetics of fluconazole in the cerebrospinal fluid of children with hydrocephalus. *Chemother.* 2005;51:370-376.
28. Trissel LA, ed. *Handbook on Injectable Drugs.* 15th ed. Bethesda, MD: American Society of Health-System Pharmacists; 2009.
29. Esch JJ, Kantoch MJ. Torsades de pointes ventricular tachycardia in a pediatric patient treated with fluconazole. *Pediatr Cardiol.* 2008;29: 210-213.
30. Fluconazole. Lexi-Comp Online with AHFS (database). Hudson, OH: Lexi-Comp Inc; updated October 13, 2009.
31. Debruyne D, Rycelynck JP. Clinical pharmacokinetics of fluconazole. *Clin Pharmacokinet.* 1993;24:10-27.
32. Seay RE, Larson TA, Toscano JP, et al. Pharmacokinetics of fluconazole in immune-compromised children with leukemia or other hematologic diseases. *Pharmacotherapy.* 1995;15:52-58.
33. Wade KC, Wu D, Kaufman DA, et al. Population pharmacokinetics of fluconazole in young infants. *Antimicrob Agents Chemother.* 2008;52:4043-4049.

References

Flumazenil

1. Available at: http://www.usp.org/hqi/similarProducts/choosy.html. Accessed October 6, 2009.
2. Flumazenil Injection USP [package insert]. Bedford, OH: Bedford Laboratories; December 2007.
3. Hoffman EJ, Warren EW. Flumazenil: a benzodiazepine antagonist. *Clin Pharm*. 1993;12:614-656.
4. Sugarman JM, Paul RI. Flumazenil: a review. *Pediatr Emerg Care*. 1994;10:37-43.
5. Jones RD, Lawson AD, Andrew LJ, et al. Antagonism of the hypnotic effect of midazolam in children: a randomized, double blind study of placebo and flumazenil administered after midazolam-induced anesthesia. *Br J Anaesth*. 1991;66:660-666.
6. Jones RDM, Chan K, Roulson CJ, et al. Pharmacokinetics of flumazenil and midazolam. *Brit J Anaesthes*. 1993;70:286-292.
7. Negus BH, Street NE. Midazolam-opioid combination and postoperative upper airway obstruction in children. *Anaesthesia Int Care*. 1994;22:232-233.
8. Shannon M, Albers G, Burkhart K, et al. Safety and efficacy of flumazenil in the reversal of benzodiazepine-induced conscious sedation. *J Pediatr*. 1997;131:582-586.
9. Peters JM, Tolia V, Simpson P, et al. Flumazenil in children after esophagogastroduodenoscopy. *Am J Gastroenterol*. 1999;94:1857-1861.
10. Baktai G, Szekely E, Marialigeti T, et al. Use of midazolam (Dormicum) and flumazenil (Anexate) in paediatric bronchology. *Curr Med Res Opin*. 1992;12:552-559.
11. American Academy of Pediatrics Committee on Drugs. Emergency drug doses for infants and children. *Pediatrics*. 1998;101:e1-e11.
12. Terri Voepel-Lewis T, Mitchell A, Malviya S. Delayed postoperative agitation in a child after preoperative midazolam. *J PeriAnesthesia Nurs*. 2007;22:303-308.
13. Collins S, Carter JA. Resedation after bolus administration of midazolam to an infant and its reversal by flumazenil. *Anaesthesia*. 1991;46:471-472.
14. Clark RF, Sage TA, Tunget CL, et al. Delayed onset lorazepam poisoning successfully reversed by flumazenil in a child: case report and review of the literature. *Pediatr Emerg Care*. 1995;11:32-34.
15. Kelly C, Egner J, Rubin J. Successful treatment of triazolam overdose with Ro 15-1788 (Anexate). *S Afr Med J*. 1988;73:442.
16. Roald OK, Dahl V. Flunitrazepam intoxication in a child successfully treated with the benzodiazepine antagonist flumazenil. *Crit Care Med*. 1989;17:1355-1356.
17. Richard P, Autret E, Bardon J, et al. The use of flumazenil in a neonate. *Clin Toxicol*. 1991;29:137-140.
18. Winkler E, Almog S, Kriger D, et al. Use of flumazenil in the diagnosis and treatment of patients with coma of unknown etiology. *Crit Care Med*. 1993;21:538-542.
19. Hojer J, Baehrendtz S, Matell G, Gustafsson LL. Diagnostic utility of flumazenil in coma with suspected poisoning: a double blind, randomised controlled study. *BMJ*. 1990;301:1308-1311.
20. Hofer P, Scollo-Lavizzari G. Benzodiazepine antagonist Ro 15-1788 in self-poisoning. Diagnostic and therapeutic use. *Arch Intern Med*. 1985;145:663-664.
21. Aronoff GR, Berns JS, Brier ME, et al. Drug prescribing in renal failure. 4th ed. Available at: http://www.kdp-baptist.louisville.edu/renalbook/. Accessed October 6, 2009.
22. Trissel LA, ed. *Handbook on Injectable Drugs*. 15th ed. Bethesda, MD: American Society of Health-System Pharmacists; 2009.
23. Haret D. Rectal flumazenil can save the day. *Paediatr Anaesth*. 2008;18:352.
24. Carbajal R, Simon N, Blanc P, etal. Rectal flumazenil to reverse midazolam sedation in children. *Anesth Analg*. 1996;82:895.

Fomepizole

1. Available at: http://ismp.org/Tools/confuseddrugnames.pdf. Accessed September 25, 2009.
2. Antizole [package insert]. Dover, DE: Paladin Labs (USA) Inc; April 2009.
3. Barceloux DG, Krenzelok EP, Olson K, Watson W. American Academy of Clinical Toxicology Practice Guidelines on the Treatment of Ethylene Glycol Poisoning. Ad Hoc Committee. *J Toxicol Clin Toxicol*. 1999;37:537-560.
4. Barceloux DG, Bond GR, Krenzelok EP, et al. American Academy of Clinical Toxicology practice guidelines on the treatment of methanol poisoning. *J Toxicol Clin Toxicol*. 2002;40:415-446.
5. Brent J. Fomepizole for ethylene glycol and methanol poisoning. *N Engl J Med*. 2009;360:2216-2223.
6. Baun CR, Langman CB, Oker EE, et al. Fomepizole treatment of ethylene glycol poisoning in an infant. *Pediatrics*. 2000;106:1489-1491.
7. Brophy PD, Tenenbein M, Gardner J, et al. Childhood diethylene glycol poisoning treated with alcohol dehydrogenase inhibitor fomepizole and hemodialysis. *Am J Kidney Dis*. 2000;35:958-962.
8. Detaille T, Wallemacq P, Clément de Cléty S, et al. Fomepizole alone for severe infant ethylene glycol poisoning. *Pediatr Crit Care Med*. 2004;5:490-491.
9. Caravati EM, Heileson HL, Jones MJ. Treatment of severe pediatric ethylene glycol intoxication without hemodialysis. *Toxicol Clin Toxicol*. 2004;42:255-259.
10. Brown MJ, Shannon MW, Woolf A, Boyer EW. Childhood methanol ingestion treated with fomepizole and hemodialysis. *Pediatrics*. 2001;108:E77.
11. Benitez JG, Swanson-Biearman B, Krenzelok EP. Nystagmus secondary to fomepizole administration in a pediatric patient. *Clin Toxicol*. 2000;38:795-798.
12. De Brabander N, Wojciechowski M, De Decker K, et al. Fomepizole as a therapeutic strategy in paediatric methanol poisoning. A case report and review of the literature. *Eur J Pediatr*. 2005;164:158-161.
13. Brent J. Current management of ethylene glycol poisoning. *Drugs*. 2001;61:979-988.
14. Mycyk MB, Leikin JB. Antidote review: fomepizole for methanol poisoning. *Am J Ther*. 2003;10:68-70.
15. Mégarbane B, Borron SW, Baud FJ. Current recommendations for treatment of severe toxic alcohol poisonings. *Intensive Care Med*. 2005;31:189-195.
16. Faessel H, Houze P, Baud FJ, et al. 4-methylpyrazole monitoring during haemodialysis of ethylene glycol intoxicated patients. *Eur J Clin Pharmacol*. 1995;49:211-213.
17. Jobard E, Harry P, Turcant A, et al. 4-Methylpyrazole and hemodialysis in ethylene glycol poisoning. *J Toxicol Clin Toxicol*. 1996;34:373-377.
18. Bestic M, Blackford M, Reed M. Fomepizole: a critical assessment of current dosing recommendations. *J Clin Pharmacol*. 2009;49:130-137.
19. Mégarbane B, Borron SW, Trout H, et al. Treatment of acute methanol poisoning with fomepizole. *Intensive Care Med*. 2001;27:1370-1378.
20. Borron SW, Mégarbane B, Baud FJ. Fomepizole in treatment of uncomplicated ethylene glycol poisoning. *Lancet*. 1999;354:831.
21. Lepik KJ, Levy AR, Sobolev BG, et al. Adverse drug events associated with the antidotes for methanol and ethylene glycol poisoning: a comparison of ethanol andfomepizole. *Ann Emerg Med*. 2009;53:439-450.

Foscarnet Sodium

1. Available at: http://ismp.org/Tools/confuseddrugnames.pdf. Accessed October 26, 2009.
2. Available at: http://www.usp.org/hqi/similarProducts/choosy.html. Accessed October 26, 2009.
3. Foscarnet sodium [package insert]. Lake Forest, IL: Hospira Inc; February 2008.
4. American Academy of Pediatrics. Pickering LK, Baker CJ, Kimberlin DW, et al., eds. *2009 Red Book: Report of the Committee on Infectious Diseases*. 28th ed. Elk Grove Village, IL: American Academy of Pediatrics; 2009.

References

5. Walton RC, Whitcup SM, Mueller BU, et al. Combined intravenous ganciclovir and foscarnet for children with recurrent cytomegalovirus retinitis. *Ophthalmology.* 1995;102:1865-1870.
6. Sastry SM, Epps CH, Walton RC, et al. Combined ganciclovir and foscarnet in pediatric cytomegalovirus retinitis. *J Natl Med Assoc.* 1996;88:661-662.
7. Tejada P, Sarmiento B, Ramos JT, et al. Report of a case of aggressive cytomegalovirus retinitis in an infant with AIDS. *Int Ophthalmol.* 1996–1997;20:333-337.
8. Khurana RN, Charonis A, Samuel MA, et al. Intravenous foscarnet in the management of acyclovir-resistant herpes simplex virus type 2 in acute retinal necrosis in children. *Med Sci Monit.* 2005;11:CS75-CS78.
9. Bryant P, Sasadeusz J, Carapetis J, et al. Successful treatment of foscarnet-resistant herpes simplex stomatitis with intravenous cidofovir in a child. *Pediatr Infect Dis J.* 2001;20:1083-1086.
10. Crassard N, Souillet AL, Morfin F, et al. Acyclovir-resistant varicella infection with atypical lesions in a non-HIV leukemic infant. *Acta Paediatr.* 2000;89:1497-1499.
11. Levin MJ, Dahl KM, Weinberg A, et al. Development of resistance to acyclovir during chronic infection with the Oka vaccine strain of varicella-zoster virus, in an immunosuppressed child. *J Infect Dis.* 2003;188:954-959.
12. Bryan CJ, Prichad MN, Daily S, et al. Acyclovir-resistant chronic verrucous vaccine strain varicella in a patient with neuroblastoma. *Pediatr Infect Dis J.* 2008;27:946-948.
13. Aronoff GR, Berns JS, Brier ME, et al. Drug prescribing in renal failure. 4th ed. Available at: http://www.kdp-baptist.louisville.edu/renalbook/. Accessed October 26, 2009.
14. Trissel LA, ed. *Handbook on Injectable Drugs.* 15th ed. Bethesda, MD: American Society of Health-System Pharmacists; 2009.
15. Hainaut M, Gerard M, Peltier CA, et al. Effectiveness of rescue antiretroviral therapy including intravenously administered zidovudine and foscarnet in a child with HIV-1 enteropathy. *Eur J Pediatr.* 2003;162:528-529.
16. Sohal A, Riordan A, Mallewa M, et al. Successful treatment of cytomegalovirus polyradiculopathy in a 9-year-old child with congenital human immunodeficiency virus infection. *J Child Neurol.* 2009;24:215-218.
17. Korr B, Kessler U, Poschl J, et al. A haemophagocytic lymphohistiocytosis (HLH)-like picture following breastmilk transmitted cytomegalovirus infection in a preterm infant. *Scand J Infect Dis.* 2007;39:173-176.

Fosphenytoin

1. Available at: http://www.usp.org/hqi/similarProducts/choosy.html. Accessed September 13, 2009.
2. Available at: http://www.fda.gov/Safety/MedWatch/SafetyInformation/SafetyAlertsforHumanMedicalProducts/ucm110509.htm. Accessed September 13, 2009.
3. Fosphenytoin. Lexi-Comp® Online with AHFS® (database). Hudson, OH: Lexi-Comp Inc; updated August 28, 2009.
4. Available at: http://www.ismp.org/Newsletters/acutecare/articles/19970827.asp. Accessed September 13, 2009.
5. Cerebyx® [package insert]. Parke-Davis, Warner Lambert LLC.
6. Bohan KH, Mansuri TF, Wilson NM. Anticonvulsant hypersensitivity syndrome: implications for pharmaceutical care. *Pharmacotherapy.* 2007;27:1425-1439.
7. Bessmerty O, Pham T. Antiepileptic hypersensitivity syndrome: clinicians beware and be aware. *Curr Allergy Asthma Rep.* 2002;2:34-39.
8. Kaur S, Sarkar R, Thami GP, Kanwar AJ. Anticonvulsant hypersensitivity syndrome. Pediatr *Dermatol.* 2002;19:142-145.
9. Boucher BA. Fosphenytoin: a novel phenytoin prodrug. *Pharmacotherapy.* 1996;16:777-791.
10. Abernethy DR, Greenblatt DJ. Phenytoin disposition in obesity: determination of loading dose. *Arch Neurol.* 1985;42:468-471.
11. Gustafson MC, Ritter FJ. Fosphenytoin loading for status epilepticus in the neonate. *Epilepsia.* 1999;40:S124.
12. Kriel RL, Cifuentes RF. Fosphenytoin in infants of extremely low birth weight. *Pediatr Neurol.* 2001;24:219-221.
13. Pellock JM. Fosphenytoin use in children. *Neurology.* 1996;46:S14-S16.
14. Meek PD, Davis SN, Collins DM, et al. Guidelines for nonemergency use of parenteral phenytoin products: proceedings of an expert panel consensus process. Panel on Nonemergency Use of Parenteral Phenytoin Products. *Arch Intern Med.* 1999;159:2639-2644.
15. Takeoka M, Krishnamoorthy KS, Soman TB, et al. Fosphenytoin in infants. *J Child Neurol.* 1998;13:537-540.
16. Koul R, Deleu D. Subtherapeutic free phenytoin levels following fosphenytoin therapy in status epilepticus. *Neurology.* 2002;58:147-148.
17. Lewis RJ, Yee L, Inkelis SH, et al. Clinical predictors of post-traumatic seizures in children with head trauma. *Ann Emerg Med.* 1993;22:1114-1118.
18. Tilford JM, Simpson PM, Yeh TS, et al. Variation in therapy and outcome for pediatric head trauma patients. *Crit Care Med.* 2001;29:1056-1061.
19. Adelson PD, Bratton SL, Carney NA, et al. Guidelines for the acute medical management of severe traumatic brain injury in infants, children, and adolescents. Chapter 19. The role of anti-seizure prophylaxis following severe pediatric traumatic brain injury. *Pediatr Crit Care Med.* 2003;4(3 suppl):S72-S75.
20. Beck DE, Farringer JA, Ravis WR, et al. Accuracy of three methods for predicting concentrations of free phenytoin. *Clin Pharm.* 1987;6:888-894.
21. Stowe CD, Lee KR, Storgion SA, et al. Altered phenytoin pharmacokinetics in children with severe, acute traumatic brain injury. *J Clin Pharmacol.* 2000;40:1452-1461.
22. Trissel LA, ed. *Handbook on Injectable Drugs.* 15th ed. Bethesda, MD: American Society of Health-System Pharmacists; 2009.
23. Pryor FM, Gidal B, Ramsay RE, et al. Fosphenytoin: pharmacokinetics and tolerance of intramuscular loading doses. *Epilepsia.* 2001;42:245-250.
24. Data on file. New York, NY: Pfizer Inc; 2000.
25. Jamerson BD, Dukes GE, Brouwer KL, et al. Venous irritation related to intravenous administration of phenytoin versus fosphenytoin. *Pharmacotherapy.* 1994;14:47-52.
26. Available at: http://www.fda.gov/Safety/MedWatch/SafetyInformation/SafetyAlertsforHumanMedicalProducts/ucm074939.htm. Accessed October 4, 2009.
27. McBryde KD, Wilcox J, Kher KK. Hyperphosphatemia due to fosphenytoin in a pediatric ESRD patient. *Pediatr Nephrol.* 2005;20:1182-1185.
28. Sjoholm I, Kober A, Odar-Cedelof I, et al. Protein binding in uremia and normal serum: the role of endogenous binding inhibitors. *Biochem Pharmacol.* 1976;25:1205-1213.
29. Liponi DL, Winter ME, Tozer TN. Renal function and therapeutic concentrations of phenytoin. *Neurology.* 1984;34:395-397.
30. Kugler AR, Annesley TM, Nordblom GD, et al. Cross-reactivity of fosphenytoin in two human plasma phenytoin immunoassays. *Clin Chem.* 1998;44:1474-1480.

Furosemide

1. Available at: http://ismp.org/Tools/confuseddrugnames.pdf. Updated April 1, 2005.
2. Available at: http://www.usp.org/hqi/similarProducts/choosy.html. Accessed June 29, 2009.
3. Furosemide. Lexi-Comp® Online with AHFS® (database). Bethesda, MD: American Society of Health-System Pharmacists; updated May 26, 2009.
4. Loggie JMH, Kleinman LI, Maanen EFV. Renal function and diuretic therapy in infants and children. Part III. *J Pediatr.* 1975;86:825-832.
5. Gallagher KL, Jones JK. Furosemide-induced ototoxicity. *Ann Intern Med.* 1979;91:744-745.
6. Eades SK, Christensen ML. The clinical pharmacology of loop diuretics in the pediatric patient. *Pediatr Nephrol.* 1998;12:603-616.
7. Mirochnick MH, Miceli JJ, Kramer PA, et al. Furosemide pharmacokinetics in very low birth weight infants. *J Pediatr.* 1988;112:653-657.

References

8. Singh NC, Kissoon N, Mofada SA, et al. Comparison of continuous versus intermittent furosemide administration in postoperative pediatric cardiac patients. *Crit Care Med.* 1992;20:17-21.
9. Luciano GB, Nichani S, Chang AC, et al. Continuous versus intermittent furosemide infusion in critically ill infants after open heart operations. *Ann Thorac Surg.* 1997;64:1133-1139.
10. Copeland JG, Campbell DW, Plachetka JR, et al. Diuresis with continuous infusion of furosemide after cardiac surgery. *Am J Surg.* 1983;146:796-799.
11. Wells TG. The pharmacology and therapeutics of diuretics in the pediatric patient. *Pediatr Clin North Am.* 1990;37:463-504.
12. Ross BS, Pollak A, Oh W. The pharmacologic effects of furosemide therapy in the low-birth-weight infant. *J Pediatr.* 1978;92:149-152.
13. Engle MA, Lewy JE, Lewy PR, et al. The use of furosemide in the treatment of edema in infants and children. *Pediatrics.* 1978;62:811-818.
14. Woo WC, Dupont C, Collinge J, et al. Effects of furosemide in the newborn. *Clin Pharmacol Ther.* 1978;23:266-271.
15. Yeh TF, Wilks A, Singh J, et al. Furosemide prevents the renal side effects of indomethacin therapy in premature infants with patent ductus arteriosus. *J Pediatr.* 1982;101:433-437.
16. Peterson RG, Simmons MA, Rumack BH. Pharmacology of furosemide in the premature newborn infant. *J Pediatr.* 1980;97:139-143.
17. Schwartz GH, David DS, Riggio RR, et al. Ototoxicity induced by furosemide. *N Engl J Med.* 1970;282:1413-1414.
18. Aranda JV, Perez J, Sitar DS, et al. Pharmacokinetic disposition and protein binding of furosemide in newborn infants. *J Pediatr.* 1978;93:507-511.
19. Chemtob S, Papageorgiou A, du Souich P, et al. Cumulative increase in serum furosemide concentration following repeated doses in the newborn. *Am J Perinatol.* 1987;4:203-205.
20. Prandota J. Pharmacodynamic determinants of furosemide diuretic effect in children. *Dev Pharmacol Ther.* 1986;9:88-101.
21. Serratto M. Diagnosis and management of heart failure in infants and children. *Comprehensive Ther.* 1992;18:11-19.
22. Dettorre MD, Stidham GL, Watson DC, et al. Enhanced diuresis with continuous furosemide infusion in post-operative pediatric cardiac surgery patients. *Crit Care Med.* 1993;22:A183.
23. Chemtob S, Doray JL, Laudignon N, et al. Alternating sequential dosing with furosemide and ethacrynic acid in drug tolerance in the newborn. *Am J Dis Child.* 1989;143:850-854.
24. Weiss RA, Schoeneman M, Greifer I. Treatment of severe nephrotic edema with albumin and furosemide. *NY State J Med.* 1984;84:384-386.
25. Melvin T, Bennett W. Management of nephrotic syndrome in childhood. *Drugs.* 1991;42:30-51.
26. Baliga R, Lewy JE. Pathogenesis and treatment of edema. *Pediatr Nephrol.* 1987;34:639-647.
27. Haws RM, Baum M. Efficacy of albumin and diuretic therapy in children with nephrotic syndrome. *Pediatrics.* 1993;91:1142-1146.
28. Kelsch RC, Sedman AB. Nephrotic syndrome. *Pediatr Rev.* 1993;14:30-38.
29. Robson WLM, Leung AKC. Nephrotic syndrome in childhood. *Adv Pediatr.* 1993;40:287-323.
30. Scala JL, Jew RK, Poon CY, et al. In vitro analysis of furosemide disposition during neonatal extracorporeal membrane oxygenation (ECMO). *Pediatr Res.* 1996;39(suppl):78A.
31. Trissel LA, ed. *Handbook on Injectable Drugs.* 15th ed. Bethesda, MD: American Society of Health-System Pharmacists; 2009.
32. Robertson CMT, Tyebkhan JM, Peliowski A, et al. Ototoxic drugs and sensorineural hearing loss following severe neonatal respiratory failure. *Acta Paediatrica.* 2006;95:214-223.
33. Green TP, Thompson TR, Johnson DE, et al. Furosemide promotes patent ductus arteriosus in premature infants with respiratory-distress syndrome. *N Engl J Med.* 1983;308:743-748.
34. Hufnagle KG, Khan SN, Penn D, et al. Renal calcifications: a complication of long term furosemide therapy in preterm infants. *Pediatrics.* 1982;70:360-363.
35. Pope JC, Trusler LA, Klein AM, et al. The natural history of nephrocalcinosis in premature infants treated with loop diuretics. *J Urol.* 1996;156:709-712.
36. Alpert SA, Noe HN. Furosemide nephrolithiasis causing ureteral obstruction and urinoma in a preterm neonate. *Urology.* 2004;64:589. e9-589.e11.
37. Saarela T, Lanning P, Koivisto M, et al. Nephrocalcinosis in full-term infants receiving furosemide treatment for congestive heart failure: a study of the incidence and 2-year follow up. *Eur J Pediatr.* 1999;158:668-772.
38. Borradori C, Fawer CL, Buelin T, et al. Risk factors of sensorineural hearing loss in preterm infants. *Biol Neonate.* 1997;71:1-10.
39. Rybak LP. Furosemide ototoxicity: clinical and experimental aspects. *Laryngoscope.* 1985;95:1-14.
40. Brummett RE, Bendrick T, Himes D. Comparative ototoxicity of bumetanide and furosemide when used in combination with kanamycin. *J Clin Pharmacol.* 1981;21:628-636.
41. Rybak LP. Pathophysiology of furosemide ototoxicity. *J Otolaryngol.* 1982;11:127-133.
42. Turmen T, Thom P, Louridas AT, et al. Protein binding and bilirubin displacing properties of bumetanide and furosemide. *J Clin Pharmacol.* 1982;22:551-556.

Ganciclovir Sodium

1. Available at: http://www.usp.org/hqi/similarProducts/choosy.html. Accessed August 27, 2009.
2. Cytovene [package insert]. Nutley, NJ: Roche Laboratories Inc; 2008.
3. Singhal S, Mehta J, Powles R, et al. Three weeks of ganciclovir for cytomegaloviraemia after allogenic bone marrow transplant. *Bone Marrow Transplant.* 1995;15:777-781.
4. Bilgrami S, Aslanzadeh J, Feingold JM, et al. Cytomegalovirus viremia, viruria, and disease after autologous peripheral blood stem cell transplantation: no need for surveillance. *Bone Marrow Transplant.* 1999;24:69-73.
5. Atkinson K, Arthur C, Bradstock K, et al. Prophylactic ganciclovir is more effective in HLA-identical family member marrow transplant recipients than in more heavily immune-suppressed HLA-identical unrelated donor marrow transplant recipients. *Bone Marrow Transplant.* 1995;15:401-405.
6. Schmidt GM, Horak DA, Niland JC, et al. A randomized controlled trial of prophylactic ganciclovir for cytomegalovirus pulmonary infection in recipients of allogeneic bone marrow transplants. *N Engl J Med.* 1991;324:1005-1011.
7. American Academy of Pediatrics. Pickering LK, Baker CJ, Kimberlin DW, et al., eds. *2009 Red Book: Report of the Committee on Infectious Diseases.* 28th ed. Elk Grove Village, IL: American Academy of Pediatrics; 2009.
8. Green M, Reyes J, Nour B, et al. Randomized trial of ganciclovir followed by high-dose oral acyclovir vs. ganciclovir alone in the prevention of cytomegalovirus disease in pediatric liver transplant recipients: preliminary analysis. *Transplant Proc.* 1994;25:173-174.
9. Prokurat S, Drabik E, Grenda R. Ganciclovir in cytomegalovirus prophylaxis in high-risk pediatric renal transplant recipients. *Transplant Proc.* 1993;24:2577.
10. Canpolat C, Culbert S, Gardner M, et al. Ganciclovir prophylaxis for cytomegalovirus infection in pediatric allogeneic bone marrow transplant recipients. *Bone Marrow Transplant.* 1996;17:589-593.
11. Seu P, Winston DJ, Holt CD, et al. Long-term ganciclovir prophylaxis for successful prevention of primary cytomegalovirus (CMV) disease in CMV-seronegative liver transplant recipients with CMV-seropositive donors. *Transplantation.* 1997;4:1614-1617.
12. Gajarski RJ, Rosenblatt HW, Schowengerdt KO, et al. Outcomes among pediatric heart transplant recipients. *Tex Heart Inst J.* 1997;24:97-104.
13. Gerbase MW, Dubois D, Rothmeier C, et al. Cost and outcomes of prolonged cytomegalovirus prophylaxis to cover the enhanced immunosuppression phase following lung transplantation. *Chest.* 1999;116:1265-1272.

References

14. Spivey JF, Jewell D, Sweet S, et al. Safety and efficacy of prolonged cytomegalovirus prophylaxi with intravenous ganciclovir in pediatric and young adult lung transplant recipients. *Pediatr Transplant.* 2007;11:312-318.
15. Gudnason T, Belani KK, Balfour HH Jr. Ganciclovir treatment of cytomegalovirus disease in immunocompromised children. *Pediatr Infect Dis J.* 1989;8:436-440.
16. King SM, Petric M, Superina R, et al. Cytomegalovirus infections in pediatric liver transplantation. *Am J Dis Child.* 1990;144:1307-1310.
17. Megison SM, Andrews WS. Combination therapy with ganciclovir and intravenous IgG for cytomegalovirus infections in pediatric liver transplant recipients. *Transplantation.* 1991;52:151-154.
18. Reusser P, Einsele H, Lee J, et al. Randomized multicenter trial of foscarnet versus ganciclovir for preemptive therapy of cytomegalovirus infection after allogeneic stem cell transplantation. *Blood.* 2002;99:1159-1164.
19. Tanaka-Kitajima N, Sugaya N, Fuatani T, et al. Ganciclovir therapy for congenital cytomegalovirus infection in six infants. *Pediatr Infect Dis J.* 2005;24:782-785.
20. Rojo P, Ramos JT. Ganciclovir treatment of children with congenital cytomegalovirus infection. *Pediatr Infect Dis J.* 2004;23:88-89.
21. Kimberlin DW, Lin CY, Sanchez PJ, et al. Effect of ganciclovir therapy on hearing in symptomatic congenital cytomegalovirus disease involving the central nervous system: a randomized, controlled trial. *J Pediatr.* 2003;143:16-25.
22. Michaels MG, Greenberg DP, Sabo DL, et al. Treatment of children with congenital cytomegalovirus infection with ganciclovir. *Pediatr Infect Dis J.* 2003;22:504-508.
23. Demmler GJ. Congenital cytomegalovirus infection treatment. *Pediatr Infect Dis J.* 2003;22:1005-1006.
24. Whitley RJ, Cloud G, Gruber W, et al. Ganciclovir treatment of symptomatic congenital cytomegalovirus infection: results of a phase II study. National Institute of Allergy and Infectious Diseases Collaborative Antiviral Study Group. *J Infect Dis.* 1997;175:1080-1086.
25. Nigro G, Scholz H, Bartmann U. Ganciclovir therapy for symptomatic congenital cytomegalovirus infection in infants: a two-regimen experience. *J Pediatr.* 1994;124:318-322.
26. Trang JM, Kidd L, Gruber W, et al. Linear single-dose pharmacokinetics of ganciclovir in newborns with congenital cytomegalovirus infections. *Clin Pharmacol Ther.* 1993;53:15-21.
27. Whitley RJ, Pass RF, Stagna SB, et al. Pharmacodynamic evaluation of ganciclovir (DHPG) in the treatment of symptomatic congenital cytomegalovirus (CMV) infection. *Pediatr Res.* 1991;29:188A. Abstract.
28. Saitoh A, Viani RM, Schrier RD, et al. Treatment of infants coinfected with HIV-1 and cytomegalovirus with combination antiretrovirals and ganciclovir. *J Allergy Clin Immunol.* 2004;114:983-985.
29. Tezer H, Devrim I, Kara A, et al. Ganciclovir therapy in an immunocompetent child with resistant fever and hepatosplenomegaly due to cytomegalovirus infection. Who and when to treat? *Int J Infect Dis.* 2008;12:340-342.
30. Tokimasa S, Hara J, Osugi Y, et al. Ganciclovir is effective for prophylaxis and treatment of human herpes-virus-6 in allogenic stem cell transplantation. *Bone Marrow Transplant.* 2002;29:595-598.
31. Janoly-Dumenil A, Galambrun C, Basset T, et al. Human herpes virus-6 encephalitis in a paediatric bone marrow recipient: successful treatment with pharmacokinetic monitoring and high doses of ganciclovir. *Bone Marrow Transplant.* 2006;38:769-770.
32. Aronoff GR, Berns JS, Brier ME, et al. Drug prescribing in renal failure. 4th ed. Available at: http://www.kdp-baptist.louisville.edu/renalbook/. Accessed October 15, 2009.
33. Trissel LA. *Handbook on Injectable Drugs.* 15th ed. Bethesda, MD: American Society of Health-Sytem Pharmacists; 2009.
34. Ghosh K, Muirhead D, Christine B, et al. Ultrastructural changes in peripheral blood neutrophils in a patient receiving ganciclovir for CMV pneumonitis following allogenic bone marrow transplantation. *Bone Marrow Transplant.* 1999;24:429-431.
35. Ozkan TB, Mistik R, Dikici B, et al. Antiviral therapy in neonatal cholestatic cytomegalovirus hepatitis. *BMC Gastroenterology.* 2007;7:9.
36. Fischler B, Casswall TH, Malmborg P, et al. Ganciclovir treatment in infants with cytomegalovirus infection and cholestasis. *J Pediatric Gastroent Nutr.* 2002;34:154-157.
37. Iwanaga M, Zaitsu M, Ishii E, et al. Protein-losing gastroenteropathy and retinitis associated with cytomegalovirus infection in an immunocompetent infant: a case report. *Eur J Pediatr.* 2004;163:81-84.
38. Rongkavilit C, Bedard M, Ang JY, et al. Severe cytomegalovirus enterocolitis in an immunocompetent infant. *Pediatr Infect Dis J.* 2004;23:579-581.
39. Abdulhannan P, Sugarman iD, Wood P, et al. Primary CMV colitis in an immunocompetent infant, successfully treated with ganciclovir. *J Pediatr Gastroenterol Nutr.* 2008;47:203-205.
40. Greco F, Garozzo R, Sorge G. Isolated abducens nerve palsy complicating cytomegalovirus infection. *Pediatr Neurol.* 2006;35:229-230.
41. Sohal A, Riordan A, Mallewa M, et al. Successful treatment of cytomegalovirus polyradiculopathy in a 9-year-old child with congenital human immunodeficiency virus infection. *J Child Neurol.* 2009;24:215-218.
42. Brady RC, Schleiss MR, Witte DP, et al. Placental transfer of ganciclovir in a woman with acquired immunodeficiency syndrome and cytomegalovirus disease. *Pediatr Infect Dis J.* 2002;21:796-797.

Gentamicin Sulfate

1. Available at: http://ismp.org/Tools/confuseddrugnames.pdf Accessed October 27, 2009.
2. Available at: http://www.usp.org/hqi/similarProducts/choosy.html. Accessed October 27, 2009.
3. Gentamicin [package insert]. Lake Forest, IL: Hospira Inc; October 2004.
4. Pannu N, Nadim MK. An overview of drug-induced acute kidney injury. *Crit Care Med.* 2008;36(4 Suppl):S216-S223.
5. Guthrie OW. Aminoglycoside induced ototoxicity. *Toxicology.* 2008;249:91-96.
6. Snavely SR, Hodges GR. The neurotoxicity of antibacterial agents. *Ann Intern Med.* 1984;101:92-104.
7. Paradelis AG. Aminoglycoside antibiotics and neuromuscular blockade. *J Antimicrob Chemother.* 1979;5:737-738.
8. Gentamicin. In: Kucer A, Crowe SM, Grayson ML, et al., eds. *The Use of Antibiotics: A Clinical Review of Antibacterial, Antifungal and Antiviral Drugs.* 5th ed. Boston, MA: Butterworth Heinemann; 1997:490-503.
9. Buchholz U, Richards C, Murthy R, et al. Pyrogenic reactions associated with single daily dosing of intravenous gentamicin. *Infect Control Hosp Epidemiol.* 2000;21:771-774.
10. Fanning MM, Wassel R, Piazza-Hepp T. Pyrogenic reactions to gentamicin therapy. *N Engl J Med.* 2000;343;1658-1659.
11. Schwartz SN, Pazin GJ, Lyon JA, et al. A controlled investigation of the pharmacokinetics of gentamicin and tobramycin in obese subjects. *Infect Dis.* 1978;138:499-505.
12. Watterberg KL, Kelly W, Angelus P, et al. The need for a loading dose of gentamicin in neonates. *Ther Drug Monit.* 1989;11:16-20.
13. Semchuk W, Borgmann J, Bowman L. Determination of a gentamicin loading dose in neonates and infants. *Ther Drug Monit.* 1993;15:47-51.
14. Glover ML, Shaffer CL, Rubino CM, et al. A multicenter evaluation of gentamicin therapy in the neonatal intensive care unit. *Pharmacotherapy.* 2001;21:7-10.
15. Prober CG, Stevenson DK, Benitz WE. The use of antibiotics in neonates weighing less than 1200 grams. *Pediatr Infect Dis J.* 1990;9:111-121.
16. American Academy of Pediatrics. Pickering LK, Baker CJ, Kimberlin DW, et al., eds. *2009 Red Book: Report of the Committee on Infectious Diseases.* 28th ed. Elk Grove Village, IL: American Academy of Pediatrics; 2009.
17. Nelson JD, Bradley JS, eds. *Nelson's Pocket Book of Pediatric Antimicrobial Therapy.* 17th ed. Chicago, IL: American Academy of Pediatrics; 2009.
18. Garfunkel JM. Use of gentamicin in newborn infants. *J Infect Dis.* 1971;124:S247-S248.
19. Paisley JW, Smith AL, Smith DH. Gentamicin in newborn infants. *Am J Dis Child.* 1973;126:473-477.
20. McCracken GH Jr, Threlkeld N, Thomas ML. Intravenous administration of kanamycin and gentamicin in newborn infants. *Pediatrics.* 1977;60:463-466.

References

21. Assael BM, Gianni V, Marini A, et al. Gentamicin dosage in preterm and term neonates. *Arch Dis Child.* 1977;52:883-886.
22. Szefler SJ, Wynn RJ, Clarke DF, et al. Relationship of gentamicin serum concentrations to gestational age in preterm and term neonates. *J Pediatr.* 1980;97:312-315.
23. Zenk KE, Miwa L, Cohen JL, et al. Effect of body weight on gentamicin pharmacokinetics in neonates. *Clin Pharm.* 1984;3:170-173.
24. Mulhall A, De Louvois J, Hurley R. Incidence of potentially toxic concentrations of gentamicin in the neonate. *Arch Dis Child.* 1983;58:897-900.
25. Koren G, Leeder S, Harding E, et al. Optimization of gentamicin therapy in very low birth weight infants. *Pediatr Pharmacol.* 1985;5:79-87.
26. Miranda JC, Schimmel MM, James LS, et al. Gentamicin kinetics in the neonate. *Pediatr Pharmacol.* 1985;5:57-61.
27. Edwards C, Low DC, Bissenden JG. Gentamicin dosage for the newborn. *Lancet.* 1986;1:508-509. Letter.
28. Dahl LB, Melby K, Gutteberg TJ, et al. Serum levels of ampicillin and gentamicin in neonates of varying gestational age. *Eur J Pediatr.* 1986;145:218-221.
29. Zarowitz BJ, Wynn RJ, Buckwald S, et al. High gentamicin trough concentrations in neonates of less than 28 weeks gestational age. *Dev Pharmacol Ther.* 1982;5:68-75.
30. Hindmarsh KW, Nation RL, Williams GL, et al. Pharmacokinetics of gentamicin in very low birth weight preterm infants. *Eur J Clin Pharmacol.* 1983;24:649-653.
31. Stolk LML, Degraeuwe PLJ, Nieman FHM, et al. Population pharmacokinetics and relationship between demographic and clinical variables and pharmacokinetics of gentamicin in neonates. *Ther Drug Monit.* 2002;24:527-531.
32. Thureen PJ, Reiter PD, Gresores A, et al. Once- versus twice-daily gentamicin dosing in neonates ≥34 weeks' gestation: cost-effectiveness analyses. *Pediatrics.* 1999;103;594-598.
33. Agarwal G, Rastogi A, Pyati S, et al. Comparison of once-daily versus twice-daily gentamicin dosing regimens in infants ≥2500 g. *J Perinatol.* 2002;22:268-274.
34. Serane TV, Zengeya S, Penford G, et al. Once daily dose gentamicin in neonates—is our dosing correct? *Acta Paediatrica.* 2009;98:1100-1105.
35. Hagen I, Oymar K. Pharmacological differences between once daily and twice daily gentamicin dosage in newborns with suspected sepsis. *Pharm World Sci.* 2009;31:18-23.
36. Nielsen EI, Sandstrom M, Honore PH, et al. Developmental pharmacokinetics of gentamicin in preterm and term neonates. *Clin Pharmacokinet.* 2009;48:253-263.
37. McAllister TA. Gentamicin in paediatrics. *Postgrad Med J.* 1974;50(suppl 7):45-52.
38. McCracken GH Jr, Eichenwald HF. Antimicrobial therapy: therapeutic recommendations and a review of the newer drugs. Part II. *J Pediatr.* 1974;85:451-456.
39. Taylor M, Keane C. Gentamicin dosage in children. *Arch Dis Child.* 1976;51:369-372.
40. Evans WE, Feldman S, Ossi M, et al. Gentamicin dosage in children: a randomized prospective comparison of body weight and body surface area as dose determinants. *J Pediatr.* 1979;94:139-143.
41. Contopoulos-Ioannidis DG, Giotis ND, Baliatsa DV, et al. Extended-Interval aminoglycoside administration for children: A META-analysis. *Pediatrics.* 2004;114:e111-e118.
42. Marik PE, Lipman J, Kobilski S, et al. A prospective randomized study comparing once- versus twice-daily amikacin dosing in critically ill adult and paediatric patients. *J Antimicrob Chemother.* 1991;28:753-764.
43. Kafetzis DA, Sianidou L, Vlachos E, et al. Clinical and pharmacokinetic study of a single daily dose of amikacin in paediatric patients with severe gram-negative infections. *J Antimicrob Chemother.* 1991;27:105-112.
44. Trujillo H, Robledo J, Robledo C, et al. Single dose amikacin in paediatric patients with severe gram-negative infections. *J Antimicrob Chemother.* 1991;27:141-147.
45. Viscoli C, Dudley M, Ferrea G, et al. Serum concentration and safety of a single daily dose of amikacin in children undergoing bone marrow transplantation. *J Antimicrob Chemother.* 1991;27:113-120.
46. Sung L, Dupuis LL, Bliss B, et al. Randomized controlled trial of once- versus thrice-daily tobramycin in febrile neutropenic children undergoing stem cell transplantation. *J Natl Cancer Inst.* 2003;95:1869-1877.
47. Dupuis LL, Sung L, Taylor T, et al. Tobramycin pharmacokinetics in children with febrile neutropenia undergoing stem cell transplantation: once-daily versus thrice-daily administration. *Pharmacotherapy.* 2004;24:564-573.
48. Bouffet E, Fuhrmann C, Frappaz D, et al. Once daily antibiotic regimen in paediatric oncology. *Arch Dis Child.* 1994;70:484-487.
49. International Antimicrobial Therapy Cooperative Group of the European Organization for Research and Treatment of Cancer. Efficacy and toxicity of single daily doses of amikacin and ceftriaxone versus multiple daily doses of amikacin and ceftazidime for infection in patients with cancer and granulocytopenia. *Ann Intern Med.* 1993;119:584-593.
50. Krivoy N, Postovsky S, Elhasid R, et al. Pharmacokinetic analysis of amikacin twice and single daily dosage in immunocompromised pediatric patients. *Infection.* 1998;26:396-398.
51. Chicella M. Once-daily aminoglycoside dosing in pediatrics. What is its role? *J Pediatr Pharm Pract.* 2000:5;98-103.
52. Asghar R, Banajeh S, Egas J, et al. Chloramphenicol versus ampicillin plus gentamicin for community acquired very severe pneumonia among children aged 2-59 months in low resource settings: multicentre randomized controlled trial (SPEAR study). *BMJ.* 2008;12:80-84. Epub 2008 Jan 8.
53. Dore-Bergeron MJ, Gauthier M, Chevalier I, et al. Urinary tract infections in 1- to 3-month old infants: ambulatory treatment with intravenous antibiotics. *Pediatrics.* 2009;124:16-22.
54. Wakkace AW, Bertino JS. Use of once-daily aminoglycosides in children—rational or inappropriate? *J Pediatr Pharmacol Ther.* 2001;6:380-383.
55. Wilson W, Taubert K, Gewitz m, et al. Prevention of infective endocarditis. Guidelines from the American Heart Association Rheumatic Fever, Endocarditis, and Kawasaki Disease Committee, Council on Cardiovascular Disease in the Young, and the Councils on Clinical Cardiology, Council on Cardiovascular Surgery and Anesthesia and the Quality of Care and Outcomes Research Interdisciplinary Working Group. *Circulation.* 2007;115:1736-1754; correction *Circulation.* 2007;116:1736-1754.
56. Baddour LM, Wilson WR, Bayer AS, et al. Infective endocarditis: diagnosis, antimicrobial therapy, and management of complications: a statement for healthcare professionals from the Committee on Rheumatic Fever, Endocarditis, and Kawasaki Disease, Council on Cardiovascular Disease in the Young, and the Councils on Clinical Cardiology, Stroke, and Cardiovascular Surgery and Anesthesia, American Heart Association: endorsed by the Infectious Diseases Society of America. *Circulation.* 2005;111:e394-e434.
57. Aronoff GR, Berns JS, Brier ME, et al. Drug prescribing in renal failure. 4th ed. Available at: http://www.kdp-baptist.louisville.edu/renalbook/. Accessed October 27, 2009.
58. Beringer PM, Vinks AA, Jelliffe RW, et al. Pharmacokinetics of tobramycin in adults with cystic fibrosis: implications for once-daily administration. *Antimicrob Agents Chemother.* 2000;44:809-813.
59. Bates RD, Nahata MC, Jones JW, et al. Pharmacokinetics and safety of tobramycin after once-daily administration in patients with cystic fibrosis. *Chest.* 1997;112:1208-1213.
60. Bragonier R, Brown NM. The pharmacokinetics and toxicity of once-daily tobramycin therapy in children with cystic fibrosis. *J Antimicrob Chemother.* 1998;42:103-106.
61. Master V, Roberts GW, Coulthard KP, et al. Efficacy of once-daily tobramycin monotherapy for acute pulmonary exacerbations of cystic fibrosis: a preliminary study. *Pediatr Pulmonol.* 2001;3:367-376.
62. Loirat P, Rohan J, Baillet A, et al. Increased glomerular filtration rate in patients with major burns and its effect on the pharmacokinetics of tobramycin. *N Engl J Med.* 1978;299:915-919.
63. Buck ML. Pharmacokinetic changes during extracorporeal membrane oxygenation. *Clin Pharmacokinet.* 2003;42:403-417.
64. Trissel LA, ed. *Handbook on Injectable Drugs.* 15th ed. Bethesda, MD: American Society of Health-System Pharmacists; 2009.
65. Robinson CA, Sawyer JE. Y-site compatibility of medications with parenteral nutrition. *J Pediatr Pharmacol Ther.* 2009;14:49-57.
66. Mendelson J, Portnoy J, Dick V, et al. Safety of the bolus administration of gentamicin. *Antimicrob Agents Chemother.* 1976;9:633-638.
67. Barza M, Brown RB, Shen D, et al. Predictability of blood levels of gentamicin in man. *J Infect Dis.* 1975;132:165-174.

References

68. Gillett AP, Falk RH, Andrews J, et al. Rapid intravenous injection of tobramycin: suggested dosage schedule and concentrations in serum. *J Infect Dis.* 1976;134:S110-S113.
69. Powell SH, Thompson WL, Luthe MA, et al. Once daily vs. continuous aminoglycoside dosing: efficacy and toxicity in animal and clinical studies of gentamicin, netilmicin and tobramycin. *J Infect Dis.* 1983;147:918-932.
70. Bodey GP, Chang HY, Rodriguez V, et al. Feasibility of administering aminoglycoside antibiotics by continuous intravenous infusion. *Antimicrob Agents Chemother.* 1975;8:328-333.
71. Giacoia GP, Schentag JJ. Pharmacokinetics and nephrotoxicity of continuous intravenous infusion of gentamicin in low birth weight infants. *J Pediatr.* 1986;109:715-719.
72. Beaubien AR, Desjardins S, Ormsby E, et al. Incidence of amikacin ototoxicity: a sigmoid function of total drug exposure independent of plasma levels. *Am J Otolaryngol.* 1989;10:234-243.
73. Beaubien AR, Ormsby E, Bayne A, et al. Evidence that amikacin ototoxicity is related to total perilymph area under the concentration-time curve regardless of concentration. *Antimicrob Agents Chemother.* 1991;35:1070-1074.
74. Brownsberger RJ, Morrelli HF. Neuromuscular blockade due to gentamicin sulfate. *West J Med.* 1988;148:215.
75. Warner WA, Sanders E. Neuromuscular blockade associated with gentamicin therapy. *JAMA.* 1971;215:1153-1154.
76. Massey KL, Hendeles L, Neims A. Identification of children for whom routine monitoring of aminoglycoside serum concentrations is not cost effective. *J Pediatr.* 1986;109:897-901.
77. Logsdon BA, Phelps SJ. Routine monitoring of gentamicin serum concentrations in pediatric patients with normal renal function is unnecessary. *Ann Pharmacother.* 1997;31:1514-1518.
78. Franson TR, Ritch PS, Quebbeman EJ. Aminoglycoside serum concentration sampling via central venous catheters: a potential source of clinical error. *JPEN J Parenter Enteral Nutr.* 1987;11:77-79.

Glycopyrrolate

1. Available at: http://ismp.org/Tools/confuseddrugnames.pdf. Updated April 1, 2005.
2. Glycopyrrolate injection, USP [package insert]. Shirley, NY: American Regent Laboratories Inc; January 2009.
3. Annila P, Rorarius M, Reonikainen P, et al. Effect of pre-treatment with intravenous atropine or glycopyrrolate on cardiac arrhythmias during halothane anaesthesia for adenoidectomy in children. *Br J Anaesth.* 1998;80:756-760.
4. Badgwell JM, Heavner JE, Cooper MW, et al. The cardiovascular effects of anticholinergic agents administered during halothane anaesthesia in children. *Acta Anaesthesiol Scand.* 1988;32:383-387.
5. Mirakhur RK, Shepherd WF, Jones CJ. Ventilation and the oculocardiac reflex. Prevention of oculocardiac reflex during surgery for squints: role of controlled ventilation and anticholinergic drugs. *Anaesthesia.* 1986;41:825-828.
6. Pokela ML, Koivisto M. Physiological changes, plasma beta-endorphin and cortisol responses to tracheal intubation in neonates. *Acta Paediatr.* 1994;83:151-156.
7. Hardy JF, Charest J, Girouard G, et al. Nausea and vomiting after strabismus surgery in preschool children. *Can Anaesth Soc J.* 1986;33:57-62.
8. Langston WT, Wathen JE, Roback MG, Bajaj L. Effect of ondansetron on the incidence of vomiting associated with ketamine sedation in children: a double-blind, randomized, placebo-controlled trial. *Ann Emerg Med.* 2008;52:30-34.
9. Rautakorpi P, Ali-Melkkila T, Kaila T, et al. Pharmacokinetics of glycopyrrolate in children. *J Clin Anesth.* 1994;6:217-220.
10. Wong Ay, Salem MR, Mani M, et al. Glycopyrrolate as a substitute for atropine in reversal of curarization in pediatric cardiac patients. *Anesth Analg.* 1974;53:412-417.
11. Goldhill DR, Pyne A, Cones CJ. Antagonism of neuromuscular blockade. The cardiovascular effects in children of the combination of edrophonium and glycopyrronium. *Anaesthesia.* 1988;43:930-934.
12. Pruitt JW, Goldwasser MS, Sabol SR, et al. Intramuscular ketamine, midazolam, glycopyrrolate for pediatric sedation in the emergency department. *J Oral Maxillofac Surg.* 1995;53:13-17.
13. Reyntjens K, Foubert L, De Wolf D, et al. Glycopyrrolate during sevoflurane-remifentanil-based anaesthesia for cardiac catheterization of children with congenital heart disease. *Br J Anaesthesia.* 2005;95:680-684.

Granisetron HCl

1. Available at: http://www.usp.org/hqi/similarProducts/choosy.html. Accessed July 27, 2009.
2. Kytril [prescribing information]. Nutley, NJ: Roche Laboratories; November 2005.
3. Buyukcavci M, Olgun H, Ceviz N. The effects of ondansetron and granisetron on electrocardiography in children receiving chemotherapy for acute leukemia. *Am J Clin Oncol.* 2005;28:201-204.
4. Boike SC, Ilson B, Zariffa N, et al. Cardiovascular effects of i.v. granisetron at two administration rates and of ondansetron in healthy adults. *Am J Health Syst Pharm.* 1997;54:1172-1176.
5. Watanabe H, Hasegawa A, Shinozaki T, et al. Possible side effects of granisetron, an antiemetic agent, inpatients with bone and soft-tissue sarcomas receiving cytotoxic chemotherapy. *Cancer Chemother Pharmacol.* 1995;35:278-282.
6. Carmichael J, Harris AL. High-dose iv granisetron for the prevention of chemotherapy-induced emesis: cardiac safety and tolerability. *Anti-Cancer Drugs.* 2003;14:739-744.
7. Miyamima Y, Numata S, Katayama I, et al. Prevention of chemotherapy-induced emesis with granisetron in children with a malignant disease. *Am J Pediatr Hematol Oncol.* 1994;16:236-241.
8. Lemerle J, Amaral D, Southall DP, et al. Efficacy and safety of granisetron in the prevention of chemotherapy-induced emesis in paediatric patients. *Eur J Cancer.* 1991;27:1081-1083.
9. Palmer R. Efficacy and safety of granisetron (Kytril) in two special patient populations: children and adults with impaired hepatic function. *Sem Oncol.* 1994;21:22-25.
10. Jacobson SJ, Shore RW, Greenberg M, et al. The efficacy and safety of granisetron in pediatric cancer patients who had failed standard antiemetic therapy during anticancer chemotherapy. *Am J Pediatr Hematol Oncol.* 1994;16:231-235.
11. Hahlen K, Quintana E, Pinkerton CR, et al. A randomized comparison of intravenously administered granisetron versus chlorpromazine plus dexamethasone in the prevention of ifosfamide-induced emesis in children. *J Pediatr.* 1995;126:309-313.
12. Craft AW, Price L, Eden OB, et al. Granisetron as antiemetic therapy in children with cancer. *Med Pediatr Oncol.* 1995;25:28-32.
13. Komada Y, Matsuyama T, Takao A, et al. A randomized dose-comparison trial of granisetron in preventing emesis in children with leukaemia receiving emetogenic chemotherapy. *Eur J Cancer.* 1999;35:1095-1101.
14. Fujii Y, Tanaka H, Ito M. Ramosetron compared with granisetron for the prevention of vomiting following strabismus surgery in children. *Br J Ophthalmol.* 2001;85:670-672.
15. Fujii Y, Tanaka H. Comparison of granisetron, droperidol, and metoclopramide for prevention of postoperative vomiting in children with a history of motion sickness undergoing tonsillectomy. *J Pediatr Surg.* 2001;36:460-462.
16. Berrak SG, Ozdemir N, Bakirel N, et al. A double-blind, crossover, randomized dose-comparison trial of granisetron for the prevention of acute and delayed nausea and emesis in children receiving moderately emetogenic carboplatin-based chemotherapy. *Support Care Cancer.* 2007;15:1163-1168.
17. Tsuchida Y, Hayashi Y, Asami K, et al. Effects of granisetron in children undergoing high-dose chemotherapy: a multi-institutional, cross-over study. *Int J Oncol.* 1999;14:673-679.

18. Orchard PJ, Rogosheske J, Burns L, et al. A prospective randomized trial of the anti-emetic efficacy of ondansetron and granisetron during bone marrow transplantation. *Biol Blood Marrow Transplant.* 1999;5:386-393.
19. Kris MG, Hesketh PJ, Somerfield MR, et al. American Society of Clinical Oncology Guideline for antiemetics in oncology: update 2006. *J Clin Oncology.* 2006;24:2932-2947.
20. Cieslak GD, Watcha MF, Phillips MB, et al. The dose-response relationship and cost-effectiveness of granisetron for the prophylaxis of pediatric postoperative emesis. *Anesthesiology.* 1996;85:1076-1085.
21. Fujii Y, Toyooka H, Tanaka H. A granisetron-droperidol combination prevents postoperative vomiting in children. *Anesth Analg.* 1998;87:761-765.
22. Fujii Y, Toyooka H, Tanaka H. Effective dose of granisetron for preventing postoperative emesis in children. *Can J Anaesth.* 1996;43:660-664.
23. Fujii Y, Tanaka H. Granisetron reduces post-operative vomiting in children: a dose-ranging study. *Eur J Anesthesiology.* 1999;16:62-65.
24. Fujii Y, Saitoh, Y, Tanaka H, et al. Prophylactic therapy with combined granisetron and dexamethasone for the prevention of post-operative vomiting in children. *Eur J Anesthesiology.* 1999;16:376-379.
25. Fujii Y, Tanaka H, Toyooka H. Granisetron and dexamethasone provide more improved prevention of postoperative emesis than granisetron alone in children. *Can J Anaesth.* 1996;43:229-232.
26. Trissel LA. *Handbook on Injectable Drugs.* 15th ed. Bethesda, MD: American Society of Health-System Pharmacists; 2009.
27. Kalaycio M, Mendez Z, Pohlman B, et al. Continuous-infusion granisetron compared to ondansetron for the prevention of nausea and vomiting after high-dose chemotherapy. *J Cancer Res Clin Oncol.* 1998;124:265-269.
28. Contu A, Olmeo N, Piro S, et al. A comparison of the antiemetic efficacy and safety of intramuscular and intravenous formulations of granisetron in patients receiving moderately emetogenic chemotherapy. *Anticancer Drugs.* 1995;6:652-656.
29. The Italian Multicenter Study Group. A double-blind randomized study comparing intramuscular (i.m.) granisetron with i.m. granisetron plus dexamethasone in the prevention of delayed emesis induced by cisplatin. *Anticancer Drugs.* 1999;10:465-470.
30. Wada I, Takeda T, Sato M, et al. Pharmacokinetics of granisetron in adults and children with malignant diseases. *Biol Pharm Bull.* 2001;244:432-435.

Haloperidol Lactate

1. Available at: http://www.usp.org/hqi/similarProducts/choosy.html. Accessed August 16, 2009.
2. Haloperidol injection, USP [prescribing information]. Schaumburg, IL: APP Pharmaceuticals LLC; November 2008.
3. Sharma ND, Rosman HS, Padhi D, et al. Torsades de pointes associated with intravenous haloperidol in critically ill patients. *Am J Cardiol.* 1998;81:238-240.
4. Harrison AM, Lugo RA, Lee WE, et al. The use of haloperidol in agitated critically ill children. *Clin Pediatr.* 2002;41:51-54.
5. Brown RL, Henke A, Greenhalgh DG, et al. The use of haloperidol in the agitated, critically ill pediatric patient with burns. *J Burn Care Rehabil.* 1996;17:34-38.
6. American Academy of Pediatrics Committee on Drugs. Drugs for pediatric emergencies. *Pediatrics.* 1998;101:e1-e11.
7. Ratcliff SL, Meyer WJ, Cuervo LJ, et al. The use of haloperidol and associated complications in the agitated, acutely ill pediatric burn patient. *J Burn Care Rehabil.* 2004;25:472-478.
8. Schieveld JN, Leentjens AF. Delirium in severely ill young children in the pediatric Intensive care unit (picu). *J Am Acad Child Adolesc Psychiatry.* 2005;44:392-394.
9. Trissel LA. *Handbook on Injectable Drugs.* 15th ed. Bethesda, MD: American Society of Health-System Pharmacists; 2009.
10. Riker RR, Fraser GL, Cox PM. Continuous infusion of haloperidol controls agitation in critically ill patients. *Crit Care Med.* 1994;22:433-439.
11. Isbister GK, Calit C, Kilham HA. Antipsychotic poisoning in young children. A systematic review. *Drug Safety.* 2005;28:1029-1044.
12. Scialli JV, Thornton WE. Toxic reactions from a haloperidol overdose in two children: thermal and cardiac manifestations. *JAMA.* 1978;239:48-49.

Heparin Sodium

1. Available at: http://ismp.org/Tools/highalertmedications.pdf. ISMP. 2008.
2. Available at: http://ismp.org/Tools/confuseddrugnames.pdf. Updated April 1, 2005.
3. Heparin [package insert]. Schaumburg, IL: APP Pharmaceuticals LLC; August 2008.
4. Lesko SM, Mitchell AA, Epstein MR, et al. Heparin use as a risk factor for intraventricular hemorrhage in low birth weight infants. *N Engl J Med.* 1986;314:1156-1160.
5. Cines DB, Kaywin P, Bina M, et al. Heparin-associated thrombocytopenia. *N Engl J Med.* 1980;303:788-795.
6. Murdoch IA, Beattie RM, Silver DM. Heparin-induced thrombocytopenia in children. *Acta Paediatr.* 1993;82:495-497.
7. Available at: http://www.fda.gov/NewsEvents/Newsroom/PressAnnouncements/ucm184674.htm. Accessed October 8, 2009.
8. Monagle P, Chalmers E, Chan A, et al. Antithrombotic therapy in neonates and children. *Chest.* 2008;133:997S-968S.
9. Andrew M, Marzinotto V, Massicotte P, et al. Heparin therapy in pediatric patients: a prospective cohort study. *Pediatr Res.* 1994;35:78-83.
10. Gal P, Ransom L. Neonatal thrombosis: treatment with heparin and thrombolytics. *DICP Ann Pharmacother.* 1991;25:853-856.
11. McDonald MM, Hathaway WE. Anticoagulant therapy by continuous heparinization in newborn and older infants. *J Pediatr.* 1982;101:451-457.
12. Coombs CJ, Richardson RW, Dowling GJ, et al. Brachial artery thrombosis in infants: an algorithm for limb salvage. *Plast Reconstr Surg.* 2006;117:1481-1488.
13. Grady RM, Eisenberg PR, Bridges ND. Rational approach to use of heparin during cardiac catheterization in children. *J Am Coll Cardiol.* 1995;25:725-729.
14. Heparin. Lexi-Comp® Online with AHFS® (database). Hudson, OH: Lexi-Comp Inc; updated August 3, 2009.
15. Schmidt B, Andrew M. Neonatal thrombotic disease: prevention, diagnosis, and treatment. *J Pediatr.* 1988;113:407-409.
16. Alpan G, Eyal F, Springer C, et al. Heparinization of alimentation solutions administered through peripheral veins in premature infants: a controlled study. *Pediatrics.* 1984;74:375-378.
17. Treas LS, Katinis-Bridges B. Efficacy of heparin in peripheral venous infusion in neonates. *J Obstet Gynecol Neonatal Nurs.* 1991;21:214-219.
18. Moclair A, Bates I. The efficacy of heparin in maintaining peripheral infusions in neonates. *Eur J Pediatr.* 1995;154:567-570.
19. Klenner AF, Fusch C, Rakow A, et al. Benefit and risk of heparin for maintaining peripheral venous catheters in neonates: a placebo-controlled trial. *J Pediatr.* 2004;143:741-745.
20. Bossert E, Peecroft PC. Peripheral intravenous lock irrigation in children: current practice. *Pediatr Nurs.* 1994;20:346-349, 355.
21. Lombardi TP, Gundersen B, Zammett LO, et al. Efficacy of 0.9% sodium chloride injection with or without heparin sodium for maintaining patency of intravenous catheters in children. *Clin Pharm.* 1988;7:832-836.
22. Kleiber C, Hanrahan K, Fagan CL, et al. Heparin vs. saline for peripheral IV locks in children. *Pediatr Nurs.* 1993;19:376, 405-409.
23. Heilskov J, Kleiber C, Johnson K, et al. A randomized trial of heparin and saline for maintaining intravenous locks in neonates. *JSPN.* 1998;3:111-116.
24. Randolph AG, Cook DJ, Gonzales CA, et al. Benefit of heparin in peripheral venous and arterial catheters: systemic review and meta-analysis of randomized controlled trials. *BMJ.* 1998;16:969-975.
25. Shah PS, Kalyn A, Satodia P, et al. A randomized, controlled trial of heparin versus placebo infusion to prolong the usability of peripherally placed percutaneous central venous catheters (PCVCs) in neonates: The HIP (heparin infusion for PCVC) study. *Pediatr.* 2007;119:e284-e291.
26. Cesaro S, Tridello G, Cavaliere M, et al. Prospective, randomized trial of two different modalities of flushing central venous catheters in pediatric patients with cancer. *J Clin Oncol.* 2009;27:2059-2065.

References

27. Rajani K, Goetzman BW, Wennberg RP, et al. Effect of heparinization of fluids infused through an umbilical artery catheter on catheter patency and frequency of complications. *Pediatrics.* 1979;63:552-556.
28. David RJ, Merten DF, Anderson JC, et al. Prevention of umbilical artery catheter clots with heparinized infusates. *Dev Pharmacol Ther.* 1981;2:117-126.
29. Edwards MS, Buffone GJ, Rench MA, et al. Effect of continuous heparin infusion on bactericidal activity for group B streptococci in neonatal sera. *J Pediatr.* 1983;103:787-790.
30. Bosque E, Weaver L. Continuous versus intermittent heparin infusion of umbilical artery catheters in the newborn infant. *J Pediatr.* 1986;108:141-143.
31. Gilhooly JT, Lindenberg JA, Reynolds JW. Survey of umbilical artery catheter practices. *Clin Res.* 1986;34:142A.
32. Chang GY, Lueder FL, DiMichele DM, et al. Heparin and the risk of intraventricular hemorrhage in premature infants. *J Pediatr.* 1997;131:362-366.
33. Ronco C, Brendolan A, Bragantini L, et al. Treatment of acute renal failure in newborns by continuous arterio-venous hemofiltration. *Kidney Int.* 1986;29:908-915.
34. Rais-Bahrami K, Short BL. The current status of neonatal extracorporeal membrane oxygenation. *Semin Perinatol.* 2000;24:406-417.
35. Zaidan H, Dhanireddy R, Hamosh M, et al. Effect of continuous heparin administration on Intralipid clearing in very low birth weight infants. *J Pediatr.* 1982;101:599-602.
36. Spear ML, Stahl GE, Hamosh M, et al. Effect of heparin dose and infusion rate on lipid clearance and bilirubin binding in premature infants receiving intravenous fat emulsions. *J Pediatr.* 1988;112:94-98.
37. Green TP, Isham-Schopf B, Irmiter RJ, et al. Inactivation of heparin during extracorporeal circulation in infants. *Clin Pharmacol Ther.* 1990;48:148-154.
38. Trissel LA. *Handbook on Injectable Drugs.* 15th ed. Bethesda, MD: American Society of Health-System Pharmacists; 2009.
39. Shah PS, Ng E, Sinha AK. Heparin for prolonging peripheral intravenous catheter use in neonates. *Cochrane Database Syst Rev.* 2005 Oct 19;(4):CD002774.

HydrALAZINE HCl

1. Available at: http://ismp.org/Tools/confuseddrugnames.pdf. Accessed August 24, 2009.
2. Available at: http://www.usp.org/hqi/similarProducts/choosy.html. Accessed August 24, 2009.
3. Hydralazine hydrochloride injection [package insert]. Lake Forest, IL: Akorn Inc; April 2009.
4. Hydralazine hydrochloride. Lexi-Comp Online with AHFS (database). Bethesda, MD: American Society of Health-System Pharmacists. 2009. Accessed October 4, 2009.
5. Adelman RD, Coppo R, Dillon MJ. The emergency management of severe hypertension. *Pediatr Nephrol.* 2000;14:422-427.
6. Young TE, Mangum B, eds. *Neofax.* 22nd ed. Montvale, NJ: Thomson Reuters; 2009.
7. Beekman RH, Rocchini AP, Rosenthal A. Hemodynamic effects of hydralazine in infants with a large ventricular septal defect. *Circulation.* 1982;65:523-528.
8. Friedman WF, George BL. Treatment of congestive heart failure by altering loading conditions of the heart. *J Pediatr.* 1985;106:697-706.
9. Fried R, Steinherz LJ, Levin AR. Use of hydralazine for intractable cardiac failure in childhood. *J Pediatr.* 1980;97:1009-1011.
10. Plumer LB, Kaplan GW, Mendoza SA. Hypertension in infants—a complication of umbilical arterial catheterization. *J Pediatr.* 1976;89:802-805.
11. Fleischmann LE. Management of hypertensive crises in children. *Pediatr Ann.* 1977;6:410-414.
12. Friedman WF, George BL. New concepts and drugs in the treatment of congestive heart failure. *Pediatr Clin North Am.* 1984;31:1197-1227.
13. Artman M, Parrish MD, Appleton S, et al. Hemodynamic effects of hydralazine in infants with idiopathic dilated cardiomyopathy and congestive heart failure. *Am Heart J.* 1987;113:144-150.
14. Farine M, Arbus GS. Management of hypertensive emergencies in children. *Pediatr Emerg Care.* 1989;5:51-55.
15. Serratto M. Diagnosis and management of heart failure in infants and children. *Comprehensive Ther.* 1992;18:11-19.
16. Miller K. Pharmacological management of hypertension in paediatric patients. *Drugs.* 1994;48:868-887.
17. American Academy of Pediatrics. Committee on Drugs. Emergency drug doses for infants and children. *Pediatrics.* 1988;81:462-465.
18. Loggie JM. Hypertension in children and adolescents. II. Drug therapy. *J Pediatr.* 1969;74:640-654.
19. Fivush B, Neu A, Furth S. Acute hypertensive crises in children: emergencies and urgencies. *Curr Opin Pediatr.* 1997;9:233-236.
20. Aronoff GR, Berns JS, Brier ME, et al. Drug prescribing in renal failure. 4th ed. Available at: http://www.kdp-baptist.louisville.edu/renalbook/. Accessed October 4, 2009.
21. Hydralazine hydrochloride. Lexi-Comp Online with AHFS (database). Hudson, OH: Lexi-Comp Inc. Accessed October 4, 2009.
22. Adelman RD. Neonatal hypertension. *Pediatr Clin North Am.* 1978;25:99-110.
23. Hanna JD, Chan JC, Gill JR. Hypertension and the kidney. *J Pediatr.* 1991;118:327-340.
24. Trissel LA, ed. *Handbook on Injectable Drugs.* 15th ed. Bethesda, MD: American Society of Health-System Pharmacists; 2009.
25. Grossman E, Ironi AN, Messerli FH. Comparative tolerability profile of hypertensive crisis treatments. *Drug Safety.* 1998;19:99-122.
26. Deal JE, Barratt TM, Dillion MJ. Management of hypertensive emergencies. *Arch Dis Child.* 1992;67:1089-1092.

Hydrochloric Acid (HCl)

1. Knutsen OH. New method for administration of hydrochloric acid in metabolic alkalosis. *Lancet.* 1983;1:953-956.
2. Galla JH. Metabolic alkalosis. *J Am Soc Nephrol.* 2000;11:369-375.
3. Adrogue HJ, Madias NE. Management of life-threatening acid-base disorders. *N Engl J Med.* 1998;338:107-111.
4. Duffy L, Kerzner B, Gebuw V, et al. Treatment of central venous catheter occlusion with HCl. *J Pediatr.* 1989;114:1002-1004.
5. Breaux CW, Duke D, Georgeson KE, et al. Calcium phosphate crystal occlusion of central venous catheters used for total parenteral nutrition in infants and children: prevention and treatment. *J Pediatr Surg.* 1987;22:829-832.
6. Shulman RJ, Reed T, Pitre D, et al. Use of hydrochloric acid to clear obstructed central venous catheters. *J Parenter Enteral Nutr.* 1988;12:509-510.
7. Holcombe BJ, Forloines-Lynn S, Garmhausen LW. Restoring patency of long-term central venous access devices. *J Intraven Nurs.* 1992;15:36-41.
8. Kerner JA, Garcia-Careaga MG, Fisher AA, et al. Treatment of catheter occlusion in pediatric patients. *J Parenter Enter Nutr.* 2006;30:S73-S81.
9. Unger A, Rhenman B, Fuller JK, et al. Treatment of severe metabolic alkalosis in a neonate with hydrochloric acid infusion. *Clin Pediatr.* 1985;24:444-448.
10. Nasimi A, Cardona J, Berthier M, et al. Hydrochloric acid infusion for treatment of severe metabolic alkalosis in a neonate. *Clin Pediatr.* 1996;35:271-272.
11. Martin WF, Matzke GR. Treating severe metabolic alkalosis. *Clin Pharm.* 1982;1:42-48.
12. Barbaric D, Curtin J, Pearson L, et al. Role of hydrochloric acid in the treatment of central venous catheter infections in children with cancer. *Cancer.* 2004;101:1866-1872.
13. Kopel RF, Durbin CG. Pulmonary artery catheter deterioration during hydrochloric acid infusion for the treatment of metabolic alkalosis. *Crit Care Med.* 1989;17:688-689.
14. Shulman RJ, Barrish JP, Hicks MJ. Does the use of hydrochloric acid damage silicone rubber central venous catheters? *J Parenter Enter Nutr.* 1995;19:407-409.

References

Hydrocortisone Sodium Succinate

1. Available at: http://www.usp.org/hqi/similarProducts/choosy.html. Accessed August 10, 2009.
2. Solu-Cortef [prescribing information]. New York, NY: Pfizer Inc; May 2008.
3. Goldstein DA, Zimmerman B, Spielberg SP. Anaphylactic response to hydrocortisone in childhood: a case report. *Ann Allergy.* 1985;55:599-600.
4. Fass B. Glucocorticoid therapy for non-endocrine disorders: withdrawal and coverage. *Pediatr Clin North Am.* 1979;26:251-256.
5. Chamberlin P, Meyer WJ. Management of pituitary-adrenal suppression secondary to corticosteroid therapy. *Pediatrics.* 1981;67:245-251.
6. Hydrocortisone. Lexi-Comp® Online with AHFS® (database). Hudson, OH: Lexi-Comp Inc; updated July 28, 2009.
7. Miller JJ. Prolonged use of large intravenous steroid pulses in the rheumatic diseases of children. *Pediatrics.* 1980;65:989-994.
8. Klevit HD. Corticosteroid therapy in the neonatal period. *Pediatr Clin North Am.* 1970;17:1003-1113.
9. MacDonald MG, Seshia MM, Mullett MD, eds. *Avery's Neonatology Pathophysiology & Management of the Newborn.* Philadelphia, PA: Lippincott Williams & Wilkins; 2005.
10. American Academy of Pediatrics, Section on Endocrinology and Committee on Genetics. Technical report: congenital adrenal hyperplasia. *Pediatrics.* 2000;106:1511-1518.
11. Seri I, Tan R, Evans J. Cardiovascular effects of hydrocortisone in preterm infants with pressor-resistant hypotension. *Pediatrics.* 2001;107:1070-1074.
12. Helbock HJ, Insoft RM, Conte FA. Glucocorticoid-responsive hypotension in extremely low birth weight newborns. *Pediatrics.* 1993;92:715-717.
13. National Asthma Education and Prevention Program. *Expert Panel Report 3: Guidelines for the Diagnosis and Management of Asthma.* Bethesda, MD: National Institutes of Health; August 2007.
14. Tepper RS, Eigen H, Stevens J, et al. Lower respiratory illness in infants and young children with cystic fibrosis: evaluation of treatment with intravenous hydrocortisone. *Pediatr Pulmonol.* 1997;24:48-51.
15. Trissel LA. *Handbook on Injectable Drugs.* 15th ed. Bethesda, MD: American Society of Health-System Pharmacists; 2009.
16. Atkinson WL, Pickering LK, Schwartz B, et al. General recommendations on immunization. Recommendations of the Advisory Committee on Immunization Practices (ACIP) and the American Academy of Family Physicians (AAFP). *MMWR Recomm Rep.* 2002;51(RR-2):1-35.
17. Botos CM, Kurlat I, Young SM, et al. Disseminated candidal infections and intravenous hydrocortisone in preterm infants. *Pediatrics.* 1995;95:883-887.
18. Watterberg KL, Gerdes JS, Cole CH, et al. Prophylaxis of early adrenal insufficiency to prevent bronchopulmonary dysplasia: a multicenter trial. *Pediatrics.* 2004;114:1649-1657.

Hydroxocobalamin

1. Available at: http://ismp.org/Tools/confuseddrugnames.pdf. Accessed August 24, 2009.
2. Available at: http://www.usp.org/hqi/similarProducts/choosy.html. Accessed August 24, 2009.
3. Hydroxocobalamin acetate injection [package insert]. Corona, CA:Watson Laboratories Inc; February 2006.
4. Hydroxocobalamin (Cyanokit) for Injection [package insert]. Columbia, MD: Meridian Medical Technologies Inc; August 2008.
5. Hydroxocobalamin. Lexi-Comp Online with AHFS (database). Hudson, OH: Lexi-Comp Inc; 1978–2009.
6. Hall AH, Saiers J, Baud F. Which cyanide antidote? *Crit Rev Toxicol.* 2009;541-552.
7. Barillo DJ. Diagnosis and treatment of cyanide toxicity. *J Burn Care Res.* 2009;30:148-152.

Ibuprofen Lysine

1. Ibuprofen lysine [package insert]. Deerfield, IL: Lundbeck Inc; May 2009.
2. Van Overmeire B, Follens I, Hartmann S, et al. Treatment of patent ductus arteriosus with ibuprofen. *Arch Dis Child Fetal Neonatal Ed.* 1997;76:F179-F184.
3. Van Overmeire B, Smets K, Lecoutere D, et al. A comparison of ibuprofen and indomethacin for closure of patent ductus arteriosus. *N Eng J Med.* 2000;343:674-681.
4. Lago P, Bettiol T, Salvadori S, et al. Safety and efficacy of ibuprofen versus indomethacin in preterm infants treated for patent ductus arteriosus: a randomised controlled trial. *Eur J Pediatr.* 2002;161:202-207.
5. Su PH, Chen JY, Su CM, et al. Comparison of ibuprofen and indomethacin therapy for patent ductus arteriosus in preterm infants. *Pediatr Int.* 2003;45:665-670.
6. Hirt D, Overmeire BV, Treluyer JM, et al. An optimized ibuprofen dosing scheme for preterm neonates with patent ductus arteriosus, based on pharmacokinetic and pharmacodynamic study. *Br J Clin Pharmacol.* 2008;65:629-636.
7. Hammerman C, Shchors I, Jacobson S, et al. Ibuprofen versus continuous indomethacin in premature neonates with patent ductus arteriosus: is the difference in the mode of administration? *Pediatr Res.* 2008;64:291-297.
8. Van Overmeire B, Allegart K, Casaer A, et al. Prophylactic ibuprofen in premature infants: a multicentre, randomized, double-blind, placebo-controlled trial. *Lancet.* 2004;364:1945-1949.
9. Shah SS, Ohlsson A. Ibuprofen for the prevention of patent ductus arteriosus in preterm and/or low birth weight infants. *Cochrane Database Syst Rev.* 2006;25:1:CD004213.
10. Ibuprofen. Lexi-Comp® Online with AHFS® (database). Hudson, OH: Lexi-Comp Inc; updated September 17, 2009.
11. Mosca F, Bray M, Lattanzio M, et al. Comparative evaluation of the effects of indomethacin and ibuprofen on cerebral perfusion and oxygenation in preterm infants with patent ductus arteriosus. *J Pediatr.* 1997;131:549-554.
12. Patel J, Roberts I, Azzopardi D, et al. Randomized double-blind controlled trial comparing the effects of ibuprofen with indomethacin on cerebral hemodynamics in preterm infants with patent ductus arteriosus. *Pediatr Res.* 2000;47:36-41.
13. Dani C, Bertini G, Pezzati M, et al. Prophylactic ibuprofen for the prevention of intraventricular hemorrhage among preterm infants: a multicenter, randomized study. *Pediatrics.* 2005;115:1529-1535.
14. Grosfeld JL, Kamman K, Gross K, et al. Comparative effects of indomethacin, prostaglandin E1, and ibuprofen on bowel ischemia. *J Pediatr Surg.* 1983;18:738-742.
15. Alpan G, Eyal F, Vinograd I, et al. Localized intestinal perforations after enteral administration of indomethacin in premature infants. *J Pediatr.* 1985;106:277-281.
16. Kuhl G, Wille L, Bolkenius M, et al. Intestinal perforation associated with indomethacin treatment in premature infants. *Eur J Pediatr.* 1985;143:213-216.
17. Fujii AM, Brown E, Mirochnick M, et al. Neonatal necrotizing enterocolitis with intestinal perforation in extremely premature infants receiving early indomethacin treatment for patent ductus arteriosus.*J Perinatol.* 200;22:535-540.
18. Pezzati M, Vangi V, Biagiotti R, et al. Effects of indomethacin and ibuprofen on mesenteric and renal blood flow in preterm infants with patent ductus arteriosus. *J Pediatr.* 1999;135:733-738.
19. Peitz GJ, Hoie EB, Hoy S, et al. Repeated bowel perforation with ibuprofen lysine: a case report. *J Pediatr Pharmacol Ther.* 2008;13:166-169.
20. Thomas RL, Parker GC, Overmeire BV, et al. A meta-analysis of ibuprofen versus indomethacin for closure of patent ductus arteriosus. *Eur J Pediatr.* 2005;164:135-140.
21. Hammerman C, Shchors I, Jacobson S, et al. Ibuprofen versus continuous indomethacin in premature neonates with patent ductus arteriosus: is the difference in the mode of administration? *Pediatr Res.* 2008;64:291-297.

References

22. Gal P. Patent ductus arteriosus: Indomethacin, ibuprofen, surgery, or not treatment? *J Pediatr Pharmacol Ther*. 2009;14:4-9.
23. Aranda JV, Varvarigou A, Beharry K, et al. Pharmacokinetics and protein binding of intravenous ibuprofen in the premature newborn infants. *Acta Pedaitr*. 1997;86:289-298.
24. Willy T, Hansen R. Ibuprofen for closure of patent ductus arteriosus: is it really safe in hyperbilirubinaemic infants? *Eur J Pediatr*. 2003;162:356.
25. Gal P, Ransom JL, Davis SA. Possible ibuprofen-induced kernicterus in a near-term infant with moderate hyperbilirubinemia. *J Pediatr Pharmacol Ther*. 2006;11:245-250.
26. Bellini C, Campone F, Serra G. pulmonary hypertension following l-lysine ibuprofen therapy in a preterm infant with patent ductus arteriosus. *CMAJ*. 2006;174:1843-1844.
27. Aithal GP, Day CP. Nonsteroidal anti-inflammatory drug induced hepatotoxicity. *Clin Liv Dis*. 2007;11:563-575.
28. Breen EG, McNichole J, Cosgrove E, et al. Fatal hepatitis associtated with diclofenac. *Gut*. 1986;27:1390-1393.

Ifosfamide

1. Available at: http://ismp.org/Tools/highalertmedications.pdf. ISMP 2008. Accessed August 24, 2009.
2. Ifosfamide [package insert]. Princeton, NJ: Bristol Myers Squibb; February 2008.
3. Ifosfamide. Lexi-Comp Online with AHFS (database). Hudson, OH: Lexi-Comp Inc; updated October 22, 2009.
4. Ninane J, Baurain R, de Kraker J, et al. Alkylating activity in serum, urine, and CSF following high-dose ifosfamide in children. *Cancer Chemother Pharmacol*. 1989;24(suppl 1):S2-S6.
5. Pinkerton CR, Rogers H, James C, et al. A phase II study of ifosfamide in children with recurrent solld tumours. *Cancer Chemother Pharmacol*. 1985;15(3):258-262.
6. Miser JS, Krailo MD, Tarbell NJ, et al. Treatment of metastatic Ewing's sarcoma or primitive neuroectodermal tumor of bone: evaluation of combination ifosfamide and etoposide—a Children's Cancer Group and Pediatric Oncology Group study. *J Clin Oncol*. 2004;22(14):2873-2876.
7. Le Deley MC, Guinebretiere JM, Gentet JC, et al. SFOP OS94: a randomised trial comparing preoperative high-dose methotrexate plus doxorubicin to high-dose methotrexate plus etoposide and ifosfamide in osteosarcoma patients. *Eur J Cancer*. 2007;43:752-761.
8. Goorin AM, Harris MB, Bernstein M, et al. Phase II/III trial of etoposide and high-dose ifosfamide in newly diagnosed metastatic osteosarcoma: a pediatric oncology group trial. *J Clin Oncol*. 2002;20(2):426-433.
9. Aronoff GR, Berns JS, Brier ME, et al. Drug prescribing in renal failure. 4th ed. Available at: http://www.kdp-baptist.louisville.edu/renalbook/. Accessed October 23, 2009.
10. Falkson G, Hunt M, Borden EC, et al. An extended phase II trial of ifosfamide plus mesna in malignant mesothelioma. *Invest New Drugs*. 1992;10(4):337-343.
11. Trissel LA, ed. *Handbook on Injectable Drugs*. 15th ed. Bethesda, MD: American Society of Health-System Pharmacists; 2009.
12. Silies H, Blaschke G, Hohenlochter B, et al. Excretion kinetics of ifosfamide side-chain metabolites in children on continuous and short-term infusion. *Int J Clin Pharmacol Ther*. 1998;36(5):246-252.
13. Boddy AV, Yule SM, Wyllie R, et al. Pharmacokinetics and metabolism of ifosfamide administered as a continuous infusion in children. *Cancer Res*. 1993;3(16):3758-3764.
14. Suarez A, McDowell H, Niaudet P, et al. Long-term follow-up of ifosfamide renal toxicity in children treated with malignant mesenchymal tumors: an International Society of Pediatric Oncology report. *J Clin Oncol*. 1991;9(12):2177-2182.
15. National Comprehensive Cancer Network (NCCN) Antiemesis Panel Members. NCCN Clinical Practice Guidelines in Oncology. Antiemesis, v.1.2006. Available at www.nccn.org. Last accessed March 29, 2006.
16. Roila F, Feyer P, Maranzamo E, et al. Antiemetics in children receiving chemotherapy. *Support Care Cancer*. 2005;13:129-131.

Imipenem–Cilastatin Sodium

1. Available at: http://www.usp.org/hqi/similarProducts/choosy.html. Accessed September 2, 2009.
2. Primaxin® IV [package insert]. Whitestation, NJ: Merck & Co; December 2007.
3. Reed MD, Kliegman RM, Yamashita TS, et al. Clinical pharmacology of imipenem and cilastatin in premature infants during the first week of life. *Antimicrob Agents Chemother*. 1990;34:1172-1177.
4. Begue PC, Challier BP, Fontaine JL, Lasfargues G. Pharmacokinetics and clinical evaluation of imipenem/Cilastatin in children and neonates. *Scand J Infec Dis*. Suppl 1987;52:40-45.
5. Ahonkhai VI, Cyhan GM, Wilson SE, et al. Imipenem–cilastatin in pediatric patients: an overview of safety and efficacy in studies conducted in the United States. *Pediatr Infect Dis J*. 1989;8:740-744.
6. Nalin DR, Hart CB, Shih WJ, et al. Imipenem/cilastatin for pediatric infections in hospitalized patients. *Scand J Infect Dis*. 1987;52:56-64.
7. Freij BJ, Kusmiesz H, Shelton S, et al. Imipenem and cilastatin in acute osteomyelitis and suppurative arthritis. Therapy in infants and children. *Am J Dis Child*. 1987;141:335-342.
8. Alpert G, Dagan R, Connor E, et al. Imipenem/cilastatin for the treatment of infections in hospitalized children. *Am J Dis Child*. 1985;139:1153-1156.
9. Riikonen P. Imipenem compared with ceftazidime plus vancomycin as initial therapy for fever in neutropenic children with cancer. *Pediatr Infect Dis J*. 1991;10:918-923.
10. Inglesby TV, O'Toole T, Henderson DA, et al., for the Working Group on Civilian Biodefense. Anthrax as a biological weapon 2002: updated recommendations for management. *JAMA*. 2002;287:2236-2252.
11. Centers for Disease Control and Prevention. Update: Investigation of bioterrorism-related anthrax and interim guidelines for exposure management and antimicrobial therapy, October 2001. *MMWR Morb Mortal Wkly Rep*. 2001;50:909-919.
12. Aronoff GR, Berns JS, Brier ME, et al. Drug prescribing in renal failure. 4th ed. Available at: http://www.kdp-baptist.louisville.edu/renalbook/. Accessed September 2, 2009.
13. Trissel LA, ed. *Handbook on Injectable Drugs*. 15th ed. Bethesda, MD: American Society of Health-System Pharmacists; 2009.
14. Robinson CA, Sawyer JE. Y-site compatibility of medications with parenteral nutrition. *J Pediatr Pharmacol Ther*. 2009;14:49-57.
15. Jacobs RF, Kearns GL, Trang JM, et al. Single-dose pharmacokinetics of imipenem in children. *J Pediatr*. 1984;105:996-1001.
16. Norrby SR. Neurotoxicity of the carbapenem antibacterials. *Drug Safety*. 1996;15:87-90.
17. Norrby SR. Carbapenems in serious infections: a risk-benefit assessment. *Drug Safety*. 2000;22:191-194.
18. Stuart RL, Turnidge J, Grayson ML. Safety of imipenem is neonates. *Pediatr Infect Dis J*. 1995;14:804-805.
19. Wong VK, Wright HT Jr, Ross LA, et al. Imipenem/cilastatin treatment of bacterial meningitis in children. *Pediatr Infect Dis J*. 1991;10:122-125.
20. Calandra G, Lydick E, Carrigan J, et al. Factors predisposing to seizures in seriously ill infected patients receiving antibiotics: experience with imipenem/cilastatin. *Am J Med*. 1988;84:911-918.
21. Mori H, Takahashi K, Mizutani T. Interaction between valproic acid and carbapenem antibiotics. *Drug Metab Rev*. 2007;39:647-657.
22. Tartaglione TA, Flint NB. Effect of imipenem-cilastatin and ciprofloxacin on tests for glycosuria. *Am J Hosp Pharm*. 1985;42:602-605.

References

Immune Globulin Intravenous

1. Available at: http://www.usp.org/hqi/similarProducts/choosy.html. Accessed September 8, 2009.
2. Carimune NF [prescribing information]. Kankakee, IL: CSL Behring LLC; October 2008.
3. Flebogamma 5% [prescribing information]. Los Angeles, CA: GRIFOLS USA Inc; December 2003.
4. GAMMAGARD LIQUID [prescribing information]. Westlake Village, CA: Baxter Healthcare Corp; April 2005.
5. GAMMAGARD S/D [prescribing information]. Westlake Village, CA: Baxter Healthcare Corp; October 2008.
6. Gamunex [prescribing information]. Research Triangle Park, NC: Talecris Biotherapeutics Inc; October 2008.
7. Octagam [prescribing information]. Centreville, VA: Octapharma USA; March 2007.
8. Privigen [prescribing information]. Kankakee, IL: CSL Behring LLC; July 2007.
9. Brennan VM, Salome-Bentley NJ, Chapel HM. Prospective audit of adverse reactions occurring in 459 primary antibody-deficient patients receiving intravenous immunoglobulin. *Clin Exp Immunol.* 2003;133:247-51.
10. ASHP Commission on Therapeutics. ASHP therapeutic guidelines for intravenous immune globulin. *Clin Pharm.* 1992;11:117-136.
11. Eijkhout HW, van Der Meer JW, Kallenberg CG, et al. The effect of two different dosages of intravenous immunoglobulin on the incidence of recurrent infections in patients with primary hypogammaglobulinemia. *Ann Intern Med.* 2001;135:165-174.
12. Dwyer JM. Manipulating the immune system with immune globulin. *N Engl J Med.* 1992;326:107-116.
13. Warrier I, Bussel JB, Valdez L, et al. Safety and efficacy of low-dose intravenous immune globulin (IVIG) treatment for infants and children with immune thrombocytopenic purpura. Low-Dose IVIG Study Group. *J Pediatr Hematol Oncol.* 1997;19:197-201.
14. George JN, Woolf SH, Raskob GE, et al. Idiopathic thrombocytopenic purpura: a practice guideline developed by explicit methods for the American Society of Hematology. *Blood.* 1996;88:3-40.
15. Gurcan HM, Ahmed AR. Efficacy of various intravenous immunoglobulin therapy protocols in autoimmune and chronic inflammatory disorders. *Ann Pharmacother.* 2007;41:812-822.
16. American Academy of Pediatrics. Kawasaki disease. In: Pickering LK, Baker CJ, Kimberlin DW, et al., eds. *2009 Red Book: Report of the Committee on Infectious Diseases.* 28th ed. Elk Grove Village, IL: American Academy of Pediatrics; 2009:413-417.
17. Newberger JW, Takahashi M, Beiser AS, et al. A single intravenous infusion of gamma globulin as compared with four infusions in the treatment of acute Kawasaki syndrome. *N Engl J Med.* 1991;324:1633-1639.
18. Rowley AH, Shulman ST. Current therapy for acute Kawasaki syndrome. *J Pediatr.* 1991;118:987-991.
19. Kawasaki T. Kawasaki disease. *Acta Paediatr.* 1995;84:713-715.
20. Tse SM, Silverman ED, McCrindle BW, et al. Early treatment with intravenous immunoglobulin in patients with Kawasaki disease. *J Pediatr.* 2002;140:450-455.
21. Sato N, Sugimura T, Akagi T, et al. Selective high dose gamma-globulin treatment in Kawasaki disease: assessment of clinical aspects and cost effectiveness. *Pediatr Internat.* 1999;41:1-7.
22. Newburger JW, Takahashi M, Gerber MA, et al. Diagnosis, treatment, and long-term management of Kawasaki disease: a statement for health professionals from the Committee on Rheumatic Fever, Endocarditis, and Kawasaki Disease, Council on Cardiovascular Disease in the Young, American Heart Association. *Pediatrics.* 2004;114:1708-1733.
23. Burns JC, Capparelli EV, Brown JA, et al. Intravenous gamma-globulin treatment and retreatment in Kawasaki disease. US/Canadian Kawasaki Syndrome Study Group. *Pediatr Infect Dis J.* 1998;17:1144-1148.
24. Immune Globulin (Intravenous). Lexi-Comp® Online with AHFS® (database). Hudson, OH: Lexi-Comp Inc; updated Augusr 13, 2009.
25. Guidelines for preventing opportunistic infections among hematopoietic stem cell transplant recipients. Recommendations of CDC, the Infectious Disease Society of America, and the American Society of Blood and Marrow Transplantation. *MMWR Recommendations and Reports.* October 20, 2000/49(RR10):1-128.
26. Korinthenberg R, Schessl J, Kirschner J, et al. Intravenously administered immunoglobulin in the treatment of childhood Guillain-Barré syndrome: a randomized trial. *Pediatrics.* 2005;116:8-14.
27. Yata J, Nihei K, Ohya T, et al. High-dose immunoglobulin therapy for Guillain-Barré syndrome in Japanese children. *Pediatr Internat.* 2003;45:543-549.
28. Spector SA, Gelber RD, McGrath N, et al. A controlled trial of intravenous immune globulin for the prevention of serious bacterial infections in children receiving zidovudine for advanced human immunodeficiency virus infection. *N Engl J Med.* 1994;331:1181-1187.
29. American Academy of Pediatrics. HIV. In: Pickering LK, Baker CJ, Kimberlin DW, et al., eds. *2009 Red Book: Report of the Committee on Infectious Diseases.* 28th ed. Elk Grove Village, IL: American Academy of Pediatrics; 2009:380-399.
30. Miqdad AM, Abdelbasit OB, Shaheed MM, et al. Intravenous immunoglobulin G (IVIG) therapy for significant hyperbilirubinemia in ABO hemolytic disease of the newborn. *J Matern Fetal Neonatal Med.* 2004;16:163-166.
31. Tanyer G, Siklar Z, Dallar Y, et al. Multiple dose IVIG treatment in neonatal immune hemolytic jaundice. *J Trop Pediatr.* 2001;47:50-53.
32. Perlmutter SJ, Leitman SF, Garvey MA, et al. Therapeutic plasma exchange and intravenous immunoglobulin for obsessive-compulsive disorder and tic disorders in childhood. *Lancet.* 1999;354:1153-1158.
33. Chirico G, Rondini G, Plebani A, et al. Intravenous gamma globulin therapy for prophylaxis of infection in high-risk neonates. *J Pediatr.* 1987;110:437-442.
34. Fischer GW, Weisman LE, Hemming VG. Directed immune globulin for the prevention or treatment of neonatal group B streptococcal infections: a review. *Clin Immunol Immunopathol.* 1992;62:S92-S97.
35. Baker CJ, Melish ME, Hall RT, et al. Intravenous immune globulin for the prevention of nosocomial infection in low-birth-weight neonates. *N Engl J Med.* 1992;327:213-219.
36. Kyllonen KS, Clapp DW, Kliegman RM, et al. Dosage of intravenously administered immune globulin and dosing interval required to maintain target levels of immunoglobulin G in low birth weight infants. *J Pediatr.* 1989;115:1013-1016.
37. Clapp DW, Kliegman RM, Baley JE, et al. Use of intravenously administered immune globulin to prevent nosocomial sepsis in low birth weight infants: report of a pilot study. *J Pediatr.* 1989;115:973-978.
38. Garvey MA, Snider LA, Leitman SF, et al. Treatment of Sydenham's chorea with intravenous immunoglobulin, plasma exchange, or prednisone. *J Child Neurol.* 2005;20:424-429.
39. Metry DW, Jung P, Levy ML. Use of intravenous immunoglobulin in children with Stevens-Johnson syndrome and toxic epidermal necrolysis: seven cases and review of the literature. *Pediatrics.* 2003;112:1430-1436.
40. Prins C, Kerdel FA, Padilla RS, et al. Treatment of toxic epidermal necrolysis with high-dose intravenous immunoglobulins. Multicenter retrospective analysis of 48 consecutive cases. *Arch Dermatol.* 2003;139:26-32.
41. Berkovitch M, Dolinski G, Tauber T, et al. Neutropenia as a complication of intravenous immunoglobulin (IVIG) therapy in children with immune thrombocytopenic purpura: common and non-alarming. *Int J Immunopharmacol.* 1999;21:411-415.
42. Nakagawa M, Watanabe N, Okuno M, et al. Severe hemolytic anemia following high-dose intravenous immunoglobulin administration in a patient with Kawasaki disease. *Am J Hematol.* 2000;63:160-161.
43. American Academy of Pediatrics. Table 3.34. Suggested intervals between immune globulin administration and measles immunization. In: Pickering LK, Baker CJ, Kimberlin DW, et al., eds. *2009 Red Book: Report of the Committee on Infectious Diseases.* 28th ed. Elk Grove Village, IL: American Academy of Pediatrics; 2009:448.

References

Inamrinone Lactate (previously amrinone)

1. Available at: http://ismp.org/Tools/highalertmedications.pdf. Accessed August 30, 2009.
2. Available at: http://www.usp.org/hqi/similarProducts/choosy.html. Accessed August 30, 2009.
3. Inamrinone [package insert]. Bedfore OH: Ben Venure Laboriesties; August 2002.
4. American Heart Association (AHA), The American Heart Association Emergency Cardiovascular Care Committee. 2005 guidelines for cardiopulmonary resuscitation (CPR) and emergency cardiovascular care (ECC)—part 7.4: monitoring and medications and part 12: pediatric advanced life support. *Circulation.* 2005;112(24 Suppl):IV72-83, 167-187.
5. Lawless ST, Burckart GJ. Amrinone pharmacokinetics in neonates and infants (reply to letter). *Crit Care Med.* 1990;18:1495.
6. Lawless ST, Zaritsky A, Miles M. The acute pharmacokinetics and pharmacodynamics of amrinone in pediatric patients. *J Clin Pharmacol.* 1991;31:800-803.
7. Allen-Webb EM, Ross MP, Pappas JB, et al. Age-related amrinone pharmacokinetics in a pediatric population. *Crit Care Med.* 1994;22:1016-1024.
8. Ross MP, Allen-Webb EM, Pappas JB, et al. Amrinone-associated thrombocytopenia: pharmacokinetic analysis. *Clin Pharmacol Ther.* 1993;53:661-667.
9. Rathmell JP, Prielipp RC, Butterworth JF, et al. A multicenter, randomized, blind comparison of amrinone with milrinone after elective cardiac surgery. *Anesth Analg.* 1998;86:683-690.
10. Bailey JM, Miller BE, Kanter KR, et al. A comparison of the hemodynamic effects of amrinone and sodium nitroprusside in infants after cardiac surgery. *Pediatr Anesth.* 1997;84:294-298.
11. Sorensen SK, Ramamoorthy C, Lynn AM, et al. Hemodynamic effects of amrinone in children after Fontan surgery. *Anesth Analg.* 1996;82:241-246.
12. Lawless S, Burckart G, Diven W, et al. Amrinone in neonates and infants after cardiac surgery. *Crit Care Med.* 1989;17:751-754.
13. Laitinen P, Happonen JM, Sairanen H, et al. Amrinone versus dopamine and nitroglycerine in neonates after arterial switch operation for transposition of the great arteries. *J Cardiothoracic Vascular Anesth.* 1999;13:186-190.
14. Aronoff GR, Berns JS, Brier ME, et al. Drug prescribing in renal failure. 4th ed. Available at: http://www.kdp-baptist.louisville.edu/renalbook/. Accessed August 30, 2009.
15. Berner M, Jaccard C, Oberhansli I, et al. Hemodynamic effects of amrinone in children after cardiac surgery. *Inten Care Med.* 1990;16:85-88.
16. Lebovitz DJ, Lawless ST, Weise KL. Fatal amrinone overdose in a pediatric patient. *Crit Care Med.* 1995;23:977-980.
17. Trissel LA, ed. *Handbook on Injectable Drugs.* 15th ed. Bethesda, MD: American Society of Health-System Pharmacists; 2009.

Indomethacin Sodium Trihydrate

1. Available at: http://www.usp.org/hqi/similarProducts/choosy.html. Accessed October 25, 2009.
2. Indomethacin [package insert]. Deerfield, IL: Merck & Co; July 2006.
3. Form Web. Black boxed warnings. Available at: http://www.formularyproductions.com/blackbox/. Accessed October 25, 2009.
4. Indometehicin, Lexi-Comp® Online with AHFS® (database). Hudson, OH: Lexi-Comp Inc; updated October 27, 2009.
5. Rennie JM, Cooke RWI. Prolonged low dose indomethacin for persistent ductus arteriosus of prematurity. *Arch Dis Child.*1991;66:55-58.
6. Rhodes PG, Ferguson MG, Reddy NS et al. Effects of prolonged verses acute indomethacin therapy in very low birth-weight infants with patent ductus arteriosus. *Eur J Pediatr.* 1988;147:481-484.
7. Hammerman C, Armaburo MJ. Prolonged indomethacin therapy for the prevention of recurrences of patent ductus arteriosus. *J Pediatr.* 1990;117:772-776.
8. Nakamura T, Tamura M, Kadowaki S. Low-dose continuous indomethacin in early days of age reduce the incidence of symptomatic patent ductus arteriosus without adverse effects. *Am J Perinatol.* 2000;17:271-275.
9. Mahony L, Carnero V, Brett C et al. Prophylactic indomethacin therapy for patent ductus arteriosus in very-low-birth-weight infants. *N Engl J Med.* 1982;306:506-510.
10. Fowlie PR, Davis PG. Prophylactic indomethacin therapy for preterm infants: a systematic review and meta-analysis. *Arch Dis Child Fetal Neonatal Ed.* 2003;88:F64-F66.
11. Gersony WM, Peckham GL, Ellison RC, et al. Effects of indomethacin in premature infants with patent ductus areteriosus: results of a national collaborative study. *J Pediatr.* 1983;102:895-906.
12. Weist DB, Pinson JB, Gal PS, et al. Population pharmacokinetics of intravenous indomethacin in neonates with symptomatic patent ductus arteriosus. *Clin Pharmacol Ther.* 1991;49:550-557.
13. Stefano JL, Abbasu, Pearlmen SA, et al. Closure of the ductus areteriosus with indomethacin in ventilated neonates with respiratory distress syndrome. *Am Rev Respir Dis.* 1991;143:236-239.
14. Hammerman C, Glaser J, Schimmel MS, et al. Continuous versus multiple rapid infusion of indomethacin: effect on cerebral blood flow velocity. *Pediatrics.* 1995;95:244-248.
15. Christmann V, Liem KD, Semmekrot BA, et al. Changes in cerebral, renal, and mesenteric blood flow velocity during continuous and bolus infusion of indomethacin. *Acta Paediatr.* 2002;91:440-46.
16. Bada HS, Green RS, Pourcyrous M, et al. Indomethacin reduces the risks of severe intraventricular hemorrhage. *J Pediatr.* 1989; 115:631-637.
17. Hanigan WC, Kenedy G, Roemisch F, et al. Administration of indomethacin for the prevention of periventricular-intraventricular hemorrhage in high-risk neonates. *J Pediatr.* 1988;112:941-947.
18. Ment LR, Oh W, Ehrenkranz RA, et al. Low-dose indomethacin and prevention of intraventricular hemorrhage: a multicenter randomized trial. *Pediatrics.* 1994;93:543-550.
19. Gal P, Ransom JL, Weaver RL, et al. Indomethacin pharmacokinetics in neonates: the value of volme of distribution as a marker of permanent patent ductus arteriosus closure. *Ther Drug Monito.* 1991;13:42-45.
20. Yeh TF, Achanti B, Patel H, et al. Indomethacin therapy in premature infants with patent ductus arteriosus—determination of therapeutic plasma levels. *Dev Pharmacol Ther.* 1989;12:169-178.
21. Sperandio M, Beedgen B, Feneberg R. Effectiveness and side effects of an escalating, stepwise approach to indomethacin treatment for symptomatic patent ductus arteriosus in premature infants below 33 weeks gestation. *Pediatrics.* 2005:116:1361-1366.
22. Trissel LA, ed. *Handbook on Injectable Drugs.* 15th ed. Bethesda, MD: American Society of Health-System Pharmacists; 2009.
23. Robinson CA, Sawyer JE. Y-site compatibility of medications with parenteral nutrition. *J Pediatr Pharmacol Ther.* 2009;14:49-57.
24. Cowan F. Indomethacin, patent ductus arteriosus, andcerebral blood flow. *J Pediatr.* 1986;109:341-344.
25. Mardoum R, Bejar R, Merritt A, et al. Controlled study of the effects of indomethacin on cerebral blood flow velocities in newborn infants. *J Pediatr.* 1991;118:112-115.
26. Coombs RC, Morgan ME, Durbin GM, et al. Gut blood flow velocities in newborn: effects of patent ductus arteriosus and parenteral indomethacin. *Arch Dis Child.* 1990;65:1067-1071.
27. Colditz P, Murphy D, Rolfe P, et al. Effect of infusion rate of indomethacin on cerebrovascular response in premature neonates. *Arch Dis Child.* 1989;64:8-12.
28. Van Bel F, Van de Bor M, Stijnen T, et al. Cerebral blood flow velocity changes in preterm infants after single dose of indomethacin: duration of its effect. *Pediatrics.* 1989;84:802-807.
29. Bada HS, Green RS, Pourcyrous M, et al. Indomethacin reduces the risks of severe intraventricular hemorrhage. *J Pediatr.* 1989;115:631-637.
30. Schmidt B, Davis P, Moddemann D, et al. Long-Term Phrophylaxis of Indomethacin in extremely-low-birth-weight infants. *N Eng J Med.* 2001;344:1966-1972.

References

31. Lee J, Rajadaurai VS, Tan KW, et al. Randomized trial of prolonged low-dose versus conventional-dose indomethacin for the treating patent ductus arteriosus in very low birth weight infants. *Pediatrics*. 2003;112:345-350.
32. Herrera CM., Holberton JR, Davis PG. Prolonged versus short course of indomethacin for the treatment of patent ductus arteriosus in preterm infants. *Cochrane Database Syst Rev*. 2007;(2):CD003480.
33. Smyth JM, Colliet PS, Darwish M, et al. Intravenous indomethacin in preterm infants with symptomatic patent ductus arteriosus. A population pharmacokinetic study. *Br J Clin Pharmacol*. 2004;58:249-258.
34. Hosono S, Ohono T, Ojima K, et al. Intractable hypoglycemia following indomethacin therapy for patent ductus arteriosus. *Pediatr Internat*. 2000;42:372-374.
35. Hosono S, Ohono T, Kimoto H, et al. Reduction in blood glucose values following indomethacin therapy for patent ductus arteriosus. *Pediatr Internat*. 1999:41:525-538.
36. Hosono S, Ohono T, Kimoto H, et al. Preventative management of hypoglycemia in very low birthweight infants following indomethacin therapy for patent ductus arteriosus. *Pediatr Internat*. 2001;43:465-468.
37. Mannila A, Kumpulainen E, Lehtonen M, et al. Plasma and cerebrospinal fluid concentrations of indomethacin in children after intravenous administration. *J Clin Pharm*. 2007;47:94-100.
38. Aithal GP, Day CP. Nonsteroidal anti-inflammatory drug induced hepatotoxicity. *Clin Liv Disease*. 2007;11:563-575.
39. Breen EG, McNichole J, Cosgrove E, et al. Fatal hepatitis associated with diclofenac. *Gut*. 1986; 27:1390-1393.
40. Jorgenson HS, Christensen HR, Kampmann JP. Interaction between digoxin and indomethacin or ibuprofen. *Br J Clin Pharmac*. 1991;31: 108-110.
41. Zarfin Y, Koren G, Maresky D. Possible indomethacin—aminoglycoside interaction in preterm infants. *J Pediatr*. 1985;106:511-513.
42. Lam BCC, Wong HN, Yeung CY. Effect of indomethacin on binding of bilirubin to albumin. *Arch Dis Child*. 1990;65:690-691.

Infliximab

1. Available at: http://www.usp.org/hqi/similarProducts/choosy.html. Accessed March 4, 2009.
2. Available at: http://ismp.org/Tools/confuseddrugnames.pdf. Updated April 1, 2005.
3. Prescribing information [Remicade]. Malvern, PA: Centocor Inc; December 2008.
4. Infliximab. Lexi-Comp® Online with AHFS® (database). Bethesda, MD: American Society of Health-System Pharmacists; updated March 10, 2009.
5. Available at: http://www.fda.gov/Drugs/DrugSafety/PostmarketDrugSafetyInformationforPatientsandProviders/ Drug SafetyInformationforPatientsandProviders/ucm109340.htm.
6. Crandall WV, Mackner LM. Infusion reactions to infliximab in children and adolescents: frequency, outcome and a predictive model. *Aliment Pharmacol Ther*. 2003;17:75-84.
7. Friesen CA, Calabro C, Christenson K, et al. Safety of infliximab treatment in pediatric patients with inflammatory bowel disease. *J Pediatr Gastroenterol Nutr*. 2004;39:265-269.
8. Jacobstein DA, Markowitz JE, Kirschner BS, et al. Premedication and infusion reactions with infliximab: results from a pediatric inflammatory bowel disease consortium. *Inflamm Bowel Dis*. 2005;11:442-446.
9. Miele E, Markowitz JE, Mamula P, et al. Human antichimeric antibody in children and young adults with inflammatory bowel disease receiving infliximab. *J Pediatr Gastroenterol Nutr*. 2004;38:502-508.
10. Lamireau T, Cezard JP, Dabadie A, et al. Efficacy and tolerance of infliximab in children and adolescents with Crohn's disease. *Inflamm Bowel Dis*. 2004;10:745-750.
11. Lionetti P, Bronzini P, Salvestrini C, et al. Response to infliximab is related to disease duration in paediatric Crohn's disease. *Aliment Pharmacol Ther*. 2003;18:425-431.
12. Serrano MS, Schmidt-Sommerfeld E, Kilbaugh TJ, et al. Use of infliximab in pediatric patients with inflammatory bowel disease. *Ann Pharmacother*. 2001;35:823-828.
13. Hyams JS, Markowitz J, Wyllie R. Use of infliximab in the treatment of Crohn's disease in children and adolescents. *J Pediatr*. 2000;137:192-196.
14. Stephens MC, Shepanski MA, Mamula P, et al. Safety and steroid-sparing experience using infliximab for Crohn's disease at a pediatric inflammatory bowel disease center. *Am J Gastroenterol*. 2003;98:104-111.
15. deRidder L, Escher JC, Bouquet J, et al. Infliximab therapy in 30 patients with refractory pediatric Crohn disease with and without fistulas in The Netherlands. *J Pediatr Gastroenterol Nutr*. 2004;39:46-52.
16. Borrelli O, Bascietto C, Viola F, et al. Infliximab heals intestinal inflammatory lesions and restores growth in children with Crohn's disease. *Dig Liver Dis*. 2004;36:342-347.
17. Cucchiara S, Romeo E, Viola F, et al. Infliximab for pediatric ulcerative colitis: a retrospective Italian multicenter study. *Dig Liver Dis*. 2008;40S:S260-S264.
18. Hyams J, Crandall W, Kugathasan S, et al. Induction and maintenance infliximab therapy for the treatment of moderate –to-severe Crohn's disease in children. *Gastroenterol*. 2007;132:863-868.
19. Cezard JP, Nouaili N, Talbotec C, et al. A prospective study of the efficacy and tolerance of a chimeric antibody to tumor necrosis factors (Remicade) in severe pediatric Crohn's disease. *J Pediatr Gastroenterol Nutr*. 2003;632-636.
20. Baldassano R, Braegger CP, Escher JC. Infliximab (Remicade) therapy in the treatment of pediatric Crohn's disease. *Am J Gastroenterol*. 2003;98:833-838.
21. Mamula P, Markowitz JE, Brown KA, et al. Infliximab as a novel therapy for pediatric ulcerative colitis. *J Pediatr Gastroenterol Nutr*. 2002;34:307-311.
22. Mamula P, Markowitz JE, Cohen LJ. Infliximab in pediatric ulcerative colitis: two-year follow up. *J Pediatr Gastroenterol Nutr*. 2004;38:298-301.
23. Eidelwein AP, Cuffari C, Abadom V, et al. Infliximab efficacy in pediatric ulcerative colitis. *Inflamm Bowel Dis*. 2005;11(3):213-218.
24. Russell AM, Katz AJ. Infliximab is effective in acute but not chronic childhood ulcerative colitis. *J Pediatr Gastroenterol Nutr*. 2004;39:166-170.
25. Lahdenne P, Vahasalo P, Honkanen V. Infliximab or etanercept in the treatment of children with refractory juvenile idiopathic arthritis: an open label study. *Ann Rheum Dis*. 2003;62:245-247.
26. Gerloni V, Pontikaki I, Gattinara M, et al. Efficacy of repeated intravenous infusions of an anti-tumor necrosis factor α monoclonal antibody, infliximab, in persistently active, refractory juvenile idiopathic arthritis. *Arthritis Rheum*. 2005;52:548-553.
27. Ruperto N, Lovell DJ, Cuttica R, et al. A randomized, placebo controlled trial of infliximab plus methotrexate for the treatment of polyarticular-course juvenile rheumatoid arthritis. *Arthritis Rheum*. 2007;56:3096-3106.
28. Richards JC, Tay-Kearney ML, Murray K, et al. Infliximab for juvenile idiopathic arthritis-associated uveitis. *Clin Experiment Ophthalmol*. 2005;33:461-468.
29. Rajaraman RT, Kimura Y, Li S, et al. Retrospective case review of pediatric patients with uveitis treated with infliximab. *Ophthalmology*. 2006;113:308-314.
30. Burns JC, Mason WH, Hauger SB, et al. Infliximab treatments for refractory Kawasaki syndrome. *J Pediatr*. 2005;146:662-667.
31. Costamagna P, Furst K, Tully K, et al. Tuberculosis associated with blocking agents against tumor necrosis factor-alpha—California, 2002–2003. *MMWR Morb Mortal Wkly Rep*. 2004;53(30):683-686.
32. Foeldvari I, Nielsen S, Kummerle-Deschner J, et al. Tumor necrosis factor-α blocker in treatment of juvenile idiopathic arthritis-associated uveitis refractory to second-line agents: results of a multinational survey. *J Rheumatol*. 2007;34:1146-1150.
33. Tynjala P, Lindal P, Vonkanen V, et al. Infliximab and etanercept in the treatment of chronic uveitis associated with refractory juvenile idiopathic arthritis. *Ann Rheum Dis*. 2007;66:548-550.

References

Insulin

1. Available at: http://ismp.org/Tools/highalertmedications.pdf. ISMP 2008.
2. Available at: http://ismp.org/Tools/confuseddrugnames.pdf. Updated April 1, 2005.
3. Available at: http://www.usp.org/hqi/similarProducts/choosy.html. Accessed July 3, 2009.
4. Insulin human. Lexi-Comp® Online with AHFS® (database). Hudson, OH: Lexi-Comp Inc; updated August 31, 2009.
5. Trissel LA. *Handbook on Injectable Drugs*. 15th ed. Bethesda. MD: American Society of Health-System Pharmacists; 2009.
6. Wolfsdorf J, Glaser N, Sperling MA. Diabetic ketoacidosis in infants, children, and adolescents. A consensus statement from the American Diabetes Association. *Diabetes Care*. 2006;29:1150-1159.
7. Kitabchi AE, Umpierrez GE, Murphy MB, et al. Management of hyperglycemic crises in patients with diabetes. *Diabetes Care*. 2001;24:131-153.
8. American Academy of Pediatrics Committee on Drugs. Emergency drug doses for infants and children. *Pediatrics*. 1998;101:e1-e11.
9. Krane EJ. Diabetic ketoacidosis: biochemistry, physiology, treatment, and prevention. *Pediatr Clin North Am*. 1987;34:935-961.
10. Kecskes SA. Diabetic ketoacidosis. *Pediatr Clin North Am*. 1993;40:355-363.
11. Trachtenbarg DE. Diabetic ketoacidosis. *Am Fam Physician*. 2005;71:1705-1714.
12. Vemgal P, Ohlsson A. Interventions for non-oliguric hyperkalemia in preterm neonates. *Cochrane Database of Systematic Reviews. Cochrane Database Syst Rev*. 2007 Jan 24;1:CD005257.
13. Levy MM, Rhodes A. The ongoing enigma of tight glucose control. *Lancet*. 2009;373:520-521. Comment.
14. Hirshberg E, Lacroix J, Sward K, et al. Blood glucose control in critically ill adults and children. *Chest*. 2008;133:1328-1335.
15. Pham TN, Warren AJ, Phan HH, et al. Impact of tight glycemic control in severely burned children. *J Trauma*. 2005;59:1148-1154.
16. Vlasselaers D, Milants I, Desmet L, et al. Intensive insulin therapy for patients in paediatric intensive care: a prospective, randomised controlled study. *Lancet*. 2009;373:547-556.
17. Beardsall K, Vanhaesebrouck S, Ogilvy-Stuart A, et al. Early insulin therapy in very-low birth-weight infants. *N Engl J Med*. 2008;359:1873-1884.
18. Collins JW Jr, Hoppe M, Brown K, et al. A controlled trial of insulin infusion and parenteral nutrition in extremely low birth weight infants with glucose intolerance. *J Pediatr*. 1991;118:921-927.
19. Binder ND, Raschko PK, Benda GI, et al. Insulin infusion with parenteral nutrition in extremely low birth weight infants with hyperglycemia. *J Pediatr*. 1989;114:273-280.
20. Goldman SL, Hirata T. Attenuated response to insulin in very low birth weight infants. *Pediatr Res*. 1980;14:50-55.
21. Fuloria M, Friedberg MA, DuRant RH, et al. Effect of flow rate and insulin priming on the recovery of insulin from microbore infusion tubing. *Pediatrics*. 1998;102:1401-1406.
22. Ng SM, May JE, Emmerson AJB. Continuous insulin infusion in hyperglycaemic extremely-low-birth-weight neonates. *Biol Neonate*. 2005;87:269-272.
23. Thabet F, Bourgeois J, Guy B, et al. Continuous insulin infusion in hyperglycaemic very-low-birth-weight infants receiving parenteral nutrition. *Clin Nutr*. 2003;22:545-547.
24. Mena P, Llanos A, Uauy R. Insulin homeostasis in the extremely low birth weight infant. *Semin Perinatol*. 2001;25:436-446.
25. Simeon PS, Feggner ME, Levin SR. Continuous insulin infusions in neonates: pharmacologic availability of insulin in intravenous solutions. *J Pediatr*. 1994;124:818-820.
26. Furberg H, Jensen AK, Salbu B. Effect of pretreatment with 0.9% sodium chloride or insulin solutions on the delivery of insulin from an infusion system. *Am J Hosp Pharm*. 1986;43:2209-2213.
27. Bull HB. Adsorption of bovine serum albumin on glass. *Biochemica et Biophysica Acta*. 1956;19:464-472.
28. Alawi KA, Morrison GC, Fraser DD, et al. Insulin infusion via an intraosseous needle in diabetic ketoacidosis. *Anaesth Intensive Care*. 2008;36:110-112.

Interferon Alfa-2b

1. Available at: http://www.usp.org/hqi/similarProducts/choosy.html. Accessed August 13, 2009.
2. Intron A [package insert]. Kenilworth, NJ: Schering Corporation; January 2009.
3. Vajro P, Tedesco M, Fontanella A, et al. Prolonged and high dose recombinant interferon alpha-2b alone or after prednisone priming accelerates termination of active viral replication in children with chronic hepatitis B infection. *Pediatr Infect Dis J*. 1996;15:223-231.
4. Gurakan F, Kocak N, Ozen H, et al. Comparison of standard and high dosage recombinant interferon alpha 2b for treatment of children with chronic hepatitis B infection. *Pediatr Infect Dis J*. 2000;19:52-56.
5. Ruiz-Moreno M, Rua MJ, Molina J, et al. Prospective, randomized controlled trial of interferon-alpha in children with chronic hepatitis B. *Hepatology*. 1991;13:1035-1039.
6. Sokal EM, Wirth S, Goyens P. Interferon alpha-2b therapy in children with chronic hepatitis B. *Gut*. 1993;17:S87-S90.
7. Sokal EM, Conjeevaram HS, Roberts EA, et al. Interferon alpha therapy for chronic hepatitis B in children: a multinational randomized controlled trial. *Gastroenterology*. 1998;114:988-995.
8. Bruguera M, Amat L, Garcia O, et al. Treatment of chronic hepatitis B in children with recombinant alpha interferon. *J Clin Gastroenterol*. 1993:17:296-299.
9. Dikici B, Bosnak M, Kara, IH, et al. Lamivudine and interferon-alpha combination treatment of childhood patients with chronic hepatitis B infection. *Pediatr Infect Dis J*. 2001;20:988-992.
10. Dikici B, Ozgenc F, Kalayci AG, et al. Current therapeutic approaches in childhood chronic hepatitis B infection: a multicenter study. *J Gastroenterol Hepatol*. 2004;19:127-133.
11. Dikici B, Bosnak M, Bosnak V, et al. Comparison of treatments of chronic hepatitis B in children with lamivudine and α-interferon combination and α-interferon alone. *Pediatr Internat*. 2002;44:517-521.
12. Di Marco V, Lo Iacono O, Almasio P, et al. Long-term efficacy of alpha-interferon in beta-thalassemics with chronic hepatitis C. *Blood*. 1997;90:2207-2212.
13. Ruiz-Moreno M, Rua MJ, Castillo I, et al. Treatment of children with chronic hepatitis C with recombinant interferon-alpha: a pilot study. *Hepatology*. 1992;16:882-885.
14. Bortolotti F, Giacchino R, Vajro P, et al. Recombinant interferon-alpha therapy in children with chronic hepatitis C. *Hepatology*. 1995;22:1623-1627.
15. Gonzalez-Peralta RP, Kelly DA, Haber B, et al. Interferon alfa-2b in combination with ribavirin for the treatment of chronic hepatitis C in children: efficacy, safety, and pharmacokinetics. *Hepatology*. 2005;42:1010-1018.
16. Matsuoka S, Mori K, Nakano Y, et al. Efficacy of interferons in treating children with chronic hepatitis C. *Eur J Pediatr*. 1997;156:704-708.
17. Navid F, Furman WL, Fleming M, et al. The feasibility of adjuvant interferon α-2b in children with high-risk melanoma. *Cancer*. 2005;103:780-787.
18. Dubois J, Hershon L, Carmant L, et al. Toxicity profile of interferon alpha-2b in children: a prospective evaluation. *J Pediatr*. 1999;135:782-785.
19. Chang E, Boyd A, Nelson CC, et al. Successful treatment of infantile hemangiomas with interferon-alpha-2b. *J Pediatr Hematol Oncol*. 1997;19:237-244.

20. Tamayo L, Oritz DM, Orozco-Covarrubias L, et al. Therapeutic efficacy of interferon alpha-2b in infants with life-threatening giant hemangiomas. *Arch Dermatol.* 1997;133:1567-1571.
21. Garmendia G, Miranda N, Borroso S, et al. Regression of infancy hemangiomas with recombinant IFN-α2b. *J Interferon Cytokine Res.* 2001;21:31-38.
22. Wananukul S, Nuchprayoon I, Seksarn P. Treatment of Kasabach-Merritt syndrome: a stepwise regimen of prednisolone, dipyridamole, and interferon. *Int J Dermatol.* 2003;42:741-748.
23. Lauer SJ, Ochs J, Pollock BH, et al. Recombinant alpha-2B interferon treatment for childhood T-lymphoblastic disease in relapse. *Cancer.* 1994;74:197-202.
24. Ochs J, Abramowitch M, Rudnick S, et al. Phase I-II study of recombinant alpha-2 interferon against advanced leukemia and lymphoma in children. *J Clin Oncol.* 1986;4:883-887.
25. Iorio R, Pasqualina P, Botta S, et al. Side effects of alpha-interferon therapy and impact on health-related quality of life in children with chronic viral hepatitis. *Pediatr Infect Dis J.* 1997;16:984-990.
26. Williams SJ, Baird-Lambert JA, Farrell GC. Inhibition of theophylline metabolism by interferon. *Lancet.* 1987;2:939-941.

Irinotecan HCl

1. Available at: http://ismp.org/Tools/highalertmedications.pdf. ISMP 2008. Accessed August 27, 2009.
2. Available at: http://www.usp.org/hqi/similarProducts/choosy.html. Accessed August 27, 2009.
3. Camptosar [package insert]. New York, NY: Pfizer; July 2008.
4. Irinotecan. Lexi-Comp® Online with AHFS® (database). Bethesda, MD: American Society of Health-System Pharmacists; updated January 2007.
5. Irinotecan. Lexi-Comp Online with AHFS (database). Hudson, OH: Lexi-Comp Inc; updated October 22, 2009.
6. Cosetti M, Wexler LH, Calleja E, et al. Irinotecan for pediatric solid tumors: the Memorial Sloan Kettering experience. *J Pediatr Hematol Oncol.* 2002;24(2):101-105.
7. Gajjar A, Chintagumpala MM, Bowers DC, et al. Effect of intrapatient dosage escalation of irinotecan on its pharmacokinetics in pediatric patients who have high-grade gliomas and receive enzyme-inducing anticonvulsant therapy. *Cancer.* 2003;97(suppl 9):2374-2380.
8. Blaney S, Berg SL, Pratt C, et al. A phase I study of irinotecan in pediatric patients: a pediatric oncology group study. *Clin Cancer Res.* 2001;7(1):32-37.
9. Vassal G, Giammarile F, Brooks M, et al. A phase II study of irinotecan in children with relapsed or refractory neuroblastoma: a European cooperation of the Societe Francaise d'Oncologie Pediatrique (SFOP) and the United Kingdom Children Cancer Study Group (UKCCSG). *Eur J Cancer.* 2008;44:2453-2460.
10. Levy AS, Meyers PA, Wexler LH, et al. Phase 1 and pharmacokinetic study of concurrent carboplatin and irinotecan in subjects aged 1 to 21 years with refractory solid tumors. *Cancer.* 2009;115:207-216.
11. Bomgaars L, Kerr J, Berg S, et al. A phase I study of irinotecan administered on a weekly schedule in pediatric patients. *Pediatr Blood Cancer.* 2006;46(1):50-55.
12. Solimando DA, ed. *Lexi-Comp's Drug Information Handbook for Oncology.* 4th ed. Hudson, OH: Lexi-Comp; 2004:475-482.
13. Trissel LA, ed. *Handbook on Injectable Drugs.* 15th ed. Bethesda, MD: American Society of Health-System Pharmacists; 2009.
14. van Riel JM, van Groeningen CJ, de Greve J, et al. Continuous infusion of hepatic arterial irinotecan in pretreated patients with colorectal cancer metastatic to the liver. *Ann Oncol.* 2004;15(1):59-63.
15. National Comprehensive Cancer Network (NCCN) Antiemesis Panel Members. NCCN Clinical Practice Guidelines in Oncology. Antiemesis, v.1.2006. Available at www.nccn.org. Last accessed October 3, 2009.
16. Roila F, Feyer P, Maranzamo E, et al. Antiemetics in children receiving chemotherapy. *Support Care Cancer.* 2005;13:129-131.

Iron Dextran

1. Available at: http://www.usp.org/hqi/similarProducts/choosy.html. Accessed August 27, 2009.
2. Dexferrum [package insert]. Shirley, NY: American Regent Inc; August 2008.
3. Fishbane S, Kowalski EA. The comparative safety of intravenous iron dextran, iron saccharate, and sodium ferric gluconate. *Seminars in Dialysis.* 2000;13:381-384.
4. Chertow GM, Mason PD, Vaage-Nilsen O, et al. On the relative safety of parenteral iron formulations. *Nephrol Dial Transplant.* 2004;19:1571-1575.
5. Baile GR, Clark JA, Lane CE, et al. Hypersensitivity reactions and deaths associated with intravenous iron preparations. *Nephrol Dial Transplant.* 2005;20:1443-1449.
6. Fishbane S. Safety in iron management. *Am J Kid Disease.* 2003;41:S18-S36.
7. National Kidney Foundation. KDOQI clinical practice guidelines and clinical practice recommendations for anemia in chronic kidney disease. *Am J Kidney Dis.* 2006;47(suppl 3):S1-S146.
8. National Kidney Foundation. NKR-DOQI clinical practice guidelines for the treatment of anemia of chronic renal failure—dialysis outcomes quality initiative. Available at: http://www.kidney.org/professionals/kdoqi/guidelines_updates/doqiupan_iii.html#8:. Accessed October 6, 2009.
9. Reed MD, Bertino JS, Halpin TC. Use of intravenous iron dextran injection in children receiving total parenteral nutrition. *Am J Dis Child.* 1981;135:829-831.
10. Halpin TC, Bertino JS, Rothstein FC, et al. Iron-deficiency anemia in childhood inflammatory bowel disease: treatment with intravenous iron–dextran. *J Parenter Enteral Nutr.* 1982;6:9-11.
11. Fridge JL, Vichinsky EP. Correction of the anemia of epidermolysis bullosa with intravenous iron and erythropoietin. *J Pediatr.* 1998;132:871-873.
12. Brandt JR, Avner ED, Hickman RO, et al. Safety and efficacy of erythropoietin in children with chronic renal failure. *Pediatr Nephrol.* 1999;13:143-147.
13. Trissel LA, ed. *Handbook on Injectable Drugs.* 15th ed. Bethesda, MD: American Society of Health-System Pharmacists; 2009.
14. Ohls RK, Harcum J, Schibler KR, et al. The effect of erythropoietin on the transfusion requirements of preterm infants <750 grams: a randomized, double-blind, placebo controlled study. *J Pediatr.* 1997;131:661-665.
15. Young TE, Mangum B, eds. *Neofax.* 22nd ed. Montvale, NJ: Thomson Reuters; 2009.
16. Ohls RK, Ehrenkranz RA, Wright LL, et al. Effects of early erythropoietin therapy on the transfusion requirements of preterm infants below 1250 grams birth weight: a multicenter, randomized controlled trial. *Pediatrics.* 2001;108:934-942.
17. Carnielli VP, da Riol R, Montini G. Iron supplementation enhances response to high doses of recombinant human erythropoietin in preterm infants. *Arch Dis Child Fetal Neonatal Ed.* 1998;79:F44-F48.
18. Pollak A, Hayde M, Hayn M, et al. Effect of intravenous iron supplementation on erythropoiesis in erythropoietin-treated premature infants. *Pediatrics.* 2001;107:78-85.
19. Meyer MP, Haworth C, Meyer JH, et al. A comparison of oral and intravenous iron supplementation in preterm infants receiving recombinant erythropoietin. *J Pediatr.* 1996;129:258-263.
20. Zlotkin SH, Stallings VA, Penchary PB. Total parenteral nutrition in children. *Pediatr Clin North Am.* 1985;32:381-400.
21. Wan KK, Tsallas G. Dilute iron dextran formulation for addition to parenteral nutrient solutions. *Am J Hosp Pharm.* 1980;37:206-210.

References

22. Norton JA, Peters ML, Wesley R, et al. Iron supplementation of total parenteral nutrition: a prospective study. *J Parenter Enteral Nutr.* 1983;7:457-461.
23. Warady BA, Kausz A, Lerner G, et al. Iron therapy in the pediatric hemodialysis population. *Pediatr Nephrol.* 2004;19:655-661.
24. Greenbaum LA, Pan CG, Caley C, et al. Intravenous iron dextran and erythropoietin use in pediatric hemodialysis patients. *Pediatr Nephrol.* 2000;14:908-911.
25. Mayhew SL, Quick MW. Compatibility of iron dextran with neonatal parenteral nutrient solutions. *Am J Health-Syst Pharm.* 1995;54:570-571.
26. Tu Y, Knox NL, Biringer JM, et al. Compatibility of iron dextran with total nutrient admixtures. *Am J Hosp Pharm.* 1992;49:2233-2235.
27. Vaughan LM, Small C, Plunkett V. Incompatibility of iron dextran and a total nutrient admixture. *Am J Hosp Pharm.* 1990;47:1745-1746.
28. Cochran EB, Phelps SJ, Helms RA. Parenteral nutrition in pediatric patients. *Clin Pharm.* 1988;7:351-366.
29. Kumpf VJ. Parenteral iron supplementation. *Nutr Clin Pract.* 1996;11:139-146.

Isoproterenol HCl

1. Available at: http://ismp.org/Tools/highalertmedications.pdf. ISMP 2008. Accessed August 27, 2009.
2. Available at: http://www.usp.org/hqi/similarProducts/choosy.html. Accessed August 27, 2009.
3. Isuprel [package insert]. Lake Forest, IL: Hospira Inc; August 2004.
4. Parry WH, Martorano F, Cotton EK. Management of life-threatening asthma with intravenous isoproterenol infusions. *Am J Dis Child.* 1976;130:39-42.
5. Wood DW, Downes JJ. Intravenous isoproterenol in the treatment of respiratory failure in childhood status asthmaticus. *Ann Allergy.* 1973;31:607-610.
6. Matson JR, Loughlin GM, Strunk RC. Myocardial ischemia complicating the use of isoproterenol in asthmatic children. *J Pediatr.* 1978;92:776-778.
7. Page R, Gay W, Friday G, et al. Isoproterenol associated myocardial dysfunction during status asthmaticus. *Ann Allergy.* 1987;57:402-404.
8. Maguire JF, O'Rourke PP, Colan SD, et al. Cardiotoxicity during treatment of severe childhood asthma. *Pediatrics.* 1991;88:1180-1186.
9. Kurland G, Williams J, Lewiston NJ. Fatal myocardial toxicity during continuous infusion intravenous isoproterenol therapy of asthma. *J Allergy Clin Immunol.* 1979;63:407.
10. Drislane FW, Samuels MA, Kozakewich H, et al. Myocardial contractions band lesions in patient with fatal asthma: possible neurocardiologic mechanism. *Am Rev Respir Dis.* 1987;135:498-501.
11. Schleien CL, Setzer NA, McLaughlin GE, et al. Postoperative management of the cardiac surgical patient. In: Rogers MC, ed. *Textbook of Pediatric Intensive Care.* 2nd ed. Baltimore, MD: Lippincott Williams & Wilkins; 1992:467-531.
12. Wetzel RC, Tobin JR. Shock. In: Rogers MC, ed. *Textbook of Pediatric Intensive Care.* 2nd ed. Baltimore, MD: Lippincott Williams & Wilkins; 1992:563-613.
13. Nakazawa M, Takahashi Y, Aiba S, et al. Acute hemodynamic effects of dopamine, dobutamine, and isoproterenol in congested infants or young children with large ventricular septal defect. *Jpn Cir J.* 1987;51:1010-1015.
14. Reyes G, Schwartz PH, Newth CJL, et al. The pharmacokinetics of isoproterenol in critically ill pediatric patients. *J Clin Pharmacol.* 1993;33:29-34.
15. Perkin RM, Anas NG. Cardiovascular evaluation and support in the critically ill child. *Pediatr Ann.* 1986;15:30-41.
16. Perkin RM, Levin DL. Shock in the pediatric patient. Part II. Therapy. *J Pediatr.* 1982;101:319-332.
17. Isoproterenol. Lexi-Comp Online with AHFS (database). Hudson, OH: Lexi-Comp Inc; updated August 13, 2009.
18. Zaritsky A, Chernow B. Use of catecholamines in pediatrics. *J Pediatr.* 1984;105:341-350.
19. National Asthma Education and Prevention Program. Expert panel report 2: guidelines for the diagnosis and management of asthma. Available at: www.nhlbi.nih.gov/guidelines/asthma/asthgdln.htm. Accessed April 20, 2006.
20. Dellinger RP, Carlet JM, Masur H, et al. Surviving Sepsis Campaign guidelines for management of severe sepsis and septic shock. *Crit Care Med.* 2004;32:858-873.
21. Tulloh R. Management and therapeutic options in pediatric pulmonary hypertension. *Expert Rev Cardiovasc Ther.* 2006;4:361-374.
22. Swissa M, Epstein M, Paz O, et al. Head-up tilt table testing in syncope: safety and efficiency of isosorbide versus isoproterenol in pediatric population. *Am Heart J.* 2008;156:477-482.
23. Vlahos AP, Tzoufi M, Katsouras CS, et al. Provocation of neurocardiogenic syncope during head-up tilt testing in children: comparison between isoproterenol and nitroglycerin. *Pediatrics.* 2007;119:e419-e425.
24. Trissel LA, ed. *Handbook on Injectable Drugs.* 15th ed. Bethesda, MD: American Society of Health-System Pharmacists; 2009.
25. Rich DS. New JCAHO medication management standards for 2004. *Am J Health-Syst Pharm.* 2004;61:1349-1358.

Itraconazole

1. Available at: http://www.usp.org/hqi/similarProducts/choosy.html. Accessed August 27, 2009.
2. Sporanox [package insert]. Raritan, NJ: Ortho Biotech Products LP; August 2004.
3. American Academy of Pediatrics. Antifungal drugs for systemic fungal infections. In: Pickering LK, Baker CJ, Kimberlin DW, et al., eds. *2009 Red Book: Report of the Committee on Infectious Diseases.* 28th ed. Elk Grove Village, IL: American Academy of Pediatrics; 2009:765-776.
4. Pandya NA, Atra AA, Riley U, et al. Role of itraconazole in haematology/oncology. *Arch Dis Child.* 2003;88:258-260.
5. Zhou H, Goldman M, Wu J, et al. A pharmacokinetic study if intravenous itraconazole followed by oral administration of itraconazole capsules in patients with advanced human immunodeficiency. *J Clin Pharmacol.* 1998;38:593-562.
6. Trotman RL, Williamson JC, Shoemaker DM, et al. Antibiotic dosing in critically ill adult patients receiving continuous renal replacement therapy. *Clin Infect Dis.* 2005;41:1159-1166.
7. Willems L, van der Geest R, de Beule K. Itraconazole oral solution and intravenous formulations: a review of pharmacokinetics and pharmacodynamics. *J Clin Pharm Ther.* 2001;26:159-169.

Kanamycin Sulfate

1. Snavely SR, Hodges GR. The neurotoxicity of antibacterial agents. *Ann Intern Med.* 1984;101;92-104.
2. Manian FA, Stone WJ, Alford RH. Adverse antibiotic effects associated with renal insufficiency. *Rev Infect Dis.* 1990;12:236-249.
3. American Academy of Pediatrics. Pickering LK, Baker CJ, Kimberlin DW, et al., eds. *2009 Red Book: Report of the Committee on Infectious Diseases.* 28th ed. Elk Grove Village, IL: American Academy of Pediatrics; 2009.
4. Schwartz SN, Pazin GJ, Lyon JA, et al. A controlled investigation of the pharmacokinetics of gentamicin and tobramycin in obese subjects. *J Infect Dis.* 1978;138:499-505.
5. Bauer LA, Blouin RA, Griffen WO, et al. Amikacin pharmacokinetics in morbidly obese patients. *Am J Hosp Pharm.* 1980;37:519-522.
6. Prober CG, Stevenson DK, Benitz WE. The use of antibiotics in neonates weighing less than 1200 grams. *Pediatr Infect Dis J.* 1990;9:111-121.
7. Howard JB, McCracken GH. Reappraisal of kanamycin usage in neonates. *J Pediatr.* 1975;86:949-956.
8. McCracken GH, Threlkeld N. Kanamycin dosage in newborn infants. *J Pediatr.* 1976;89:313-314.

References

9. Kanamycin. In: Kucer A, Crowe SM, Grayson ML, et al., eds. *The Use of Antibiotics: A Clinical Review of Antibacterial, Antifungal and Antiviral Drugs.* 5th ed. Boston, MA: Butterworth Heinemann; 1997:439-449.
10. Aronoff GR, Berns JS, Brier ME, et al. Drug prescribing in renal failure. 4th ed. Available at: http://www.kdpbaptist.louisville.edu/renalbook/. Accessed June 19, 2009.
11. Yow MD, Tengg NE, Bangs J. The ototoxic effects of kanamycin sulfate in infants and children. *J Pediatr.* 1962;60:230-242.
12. Horrevorts AM, de Witte J, Degener JE, et al. Tobramycin in patients with cystic fibrosis. Adjustments in dosing interval for effective treatment. *Chest.* 1987;92:844-848.
13. Kelly HB, Menendez R, Fan L, et al. Pharmacokinetics of tobramycin in cystic fibrosis. *J Pediatr.* 1982;100:318-321.
14. Loirat P, Rohan J, Baillet A, et al. Increased glomerular filtration rate in patients with major burns and its effect on the pharmacokinetics of tobramycin. *N Engl J Med.* 1978;299:915-919.
15. Kanamycin. Lexi-Comp® Online with AHFS® (database). Bethesda, MD: American Society of Health-System Pharmacists; updated March 19, 2009.
16. Trissel LA, ed. *Handbook on Injectable Drugs.* 15th ed. Bethesda, MD: American Society of Health-System Pharmacists; 2009.
17. McLaughlin JE, Reeves DS. Clinical and laboratory evidence for inactivation of gentamicin by carbenicillin. *Lancet.* 1971;1(7693):261-264.
18. Riff LJ, Jackson GG. Laboratory and clinical conditions for gentamicin inactivation by carbenicillin. *Arch Intern Med.* 1972;130:887-981.
19. Manian FA, Stone WJ, Alford RH. Adverse antibiotic effects associated with renal insufficiency. *Rev Infect Dis.* 1990;12:236-249.
20. Davies M, Morgan JR, Anand C. Interactions of carbenicillin and ticarcillin with gentamicin. *Antimicrob Agents Chemother.* 1975;7:431-434.
21. Weibert R, Keane W, Shapiro F. Carbenicillin inactivation of aminoglycosides in patients with severe renal failure. *Trans Amer Soc Artif Int Organs.* 1976;22:439-443.
22. Robinson CA, Sawyer JE. Y-site compatibility of medications with parenteral nutrition. *J Pediatr Pharmacol Ther.* 2009;14:49-57.
23. Gillett AP, Falk RH, Andrews J, et al. Rapid intravenous injection of tobramycin: suggested dosage schedule and concentrations in serum. *J Infect Dis.* 1976;134:S110-S113.
24. Dobbs SM, Mawer GE. Intravenous injection of gentamicin and tobramycin without impairment of hearing. *J Infect Dis.* 1976;134 (Suppl):S114-S117.
25. Mendelson J, Portnoy J, Dick V, et al. Safety of the bolus administration of gentamicin. *Antimicrob Agents Chemother.* 1976;9:633-638.
26. Bodey GP, Chang HY, Rodriguez V, et al. Feasibility of administering aminoglycoside antibiotics by continuous intravenous infusion. *Antimicrob Agents Chemother.* 1975;8:328-333.
27. Powell SH, Thompson WL, Luthe MA, et al. Once daily vs. continuous aminoglycoside dosing: efficacy and toxicity in animal and clinical studies of gentamicin, netilmicin and tobramycin. *J Infect Dis.* 1983;147:918-932.
28. Giacoia GP, Schentag JJ. Pharmacokinetics and nephrotoxicity of continuous intravenous infusion of gentamicin in low birth weight infants. *J Pediatr.* 1986;109:715-719.
29. Hieber JP, Kusmiesz H, Nelson JD. Kanamycin in children: pharmacology and lack of toxicity of an increased dosage regimen. *J Pediatr.* 1980;96:1089-1091.
30. McCracken GH Jr, Threlkeld N, Thomas ML. Intravenous administration of kanamycin and gentamicin in newborn infants. *Pediatrics.* 1977;60:463-466.
31. Massey KL, Hendeles L, Neims A. Identification of children for whom routine monitoring of aminoglycoside serum concentrations is not cost effective. *J Pediatr.* 1986;109:897-901.
32. Logsdon BA, Phelps SJ. Routine monitoring of gentamicin serum concentrations in pediatric patients with normal renal function is unnecessary. *Ann Pharmacother.* 1997;31:1514-1518.
33. Beaubien AR, Desjardins S, Ormsby E, et al. Incidence of amikacin ototoxicity: a sigmoid function of total drug exposure independent of plasma levels. *Am J Otolaryngol.* 1989;10:234-243.
34. Beaubien AR, Ormsby E, Bayne A, et al. Evidence that amikacin ototoxicity is related to total perilymph area under the concentration-time curve regardless of concentration. *Antimicrob Agents Chemother.* 1991;35:1070-1074.
35. Franson TR, Ritch PS, Quebbeman EJ. Aminoglycoside serum concentration sampling via central venous catheters: a potential source of clinical error. *JPEN J Parenter Enteral Nutr.* 1987;11:77-79.

Ketamine HCl

1. Available at: http://ismp.org/Tools/confuseddrugnames.pdf. Updated April 1, 2005.
2. Ketamine hydrochloride injection, USP [product information]. Bedford, OH: Ben Venue Laboratories Inc; January 2008.
3. Green SM, Nakamura R, Johnson NE. Ketamine for sedation for pediatric procedures: part 2, review and implications. *Ann Emerg Med.* 1990;19:1033-1046.
4. Singh A, Girotra S, Mehta Y, et al. Total intravenous anesthesia with ketamine for pediatric interventional cardiac procedures. *J Cardiothorac Vasc Anesth.* 2000;14:36-39.
5. Smith JA, Santer LJ. Respiratory arrest following intramuscular ketamine injection in a 4-year-old child. *Ann Emerg Med.* 1993;22:613-615.
6. American Academy of Pediatrics Committee on Drugs. Emergency drug doses for infants and children. *Pediatrics.* 1998;101:e1-e11.
7. Slonim AD, Ognibene FP. Amnestic agents in pediatric bronchoscopy. *Chest.* 1999;116:1802-1808.
8. Hostetler MA, Davis CO. Prospective age-based comparison of behavioral reactions occurring after ketamine sedation in the ED. *Am J Emerg Med.* 2002;20:463-468.
9. Tobias JD. Sedation and analgesia in paediatric intensive care units. *Paediatr Drugs.* 1999;1:109-126.
10. Lin C, Durieux ME. Ketamine and kids: an update. *Paediatr Anaesth.* 2005;15:91-97.
11. Tugrul M, Camci E, Pembeci K, et al. Ketamine infusion versus isoflurane for the maintenance of anesthesia in the pre bypass period in children with tetralogy of Fallot. *J Cardiothorac Vasc Anesth.* 2000;14:557-561.
12. Aouad MT, Moussa AR, Dagher CM, et al. Addition of ketamine to propofol for initiation of procedural anesthesia in children reduces propofol comsumption and preserves hemodynamic stability. *Acta Anaesthesiol Scand.* 2008;52:561-565.
13. Langston WT, Wathen JE, Roback MG, Bajaj L. Effect of ondansetron on the incidence of vomiting associated with ketamine sedation in children: a double-blind, randomized, placebo-controlled trial. *Ann Emerg Med.* 2008;52:30-34.
14. Ramchandra DS, Anisya V, Gourie-Devi M. Ketamine monoanaesthesia for diagnostic muscle biopsy in neuromuscular disorders in infancy and childhood: floppy infant syndrome. *Can J Anaesth.* 1990;37:474-476.
15. Pruitt JW, Goldwasser MS, Sabol SR, et al. Intramuscular ketamine, midazolam, glycopyrrolate for pediatric sedation in the emergency department. *J Oral Maxillofac Surg.* 1995;53:13-17.
16. Petrack EM, Marx CM, Wright MS. Intramuscular ketamine is superior to meperidine, promethazine and chlorpromazine for pediatric emergency department sedation. *Arch Pediatr Adolesc Med.* 1996;150:676-681.
17. Epstein FB. Ketamine dissociative sedation in pediatric emergency medical practice. *Am J Emerg Med.* 1993;11:180-182.
18. Hartvig P, Larsson E, Joachimsson PO. Postoperative analgesia and sedation following pediatric cardiac surgery using a constant infusion of ketamine. *J Cardiothorac Vasc Anesth.* 1993;7:148-153.
19. Tobias JD, Martin LD, Wetzel RC. Ketamine by continuous infusion for sedation in the pediatric intensive care unit. *Crit Care Med.* 1990;18:819-821.
20. Nehama I, Pass R, Bech Her-Karsch A, et al. Continuous ketamine infusion for the treatment of refractory asthma in a mechanically ventilated infant: case report and review of the pediatric literature. *Pediatr Emerg Care.* 1996;12:294-297.

References

21. Youssef-Ahmed MZ, Silver P, Nimkoff L, et al. Continuous infusion of ketamine in mechanically ventilated children with refractory bronchospasm. *Intensive Care Med.* 1996;22:972-976.
22. Denmark TK, Crane HA, Brown L. Ketamine to avoid mechanical ventilation in severe pediatric asthma. *J Emerg Med.* 2006;30(2):163-166.
23. Ito H, Sobue K, Hirate J, et al. Use of ketamine to facilitate opioid withdrawal in a child. *Anethesiology.* 2006;104:1113.
24. Reich DL, Silvay G. Ketamine: an update on the first twenty-five years of clinical experience. *Can J Anaesth.* 1989;36:2:186-197.
25. Aronoff GR, Berns JS, Brier ME, et al. Drug prescribing in renal failure. 4th ed. Available at: http://www.kdp-baptist.louisville.edu/renalbook/pediatric/. Accessed October 12, 2009.
26. Trissel LA, ed. *Handbook on Injectable Drugs.* 15th ed. Bethesda, MD: American Society of Health-System Pharmacists; 2009.
27. Klepstad P, Borchgrevink P, Hval B, et al. Long-term treatment with ketamine in a 12-year-old girl with severe neuropathic pain caused by a cervical spinal tumor. *J Pediatr Hematol Oncol.* 2001;23:616-619.
28. Green SM, Rothrock SG, Lynch EL, et al. Intramuscular ketamine for pediatric sedation in the emergency department: safety profile in 1,022 cases. *Ann Emerg Med.* 1998;31:688-697.
29. Melendez E, Bachur R. Serious adverse events during procedural sedation with ketamine. *Pediatr Emerg Care.* 2009;25:325-328.
30. Thorp AW, Brown L, Green SM. Ketamine-associated vomiting. Is it dose-related? *Pediatr Emerg Care.* 2009;25:15-18.
31. Roback MG, Wathen JE, Bajaj L, Bothner JP. Adverse events associated with procedural sedation and analgesia in a pediatric emergency department: a comparison of common parenteral drugs. *Acad Emerg Med.* 2005;12:508-513.
32. Pandey CK, Mathur N, Singh N, et al. Fulminant pulmonary edema after intramuscular ketamine. *Can J Anesth.* 2000;47:894-896.

Ketorolac Tromethamine

1. Available at: http://www.usp.org/hqi/similarProducts/choosy.html. Accessed October 12, 2009.
2. Available at: http://ismp.org/Tools/confuseddrugnames.pdf. Updated April 1, 2005.
3. Ketorolac tromethamine injection, USP [prescribing information]. Schaumburg, IL: APP Pharmaceuticals LLC; April 2008.
4. Forrest JB, Heitlinger EL, Revell S. Ketorolac for postoperative pain management in children. *Drug Safety.* 1997;16:309-329.
5. Dsida RM, Wheeler M, Birmingham PK, et al. Age-stratified pharmacokinetics of ketorolac tromethamine in pediatric surgical patients. *Anesth Analg.* 2002;94:266-270.
6. Munro HM, Walton S, Malviya S, et al. Low-dose ketorolac improves analgesia and reduces morphine requirements following posterior or spinal fusion in adolescents. *Can J Anesth.* 2002;49:461-466.
7. Hackmann T. Smaller dose of 0.5 mg/kg IV ketorolac is sufficient to provide pain relief in children. *Anesth Analg.* 2004;98:275-276.
8. Watcha MF, Jones MB, Lagueruela RG, et al. Comparison of ketorolac and morphine as adjuvants during pediatric surgery. *Anesthesiology.* 1992;76:368-372.
9. Bean JD, Hunt R, Custer MD. Effects of ketorolac on postoperative analgesia and bleeding time in children. *Anesthesiology.* 1993;79:A1190.
10. Vetter TR, Heiner EJ. Intravenous ketorolac as an adjuvant to pediatric patient-controlled analgesia with morphine. *J Clin Anesth.* 1994;6:110-113.
11. Richter RL, Valley RD, Bailey AG, et al. A comparison of intraoperative ketorolac, morphine and saline on postoperative analgesia in the pediatric patient. *Anesthesiology.* 1992;77:A1161.
12. Splinter WM, Reid CW, Roberts DJ, et al. Reducing pain after inguinal hernia repair in children. *Anesthesiology.* 1997;87:542-546.
13. Romsing J, Ostergaard D, Walther-Larsen S, et al. Analgesic efficacy and safety of preoperative versus postoperative ketorolac in paediatric tonsillectomy. *Acta Anaesthesiol Scand.* 1998;42:770-775.
14. Shende D, Das K. Comparative effects of intravenous ketorolac and pethidine on perioperative analgesia and postoperative nausea and vomiting (PONV) for pediatric strabismus surgery. *Acta Anaesthesiol Scand.* 1999;43:265-269.
15. Maunuksela EL, Kokki H, Bullingham RES. Comparison of intravenous ketorolac with morphine for postoperative pain in children. *Clin Pharmacol Ther.* 1992;52:436-443.
16. Olkkola KT, Maunuksela EL. The pharmacokinetics of postoperative intravenous ketorolac tromethamine in children. *Br J Clin Pharmacol.* 1991;31:182-184.
17. Lieh-Lai, MW, Kaufmann RE, Uy HG, et al. A randomized comparison of ketorolac tromethamine and morphine for postoperative analgesia in critically ill children. *Crit Care Med.* 1999;27:2786-2791.
18. Gunter JB, Varughese AM, Harrington JF, et al. Recovery and complications after tonsillectomy in children: a comparison of ketorolac and morphine. *Anesth Analg.* 1995;81:1136-1141.
19. Rusy LM, Houck CS, Sullivan LJ, et al. A double-blind evaluation of ketorolac tromethamine versus acetaminophen in pediatric tonsillectomy: analgesia and bleeding. *Anesth Analg.* 1995;80:226-229
20. Papacci P, De Francisci G, Iacobucci T, et al. Use of intravenous ketorolac in the neonate and premature babies. *Paediatr Anaesth.* 2004;14:487-492.
21. Buck ML. Clinical experience with ketorolac in children. *Ann Pharmacother.* 1994;28:1009-1013.
22. Burd RS, Tobias JS. Ketorolac for pain management after abdominal surgical procedures in infants. *South Med J.* 2002;95:331-333.
23. Gerhardt RT, Gerhardt DM. Intravenous ketorolac in the treatment of fever. *Am J Emerg Med.* 2000;18:500-501.
24. Park JM, Houck CS, Sethna NF, et al. Ketorolac suppresses postoperative bladder spasms after pediatric ureteral reimplantation. *Anesth Analg.* 2000;91:11-15.
25. Brousseau DC, Duffy SJ, Anderson AC, et al. Treatment of pediatric migraine headaches: a randomized, double-blind trial of prochlorperazine versus ketorolac. *Ann Emerg Med.* 2004;43:256-262.
26. Harwick WE Jr, Givens TG, Monroe KW, et al. Effect of ketorolac in pediatric sickle cell vaso-occlusive pain crisis. *Pediatr Emerg Care.* 1999;15:179-182.
27. Suresh S, Wheeler M, Patel A. Case series: IV regional anesthesia with ketorolac and lidocaine: is it effective for the management of complex regional pain syndrome 1 in children and adolescents? *Anesth Analg.* 2003;96:694-695
28. Aronoff GR, Berns JS, Brier ME, et al. Drug prescribing in renal failure. 4th ed. Available at: http://www.kdp-baptist.louisville.edu/renalbook/pediatric/. Accessed October 12, 2009.
29. Trissel LA, ed. *Handbook on Injectable Drugs.* 15th ed. Bethesda, MD: American Society of Health-System Pharmacists; 2009.
30. Jung D, Mroszczak E, Bynum L. Pharmacokinetics of ketorolac tromethamine in humans after intravenous, intramuscular, and oral administration. *Eur J Clin Pharmacol.* 1988;35:423-425.

L-Cysteine HCl

1. L-cysteine hydrochloride injection [USP package insert] Irvine, CA: Gensia Sicor Pharmaceuticals Inc; July 2004.
2. Helms RA, Storm MC, Christensen ML, et al. Cysteine supplementation results in normalization of plasma taurine concentrations in children receiving home parenteral nutrition. *J Pediatr.* 1999;134:358-361.
3. Shew SB, Keshen TH, Jahoor F, et al. Assessment of cysteine synthesis in very low-birth weight neonates using a [$^{13}C_6$]glucose tracer. *J Pediatr Surg.* 2005;40:52-56.
4. Heird WC, Hay W, Helms RA, et al. Pediatric parenteral amino acid mixture in low birth weight infants. *Pediatrics.* 1988;81:41-50.
5. Laine L, Shulman RJ, Pitre D, et al. Cysteine usage increases the need for acetate in neonates who receive parenteral nutrition. *Am J Clin Nutr.* 1991;54:565-567.

6. Schmidt GL, Baumgartner TG, Fischlschweiger W, et al. Cost containment using cysteine HCl acidification to increase calcium/phosphate solubility in hyperalimentation solutions. *JPEN J Parenter Enteral Nutr.* 1986;10:203-207.

Labetalol HCl

1. Available at: http://ismp.org/Tools/highalertmedications.pdf. Accessed June 19, 2009.
2. Available at: http://www.usp.org/hqi/similarProducts/choosy.html. Accessed June 19, 2009.
3. Labetalol. Lexi-Comp® Online with AHFS® (database). Bethesda, MD: American Society of Health-System Pharmacists; updated March 19, 2009.
4. Hanna JD, Chan JC, Gill JR. Hypertension and the kidney. *J Pediatr.* 1991;118:327-340.
5. National High Blood Pressure Education Program Working Group on High Blood Pressure in Children and Adolescents. The fourth report on the diagnosis, evaluation, and treatment of high blood pressure in children and adolescents. *Pediatrics.* 2004:114(2 suppl 4th Report):555-576.
6. Bunchman TE, Lynch RE, Wood EG. Intravenously administered labetalol for treatment of hypertension in children. *J Pediatr.* 1992;120:140-144.
7. Deal JE, Barratt TM, Dillion MJ. Management of hypertensive emergencies. *Arch Dis Child.* 1992;67:1089-1092.
8. Ishisaka DY, Toman CS, Housel BF. Labetalol treatment of hypertension in a child. *Clin Pharm.* 1991;10:500-501.
9. Michael J, Groshong T, Tobuas JD. Nicardipine for hypertensive emergencies in children with renal disease. *Pediatr Nephrol.* 1998;12:40-42.
10. Trissel LA, ed. *Handbook on Injectable Drugs.* 15th ed. Bethesda, MD: American Society of Health-System Pharmacists; 2009.

Lansoprazole

1. Available at: http://www.usp.org/hqi/similarProducts/choosy.html. Accessed August 17, 2009.
2. Prevacid IV for Injection [package insert]. Deerfield, IL: Takeda Pharmaceuticals America Inc; July 2008.
3. Kovacs TO, Lee CQ, Chiu YL, et al. Intravenous and oral lansoprazole are equivalent in suppressing stimulated acid output in patient volunteers with erosive esophagitis. *Aliment Pharmacol Ther.* 2004;20:883-889.
4. Faure C, Michaud L, Shaghaghi EK, et al. Lansoprazole in children: pharmacokinetics and efficacy in reflux oesophagitis. *Aliment Pharmacol Ther.* 2001;15:1397-1402.
5. Franco MT, Salvia G, Terrin G, et al. Lansoprazole in the treatment of gastro-oesophageal reflux disease in childhood. *Dig Liver Dis.* 2000;32(8):660-666.
6. Gibbons TE, Gold BD. The use of proton pump inhibitors in children: a comprehensive review. *Pediatr Drugs.* 2003;5(1):25-40.
7. Heyman MB, Zhang W, Huang B, et al. Pharmacokinetics and pharmacodynamics of lansoprazole in children 13 to 24 months old with gastroesophageal reflux disease. *J Pediatr Gastroenterol Nutr.* 2007;44:35-40.
8. Tran A, Rey E, Pons G. Pharmacokinetic-pharmacodynamic study of oral lansoprazole in children. *Clin Pharmacol Ther.* 2002;71:359-367.
9. Zhang W, Kukulka M, Atkinson S, et al. Age-dependent pharmacokinetics of lansoprazole in neonates and infants. *Pediatr Drugs.* 2008;10(4):265-274.
10. Springer M, Atkinson, S, Raanan M, et al. Safety and pharmacodynamics of lansoprazole in patients with gastroesophageal reflux disease aged <1 year. *Pediatr Drugs.* 2008;10(4):255-263.
11. Khoshoo V, Dhume P. Clinical response to 2 dosing regimens of lansoprazole in infants with gastroesophageal reflux. *J Pediatr Gastroenterol Nutr.* 2008;46:352-354.
12. Orenstein SR, Hassall E, Furmaga-Jablonska W, et al. Multicenter, double-blind, randomized, placebo-controlled trial assessing the efficacy and safety of proton pump inhibitor lansoprazole in infants with symptoms of gastroesophageal reflux disease. *J Pediatr.* 2009;154:514-520.
13. Aronoff GR, Berns JS, Brier ME, et al. Drug prescribing in renal failure. 4th ed. Available at: http://www.kdp-baptist.louisville.edu/renalbook/. Accessed October 27, 2009.
14. Haber M, Hassall E, Hayman MB, et al. Correlation of endoscopic and histologic findings in children with erosive and nonerosive esophagitis pre- and post-treatment. *J Pediatr Gastroenterol Nutr.* 2001;33(3):423.
15. Tolia V, Fitzgerald J, Hassall E, et al. Safety of lansoprazole in the treatment of gastroesophageal reflux disease in children. *J Pediatr Gastroenterol Nutr.* 2002;35(4):S300-S307.
16. Tolia V, Ferry G, Gunasekaran T, et al. Efficacy of lansoprazole in the treatment of gastroesophageal reflux disease in children. *J Pediatr Gastroenterol Nutr.* 2002;35(4):S308-S318.
17. Croom KF, Scott LJ. Lansoprazole in the treatment of gastro-oesophageal reflux disease in children and adolescents. *Drugs.* 2005;65(15):2129-2135.
18. Scott LJ. Lansoprazole in the management of gastroesophageal reflux disease in children. *Pediatr Drugs.* 2003;5(1)57-61.
19. Gremse D, Winter H, Tolia V, et al. Pharmacokinetics and pharmacodynamics of lansoprazole in children with gastroesophageal reflux disease. *J Pediatr Gastro Nutr.* 2002;35:S319-S326.
20. Fiedorek S, Tolia V, Gold BD, et al. Efficacy and safety of lansoprazole in adolescents with symptomatic erosive and non-erosive gastroesophageal reflux disease. *J Pediatr Gastroenterol Nutr.* 2005;40:319-327.
21. Litalien C, Theoret Y, Faure C. Pharmacokinetics of proton pump inhibitors in children. *Clin Pharmacokinet.* 2005;44:441-466.
22. Metz DC, Amer F, Hunt B, et al. Lansoprazole regimens that sustain intragastric pH >6.0: an evaluation of intermittent oral and continuous intravenous infusion dosages. *Aliment Pharmacol Ther.* 2006;23:985-995.
23. Canani RB, Cirillo P, Roggero P, et al. Therapy with gastric acidity inhibitors increases the risk of acute gastroenteritis and community-acquired pneumonia in children. *Pediatrics.* 2006;117:817-820.
24. Hirschowitz BI, Worthington J, Mohnen J. Vitamin B12 deficiency in hypersecretors during long-term acid suppression with proton pump inhibitors. *Aliment Pharmacol Ther.* 2008;27:1110-1121.
25. Last EJ, Sheehan AH. Review of recent evidence: potential interaction between clopidogrel and proton pump inhibitors. *Am J Health-Syst Pharm* .2009;66:e11-e16.

Levetiracetam

1. Available at: http://www.usp.org/hqi/similarProducts/choosy.html.
2. Levetiracetam. Lexi-Comp® Online with AHFS® (database). Hudson, OH: Lexi-Comp Inc; updated September 15, 2009.
3. Levetiracetam [package insert]. Smyrna, GA: UCB Inc; 2008.
4. Michaelides C, Thibert RL, Shapiro MJ, et al. Tolerability and dosing experience of intravenous levetiracetam in children and infants. *Epilepsy Res.* 2008;81:143-147.
5. Kirmani BF, Crisp ED, Kayani S, Rajab H. Role of intravenous levetiracetam in acute seizure management of children. *Pediatr Neurol.* 2009;41:37-39.
6. Goraya JS, Khurana DS, Valencia I, et al. Intravenous levetiracetam in children with epilepsy. *Pediatr Neurol.* 2008;38:177-180.
7. Cilio MR, Bianchi R, Balestri M, et al. Intravenous levetiracetam terminates refractory status epilepticus in two patients with migrating partial seizures in infancy. *Epilepsy Res.* 2009;86:66-71.
8. Abend NS, Monk HM, Licht DJ, Dlugos DJ. Intravenous levetiracetam in critically ill children with status epilepticus or acute repetitive seizures. *Pediatr Crit Care Med.* 2009;10:505-510.

References

9. Aronoff GR, Berns JS, Brier ME, et al. Drug prescribing in renal failure. 4th ed. Available at: http://www.kdp-baptist.louisville.edu/renalbook/. Accessed October 31, 2009.
10. Available at: http://www.fda.gov/Safety/MedWatch/SafetyInformation/SafetyAlertsforHumanMedicalProducts/ucm074939.htm. Accessed October 31, 2009.
11. French J, Edrich P, Cramer JA. A systematic review of the safety profile of levetiracetam: a new antiepileptic drug. *Epilepsy Res.* 2001;47: 77-90.
12. Arroyo S, Crawford P. Safety profile of levetiracetam. *Epileptic Disor.* 2003;5 (Suppl 1):S57-S63.
13. Patsalos PN. Pharmacokinetic profile of levetiracetam: toward ideal characteristics. *Pharmacol Ther.* 2000;85:77-85.

Levocarnitine

1. Available at: http://www.usp.org/hqi/similarProducts/choosy.html. Accessed August 27, 2009.
2. Carnitor [package insert]. Gaithersburg, MD: Sigma-Tau Pharmaceuticals Inc; March 2004.
3. Crill CM, Helms RA. The use of carnitine in pediatric nutrition. *Nutr Clin Pract.* 2007;22:204-213.
4. Goa, KL, Brogden RN. L-carnitine, a preliminary review of its pharmacokinetics, and its therapeutic use in ischemic cardiac disease and primary and secondary carnitine deficiencies in relationship to its role in fatty acid metabolism. *Drugs.* 1987;34:1-24.
5. Zachwieja J, Duran M, Joles JA, et al. Amino acid and carnitine supplementation in haemodialysed children. *Pediatr Nephrol.* 1994;8:739-743.
6. Berard E, Iordache A, Barrillon D, et al. L-carnitine in dialysed patients: the choice of dosage regimen. *Int J Clin Pharmacol Res.* 1995;15:127-133.
7. Berard E, Iordache A. Effect of low doses of L-carnitine on the response to recombinant human erythropoietin in hemodialyzed children: about two cases. *Nephron.* 992;62:368-369.
8. Gloggler A, Bulla M, Furst P. Effect of low dose supplementation of L-carnitine on lipid metabolism in hemodialyzed children. *Kidney Int Suppl.* 1989;27:256-258.
9. National Kidney Foundation. Clinical practice recommendations for anemia in chronic kidney disease in children. *Am J Kidney Dis.* 2006;47:S86-S108.
10. Van Hove JLK, Kahler D, Millington DS, et al. Intravenous L-carnitine and acetyl-L-carnitine in medium chain acyl-coenzyme A dehydrogenase deficiency and isovaleric acidemia. *Pediatr Res.* 1994;35:96-101.
11. Schmidt-Sommerfeld E, Penn D, Wolf H. Carnitine deficiency in premature infants receiving total parenteral nutrition: effect of L-carnitine supplementation. *J Pediatr.* 1983;102:931-935.
12. Bonner CM, DeBrie KL, Hug G, et al. Effects of parenteral L-carnitine supplementation on fat metabolism and nutrition in premature neonates. *J Pediatr.* 1995;126:287-292.
13. Helms RA, Mauer EC, Hay WW, et al. Effect of intravenous L-carnitine on growth parameters and fat metabolism during parenteral nutrition in premature neonates. *J Parenter Enteral Nutr.* 1990;14:448-453.
14. Shortland GJ, Walter JH, Stroud C, et al. Randomised controlled trial of L-carnitine as a nutritional supplement in preterm infants. *Arch Dis Child Fetal Neonatal Ed.* 1998;78:185-188.
15. O'Donnell, Finer NN, Rich W, et al. Role of L-carnitine in apnea of prematurity: a randomized, controlled trial. *Pediatrics.* 2002;109:622-626.
16. Whitfield J, Smith T, Sollohub H, et al. Clinical effects of L-carnitine supplementation on apnea and growth in very low birth weight infants. *Pediatrics.* 2003;111:477-482.
17. Pande S, Brio LP, Campbell DE, et al. Lack of effect of L-carnitine supplementation on weight gain in very preterm infants. *J Perinatol.* 2005;25:470-477.
18. Crill CM, Storm MC, Christensen ML, et al. Carnitine supplementation in premature neonates: effect on plasma and red blood cell total carnitine concentrations, nutrition parameters and morbidity. *Clin Nutr.* 2006;25:886-896.
19. DeVivo DC, Bohan TP, Coulter DL, et al. L-Carnitine supplementation in childhood epilepsy: current perspectives. *Epilepsia.* 1998;1216-1225.
20. Raskind JY, El-Chaar GM. The role of carnitine supplementation during valproic acid therapy. *Ann Pharmacother.* 2000;34:630-638.
21. Bohles H, Sewell AC, Wenzel D, et al. The effect of carnitine supplementation in valproate-induced hyperammonaemia. *Acta Paediatr.* 1996;85:446-449.
22. Sulkers EJ, Lafeber HN, Degenhart HJ, et al. Effects of high carnitine supplementation on substrate utilization in low-birth-weight infants receiving total parenteral nutrition. *Am J Clin Nutr.* 1990;52:889-894.
23. Storm MC, Wang B, Helms RA. Stability of carnitine in pediatric TPN and TNA formulations. *J Parenter Enteral Nutr.* 1998;22:S18.
24. Bullock L, Fitzgerald JF, Walter WV. Emulsion stability in total nutrient admixtures containing a pediatric amino acid formulation. *J Parenter Enteral Nutr.* 1992;16:64-68.
25. Helton E, Darragh R, Francis P, et al. Metabolic aspects of myocardial disease and a role for L-carnitine in the treatment of childhood cardiomyopathy. *Pediatrics.* 2000;105:1260-1270.
26. Carter RW, Singh J, Archambault C, et al. Severe lactic acidosis in association with reverse transcriptase inhibitors with potential response to L-carnitine in a pediatric HIV-positive patient. *AIDS Patient Care STDS.* 2004;18:131-134.

Levothyroxine Sodium

1. Available at: http://ismp.org/Tools/confuseddrugnames.pdf. Accessed August 27, 2009.
2. Available at: http://www.usp.org/hqi/similarProducts/choosy.html. Accessed August 27, 2009.
3. Levothyroxine sodium [package insert]. Schaumberg, IL: APP Pharmaceuticals LLC; January 2008.
4. Levothyroxine sodium. Lexi-Comp Online with AHFS (database). Bethesda, MD: American Society of Health-System Pharmacists; 2009. Accessed September 13, 2009.
5. Young TE, Mangum B, eds. *Neofax.* 22nd ed. Montvale, NJ: Thomson Reuters; 2009.
6. American Academy of Pediatrics. Update of newborn screening and therapy for congenital hypothyroidism. *Pediatrics.* 2006;117:2290-2303.
7. Trissel LA, ed. *Handbook on Injectable Drugs.* 15th ed. Bethesda, MD: American Society of Health-System Pharmacists; 2009.
8. Pagliaro LA, Pagliaro AM, eds. *Problems in Pediatric Drug Therapy.* 2nd ed. Hamilton, IL: Drug Intelligence Publications; 1987.
9. Raghavan S, DiMartino J, Saenger P, et al. Pseudotumor cerebri in an infant and l-thyroxine therapy for transient neonatal hypothyroidism. *J Pediatr.* 1997;120:481-483.
10. Fisher DA. The importance of early management in optimizing IQ in infants with congenital hypothyroidism. *J Pediatr.* 2000;136:273-274.
11. Dubuis JM, Glorieux J, Richer F, et al. Outcome of severe congenital hypothyroidism: closing the developmental gap with early high dose levothyroxine treatment. *J Clin Endocrin Meta.* 1996;81:222-227.
12. Zuppa AF, Nadkarni V, Davis L, et al. The effect of a thyroid hormone infusion on vasopressor support in critically ill children with cessation of neurologic function. *Crit Care Med.* 2004;32:2318-2322.

Lidocaine HCl

1. Available at: http://ismp.org/Tools/highalertmedications.pdf. Accessed September 19, 2009.
2. Available at: http://www.usp.org/hqi/similarProducts/choosy.html. Accessed September 19, 2009.

References

3. Lidocaine [package insert]. Lake Forest, IL; Hospira Inc; 2004.
4. American Heart Association. Guidelines 2005 for cardiopulmonary resuscitation and emergency cardiovascular care.—part 12: pediatric advanced life support. *Circulation*. 2005;112:167-187.
5. American Academy of Pediatrics Committee on Drugs. Emergency drug doses for infants and children. *Pediatrics*.1998;101:e1-e11.
6. Lidocaine. Lexi-Comp® Online with AHFS® (database). Hudson, OH: Lexi-Comp Inc; updated September 17, 2009.
7. Ramsey RE. Treatment of status epilepticus. *Epilepsia*. 1993;34:S71-S81.
8. Aggarwal P, Wali JP. Lidocaine in refractory status epilepticus: a forgotten drug in the emergency department. *Am J Emerg Med*. 1993;2:243-244.
9. van Rooij LG, Toet MC, Rademaker KM, et al. Cardiac arrhythmias in neonates receiving lidocaine as anticonvulsive treatment. *Eur J Pediatr*. 2004;163:637-641.
10. Sawaishi Y, Yano T, Enoki M, et al. Lidocaine-dependent early infantile status epilepticus with highly suppressed EEG. *Epilepsia*. 2002;43:201-204.
11. Kobayashi K, Ito M, Miyajima T, et al. Successful management of intractable epilepsy with intravenous lidocaine and lidocaine tapes. *Pediatr Neurol*. 1999;21:476-480.
12. Hellstrom-Westas L, Westgren U, Svenningsen NW, et al. Lidocaine for treatment of severe seizures in newborn infants. *Acta Pediatr Scand*. 1988;77:79-84.
13. Hamano S, Sugiyama N, Yamashita S, et al. Intravenous lidocaine for status epilepticus during childhood. *Dev Med Child Neurol*. 2006;48:220-222.
14. Pascual J, Ciudad J, Berciano J. Role of lidocaine (lignocaine) in managing status epilepticus. *J Neurol Neurosurg Psychiatry*. 1992;55:49-51.
15. Shany E, Benzaquen O, Watermberg N. Comparison of continuious drip midazolam or lidocaine in the treatment of intractable neonatal seizures. *J Child Neurol*. 2007;22:255-259.
16. Hattori H, Yamano T, Hayashi K, et al. Effectiveness of lidocaine infusion for status epilepticus in childhood: a retrospective multi-institutional study in Japan. *Brain Dev*. 2008;30:504-512.
17. Bedford RF, Persing JA, Pobereskin L, et al. Lidocaine or thiopental for rapid control of intracranial hypertension. *Anesth Analg*. 1980;59:435-437.
18. Brucia JJ, Owen DC, Rudy EB. The effects of lidocaine on intracranial hypertension. *J Neurosci Nurs*. 1992;24:205-214.
19. Wallace MS, Lee J, Sorkin L, et al. Intravenous lidocaine: effects on controlling pain after Anti-GD2 antibody therapy in children with neuroblastoma—a report of a series. *Anesth Analg*. 1997;85:794-796.
20. Pentel P, Benowitz N. Pharmacokinetic and pharmacodynamic considerations in drug therapy of cardiac emergencies. *Clin Pharmacokinet*. 1984;9:273-308.
21. Thomson PD, Melmon KL, Richardson JA, et al. Lidocaine pharmacokinetics in advanced heart failure, liver disease, and renal failure in humans. *Ann Intern Med*. 1973;78:499-508.
22. Aronoff GR, Berns JS, Brier ME, et al. Drug prescribing in renal failure. 4th ed. Available at: http://www.kdp-baptist.louisville.edu/renalbook/. Accessed September 19, 2009.
23. Orlowski JP. Cardiopulmonary resuscitation in children. *Pediatr Clin North Am*. 1980;27:495-512.
24. Trissel LA, ed. *Handbook on Injectable Drugs*. 15th ed. Bethesda, MD: American Society of Health-System Pharmacists; 2009.
25. Robinson CA, Sawyer JE. Y-site compatibility of medications with parenteral nutrition. *J Pediatr Pharmacol Ther*. 2009;14:49-57.
26. Berger I, Steinberg A, Schlesinger Y, et al. Neonatal mydriasis: intravenous lidocaine adverse reaction. *J Child Neurol*. 2002;17:400-401.
27. Burches BR, Jr. Warner DO. Brochospasm after intravenous lidocaine. *Anesth Analg*. 2008;107:1260-1262.

Linezolid

1. Available at: http://www.usp.org/hqi/similarProducts/choosy.html. Accessed October 18, 2009.
2. Linezolid [package insert]. New York, NY: Pharmacia and Upjohn Company, Division of Pfizer; July 2008.
3. American Academy of Pediatrics. In: Pickering LK, ed. *2009 Red Book: Report of the Committee on Infectious Diseases*. 28th ed. Elk Grove Village, IL: American Academy of Pediatrics; 2009:746, 753.
4. Kearns GL, Jungbluth GL, Abdel-Rahman SM, et al. Impact of ontogeny on linezolid and disposition in neonates and infants. *Clin Pharmacol Ther*. 2003;74:413-422.
5. Nelson JD, Bradley JS, eds. *Nelson's Pocket Book of Pediatric Antimicrobial Therapy*. 17th ed. Chicago, IL: American Academy of Pediatrics; 2009.
6. Kaplan SL, Deville JG, Yogev R, et al. Linezolid versus vancomycin for treatment of Gram-positive infections in children. *Pediatr Infect Dis J*. 2003;22:677-686.
7. Deville JG, Adler S, Azimi PH, et al. Linezolid versus vancomycin in the treatment of known or suspected resistant Gram-positive infections or neonates. *Pediatr Infect Dis J*. 2003;22:S158-S163.
8. Kaplan SL, Afghani B, Lopez P, et al. Linezolid for the treatment of methacillin-resistant Staphylococcus aureus infections in children. *Pediatr Infect Dis J*. 2003;22:S178-S185.
9. Jantausch BA, Deville J, Adler S, et al. Linezolid for the treatment of children with bacteremia or nosocomial pneumonia caused by resistant Gram-positive bacterial pathogens. *Pediatr Infect Dis J*. 2003;22:S164-171.
10. Kaplan SL, Patterson L, Edwars KM, et al. the Linezolid Pediatric Study Group. Linezolid for the treatment of community-acquired pneumonia in hospitalized children. *Pediatr Infect Dis J*. 2001;20:488-494.
11. Meissner HC, Townsend T, Wenman W, et al. Hematologic effects of linezolid in young children. *Pediatr Infect Dis J*. 2003;22:S186-S192.
12. Lucas da Silva PS, Neto HM, Sejas LM. Successful treatment of vancomycin-resistant Enterococcus ventriculitis in a child. *Brazilian J Infect Dis*. 2007;11:297-299.
13. Vigano SM, Edefonti A, Ferraresso M, et al. Successful medical treatment of multiple brain abcesses due to *Nocardia farcinica* in a paediatric renal recipient. *Pediatr Nephrol*. 2005;20:1186-1188.
14. Baddour LM, Wilson WR, Bayer AS, et al. Infective endocarditis: diagnosis, antimicrobial therapy, and management of complications: a statement for healthcare professionals from the Committee on Rheumatic Fever, Endocarditis, and Kawasaki Disease, Council on Cardiovascular Disease in the Young, and the Councils on Clinical Cardiology, Stroke, and Cardiovascular Surgery and Anesthesia, American Heart Association: endorsed by the Infectious Diseases Society of America. *Circulation*. 2005;111:e394-e434.
15. Ang JY, Lua JL, Turner DR, Asmar BI. Vancomycin-resistant Enterococcus facium endocarditis in a premature infant successfully treated wth linezolid. *Pediatr Infect Dis J*. 2003;22:1101-1103.
16. Graham PL, Ampofo K, Saiman L. Linezolid treatment of vancomycin-resistant Enterococcus faecium ventriculitis. *Pediatr Infect Dis J*. 2002;21:798-800.
17. Castagnola E, Gandullia P, Oddone M, Peri C, et al. Catheter lock and systemic infusion of linezolid for the treatment of Broviac catheter-related Staphylococcal bacteremia. *Antimicrob Agents Chemother*. 2006;50:1120-1121.
18. Fennell JP, O'Donohoe M, Cormican M, Lynch M. Linezolid lock prophylaxis of central venous catheter infection. *J Med Microbiol*. 2008;57:534-535.
19. Aronoff GR, Berns JS, Brier ME, et al. Drug prescribing in renal failure. 4th ed. Available at: http://www.kdp-baptist.louisville.edu/renalbook/. Accessed October 20, 2009.
20. Trissel LA, ed. *Handbook on Injectable Drugs*. 15th ed. Bethesda, MD: American Society of Health-System Pharmacists; 2009.
21. Robinson CA, Sawyer JE. Y-site compatibility of medications with parenteral nutrition. *J Pediatr Pharmacol Ther*. 2009;14:49-57.
22. Apodaca AA, Rakita RM. Linezolid-induced lactic acidosis. *N Eng J Med*. 2003;348:86-87.
23. Narita M, Tsuji B, Yu VL. Linezolid-associated peripheral and optic neuropathy, lactic acidosis, and serotonin syndrome. *Pharmacotherapy*. 2007;27:1189-1197.
24. Brennan K, Jones BL, Jackson L. Auditory nerve neuropathy in a neonate after linezolid treatment. *Pediatr Infect Dis J*. 2009;28:169.

References

25. Huang V, Gortney JS. Risk of serotonin syndrome with concomitant administration of linezolid and serotonin agonists. *Pharmacotherapy*. 2006;26:1784-1793.
26. Bergeron L, Boule M, Perreault S. Serotonin toxicity associated with concomitant use of linezolid. *Ann Pharmacother*. 2005;39:956-961.
27. Morales-Molina JA, Mateu-de Antonio J, Marin-Casino M, Grau S. Linezolid-associated serotonin syndrome: what we can learn from cases reported so far. *J Antimicrob Chemother*. 2005;56:1176-1178.
28. Thomas CR, Rosenberg M, Blythe V, Meyer WJ. Serotonin syndrome and linezolid. *J Am Aca Child Adolesc Psychiatry*. 2004;43:790.
29. Ma JS. Teeth and tongue discoloration during linezolid therapy. *Pediatr Infect Dis J*. 2009;28:345-346.
30. Matson KL, Miller SE. Tooth discoloration after treatment with linezolid. *Pharmacotherapy*. 2003;23:682-685.
31. Shneker BF, Baylin PD, Nakhla ME. Linezolid inducing complex partial status epilepticus in a patient with epilepsy. *Neurology*. 2009;72: 378-379.
32. Taketani T, Kanai R, Fukuda S, Uchida Y, et al. Pure red cell precursor toxicity by linezolid in a pediatric case. *J Pediatr Hematol Oncol*. 2009;31:684-686.
33. Attassi K, Hershberger E, Alam R, Zervos MJ. Thrombocytopenia associated with linezolid therapy. *CID*. 2002;34:695-698.
34. Pfizer. Linezolid vs vancomycin/oxacillin/dicloxacillin in the treatment of catheter-related gram-positive bloodstream infections. Protocol M12600080. PhRMA Web Synopsis 8 June 2007. Available at: http://pdf.clinicalstudyresults.org/documents/company-study_1480_0.pdf. Accessed October 22, 2009.

LORazepam

1. Available at: http://ismp.org/Tools/highalertmedications.pdf. Accessed October 9, 2009.
2. Available at: http://www.ismp.org/Tools/tallmanletters.pdf. Accessed October 9, 2009.
3. Available at: http://www.usp.org/hqi/similarProducts/choosy.html. Accessed October 9, 2009.
4. Lorazepam [package insert]. Deerfield, IL: Baxter Healthcare Corp; MLT-01086/1.0.
5. Khalil SN, Berry JM, Howard G, et al. The antiemetic effect of lorazepam after outpatient strabismus surgery in children. *Anesthesiology*. 1992;77:915-919.
6. Relling RV, Mulhern RK, Fairclough D, et al. Chlorpromazine with and without lorazepam as antiemetic therapy in children receiving uniform chemotherapy. *J Pediatr*. 1993;12:811-816.
7. Relling MV, Mulhern RK, Johnson D, et al. Lorazepam pharmacodynamics in children with cancer. *J Pediatr*. 1989;114:641-646.
8. American Academy of Pediatrics Committee on Drugs. Emergency drug doses for infants and children. *Pediatrics*. 1998;101:e1-e11.
9. Nahata MC. Sedation in pediatric patients undergoing diagnostic procedures. *Drug Intell Clin Pharm*. 1988;22:711-715.
10. Shankar V, Deshpande JK. Procedural sedation in the pediatric patient. *Anesthesiol Clin N Am*. 2005;23:635-654, viii.
11. Flood RG, Krauss B. Procedural sedation and analgesia for children in the emergency department. *Emerg Med Clin North Am*. 2003;21:121-139.
12. Krauss B, Green S. Procedural sedation and analgesia in children. *Lancet*. 2006;367:766-780.
13. Tobias JD. Sedation analgesia in paediatric intensive care units. *Pediatr Drugs*. 1999;1:109-126.
14. Eberly AL, Anderson GD, Bubalo JS, et al. Optimal prevention of seizures induced by high-dose busulfan. *Pharmacotherapy*. 2008;28:1502-1510.
15. Chan KW, Mullen CA, Worth LL, et al. Lorazepam for seizure prophylaxis during high dosebusulfan administration. *Bone Marrow Transplant*. 2002;29:963-965.
16. Caselli D, Ziino O, Bartoli A, et al. Continuous intravenous infusion of lorazepan as seixure prophylaxis In children treated with high-dose busulfan. *Bone Marrow Transplant*. 2008;42:135-136.
17. Bartha AI, Shen J, Katz KH, et al. Neonatal seizures: multicenter variability in current treatment practices. *Pediatr Neurol*. 2007;37:85-90.
18. Deshmukh A, Wittert W, Schnitzler E, et al. Lorazepam in the treatment of refractory neonatal seizures. *Am J Dis Child*. 1986;140:1042-1044.
19. Maytal J, Novak GP, King KC. Lorazepam in the treatment of refractory neonatal seizures. *J Child Neurol*. 1991;6:319-323.
20. Roddy SM, McBride MC, Torres CF. Treatment of neonatal seizures with lorazepam. *Ann Neurol*. 1987;22:412. Abstract.
21. McDermott CA, Kowalczyk AL, Schnitzler ER, et al. Pharmacokinetics of lorazepam in critically ill neonates with seizures. *J Pediatr*. 1992;120:479-483.
22. Lacey DJ, Singer WD, Horwitz SJ, et al. Clinical and laboratory observations: lorazepam therapy of status epilepticus in children and adolescents. *J Pediatr*. 1986;108:771-774.
23. Crawford TO, Mitchell WG, Snodgrass SR. Lorazepam in childhood status epilepticus and serial seizures: effectiveness and tachyphylaxis. *Neurology*. 1987;37:190-195.
24. Giang DW, McBride MC. Lorazepam versus diazepam for the treatment of status epilepticus. *Pediatr Neurol*. 1988;4:358-361.
25. Appleton R, Sweeney A, Shoonara I, et al. Lorazepam versus diazepam in the acute treatment of epileptic seizures and status epilepticus. *Dev Med Child Neurol*. 1995;37:682-688.
26. Aronoff GR, Berns JS, Brier ME, et al. Drug prescribing in renal failure. 4th ed. Available at: http://www.kdp-baptist.louisville.edu/renalbook/. Accessed October 9, 2009.
27. Maloley PA, Gal P, Mize R, et al. Lorazepam dosing in neonates; application of objective sedation scores. *DICP Ann Pharmacother*. 1990;24:326-327. Letter.
28. Reincke HM, Gilmore RL, Kuhn RJ. High-dose lorazepam therapy for status epilepticus in a pediatric patient. *Drug Intell Clin Pharm*. 1988;22:889-890.
29. Trissel LA, ed. *Handbook on Injectable Drugs*. 15th ed. Bethesda, MD: American Society of Health-System Pharmacists; 2009.
30. Robinson CA, Sawyer JE. Y-site compatibility of medications with parenteral nutrition. *J Pediatr Pharmacol Ther*. 2009;14:49-57.
31. McCollam JS, O'Neil MG, Norcross ED, et al. Continuous infusion of lorazepam, midazolam, and propofol for sedation of the critically ill surgery trauma patient: a prospective, randomized comparison. *Crit Care Med*. 1999;27:2454-2458.
32. Pohlman AS, Simpson KP, Hall JB. Continuous intravenous infusions of lorazepam versus midazolam for sedation during mechanical ventilatory support: a prospective, randomized study. *Crit Care Med*. 1994;22:1241-1247.
33. Watling SM, Johnson M, Yanos J. A method to produce sedation in critically ill patients. *Ann Pharmacother*. 1996;30:1227-1231.
34. Swart EL, Schijndel RJ, van Loenen AC, et al. Continuous infusion of lorazepam versus midazolam in patients in the intensive care unit: sedation with lorazepam is easier to manage and is more cost-effective. *Crit Care Med*. 1999;27:1461-1465.
35. Walker JE, Homan RW, Vasko MR, et al. *Ann Neurol*. 1979;6:207-213.
36. Neale BW, Mesler EL, Young M, et al. Proylene glycol-induced lactic acidosis in a patient with normal renal function: a proposed mechanism and monitoring recommendations. *Ann Pharmacother*. 2005;39:1732-1736.
37. Chicella M, Jansen P, Parthiban A, et al. Propylene glycol accumulation associated with continuous infusion of lorazepam in pediatric intensive care patients. *Crit Care Med*. 2002;30:2752-2756.
38. Yaucher NE, Fish JT, Smith HW, et al. Propylene glycol-associated renal toxicity from lorazapam infusion. *Pharmacotherapy*. 2003;23:1094-1099.
39. MacDonald MG, Getson PR, Glasgow AM, et al. Propylene glycol: increased incidence of seizures in low birth weight infants. *Pediatrics*. 1987;79:622-625.
40. Cronin CM. Neurotoxicity of lorazepam in a premature infant. *Pediatrics*. 1992;89:1129.
41. Reiter PD, Stiles AD. Lorazepam toxicity in a premature infant. *Ann Pharmacother*. 1993; 27:727-729.
42. Chess PR, D'Angio CT. Clonic movement following lorazepam administration in full-term infants. *Arch Pediatr Adolesc Med*. 1998;152:98-99.

References

43. Straaten HL, Rademaker CM, de Vries LS. Comparison of the effect of midazolam or vecuronium on blood pressure and cerebral blood flow velocity in premature newborns. *Dev Pharmacol Ther.* 1992;19:191-195.
44. Hoffman EJ, Warren EW. Flumazenil: a benzodiazepine antagonist. *Clin Pharm.* 1993;12:614-656.
45. Flumazenil Injection USP [package insert]. Bedford, OH: Bedford Laboratories; December 2007.
46. Bhatt-Mehta V, Annich G. Sedative clearance during extracorporeal membrane oxygenation. *Perfusion.* 2005;20:309-315.

Lymphocyte Immune Globulin–Antithymocyte Globulin (equine)

1. Atgam [product information]. Kalamazoo, MI: Pharmacia & Upjohn Company; January 2003.
2. Whitehead B, James I, Helms P, et al. Intensive care management of children following heart and heart-lung transplantation. *Inten Care Med.* 1990;16:426-430.
3. Uittenbogaart CH, Robinson BJ, Malekzadeh MH, et al. Use of antithymocyte globulin (dose by rosette protocol) in pediatric renal allograft recipients. *Transplantation.* 1979;28:291-293.
4. Bunchman TE, Ham JM, Sedman AB, et al. Superior allograft survival in pediatric renal transplant recipients. *Transplant Proc.* 1994;26:24-25.
5. Leichter HE, Ettenger RB, Jordan SC, et al. Short-course antithymocyte globulin for treatment of renal transplant rejection in children. *Transplantation.* 1985;41:133-135.
6. Conley SB, al-Urzi A, So S, et al. Prevention of rejection and graft loss with an aggressive quadruple immunosuppressive therapy regimen in children and adolescents. *Transplantation.* 1994;57:540-544.
7. Khositseth S, Matas A, Cook ME, et al. Thymoglobulin versus ATGAM induction therapy in pediatric kidney transplant recipients: a single-center report. *Transplantation.* 2005;8:958-963.
8. Kawahara K, Storb R, Sanders J, et al. Successful allogeneic bone marrow transplantation in a 6.5-year-old male for severe aplastic anemia complicating orthotopic liver transplantation for fulminant non-A non-B hepatitis. *Blood.* 1991;78:1140-1143.
9. Zander AR, Zabelina T, Kroger N, et al. Use of a five-agent GVHD prevention regimen in recipients of unrelated donor marrow. *Bone Marrow Transplant.* 1999;23:889-893.
10. Ayas M, Al-Jefri A, Al-Mahr M, et al. Stem cell transplantation for patients with Fanconi anemia with low-dose cyclophosphamide and antithymocyte globulins without the use of radiation therapy. *Bone Marrow Transplant.* 2005;35:463-466.
11. Abdelkefi A, Othman TB, Ladeb S, et al. Bone marrow transplantation for patients with acquired severe aplastic anemia using cyclophosphamide and antithymocyte globulin: the experience from a single center. *Hemtaol J.* 2003;4:208-213.
12. Lynch BA, Vasef MA, Comito M, et al. Effect of *in vivo* lymphocyte-depleting strategies on development of lymphoproliferative disorders in children post allogeneic bone marrow transplantation. *Bone Marrow Transplant.* 2003;32:527-533.
13. Whitehead B, Helms P, Goodwin M, et al. Heart-lung transplantation for cystic fibrosis. 2: outcome. *Arch Dis Child.* 1991;66:1022-1026.
14. Bernstein D, Baum D, Berry G, et al. Neoplastic disorders after pediatric heart transplantation. *Circulation.* 1993;5(part 2):230-237.
15. Wall DA, Carter SL, Kernan NA, et al. Busulfan/melphalan/antithymocyte globulin followed by unrelated donor cord blood transplantation for treatment of infant leukemia and leukemia in young children: the cord blood transplantation study (COBLT) experience. *Biol Blood Marrow Transplant.* 2005;11:637-646.
16. Matloub YH, Bostrom B, Golembe B, et al. Antithymocyte globulin, cyclosporine, and prednisone for the treatment of severe aplastic anemia in children. *Am J Pediatr Hematol Oncol.* 1994;16:104-106.
17. Fang JP, XU HG, Huang SL, et al. Immunosuppressive treatment of aplastic anemia in Chinese children with antithymocyte globulin and cyclosporine. *Pediatr Hematol Oncol.* 2006;23:45-50.
18. Rosenfeld S, Follman D, Nunez O, et al. Antithymocyte globulin and cyclosporine for severe aplastic anemia. *JAMA.* 2003;289:1130-1135.
19. Goldenberg NA, Graham DK, Liang X, et al. Successful treatment of severe aplastic anemia in children using standardized immunosuppressive therapy with antithymocyte globulin and cyclosporine A. *Pediatr Blood Cancer.* 2004;43:718-722.
20. Scheinberg P, Fischer SH, Li L, et al. Distinct EBC and CMV reactivation patterns following antibody-based immunosuppressive regimens in patients with severe aplastic anemia. *Blood.* 2007;109:3219-3224.
21. Rosenfeld SJ, Kimball J, Vining D, et al. Intensive immunosuppression with antithymocyte globulin and cyclosporine as treatment for severe acquired aplastic anemia. *Blood.* 1995;85:3058-3065.
22. MacMillan ML, Couriel D, Weisdorf DJ, et al. A phase 2/3 multicenter randomized clinical trial of ABX-CBL versus ATG as secondary therapy for steroid-resistant acute graft-versus-host disease. *Blood.* 2007;109:2657-2662.
23. MacMillan ML, Weisdorf DJ, Davies SM, et al. Early antithymocyte globulin therapy improves survival in patients with steroid-resistant acute graft-versus-host disease. *Biol Blood Marrow Transplant.* 2002;8:40-46.
24. Rahman GF, Hardy MA, Cohen DJ. Administration of equine anti-thymocyte globulin via peripheral vein in renal transplant recipients. *Transplantation.* 2000;69:1958-1960.
25. Monchon M, Kaiser B, Palmer JA, et al. Evaluation of OKT3 monoclonal antibody and anti-thymocyte globulin in the treatment of steroid-resistant acute allograft rejection in pediatric renal transplants. *Pediatr Nephrol.* 1993;7:259-262.
26. Dearden C, Foukaneli T, Lee P, et al. The incidence and significance of fevers during treatment with antithymocyte globulin for aplastic anemia. *Br J Hematol.* 1998;103:846-848.

Lymphocyte Immune Globulin–Antithymocyte Globulin (rabbit)

1. Thymoglobulin [package insert]. Cambridge, MA: Genzyme Corporation; September 2007.
2. Ault BH, Honaker MR, Gaber AO, et al. Short-term outcomes of Thymoglobulin induction in pediatric renal transplant recipients. *Pediatr Nephrol.* 2002;17:815-818.
3. Brophy PD, Thomas SE, McBryde KD, et al. Comparison of polyclonal induction agents in pediatric renal transplantation. *Pediatr Transplant.* 2001;5:174-178.
4. Khositseth S, Matas A, Cook ME, et al. Thymoglobulin versus ATGAM induction therapy in pediatric kidney transplant recipients: a single-center report. *Transplantation.* 2005;79:958-963.
5. Bell L, Girardin C, Sharma A, et al. Lymphocyte subsets during and after rabbit anti-thymocyte globulin induction in pediatric renal transplantation: sustained T cell depletion. *Transplant Proc.* 1997;29:6S-9S.
6. Kamel MH, Mohan P, Little DM, et al. Rabbit antithymocyte globulin as induction immunotherapy for pediatric deceased donor kidney transplantation. *J Urol.* 2005;174:703-707.
7. Bond GJ, Mazariegos GV, Sindhi R, et al. Evolutionary experience with immunosuppression in pediatric intestinal transplantation. *J Pediatr Surg.* 2005;40:274-280.
8. Reyes J, Mazariegos GV, Abu-Elmagd K, et al. Intestinal transplantation under tacrolimus monotherapy after perioperative lymphoid depletion with rabbit anti-thymocyte globulin (Thymoglobulin). *Am J Transplant.* 2005;5:1430-1436.
9. Sindhi R, Magill A, Bentlejewski C, et al. Enhanced donor-specific alloreactivity occurs independently of immunosuppression in children with early liver rejection. *Am J Transplant.* 2005;5:96-102.
10. Remberger M, Storer, B, Ringden O, et al. Association between pretransplant Thymoglobulin and reduced non-relapse mortality rate after marrow transplantation from unrelated donors. *Bone Marrow Transplant.* 2002;29:391-397.
11. Seidel MG, Fritsch G, Matthes-Martin S, et al. Antithymocyte globulin pharmacokinetics in pediatric patients after hematopoietic stem cell transplantation. *J Pediatr Hematol Oncol.* 2005;27:532-536.

References

12. Di Filippo S, Boissonnat P, Sassolas F, et al. Rabbit antithymocyte globulin as induction immunotherapy in pediatric heart transplantation. *Transplantation.* 2003;75:354-358.
13. Parisi F, Danesi H, Squitieri C, et al. Thymoglobuline use in pediatric heart transplantation. *J Heart Lung Transplant.* 2003;22:591-593.
14. DiBona E, Rodeghiero F, Bruno B, et al. Rabbit antithymocyte globulin (r-ATG) plus cyclosporine and granulocyte colony stimulating factor is an effective treatment for aplastic anaemia patients unresponsive to a first course of intensive immunosuppressive therapy. *Br J Haematol.* 1999;107:330-334.
15. Fang JP, Xu HG, Huang SL, et al. Immunosuppressive treatment of aplastic anemia in Chinese children with antithymocyte globulin and cyclosporine. *Pediatr Hematol Oncol.* 2006;23:45-50.
16. Scheinberg P, Fischer SH, Nunez O, et al. Distinct EBV and CMV reactivation patterns following antibody-based immunosuppressive regimens in patients with severe aplastic anemia. *Blood.* 2007;109:3219-3224
17. Trissel LA. *Handbook on Injectable Drugs.* 15th ed. Bethesda, MD: American Society of Health-System Pharmacists; 2009.

Magnesium Sulfate

1. Available at: http://ismp.org/Tools/highalertmedications.pdf. ISMP 2008.
2. Magnesium sulfate injection USP [package insert]. Schaumburg, IL: American Pharmaceutical Partners Inc; January 2008.
3. Tsang RC. Neonatal magnesium disturbances. *Am J Dis Child.* 1972;124:282-283.
4. Maggioni A, Orzalesi M, Mimouni FB. Intravenous correction of neonatal hypomagnesemia: effect on ionized magnesium. *J Pediatr.* 1998;132:652-655.
5. Magnesium sulfate. Lexi-Comp® Online with AHFS® (database). Hudson, OH: Lexi-Comp Inc; updated September 25, 2009.
6. Slayton W, Anstine D. Tetany in a child with AIDS receiving intravenous tobramycin. *S Med J.* 1996;89:1108-1111.
7. 2005 American Heart Association guidelines for cardiopulmonary resuscitation and emergency cardiovascular care: Part 12: Pediatric advanced life support. *Circulation.* 2005;112(suppl 24):IV167-IV187.
8. DiNicola LK, Monem GF, Gayle MO, et al. Treatment of critical status asthmaticus in children. In: Respiratory medicine 1: current issues. *Pediatr Clin North Am.* 1994;41:1293-1324.
9. Ciarallo L, Sauer AH, Shannon MW. Intravenous magnesium therapy for moderate to severe pediatric asthma: results of a randomized placebo-controlled trial. *J Pediatr.* 1996;129:809-814.
10. Dib JG, Engstrom FM, Sisca TS, et al. Intravenous magnesium sulfate treatment in a child with status asthmaticus. *Am J Health-Syst Pharm.* 1999;56:997-1000.
11. Scarfone RJ, Loiselle JM, Joffe MD, et al. A randomized trial of magnesium in the emergency department treatment of children with asthma. *Ann Emerg Med.* 2000;36:572-578.
12. National Asthma Education and Prevention Program. *Expert Panel Report 3 (EPR3): Guidelines for the Diagnosis and Management of Asthma.* Bethesda, MD: National Institutes of Health; August 2007.
13. Dorman BH, Sade RM, Burnette JS, et al. Magnesium supplementation in the prevention of arrhythmias in pediatric patients undergoing surgery for congenital heart defects. *Am Heart J.* 2000; 139:522-528.
14. Abu-Osba YK, Galal O, Manasra K, et al. Treatment of severe persistent pulmonary hypertension of the newborn with magnesium sulfate. *Arch Dis Child.* 1992;67:31-35.
15. Trissel LA, ed. *Handbook on Injectable Drugs.* 15th ed. Bethesda, MD: American Society of Health-System Pharmacists; 2009.
16. Levene M, Blennow M, Witelaw A, et al. Acute effects of two different doses of magnesium sulphate in infants with birth asphyxia. *Arch Dis Child.* 1995;73:F174-F177.

Mannitol

1. Mannitol injection, USP [package insert]. Schaumburg, IL: APP Pharmaceuticals LLC; April 2008.
2. American Academy of Pediatrics Committee on Drugs. Emergency drug doses for infants and children. *Pediatrics.* 1998;101:e1-e11.
3. Adelson PD, Bratton SL, Carney NA, et al. Guidelines for the acute medical management of severe traumatic brain injury in infants, children, and adolescents. Chapter 11. Use of hyperosmolar therapy in the management of severe pediatric traumatic brain injury. *Pediatr Crit Care Med.* 2003;4:S40-S44.
4. Marshall LF, Smith RW, Rauscher LA, et al. Mannitol dose requirements in brain-injured patients. *J Neurosurg.* 1978;48:169-172.
5. Shaywitz BA, Rothstein P, Venes JL. Monitoring and management of increased intracranial pressure in Reyes syndrome: results in 29 children. *Pediatrics.* 1980;66:198-204.
6. Soriano SG, McManus ML, Sullivan LJ, et al. Cerebral blood flow velocity after mannitol infusion in children. *Can J Anaesth.* 1996;43:461-466.
7. James HE. Methodology for the control of intracranial pressure with hypertonic mannitol. *Acta Neurochir.* 1980;51:161-172.
8. Lewis MA, Awan A. Mannitol and furosemide in the treatment of diuretic resistant oedema in nephrotic syndrome. *Arch Dis Child.* 1999;80:184-185.
9. Trissel LA, ed. *Handbook on Injectable Drugs.* 15th ed. Bethesda, MD: American Society of Health-System Pharmacists; 2009.
10. Jaques A, Daviskas E, Turton JA, et al. Inhaled mannitol improves lung function in cystic fibrosis. *Chest.* 2008;133:1388-1396.
11. Cottrell JE, Robustelli A, Post K, et al. Furosemide-and mannitol-induced changes in intracranial pressure and serum osmolality and electrolytes. *Anesthesiology.* 1977;47:28-30.
12. Goldwasser P, Fotino S. Acute renal failure following massive mannitol infusion. Appropriate response of tubuloglomerular feedback? *Arch Intern Med.* 1984;144:2214-2216.

Meperidine HCl

1. Available at: http://ismp.org/Tools/highalertmedications.pdf. ISMP 2008.
2. Available at: http://www.usp.org/hqi/similarProducts/choosy.html. Accessed October 13, 2009.
3. Meperidine hydrochloride injection, USP [package insert]. Deerfield, IL: Baxter Healthcare Corporation; October 2006.
4. Levy JH, Rockoff MA. Anaphylaxis to meperidine. *Anesth Analg.* 1982;61:301-303.
5. Tobias JD. Sedation and analgesia in paediatric intensive care units. A guide to drug selection and use. *Paediatr Drugs.* 1999;1:109-126.
6. Nahata MC, Clotz MA, Krogg EA. Adverse effects of meperidine, promethazine, and chlorpromazine for sedation in pediatric patients. *Clin Pediatr.* 1985;24:558-560.
7. Nahata MC. Sedation in pediatric patients undergoing diagnostic procedures. *Drug Intell Clin Pharm.* 1988;22:711-715.
8. Snodgrass WR, Dodge WF. Lytic/DPT cocktail: time for rational and safer alternatives. *Pediatr Clin North Am.* 1989;36:1285-1291.
9. American Academy of Pediatrics. Committee on Drugs. Reappraisal of lytic cocktail/demerol, phenergan, and thorazine (DPT) for the sedation of children. *Pediatrics.* 1995;95:598-602.
10. Auden SM, Sobczyk WL, Solinger RE, et al. Oral ketamine/midazolam is superior to intramuscular meperidine, promethazine, and chlorpromazine for pediatric cardiac catheterization. *Anesth Analg.* 2000;90:299-305.
11. Pokela ML, Olkkola KT, Koivisto ME, et al. Pharmacokinetics and pharmacodynamics of intravenous meperidine in neonates and infants. *Clin Pharmacol Ther.* 1992;52:342-349.

References

12. Bhatt-Mehta V, Rosen DA. Management of acute pain in children. *Clin Pharm*. 1991;10:667-685.
13. Fixler DE, Carrell T, Browne R, et al. Oxygen consumption in infants and children during cardiac catheterization under different sedation regimens. *Circulation*. 1974;50:788-794.
14. American Academy of Pediatrics Committee on Drugs. Emergency drug doses for infants and children. *Pediatrics*. 1998;101:e1-e11.
15. Cole TB, Sprinkle RH, Smith SJ, et al. Intravenous narcotic therapy for children with severe sickle cell pain crisis. *Am J Dis Child*. 1986;140:1255-1259.
16. Stanger P, Heymann MA, Tarnoff H, et al. Complications of cardiac catheterization of neonates, infants, and children. A three-year study. *Circulation*. 1974;50:595-608.
17. Atwood GF, Evans MA, Harbison RD. Pharmacokinetics of meperidine in infants. *Pediatr Res*. 1976;10:328. Abstract.
18. Martinez JL, Sutters KA, Waite S, et al. A comparison of oral diazepam versus midazolam, administered with intravenous meperidine, as premedication to sedation for pediatric endoscopy. *J Pediatr Gastroenterol Nutr*. 2002;35:51-58.
19. Aronoff GR, Berns JS, Brier ME, et al. Drug prescribing in renal failure. 4th ed. Available at: http://www.kdp-baptist.louisville.edu/renalbook/pediatric/. Accessed October 13, 2009.
20. Szeto HH, Inturrisi CE, Houde R. Accumulation of normeperidine, an active metabolite of meperidine, in patients with renal failure or cancer. *Ann Intern Med*. 1977;86:738-741.
21. Trissel LA, ed. *Handbook on Injectable Drugs*. 15th ed. Bethesda, MD: American Society of Health-System Pharmacists; 2009.
22. Thomas R. Meperidine HCl and heparin sodium precipitation. *Hosp Pharm*. 1974;9:356. Letter.
23. Kaiko RF, Foley KM, Grabinski PY, et al. Central nervous system excitatory effects of meperidine in cancer patients. *Ann Neurol*. 1983;13:180-185.
24. Goetting MG, Thirman MJ. Neurotoxicity of meperidine. *Ann Emerg Med*. 1985;14:1007-1009.
25. Kyff JV, Rice TL. Meperidine-associated seizures in a child. *Clin Pharm*. 1990;9:337-338.
26. Saneto RP, Fitch JA, Cohen BH. Acute neurotoxicity of meperidine in an infant. *Pediatr Neurol*. 1996;14:339-341.

Meropenem

1. Available at: http://www.usp.org/hqi/similarProducts/choosy.html. Accessed August 27, 2009.
2. Meropenem [package insert].Wilmington, DE: AstraZeneca Pharmaceuticals LP; November 2007.
3. van Enk JG, Touw DJ, Lafeber HN. Pharmacokinetics of meropenem in preterm neonates. *Ther Drug Monit*. 2001;23:198-201.
4. Nair PM. Meropenem in neonates. *Indian Pediatr*. 2005;42:963. Letter.
5. Vartzelis G, Theodoridou M, Daikos GL, et al. Brain abscesses complicating Staphylococcus aureus sepsis in a premature infant. *Infection*. 2005;33:36-38.
6. American Academy of Pediatrics Committee on Infectious Diseases. Therapy for children with invasive pneumococcal infections. *Pediatrics*. 1997;99:289-299.
7. Tunkel AR, Hartman BJ, Kaplan SL, et al. Practice guidelines for the management of bacterial meningitis. *Clin Infect Dis*. 2004;39:1267-1284.
8. Klugman KP, Dagan R. The Meropenem Meningitis Study Group. Randomized comparison of meropenem with cefotaxime for treatment of bacterial meningitis. *Antimicrob Agents Chemother*. 1995;39:1140-1146.
9. Aronoff GR, Berns JS, Brier ME, et al. Drug prescribing in renal failure. 4th ed. Available at: http://www.kdp-baptist.louisville.edu/renalbook/. Accessed September 1, 2009.
10. Trissel LA, ed. *Handbook on Injectable Drugs*. 15th ed. Bethesda, MD: American Society of Health-System Pharmacists; 2009.
11. Robinson CA, Sawyer JE. Y-site compatibility of medications with parenteral nutrition. *J Pediatr Pharmacol Ther*. 2009;14:49-57.
12. Capitano B, Nicolau DP, Potoski BA, et al. Meropenem administered as a prolonged infusion to treat serious gram-negative central nervous system infections. *Pharmacotherapy*. 2004;24:803-807.
13. Thalhammer F, Traunmuller F, El Menyawi I, et al. Continuous infusion versus intermittent administration of meropenem in critically ill patients. *J Antimicrob Chemother*. 1999;43:523-527.
14. Romanelli G, Cravarezza P. Intramuscular meropenem in the treatment of bacterial infections of the urinary and lower respiratory tracts. *J Antimicrob Chemother*. 1995;36 (supplement A):109-119.
15. Norrby SR. Neurotoxicity of the carbapenem antibacterials. *Drug Safety*. 1996;15:87-90.
16. Norrby SR. Carbapenems in serious infections: a risk-benefit assessment. *Drug Safety*. 2000;22:191-194.
17. Calandra G, Lydick E, Carrigan J, et al. Factors predisposing to seizures in seriously ill infected patients receiving antibiotics: experience with imipenem/cilastatin. *Am J Med*. 1988;84:911-918.
18. Latzin P, Fehling M, Bauernfeind, et al. Efficacy and safety of intravenous meropenem and tobramycin verses ceftazidime and tobramycin in cystic fibrosis. *Journal of Cystic Fibrosis*. 2008;7:142-146.
19. Fudio S, Carcas A, Piñana E, et al. Epileptic seizures caused by low valproic acid levels from an interaction with meropenem. *J Clin Pharm Ther*. 2006;31:393-396.
20. Lexi-Comp® Online with AHFS® (database). Hudson, OH: Lexi-Comp Inc; updated August 13, 2009.

Methotrexate

1. Available at: http://ismp.org/Tools/highalertmedications.pdf. ISMP 2008. Accessed August 29, 2009.
2. Available at: http://www.usp.org/hqi/similarProducts/choosy.html. Accessed August 29, 2009.
3. Available at: http://ismp.org/Tools/confuseddrugnames.pdf. Accessed August 29, 2009.
4. Methotrexate [package insert]. Lake Forest, IL: Hospira Inc; August 2007.
5. Methotrexate. Lexi-Comp ®Online with AHFS® (database). Bethesda, MD: American Society of Health-System Pharmacists; updated May 26, 2009.
6. Goldberg NH, Romolo JL, Austin EH, et al. Anaphylactoid type reactions in two patients receiving high-dose intravenous methotrexate. *Cancer*. 1978;41:52-55.
7. Evans WE, Crom WR, Abromowitch M, et al. Clinical pharmacodynamics of high-dose methotrexate in acute lymphocytic leukemia: identification of a relation between concentration and effect. *N Engl J Med*. 1986;314:471-477.
8. Evans WE, Hutson PR, Stewart CF, et al. Methotrexate cerebrospinal fluid and serum concentrations after intermediate dose methotrexate infusion. *Clin Pharmacol Ther*. 1983;33:301-307.
9. Christensen ML, Rivera, GK, Crom WR, et al. Effect of hydration on methotrexate plasma concentrations in children with acute leukemia. *J Clin Oncol*. 1988;6:797-801.
10. Reiter A, Schrappe M, Ludwig WD, et al. Intensive ALL-type therapy without local radiotherapy provides a 90% event-free survival for children with T-cell lymphoblastic lymphoma: a BFM group report. *Blood*. 2000;95:416-421.
11. Poplack DG, Reaman GH, Bleyer WA, et al. Central nervous system (CNS) preventive therapy with high dose methotrexate (HDMTX) in acute lymphoblastic leukemia (ALL); a preliminary report. *Proc Am Soc Clin Oncol*. 1984;3:204-206.
12. Balis FM, Savitch JL, Bleyer WA, et al. Remission induction meningeal leukemia with high dose intravenous methotrexate. *J Clin Oncol*. 1985;3:485-489.
13. Relling MV, Fairclough D, Ayers D, et al. Patient characteristics associated with high risk methotrexate concentrations and toxicity. *J Clin Oncol*. 1994;12:1667-1672.
14. Evans WE, Crom WR, Stewart CF, et al. Methotrexate systemic clearance influences the probability of relapse in children with standard-risk acute lymphocytic leukemia. *Lancet*. 1984;1:359-362.

References

15. Horning SJ, Hoppe RT, Hancock SL, et al. Vinblastine, bleomycin, and methotrexate: an effective adjuvant in favorable Hodgkin's disease. *J Clin Oncol.* 1988;6:1822-1831.
16. Djerassi I, Sun Kim J. Methotrexate and citrovorum factor rescue in the management of childhood lymphosarcoma and reticulum cell sarcoma (non-Hodgkin's lymphoma). *Cancer.* 1976;38:1043-1051.
17. Murphy SB, Bowman WP, Abromowitch M, et al. Results of treatment of advanced stage Burkitt's lymphoma and B cell (SIg+) acute lymphoblastic leukemia with high dose fractionated cyclophosphamide and coordinated high dose methotrexate and cytarabine. *J Clin Oncol.* 1986;4:1732-1739.
18. Patte C, Bernard A, Hartmann O, et al. High-dose methotrexate and continuous infusion ara-c in children's non-Hodgkin's lymphoma: phase II studies and their use in further protocols. *Pediatric Hematol Oncol.* 1986;3:11-18.
19. Ramirez I, Sullivan MP, Wang Y, et al. Effective therapy for Burkitt's lymphoma: high dose cyclophosphamide + high dose methotrexate with coordinated intrathecal therapy. *Cancer Chemother Pharmacol.* 1979;3:103-109.
20. Bleyer WA. Clinical pharmacology of intrathecal methotrexate. II: an improved dosage regimen derived from age-related pharmacokinetics. *Cancer Treat Rep.* 1977;61:1419-1425.
21. Trissel LA, ed. *Handbook on Injectable Drugs.* 15th ed. Bethesda, MD: American Society of Health-System Pharmacists; 2009.
22. Jaffe N, Robertson R, Ayala A, et al. Comparison of intra-arterial cis-diamminedichloroplatinum II with high dose methotrexate and citrovorum factor rescue in the treatment of primary osteosarcoma. *J Clin Oncol.* 1985;3:1101-1104.
23. Rosen G, Caparros B, Huvos AG, et al. Preoperative chemotherapy for osteogenic sarcoma: selection of postoperative adjuvant chemotherapy based on the response of the primary tumor to preoperative chemotherapy. *Cancer.* 1979;43:1221-1230.
24. Pratt CB, Howarth C, Ransom JL, et al. High dose methotrexate used alone and in combination for measurable primary or metastatic osteosarcoma. *Cancer Treat Rep.* 1980;64:11-20.
25. Jaffe N, Traggis D. Toxicity of high dose methotrexate (NSC-740) and citrovorum factor (NSC-3590) in osteogenic sarcoma. *Cancer Chemother Rep.* 1975;6:31-36.
26. Wallace CA, Sherry DD. Preliminary report of higher dose methotrexate treatment in juvenile rheumatoid arthritis. *J Rheumatol.* 1992;19:1604-1607.
27. Reiff A, Shaham B, Wood BP, et al. High dose methotrexate in the treatment of refractory juvenile rheumatoid arthritis. *Clin and Exper Rheum.* 1995;13:113-118.
28. Gabriel S, Creagan E, O'Fallon WM, et al. Treatment of rheumatoid arthritis with higher dose intravenous methotrexate. *J Rheumatol.* 1990;17:460-465.
29. Aronoff GR, Berns JS, Brier ME, et al. Drug prescribing in renal failure. 4th ed. Available at: http://www.kdp-baptist.louisville.edu/renalbook/. Accessed October 23, 2009.
30. Shapiro WR, Young DF, Mehta BM, et al. Methotrexate: distribution in cerebrospinal fluid after intravenous, ventricular and lumbar injections. *N Engl J Med.* 1975;293:161-166.
31. Gregory RE, Pui CH, Crom WR. Raised plasma methotrexate concentrations following intrathecal administration in children with renal dysfunction. *Leukemia.* 1991;5:999-1003.
32. Hande KR, Balow JE, Drake JC, et al. Methotrexate and hemodialysis. *Ann Intern Med.* 1977;87:495-496.
33. Relling MV, Stapelton FB, Ochs J, et al. Removal of methotrexate, leucovorin, and their metabolites by combined hemodialysis and hemoperfusion. *Cancer.* 1988;62:884-888.
34. Gadgil SD, Damle SR, Advani SH, et al. Effect of activated charcoal on the pharmacokinetics of high-dose methotrexate. *Cancer Treat Rep.* 1982;66:1169-1171.
35. Crom WR, Evans WE. Methotrexate. In: Evans WE, Schentag JJ, Jusko WJ, eds. *Applied Pharmacokinetics: Principles of Therapeutic Drug Monitoring.* 3rd ed. Vancouver, WA: Applied Therapeutics Inc; 1992:1-42.
36. Lascari AD, Strano AJ, Johnson WW, et al. Methotrexate-induced sudden fatal pulmonary reaction. *Cancer.* 1977;40:1393-1397.
37. Doyle LA, Berg C, Bottino G, et al. Erythema and desquamation after high-dose methotrexate. *Ann Intern Med.* 1983;98:611-612.
38. Von Hoff DD, Penta JS, Helman LJ, et al. Incidence of drug-related deaths secondary to high-dose methotrexate and citrovorum factor administration. *Cancer Treat Rep.* 1977;61:745-748.
39. Ackland SP, Schilsky RL. High-dose methotrexate: a critical reappraisal. *J Clin Oncol.* 1987;5:2017-2031.
40. Nirenberg A, Mosende C, Mehta BM, et al. High-dose methotrexate with citrovorum factor rescue: predictive values of serum methotrexate concentration and corrective measures to avert toxicity. *Cancer Treat Rep.* 1977;61:779-783.
41. Chan H, Evans WE, Pratt CB. Recovery from toxicity associated with high dose methotrexate prognostic factors. *Cancer Treat Rep.* 1977;61:797-804.
42. Stoller RG, Jacobs SA, Drake JC, et al. Pharmacokinetics of high-dose methotrexate (NSC-740). *Cancer Chemother Rep.* 1975;6:19-24.
43. Romolo JL, Goldberg NH, Hande KR, et al. The effect of hydration on plasma methotrexate levels. *Cancer Treat Rep.* 1977;61:1393-1396.
44. Stoller RC, Hande KR, Jacobs SA, et al. Use of plasma pharmacokinetics to predict and prevent methotrexate toxicity. *N Engl J Med.* 1977;297:630-634.
45. Van Den Berg HW, Murphy RF, Kennedy DG, et al. Rapid plasma clearance and reduced rate and extent of urinary elimination of parenterally administered methotrexate as a result of severe vomiting and diarrhea. *Cancer Chemother Pharmacol.* 1980;4:47-48.
46. Sand TE, Jacobsen S. Effect of urine pH and flow on renal clearance of methotrexate. *Eur J Clin Pharmacol.* 1981;19:453-456.
47. Evans WE, Pratt CB. Effect of pleural effusions on high-dose methotrexate kinetics. *Clin Pharmacol Ther.* 1978;23:68-72.
48. Chabner BA, Stoller RG, Hande K, et al. Methotrexate disposition in humans: case studies in ovarian cancer and following high dose infusion. *Drug Metab Rev.* 1978;8:107-117.
49. Evans WE, Tsiatis A, Crom WR, et al. Pharmacokinetics of sustained serum methotrexate concentrations secondary to gastrointestinal obstruction. *J Pharm Sci.* 1981;70:1194-1198.
50. Crom WR, Pratt CB, Green AA, et al. The effect of prior cisplatin therapy on the pharmacokinetics of high-dose methotrexate. *J Clin Oncol.* 1984;2:655-661.
51. Garré ML, Relling MV, Kalwinsky D, et al. Pharmacokinetics and toxicity of methotrexate in children with Down's syndrome and acute lymphocytic leukemia. *J Pediatr.* 1987;111:606-612.
52. Leigler DG, Henderson ES, Hahn MA, et al. The effect of organic acids on renal clearance of methotrexate in man. *Clin Pharmacol Ther.* 1970;10:849-857.
53. Reid T, Yuen A, Catilico M, et al. Impact of omeprazole on the plasma clearance of methotrexate. Cancer Chemother Pharmacol. 1993;33: 82-84.
54. Furst DE. Practical clinical pharmacology and drug interactions of low-dose methotrexate therapy in rheumatoid arthritis. *Br J Rheum.* 1995;34:20-25.
55. DuPuis LL, Koren G, Shore A, et al. Methotrexate-nonsteroidal antiinflammatory drug interaction in children with arthritis. *J Rheumatol.* 1990;17:1469-1473.
56. Wallace CA, Smith AL, Sherry DD. Pilot investigation of naproxen/methotrexate interaction in patients with juvenile rheumatoid arthritis. *J Rheumatol.* 1993;20:1764-1768.
57. Ferrazzini G, Klein J, Sulh H, et al. Interaction between trimethoprim-sulfamethoxazole and methotrexate in children with leukemia. *J Pediatr.* 1990;117:823-826.
58. Aherne GW, Piall E, Marks V, et al. Prolongation and enhancement of serum methotrexate concentrations by probenecid. *Br Med J.* 1978;1:1097.
59. Ronchera CL, Hernandez T, Peris E, et al. Pharmacokinetic interaction between high-dose methotrexate and amoxicillin. *Ther Drug Monit.* 1993;15:375-379.

60. National Comprehensive Cancer Network (NCCN) Antiemesis Panel Members. NCCN Clinical Practice Guidelines in Oncology. Antiemesis, v.1.2006. Available at www.nccn.org. Accessed September 15, 2006.
61. Roila F, Feyer P, Maranzamo E, et al. Antiemetics in children receiving chemotherapy. *Supportive Care Cancer.* 2005;13:129-131.
62. Evans WE, Pratt CB, Taylor RH, et al. Pharmacokinetic monitoring of high-dose methotrexate: early recognition of high risk patients. *Cancer Chemother Pharmacol.* 1979;3:161-166.

Methyldopate HCl

1. Available at: http://www.usp.org/hqi/similarProducts/choosy.html. Accessed August 29, 2009.
2. Methyldopate hydrochloride injection [package insert]. Shirley, NY: American Regent Laboratories Inc; December 2002.
3. Methyldopate hydrochloride. Lexi-Comp Online with AHFS (database). Bethesda, MD: American Society of Health-System Pharmacists; updated January 2009.
4. Loggie JM. Hypertension in children and adolescents. II. Drug therapy. *J Pediatr.* 1969;74:640-654.
5. Adelman RD. Neonatal hypertension. *Pediatr Clin North Am.* 1978;25:99-110.
6. Fivush B, Neu A, Furth S. Acute hypertensive crises in children: emergencies and urgencies. *Curr Opin Pediatr.* 1997;9;233-236.
7. Adelman RD, Coppo R, Dillon MJ. The emergency management of severe hypertension. *Pediatr Nephrol.* 2000;14:422-427.
8. Aronoff GR, Berns JS, Brier ME, et al. Drug prescribing in renal failure. 4th ed. Available at: http://www.kdp-baptist.louisville.edu/renalbook/. Accessed August 17, 2009.
9. Pagliaro LA, Pagliaro AM, eds. *Problems in Pediatric Drug Therapy.* 2nd ed. Hamilton, IL: Drug Intelligence Publications Inc; 1987.
10. Trissel LA, ed. *Handbook on Injectable Drugs.* 15th ed. Bethesda, MD: American Society of Health-System Pharmacists; 2009.

MethylPREDNISolone Sodium Succinate

1. Available at: http://ismp.org/Tools/confuseddrugnames.pdf. Updated April 1, 2005.
2. Available at: http://www.usp.org/hqi/similarProducts/choosy.html. Accessed August 11, 2009.
3. Solu-Medrol [prescribing information]. New York, NY: Pfizer; May 2009.
4. Bocanegra TS, Castaneda MO, Espinoza LR, et al. Sudden death after methylprednisolone pulse therapy. *Ann Intern Med.* 1981;95:122.
5. Moses RE, McCormick A, Nickey W. Fatal arrhythmia after pulse methylprednisolone therapy. *Ann Intern Med.* 1981;95:781-782.
6. Freedman MD, Schoket AL, Chapel N, et al. Anaphylaxis after methylprednisolone therapy. *JAMA.* 1981;245:607-608.
7. Schonwald S. Methylprednisolone anaphylaxis. *Am J Emerg Med.* 1999;17:583-585.
8. Fass B. Glucocorticoid therapy for non-endocrine disorders: withdrawal and coverage. *Pediatr Clin North Am.* 1979;26:251-256.
9. Chamberlin P, Meyer WJ. Management of pituitary-adrenal suppression secondary to corticosteroid therapy. *Pediatrics.* 1981;67:245-251.
10. Bone RC, Fisher CJ, Clemmer TP, et al. A controlled clinical trial of high dose methylprednisolone in the treatment of severe sepsis and septic shock. *N Engl J Med.* 1987;317:653-658.
11. The Veterans Administration Systemic Sepsis Cooperative Study Group. Effect of high-dose glucocorticoid therapy on mortality in patients with clinical signs of systemic sepsis. *N Engl J Med.* 1987;317:659-665.
12. MethylPREDNISolone. Lexi-Comp® Online with AHFS® (database). Hudson, OH: Lexi-Comp Inc; updated August 3, 2009.
13. Thompson JF, Chalmers DHK, Wood RFM, et al. Sudden death following high-dose intravenous methylprednisolone. *Transplantation.* 1983;36:594-596.
14. McDougal BA, Whittier FC, Cross DE. Sudden death after bolus steroid therapy for acute rejection. *Transplant Proc.* 1976;8:493-496.
15. Miller JJ. Prolonged use of large intravenous steroid pulses in the rheumatic diseases of children. *Pediatrics.* 1980;65:989-994.
16. Ferraris JR, Gallo GE, Ramirez J, et al. Pulse methylprednisolone therapy in the treatment of acute crescentic glomerulonephritis. *Nephron.* 1983;34:207-208.
17. Bolton WK, Couser WG. Intravenous pulse methylprednisolone therapy of acute crescentic rapidly progressive glomerulonephritis. *Am J Med.* 1979;66:495-502.
18. Cole BR, Brocklebank JT, Kienstra RA, et al. Pulse methylprednisolone therapy in the treatment of severe glomerulonephritis. *J Pediatr.* 1976;88:307-314.
19. Kimberly RP, Lockshin MD, Sherman RL, et al. High dose intravenous methylprednisolone pulse therapy in systemic lupus erythematosus. *Am J Med.* 1981;70:817-824.
20. Tunc B, Oner AF, Hicsonmez G. The effect of short-course high-dose methylprednisolone on peripheral blood lymphocyte subsets in children with acute leukemia during remission induction treatment. *Leuk Res.* 2003;27:19-21.
21. Orta-Sibu N, Chantler C, Bewick M, et al. Comparison of high-dose intravenous methylprednisolone with low-dose oral prednisolone in acute renal allograft rejection in children. *Br Med J.* 1982;285:258-260.
22. National Education and Prevention Program. *Expert Panel Report 3 (EPR3): Guidelines for the Diagnosis and Management of Asthma.* Bethesda, MD: National Institutes of Health; August 2007.
23. Ancona KG, Parker RI, Atlas MP, et al. Randomized trial of high-dose methylprednisolone versus intravenous immunoglobulin for the treatment of acute idiopathic thrombocytopenic purpura in children. *J Pediatr Hematol Oncol.* 2002;24:540-544.
24. Plebani A, Clerici Schoeller M, Pietrogrande MC, et al. Steroids in Pneumocystis carinii pneumonia in HIV seropositive infants. *Eur J Pediatr.* 1989;148:579-584.
25. Kline MW, Shearer WT. A national survey on the care of infants and children with human immunodeficiency virus infection. *J Pediatr.* 1991;118:817-821.
26. Sleasman JW, Hemenway C, Klein AS, et al. Corticosteroids improve survival of children with AIDS and Pneumocystis carinii pneumonia. *Am J Dis Child.* 1993;147:30-34.
27. National Institutes of Health, University of California. Expert Panel for corticosteroids as adjunctive therapy for pneumocystis pneumonia. Consensus statement on the use of corticosteroids as adjunctive therapy for pneumocystis pneumonia in the acquired immunodeficiency syndrome. *N Engl J Med.* 1990;323:1500-1504.
28. Bracken MB, Shepard MJ, Collins WF, et al. A randomized, controlled trial of methylprednisolone or naloxone in the treatment of acute spinal-cord injury. *N Engl J Med.* 1990;322:1405-1411.
29. Bracken MB, Shepard MJ, Holford TR, et al. Administration of methylprednisolone for 24 or 48 hours or tirilazad mesylate for 48 hours in the treatment of acute spinal cord injury. *JAMA.* 1997;277:1597-1604.
30. Jaffe K, Weddon D. Emergency management of blunt trauma in children. *N Engl J Med.* 1991;324:1477.
31. Fackler JC, Yaster M. Multiple trauma in the pediatric patient. In: Rogers MC, ed. *Textbook of Pediatric Intensive Care.* 2nd ed. Baltimore, MD: Lippincott Williams & Wilkins; 1992:1468.
32. Ino T, Okubo M, Akimoto K, et al. Corticosteroid therapy for ventricular tachycardia in children with silent lymphocytic myocarditis. *J Pediatr.* 1995;126:304-308.
33. Desmarquest P, Tamalet A, Fauroux B, et al. Chronic interstitial lung disease in children: response to high-dose intravenous methylprednisone pulses. *Pediatr Pulmonol.* 1998;26:332-338.
34. Delesalle F, Staumont D, Houmany MA, et al. Pulse methylprednisolone therapy for threatening periocular haemangiomas of infancy. *Acta Derm Venereol.* 2006;86:429-432.
35. Pope E, Krafchik BR, Macarthur C, et al. Oral versus high-dose pulse corticosteroids for problematic infantile hemangiomas: a randomized, controlled trial. *Pediatr.* 2007;119:e1239-e1247.

References

36. Raymond G, Day P, Rabb M. Sodium content of commonly administered intravenous drugs. *Hosp Pharm*. 1982;17:560-561.
37. Trissel LA, ed. *Handbook on Injectable Drugs*. 15th ed. Bethesda, MD: American Society of Health-System Pharmacists; 2009.
38. Sundel RP, Baker AL, Fulton DR, et al. Corticosteroids in the initial treatment of Kawasaki Disease: report of a randomized trial. *J Pediatr*. 2003;142:611-616.
39. Newburger J, Sleeper LA, McCrindle BW, et al. Randomized trial of pulsed corticosteroid therapy for primary treatment of Kawasaki disease. *N Engl J Med*. 2007;356:663-675.
40. Falcini F, Ricci L, Poggi GM, et al. Severe cutaneous manifestations in a child with refractory Kawasaki disease. *Rheumatology*. 2006;45:1445-1446.
41. Baethge BA, Lidsky MD. Intractable hiccups associated with high dose intravenous methylprednisolone therapy. *Ann Intern Med*. 1986;104:58-59.
42. Klein-Gitelman MS, Pachman LM. Intravenous corticosteroids: adverse reactions are more variable than expected in children. *J Rheumatol*. 1998;25:1995-2002.
43. Sheth A, Reddymasu S, Jackson R. Worsening of asthma with systemic corticosteroids: a case report and review of literature. *J Gen Intern Med*. 2006;21:C11-C13.
44. Ueda N, Yoshikawa T, Chihara M, et al. Atrial fibrillation following methylprednisone pulse therapy. *Pediatr Nephrol*. 1988;2:29-31.
45. Bettinelli A, Paterlini G, Mazzucchi E, et al. Seizures and transient blindness following intravenous pulse methylprednisone in children with primary glomerulonephritis. *Child Nephrol Urol*. 1991;11:41-43.
46. Kasper WJ, Howe PM. Fatal varicella after a single course of corticosteroids. *Pediatr Infect Dis J*. 1990;9:729-732.
47. Siomou E, Challa A, Tzoufi M, et al. Biochemical markers of bone metabolism in infants and children under intravenous corticosteroid therapy. *Calcif Tissue Int*. 2003;73:319-325.
48. Sun Jo D, Yang JW, Han Hwang P, et al. Stevens-Johnson syndrome in a boy with nephrotic syndrome during prednisolone therapy. *Pediatr Nephrol*. 2003;18:959-961.

Metoclopramide HCl

1. Available at: http://www.usp.org/hqi/similarProducts/choosy.html. Accessed August 29, 2009.
2. Available at: http://www.fda.gov/NewsEvents/Newsroom/PressAnnouncements/ucm149533.htm. Accessed September 13, 2009.
3. Metoclopramide hydrochloride injection [package insert]. Lake forest, IL: Hospira Inc; October 2006.
4. Marshall G, Kerr S, Vowels M, et al. Antiemetic therapy for chemotherapy-induced vomiting: metoclopramide, benztropine, dexamethasone, and lorazepam regimens compared with chlorpromazine alone. *J Pediatr*. 1989;115:156-160.
5. Gralla RJ, Tyson LB, Kris MG, et al. The management of chemotherapy induced nausea and vomiting. *Med Clin North Am*. 1987;71:289-301.
6. Kohli-Kumar M, Pearson ADJ, Sharkey I, et al. Urinary retention—an unusual dystonic reaction to continuous metoclopramide infusion. *DICP Ann Pharmacother*. 1991;25:469-470.
7. De Mulder PHM, Seynaeve C, Vermorken JB, et al. Ondansetron compared with high-dose metoclopramide in prophylaxis of acute and delayed cisplatin-induced nausea and vomiting. *Ann Intern Med*. 1990;113:834-840.
8. Brechot JM, Dupeyron JP, Delattre C, et al. Continuous infusion of high-dose metoclopramide: comparison of pharmacokinetically adjusted and standard doses for the control of cisplatin-induced acute emesis. *Eur J Clin Pharmacol*. 1991;40:283-286.
9. Kearns GL, Fiser DH. Metoclopramide-induced methemoglobinemia. *Pediatrics*. 1988;82:364-366.
10. Robertson J, Shilkofski N, eds. *The Harriet Lane Handbook*. 17th ed. Philadelphia, PA: Elsevier Mosby; 2005.
11. Benitz WE, Tatro DS. *The Pediatric Drug Handbook*. Chicago, IL: Year Book; 1988:14.
12. Furst SR, Rodarte A. Prophylactic antiemetic treatment with ondansetron in children undergoing tonsillectomy. *Anesthesiol*. 1994;81:799-803.
13. Lin DM, Furst ST, Rodarte A. A double-blinded comparison of metoclopramide and droperidol for prevention of emesis following strabismus surgery. *Anesthesiol*. 1992;76:357-361.
14. Ferrari LR, Donlon JV. Metoclopramide reduces the incidence of vomiting after tonsillectomy in children. *Anesth Analg*. 1992;75:351-354.
15. Shende D, Mandal NG. Efficacy of ondansetron and metoclopramide for preventing postoperative emesis following strabismus surgery in children. *Anaesthesia*. 1997;52:496-500.
16. Kathirvel S, Shende D, Madan R. Comparison of anti-emetic effects of ondansetron, metoclopromidine or a combination of both in children undergoing surgery for strabismus. *Eur J Anaesthesiol*. 1999;16:761-765.
17. Stene FN, Seay RE, Young LA, et al. Prospective, randomized, double-blind, placebo-controlled comparison of metoclopramide and ondansetron for prevention of posttonsillectomy or adenotonsillectomy emesis. *J Clin Anesth*. 1996;8:540-544.
18. Bolton AM, Myles PS, Carlin JB, et al. Randomized, double-blind study comparing the efficacy of moderate-dose metoclopramide and ondansetron for the prophylactic control of postoperative vomiting in children after tonsillectomy. *Br J Anaesth*. 2007;99:699-703.
19. Aronoff GR, Berns JS, Brier ME, et al. Drug prescribing in renal failure. 4th ed. Available at: http://www.kdp-baptist.louisville.edu/renalbook/. Accessed September 13, 2009.
20. Roila F, Basurto C, Bracarda S, et al. Double-blind crossover trial of single vs divided dose of metoclopramide in a combined regimen for treatment of cisplatin-induced emesis. *Eur J Cancer*. 1991;27:119-121.
21. Gralla RJ, Itri LM, Pisko SE, et al. Antiemetic efficacy of high-dose metoclopramide: randomized trials with placebo and prochlorperazine in patients with chemotherapy-induced nausea and vomiting. *N Engl J Med*. 1981;305:905-909.
22. Trissel LA, ed. *Handbook on Injectable Drugs*. 15th ed. Bethesda, MD: American Society of Health-System Pharmacists; 2009.
23. Allen JC, Gralla RJ, Reilly C, et al. Metoclopramide: dose-related toxicity and preliminary antiemetic studies in children receiving cancer chemotherapy. *J Clin Oncol*. 1985;3:1135-1141.
24. Terrin BN, McWilliams NB, Maurer HM. Side effects of metoclopramide as an antiemetic in childhood cancer chemotherapy. *J Pediatr*. 198;104:138-140.
25. Howrie DL, Felix C, Wollman M, et al. Metoclopramide as an antiemetic agent in pediatric oncology patients. *Drug Intell Clin Pharm*. 1986;20:122-124.
26. Madani S, Tolia V. Gynecomastia with metoclopramide use in pediatric patients. *J Clin Gastroenterol*. 1997;24:79-81.
27. Chellis MJ, Sanders SV, Dean JM, et al. Bedside transpyloric tube placement in the pediatric intensive care unit. *J Parenter Enteral Nutr*. 1996;20:88-90.
28. Ozucelik DN, Karaca MA, Sivri B. Effectiveness of pre-emptive metoclopramide infusion in alleviating pain, discomfort and nausea associated with nasogastric tube insertion: a randomized, double-blind placebo-controlled trial. *Int J Clin Pract*. 2005;59:1422-1427.
29. Harlev D, Mimouni F, Dollberg S. A clinical pilot trial of metoclopramide therapy for gastric residuals in preterm infants. *Acta Paediatrica*. 2007;96:1238-1244.

metroNIDAZOLE/metroNIDAZOLE HCl

1. Available at: http://www.ismp.org/Tools/tallmanletters.pdf. Accessed November 11, 2009.
2. Available at: http://ismp.org/Tools/confuseddrugnames.pdf. Accessed November 27, 2009.
3. Available at: http://www.usp.org/hqi/similarProducts/choosy.html. Accessed November 11, 2009.
4. Metronidazole [package insert]. Deerfield, IL: Baxter Pharmaceuticals.
5. Prober CG, Stevenson DK, Benitz WE. The use of antibiotics in neonates weighing less than 1200 grams. *Pediatr Infect Dis J*. 1990;9: 111-121.

6. Jager-Roman E, Doyle PE, Baird-Lambert J, et al. Pharmacokinetics and tissue distribution of metronidazole in the new born infant. *J Pediatr.* 1982;100:651-654.
7. Nelson JD, Bradley JS, *eds. Nelson's Pocket Book of Pediatric Antimicrobial Therapy.* 17th ed. Chicago, IL: American Academy of Pediatrics; 2009.
8. American Academy of Pediatrics. Pickering LK, Baker CJ, Kimberlin DW, et al., eds. *2009 Red Book: Report of the Committee on Infectious Diseases.* 28th ed. Elk Grove Village, IL: American Academy of Pediatrics; 2009.
9. Hall P, Kaye CM, McIntosh N, et al. Intravenous metronidazole in the newborn. *Arch Dis Child.* 1983;58:529-531.
10. Upadhyaya P, Bhatnagar V, Basu N. Pharmacokinetics of intravenous metronidazole in neonates. *J Pediatr Surg.* 1988;23:263-265.
11. Brook I. Treatment of anaerobic infections in children with metronidazole. *Dev Pharmacol Ther.* 1983;6:187-198.
12. Oldenburg B, Speck WT. Metronidazole. *Pediatr Clin North Am*. 1983;30:71-75.
13. Grundfest-Broniatowski S, Quader M, Alexander F, et al. Clostridium difficile colitis in the critically ill. *Dis Colon Rectum.* 1996;39:619-623.
14. Bouza E, Munoz P, Alonso R. Clinical manifestations, treatment and control of infections caused by Clostridium difficile. *Clin Microbiol Infect.* 2005;11 suppl 4:57-64.
15. Emil S, Laberge JM, Mikhail P, et al. Appendicitis in children: a ten-year update of therapeutic recommendations. *J Pediatr Surg.* 2003;38: 236-242.
16. Arnoff GR, Berns JS, Brier ME, et al. *Drug Prescribing in Renal Failure: Dosing Guidelines for Adults.* 4th ed. Philadelphia, PA: American College of Physicians; 1999.
17. Trissel LA, ed. *Handbook on Injectable Drugs.* 15th ed. Bethesda, MD: American Society of Health-System Pharmacists; 2009.
18. Robinson CA, Sawyer JE. Y-site compatibility of medications with parenteral nutrition. *J Pediatr Pharmacol Ther.* 2009;14:49-57.
19. Bailes J, Willis J, Piebe, C, et al. Encephelopathy with metronidazole in a child. *Am J Dis Child.* 1983 Mar;137:290-291.
20. Halloran T. Convulsions associated with high cumulative doses of metronidazole. *Drug Intell Clin Pharm.* 1982;16:409.
21. Duffy L, Daum F, Fisher S, et al. Peripheral neuropathy in crohn's disease patients treated with metronidazole. *Gastroenterology.* 1985;88:681-684.
22. Hobson-Webb L, Roach S, Donofrio D. Metronidazole: newly recognized cause of autonomic neuropathy. *J Child Neurol* 2006;21:429-431.

Micafungin

1. Available at: http://ismp.org/Tools/highalertmedications.pdf. ISMP 2008. Accessed August 24, 2009.
2. Available at: http://ismp.org/Tools/confuseddrugnames.pdf. Accessed August 24, 2009.
3. Available at: http://www.usp.org/hqi/similarProducts/choosy.html. Accessed August 24, 2009.
4. Mycamine [package insert]. Deerfield, IL: Astellas Pharma US Inc; January 2008.
5. American Academy of Pediatrics. Antifungal drugs for systemic fungal infections. Pickering LK, Baker CJ, Kimberlin DW, et al., eds. *2009 Red Book: Report of the Committee on Infectious Diseases.* 28th ed. Elk Grove Village, IL: American Academy of Pediatrics; 2009:765-776.
6. Heresi GP, Gerstmann DR, Reed MD, et al. The pharmacokinetics and safety of micafungin, a novel echinocandin, in premature neonates. *Pediatr Infect Dis J.* 2006;25:1110-1115.
7. Pannaraj PS, Walsh TJ, Baker CJ. Advances in antifungal therapy. *Pediatr Infect Dis J.* 2005;24:921-922.
8. Ostrosky-Zeichner L, Kontoyiannis D, Raffalli J, et al. International, open-label, noncomparative, clinical trial of micafungin alone and in combination for treatment of newly diagnosed and refractory candidemia. *Eur J Clin Microbiol Infect Dis.* 2005;24:654-661.
9. Tabata K, Katashima M, Kawamura A, et al. Linear pharmacokinetics of micafungin and its active metabolites in Japanese pediatric patients with fungal infections. *Biol Pharm Bull.* 2006;29:1706-1711.
10. Kobayashi S, Murayama S, Tatsuzawa, et al. X-linked severe combined immunodeficiency (X-SCID) with high blood levels of immunoglobulins and *Aspergillus* pneumonia successfully treated with micafangin followed by unrelated cord blood stem cell transplantation. *Eur J Pediatr.* 2007;166:207-210.
11. Denning DW, Marr KA, Lau WM, et al. Micafungin (FK463), alone or in combination with other systemic antifungal agents, for the treatment of acute invasive aspergillosis. *J Infect.* 2006;53:337-349.
12. Singer MS, Seibel N, Vezina G, et al. Successful treatment of invasive aspergillosis in two patients with acute myelogenous leukemia. *J Pediatr Hematol Oncol.* 2003;25:252-256.
13. Fallon RM, Girotto JE. A review of clinical experience with newer antifungals in children. *J Pediatr Pharmacol Ther.* 2008;13:124-140.
14. Queiroz-Telles F, Berezin E, Leverger G, et al. Micafungin versus liposomal amphotericin B for pediatric patients with invasive candidiasis. *Pediatr Infect Dis J.* 2008;27:820-826.
15. Seibel NL, Schwartz C, Arrieta A, et al. Safety, tolerability, and pharmacokinetics of micafungin (FK463) in febrile neutropenic pediatric patients. *Antimicrob Agent Chemother.* 2005;49:3317-3324.
16. Steinbach WJ, Benjamin DK. New antifungal agents under development in children and neonates. *Curr Opin Infect Dis.* 2005;18:484-489.
17. van Burik JA, Ratanatharathorn V, Stepan DE., et al. Micafungin versus fluconazole for prophylaxis against invasive fungal infections during neutropenia in patients undergoing hematopoietic stem cell transplantation. *Clin Infect Dis.* 2004;39:1407-1416.
18. Kishino S, Ohno K, Shimanura T, et al. Optimal prophylactic dosage and disposition of micafungin in living donor liver recipients. *Clin Transplant.* 2004;18:676-680.
19. Carver PL. Micafungin. *Ann Pharmacother.* 2004;38:1707-1721.
20. Herbert MF, Smith HE, Marbury TC, et al. Pharmacokinetics of micafungin in healthy volunteers, volunteers with moderate liver disease, and volunteers with renal dysfunction. *J Clin Pharm.* 2005;45:1145.
21. Aronoff GR, Berns JS, Brier ME, et al. Drug prescribing in renal failure. 4th ed. Available at: http://www.kdp-baptist.louisville.edu/renalbook/. Accessed November 9, 2009.
22. Trissel LA, ed. *Handbook on Injectable Drugs.* 15th ed. Bethesda, MD: American Society of Health-System Pharmacists; 2009.

Midazolam HCl

1. Available at: http://ismp.org/Tools/highalertmedications.pdf. Accessed October 9, 2009.
2. Available at: http://www.usp.org/hqi/similarProducts/choosy.html. Accessed October 9, 2009.
3. Midazolam hydrochloride [package insert]. Lake Forest, IL: Hospira Inc; December 2004.
4. Midazolam. Lexi-Comp® Online with AHFS® (database). Hudson, OH: Lexi-Comp Inc; updated September 8, 2009.
5. Yaster M, Nichols DG, Deshpande JK, et al. Midazolam–fentanyl intravenous sedation in children: case report of respiratory arrest. *Pediatrics.* 1990;86:463-467.
6. Cole WHJ. Midazolam in paediatric anaesthesia. *Anaesth Intensive Care.* 1982;10:36-39.
7. Holloway AM, Jordaan DG, Brock-Utne JG. Midazolam for the intravenous induction of anaesthesia in children. *Anaesth Intensive Care.* 1982;10:340-343.
8. Salonen M, Kanto J, Iisalo E, et al. Midazolam as an induction agent in children: a pharmacokinetic and clinical study. *Anesth Analg.* 1987;66:625-628.
9. Shankar V, Deshpande JK. Procedural sedation in the pediatric patient. *Anesthesiol Clin N Am.* 2005;23:635-654.
10. Flood RG, Krauss B. Procedural sedation and analgesia for children in the emergency department. *Emerg Med Clin North Am.* 2003;21:121-139.
11. Krauss B, Green S. Procedural sedation and analgesia in children. *Lancet.* 2006;367:766-780.
12. Sandler ES, Weyman C, Conner K, et al. Midazolam versus fentanyl as premedication for painful procedures in children with cancer. *Pediatrics.* 1992;89:631-634.
13. Tobias JD. Sedation and analgesia in paediatric intensive care units. *Pediatr Drugs.* 1999;109-125.

References

14. Sievers TD, Yee JD, Foley ME, et al. Midazolam for conscious sedation during pediatric oncology procedures: safety and recovery parameters. *Pediatrics.* 1992;88:1172-1179.
15. Manzi SF, Shannon WM. Drug therapy in the pediatric emergency department. In: Yaffe SJ, Aranda JV, eds. *Neonatal and Pediatric Pharmacology.* 3rd ed. Philadelphia, PA: Lippincott Williams & Wilkins; 2005:288-289.
16. Slovis TL, Parks C, Reneau D, et al. Pediatric sedation: short-term effects. *Pediatric Radiology.* 1993;23:345-348.
17. Di Liddo L, D'Angelo A, Nguyen B, et al. Etomidate versus midazolam for procedural sedation in pediatric outpatients: a randomized controlled trial. *Ann Emerg Med.* 2006;48:433-440.
18. Pershad J, Wan J, Anghelescu DL. Comparison of propofol with pentobarbital/midazolam/fentanyl sedation for magnetic resonance imaging of the brain in children. *Pediatrics.* 2007;120:e629-e636.
19. Heard C, Burrows F, Johnson K, et al. A comparison of dexmedetomidine-midazolam with propofol for maintenance of anesthesia in children undergoing magnetic resonance imaging. *Anesth Analg.* 2008;107:1832-1839.
20. Hartwig S, Roth B, Theisohn M. Clinical experience with continuous intravenous sedation using midazolam and fentanyl in the paediatric intensive care unit. *Eur J Pediatr.* 1991;150:784-788.
21. Jacqz-Aigrain E, Daoud P, Burtin P, et al. Pharmacokinetics of midazolam during continuous infusion in critically ill neonates. *Eur J Clin Pharmacol.* 1992;42:329-332.
22. Silvasi DL, Rosen DA, Rosen KR. Continuous intravenous midazolam infusion for sedation in the pediatric intensive care unit. *Anesth Analg.* 1988;67:286-288.
23. Lloyd-Thomas AR, Booker PD. Infusion of midazolam in paediatric patients after cardiac surgery. *Br J Anaesth.*1986;58:1109-1115.
24. Jacqz-Aigrain E, Daoud P, Burtin P, et al. Placebo-controlled trial of midazolam sedation in mechanically ventilated newborn babies. *Lancet.* 1994;344:646-650.
25. Rigby-Jones AE, Priston MJ, Sneyd JR, et al. Remifentanil-midazolam sedation for paediatric patients receiving mechanical ventilation after cardiac surgery. *Br J Anaesth.* 2007;99:252-261.
26. Booker PD, Beechey A, Lloyd-Thomas AR. Sedation of children requiring artificial ventilation using an infusion of midazolam. *Br J Anaesth.* 1986;58:1104-1108.
27. Rivera R, Segnini M, Baltodano A, et al. Midazolam in the treatment of status epilepticus in children. *Crit Care Med.* 1993;21:991-994.
28. Kumar A, Bleck TP. Intravenous midazolam for the treatment of refractory status epilepticus. *Crit Care Med.* 1992;20:483-388.
29. Parent JM, Lowenstein DH. Treatment of refractory generalized status epilepticus with continuous infusion of midazolam. *Neurology.* 1994;44:1837-1840.
30. Igartua J, Silver P, Maytal J, et al. Midazolam coma for refractory status epilepticus in children. *Crit Care Med.* 1999;27:1982-1985.
31. Ozdemir D, Gulez P, Uran N, et al. Efficacy of continuous midazolam infusion and mortality in childhood refractory generalized convulsive status epilepticus. *Seizure.* 2005;14:129-132.
32. Holmes GL, Riviello JJ. Midazolam and pentobarbital for refractory status epilepticus. *Pediatr Neurol.* 1999;20:259-264.
33. Marik PE, Varon J. The management of status epilepticus. *Chest.* 2004;126:582-591.
34. Conde Castro JR, Borges AA, Martinez ED, et al. Midazolam in neonatal seizures with no response to phenobarbital. *Neurology.* 2005;64:876-879.
35. Shany E, Benzaqen O, Watemberg N. Comparison of continuous drip of midazolam or lidocaine in the treatment of intractable neonatal seizures. *Child Neurol.* 2007;22:255-259.
36. Morrison G, Gibbons E, Whitehouse WP. High-dose midazolam therapy for refractory status epilepticus in children. *Intensive Care Med.* 2006;32:2070-2076.
37. Hayashi K, Osawa M, Aihara M, et al. Efficacy of intravenous midazolam for status epilepticus in childhood. *Pediatr Neurol.* 2007;36:366-372.
38. Morrison GC, Whitehouse WP. High-dose midazolam in convulsive status epilepticus. *Pediatr Neurol.* 2008;39:221.
39. Aronoff GR, Berns JS, Brier ME, et al. Drug prescribing in renal failure. 4th ed. Available at: http://www.kdp-baptist.louisville.edu/renalbook/. Accessed October 10, 2009.
40. Robinson CA, Sawyer JE. Y-site compatibility of medications with parenteral nutrition. *J Pediatr Pharmacol Ther.* 2009;14:49-57.
41. Chamberlain JM, Altieri MA, Futterman C, et al. A prospective randomized study comparing intramuscular midazolam with intravenous diazepam for the treatment of seizures in children. *Pediatr Emerg Care.* 1997;13:92-94.
42. Vilke GM, Sharieff GQ, Marino A, et al. Midazolam for the treatment of out-of-hospital pediatric seizures. *Prehosp Emerg Care.* 2002;6:215-217.
43. van den Anker JN, Sauer PJJ. The use of midazolam in the premature neonate. *Eur J Pediatr.* 1992;151:152.
44. Magny JF, Zupan V, Dehan M, et al. Midazolam and myoclonus in neonate. *Eur J Pediatr.* 1992;153:389-390.
45. Cronin CM. Neurotoxicity of lorazepam in a premature infant. *Pediatrics.* 1992;89:1129.
46. Reiter PD, Stiles AD. Lorazepam toxicity in a premature infant. *Ann Pharmacother.* 1993; 27:727-729.
47. Chess PR, D'Angio CT. Clonic movement following lorazepam administration in full-term infants. *Arch Pediatr Adolesc Med.* 1998;152:98-99.
48. Cronin CM. Neurotoxicity of lorazepam in a premature infant. *Pediatrics.* 1992;89:1129.
49. Reiter PD, Stiles AD. Lorazepam toxicity in a premature infant. *Ann Pharmacother.* 1993; 27:727-729.
50. Chess PR, D'Angio CT. Clonic movement following lorazepam administration in full-term infants. *Arch Pediatr Adolesc Med.* 1998;152:98-99.
51. Ng E, Klinger G, Shah V, et al. Safety of benzodiazepines in newborns. *Ann Pharmacother.* 2002;36:1150-1155.
52. Bergman I, Steeves M, Burckart G, et al. Reversible neurologic abnormalities associated with prolonged intravenous midazolam and fentanyl administration. *J Pediatr.* 1991;119:644-649
53. Sury MR, Billingham I, Russell GN, et al. Acute benzodiazepine withdrawal syndrome after midazolam infusions in children. *Crit Care Med.* 1989;17:301-302.
54. Conway EE Jr, Singer LP. Acute benzodiazepine withdrawal after midazolam in children. *Crit Care Med.* 1990;18:461. Letter.
55. Fonsmark L, Rasmussen YH, Carl P. Occurrence of withdrawal in critically ill children. *Crit Care Med.* 1999;27:196-199.
56. Lieh-Lai M, Sarnaik AP. Therapeutic applications in pediatric intensive care. In: Yaffe SJ, Aranda JV, eds. *Neonatal and Pediatric Pharmacology.* 3rd ed. Philadelphia, PA: Lippincott Williams & Wilkins; 2005:261-277.
57. Hoffman EJ, Warren EW. Flumazenil: a benzodiazepine antagonist. *Clin Pharm.* 1993;12:614-656.

Milrinone Lactate

1. Available at: http://ismp.org/Tools/highalertmedications.pdf. Accessed October 13, 2009.
2. Available at: http://www.usp.org/hqi/similarProducts/choosy.html. Accessed October 13, 2009.
3. Milrinone [package insert]. Bedford OH: Bedford Laboratories; July 2007.
4. Chang AC, Atz AM, Wernovsky G, et al. Milrinone: systemic and pulmonary hemodynamic effects in neonates after cardiac surgery. *Crit Care Med.* 1995;23:1907-1914.
5. Barton P, Garcia J, Kouatli A, et al. Hemodynamic effects of IV milrinone lactate in pediatric patients with septic shock. *Chest.* 1996;109:302-312.
6. Lindsay CA, Barton P, Lawless S, et al. Pharmacokinetics and pharmacodynamics of milrinone lactate in pediatric patients with shock. *J Pediatr.* 1998;132:329-334.
7. Zuppa AF, Nicolson SC, Adamson PC, et al. Population pharmacokinetics of milrinone in neonates with hypoplastic left heart syndrome undergoing stage I reconstruction. *Anesth Analg.* 2006;102:1062-1069.
8. De Oliveira NC, Ashburn DA, Khalid F, et al. Prevention of early sudden circulatory collapse after the Norwood operation. *Circulation.* 2004;110(11 suppl 1):II133-138.
9. Bailey JM, Miller BE, Lu W, et al. The pharmacokinetics of milrinone in pediatric patients after cardiac surgery. *Anesthesiology.* 1999;90:1012-1018.
10. Ramamoorthy C, Anderson GD, Williams GD, et al. Pharmacokinetics and side effects of milrinone in infants and children after open heart surgery. *Anesth Analg.* 1998;86:283-289.

11. American Heart Association. Guidelines 2005 for cardiopulmonary resuscitation and emergency cardiovascular care—part 12: pediatric advanced life support. *Circulation.* 2005;112:167-187.
12. Paradisis M, Evans N, Kluckow M, et al. Pilot study of milrinone for low systemic blood flow in very preterm infants. *J Pediatr.* 2006;148:306-313.
13. Paradisis M, Jiang X, McLachlan AJ, et al. Population pharmacokinetics and dosing regimen design of milrinone in preterm infants. *Arch Dis Child Fetal Neonatal Ed.* 2007;92:F204-F209.
14. Paradisis M, Evans N, Kluckow M, et al. Randomized trial of milrinone versus placebo for prevention of low systemic blood flow in very preterm infants. *J Pediatr.* 2009;154:189-195.
15. Cai J, Su Z, Shi Z, et al. Nitric oxide and milrinone: combined effect on pulmonary circulation after Fontan-type procedure: a prospective, randomized study. *Ann Thorac Surg.* 2008;86:882-888.
16. Watson S, Christian K, Churchwell KB. Use of milrinone in the pediatric critical care unit. *Pediatrics.* 1999;104:S681-S682.
17. Rich N, West N, McMaster P, et al. Milrinone in meningococcal sepsis. *Pediatr Crit Care Med.* 2003;4:394-395.
18. Trissel LA, ed. *Handbook on Injectable Drugs.* 15th ed. Bethesda, MD: American Society of Health-System Pharmacists; 2009.
19. Akkerman SR, Zhang H, Mullins RE, et al. Stability of milrinone lactate in the presence of 29 critical care drugs and 4 i.v. solutions. *Am J Health-Syst Pharm.* 1999;56:63-68.
20. Robinson CA, Sawyer JE. Y-site compatibility of medications with parenteral nutrition. *J Pediatr Pharmacol Ther.* 2009;14:49-57.
21. Milrinone. Lexi-Comp® Online with AHFS® (database). Bethesda, MD: American Society of Health-System Pharmacists; updated August 13, 2009.
22. Young RA, Ward A. Milrinone: a preliminary review of its pharmacological properties and therapeutic use. *Drugs.* 1988;36:158-192.

Mivacurium

1. Available at: http://ismp.org/Tools/highalertmedications.pdf. ISMP 2008. Accessed August 24, 2009.
2. Mivacron [package insert]. Lake Forest, IL: Hospira Inc.
3. Rowlee SC. Monitoring neuromuscular blockade in the intensive care unit: the peripheral nerve stimulator. *Heart Lung.* 1999;28:352-362.
4. Martin LD, Bratton SL, O'Rourke PP. Clinical uses and controversies of neuromuscular blocking agents in infants and children. *Crit Care Med.* 1999;27:1358-1368.
5. McCluskey A, Meakin G. Dose-response and minimum time to satisfactory intubation conditions after mivacurium in children. *Anaesthesia.* 1996;51:438-441.
6. Markakis DA, Lau M, Brown R, et al. The pharmacokinetics and steady state pharmacodynamics of mivacurium in children. *Anesthesiology.* 1998;88:978-983.
7. Ostergaard D, Gatke MR, Berg H, et al. The pharmacodynamics and pharmacokinetics of mivacurium in children. *Acta Anaesthiol Scand.* 2002;46:512-518.
8. Fox MH, Hunt PC. Prolonged neuromuscular block associated with mivacurium. *Br J Anaesth.* 1995;74:237-238.
9. Kendrick K. Prolonged paralysis related to mivacurium: a case study. *J Perianesth Nur.* 2005;20:7-12.

Morphine Sulfate

1. Available at: http://ismp.org/Tools/highalertmedications.pdf. ISMP 2008.
2. Available at: http://ismp.org/Tools/confuseddrugnames.pdf. Updated April 1, 2005.
3. Available at: http://www.usp.org/hqi/similarProducts/choosy.html. Accessed October 16, 2009.
4. Astromorph/PF (morphine sulfate injection, USP) Preservative-Free. Wilmington, DE: Astra Zeneca; August 2005.
5. Morphine sulfate injection, USP. Deerfield, IL: Baxter; December 2003.
6. Trissel LA. *Handbook on Injectable Drugs.* 10th ed. Bethesda, MD: American Society of Health-System Pharmacists; 1998.
7. Vicente KJ, Kada-Bekhaled K, Hillel G, et al. Programming errors contribute to death from patient-controlled analgesia: case report and estimate of probability. *Can J Anesth.* 2003;50:328-332.
8. Morphine. Lexi-Comp® Online with AHFS® (database). Hudson, OH: Lexi-Comp Inc; updated September 25, 2009.
9. Anand KJS. Pharmacological approaches to the management of pain in the neonatal intensive care unit. *J Perinatol.* 2007;27:S4-S11.
10. Lynn AM, Slattery JT. Morphine pharmacokinetics in early infancy. *Anesthesiology.* 1987;66:136-139.
11. Koren G, Butt W, Chinyanga H, et al. Postoperative morphine infusion in newborn infants: assessment of disposition characteristics and safety. *J Pediatr.* 1985;107:963-967.
12. Farrington EA, McGuiness GA, Johnson GF, et al. Continuous intravenous morphine infusion in postoperative newborn infants. *Am J Perinatol.* 1993;10:84-87.
13. Scott CS, Riggs KW, Ling EW, et al. Morphine pharmacokinetics and pain assessment in premature newborns. *J Pediatr.* 1999;135:423-329.
14. Lynn A, Nespeca MK, Bratton SL, et al. Clearance of morphine in postoperative infants during intravenous infusion: the influence of age and surgery. *Anesth Analg.* 1998;86:958-963.
15. Saarenmaa E, Neuvonen PJ, Rosenberg P, et al. Morphine clearance and effects in newborn infants in relation to gestational age. *Clin Pharmacol Ther.* 2000;68:160-166.
16. Anderson BJ, Palmer GM. Recent pharmacological advances in paediatric analgesics. *Br J Anaesth.* 2006;60:303-309.
17. Bouwmeester NJ, Anderson BJ, Tibboel D, Holford NHG. Developmental pharmacokinetics of morphine and its metabolites in neonates, infants and young children. *Br J Anaesth.* 2004;92:208-217.
18. American Academy of Pediatrics Committee on Drugs. Emergency drug doses for infants and children. *Pediatrics.* 1998;101:e1-e11.
19. Bray RJ. Postoperative analgesia provided by morphine infusion in children. *Anaesthesia.* 1983;38:1075-1078.
20. Lynn AM, Opheim KE, Tyler DC. Morphine infusion after pediatric cardiac surgery. *Crit Care Med.* 1984;12:863-866.
21. Dahlstrom B, Bolme P, Feychting H, et al. Morphine kinetics in children. *Clin Pharmacol Ther.* 1979;26:354-365.
22. Cole TB, Sprinkle RH, Smith SJ, et al. Intravenous narcotic therapy for children with severe sickle cell pain crisis. *Am J Dis Child.* 1986;140:1255-1259.
23. Dampier CD, Setty BNY, Logan J, et al. Intravenous morphine pharmacokinetics in pediatric patients with sickle cell disease. *J Pediatr.* 1995;126:461-467.
24. Miser AW, Miser JS, Clark BS. Continuous intravenous infusion of morphine sulfate for control of severe pain in children with terminal malignancy. *J Pediatr.* 1980;96:930-932.
25. Eschertzhuber S, Hohlrieder M, Keller C, et al. Comparison of high- and low-dose intrathecal morphine for spinal fusion in children. *Br J Anaesth.* 2008;100:538-543.
26. Aronoff GR, Berns JS, Brier ME, et al. Drug prescribing in renal failure. 4th ed. Available at: http://www.kdp-baptist.louisville.edu/renalbook/pediatric/. Accessed October 19, 2009.
27. Buck ML. Pharmacokinetic changes during extracorporeal membrane oxygenation. Implications for drug therapy of neonates. *Clin Pharmacokinet.* 2003;42:403-417.
28. Bhatt-Meta V, Annich G. Sedative clearance during extracorporeal membrane oxygenation. *Perfusion.* 2005;20:309-315.
29. Hartley R, Green M, Quinn M, et al. Pharmacokinetics of morphine infusion in premature neonates. *Arch Dis Child.* 1993;69:55-58.
30. Chay PC, Duffy BJ, Walker JS. Pharmacokinetic pharmacodynamic relationships of morphine in neonates. *Clin Pharmacol Ther.* 1992;51:334-342.

References

31. Bouwmeester NJ, van den Anker JN, Hop WCJ, et al. Age- and therapy-related effects on morphine requirements and plasma concentrations of morphine and its metabolites in postoperative infants. *Br J Anaesth*. 2003;90:642-652.

Multivitamins (Adult)

1. MVI Adult [package insert]. Lake Forest, IL: Hospira; October 2007.
2. Infuvite ADULT [package insert]. Deerfield, IL: Baxter Healthcare Corporation; May 2004.
3. Intravenous multivitamin shortage information. Available at: http://www.nutritioncare.org/wcontent.aspx?id=218. September 2007.
4. Multivitamin preparations for parenteral use. A statement by the Nutrition Advisory Group. American Medical Association—Department of Foods and Nutrition, 1975. *J Parenter Enteral Nutr*. 1979;3:258-262.
5. Trissel LA. *Handbook on Injectable Drugs*. 15th ed. Bethesda, MD: American Society of Health-System Pharmacists; 2009.
6. Scheiner JM, Araujo MM, DeRitter E. Thiamine destruction by sodium bisulfite in infusion solutions. *Am J Hosp Pharm*. 1981;38:1911-1913.
7. Glockling MR, Lutomski DM, Youngs CH, et al. Small volume infusion of multiple vitamins. *Clin Pharm*. 984;3:516-518.
8. Shils ME, Baker H, Frank O. Blood vitamin levels of long-term adult home total parenteral nutrition patients: the efficacy of the AMA–FDA parenteral multivitamin formulation. *J Parenter Enteral Nutr*. 1985;9:179-188.

Multivitamins (Pediatric)

1. MVI Pediatric [package insert]. Lake Forest, IL: Hospira; August 2007.
2. Infuvite Pediatric [package insert]. Deerfield, IL: Baxter Healthcare Corporation; September 2007.
3. Greene HL, Phillips BL. Vitamin dosages in premature infants. *Pediatrics*. 1987;79:655. Letter.
4. Greene HL, Hambidge KM, Schanler R, et al. Guidelines for the use of vitamins, trace elements, calcium, magnesium, and phosphorus in infants and children receiving total parenteral nutrition. Report of the Subcommittee on Pediatric Parenteral Nutrient Requirements from the Committee on Clinical Practice Issues of the American Society for Clinical Nutrition. *Am J Clin Nutr*. 1988;48:1324-1342.
5. Moore MC, Greene HL, Phillips B, et al. Evaluation of a pediatric multiple vitamin preparation for total parenteral nutrition in infants and children I. Blood levels of water soluble vitamins. *Pediatrics*. 1986;77:530-538.
6. Greene HL, Moore ME, Phillips B, et al. Evaluation of a pediatric multiple vitamin preparation for total parenteral nutrition II. Blood levels of vitamins A, D, and E. *Pediatrics*. 1986;77:539-547.
7. Intravenous multivitamin shortage information. Available at: http://www.nutritioncare.org/wcontent.aspx?id=218. September 2007.
8. Trissel LA. *Handbook on Injectable Drugs*. 15th ed. Bethesda, MD: American Society of Health-System Pharmacists; 2009.
9. Scheiner JM, Araujo MM, DeRitter E. Thiamine destruction by sodium bisulfite in infusion solutions. *Am J Hosp Pharm*. 1981;38:1911-1913.
10. Collier S, Crouch J, Hendricks K, et al. Use of cyclic parenteral nutrition in infants less than 6 months of age. *Nutr Clin Pract*. 1994;9:65-68.
11. Franck LS, Greene HL, Phillips BL. Alpha tocopheral (E) levels in premature infants during and after intravenous multivitamin supplementation. *Clin Res*. 1987;34:115A.
12. Greene HL, Porchelli P, Adcock E, et al. Vitamins for newborn infant formulas: a review of recommendations with emphasis on data from low birth-weigh infants. *Eur J Clin Nutr*. 1992;46(suppl 4):S1-S8.
13. Levy R, Herzberg GR, Andrews WL, et al. Thiamine, riboflavin, folate, and vitamin B12 status of low birth weight infants receiving parenteral and enteral nutrition. *J Parenter Enteral Nutr*. 1992;16:241-247.
14. Lavoie JC, Bélanger S, Spalinger M, et al. Admixture of a multivitamin preparation to parenteral nutrition: the major contributor to invitro generation of peroxides. *Pediatrics*. 1997 Mar;99:E6.
15. Laborie S, Lavoie JC, Pineeault M, et al. Protecting solutions of parenteral nutrition from peroxidatiion. *JPEN*. 1999;23:104-108.

Muromonab-CD3

1. Orthoclone OKT3 [prescribing information]. Raritan, NJ; Ortho Biotech; November 2004.
2. Schroeder TJ, Ryckman FC, Hurtabaise PE, et al. Immunological monitoring during and following OKT3 therapy in children. *Clin Transplantation*. 1991;5:191-196.
3. Schroeder TJ. Monoclonal antibody therapy in pediatric transplantation. *Transplantation Proc*. 1992;24(suppl 1):2-10.
4. Ettenger RB, Marik J, Rosenthal JT, et al. OKT3 for rejection reversal in pediatric renal transplantation. *Clin Transplantation*. 1988;2:180-184.
5. McDiarmid SV, Millis M, Terashita G, et al. Low serum OKT3 levels correlate with failure to prevent rejection in orthotopic liver transplant patients. *Transplantation Proc*. 1990;22:1774-1776.
6. Piatosa B, Grenda R, Prokurat S. Comparison of adjusted-dose vs. standard-dose OKT3 therapy of acute rejection in pediatric kidney transplant recipients. *Transplantation Proc*. 1993;25:2574.
7. Wilmot I, Kanter KR, Vincent RN, et al. OKT3 treatment in refractory pediatric heart transplant rejection. *J Heart Lung Transplant*. 2005;24:1793-1797.
8. Younes B, McDiarmid S, Martin M, et al. The effect of immunosuppression on post-transplant lymphoproliferative disease in pediatric liver transplant patients. *Transplant*. 2000;71:94-99.
9. Leone MR, Barry JM, Alexander SR, et al. Monoclonal antibody OKT3 therapy in pediatric kidney transplant recipients. *J Pediatr*. 1990;116:S86-S91.
10. McOmber D, Ibrahim J, Lublin DM, et al. Non-ischemic left ventricular dysfunction after pediatric cardiac transplantation: treatment with plasmapheresis and OKT3. *J Heart Lung Transplant*. 2004;23:552-557.
11. Benekli M, Hahn T, Williams BT, et al. Muromonab-CD3 (Orthoclone OKT3), methylprednisolone and cyclosporine for acute graft-versus-host disease prophylaxis in allogenic bone marrow transplantation. *Bone Marrow Transplantation*. 2006:38:365-370.
12. Chin C, Pittson SK, Luikart H, et al. Induction therapy for pediatric and adult heart transplantation: comparison between OKT3 and daclizumab. *Transplantation*. 2005;80:477-481.
13. Ahdoot J, Galindo A, Alejos JC, et al. Use of OKT3 for acute myocarditis in infants and children. *J Heart Lung Transplant*. 2000;19:1118-1121.
14. Jeyarajah DR, Thistlethwaite JR. General aspects of cytokine-release syndrome: timing and incidence of symptoms. *Transplantation Proc*. 1993;25(suppl 1):16-20.
15. Ryckman FC, Schroeder TJ, Pederson SH, et al. Use of monoclonal antibody immunosuppressive therapy in pediatric renal and liver transplantation. *Clin Transplantation*. 1991;5:186-190.

Nafcillin Sodium

1. Available at: http://www.usp.org/hqi/similarProducts/choosy.html. Accessed June 19, 2009.
2. Nafcillin. Lexi-Comp® Online with AHFS® (database). Bethesda, MD: American Society of Health-System Pharmacists; updated March 10, 2009.
3. Feldman WE, Nelson JD, Stanberry LR. Clinical and pharmacokinetic evaluation of nafcillin in infants and children. *J Pediatr*. 1978;93:1029-1033.
4. Zenk KE, Dungy CI, Greene GR. Nafcillin extravasation injury. *Am J Dis Child*. 1981;135:1113-1114.

References

5. Tilden SJ, Craft JC, Cano R, et al. Cutaneous necrosis associated with intravenous nafcillin therapy. *Am J Dis Child*. 1980;134:1046-1048.
6. MacCara ME. Extravasation: a hazard of intravenous therapy. *Drug Intell Clin Pharm*. 1983;17:713-717.
7. American Academy of Pediatrics. Pickering LK, Baker CJ, Kimberlin DW, et al., eds. *2009 Red Book: Report of the Committee on Infectious Diseases*. 28th ed. Elk Grove Village, IL: American Academy of Pediatrics; 2009.
8. Prober CG, Stevenson DK, Benitz WE. The use of antibiotics in neonates weighing less than 1200 grams. *Pediatr Infect Dis J*. 1990;9:111-121.
9. Greene GR, Cohen E. Nafcillin-induced neutropenia in children. *Pediatrics*. 1978;61:94-97.
10. Kancir LM, Tuazon CU, Cardella TA, et al. Adverse reactions to methicillin and nafcillin during treatment of serious Staphylococcus aureus infections. *Arch Intern Med*. 1978;138:909-911.
11. Rhodes KH, Henry NK. Antibiotic therapy for severe infections in infants and children. *Mayo Clin Proc*. 1992;67:59-68.
12. Baddour LM, Wilson WR, Bayer AS, et al. Infective endocarditis: diagnosis, antimicrobial therapy, and management of complications: a statement for healthcare professionals from the Committee on Rheumatic Fever, Endocarditis, and Kawasaki Disease, Council on Cardiovascular Disease in the Young, and the Councils on Clinical Cardiology, Stroke, and Cardiovascular Surgery and Anesthesia, American Heart Association: endorsed by the Infectious Diseases Society of America. *Circulation*. 2005;111:e394-e434.
13. Tunkel AR, Hartman BJ, Kaplan SL, et al. Practice guidelines for the management of bacterial meningitis. *Clin Infect Dis*. 2004;39:1267-1284.
14. Klein JO, Feigin RD, McCracken GH. Report of American Academy of Pediatrics task force on diagnosis and management of meningitis. *Pediatrics*. 1986;78(suppl):959-982.
15. American Academy of Pediatrics, Committee on Infectious Diseases. Treatment of bacterial meningitis. *Pediatrics*. 1988;6:904-907.
16. Eickhoff TC, Kislak JW, Finland M. Clinical evaluation of nafcillin in patients with severe staphylococcal disease. *N Engl J Med*. 1965; 272:699-708.
17. Trissel LA, ed. *Handbook on Injectable Drugs*. 15th ed. Bethesda, MD: American Society of Health-System Pharmacists; 2009.
18. Robinson DC, Cookson TL, Frisafe JA. Concentration guidelines for parenteral antibiotics in fluid-restricted patients. *Drug Intell Clin Pharm*. 1987;21:985-989.
19. McLaughlin JE, Reeves DS. Clinical and laboratory evidence for inactivation of gentamicin by carbenicillin. *Lancet*. 1971;1:261-264.
20. Riff LJ, Jackson GG. Laboratory and clinical conditions for gentamicin inactivation by carbenicillin. *Arch Intern Med*. 1972;130:887-981.
21. Manian FA, Stone WJ, Alford RH. Adverse antibiotic effects associated with renal insufficiency. *Rev Infect Dis*. 1990;12:236-249.
22. Davies M, Morgan JR, Anand C. Interactions of carbenicillin and ticarcillin with gentamicin. *Antimicrob Agents Chemother*. 1975;7:431-434.
23. Weibert R, Keane W, Shapiro F. Carbenicillin inactivation of aminoglycosides in patients with severe renal failure. *Trans Amer Soc Artif Int Organs*. 1976;22:439-443.
24. Robinson CA, Sawyer JE. Y-site compatibility of medications with parenteral nutrition. *J Pediatr Pharmacol Ther*. 2009;14:49-57.
25. Knoderer CA, Morris JL, Cox EG. Continuous infusion nafcillin for sterna osteomyelitis in an infant after cardiac surgery. *J. Pediatr Pharmacol Ther*. 2010;15:49-54.

Naloxone HCl

1. Available at: http://ismp.org/Tools/confuseddrugnames.pdf. Accessed September 30, 2009.
2. Available at: http://www.usp.org/hqi/similarProducts/choosy.html. Accessed September 30, 2009.
3. Naloxone [package insert]. Lake Forest, IL: Hospira Inc; January 2008.
4. Naloxone. Lexi-Comp® Online with AHFS® (database). Hudson, OH: Lexi-Comp Inc; updated September 9, 2009.
5. McGuire W, Fowie PW. Naloxone for narcotic exposed newborn infants. Systematic review. *Arch Dis Child Fetal Neonatal Ed*. 2003;88:F308-F311.
6. American Heart Association. Guidelines 2005 for cardiopulmonary resuscitation and emergency cardiovascular care—part 12: pediatric advanced life support. *Circulation*. 2005;112:167-187.
7. American Academy of Pediatrics Committee on Drugs. Emergency drug doses for infants and children. *Pediatrics*.1998;101:e1-e11.
8. Standards and guidelines for cardiopulmonary resuscitation (CPR) and emergency cardiac care (ECC)—part VI: neonatal advanced life support. *JAMA*. 1986;255:2969-2973.
9. American Academy of Pediatrics, Committee on Drugs. Naloxone use in newborns. *Pediatrics*. 1980;65:667-669.
10. Handal KA, Schauben JL, Salamone FR. Naloxone. *Ann Emerg Med*. 1983;12:438-445.
11. American Academy of Pediatrics, Committee on Drugs. Emergency drug doses for infants and children and naloxone use in newborns: clarification. *Pediatrics*. 1989;83:803.
12. American Academy of Pediatrics, Committee on Drugs. Naloxone dosage and route of administration for infants and children: addendum to emergency drug doses for infants and children. *Pediatrics*. 1990;86:484-485.
13. Bowden CA, Krenzelok EP. Clinical applications of commonly used contemporary antidotes. *Drug Safety*. 1997;16:9-47.
14. Lewis JM, Klein-Schwartz W, Benson BE, et al. Continuous naloxone infusion in pediatric narcotic overdose. *Am J Dis Child*. 1984;138:944-946.
15. Moore RA, Rumack BH, Conner CS, et al. Naloxone: underdosage after narcotic poisoning. *Am J Dis Child*. 1980;134:156-158.
16. Tenenbein M. Continuous naloxone infusion for opiate poisoning in infancy. *J Pediatr*. 1984;105:645-648.
17. Furman WL, Menke JA, Barson WJ, et al. Continuous naloxone infusion in two neonates with septic shock. *J Pediatr*. 1984;105:649-651.
18. Fischer CG, Cook DR. The respiratory and narcotic antagonistic effects of naloxone in infants. *Anesth Analg*. 1974;53:849-852.
19. Groeger JS, Carlon GC, Howland WS. Naloxone in septic shock. *Crit Care Med*. 1983;11:650-654.
20. Hackshaw KV, Parker GA, Roberts JW. Naloxone is septic shock. *Crit Care Med*.1990;18:47-51.
21. Shenep JL. Septic shock. *Adv Pediatr Infect Dis*. 1996;12:209-241.
22. Boeuf B, Gauvin G, Guerguerian AM, et al. Therapy of shock with naloxone: a meta-analysis. *Crit Care Med*. 1998;26:1910-1916.
23. Tiengo M. Naloxone in irreversible shock. *Lancet*. 1980;2:690.
24. Cocchi P, Silenzi M, Calabri G, et al. Naloxone in fulminant meningococcemia. *Pediatr Infect Dis*. 1984;3:187.
25. Aronoff GR, Berns JS, Brier ME, et al. Drug prescribing in renal failure. 4th ed. Available at: http://www.kdp-baptist.louisville.edu/renalbook/. Accessed September 30, 2009.
26. Chernick V, Manfreda J, DeBooy V, et al. Clinical trial of naloxone in birth asphyxia. *J Pediatr*. 1988;113:519-525.
27. Gober AE, Kearns GL, Yokel RA, et al. Repeated naloxone administration for morphine overdose in a 1-month-old infant. *Pediatrics*. 1979;63:606-608.
28. Romac DR. Safety of prolonged high-dose infusion of naloxone hydrochloride for severe methadone overdose. *Clin Pharm*. 1986;5:251-254.
29. Waldron VD: Methadone overdose treated with naloxone infusion. *JAMA*. 1973;225:53.
30. Trissel LA, ed. *Handbook on Injectable Drugs*. 15th ed. Bethesda, MD: American Society of Health-System Pharmacists; 2009.
31. Prough DS, Roy R, Bumgarner J, et al. Acute pulmonary edema in healthy teenagers following conservative doses of intravenous naloxone. *Anesthesiology*. 1984;60:485-486.

Nesiritide

1. Available at: http://ismp.org/Tools/highalertmedications.pdf. ISMP 2008.
2. Available at: http://www.usp.org/hqi/similarProducts/choosy.html. Accessed August 29, 2009.
3. Natrecor [package insert]. Mountain View, CA: Scios Inc; January 2007.

References

4. BNP Consensus Panel 2004: A clinical approach for the diagnostic, prognostic, screening, treatment monitoring, and therapeutic roles of natriuretic peptides in cardiovascular disease. *Cong Heart Fail.* 2004;10:1-30.
5. Costello JM, Goodman DM, Green TP. A review of the natriuretic hormone system's diagnostic and therapeutic potential in critically ill children. *Pediatr Crit Care Med.* 2006;7:308-318.
6. Mahle WT, Cuadarado AR, Kirshbom PM, et al. Nesiritide in infants and children with congestive heart failure. *Pediatr Crit Care Med.* 2005;6:543-546.
7. Moffett BS, Jefferies JL, Price JF, et al. Administration of a large nesiritide bolus dose in a pediatric patient: case report and review of nesiritide use in pediatrics. *Pharmacotherapy.* 2006;26:277-280.
8. Simsic JM, Reddy VS, Kanter et al. Use of nesiritide (human B-type natriuretic peptide) in infants following cardiac surgery. *Pediatr Cardiol.* 2004;25:668-670.
9. Feingold B, Law YW. Nesiritide use in pediatric patients with congestive heart failure. *J Heart Lung Transplant.* 2004;23:1455-1459.
10. Simsic JM, Scheurer M, Tobias JD, et al. Perioperative effects and safety of nesiritide following cardiac surgery in children. *J Intensive Care Med.* 2006;21:22-26.
11. Smith T, Rose DA, Russo P, et al. Nesiritide during extracorporeal membrane oxygenation. *Pediatr Anesthesia.* 2005;15:152-157.
12. Ivy DD, Kinsella JP, Wolfe RR, et al. Atrial natriuretic peptide and nitric oxide in children with pulmonary hypertension after surgical repair of congenital heart disease. *Am J Cardiol.* 1996;77:102-105.
13. Marshall J, Berkenbosch JW, Russo P, et al. Preliminary experience with nesiritide in the pediatric population. *J Intensive Care Med.* 2004;19:164-170.
14. Sehra R, Underwood K. Nesiritide improves urine output in severely ill pediatric patients awaiting heart transplant [abstract]. *J Card Fail.* 2003;254.
15. Wheeler AD, Tobias JD. Nesiritide in a pediatric oncology patient with renal insufficiency and myocardial dysfunction following septic shock. *Pediatr Hem Oncol.* 2005;22:323-333.
16. Trissel LA, ed. *Handbook on Injectable Drugs.* 15th ed. Bethesda, MD: American Society of Health-System Pharmacists; 2009.
17. Food and Drug Administration. MedWatch Program. *2005 Safety Alert: Natrecor (nesiritide).* Available at: http://www.fda.gov/medwatch/SAFETY/2005/natrecor2_DHCP.htm. Accessed July 15, 2006.
18. Moffett BS, Jefferies JL, Rossano J, et al. Nesiritide therapy in a term neonate with renal disease. *Pharmacotherapy.* 2006;26:281-284.
19. Price JF, Mott AR, Dickerson HA, et al. Worsening renal function in children hospitalized with decompensated heart failure: evidence for a pediatric cardiorenal syndrome? *Pediatr Crit Care Med.* 2008;9:279-284.
20. Behera SK, Zuccaro JC, Wetzel GT, et al. Nesiritide improves hemodynamics in children with dilated cardiomyopathy: a pilot study. *Pediatr Cardiol.* 2009;30:26-34.

NiCARdipine

1. Available at: http://ismp.org/Tools/confuseddrugnames.pdf. Accessed August 29, 2009.
2. Available at: http://www.usp.org/hqi/similarProducts/choosy.html. Accessed August 29, 2009.
3. Cardene [package insert]. Deerfield, IL: Baxter Healthcare Corp; January 2006.
4. Temple ME, Nahata MC. Treatment of pediatric hypertension. *Pharmacotherapy.* 2000;20:140-150.
5. Trissel LA, ed. Handbook on Injectable Drugs. 15th ed. Bethesda, MD: American Society of Health-System Pharmacists; 2009.
6. Milou C, Debuche-Benouachkou V, Semama DS, et al. Intravenous nicardipine as a first-line antihypertensive drug in neonates. *Intensive Care Med.* 2000;26:956-958.
7. Gouyon JB, Geneste B, Semama DS, et al. Intravenous nicardipine in hypertensive preterm infants. *Arch Dis Child Fetal Neonatal Ed.* 1997;76:F126-F127.
8. Treluyer JM, Hubert P, Jouvet P, et al. Intravenous nicardipine in hypertensive children. *Eur J Pediatr.* 1993;152:712-714.
9. Flynn JT, Mottes TA, Brophy PD, et al. Intravenous nicardipine for treatment of severe hypertension in children. *J Pediatr.* 2001;139:38-43.
10. McBride BF, White CM, Campbell M, et al. Nicardipine to control neonatal hypertension during extracorporeal membrane oxygen support. *Ann Pharmacother.* 2003;37:667-670.
11. Tobias JD. Nicardipine to control mean arterial pressure after cardiothoracic surgery in infants and children. *Am J Ther.* 2001;8:3-6.
12. Michael J, Groshong T, Tobias JD. Nicardipine for hypertensive emergencies in children with renal disease. *Pediatr Nephrol.* 1998;12:40-42.
13. Tobias JD, Hersey S, Mencio GA, et al. Nicardipine for controlled hypotension during spinal surgery. J Pediatr Ortho 1996;16:370-373.
14. Tobias JD, Pietsch JB, Lynch A. Nicardipine to control mean arterial pressure during extracorporeal membrane oxygenation. *Paediatr Anaesth.* 1996;6:51-60.
15. Tenney F, Sakarcan A. Nicardipine is a safe and effective agent in pediatric hypertensive emergencies. *Am J Kidney Dis.* 2000;35:1-3.
16. US Department of Health and Human Services, National Institutes of Health, National Heart, Lung, and Blood Institute. Diagnosis, evaluation, and treatment of high blood pressure in children and adolescents. 4th report. NIH Publication 05-5267. Revised May 2005.
17. Adelman RD, Coppo R, Dillon MJ. The emergency management of severe hypertension. *Pediatr Nephrol.* 2000;14:422-427.
18. Strauser LM, Groshong T, Tobias JD. Initial experience with isradipine for the treatment of hypertension in children. *South Med J.* 2000;93:287-293.
19. Flynn JT, Pasko DA. Calcium channel blockers: pharmacology and place in therapy of pediatric hypertension. *Pediatr Nephrol.* 2000;15:302-316.
20. Ingu A, Morikawa M, Fuse S, et al. Acute occlusion of a simple aortic coarctation presenting as abdominal angina. *Pediatr Cardiol.* 2003;24:488-489.
21. Nakagawa TA, Sartori SC, Morris A, et al. Intravenous nicardipine for treatment of postcoarctectomy hypertension in children. *Pediatr Cardiol.* 2004;25:26-30.
22. Madre C, Orbach D, Baudouin V, et al. Hypertension in childhood cancer. *J Pediatr Hematol Oncol.* 2006;28:659-664.
23. Nicardipine. Lexi-Comp Online with AHFS (database). Bethesda, MD: American Society of Health-System Pharmacists; updated May 26, 2009.
24. Fivush B, Neu A, Furth S. Acute hypertensive crises in children: emergencies and urgencies. *Curr Opin Pediatr.* 1997;9:233-236.
25. Aronoff GR, Berns JS, Brier ME, et al. Drug prescribing in renal failure. 4th ed. Available at: http://www.kdp-baptist.louisville.edu/renalbook/. Accessed October 18, 2009.
26. Larson A, Tobias JD. Nicardipine for the treatment of hypertension following cardiac transplantation in a 14-year-old boy. *Clin Pediatr.* 1994;25:309-311.
27. Levene MI, Gibson NA, Fenton AC, et al. The use of a calcium-channel blocker, nicardipine, for severely asphyxiated newborn infants. *Dev Med Child Neurol.* 1990;32:567-574.
28. Aya AG, Bruelle P, Lefrant JY, et al. Accidental nicardipine overdosage without serious maternal or neonatal consequence. *Anaesth Intensive Care.* 1996;24:99-101.

Nitroglycerin

1. Available at: http://www.usp.org/hqi/similarProducts/choosy.html. Accessed August 29, 2009.
2. Nitroglycerin injection, USP [package insert]. Shirley, NY: American Regent Laboratories Inc; October 2002.
3. Nitroglycerin. Lexi-Comp Online with AHFS (database). Bethesda, MD: American Society of Health-System Pharmacists; updated January 2009.
4. Friedman WF, George BL. New concepts and drugs in the treatment of congestive heart failure. *Pediatr Clin North Am.* 1984;31:1197-1227.

5. Benson LN, Bohn D, Edmonds JF, et al. Nitroglycerin therapy in children with low cardiac index after heart surgery. *Cardiovasc Med.* 1979;4:207-215.
6. Ilbawi MN, Idriss FS, DeLeon SY, et al. Hemodynamic effects of intravenous nitroglycerin in pediatric patients after heart surgery. *Circulation.* 1985;72:101-107.
7. Schleien CL, Setzer NA, McLaughlin GE, et al. Postoperative management of the cardiac surgical patient. In: Rogers MC, ed. *Textbook of Pediatric Intensive Care.* Baltimore, MD: Williams & Wilkins; 1992:467-531.
8. American Academy of Pediatrics and American Heart Association. *Pediatric Advanced Life Support. Provider Manual.* Dallas, TX: American Heart Association; 2006.
9. Adelman RD, Coppo R, Dillon MJ. The emergency management of severe hypertension. *Pediatr Nephrol.* 2000;14:422-427.
10. Nitroglycerin injection, USP [package insert]. Lake Forest, IL: Hospira Inc; 2004.
11. Trissel LA, ed. *Handbook on Injectable Drugs.* 15th ed. Bethesda, MD: American Society of Health-System Pharmacists; 2009.
12. Herling IM. Intravenous nitroglycerin: clinical pharmacology and therapeutic considerations. *Am Heart J.* 1984;108:141-149.
13. Gibson GR, Hunter JB, Raabe DS, et al. Methemoglobinemia induced by high-dose intravenous nitroglycerin. *Ann Intern Med.* 1982;96:615-616.
14. Williams RS, Mickell JJ, Young ES, et al. Methemoglobin levels during prolonged combination nitroglycerin and sodium nitroprusside infusion in infants after cardiac surgery. *J Cardiothorac Vasc Anesth.* 1994;8:658-662.
15. Elkayam U. Tolerance to organic nitrates: evidence, mechanisms, clinical relevance, and strategies for prevention. *Ann Intern Med.* 1991;114:667-677.

Norepinephrine Bitartrate

1. Available at: http://ismp.org/Tools/highalertmedications.pdf. ISMP 2008. Accessed August 29, 2009.
2. Available at: http://www.usp.org/hqi/similarProducts/choosy.html. Accessed August 29, 2009.
3. Levophed [package insert]. Lake Forest, IL: Hospira Inc. June 2007.
4. Zaritsky A, Chernow B. Use of catecholamines in pediatrics. *J Pediatr.* 1984;105:341-350.
5. MacCara ME. Extravasation: a hazard of intravenous therapy. *Drug Intell Clin Pharm.* 1983;17:713-717.
6. Gaze NR. Tissue necrosis caused by commonly used intravenous infusions. *Lancet.* 1978;2:417-419.
7. American Academy of Pediatrics and American Heart Association. *Pediatric Advanced Life Support. Provider Manual.* Dallas, TX: American Heart Association; 2006.
8. Hegenbarth MA, American Academy of Pediatrics Committee on Drugs. Preparing for pediatric emergencies: drugs to consider. *Pediatrics.* 2008;121:433-443.
9. Trissel LA, ed. Handbook on Injectable Drugs. 15th ed. Bethesda, MD: American Society of Health-System Pharmacists; 2009.
10. Schleien CL, Kuluz JW, Shaffner DH, et al. Cardiopulmonary resuscitation. In: Rogers MC, ed. *Textbook of Pediatric Intensive Care.* Baltimore, MD: Williams & Wilkins; 1992.
11. Norepinephrine bitartrate. Lexi-Comp Online with AHFS (database). Hudson, OH: Lexi-Comp Inc; updated August 13, 2009.
12. Buck ML, Wiggins BS, Sesler JM. Intraosseous Drug Administration in Children and Adults During Cardiopulmonary Resuscitation. *Ann Pharmacother.* 2007;41:1679-1686.
13. Norepinephrine bitartrate. Lexi-Comp Online with AHFS (database). Bethesda, MD: American Society of Health-System Pharmacists; updated May 26, 2009.

Octreotide Acetate

1. Sandostatin [package insert]. East Hanover, NJ: Novartis Pharmaceuticals Corp; September 2005.
2. Available at: http://ismp.org/Tools/confuseddrugnames.pdf. Accessed August 29, 2009.
3. Available at: http://www.usp.org/hqi/similarProducts/choosy.html. Accessed August 29, 2009.
4. Roehr CC, Jung A, Proquitte H, et al. Somatostatin or octreotide as treatment options for chylothorax in young children: a systematic review. *Intensive Care Med.* 2006;32:650-657.
5. Rosti L, De Battisti F, Butera G, et al. Octreotide in the management of postoperative chylothorax. *Pediatr Cardiol.* 2005;26:440-443.
6. Mohseni-Bod H, Macrae D, Slavik Z. Somatostatin analog (octreotide) in management of neonatal postoperative chylothorax: is it safe? *Pediatr Crit Care Med.* 2004;5:356-357.
7. Lauterbach R, Sczaniecka B, Koziol J, et al. Somatostatin treatment of spontaneous chylothorax in an extremely low birth weight infant. *Eur J Pediatr.* 2005;164:195-196.
8. Lam JC, Aters S, Tobias JD. Initial experience with octreotide in the pediatric population. *Am J Ther.* 2001;8:409-415.
9. Bhatia C, Pratap U, Slavik Z. Octreotide therapy: a new horizon in treatment of iatrogenic chyloperitoneum. *Arch Dis Child.* 2001;85:234-235.
10. Andreou A, Papouli M, Papavasasiliou V, et al. Postoperative chylous ascites in a neonate treated successfully with octreotide: bile sludge and cholestasis. *Am J Perinatol.* 2005;8:401-404.
11. Hwang JB, Choi SO, Park WH. Resolution of refractory chylous ascites after Kasai portoenterostomy using octreotide. *J Pediatr Surg.* 2004;39:1806-1807.
12. Goyal A, Smith NP, Jesudason EC, et al. Octreotide for treatment of chylothorax after repair of congenital diaphragmatic hernia. *J Pediatr Surg.* 2003;38:1-2.
13. Cheung YF, Leung MP, Yip MM. Octreotide for treatment of postoperative chylothorax. *J Pediatr.* 2001;139:157-159.
14. Helin RD, Angeles STV, Bhat R. Octreotide therapy for chylothorax in infants and children: a brief review. *Pediatr Crit Care Med.* 2006;7:576-579.
15. Koçyildirim E, Yörükoğlu Y, Ekici E, et al. High-dose octreotide treatment for persistent pleural effusion after the extracardiac Fontan procedure. *Anadolu Kardiyol Derg.* 2008;8:75-76.
16. Jaros W, Biller J, Greer S, et al. Successful treatment of idiopathic secretory diarrhea of infancy with the somatostatin analogue SMS 201-995. *Gastroenterology.* 1988;94:189-193.
17. Ohlbaum P, Galperine RI, Demarquez JL, et al. Use of a long-acting somatostatin analogue (SMS 201-995) in controlling a significant ileal output in a 5-year-old child. *J Pediatr Gastroenterol Nutr.* 1987;6:466-470.
18. Smith SS, Shulman DI, O'Dorisio TM, et al. Watery diarrhea, hypokalemia, achlorhydria syndrome in an infant: effect of the long-acting somatostatin analogue SMS 201-995 on the disease and linear growth. *J Pediatr Gastroenterol Nutr.* 1987;6:710-716.
19. Lamireau T, Galperine RI, Ohlbaum P, et al. Use of a long acting somatostatin analogue in controlling ileostomy diarrhea in infants. *Acta Paediatr Scand.* 1990;79:871-872.
20. Couper RT, Berzen A, Berall G, et al. Clinical response to the long acting somatostatin analogue SMS 201-995 in a child with congenital microvillus atrophy. *Gut.* 1989;30:1020-1024.
21. Tauber MT, Harris AG, Rochiccioli P. Clinical use of the long acting somatostatin analogue octreotide in pediatrics. *Eur J Pediatr.* 1994;153:304-310.
22. Beckman RA, Siden R, Yanik GA, et al. Continuous octreotide infusion for the treatment of secretory diarrhea caused by acute intestinal graft-versus-host disease in a child. *J Pediatr Hematol Oncol.* 2000;22:344-350.
23. Wallace AM, Newman K. Successful closure of intestinal fistulae in an infant using the somatostatin analogue SMS 201-995. *J Pediatr Surg.* 1991;26:1097-1100.

References

24. Inamdar S, Slim MS, Bostwick H, et al. Treatment of duodenocutaneous fistula with somatostatin analog in a child with dermatomyositis. *J Pediatr Gastroenterol Nutr.* 1990;10:402-404.
25. Mahomed A. Subcutaneously administered somatostatin analogue in traumatic pancreatic fistula. *Pediatr Surg Int.* 1997;12:231. Letter.
26. Siafakas C, Fox VL, Nurko S. Use of octreotide for the treatment of severe gastrointestinal bleeding in children. *J Pediatr Gastroenterol Nutr.* 1998;26:356-359.
27. Eroglu Y, Emerick KM, Whitington PF, et al. Octreotide therapy for control of acute gastrointestinal bleeding in children. *J Pediatr Gastroenterol Nutr.* 2004;38:41-47.
28. Heikenen JB, Pohl JF, Werlin SL, et al. Octreotide in pediatric patients. *J Pediatr Gastroenterol Nutr.* 2002;35:600-609.
29. Zellos A, Schwartz KB. Efficacy of octreotide in children with chronic gastrointestinal bleeding. *J Pediatr Gastroenterol Nutr.* 2000;30:442-446.
30. Glaser B, Hirsch HJ, Landau H. Persistent hyperinsulinemic hypoglycemia of infancy: long-term octreotide treatment without pancreatectomy. *J Pediatr.* 1993;123:644-650.
31. Thornton PS, Alter CA, Katz LE, et al. Short and long-term use of octreotide in the treatment of congenital hyperinsulinism. *J Pediatr.* 1993;123:637-643.
32. Barrons RW. Octreotide in hyperinsulinism. *Ann Pharmacotherapy.* 1997;31:239-241.
33. Stanley CA. Hyperinsulinism in infants and children. *Ped Clin N Am.* 1997;44:363-373.
34. Apak RA, Yurdakok M, Oran O, et al. Preoperative use of octreotide in a newborn with persistent hyperinsulinemic hypoglycemia of infancy. *J Pediatr Endocrinol Metab.* 1998;11:143-145.
35. Jackson JA, Hahn HB, Oltorf CE. Long-acting somatostatin analog in refractory neonatal hypoglycemia: follow-up information. *J Pediatr.* 1988;113:1118.
36. Jackson JA, Hahn HB, Oltorf CE, et al. Long-term treatment of refractory neonatal hypoglycemia with long-acting somatostatin analog. *J Pediatr.* 1987;111:548-551.
37. DeClue TJ, Malone JI, Bercu BB. Linear growth during long-term treatment with somatostatin analog (SMS 201-995) for persistent hyperinsulinemic hypoglycemia of infancy. *J Pediatr.* 1990;116:747-749.
38. Bosman-Vermeeren JM, Veereman-Wauters G, Broos P, et al. Somatostatin in the treatment of a pancreatic pseudocyst in a child. *J Pediatr Gastroenterol Nutr.* 1996;23:422-425.
39. Yaffe MR, Gutenberger JE. Chronic pancreatitis and pancreas divisum in an infant: diagnosed by endoscopic retrograde cholangiopancreatography and treated with somatostatin analog. *J Pediatr Gastroenterol Nutr.* 1989;9:108-111.
40. Zarina AL, Hamidah A, Zulkifli SZ, et al. Malignant pancreatic carcinoid tumour. *Singapore Med J.* 2007;48:e320-e322.
41. Spiller HA. Management of sulfonylurea ingestions. *Pediatr Emerg Care.* 1999;15:227-230.
42. Tenenbein M. Recent advancements in pediatric toxicology. *Ped Clin N Am.* 1999;46:1179-1188.
43. Mordel A, Sivilotti ML, Old AC, et al. Octreotide for pediatric sulfonylurea poisoning. *J Clin Toxicol.* 1998;36:437.
44. Little GL, Boniface KS. Are one or two dangerous? Sulfonylurea exposure in toddlers. *J Emerg Med.* 2005;28:305-310.
45. Carr R, Zed PJ. Octreotide for sulfonylurea-induced hypoglycemia following overdose. *Ann Pharmacother.* 2002;36:1727-1732.
46. Rath S, Bar-Zeev N, Anderson K, et al. Octreotide in children with hypoglycaemia due to sulfonylurea ingestion. *J Paediatr Child Health.* 2008;44:383-384.
47. Nanto-Salonen K, Koskinen P, Sonninen P, et al. Suppression of GH secretion in pituitary gigantism by continuous subcutaneous octreotide infusion in a pubertal boy. *Acta Paediatr.* 1999;88:29-33.
48. Hindmarsh PC, Pringle PJ, Di Silvio L, et al. A preliminary report on the role of somatostatin analogue (SMS 201-995) in the management of children with tall stature. *Clinical Endocrinology.* 1990;32:83-91.
49. Trissel LA, ed. *Handbook on Injectable Drugs.* 15th ed. Bethesda, MD: American Society of Health-System Pharmacists; 2009.
50. Seidner DL, Speerhas R. Can octreotide be added to parenteral nutrition solutions? *Point-Counterpoint. Nutr Clin Pract.* 1998;13:84-88.
51. Batra YK, Rajeev S, Samra T, et al. Octreotide-induced severe paradoxical hyperglycemia and bradycardia during subtotal pancreatectomy for congenital hyperinsulinism in an infant. *Pediatr Anesthesia.* 2007;17:1111-1121.
52. Hunziker UA, Superti-Furga A, Zachmann M, et al. Effects of the long-acting somatostatin analogue SMS 201-995 in an infant with intractable diarrhea. *Helv Paediatr Acta.* 1988;43:103-109.
53. Reck-Burneo CA, Parekh A, Velcek FT. Is octreotide a risk factor in necrotizing enterocolitis? *J Pediatr Surg.* 2008;43:1209-1210.
54. Watanabe H, Inoue Y, Uchida K, et al. Octreotide improved the quality of life in a child with malignant bowel obstruction caused by peritoneal dissemination of colon cancer. *J Pediatr Surg.* 2007;42:259-260.

Ondansetron HCl

1. Available at: http://www.usp.org/hqi/similarProducts/choosy.html. Accessed July 31, 2009.
2. Zofran [prescribing information]. Research Triangle Park, NC: GlaxoSmithKline Inc; February 2006.
3. Ross AK, Ferrero-Conover D. Anaphylactoid reaction due to the administration of ondansetron in a pediatric neurosurgical patient. *Anesth Analg.* 1998;87:779-780.
4. Boike SC, Ilson B, Zariffa N, et al. Cardiovascular effects of i.v. granisetron at two administration rates and of ondansetron in healthy adults. *Am J Health-Syst Pharm.* 1997;54:1172-1176.
5. Alvarez O, Freeman A, Bedros AM, et al. Randomized double-blind crossover ondansetron-dexamethasone versus ondansetron-placebo study for the treatment of chemotherapy-induced nausea and vomiting in pediatric patients with malignancies. *J Pediatr Hematol Oncol.* 1995;17:145-150.
6. Vermeulen LC, Matsuzewski KA, Ratko TA, et al. Evaluation of ondansetron prescribing in U.S. academic medical centers. *Arch Intern Med.* 1994;154:1733-1740.
7. Holdsworth MT, Raisch DW, Duncan MH, et al. Assessment of chemotherapy-induced emesis and evaluation of a reduced-dose intravenous ondansetron regimen in pediatric patients. *Ann Pharmacother.* 1995;29:16-21.
8. McQueen KD, Milton JD. Multicenter postmarketing surveillance of ondansetron therapy in pediatric patients. *Ann Pharmacother.* 1994;28:8-92.
9. Sandoval C, Corbi D, Strobino B, et al. Randomized double-blind comparison of single high-dose ondansetron and multiple standard-dose ondansetron in chemotherapy-naïve pediatric oncology patients. *Cancer Invest.* 1999;17:309-313.
10. Nahata MC, Nui LN, Koepke J. Efficacy and safety of ondansetron in pediatric patients undergoing bone marrow transplantation. *Clin Ther.* 1996;18:466-476.
11. Brock P, Brichard B, Reichnitzer C, et al. An increasing loading dose of ondansetron: a North European double-blind randomized study in children, comparing 5 mg/m2 with 10 mg/m2. *Eur J Cancer.* 1996;32A:1744-1748.
12. Kris MG, Hesketh PJ, Somerfield MR, et al. American Society of Clinical Oncology guideline for antiemetics in oncology: update 2006. *J Clin Oncology.* 2006;24:2932-2947.
13. Parker RI, Prakash D, Mahan RA, et al. Randomized, double-blind, crossover, placebo-controlled trial of intravenous ondansetron for the prevention of intrathecal chemotherapy-induced vomiting in children. *J Pediatr Hematol Oncol.* 2001;23:578-581.
14. Khalil SN, Roth AG, Cohen IT, et al. A double-blind comparison of intravenous ondansetron and placebo for preventing postoperative emesis in 1- to 24-month-old pediatric patients after surgery under general anesthesia. *Anesth Analg.* 2005;101:356-361.
15. Furst SR, Rodarte A. Prophylactic antiemetic treatment with ondansetron in children undergoing tonsillectomy. *Anesthesiol.* 1994;81:799-803.
16. Watcha MF, Bras PJ, Cieslak GD, et al. The dose-response relationship of ondansetron in preventing postoperative emesis in pediatric patients undergoing ambulatory surgery. *Anesthesiology.* 1995;82:47-52.
17. Ummenhofer W, Frei FJ, Urwyler A, et al. Effect of ondansetron in the prevention of postoperative nausea and vomiting in children. *Anesthesiology.* 1994;81:804-810.

18. Rose JB, Martin TM, Corddry DH, et al. Ondansetron reduced the incidence and severity of poststrabismus repair vomiting in children. *Anesth Analg.* 1994;79:486-489.
19. Spahr-Schopfer IA, Lerman J, Sikich N, et al. Pharmacokinetics of intravenous ondansetron in healthy children undergoing ear, nose, and throat surgery. *Clin Pharm Ther.* 1995;58:316-321.
20. Patel RI, Davis PJ, Orr RJ, et al. Single-dose ondansetron prevents postoperative vomiting in pediatric outpatients. *Anesth Analg.* 1997;85:538-545.
21. Sadhasivam S, Shende D, Madan R. Prophylactic ondansetron in prevention of postoperative nausea and vomiting following pediatric strabismus surgery. *Anesthesiology.* 2000;92:1035-1042.
22. Sukhani R, Pappas AL, Lurie J, et al. Ondansetron and dolasetron provide equivalent postoperative vomiting control after ambulatory tonsillectomy in dexamethasone-pretreated children. *Anesth Analg.* 2002;95:1230-1235.
23. Langston WT, Wathen JE, Roback MG, et al. Effect of ondansetron on the incidence of vomiting associated with ketamine sedation iin children: a double-blind, randomized, placebo-controlled trial. *Ann Emerg Med.* 2008;2:30-34.
24. Reeves JJ, Shannon MW, Fleisher GR. Ondansetron decreases vomiting associated with acute gastroenteritis: a randomized, controlled trial. *Pediatrics.* 2002;109:1-6.
25. Trissel LA. *Handbook on Injectable Drugs.* 15th ed. Bethesda, MD: American Society of Health-System Pharmacists; 2009.
26. Kalaycio M, Mendez Z, Pohlman B, et al. Continuous-infusion granisetron compared to ondansetron for the prevention of nausea and vomiting after high-dose chemotherapy. *J Cancer Res Clin Oncol.* 1998;124:265-269.

Oxacillin Sodium

1. Available at: http://www.usp.org/hqi/similarProducts/choosy.html. Accessed September 19, 2009.
2. Oxacillin [package insert]. Bloomfield, CO: Sandoz Inc; January 2004.
3. Prober CG, Stevenson DK, Benitz WE. The use of antibiotics in neonates weighing less than 1200 grams. *Pediatr Infect Dis J.* 1990;9:111-121.
4. American Academy of Pediatrics. Pickering LK, Baker CJ, Kimberlin DW, et al., eds. *2009 Red Book: Report of the Committee on Infectious Diseases.* 28th ed. Elk Grove Village, IL: American Academy of Pediatrics; 2009.
5. Nelson JD, Bradley JS, eds. *Nelson's Pocket Book of Pediatric Antimicrobial Therapy.* 17th ed. Chicago, IL: American Academy of Pediatrics; 2009.
6. McCracken GH Jr, Nelson JD, eds. *Antimicrobial Therapy for Newborns: Practical Application.* 2nd ed. New York, NY: Grune and Stratton; 1983.
7. Leventhal JM, Silken AB. Oxacillin-induced neutropenia in children. *J Pediatr.* 1976; 89:769-771.
8. Howrie DL, Felix C, Wollman M, et al. Metoclopramide as an antiemetic agent in pediatric oncology patients. *Drug Intell Clin Pharm.* 1986;20:122-124.
9. McCracken GH, Eichenwald HF. Antimicrobial therapy: therapeutic recommendations and a review of newer drugs—part I: therapy of infectious conditions. *J Pediatr.* 1974;85:297-312.
10. Bulger RJ, Lindholm DD, Murray JS, et al. Effect of uremia on methicillin and oxacillin blood levels. *JAMA.* 1964;187:319-322.
11. Klein JO, Sabath LD, Steinhauer BW, et al. Oxacillin treatment of severe staphylococcal infection. *N Engl J Med.* 1963;269:1215-1225.
12. Olans RN, Weiner LB. Reversible oxacillin hepatotoxicity. *J Pediatr.* 1976;89:835-838.
13. Trissel LA, ed. *Handbook on Injectable Drugs.* 15th ed. Bethesda, MD: American Society of Health-System Pharmacists; 2009.
14. Robinson CA, Sawyer JE. Y-site compatibility of medications with parenteral nutrition. *J Pediatr Pharmacol Ther.* 2009;14:49-57.
15. Dahlgren AF. Adverse drug reactions in home care patients receiving nafcillin or oxacillin. *Am J Health-Syst Pharm.* 1997;54:1176-1179.
16. Al-Homaidhi H, Abdel-Haq NM, El-Baba M, Asmar BI. Severe hepatitis associated with oxacillin therapy. *South Med J.* 2002;95:650-652.
17. Maraqa NF, Gomez MM, Rathore MH, Alvarez AM. Higher occurrence of hepatotoxicity and rash in patients treated with oxacillin, compared with those treated with nafcillin and other commonly used antimicrobials. *Clin Infect Dis.* 2002;34:50-54.
18. D'Angelo LJ. Oxacillin and hepatotoxicity. *Ann Intern Med.* 1979;90:442.
19. Barrons RW, Murray KM, Richey RM. Populations at risk for penicillin-induced seizures. *Ann Pharmacother.* 1992;26:26-29.

Palivizumab

1. Palivizumab [package insert]. Gaithersburg, MD: Medimmune Inc; March 2009.
2. Groothius JR. Safety of palivizumab in preterm infants 29 to 32 weeks' gestational age without chronic lung disease to prevent serious respiratory syncytial virus infection. *Eur J Clin Microbiol Infect Dis.* 2003;22:414-417.
3. Null D, Poliara B, Dennehy PH, et al. Safety and immunogenicity of palivizumab (Synagis) administered for two seasons. *Pediatr Infect Dis J.* 2005;24:1021-1023.
4. Groothuis JR. Safety and tolerance of palivizumab administration in a large northern hemisphere trial. *Pediatr Infect Dis J.* 2001;20:628-630.
5. The IMpact-RSV Study Group. Palivizumab, a humanized respiratory syncytial virus monoclonal antibody, reduces hospitalization from respiratory syncytial virus infection in high-risk infants. *Pediatrics.* 1998;102:531-537.
6. Saez-Llorens X, Castano E, Null D, et al. Safety and pharmacokinetics of an intramuscular humanized monoclonal antibody to respiratory syncytial virus in premature infants and infants with bronchopulmonary dysplasia. *Pediatr Infect Dis J.* 1998;17:787-791.
7. Feltes TF, Cabalka AK, Meissner C, et al. Palivizumab prophylaxis reduces hospitalization due to respiratory syncytial virus in young children with hemodynamically significant congenital heart disease. *J Pediatr.* 2003;143:532-540.
8. AAP Subcommittee on the Diagnosis and Management of Bronchiolitis. Diagnosis and management of bronchiolitis. *Pediatrics.* 2006;118:1774-1793.
9. Cox RA, Rao P, Brandon-Cox C. The use of palivizumab monoclonal antibody to control an outbreak of respiratory syncytial virus infection in a special care baby unit. *J Hosp Infect.* 2001;48:186-192.
10. Abadesso C, Almeida HI, Virella D, et al. Use of palivizumab to control an outbreak of syncytial respiratory virus in a neonatal intensive care unit. *J Hosp Infect.* 2004;58:38-41.
11. Wu SY, Bonaparte J, Pyati S. Palivizumab use in very premature infants in the neonatal intensive care unit. *Pediatrics.* 2004;114:554-556.
12. Subramanian KNS, Weisman LE, Rhodes T, et al. Safety, tolerance, and pharmacokinetics of a humanized monoclonal antibody to respiratory syncytial virus in premature infants and infants with bronchopulmonary dysplasia. *Pediatr Infect Dis J.* 1998;17:110-115.
13. Saez-Llorens X, Moreno MT, Ramilo O, et al. Safety and pharmacokinetics of palivizumab therapy in children hospitalized with respiratory syncytial virus infection. *Pediatr Infect Dis J.* 2004;23:707-712.
14. Malley R, DeVincenzo J, Ramilo O. Reduction of respiratory syncytial virus (RSV) in tracheal aspirates in intubated infants by use of humanized monoclonal antibody to RSV F protein. *J Infect Dis.* 1998;178:1555-1561.
15. Carbajal R, Biran V, Lenclen R, et al. EMLA cream and nitrous oxide to alleviate pain induced by palivizumab (Synagis) intramuscular injections in infants and young children. *Pediatrics.* 2008;121:e1591-e1598.

Pamidronate

1. Available at: www.usp.org/hqi/similarProducts/choosy.html.
2. Aredia, pamidronate disodium injection [package insert]. East Hanover, NJ: Novartis Pharmaceuticals Corp; November 2008.
3. Glorieux FH, Bishop NJ, Plotkin H, et al. Cyclic administration of pamidronate in children with severe osteogenesis imperfecta. *N Engl J Med.* 1998;339:947-952.

References

4. Fujiwara I, Ogawa E, Igarashi Y, et al. Intravenous pamidronate treatment in osteogenesis imperfecta. *Eur J Pediatr.* 1998;157:261-262.
5. Bembi B, Parma A, Bottega M, et al. Intravenous pamidronate treatment in osteogenesis imperfecta. *J Pediatr.* 1997;131:662-665.
6. Astrom E, Soderhall S. Beneficial effect of biphosphonate during five years of treatment of severe osteogenesis imperfecta. *Acta Paediatr.* 1998;87:64-68.
7. Zacharin M, Kanumakala S. Pamidronate treatment of less severe forms of osteogenesis imperfecta in children. *J Pediatr Endocrinol Metabol.* 2004;17:1511-1517.
8. Falk MJ, Heeger S, Lynch KA, et al. Intravenous bisphosphonate therapy in children with osteogenesis imperfecta. *Pediatrics.* 2003;111:573-578.
9. Lee YS, Low SL, Lim LA, et al. Cyclic pamidronate infusion improves bone mineralization and reduces fracture incidence in osteogenesis imperfecta. *Eur J Pediatr.* 2001;160:641-644.
10. Rauch F, Munns C, Land C, et al. Pamidronate in children and adolescents with osteogenesis imperfecta: effect of treatment discontinuation. *J Clin Endocrinol Metabol.* 2006;91:1268-1274.
11. Shaw NJ, White CP, Fraser WB, et al. Osteopenia in cerebral palsy. *Arch Dis Child.* 1994;71:235-238.
12. Henderson RC, Lark RK, Kecskemetby HH, et al. Bisphosphonates to treat osteopenia in children with quadriplegic cerebral palsy: a randomized, placebo-controlled clinical trial. *J Pediatr.* 2002;141:644-651.
13. Acott PD, Wong JA, Lang BA, et al. Pamidronate treatment of pediatric fracture patients on chronic steroid therapy. *Pediatr Nephrol.* 2005;20:368-373.
14. Lteif AN, Zimmerman D. Biphosphonates for treatment of childhood hypercalcemia. *Pediatrics.* 1998;102:990-993.
15. Profumo RJ, Reese JC, Foy TM, et al. Severe immobilization-induced hypercalcemia in a child after liver transplantation successfully treated with pamidronate. *Transplantation.* 1994;57:301-303.
16. Schmid I, Stachel D, Schon C, et al. Pamidronate and calcitonin as therapy of acute cancer-related hypercalcemia in children. *Klin Padiatr.* 2001;213:30-34.
17. De Schepper J, de Pont S, Smitz J, et al. Metabolic disturbances after a single dose of 30 mg pamidronate for leukaemia-associated hypercalcemia in a 11-year-old boy. *Eur J Pediatr.* 1999;158:765-766.
18. Khan N, Licata A, Rogers D. Intravenous bisphosphonate for hypercalcemia accompanying subcutaneous fat necrosis: a novel treatment approach. *Clin Pediatr.* 2001;40:217-219.
19. Attard TM, Dhawan A, Kaufman SS, et al. Use of disodium pamidronate in children with hypercalcemia awaiting liver transplantation. *Pediatr Transplant.* 1998;2:157-159.
20. Boudailliez BR, Pautard BJ, Sebert JL, et al. Leukaemia-associated hypercalcemia in a 10-year-old boy: effectiveness of aminohydroxypropylidene biphosphonate. *Pediatr Nephrol.* 1990;4:510-511.
21. Isaia GC, Lala R, Defilippi C, et al. Bone turnover in children and adolescents with McCune-Albright Syndrome treated with pamidronate for bone fibrous dysplasia. *Calcif Tissue Int.* 2002;71:121-128.
22. Zacharin M, O'Sullivan M. Intravenous pamidronate treatment of polyostotic fibrous dysplasia associated with the McCune Albright syndrome. *J Pediatr.* 2000;137:403-409.
23. Sellers E, Sharma A, Rodd C. The use of pamidronate in three children with renal disease. *Pediatr Nephrol.* 1998;12:778-781.
24. Malmgren B, Astrom E, Soderhall S. No osteonecrosis in jaws of young patients with osteogenesis imperfecta treated with bisphosphonates. *J Oral Pathol Med.* 2008;37:196-200.

Pancuronium Bromide

1. Available at: http://ismp.org/Tools/highalertmedications.pdf. ISMP 2008. Accessed August 29, 2009.
2. Available at: http://www.usp.org/hqi/similarProducts/choosy.html. Accessed August 29, 2009.
3. Available at: http://ismp.org/Tools/confuseddrugnames.pdf. Accessed August 29, 2009.
4. Pancuronium bromide injection [package insert]. Lake Forest, IL: Hospira Inc; November 2004.
5. Perlman JM, Goodman S, Kreusser KL, et al. Reduction in intraventricular hemorrhage by elimination of fluctuating cerebral blood-flow velocity in preterm infants with respiratory distress syndrome. *N Engl J Med.* 1985;312:1353-1357.
6. Maunuksela EL, Fattiker RI. Use of pancuronium in children with congenital heart disease. *Anesth Analg.* 1981;60:798-801.
7. Cabal LA, Siassi B, Artel R, et al. Cardiovascular and catecholamine changes after administration of pancuronium in distressed neonates. *Pediatrics.* 1985;75:284-287.
8. Sinha SK, Levene MI. Pancuronium bromide induced joint contractures in the newborn. *Arch Dis Child.* 1984;59:73-75.
9. Mishima S, Yamamura T. Anaphylactoid reaction to pancuronium. *Anesth Analg.* 1984;63:865-866.
10. Martin LD, Bratton SL, O'Rourke PP. Clinical uses and controversies of neuromuscular blocking agents in infant and children. *Crit Care Med.* 1999;27:1358-1368.
11. Levene MI, Quinn MW. Use of sedatives and muscle relaxants in newborn babies receiving mechanical ventilation. *Arch Dis Child.* 1992;67:870-873.
12. Shaw NJ, Cooke RW, Gill AB, et al. Randomized trial of routine versus selective paralysis during ventilation for neonatal respiratory syndrome. *Arch Dis Child.* 1993;69:479-482.
13. Stark AR, Bascom R, Frantz ID. Muscle relaxation in mechanically ventilated infants. *J Pediatr.* 1979;94:439-433.
14. Runkle B, Bancalari E. Acute cardiopulmonary effects of pancuronium bromide in mechanically ventilated newborn infants. *J Pediatr.* 1984;104:614.
15. Piotrowski A. Comparison of atracurium and pancuronium in mechanically ventilated neonates. *Intensive Care Med.* 1993;19:401-405.
16. Yamamoto T, Baba H, Shiratsuchi T. Clinical experience with pancuronium bromide in infants and children. *Anesth Analg.* 1973;51:919-924.
17. Cunliffe M, Lucero VM, McLeod ME, et al. Neuromuscular blockade for rapid tracheal intubation in children: comparison of succinylcholine and pancuronium. *Can Anaesth Soc J.* 1986;33:760-764.
18. Bennett EJ, Daugherty MJ, Bowyer DE, et al. Pancuronium bromide: experiences in 100 pediatric patients. *Anesth Analg.* 1971;50:798-807.
19. Aronoff GR, Berns JS, Brier ME, et al. Drug prescribing in renal failure. 4th ed. Available at: http://www.kdp-baptist.louisville.edu/renalbook/. Accessed August 17, 2009.
20. Somogyi AA, Shanks CA, Triggs EJ. The effect of renal failure on the disposition and the neuromuscular blocking action of pancuronium bromide. *Eur J Clin Pharmacol.* 1977;12:23-29.
21. Nana A, Cardan E, Leitersdorfer T. Pancuronium bromide: its use in asthmatics and patients with liver disease. *Anaesthesia.* 1972;27:154-158.
22. Costakos DT, Blackwell CE, Krauss AN, et al. Aortic root blood flow increases after pancuronium in neonates with hyaline membrane disease. *Crit Care Med.* 1991;19:187-190.
23. Pancuronium bromide. Lexi-Comp Online with AHFS (database). Bethesda, MD: American Society of Health-System Pharmacists; updated 2009.
24. Trissel LA, ed. *Handbook on Injectable Drugs.* 15th ed. Bethesda, MD: American Society of Health-System Pharmacists; 2009.
25. Pancuronium bromide. Lexi-Comp Online with AHFS (database). Hudson, OH: Lexi-Comp; updated September 25, 2009.
26. Haas JL, Shaefer MS, Miwa LJ, et al. Prolonged paralysis associated with long-term pancuronium use. *Pharmacotherapy.* 1989;9:154-157.
27. Op de Coul AA, Lambregts PC, Koeman J, et al. Neuromuscular complications in patients given pavulon (pancuronium bromide) during artificial ventilation. *Clin Neurol Neurosurg.* 1985;87:17-22.
28. Watling SM, Dasta JF. Prolonged paralysis in intensive care unit patients after the use of neuromuscular blocking agents: a review of the literature. *Crit Care Med.* 1994;22:884-893.
29. Panacek EA, Sherman B. Hydrocortisone and pancuronium bromide: acute myopathy during status asthmaticus. *Crit Care Med.* 1988;16:732.

References

Pantoprazole

1. Available at: http://www.usp.org/hqi/similarProducts/choosy.html. Accessed October 27, 2009.
2. Available at: http://ismp.org/Tools/confuseddrugnames.pdf. Accessed October 27, 2009.
3. Protonix [package insert]. Philadelphia, PA: Wyeth Pharmaceuticals; April 2007.
4. Litalien C, Theoret Y, Faure C. Pharmacokinetics of proton pump inhibitors in children. *Clin Pharmacokinet*. 2005;44(5):441-466.
5. Ferron G, Schexnayder S, Marshall JD, et al. Pharmacokinetics of IV pantoprazole in pediatric patients. [abstract PII-30]. *Clin Pharmacol Ther*. 2003;73:P37.
6. Kearns GL, Blumer J, Schexnayder S, et al. Single-dose pharmacokinetics of oral and intravenous pantoprazole in children and adolescents. *J Clin Pharmacol*. 2008;48:1356-65.
7. Madrazo de la Garza A, Dibildox M, Vargas A, et al. Efficacy and safety of oral pantoprazole 20 mg given once daily for reflux esophagitis in children. *J Pediatr Gastroenterol Nutr*. 2003;36(2):261-265.
8. Morgan D. Intravenous proton pump inhibitors in the critical care setting. *Crit Care Med*. 2002;30(6):S369-S372.
9. Metz DC, Amer F, Hunt B, et al. Lansoprazole regimens that sustain intragastric pH >6.0: an evaluation of intermittent oral and continuous intravenous infusion dosages. *Aliment Pharmacol Ther*. 2006;23:985-995.
10. Van Rensburg CJ, Hartmann M, Thorpe A, et al. Intragastric pH during continuous infusion with pantoprazole in patients with bleeding peptic ulcer. *Amer J Gastroenterol*. 2003;98(12):2635-2641.
11. Somberg L, Karlstadt R, Blatcher D, et al. Intermittent intravenous pantoprazole maintains control of gastric pH in intensive care unit patients (abstract). *Am J Gastroenterol*. 2002;97:S42.
12. Aronoff GR, Berns JS, Brier ME, et al. Drug prescribing in renal failure. 4th ed. Available at: http://www.kdp-baptist.louisville.edu/renalbook/. Accessed October 27, 2009.
13. Devlin JW, Walage LS, Olsen KM. Proton pump inhibitor formulary considerations in the acutely ill. Part 1: pharmacology, pharmacodynamics, and available formulations. *Ann Pharmacother*. 2005;39:1667-1677.
14. Trissel LA, ed. *Handbook on Injectable Drugs*. 15th ed. Bethesda, MD: American Society of Health-System Pharmacists; 2009.
15. Canani RB, Cirillo P, Roggero P, et al. Therapy with gastric acidity inhibitors increases the risk of acute gastroenteritis and community-acquired pneumonia in children. *Pediatrics*. 2006;117:817-820.
16. Hirschowitz BI, Worthington J, Mohnen J. Vitamin B12 deficiency in hypersecretors during long-term acid suppression with proton pump inhibitors. *Aliment Pharmacol Ther*. 2008;27:1110-1121.
17. Sennaroglu E, Karakan S, Kayatas M, et al. Reversible edema in a male patient taking parenteral pantoprazole infusion for pyloric stenosis. *Dig Dis Sci*. 2006;51(1):121-122.
18. Last EJ, Sheehan AH. Review of recent evidence: potential interaction between clopidogrel and proton pump inhibitors. *Am J Health-Syst Pharm* .2009;66:e11-e16.
19. Pettersen G, Mouksassi MS, Theoret Y, et al. Population pharmacokinetics of intravenous pantoprazole in paediatric intensive care patients. *Br J Clin Pharmacol*. 2009;67:216-227.

Papaverine HCl

1. Available at: http://www.usp.org/hqi/similarProducts/choosy.html. Accessed August 26, 2009.
2. Papaverine hydrochloride injection [USP package insert]. West Columbia, SC: Parenta pharmaceuticals; February 2006.
3. Papaverine. Lexi-Comp® Online with AHFS® (database). Hudson, OH: Lexi-Comp Inc; updated August 13, 2009.
4. Griffin MP, Siadaty MS. Papaverine prolongs patency of peripheral arterial catheters in neonates. *J Pediatr*. 2005;146:62-65.
5. Heulitt MJ, Farrington EA, O'Shea TM, et al. Double-blind randomized controlled trial of papaverine-containing solutions to prevent failure of arterial catheters in pediatric patients. *Crit Care Med*. 1993;21:825-829.
6. Boris JR, Harned RK, Logan LA, et al. The use of papaverine in arterial sheaths to prevent loss of femoral artery pulse in pediatric cardiac catheterization. *Pediatr Cardiol*. 1998;19:390-397.
7. Trissel LA. *Handbook on Injectable Drugs*. 15th ed. Bethesda, MD: American Society of Health-System Pharmacists; 2009.

Peginterferon Alfa (alpha-2a, alpha-2b)

1. PEGASYS [package insert]. Nutley, NJ: Hoffman-La Roche Inc; October 2008.
2. PEG-Intron [package insert]. Kenilworth, NJ: Schering Corporation; February 2005.
3. Schwarz KB, Mohan P, Narkewicz, et al. Safety, efficacy and pharmacokinetics of peginterferon α-2a (40 kd) in children with chronic hepatitis C. *J Pediatr Gastroenterol Nutr*. 2006;43:499-505.
4. Castellino S, Lensing S, Riely C, et al. The epidemiology of chronic hepatitis C infection in survivors of childhood cancer: an update of the St Jude Children's Research Hospital hepatitis C seropositive cohort. *Blood*. 2004;103:2460-2466.
5. Inati A, Taher A, Ghorra S, et al. Efficacy and tolerability of peginterferon alpha-2a with or without ribavirin in thalassemia major patients with chronic hepatitis C virus infection. *Br J Haematol*. 2005;130:644-646.
6. Kowala-Paskowska A, Sluzewski W, Figlerowicz M, et al. Factors influencing early virological response in children with chronic hepatitis C treated with pegylated interferon and ribavirin. *Hep Res*. 2005;32:224-226.
7. Wirth S, Peper-Boustani H, Lang T, et al. Peginterferon alpha-2b plus ribavirin treatment in children and adolescents with chronic hepatitis C. *Hepatology*. 2005;41:1013-1018.
8. Baker RD, Dee D, Baker SS. Response to pegylated interferon-α2b and ribavirin in children with chronic hepatitis C. *J Clin Gastroenterol*. 2007;41:111-114.
9. Jara P, Hierro L, de la Vega A, et al. Efficacy and safety of peginterferon-α2b and ribavirin combination therapy in children with chronic hepatitis C infection. *Pediatr Infect Dis J*. 2008;27:142-148.

Penicillin G Potassium/Sodium

1. Available at: http://www.usp.org/hqi/similarProducts/choosy.html. Accessed October 12, 2009.
2. Penicillin g potassium [package insert]. Schaumburg, IL: APP Pharmaceutical LLC; May 2009.
3. Nelson JD, Bradley JS, eds. *Nelson's Pocket Book of Pediatric Antimicrobial Therapy*. 17th ed. Chicago, IL: American Academy of Pediatrics; 2009.
4. Available at: http://www.cdc.gov/STD/treatment/2006/congenital-syphilis.htm#congenitalfirstmonth Accessed October 12, 2009.
5. American Academy of Pediatrics. Pickering LK, Baker CJ, Kimberlin DW, et al., eds. *2009 Red Book: Report of the Committee on Infectious Diseases*. 28th ed. Elk Grove Village, IL: American Academy of Pediatrics; 2009.
6. Azimi PH, Janner D, Berne P, et al. Concentrations of procaine and aqueous penicillin in the cerebrospinal fluid of infants treated for congenital syphilis. *J Pediatr*. 1994;124:649-653.
7. Prober CG, Stevenson DK, Benitz WE. The use of antibiotics in neonates weighing less than 1200 grams. *Pediatr Infect Dis J*. 1990;9:111-121.
8. Penicillin G potassium. Pediatric Lexi-Comp® Online with AHFS® (database). Hudson, OH: Lexi-Comp Inc; updated September 8, 2009.
9. Tunkel AR, Hartman BJ, Kaplan SL, et al. Practice guidelines for the management of bacterial meningitis. *Clin Infect Dis*. 2004;39:1267-1284.

References

10. Baddour LM, Wilson WR, Bayer AS, et al. Infective endocarditis: diagnosis, antimicrobial therapy, and management of complications: a statement for healthcare professionals from the Committee on Rheumatic Fever, Endocarditis, and Kawasaki Disease, Council on Cardiovascular Disease in the Young, and the Councils on Clinical Cardiology, Stroke, and Cardiovascular Surgery and Anesthesia, American Heart Association: endorsed by the Infectious Diseases Society of America. *Circulation.* 2005;111:e394-e434.
11. Aronoff GR, Berns JS, Brier ME, et al. Drug prescribing in renal failure. 4th ed. Available at: http://www.kdp-baptist.louisville.edu/renalbook/. Accessed October 12, 2009.
12. Penicillin. In: Kucer A, Crowe SM, Grayson ML, et al., eds. *The Use of Antibiotics: A Clinical Review of Antibacterial, Antifungal and Antiviral Drugs.* 5th ed. Boston, MA: Butterworth Heinemann; 1997;3-21.
13. Trissel LA, ed. *Handbook on Injectable Drugs.* 15th ed. Bethesda, MD: American Society of Health-System Pharmacists; 2009.
14. Robinson DC, Cookson TL, Frisafe JA. Concentration guidelines for parenteral antibiotics in fluid-restricted patients. *Drug Intell Clin Pharm.* 1987;21:985-989.
15. Robinson CA, Sawyer JE. Y-site compatibility of medications with parenteral nutrition. *J Pediatr Pharmacol Ther.* 2009;14:49-57.
16. Stumpf JL. Cardiac arrest apparently induced by penicillin. *Drug Intell Clin Pharm.* 1987;21:292.
17. Bierman CW, Van Arsdel PP Jr. Penicillin allergy in children: the role of immunological tests in its diagnosis. *J Allergy Clin Immunol.* 1969;43:267-272.
18. Neftel KA, Walti M, Spengler H, et al. Effect of storage of penicillin-G solutions on sensitization to penicillin-G after intravenous administration. *Lancet.* 1982;1:986-988.
19. Kurtzman NA, Rogers PW, Harter HR. Neurotoxic reaction to penicillin and carbenicillin. *JAMA.* 1970;214:1320-1321.
20. Smith H, Lerner PI, Weinstein L. Neurotoxicity and massive intravenous therapy with penicillin: a study of possible predisposing factors. *Arch Intern Med.* 1967;120:47-53.
21. Barrons RW, Murray KM, Richey RM. Populations at risk for penicillin-induced seizures. *Ann Pharmacother.* 1992;26:26-29.
22. Manian FA, Stone WJ, Alford RH. Adverse antibiotic effects associated with renal insufficiency. *Rev Infect Dis.* 1990;12:236-249.
23. Inglesby TV, O'Toole T, Henderson DA, et al., Working Group on Civilian Biodefense. Anthrax as a biological weapon 2002: updated recommendations for management. *JAMA.* 2002;287:2236-2252.
24. Centers for Disease Control and Prevention. Update: Investigation of bioterrorism-related anthrax and interim guidelines for exposure management and antimicrobial therapy, October 2001. *MMWR Morb Mortal Wkly Rep.* 2001;50:909-919.

Pentamidine Isethionate

1. Pentam 300 [prescribing information]. Schaumburg, IL: APP Pharmaceuticals LLC; March 2008.
2. American Academy of Pediatrics. *Pneumocystis jiroveci.* In: Pickering LK, Baker CJ, Kimberlin DW, et al., eds. *2009 Red Book: Report of the Committee on Infectious Diseases.* 28th ed. Elk Grove Village, IL: American Academy of Pediatrics; 2009:536-540.
3. Loescher T, Loeschke K, Niebel J. Severe ventricular arrhythmia during pentamidine treatment of AIDS associated Pneumocystis carinii pneumonia. *Infection.* 1987;15:455.
4. Miller HC. Cardiac arrest after intravenous pentamidine in an infant. *Pediatr Infect Dis J.* 1993;12:694-696.
5. Harel Y, Scott WA, Szeinberg A, et al. Pentamidine-induced torsades de pointes. *Pediatr Infect Dis J.* 1993;12:692-694.
6. Trivedi CD, Pitchumoni CS. Drug-induced pancreatitis. An update. *J Clin Gastroenterol.* 2005;39:709-716.
7. Drake S, Lampasona V, Nicks HL, et al. Pentamidine isethionate in the treatment of Pneumocystis carinii pneumonia. *Clin Pharm.* 1985;4:507-516.
8. Das VNR, Ranjan A, Sinha AN, et al. A randomized clinical trial of low dosage combination of pentamidine and allopurinol in the treatment of antimony unresponsive cases of visceral leishmaniasis. *J Assoc Physicians India.* 2001;49:605-608.
9. Centers for Disease Control and Prevention. Guidelines for the prevention and treatment of opportunistic infections among HIV-exposed and HIV-infected children. Recommendations from CDC, the National Institutes of Health, the HIV medicine association of the Infectious Diseases Society of America, the Pediatric Infectious Diseases Society, and the American Academy of Pediatrics. *MMWR.* 2009;58(No.RR-11):45-50.
10. Kim SY, Dabb AA, Glenn DJ, et al. Intravenous pentamidine is effective as second line Pneumocystis pneumonia prophylaxis I pediatric oncology patients. *Pediatr Blood Cancer.* 2008;50:779-783.
11. Soto-Mancipe J, Grogl M, Berman JD. Evaluation of pentamidine for the treatment of cutaneous leishmaniasis in Colombia. *Clin Infect Dis.* 1993:16:417-425.
12. American Academy of Pediatrics. *Leishmaniasis.* In: Pickering LK, Baker CJ, Kimberlin DW, et al., eds. *2009 Red Book: Report of the Committee on Infectious Diseases.* 28th ed. Elk Grove Village, IL: American Academy of Pediatrics; 2009:421-422.
13. Aronoff GR, Berns JS, Brier ME, et al. Drug prescribing in renal failure. 4th ed. Available at: http://www.kdp-baptist.louisville.edu/renalbook/pediatric/. Accessed September 7, 2009.
14. Trissel LA. *Handbook on Injectable Drugs.* 15th ed. Bethesda, MD: American Society of Health-System Pharmacists; 2009.

PENTobarbital Sodium

1. Available at: http://ismp.org/Tools/highalertmedications.pdf. Accessed September 20, 2009.
2. Available at: http://www.ismp.org/tools/tallmanletters.pdf. Accessed September 20, 2009.
3. Available at: http://www.usp.org/hqi/similarProducts/choosy.html. Accessed September 20, 2009.
4. Pentobarbital sodium [package insert]. Deerfield, IL: Ovation Pharmaceuticals; July 2003.
5. Slovis TL, Parks C, Reneau D, et al. Pediatric sedation: short-term effects. *Pediatr Radiol.* 1993;23:345-348.
6. Pereira JK, Burrows PE, Richards HM, et al. Comparison of sedation regimens for pediatric outpatient CT. *Pediatr Radiol.* 1993;23:341-344.
7. Bloomfield EL, Masaryk TJ, Caplin A, et al. Intravenous sedation for MR imaging of the brain and spine in children: pentobarbital versus propofol. *Radiology.* 1993;186:93-97.
8. Pershad J, Wan J, Anghelescu. Comparison of proprfol with pentobarbital/midazolam/fentanyl sedation for magnetic resonance imaging of the brain in children. *Pediatrics.* 2007;120:e629-e636.
9. Flood RG, Krauss B. Procedural sedation and analgesia for children in the emergency department. *Emerg Med Clin North Am.* 2003;21:121-139.
10. Malviya S, Voepel-Lewis T, Tait AR, et al. Pentobarbital vs. chloral hydrate for sedation of children undergoing MRI: efficacy and recovery characteristics. *Paediatr Anaesth.* 2004;14:589-595.
11. Mason KP, Zurakowski D, Connor L et al. Infant sedation for MR imaging and CT: oral versus intravenous pentobarbital. *Radiology.* 2004;233:723-728.
12. Sanborn PA, Michna E, Zurakowski D, et al. Adverse cardiovascular and respiratory events during sedation of pediatric patients for imaging examinations. *Radiology.* 2005;237:288-294.
13. Tobias JD, Deshpande JK, Pietsch JB, et al. Pentobarbital sedation for patients in the pediatric intensive care unit. *S Med J.* 1995;88:290-294.
14. Tobias JD. Sedation and analgesia in paediatric intensive care units. *Pediatr Drugs.* 1999;1:109-125.
15. Schaible DH, Cupit GC, Rocci ML. High-dose pentobarbital pharmacokinetics in hypothermic brain-injured children. *J Pediatr.* 1982;100:655-660.
16. Rockoff MA, Marshall LF, Shapiro HM. High-dose barbiturate therapy in humans: a clinical review of 60 patients. *Ann Neurol.* 1979;6:194-199.
17. Holmes GL, Riviello JJ. Midazolam and pentobarbital for refractory status epilepticus. *Pediatr Neurol.* 1999;20:259-264.

References

18. Marik PE, Varon J. The management of status epilepticus. *Chest.* 2004;126:582-591.
19. Lowenstein DH, Alldredge BK. Status epilepticus. *New Engl J Med.* 1998;338:970-976.
20. Claassen J, Hirsch LJ, Emerson RG, Mayer SA. Treatment of refractory status epilepticus with pentobarbital, propofol, or midazolam: a systematic review. *Epilepsia.* 2002;43:146-153.
21. Aronoff GR, Berns JS, Brier ME, et al. Drug prescribing in renal failure. 4th ed. Available at: http://www.kdp-baptist.louisville.edu/renalbook/. Accessed August 28, 2009.
22. Wermeling DP, Blouin RA, Porter WH, et al. Pentobarbital pharmacokinetics in patients with severe head injury. *Drug Intell Clin Pharm.* 1987;21:459-463.
23. Quandt CM, de los Reyes RA. Pharmacologic management of acute intracranial hypertension. *Drug Intell Clin Pharm.* 1984;18:105-112.
24. Trissel LA, ed. *Handbook on Injectable Drugs.* 15th ed. Bethesda, MD: American Society of Health-System Pharmacists; 2009.
25. Pentobarbital. Lexi-Comp® Online with AHFS® (database). Bethesda, MD: American Society of Health-System Pharmacists; updated August 28, 2009.
26. Robinson CA, Sawyer JE. Y-site compatibility of medications with parenteral nutrition. *J Pediatr Pharmacol Ther.* 2009;14:49-57.
27. Young RS, Ropper AH, Hawkes D, et al. Pentobarbital in refractory status epilepticus. *Pediatr Pharmacol.* 1983;3:62-67.
28. Kinoshita H, Nakagawa E, Hanaoka S, et al. Pentobarbital therapy for status epilepticus in children: Timing of tapering. *Pediatr Neurol.* 1995;13:164-168.
29. Bohan KH, Mansuri TF, Wilson NM. Anticonvulsant hypersensitivity syndrome: implications for pharmaceutical care. *Pharmacotherapy.* 2007;27:1425-1439.
30. Bessmerty O, Pham T. Antiepileptic hypersensitivity syndrome: clinicians beware and be aware. *Curr Allergy Asthma Rep.* 2002;2:34-39.
31. Kaur S, Sarkar R, Thami GP, et al. Anticonvulsant hypersensitivity syndrome. *Pediatr Dermatol.* 2002;19:142-145.
32. Kim SJ, Lee DY, Kim JS. Neurologic outcomes of pediatric epileptic patients with pentobarbital coma. *Pediatr Neurol.* 2001;25:217-220.
33. Butte MJ, Dodson B, Dioun A. Pentobarbital desensitization in a 3-month-old child. *Allergy Asthma Proc.* 2004;25:225-227.

Phenobarbital Sodium

1. Available at: http://ismp.org/Tools/highalertmedications.pdf. Accessed September 19, 2009.
2. Available at: http://www.ismp.org/Tools/tallmanletters.pdf. Accessed September 19, 2009.
3. Available at: http://www.usp.org/hqi/similarProducts/choosy.html. Accessed September 19, 2009.
4. Phenobarbital sodium injection USP [package insert]. Cherry Hill, NJ: Elkins-Sinn Inc; August 1987.
5. Phenobarbital, Lexi-Comp® Online with AHFS® (database). Hudson, OH: Lexi-Comp Inc; updated September 3, 2009.
6. Kumar R, Narang A, Kumar P, et al. Phenobarbitone prophylaxis for neonatal jaundice in babies with birth weight 1000–1499 grams. *Indian Pediatr.* 2002;39:945-951.
7. Murki S, Dutta S, Narang A, et al. randomized, triple-blind, placebo-controlled trial of prophylactic oral phenobarbital to reduce the need for phototherapy in G6PD-deficient neonates. *J Perinato.* 2005;25:325-330.
8. Wallin A, Boreus LO. Phenobarbital prophylaxis for hyperbilirubinemia in preterm infants. A controlled study of bilirubin disappearance and infant behavior. *Acta Paediatr Scand.* 1984;73:488-497.
9. Anwar M, Valdivieso J, Hiatt IM, et al. The course of hyperbilirubinemia in the very low birth weight infant treated with phenobarbital. *J Perinatol.* 1987;7:145-148.
10. Osborn DA, Cole MJ, Jeffery HE. Opiate treatment for opiate withdrawal in newborn infants. *Cochrane Database Syst Rev.* 2002;(3):CD002059.
11. Osborn DA, Jeffery HE, Cole MJ. Sedatives for opiate withdrawal in newborn infants. *Cochrane Database Syst Rev.* 2002;(3):CD002053.
12. Finnegan L, Kandall SR. Neonatal abstinence syndrome. In: Yaffe SJ, Aranda JV, eds. *Neonatal and Pediatric Pharmacology.* 3rd ed. Philadelphia, PA: Lippincott Williams & Wilkins; 2005:848-857.
13. Evans DJ, Levene MI. Anticonvulsants for preventing mortality and morbidity in full term newborns with perinatal asphyxia. *Cochrane Database Syst Rev.* 2001;(3):CD001240.
14. Hall RT, Hall FK, Daily DK. High-dose phenobarbital therapy in term newborns infants with severe perinatal asphyxia: a randomized, prospective study with three-year follow-up. *J Pediatr.* 1998;132:345-348.
15. Nahata MC, Masuoka T, Edwards RC. Developmental aspects of phenobarbital dosage requirements in newborn infants with seizures. *J Perinatol.* 1988;8:318-320.
16. Gal P, Toback J, Erkan NV, et al. The influence of asphyxia on phenobarbital dosing requirements in neonates. *Dev Pharmacol Ther.* 1984;7:145-152.
17. Painter MJ, Pippenger C, MacDonald H, et al. Phenobarbital and diphenylhydantoin levels in neonates with seizures. J Pediatr. 1978;92:315-319.
18. Gal P, Toback J, Boer HR, et al. Efficacy of phenobarbital monotherapy in treatment of neonatal seizures—relationship to blood levels. *Neurology.* 1982;32:1401-1404.
19. Suzuki Y, Cox S, Hayes J, et al. Phenobarbital doses necessary to achieve "therapeutic" concentration in children. *Dev Pharmacol The.* 1991;17:79-87.
20. Davis AG, Mutchie KD, Thompson JA, et al. Once-daily dosing with phenobarbital in children with seizure disorders. *Pediatrics.* 1981;68:824-827.
21. Walson PD, Mimaki T, Curless R, et al. Once daily doses of phenobarbital in children. J Pediatr. 1980;97:303-305.
22. Zupanc ML. Neonatal seizures. *Pediatr Clin North Am.* 2004;51:961-978.
23. Pippenger CE, Rosen TS. Phenobarbital plasma levels in neonates. *Clin Perinatol.* 1975;2:111-115.
24. Gilman JT, Gal P, Duchowny MS, et al. Rapid sequential phenobarbital treatment of neonatal seizures. *Pediatrics.* 1989;83:674-678.
25. Donn SM, Grasela TH, Goldstein GW. Safety of a higher loading dose of phenobarbital in the term newborn. *Pediatrics.* 1985;75:1061-1064.
26. Lowenstein DH, Alldredge BK. Status epilepticus. *N Engl J Med.* 1998;338:970-976.
27. American Academy of Pediatrics Committee on Drugs. Emergency drug doses for infants and children. *Pediatrics.* 1998;101:e1-e11.
28. Appleton R, Choonara I, Martland T, et al. The treatment of convulsive status epilepticus in children. The Status Epilepticus Working Party, Members of the Status Epilepticus Working Party. *Arch Dis Child.* 2000;83:415-419.
29. Crawford TO, Mitchell WG, Fishman LS, et al. Very-high-dose phenobarbital for refractory status epilepticus in children. *Neurology.* 1988;38:1035-1040.
30. Lee WK, Liu KT, Young BW. Very-high-dose phenobarbital for childhood refractory status epilepticus. *Pediatr Neurol.* 2006;34:63-65.
31. Aronoff GR, Berns JS, Brier ME, et al. Drug prescribing in renal failure. 4th ed. Available at: http://www.kdp-baptist.louisville.edu/renalbook/. Accessed August 28, 2009.
32. Porto I, John EG, Heilliczer J. Removal of phenobarbital during continuous cycling peritoneal dialysis in a child. *Pharmacotherapy.* 1997;17:832-835.
33. Elliott ES, Buck ML. Phenobarbital dosing and pharmacokinetics in a neonate receiving extracorporeal membrane oxygenation. *Ann Pharmacother.* 1999;33:419-422.
34. Dagan O, Kleini J, Gruenwald C, et al. Preliminary studies of the effects of extracorporeal membrane oxygenator on the disposition of common pediatric drugs. *Ther Drug Monitor.* 1993;15:263-266.
35. Trissel LA, ed. *Handbook on Injectable Drugs.* 15th ed. Bethesda, MD: American Society of Health-System Pharmacists; 2009.
36. Robinson CA, Sawyer JE. Y-site compatibility of medications with parenteral nutrition. *J Pediatr Pharmacol Ther.* 2009;14:49-57.
37. Lehy VT, Chugami HT, Aranda JV. Anticonvulsants. In: Yaffe SJ, Aranda JV, eds. *Neonatal and Pediatric Pharmacology.* 3rd ed. Philadelphia, PA: Lippincott Williams & Wilkins; 2005:504-519.

References

38. Bohan KH, Mansuri TF, Wilson NM. Anticonvulsant hypersensitivity syndrome: implications for pharmaceutical care. *Pharmacotherapy.* 2007;27:1425-1439.
39. Bessmerty O, Pham T. Antiepileptic hypersensitivity syndrome: clinicians beware and be aware. *Curr Allergy Asthma Rep.* 2002;2:34-39.
40. Kaur S, Sarkar R, Thami GP, et al. Anticonvulsant hypersensitivity syndrome. *Pediatr Dermatol.* 2002;19:142-145.
41. Available at: http://www.fda.gov/Safety/MedWatch/SafetyInformation/SafetyAlertsforHumanMedicalProducts/ucm074939.htm Accessed October 4, 2009.

Phenytoin Sodium

1. Available at: http://www.usp.org/hqi/similarProducts/choosy.html. Accessed October 4, 2009.
2. Phenytoin sodium [package insert]. Deerfield, IL: Baxter Healthcare Corp; no date specified.
3. Available at: http://www.fda.gov/Drugs/DrugSafety/PostmarketDrugSafetyInformationforPatientsandProviders/ucm124788.htm Accessed October 4, 2009.
4. Snelson C, Dieckman B. Recognizing and managing purple glove syndrome. *Crit Care Nurse.* 2000;20:54-61.
5. Abernethy DR, Greenblatt DJ. Phenytoin disposition in obesity: determination of loading dose. *Arch Neuro.* 1985;42:468-471.
6. Zalzstein W, Gorodischer R. Cardiovascular drugs. In: Yaffe SJ, Aranda JV, eds. *Neonatal and Pediatric Pharmacology.* 3rd ed. Philadelphia, PA: Lippincott Williams & Wilkins; 2005:574-594.
7. Tilford JM, Simpson PM, Yeh TS, et al. Variation in therapy and outcome for pediatric head trauma patients. *Crit Care Med.* 2001;29:1056-1061.
8. Adelson PD, Bratton SL, Carney NA, et al. Guidelines for the acute medical management of severe traumatic brain injury in infants, children, and adolescents. Chapter 19. The role of anti-seizure prophylaxis following severe pediatric traumatic brain injury. *Pediatr Crit Care Med.* 2003;4(3 suppl):S72-S75.
9. Stowe CD, Lee KR, Storgion SA, et al. Altered phenytoin pharmacokinetics in children with severe, acute traumatic brain injury. Status epilepticus. *J Clin Pharmacol.* 2000;40:1452-1461.
10. Griebel ML, Kearns GL, Fisher DH, et al. Phenytoin protein binding in pediatric patients with acute traumatic injury. *Crit Care Med.* 1990;18:385-391.
11. Loughnan PM, Greenwald A, Purton W, et al. Pharmacokinetic observation of phenytoin disposition in the newborn and young infant. *Arch Dis Child.* 1977;52:302-309.
12. Bourgeois BFD, Dodson WE. Phenytoin elimination in newborns. *Neurology.* 1983;33:173-178.
13. Leff RD, Fisher LJ, Roberts RJ. Phenytoin metabolism in infants following intravenous and oral administration. *Dev Pharmacol Ther.* 1986;9:217-223.
14. Lehr VT, Chugani HT, Aranda JV. Anticonvulsants. In: Yaffe SJ, Aranda JV, eds. *Neonatal and Pediatric Pharmacology.* 3rd ed. Philadelphia, PA: Lippincott Williams & Wilkins; 2005:504-519.
15. Curless RG, Walson PD, Carter DE. Phenytoin kinetics in children. *Neurology.* 1976;26:715-720.
16. Dodson WE. Nonlinear kinetics of phenytoin in children. *Neurology.* 1982;32:42-48.
17. Painter MJ, Pippenger C, MacDonald H, et al. Phenobarbital and diphenylhydantoin levels in neonates with seizures. *J Pediatr.* 1978;92:315-319.
18. Phelps SJ, Baldree LA, Boucher BA, et al. Neuropsychiatric toxicity of phenytoin. Importance of monitoring phenytoin levels. *Clin Pediatr.* 1993;32:107-110.
19. Liponi DL, Winter ME, Tozer TN. Renal function and therapeutic concentrations of phenytoin. *Neurology.* 1984;34:395-397.
20. Drugs for epilepsy. *Med Lett Drugs Ther.* 1983;25:81-84.
21. American Academy of Pediatrics Committee on Drugs. Emergency drug doses for infants and children. *Pediatrics.* 1998;101:e1-e11.
22. Shields WD. Status epilepticus. *Pediatr Clin North Am.* 1989;36:383-393.
23. Trissel LA, ed. *Handbook on Injectable Drugs.* 15th ed. Bethesda, MD: American Society of Health-System Pharmacists; 2009.
24. Robinson CA, Sawyer JE. Y-site compatibility of medications with parenteral nutrition. *J Pediatr Pharmacol Ther.* 2009;14:49-57.
25. Pagliaro LA, Pagliaro AM, eds. *Problems in Pediatric Drug Therapy.* 2nd ed. Hamilton, IL: Drug Intelligence Publications Inc; 1987.
26. Wheless JW. Pediatric use of intravenous and intramuscular phenytoin: lessons learned. *J Child Neurol.* 1998;13:S11-14, discussion S30-S32.
27. Walsh-Kelly CM, Berens RJ, Glaeser PW, Losek JD. Intraosseous infusion of phenytoin. *Am J Emerg Med.* 1986;4:523-524.
28. Bohan KH, Mansuri TF, Wilson NM. Anticonvulsant hypersensitivity syndrome: implications for pharmaceutical care. *Pharmacotherapy.* 2007;27:1425-1439.
29. Bessmerty O, Pham T. Antiepileptic hypersensitivity syndrome: clinicians beware and be aware. *Curr Allergy Asthma Rep.* 2002;2:34-39.
30. Kaur S, Sarkar R, Thami GP, et al. Anticonvulsant hypersensitivity syndrome. *Pediatr Dermatol.* 2002;19:142-145.
31. Available at: http://www.fda.gov/Safety/MedWatch/SafetyInformation/SafetyAlertsforHumanMedicalProducts/ucm074939.htm Accessed October 4, 2009.
32. Anderson GD. A mechanistic approach to antiepileptic drug interactions. *Ann Pharmacother.* 1998;32:554-563.

Physostigmine Salicylate

1. Available at: http://www.usp.org/hqi/similarProducts/choosy.html. Accessed August 29, 2009.
2. Physostigmine salicylate injection [package insert]. Lake Forest, IL: Akorn Inc; November 2008.
3. Rumack BH. Anticholinergic poisoning: treatment with physostigmine. *Pediatrics.* 1973;52:449-451.
4. Bowden CA, Krenzelok EP. Clinical applications of commonly used contemporary antidotes. *Drug Safety.* 1997;16:9-47.
5. Shannon M. Toxicology reviews: physostigmine. *Pediatr Emergency Care.* 1998;14:224-226.
6. Wright SP. Usefulness of physostigmine in imipramine poisoning. *Clin Pediatr.* 1976;15:1123-1128.
7. Ceha LJ, Presperin C, Young E, et al. Anticholinergic toxicity from Nightshade berry poisoning responsive to physostigmine. *J Emerg Med.* 1997;15:65-69.
8. Van Herreweghe I, Mertens K, Maes V, et al. Orphenadrine poisoning in a child: clinical and analytical data. *Intensive Care Med.* 1999;25:1134-1136.
9. Arnold SM, Arnholz D, Garyfallou GT, et al. Two siblings poisoned with diphenhydramine: a case of fictitious disorder by proxy. *Ann Emerg Med.* 1998;32:256-259.
10. Tobis J, Das BN. Cardiac complications in amitriptyline poisoning. Successful treatment with physostigmine. *JAMA.* 1976;235:1474-1476.
11. Physostigmine. Drugdex Evaluations with Micromedex Online (database), 1974–2009. Montvale, NJ: Thomson Reuters; updated February 6, 2009.
12. Stern TA. Continuous infusion of physostigmine in anticholinergic delirium: case report. *J Clin Psychiatry.* 1983;44:463-464.
13. Pentel P, Peterson CD. Asystole complicating physostigmine treatment of tricyclic antidepressant overdose. *Ann Emerg Med.* 1980;9:588-590.
14. Snyder BD, Blonde L, McWhirter WR. Reversal of amitriptyline intoxication by physostigmine. *JAMA.* 1974;230:1433-1434.
15. Physostigmine. Poisondex for Micromedex Online (database), 1974–2009. Montvale, NJ: Thomson Reuters; accessed October 1, 2009.
16. Schultz U, Idelberger R, Rossaint R, et al. Central anticholinergic syndrome in a child undergoing circumcision. *Acta Anaesthesiol Scand.* 2002;46:224-226.
17. Kulka PJ, Toker H, Heim J, et al. Suspected central anticholinergic syndrome in a 6-week-old infant. *Anesth Analg.* 2004;99:1376-1378.
18. Funk W, Hollnberger H, Geroldinger J. Physostigmine and anaesthesia emergence delirium in preschool children: a randomized blinded trial. *Eur J Anaesthesiol.* 2008;25:37-42.

References

Piperacillin Sodium

1. Available at: http://www.usp.org/hqi/similarProducts/choosy.html. Accessed September 19, 2009.
2. Piperacillin [package insert]. Philadelphia, PA: Wyeth Pharmaceuticals; March 2007.
3. Placzek M, Whitelaw A, Want S, et al. Piperacillin in early neonatal infection. *Arch Dis Child.* 1983;58:1006-1009.
4. Kacet N, Roussel-Delvallez M, Gremillet C, et al. Pharmacokinetic study of piperacillin in newborns relating to gestational and postnatal age. *Pediatr Infect Dis. J.* 1992;11:365-369.
5. American Academy of Pediatrics. Pickering LK, Baker CJ, Kimberlin DW, et al., eds. *2009 Red Book: Report of the Committee on Infectious Diseases.* 28th ed. Elk Grove Village, IL: American Academy of Pediatrics; 2009.
6. Wilson CB, Koup JR, Opheim KE, et al. Piperacillin pharmacokinetics in pediatric patients. *Antimicrob Agents Chemother.* 1982;22:442-447.
7. Thirumoorthi MC, Asmar BI, Buckley JA, et al. Pharmacokinetics of intravenously administered piperacillin in preadolescent children. *J Pediatr.* 1983;102:941-946.
8. Ciftci AO, Tanyel C, Buyukpamucu N, et al. Comparative trial of four antibiotic combinations for perforated appendicitis in children. *Eur J Surg.* 1997;163:591-596.
9. Prince AS, Neu HC. Use of piperacillin, a semisynthetic penicillin, in the therapy of acute exacerbations of pulmonary disease in patients with cystic fibrosis. *J Pediatr.* 1980;97:148-151.
10. Jackson MA, Kusmiesz H, Shelton S, et al. Comparison of piperacillin vs. ticarcillin plus tobramycin in the treatment of acute pulmonary exacerbation of cystic fibrosis. *Pediatr Infect Dis J.* 1986;5:440-443.
11. Bernig T, Weigel S, Mukodzi S. Antibiotic sequential therapy for febrile neutropenia in pediatric patients with malignancy. *Pediatr Hematol Oncol.* 2000;17:93-98.
12. Mahmood S, Revesz T, Mpofu C. Ferile episodes in children with cancer in the United Arab Emirates. *Pediatr Hematol Oncol.* 1996;13:135-142.
13. Salam IM, Galala KH, Ashaal YI, et al. A randomized prospective study of cefoxitin versus piperacillin in appendectomy. *J Hosp Infect.* 1994;26:133-136.
14. DeSchepper PJ, Tjandramaga TB, Mullie A, et al. Comparative pharmacokinetics of piperacillin in normals and in patients with renal failure. *J Antimicrob Chemother.* 1982;9(suppl B):49-57.
15. Aronoff GR, Berns JS, Brier ME, et al. Drug prescribing in renal failure. 4th ed. Available at: http://www.kdp-baptist.louisville.edu/renalbook/. Accessed August 28, 2009.
16. Trissel LA, ed. *Handbook on Injectable Drugs.* 15th ed. Bethesda, MD: American Society of Health-System Pharmacists; 2009.
17. Robinson DC, Cookson TL, Frisafe JA. Concentration guidelines for parenteral antibiotics in fluid-restricted patients. *Drug Intell Clin Pharm.* 1987;21:985-989.
18. McLaughlin JE, Reeves DS. Clinical and laboratory evidence for inactivation of gentamicin by carbenicillin. *Lancet.* 1971;1:261-264.
19. Riff LJ, Jackson GG. Laboratory and clinical conditions for gentamicin inactivation by carbenicillin. *Arch Intern Med.* 1972;130:887-891.
20. Manian FA, Stone WJ, Alford RH. Adverse antibiotic effects associated with renal insufficiency. *Rev Infect Dis.* 1990;12:236-249.
21. Davies M, Morgan JR, Anand C. Interactions of carbenicillin and ticarcillin with gentamicin. *Antimicrob Agents Chemother.* 1975;7:431-434.
22. Weibert R, Keane W, Shapiro F. Carbenicillin inactivation of aminoglycosides in patients with severe renal failure. *Trans Amer Soc Artif Int Organs.* 1976;22:439-443.
23. Robinson CA, Sawyer JE. Y-site compatibility of medications with parenteral nutrition. *J Pediatr Pharmacol Ther.* 2009;14:49-57.
24. Burgess DS, Waldrep T. Pharmacokinetics and pharmacodynamics of piperacillin/tazobactam when administered by continuous infusion and intermittent dosing. *Clin Ther.* 2002;24:1090-1104.
25. Grant EM, Kuti JL, Nicolau DP, et al. Clinical efficacy and pharmacoeconomics of a continuous-infusion piperacillin-tazobactam program in a large community teaching hospital. *Pharmacotherapy.* 2002;22:471-483.
26. Florea NR, Kotapati S, Kuti JL, et al. Cost analysis of continuous versus intermittent infusion of piperacillin-tazobactam: a time-motion study. *Am J Health-Syst Pharm.* 2003;60:2321-2327.
27. Craig WA, Ebert SC. Continuous infusion of beta-lactam antibiotics. *Antimicrob Agents Chemother.* 1992;36:2577-2583.
28. Wills R, Henry RL, Francis JL. Antibiotic hypersensitivity reactions in cystic fibrosis. *J Paediatr Child Health.* 1998;34:325-329.
29. Rye PJ, Roberts G, Staugas RE, et al. Coagulopathy with piperacillin administration in cystic fibrosis: two case reports. *J Paediatr Child Health.* 1994;30:278-279.
30. Malanga CJ, Kojontis L, Mauzy S. Piperacillin-induced seizures. *Clin Pediatr.* 1997;36:475-478.
31. Piperacillin. Lexi-Comp® Online with AHFS® (database). Hudson, OH: Lexi-Comp Inc; updated July 25, 2009.
32. Zarychanski R, Wlodarczyk K, Ariano R, et al. Pharmacokinetic interaction between methotrexate and piperacillin/tazobactam resulting in prolonged toxic concentrations of methotrexate. *J Antimicrob Chemother.* 2006;58:228-230.
33. Mackie K, Pavlin EG. Recurrent paralysis following piperacillin administration. *Anesthesiology.* 1990;72:561-563.

Piperacillin Sodium–Tazobactam Sodium

1. Available at: http://www.usp.org/hqi/similarProducts/choosy.html. Accessed September 19, 2009.
2. Piperacillin Sodium–Tazobactam Sodium [package insert]. Philadelphia, PA: Wyeth Pharmaceuticals; November 2007.
3. Flidel-Rimon O, Friedman S, Leibovitz E, et al. The use of piperacillin/tazobactam (in association with amikacin) in neonatal sepsis: efficacy and safety data. *Scand J Infect Dis.* 2006;38:36-42.
4. Berger A, Kretzer V, Apfalter P, et al. Safety evaluation of piperacillin/tazobactam in very low birth weight infants. *J Chemother.* 2004;16:166-171.
5. Pillay T, Pillay DG, Adhikari M, et al. Piperacillin/tazobactam in the treatment of Klebsiella pneumoniae infections in neonates. *Am J Perinatol.* 1998;15:47-51.
6. American Academy of Pediatrics. Pickering LK, Baker CJ, Kimberlin DW, et al., eds. *2009 Red Book: Report of the Committee on Infectious Diseases.* 28th ed. Elk Grove Village, IL: American Academy of Pediatrics; 2009.
7. Reed MD, Goldfarb J, Yamashita TS, et al. Single-dose pharmacokinetics of piperacillin and tazobactam in infants and children. *Antimicrob Agents Chemother.* 1994;36:2817-2826.
8. Reed MD. The pathophysiology and treatment of cystic fibrosis. *J Pediatr Pharm Pract.* 1997;2:285-305.
9. Manno G, Cruciani M, Romano L, et al. Antimicrobial use and Pseudomonas aeruginosa susceptibility profile in a cystic fibrosis centre. *Int J Antimicrob Agents.* 2005;25:193-197.
10. Aronoff GR, Berns JS, Brier ME, et al. Drug prescribing in renal failure. 4th ed. Available at: http://www.kdp-baptist.louisville.edu/renalbook/. Accessed Sptember 19, 2009.
11. Schoonover LL, Occhipinti DJ, Rodvoid EA, et al. Piperacillin/tazobactam: a new beta-lactam/beta-lactamase inhibitor combination. *Ann Pharmacother.* 1995;29:501-513.
12. Trissel LA, ed. *Handbook on Injectable Drugs.* 15th ed. Bethesda, MD: American Society of Health-System Pharmacists; 2009.
13. McLaughlin JE, Reeves DS. Clinical and laboratory evidence for inactivation of gentamicin by carbenicillin. *Lancet.* 1971;1:261-264.
14. Riff LJ, Jackson GG. Laboratory and clinical conditions for gentamicin inactivation by carbenicillin. *Arch Intern Med.* 1972;130:887-891.
15. Manian FA, Stone WJ, Alford RH. Adverse antibiotic effects associated with renal insufficiency. *Rev Infect Dis.* 1990;12:236-249.
16. Davies M, Morgan JR, Anand C. Interactions of carbenicillin and ticarcillin with gentamicin. *Antimicrob Agents Chemother.* 1975;7:431-434.
17. Weibert R, Keane W, Shapiro F. Carbenicillin inactivation of aminoglycosides in patients with severe renal failure. *Trans Amer Soc Artif Int Organs.* 1976;22:439-443.
18. Robinson CA, Sawyer JE. Y-site compatibility of medications with parenteral nutrition. *J Pediatr Pharmacol Ther.* 2009;14:49-57.

References

19. Burgess DS, Waldrep T. Pharmacokinetics and pharmacodynamics of piperacillin/tazobactam when administered by continuous infusion and intermittent dosing. *Clin Ther.* 2002;24:1090-1104.
20. Grant EM, Kuti JL, Nicolau DP, et al. Clinical efficacy and pharmacoeconomics of a continuous-infusion piperacillin-tazobactam program in a large community teaching hospital. *Pharmacotherapy.* 2002;22:471-483.
21. Florea NR, Kotapati S, Kuti JL, et al. Cost analysis of continuous versus intermittent infusion of piperacillin-tazobactam: a time-motion study. *Am J Health-Syst Pharm.* 2003;60:2321-2327.
22. Wills R, Henry RL, Francis JL. Antibiotic hypersensitivity reactions in cystic fibrosis. *J Paediatr Child Health.* 1998;34:325-329.
23. Rye PJ, Roberts G, Staugas RE, et al. Coagulopathy with piperacillin administration in cystic fibrosis: two case reports. *J Paediatr Child Health.* 1994;30:278-279.
24. Malanga CJ, Kojontis L, Mauzy S. Piperacillin-induced seizures. *Clin Pediatr.* 1997;36:475-478.
25. Zarychanski R, Wlodarczyk K, Ariano R, et al. Pharmacokinetic interaction between methotrexate and piperacillin/tazobactam resulting in prolonged toxic concentrations of methotrexate. *J Antimicrob Chemother.* 2006;58:228-230.
26. Piperacillin. Lexi-Comp® Online with AHFS® (database). Hudson, OH: Lexi-Comp Inc; updated July 25, 2009.
27. Mackie K, Pavlin EG. Recurrent paralysis following piperacillin administration. *Anesthesiology.* 1990;72:561-563.

Potassium Chloride

1. Available at: http://ismp.org/Tools/highalertmedications.pdf. ISMP 2008.
2. Available at: http://www.usp.org/hqi/similarProducts/choosy.html. Accessed February 27, 2009.
3. Fisch C, Knoebel SB, Feigen H, et al. Potassium and the monophasic action potential, electrocardiogram, conduction, and arrhythmias. *Prog Cardiovasc Dis.* 1966;8:387-418.
4. Ash SR. The perils of i.v. potassium: are they exaggerated? *Parenterals.* 1987;(Dec/Jan):1, 5-8.
5. Schaber DE, Uden DL, Stone FM, et al. Intravenous KCl supplementation in pediatric cardiac surgical patients. *Pediatr Cardiol.* 1985;6:25-28.
6. DeFronza RA, Bia M. Intravenous potassium chloride therapy. *JAMA.* 1981;245:2446. Questions and Answers.
7. Trachtenbarg DE. Diabetic ketoacidosis. *Am Fam Physician.* 2005;71:1705-1714.
8. Potassium chloride. Lexi-Comp® Online with AHFS® (database). Hudson, OH: Lexi-Comp Inc; updated March 5, 2009.
9. Potassium supplements. Lexi-Comp® Online with AHFS® (database). Bethesda, MD: American Society of Health-System Pharmacists; updated May 26, 2009.
10. Potassium chloride [package insert]. Schaumburg, IL: American Pharmaceutical Partners LLC; April 2008.
11. Upton J, Mulliken JB, Murray JE. Major intravenous extravasation injuries. *Am J Surg.* 1979;137:497-506.
12. DeFronzo RA, Taufield PA, Black H, et al. Impaired renal tubular potassium secretion in sickle cell disease. *Ann Intern Med.* 1979;90:310-316.
13. Trissel LA. *Handbook on Injectable Drugs.* 15th ed. Bethesda, MD: American Society of Health-System Pharmacists; 2009.
14. Kruse JA, Carlson RW. Rapid correction of hypokalemia using concentrated intravenous potassium chloride infusions. *Arch Intern Med.* 1990;150:613-617.
15. Pucino F, Danielson BD, Carlson JD, et al. Patient tolerance to intravenous potassium chloride with and without lidocaine. *Drug Intell Clin Pharm.* 1988;22:676-679.

Potassium Phosphates

1. Available at: http://ismp.org/Tools/highalertmedications.pdf. ISMP 2008.
2. Available at: http://www.usp.org/hqi/similarProducts/choosy.html. Accessed February 27, 2009.
3. Potassium phosphates [package insert]. Schaumburg, IL: American Pharmaceutical Partners Inc; September 2003.
4. Potassium supplements. Lexi-Comp® Online with AHFS® (database). Bethesda, MD: American Society of Health-System Pharmacists; updated May 26, 2009.
5. Ash SR. The perils of iv potassium: are they exaggerated? *Parenterals.* 1987;(Dec/Jan):1, 5-8.
6. Upton J, Mulliken JB, Murray JE. Major intravenous extravasation injuries. *Am J Surg.* 1979;137:497-506.
7. Potassium phosphates. Lexi-Comp® Online with AHFS® (database). Hudson, OH: Lexi-Comp Inc; updated June 10, 2009.
8. Trissel LA. *Handbook on Injectable Drugs.* 15th ed. Bethesda, MD: American Society of Health-System Pharmacists; 2009.
9. Trachtenbarg DE. Diabetic ketoacidosis. *Am Fam Physician.* 2005;71:1705-1714.
10. White NH. Diabetic ketoacidosis in children. *Endocrinol Metab Clin North Am.* 2000; 29:657-682.
11. Clark CL, Sacks GS, Dickerson RN, et al. Treatment of hypophosphatemia in patients receiving specialized nutrition support using a graduated dosing scheme: results from a prospective clinical trial. *Crit Care Med.* 1995;23:1504-1511.
12. Prestridge LL, Schanler RJ, Shulman RJ, et al. Effect of parenteral calcium and phosphorus therapy on mineral retention and bone mineral content in very low birth weight infants. *J Pediatr.* 1993;122:761-768.
13. Pelegano JF, Rowe JC, Carey DE, et al. Simultaneous infusion of calcium and phosphorus in parenteral nutrition for premature infants: use of physiologic calcium/phosphorus ratio. *J Pediatr.* 1989;114;115-119.

Pralidoxime Chloride (2-PAM Chloride)

1. Available at: http://ismp.org/Tools/confuseddrugnames.pdf. Accessed August 29, 2009.
2. Available at: http://www.usp.org/hqi/similarProducts/choosy.html. Accessed August 29, 2009.
3. Protopam Chloride–pralidoxime chloride injection [package insert]. Deerfield, IL: Baxter Healthcare Corporation; May 2004.
4. Ellenhorn MJ, Barceloux DG. *Medical Toxicology Diagnosis and Treatment of Human Poisoning.* New York, NY: Elsevier; 1988:81-82,1071-1077.
5. Farrar HC, Wells TG, Kearns GL. Use of continuous infusion of pralidoxime for treatment of organophosphate poisoning in children. *J Pediatr.* 1990;116:658-661.
6. Pralidoxime. Lexi-Comp Online with AHFS (database). Bethesda, MD: American Society of Health-System Pharmacists; updated January 2009.
7. Mortensen ML. Management of acute childhood poisonings caused by selected insecticides and herbicides. *Pediatr Clin North Am.* 1986;33:421-445.
8. Bowden CA, Krenzelok EP. Clinical applications of commonly used contemporary antidotes. *Drug Safety.* 1997;16:9-47.
9. Zwiener RJ, Ginsburg CM. Organophosphate and carbamate poisoning in infants and children. *Pediatrics.* 1988;81:121-125.
10. Benitz WE, Tatro DS. *The Pediatric Drug Handbook.* Chicago, IL: Year Book; 1988:14.
11. Schexnayder S, James LP, Kearns GL, et al. The pharmacokinetics of continuous infusion pralidoxime in children with organophosphate poisoning. *Clin Toxicol.* 1998;36:549-555.
12. Namba T, Nolte CT, Jackrel J, et al. Poisoning due to organophosphate insecticides. *Am J Med.* 1971;50:475-492.

Procainamide HCl

1. Available at: http://ismp.org/Tools/highalertmedications.pdf. Accessed June 19, 2009.
2. Available at: http://www.usp.org/hqi/similarProducts/choosy.html. Accessed June 19, 2009.

References

3. Procainamide. Lexi-Comp® Online with AHFS® (database). Bethesda, MD: American Society of Health-System Pharmacists; updated August 13, 2009.
4. American Academy of Pediatrics Committee on Drugs. Emergency drug doses for infants and children. *Pediatrics.* 1998;101:e1-e11.
5. American Heart Association. Guidelines 2005 for cardiopulmonary resuscitation and emergency cardiovascular care—part 12: pediatric advanced life support. *Circulation.* 2005;112:167-187.
6. Mandapati R, Byrum CJ, Kavey RE, et al. Procainamide of rate control of postsurgical junctional tachycardia. *Pediatr Cardiol.* 2000;21:123-128.
7. Luedtke SA, Kuhn RJ, McCaffrey FM. Pharmacologic management of supraventricular tachycardias in children. *Ann Pharmacother.* 1997;21:1347-1359.
8. Trissel LA, ed. *Handbook on Injectable Drugs.* 15th ed. Bethesda, MD: American Society of Health-System Pharmacists; 2009.
9. Bryson SM, Leson CL, Irwin DB, et al. Therapeutic monitoring and pharmacokinetic evaluation of procainamide in neonates. *DICP Ann Pharmacother.* 1991;25:68-71.
10. Trujillo TC, Nolan PE. Antiarrhythmic agents: drug interactions of clinical significance. *Drug Safety.* 2000;23:509-532.

Promethazine HCl

1. Available at: http://ismp.org/tools/highalertmedications.pdf. Accessed August 29, 2009.
2. Available at: http://www.usp.org/hqi/similarProducts/choosy.html. Accessed August 29, 2009.
3. Phenergan [package insert]. Deerfield, IL: Baxter Healthcare Corp; August 2005.
4. Mostafavi H, Samimi M. Accidental intra-arterial injection of promethazine HCl during general anesthesia: report of a case. *Anesthesiology.* 1971;35:645-646.
5. *ISMP Safety Newsletter.* August 10, 2006.
6. Ruckman RN, Keane JF, Freed MD, et al. Sedation for cardiac catheterization: a controlled study. *Pediatr Cardiol.* 1980;1:263-268.
7. Fixler DE, Carrell T, Browne R, et al. Oxygen consumption in infants and children during cardiac catheterization under different sedation regimens. *Circulation.* 1974;50:788-794.
8. Khalil S, Philrook L, Rabb M, et al. Ondansetron/promethazine combination or promethazine alone reduces nausea and vomiting after middle ear surgery. *J Clin Anesth.* 1999;11:596-600.
9. Aronoff GR, Berns JS, Brier ME, et al. Drug prescribing in renal failure. 4th ed. Available at: http://www.kdp-baptist.louisville.edu/renalbook/. Accessed August 17, 2009.
10. Trissel LA, ed. *Handbook on Injectable Drugs.* 15th ed. Bethesda, MD: American Society of Health-System Pharmacists; 2009.
11. Starke PR, Weaver J, Chowdhury BA. Boxed warning added to promethazine labeling for pediatric use. *N Engl J Med.* 2005;352:2653.
12. Nahata MC, Clotz MA, Krogg EA. Adverse effects of meperidine, promethazine, and chlorpromazine for sedation in pediatric patients. *Clin Pediatr.* 1985;24:558-560.
13. Nahata MC. Sedation in pediatric patients undergoing diagnostic procedures. *Drug Intell Clin Pharm.* 1988;22:711-715.
14. Cook BA, Bass JW, Nomizu S, et al. Sedation of children for technical procedures: current standards of practice. *Clin Pediatr.* 1992;31:137-142.
15. American Academy of Pediatrics. Committee on Drugs. Reappraisal of lytic cocktail/demerol, phenergan, and thorazine (DPT) for the sedation of children. *Pediatrics.* 1995;95:598-602.
16. Brown ET, Corbett SW, Green SM. Iatrogenic cardiopulmonary arrest during pediatric sedation with meperidine, promethazine, and chlorpromazine. *Pediatr Emerg Care.* 2001;17:351-353.
17. Snodgrass WR, Dodge WF. Lytic/DPT cocktail: time for rational and safer alternatives. *Pediatr Clin North Am.* 1989;36:1285-1291.
18. Ingram DG, Hagemann TM. Promethazine treatment of steroid-induced psychosis in a child. *Ann Pharmacother.* 2003;37:1036-1039.

Propofol

1. Available at: http://ismp.org/Tools/highalertmedications.pdf. Accessed November 14, 2009.
2. Available at: http://ismp.org/Tools/confuseddrugnames.pdf. Accessed November 14, 2009.
3. Available at: http://www.usp.org/hqi/similarProducts/choosy.html. Accessed November 14, 2009.
4. Propofol [package insert]. Wilmington, DE. AstraZeneca Pharmaceuticals; May 2008.
5. Rochette A, Hocquet AF, Dadure C, et al. Avoiding propofol injection pain in children: a prospective,randomized, double-blinded, placebo-controlled study. *Brit J Anaesth.* 2008;101:390-394.
6. Morton NS, Wee M, Christie G, et al. Propofol for induction of anaesthesia in children. *Anaesthesia.* 1988;43:350-355.
7. Mirakhur RK. Induction characteristics of propofol in children: comparison with thiopentone. *Anaesthesia.* 1988;43:593-598.
8. Patel DK, Keeling PA, Newman GB, et al. Induction dose of propofol in children. *Anaesthesia.* 1988;43:949-952.
9. Martin TM, Nicolson SC, Bargas MS. Propofol anesthesia reduces emesis and airway obstruction in pediatric outpatients. *Anesth Analg.* 1993;76:144-148.
10. Hannallah RS, Britton JT, Schafer PG, et al. Propofol anaesthesia in paediatric ambulatory patients: a comparison with thiopentone and halothane. *Can J Anaesth.* 1994;41:12-18.
11. Borgeat A, Fuchs T, Tassonyi E. Induction characteristics of 2% propofol solution. *Br J Anaesth.* 1997;78:433-435.
12. Pessenbacher K, Gutmann A, Eggenreich U, et al. Two propofol formulations are equivalent in small children aged 1 month to 3 years. *Acta Anaesthesiol Scand.* 2002;46:257-263.
13. Rocca GD, Costa MG, Bruno K, et al. Pediatric renal transplantation: anesthesia and perioperative complications. *Pediatr Surg Int.* 2001;17:175-179.
14. Uezono S, Goto T, Terui K, et al. Emergence agitation after sevoflurane versus propofol in pediatric patients. *Anesth Analg.* 2000;91: 563-566.
15. Saricaoglu F, Celebi N, Celik M, et al. The evaluation of propofol dosage for anesthesia induction in children with cerebral palsy with bispectral index (BIS) monitoring. *Paediatr Anaesth.* 2005;15:1048-1052.
16. Cohen IT, Hannallah RS, Goodale DB. The clinical and biochemical effects of propofol infusion with and without EDTA for maintenance anesthesia in healthy children undergoing ambulatory surgery. *Anesth Analg.* 2001;93:106-111.
17. Exil G, Clancy RR, Hyder DJ. Propofol treatment of refractory status epilepticus: a report of five pediatric cases. *Epilepsia.* 1995;36:124.
18. Harrison AM, Lugo RA, Schunk JE. Treatment of convulsive status epilepticus with propofol: a case report. *Pediatr Emer Care.* 1997;13: 420-422.
19. Rossetti AO, Logroscino G, Bromfield EB. Refractory status epilepticus: effect of treatment aggressiveness on prognosis. *Arch Neurol.* 2005;62:1698-1702.
20. Harrison AM, Lugo RA, Schunk JE. Treatment of convulsive status epilepticus with propofol: case report. *Pediatr Emerg Care.* 1997;13: 420-422.
21. van Gestel JP, Blusse van Oud-Alblas HJ, Malingre M, et al. Propofol and thiopental for refractory status epilepticus in children. *Neurology.* 2005;23:591-592.
22. Dial S, Silver P, Bock K, Sagy M. Pediatric sedation for procedures titrated to a desired degree of immobility results in unpredictable depth of sedation. *Pediatr Emerg Care.* 2001;17:414-420.

References

23. Vardi A, Salen Y, Padeh S, et al. Is propofol safe for procedural sedation in children? A prospective evaluation of propofol versus ketamine in pediatric critical care. *Crit Care Med.* 2002;30:1231-1236.
24. Gozol D, Rein AJ, Nir A, et al. Propofol does not modify the hemodynamic status of children with intracardiac shunts undergoing cardiac catheterization. *Pediatr Cardiol.* 2001;22:488-490.
25. Hertzog JH, Campbell JK, Dalton HJ, et al. Propofol anesthesia for invasive procedures in ambulatory and hospitalized children: experience in the pediatric intensive care unit. *Pediatrics.* 1999 Mar;103(3):E30. Available at: http://www.pediatrics.org/cgi/content/full/103/3/e30.
26. Timpe EM, Eichner SF, Phelps SJ. Propofol-related infusion syndrome in critically ill pediatric patients: coincidence, association, or causation? *J Pediatr Pharmacol Ther.* 2006;11:17-42.
27. Aronoff GR, Berns JS, Brier ME, et al. Drug prescribing in renal failure. 4th ed. Available at: http://www.kdp-baptist.louisville.edu/renalbook/. Accessed November 14, 2009.
28. Trissel LA, ed. *Handbook on Injectable Drugs.* 15th ed. Bethesda, MD: American Society of Health-System Pharmacists; 2009.
29. Hofer KN, McCarthy MW, Buck ML, et al. Possible anaphylaxis after propofol in a child with food allergy. *Ann Pharmacother.* 2003;37:398-401.
30. Bennett SN, McNeil MM, Bland LA, et al. Postoperative infections traced to contamination of intravenous anesthetic, propofol. *N Engl J Med.* 1995;333:147-154.
31. McHugh GJ, Roper GM. Propofol emulsion and bacterial contamination. *Can J Anaesth.* 1995;42:801-804.
32. Reiter PD, Robles J, Dowell EB. Effect of 24-hour intravenous tubing set change on the sterility of repackaged fat emulsion in neonates. *Ann Pharmacother.* 2004;38:1603-1607.
33. Bragonier R, Bartle D, Langton-Hewer S. Acute dystonia in a 14-yr-old following propofol and fentanyl anaesthesia. *Br J Anaesth.* 2000;84:828-829.
34. Collier C, Kelly K. Propofol and convulsions—the evidence mounts. *Anaesth Intensive Care.* 1991;19:573-575.
35. Harrigan PW, Browne SM, Quail AW. Multiple seizures following re-exposure to propofol. *Anaesth Intensive Care.* 1996;24:261-264.
36. Gelber O, Gal M, Katz Y. Clonic convulsions in a neonate after propofol anaesthesia. *Paediatr Anaesth.* 1997;7:88.
37. Walder B, Tramer MR, Seeck M. Seizure-like phenomena and propofol: a systematic review. *Neurology.* 2002;58:1327-1332.
38. Gottschling S, Larsen R, Meyer S, et al. Acute pancreatitis induced by short-term propofol administration. *Paediatr Anaesth.* 2005;15:1006-1008.
39. Devlin JW, Lau AK, Tanios MA. Propofol-associated hypertriglyceridemia and pancreatitis in the intensive care unit: an analysis of frequency and risk factors. *Pharmacotherapy.* 2005;25:1348-1352.
40. Gottschling S, Meyer S, Krenn T, et al. Effects of short-term propofol administration on pancreatic enzymes and triglyceride levels in children. *Anaesthesia.* 2005;60:660-663.
41. Robinson JD, Melman Y, Walsh EP. Cardiac conduction disturbances and ventricular tachycardia after prolonged propofol infusion in an infant. *PACE.* 2008;31:1070-1073.
42. Propofol. Lexi-Comp® Online with AHFS ® (database). Bethesda, MD: American Society of Health-System Pharmacists; updated September 17, 2009.

Propranolol HCl

1. Available at: http://ismp.org/Tools/highalertmedications.pdf. Accessed June 19, 2009.
2. Available at: http://www.ismp.org/Tools/confuseddrugnames.pdf. Accessed June 19, 2009.
3. Available at: http://www.usp.org/hqi/similarProducts/choosy.html. Accessed June 19, 2009.
4. Propranolol [package insert]. Bedford, OH: Bedford Laboratories; September 2006.
5. Propranolol. Lexi-Comp® Online with AHFS® (database). Hudson, OH: Lexi-Comp Inc; updated August 28, 2009.
6. Silberbach M, Dunnigan A, Benson W Jr. Effect of intravenous propranolol or verapamil on infant orthodromic reciprocating tachycardia. *Am J Cardiol.* 1989;63:438-442.
7. American Academy of Pediatrics Committee on Drugs. Emergency drug doses for infants and children. *Pediatrics.* 1998;101:e1-e11.
8. Gelband H, Rosen MR. Pharmacologic basis for the treatment of cardiac arrhythmias. *Pediatrics.* 1975;55:59-67.
9. Roberts RJ, Mueller S, Lauer RM. Propranolol in the treatment of cardiac arrhythmias associated with amitriptyline intoxication. *J Pediatr.* 1973;82:65-67.
10. Guntheroth WG. Disorders of heart rate and rhythm. *Pediatr Clin North Am.* 1978;25:869-890.
11. Herndon DN, Barrow RE, Rutan TC, et al. Effect of propranolol on hemodynamic and metabolic response of burned pediatric patients. *Ann Surg.* 1988;208:484-492.
12. Baron PW, Barrow RE, Pierre EJ, et al. Prolonged use of propranolol safely decreases cardiac work in burned children. *J Burn Rehabil.* 1997;18:223-227.
13. National High Blood Pressure Education Program Working Group on High Blood Pressure in Children and Adolescents. The fourth report on the diagnosis, evaluation, and treatment of high blood pressure in children and adolescents. *Pediatrics.* 2004:114(2 suppl 4th Report):555-576.
14. Temple ME, Nahata MC. Treatment of pediatric hypertension. *Pharmacotherapy.* 200;20:140-150.
15. American Academy of Pediatrics Committee on Drugs. Drugs for pediatric emergencies. *Pediatrics.* 1998;101:1-11.
16. Wensley DF, Karl T, Deanfield JE, et al. Assessment of residual right ventricular outflow tract obstruction following surgery using the response to intravenous propranolol. *Ann Thorac Surg.* 1987;44:633-636.
17. Eades SK. Pharmacotherapy of congenital heart defects. *J Pediatr Pharmacol Ther.* 2004;9:160-178.
18. Aronoff GR, Berns JS, Brier ME, et al. Drug prescribing in renal failure. 4th ed. Available at: http://www.kdp-baptist.louisville.edu/renalbook/. Accessed June 19, 2009.
19. Trissel LA, ed. *Handbook on Injectable Drugs.* 15th ed. Bethesda, MD: American Society of Health-System Pharmacists; 2009.

Protamine Sulfate

1. Available at: http://ismp.org/Tools/confuseddrugnames.pdf. Updated April 1, 2005.
2. Available at: http://www.usp.org/hqi/similarProducts/choosy.html. Accessed October 18, 2009.
3. Protamine sulfate injection, USP [package insert]. Schaumburg, IL: American Pharmaceutical Partners Inc; January 2008.
4. Nordstrom L, Fletcher R, Pavek K. Shock of anaphylactoid type induced by protamine: a continuous cardiorespiratory record. *Acta Anaesthesiol Scand.* 1978;22:195-201.
5. Westaby S, Turner MW, Stark J. Complement activation and anaphylactoid response to protamine in a child after cardio-pulmonary bypass. *Br Heart J.* 1985;53:574-576.
6. Monagle P, Chalmers E, Chan A, et al. Antithrombotic therapy in neonates and children. *Chest.* 2008;133:997S-968S.
7. Protamine. Lexi-Comp® Online with AHFS® (database). Hudson, OH: Lexi-Comp Inc; updated August 13, 2009.
8. Trissel LA, ed. *Handbook on Injectable Drugs*. 15th ed. Bethesda, MD: American Society of Health-System Pharmacists; 2006.
9. Available at: http://www.fda.gov/NewsEvents/Newsroom/PressAnnouncements/ucm184674.htm Accessed October 8, 2009.
10. Boigner H, Lechner E, Brock H, et al. Life threatening cardiopulmonary failure in an infant following protamine reversal of heparin after cardiopulmonary bypass. *Paediatr Anaesth.* 2001;11:729-732.
11. Sakhai H, Casta A. Use of nitric oxide for treatment of pulmonary hypertensive crisis in a child after protamine administration. *J Cardiothor Vasc Anesth.* 2006;20:719-721.
12. Mayumi H, Toshima Y, Tokunaga K. Pretreatment with H2 blocker famotidine to ameliorate protamine-induced hypotension in open-heart surgery. *J Cardiovasc Surg.* 1992;33:738-745.

References

Protein C Concentrate (Human)

1. Available at: http://ismp.org/Tools/highalertmedications.pdf. Accessed November 22, 2009.
2. Available at: http://ismp.org/Tools/confuseddrugnames.pdf. Accessed November 22, 2009.
3. Available at: http://www.usp.org/hqi/similarProducts/choosy.html. Accessed November 22, 2009.
4. Ceprotin [package insert]. Westlake Village, CA: Baxter Healthcare Corporation; March 2007.
5. Protein C Concentrate. Lexi-Comp Online with AHFS (database). Hudson, OH: Lexi-Comp Inc; updated July 17, 2009.
6. Protein C Concentrate. Lexi-Comp Online with AHFS (database). Bethesda, MD: American Society of Health-System Pharmacists; updated December 2008.
7. Tcheng WY, Dovat S, Gurel Z, et al. Sever congenital protein C deficiency: description of a new mutation and prophylactic protein C therapy and in vivo pharmacokinetics. *J Pediatr Hematol Oncol.* 2008;30:166-171.

Ranitidine

1. Available at: http://ismp.org/Tools/confuseddrugnames.pdf. Accessed August 29, 2009.
2. Available at: http://www.usp.org/hqi/similarProducts/choosy.html. Accessed August 29, 2009.
3. Zantac [package insert]. Research Triangle Park, NC: GlaxoSmithKline; April, 2009.
4. Smith CL, Bardgett DM, Hunter JM. Haemodynamic effects of the IV administration of cimetidine or ranitidine in the critically ill patient. A double-blind prospective study. *Br J Anaesth.* 1987;59:1397-1402.
5. Blumer JL, Rothstein FC, Kaplan BS, et al. Pharmacokinetic determination of ranitidine pharmacodynamics in pediatric ulcer disease. *J Pediatr.* 1985;107:301-306.
6. Sarna MS, Saili A, Dutta AK, et al. Stress associated gastric bleeding in newborns: role of ranitidine. *Indian Pediatr.* 1991;28:1305-1308.
7. Rosenthal M, Miller PW. Ranitidine in the newborn. *Arch Dis Child.* 1988;63:88-89.
8. Kelly EJ, Chatfield SL, Brownlee KG, et al. The effect of intravenous ranitidine on the intragastric pH of preterm infants receiving dexamethasone. *Arch Dis Child.* 1993;69:37-39.
9. Kuusela AL. Long term gastric pH monitoring for determining optimal dose of ranitidine for critically ill preterm and term neonates. *Arch Dis Child Fetal Neonatal Ed.* 1998;78:F151-F153.
10. Wells TG, Heulitt MJ, Taylor BJ, et al. Pharmacokinetics and pharmacodynamics of ranitidine in neonates treated with extracorporeal membrane oxygenation. *J Clin Pharmacol.* 1998;38:402-407.
11. Cid JL, Velasco LA, Codoceo R, et al. Ranitidine prophylaxis in acute gastric mucosal damage in critically ill pediatric patients. *Crit Care Med.* 1988;16:591-593.
12. Wiest DB, O'Neal W, Reigart JR, et al. Pharmacokinetics of ranitidine in critically ill infants. *Dev Pharmacol Ther.* 1989;12:7-12.
13. Cochran EB, Storgion SA, Reiter PR, et al. Effects of continuous vs intermittent ranitidine on gastric pH in critically ill pediatric patients. *Clin Res.* 1991;39:833A. Abstract.
14. Gedeit RG, Weigle CG, Havens PL, et al. Control and variability of gastric pH in critically ill children. *Crit Care Med.* 1993;21:1850-1855.
15. Lugo RA, Harrison M, Cash J, et al. Pharmacokinetics and pharmacodynamics of ranitidine in critically ill children. *Crit Care Med.* 2001;29:759-764.
16. Crill CM, Hak EB. Upper gastrointestinal bleeding in critically ill pediatric patients. *Pharmacotherapy.* 1999;19:162-180.
17. Harrison AM, Lugo RA, Vernon DD. Gastric pH control in critically ill children receiving intravenous ranitidine. *Crit Care Med.* 1998;26:1433-1436.
18. Osteyee JL, Banner W. Effect of two dosing regimens on intravenous ranitidine on gastric pH in critically ill children. *J Crit Care.* 1994;3:267-272.
19. Hyman PE, Garvey TQ III, Abrams CE. Tolerance to intravenous ranitidine. *J Pediatr.* 1987;110:794-796.
20. Dimand RJ, Burckart G, Concepcion W, et al. Continuous infusion ranitidine in post-operative pediatric liver transplant patients: effects on intragastric pH, bleeding and metabolic alkalosis. *Crit Care Med.* 1989;S116. Abstract.
21. Eddleston JM, Booker PD, Green JR. Use of ranitidine in children undergoing cardiopulmonary bypass. *Crit Care Med.* 1989;17:26-29.
22. Aronoff GR, Berns JS, Brier ME, et al. Drug prescribing in renal failure. 4th ed. Available at: http://www.kdp-baptist.louisville.edu/renalbook/. Accessed August 17, 2009.
23. Trissel LA, ed. *Handbook on Injectable Drugs.* 15th ed. Bethesda, MD: American Society of Health-System Pharmacists; 2009.
24. Hatton J, Leur M, Hirsch J, et al. Histamine receptor antagonists and lipid stability in total nutrient admixtures. *JPEN.* 1994;18:308-312.
25. Allwood MC, Martin H. Factors influencing the stability of ranitidine in TPN mixtures. *Clin Nutr.* 1995;14:171-176.
26. Bullock L, Parks RB, Lampasona V, et al. Stability of ranitidine hydrochloride and amino acids in parenteral nutrient solutions. *Am J Hosp Pharm.* 1985;42:2683-2687.
27. Nahum E, Relsh O, Naor N, et al. Ranitidine-induced bradycardia in a neonate—a first report. *Eur J Pediatr.* 1993;152:933-934.
28. Bush A, Busst CM, Shinebourne EA. Cardiovascular effects of tolazoline and ranitidine. *Arch Dis Childhood.* 1987;62:241-246.
29. Guillet R, Stoll BJ, Cotton CM, et al. Association of H2-blocker therapy and higher incidence of necrotizing enterocolitis in very low birth weight infants. *Pediatrics.* 2006;117:e137-e142.

Rasburicase

1. Elitek [package insert]. New York, NY: Sanofi-Synthelabo Inc; July 2002.
2. Rasburicase. Lexi-Comp® Online with AHFS® (database). Bethesda, MD: American Society of Health-System Pharmacists; updated March 19, 2009.
3. Pui CH, Jeha S, Irwin D, et al. Recombinant urate oxidase (rasburicase) in the prevention and treatment of malignancy-associated hyperuricemia in pediatric and adult patients: results of a compassionate-use trial. *Leukemia.* 2001;15:1505-1059.
4. Pui CH, Mahmoud HH, Wiley JM, et al. Recombinant urate oxidase for the prophylaxis or treatment of hyperuricemia in patients with leukemia or lymphoma. *J Clin Oncol.* 2001;19(3):697-704.
5. Goldman SC, Holcengerg JS, Finklestein JZ, et al. A randomized comparison between rasburicase and allopurinol in children with lymphoma or leukemia at high risk for tumor lysis. *Blood.* 2001;97(10):2998-3003.
6. Bosly A, Sonet A, Pinkerton CR, et al. Rasburicase (recombinant urate oxidase) for the management of hyperuricemia in patients with cancer. *Cancer.* 2003;98:1048-1054.
7. Jeha S, Kantarjian, Irwin D, et al. Efficacy and safety of rasburicase, a recombinant urate oxidase (Elitek), in the management of malignancy-associated hyperuricemia in pediatric and adult patients: final results of a multicenter compassionate use trial. *Leukemia.* 2005;19:34-38.
8. Wang LY, Shih LY, Chang H, et al. Recombinant urate oxidase (rasburicase) for the prevention and treatment of tumor lysis syndrome in patients with hematologic malignancies. *Acta Haematol.* 2006;115:35-38.
9. Shin HY, Kang JH, Park ES, et al. Recombinant urate oxidase (Rasburicase) for the treatment of hyperuricemia in pediatric patients with hematologic malignancies: results of a compassionate prospective multicenter study in Korea. *Pediatr Blood Cancer.* 2006;46(4):439-445.
10. Liu CY, Sims-McCallum RP, Schiffer CA. A single dose of rasburicase is sufficient for the treatment of hyperuricemia in patients receiving chemotherapy. *Leukemia Res.* 2005;29:463-465.

References

11. Hutcherson DA, Gammon DC, Bhatt MS, et al. Reduced-dose rasburicase in the treatment of adults with hyperuricemia associated with malignancy. *Pharmacotherapy.* 2006;26(2):242-247.
12. Van den Berg H, Reintsema AM. Renal tubular damage in rasburicase: risks of alkalinisation. *Ann Oncol.* 2004;15:175-176.

Rifampin

1. Available at: http://ismp.org/Tools/confuseddrugnames.pdf. Accessed November 10, 2009.
2. Available at: http://www.usp.org/hqi/similarProducts/choosy.html. Accessed November 10, 2009.
3. Rifampin [package insert]. Bedford, OH: Bedford Laboratories; February 2004.
4. Tan TQ, Mason EO, Ou CN, et al. Use of intravenous rifampin in neonates with persistent staphylococcal bacteremia. *Antimicrob Agents Chemother.* 1993;37:2401-2406.
5. Shama A, Patole SK, Whitehall JS. Intravenous rifampicin in neonates with persistent staphylococcal bacteraemia. *Acta Paediatr.* 2002;91:670-673.
6. Nelson JD, Bradley JS, eds. *Nelson's Pocket Book of Pediatric Antimicrobial Therapy.* 17th ed. Chicago, IL: American Academy of Pediatrics; 2009.
7. American Academy of Pediatrics. Pickering LK, Baker CJ, Kimberlin DW, et al., eds. *2009 Red Book: Report of the Committee on Infectious Diseases.* 28th ed. Elk Grove Village, IL: American Academy of Pediatrics; 2009.
8. American Academy of Pediatrics Committee on Infectious Diseases. Therapy for children with invasive pneumococcal infections. *Pediatrics.* 1997;99:289-299.
9. Koup HR, Williams WJ, Weber A, et al. Pharmacokinetics of rifampin in children. I. Multiple dose intravenous infusion. *Ther Drug Monit.* 1986;8:11-16.
10. Stover BH, Duff A, Adams G, et al. Emergence and control of methicillin-resistant Staphylococcus aureus in a children's hospital and pediatric long-term care facility. *Am J Infect Control.* 1992;20:248-255.
11. Santos Sanches I, Mato R, de Lencastre H, et al. Patterns of multidrug resistance among methicillin-resistant hospital isolates of coagulase-positive and coagulase-negative staphylococci collected in the international multicenter study. RESIST in 1997 and 1998. *Microb Drug Resist.* 2000;6:199-211.
12. Inglesby TV, O'Toole T, Henderson DA, et al. For the Working Group on Civilian Biodefense. Anthrax as a biological weapon 2002: updated recommendations for management. *JAMA.* 2002;287:2236-2252.
13. Centers for Disease Control and Prevention. Update: Investigation of bioterrorism-related anthrax and interim guidelines for exposure management and antimicrobial therapy, October 2001. *MMWR Morb Mortal Wkly Rep.* 2001;50:909-919.
14. Nahata MC, Fan-Harvard P, Barson WJ, et al. Pharmacokinetics, cerebral fluid concentration, and safety of intravenous rifampin in pediatric patients undergoing shunt placement. *Eur J Clin Pharmacol.* 1990;38:515-517.
15. Aronoff GR, Berns JS, Brier ME, et al. Drug prescribing in renal failure. 4th ed. Available at: http://www.kdp-baptist.louisville.edu/renalbook/. Accessed November 9, 2009.
16. Holmberg RE, Pavia AT, Montgomery D, et al. Nosocomial legionella pneumonia in the neonate. *Pediatrics.* 1993;92:450-453.
17. Yzerman EP, Boelens HA, Vogel M, et al. Efficacy and safety of teicoplanin plus rifampicin in the treatment of bacteraemic infections caused by Staphylococcus aureus. *J Antimicrob Chemotherapy.* 1998;42:233-239.
18. Trissel LA, ed. *Handbook on Injectable Drugs.* 15th ed. Bethesda, MD: American Society of Health-System Pharmacists; 2009.
19. Chang AB, Grimwood K, Harvey AS, et al. Central nervous system tuberculosis after resolution of miliary tuberculosis. *Pediatr Infect Dis J.* 1998;17:519-523.
20. Gupta R, Wargo KA. Rifampin-induced thrombotic thrombocytopenic purpura. *Ann Pharmacother.* 2005;39:1761-1762.
21. Martínez E, Collazos J, Mayo J. Hypersensitivity reactions to rifampin. Pathogenetic mechanisms, clinical manifestations, management strategies, and review of the anaphylactic-like reactions. *Medicine.* 1999;78:361-369.
22. Baciewicz AM, Chrisman CR, Finch CK, et al. Update on rifampin and rifabutin drug interactions. *Am J Med Sci.* 2008;335:126-136.

RiTUXimab

1. Available at: http://ismp.org/Tools/highalertmedications.pdf. ISMP 2008. Accessed August 29, 2009.
2. Available at: http://ismp.org/Tools/confuseddrugnames.pdf. Accessed August 29, 2009.
3. Available at: http://www.usp.org/hqi/similarProducts/choosy.html. Accessed August 29, 2009.
4. Rituxan [package insert]. South San Francisco, CA: Genentech Inc; February 2007.
5. Colombat P, Salles G, Brousee N, et al. Rituximab (anti-CD20 monoclonal antibody) as single first-line therapy for patients with follicular lymphoma with a low tumor burden: clinical and molecular evaluation. *Blood.* 2001;97(1):101-106.
6. Jetsrisuparb A, Wiangnon S, Komvilaisak P, et al. Rituximab combined with CHOP for successful treatment of aggressive recurrent, pediatric B-cell large cell non-Hodgkin's lymphoma. *J Pediatr Hematol Oncol.* 2005;27(4):223-226.
7. Hainsworth JD, Litchy S, Shaffer DW, et al. Maximizing therapeutic benefit of rituximab: maintenance therapy versus re-treatment at progression in patients with indolent non-Hodgkin's lymphoma—a randomized phase II trial of the Minnie Pearl Cancer Research Network. *J Clin Oncol.* 2005;23(6):1088-1095.
8. Kewalramani T, Zelenetz AD, Nimer SD, et al. Rituximab and ICE as second-line therapy before autologous stem cell transplantation for relapsed or primary refractory diffuse large B-cell lymphoma. *Blood.* 2004;103(10):3684-3688.
9. Claviez A, Eckert C, Seeger K, et al. Rituximab plus chemotherapy in children with relapsed or refractory CD20-positive B-cell precursor acute lymphoblastic leukemia. *Haematologica.* 2006;91:272-273.
10. Wiseman GA, Leigh BR, Erwin WD, et al. Radiation dosimetry results from a phase II trial of ibritumomab tiuxetan (Zevalin) radioimmunotherapy for patients with non-Hodgkin's lymphoma and mild thrombocytopenia. *Cancer Biother Radiopharm.* 2003;18(2):165-178.
11. Herman J, Vandenberghe P, van den Heuvel I, et al. Successful treatment with rituximab of lymphoproliferative disorder in a child after cardiac transplantation. *J Heart Lung Transplant.* 2002;21(12):1304-1309.
12. Berney T, Delis S, Kato T, et al. Successful treatment of post-transplant lymphoproliferative disease with prolonged rituximab treatment in intestinal transplant recipients. *Transplantation.* 2002;74(7):1000-1006.
13. Zecca M, Nobili B, Ramenghi U, et al. Rituximab for the treatment of refractory autoimmune hemolytic anemia in children. *Blood.* 2003;101(10):3857-3861.
14. Motto DG, Williams JA, Boxer LA. Rituximab for refractory childhood autoimmune hemolytic anemia. *Isr Med Assoc J.* 2002;4(11):1006-1008.
15. National Comprehensive Cancer Network (NCCN) Antiemesis Panel Members. NCCN Clinical Practice Guidelines in Oncology. Antiemesis, v.1.2006. Available at www.nccn.org. Last accessed March 29, 2006.
16. Roila F, Feyer P, Maranzamo E, et al. Antiemetics in children receiving chemotherapy. *Support Care Cancer.* 2005;13:129-131.
17. Rituximab. Lexi-Comp® Online with AHFS® (database). Bethesda, MD: American Society of Health-System Pharmacists; updated October 2008.

Rocuronium Bromide

1. Available at: http://ismp.org/Tools/highalertmedications.pdf. ISMP 2008. Accessed August 29, 2009.
2. Available at: http://www.usp.org/hqi/similarProducts/choosy.html. Accessed August 29, 2009.
3. Zemuron [package insert]. Bloomington, IN: Baxter Pharmaceutical Solutions LLC; September 2008.

References

4. Rowlee SC. Monitoring neuromuscular blockade in the intensive care unit: the peripheral nerve stimulator. *Heart Lung.* 1999;28:352-362.
5. Woloszczuk-Gebicka B, Lapczynski T, Wierzejski W. The influence of halothane, isoflurane and sevoflurane on rocuronium infusions in children. *Acta Anaesthesiol Scand.* 2001;45:73-77.
6. Eikermann M, Kunkemoller I, Peine L, et al. Optimal rocuronium dose for intubation during induction with sevoflurane in children. *Br J Anaesth.* 2002;89:277-281.
7. Martin LD, Bratton SL, O'Rourke PP. Clinical uses and controversies of neuromuscular blocking agents in infants and children. *Crit Care Med.* 1999;27:1358-1368.
8. Wierda JM, Meretoja OA, Taivainen T, et al. Pharmacokinetics and pharmacodynamic modeling of rocuronium in infants and children. *Br J Anaesth.* 1997;78:690-695.
9. Ross AK, Dear GL, Dear RB, et al. Onset and recovery of neuromuscular blockade after two doses of rocuronium in children. *J Clin Anesth.* 1998;10:631-635.
10. Mendez DR, Goto CS, Abramo TJ, et al. Safety and efficacy of rocuronium for controlled intubation with paralytics in the pediatric emergency department. *Pediatr Emerg Care.* 2001;17:233-236.
11. Tobias JD. Continuous infusion of rocuronium in a paediatric intensive care unit. *Can J Anaesth.* 1996;43:353-357.
12. Driessen JJ, Robertson EN, Van Egmond J, Booij LH. Time-course of action of rocuronium 0.3 mg.kg-1 in children with and without endstage renal failure. *Paediatr Anaesth.* 2002;12:507-510.
13. Trissel LA, ed. *Handbook on Injectable Drugs.* 15th ed. Bethesda, MD: American Society of Health-System Pharmacists; 2009.
14. Rocuronium. Lexi-Comp Online with AHFS (database). Hudson, OH: Lexi-Comp Inc; updated September 25, 2009.
15. Kaplan RF, Uejima T, Lobel G, et al. Intramuscular rocuronium in infants and children: a multicenter study to evaluate tracheal intubating conditions, onset, and duration of action. *Anesthesiology.* 1999;91:633-638.
16. Reynolds LM, Lau M, Brown R, et al. Bioavailability of intramuscular rocuronium in infants and children. *Anesthesiology.* 1997;87:1096-1105.

Ropivacaine HCl

1. Available at: http://ismp.org/Tools/highalertmedications.pdf. ISMP 2008. Accessed August 29, 2009.
2. Available at: http://www.usp.org/hqi/similarProducts/choosy.html. Accessed August 29, 2009.
3. Naropin [package insert]. Schaumburg, IL: APP Pharmaceuticals LLC; November 2008.
4. Ropivacaine. Lexi-Comp Online with AHFS (database). Hudson, OH: Lexi-Comp Inc; updated November 16, 2009.
5. Available at: http://www.fda.gov/Drugs/DrugSafety/PostmarketDrugSafetyInformationforPatientsandProviders/ucm190302.htm. Accessed November 20, 2009.
6. Trissel LA, ed. *Handbook on Injectable Drugs.* 15th ed. Bethesda, MD: American Society of Health-System Pharmacists; 2009.
7. Simpson D, Curran MP, Oldfield V, et al. Ropivacaine: a review of its use in regional anaesthesia and acute pain management. *Drugs.* 2005;65:2675-2717.
8. Wulf H, Peters C, Behnke H. The pharmacokinetics of caudal ropivacaine 0.2% in children: a study of infants aged less than 1 year and toddlers aged 1–5 years undergoing inguinal hernia repair. *Anaesthesia.* 2000;55:757-760.
9. De Negri P, Ivani G, Tirri T, et al. A comparison of epidural bupivacaine, levobupivacaine, and ropivacaine on postoperative analgesia and motor blockage. *Anesth Analg.* 2004;99:45-48.
10. Hansen TG, Ilett KF, Reid C, et al. Caudal ropivacaine in infants: population pharmacokinetics and plasma concentrations. *Anesthesiology.* 2001;94:579-584.
11. Aguirre-Garay FT, Garcia R, Nava-Ocampo AA. Dose-response of ropivacaine administered caudally to children undergoing surgical procedures under sedation with midazolam. *Clin Exp Pharmacol Physiol.* 2004;31:462-465.
12. Bozkurt P, Arslan I, Bakan M, et al. Free plasma levels of bupivacaine and ropivacaine when used for caudal block in children. *Eur J Anaesth.* 2005;22:634-643.
13. Hansen TG, Ilett KF, Lim SI, et al. Pharmacokinetics and clinical efficacy of long-term epidural ropivacaine infusion in children. *Br J Anaesth.* 2000;85:347-353.
14. Khalil S, Campos C, Farag AM, et al. Caudal block in children: ropivacaine compared with bupivacaine. *Anesthesiology.* 1999;91:1279-1284.
15. Lonnqvist PA, Westrin P, Larsson BA, et al. Ropivacaine pharmacokinetics after caudal block in 1–8-year-old children. *Br J Anaesth.* 2000;85:506-511.
16. Antok E, Bordet F, Duflo F, et al. Patient-controlled epidural analgesia versus continuous epidural infusion with ropivacaine for postoperative analgesia in children. *Anesth Analg.* 2004;97:1608-1611.

Sargramostim

1. Available at: http://www.usp.org/hqi/similarProducts/choosy.html. Accessed August 15, 2009.
2. Leukine [prescribing information]. Seattle, WA: Bayer HealthCare Pharmaceuticals; April 2008.
3. Furman WL, Fairclough DL, Huhn RD, et al. Therapeutic effects and pharmacokinetics of recombinant human granulocyte-macrophage colony-stimulating factor in childhood cancer patients receiving myelosuppressive chemotherapy. *J Clin Oncol.* 1991;9:1022-1028.
4. Furman WL, Crist WM. Biology and clinical applications of hemopoietins in pediatric practice. *Pediatrics.* 1992;90:716-728.
5. Riikonen P, Saarinen UM, Makipernaa A, et al. Recombinant human granulocyte-macrophage colony-stimulating factor in the treatment of febrile neutropenia: a double blind placebo-controlled study in children. *Pediatr Infect Dis J.* 1994;13:197-202.
6. Luksch R, Massimino M, Cefalo G, et al. Effects of recombinant human granulocyte-macrophage colony-stimulating factor in an intensive treatment program for children with Ewing's sarcoma. *Haematologica.* 2001;86:753-760.
7. Saarinen-Pihkala UM, Lanning M, Perkkio M, et al. Granulocyte-macrophage colony-stimulating factor support in therapy of high-risk acute lymphoblastic leukemia in children. *Med Pediatr Oncol.* 2000;34:319-327.
8. Trigg ME, Peters C, Zimmerman MB. Administration of recombinant human granulocyte-macrophage colony-stimulating factor to children undergoing allogenic marrow transplantation: a prospective, randomized, double-masked, placebo-controlled trial. *Pediatr Transplant.* 2000;4:123-132.
9. Welte K, Zeidler C, Reiter A, et al. Differential effects of granulocyte-macrophage colony-stimulating factor and granulocyte colony-stimulating factor in children with severe congenital neutropenia. *Blood.* 1990;75:1056-1063.
10. Venkateswaran L, Wilimas JA, Dancy R, et al. Granulocyte-macrophage colony-stimulating factor in the treatment of neonates with neutropenia and sepsis. *Pediatr Hematol Oncol.* 2000;17:469-473.
11. Ahmad A, Laborada G, Bussel J, et al. Comparison of recombinant granulocyte colony-stimulating factor, recombinant human granulocyte-macrophage colony-stimulating factor and placebo for treatment of septic preterm infants. *Pediatr Infect Dis J.* 2002;21:1061-1065.
12. Carr R, Brocklehurst P, Dore CJ, Modi N. Granulocyte-macrophage colony stimulating factor administered as prophylaxis for reduction of sepsis in extremely preterm, small for gestational age neonates (the PROGRAMS trial): a single-blind, multicentre, randomized controlled trial. *Lancet.* 2009;373:226-233.
13. Guinan EC, Sieff CA, Oette DH, et al. A phase I/II trial of recombinant granulocyte-macrophage colony-stimulating factor in children with aplastic anemia. *Blood.* 1990;76:1077-1082.
14. Jeng MR, Naidu PE, Reiman MD, et al. Granulocyte-macrophage colony stimulating factor and immunosuppression in the treatment of pediatric acquired severe aplastic anemia. *Pediatr Blood Cancer.* 2005;45:170-175.

References

15. Sasse EC, Sasse AD, Brandalise ST, et al. Colony-stimulating factors for prevention of myelosupressive therapy induced febrile neutropenia in children with acute lymphoblastic leukemia. *Cochrane Database Syst Rev*. 2005 Jul 20;(3):CD004139.
16. Bonig H, Burdach S, Gobel U, et al. Growth factors and hemostasis: differential effects of GM-CSF and G-CSF on coagulation activation—laboratory and clinical evidence. *Ann Hematol*. 2001;80:525-530.

Sodium Bicarbonate

1. Available at: http://www.usp.org/hqi/similarProducts/choosy.html. Accessed November 13, 2009.
2. Sodium bicarbonate injection, USP. Lake Forest, IL: Hospira Inc; October 2005.
3. Sodium bicarbonate. Lexi-Comp® Online with AHFS® (database). Hudson, OH: Lexi-Comp Inc; updated July 16, 2009.
4. Finberg L. Dangers to infants caused by changes in osmolal concentration. *Pediatrics*. 1967;40:1031-1034.
5. Simmons MA, Adcock EW, Bard H, et al. Hypernatremia and intracranial hemorrhage in neonates. *N Engl J Med*. 1974;291:6-10.
6. Gaze NR. Tissue necrosis caused by commonly used intravenous infusions. *Lancet*. 1978; 2:417-419.
7. 2005 American Heart Association guidelines for cardiopulmonary resuscitation and emergency cardiovascular care. Part 12: pediatric advanced life support. *Circulation*. 2005;112(24 suppl):IV-167 to IV-187.
8. American Academy of Pediatrics Committee on Drugs. Emergency drug doses for infants and children. *Pediatrics*. 1998;101:e1-e11.
9. Trachtenbarg DE. Diabetic ketoacidosis. *Am Fam Physician*. 2005;71:1705-1714.
10. Green SM, Rothrock SG, Ho JD, et al. Failure of adjunctive bicarbonate to improve outcome in severe pediatric diabetic ketoacidosis. *Ann Emerg Med*. 1998;31:41-48.
11. Proudfoot AT, Krenzelok EP, Vale JA. Position paper on urine alkalinization. *J Toxicol*. 2004;42:1-26.
12. Kelly KM, Lange B. Oncologic emergencies. *Pediatr Clin NA*. 1997;44:809-830.
13. Brown CVR, Rhee P, Chan L, et al. Preventing renal failure in patients with rhabdomyolysis: do bicarbonate and mannitol make a difference? *J Trauma*. 2004;56:1191-1196.
14. Trissel LA, ed. *Handbook on Injectable Drugs*. 13th ed. Bethesda, MD: American Society of Health-System Pharmacists; 2005.

Sodium Chloride

1. Available at: http://ismp.org/Tools/highalertmedications.pdf. ISMP 2008.
2. Available at: http://www.usp.org/hqi/similarProducts/choosy.html. Accessed November 8, 2009.
3. Available at: http://www.ismp.org/Newsletters/acutecare/articles/20090813.asp Accessed November 10, 2009.
4. Concentrated sodium chloride injection, USP [package insert]. Shirley, NY: American Regent Laboratories Inc; February 2000.
5. Greenbaum L. Chapter 52. Electrolyte and acid-base disorders. In: Behrman RE, Kliegman RM, Jensen HB, eds. *Nelson Textbook of Pediatrics*. 18th ed. Philadelphia, PA: Saunders; 2007.
6. Greenbaum L. Chapter 54. Deficit therapy. In: Behrman RE, Kliegman RM, Jensen HB, eds. *Nelson Textbook of Pediatrics*. 18th ed. Philadelphia, PA: Saunders; 2007.
7. Choski R, Roach ES. Ring-enhancing lesion in central pontine myelinolysis. *Arch Neurol*. 2005;62:1016-1017.
8. Tan H, Onbas O. Central pontine myelinolysis manifesting with massive myoclonus. *Pediatr Neurol*. 2004;31:64-66.
9. Haspolat S, Duman O, Senol U, et al. Extrapontine myelinolysis in infancy: report of a case. *J Child Neurol*. 2004;19:913-15.
10. Lin M, Liu SJ, Lim IT. Disorders of water imbalance. *Emerg Med Clin N Am*. 2005;23:749-770.
11. Frankel LR, Kache S. Chapter 68. Shock. In: Behrman RE, Kliegman RM, Jensen HB, eds. *Nelson Textbook of Pediatrics*. 18th ed. Philadelphia, PA: Saunders; 2007.
12. Dellinger RP, Levy MM, Carlet J, et al. Surviving sepsis campaign: international guidelines for management of severe sepsis and septic shock: 2008. Intensive Care Med. 2008;34:17-60.
13. Simma B, Burger R, Falk M, et al. A prospective, randomized, and controlled study of fluid management in children with severe head injury: lactated Ringer's solution versus hypertonic saline. *Crit Care Med*. 1998;26:1265-1270.
14. Khanna S, Davis D, Peterson B, et al. Use of hypertonic saline in the treatment of severe refractory posttraumatic intracranial hypertension in pediatric traumatic brain injury. *Crit Care Med*. 2000;28:1144-1152.
15. Peterson B, Khanna S, Fisher B, et al. Prolonged hypernatremia controls elevated intracranial pressure in head-injured pediatric patients. *Crit Care Med*. 2000;28:1136-1143.
16. Adelson PD, Bratton SL, Carney NA, et al. Guidelines for the acute medical management of severe traumatic brain injury in infants, children, and adolescents. Chapter 11. Use of hyperosmolar therapy in the management of severe pediatric traumatic brain injury. *Pediatr Crit Care Med*. 2003 Jul;4(3 suppl):S40-4.
17. Sodium chloride. Lexi-Comp® Online with AHFS® (database). Hudson, OH: Lexi-Comp Inc; updated September 11, 2009.

Sodium Nitroprusside

1. Available at: http://ismp.org/Tools/highalertmedications.pdf. ISMP 2008.
2. Available at: http://www.usp.org/hqi/similarProducts/choosy.html. Accessed November 2, 2009.
3. Nitropress [package insert]. Lake Forest, IL: Hospira Inc; March 2006.
4. Nitroprusside. Lexi-Comp® Online with AHFS® (database). Hudson, OH: Lexi-Comp Inc; updated September 25, 2009.
5. Deal JE, Barratt TM, Dillon MJ. Management of hypertensive emergencies. *Arch Dis Child*. 1992;67:1089-1092.
6. American Academy of Pediatrics Committee on Drugs. Drugs for Pediatric Emergencies. *Pediatrics*. 1998;101:e1-e11.
7. Patel HP, Mitsnefes M. Advances in the pathogenesis and management of hypertensive crisis. *Curr Opin Pediatr*. 2005;17:210-214.
8. National High Blood Pressure Education Program Working Group on High Blood Pressure in Children and Adolescents. The Fourth Report on the Diagnosis, Evaluation, and Treatment of High Blood Pressure in Children and Adolescents. *Pediatrics*. 2004;114:555-576.
9. American Heart Association Guidelines for Cardiopulmonary Resuscitation and Emergency Cardiovascular Care. Part 12: Pediatric Advanced Life Support. *Circulation*. 2005;112(suppl 1):167-187.
10. Adelman RD, Coppo R, Dillon MJ. The emergency management of severe hypertension. *Pediatr Nephrol*. 2000;14:422-427.
11. Benitz WE, Malachowski N, Cohen RS, et al. Use of sodium nitroprusside in neonates: efficacy and safety. *J Pediatr*. 1985;106:102-110.
12. Fleischmann LE. Management of hypertensive crises in children. *Pediatr Ann*. 1977;6:410-414.
13. Gordillo-Paniagua G, Velasquez-Jones L, Martini R, et al. Sodium nitroprusside treatment of severe arterial hypertension in children. *J Pediatr*. 1975; 87:799-802.
14. Dillon TR, Janos GG, Meyer RA, et al. Vasodilator therapy for congestive heart failure. *J Pediatr*. 1980;96:623-629.
15. Beverley DW, Hughes CA, Davies DP, et al. Early use of sodium nitroprusside in respiratory distress syndrome. *Arch Dis Child*. 1979;54:403-407.
16. Beekman RH, Rocchini AP, Dick M, et al. Vasodilator therapy in children: acute and chronic effects in children with left ventricular dysfunction or mitral regurgitation. *Pediatrics*. 1984;73:43-51.
17. Kunathai S, Sholler GF, Celermajer JM, et al. Nitroprusside in children after cardiopulmonary bypass: a study of thiocyanate toxicity. *Pediatr Cardiol*. 1989;10:121-124.

18. Miller K. Pharmacological management of hypertension in paediatric patients. *Drugs.* 1994;48:868-887.

19. Grossman E, Ironi AN, Messerli FH. Comparative tolerability profile of hypertensive crisis treatments. *Drug Safety.* 1998;19:99-122. Review

20. Moffett BS, Price JF. Evaluation of sodium nitroprusside toxicity in pediatric cardiac surgical patients. *Ann Pharmacother.* 2008;42:1600-1604.

21. Palmer RF, Lasseter KC. Sodium nitroprusside. *N Engl J Med.* 1975;292:294-297.

22. Trissel LA, ed. *Handbook on Injectable Drugs.* 15th ed. Bethesda, MD: American Society of Health-System Pharmacists; 2009.

23. Raymond G, Day P, Rabb M. Sodium content of commonly administered intravenous drugs. *Hosp Pharm.* 1982;17:560-561.25.

24. Sodorff MM, Galt KA, Galt M, et al. Recommended maximum concentrations of common acute care parenteral admixtures. *Hosp Pharm.* 1999;34:937-942.

25. Friedman WF, George BL. New concepts and drugs in the treatment of congestive heart failure. *Pediatr Clin North Am.* 1984;31:1197-1227.

26. Rindone JP, Sloane EP. Cyanide toxicity from sodium nitroprusside: risk and management. *Ann Pharmacother.* 1992;26:515-519.

27. Linakis JG, Lacouture PG, Woolf A. Monitoring cyanide and thiocyanate concentrations during infusion of sodium nitroprusside in children. *Pediatr Cardiol.* 1991;12:214-218.

Succinylcholine Chloride

1. Available at: http://ismp.org/Tools/highalertmedications.pdf. Accessed October 15, 2009.

2. Succinylcholine [package insert]. Broomfield, CO: Sandoz; January 2005.

3. Martin LD, Bratton SL, O'Rourke PP. Clinical uses and controversies of neuromuscular blocking agents in infants and children. *Crit Care Med.* 1999;27:1358-1368.

4. Zelicof-Paul A, Smith-Lockridge A, Schnadower D, et al. Controversies in rapid sequence intubation in children. *Curr Opin Pediatr.* 2005;17:355-362.

5. Sullivan M, Thompson WK. Succinylcholine-induced cardiac arrest in children with undiagnosed myopathy. *Can J Anaesth.* 1994;41:497-501.

6. Succinylcholine. Lexi-Comp® Online with AHFS® (database). Hudson, OH: Lexi-Comp Inc; updated September 4, 2009.

7. Rose JB, Theroux MC, Katz MS. The potency of succinylcholine in obese adolescents. *Anesth Analg.* 2000;90:576-578.

8. Levy G. Pharmacokinetics of succinylcholine in newborns. *Anesthesiology.* 1970;32:551-552.

9. Cook DR, Fisher CG. Neuromuscular blocking effects of succinylcholine in infants and children. *Anesthesiology.* 1975;42:662-665.

10. Cook DR, Wingard L, Taylor F. Pharmacokinetics of succinylcholine in infants, children and adults. *Clin Pharmacol Ther.* 1976;20:493-498.

11. Rowlee SC. Monitoring neuromuscular blockade in the intensive care unit: the peripheral nerve stimulator. *Heart Lung.* 1999;28:352-362.

12. Trissel LA, ed. *Handbook on Injectable Drugs.* 15th ed. Bethesda, MD: American Society of Health-System Pharmacists; 2009.

13. Goudsouzian NG, Liu LM. The neuromuscular response of infants to a continuous infusion of succinylcholine. *Anesthesiology.* 1984;60:97-101.

14. Al-Takrouri H, Martin TW, Mayhew JF. Hyperkalemic cardiac arrest following succinylcholine administration: The use of extracorporeal membrane oxygenation in an emergency situation. *J Clin Anesth.* 2004;16:449-451.

15. Rosenberg H. Intractable cardiac arrest in children given succinylcholine. *Anesthesiology.* 1992;77:105.

16. Larsen U, Juhl B, Hein-Sorenson O, et al. Complications during anesthesia in patients with Duchenne's muscular dystrophy (a retrospective study). *Can J Anaesth.* 1989;36:418-422.

17. Nugent SK, Laravuso R, Rogers MC. Pharmacology and use of muscle relaxants in infants and children. *J Pediatr.* 1979;94:481-487.

18. Martyn JA, Richtsfeld M. Succinylcholine-induced hyperkalemia in acquired pathologic states: etiologic factors and molecular mechanisms. *Anesthesiology.* 2006;104:158-169.

19. Huggins RM, Kennedy WK, Melroy MJ, et al. Cardiac arrest from succinylcholine-induced hyperkalemia. *Am J Health Syst Pharm.* 2003;60:694-697.

20. Rosenberg H, Davis M, James D, et al. Malignant hyperthermia. *Orphanet J Rare Dis.* 2007;2:21.

21. Benzer A, Luz G, Oswald E, et al. Succinylcholine-induced prolonged apnea in a 3-week old newborn: treatment with human plasma cholinesterase. *Anesth Analg.* 1992;74:137-138.

22. Snavely SR, Hodges GR. The neurotoxicity of antibacterial agents. *Ann Intern Med.* 1984;101:92-104.

SUFentanil Citrate

1. Available at: http://ismp.org/Tools/highalertmedications.pdf. ISMP 2008. Accessed August 29, 2009.

2. Available at: http://ismp.org/Tools/confuseddrugnames.pdf. Accessed August 29, 2009.

3. Available at: http://www.usp.org/hqi/similarProducts/choosy.html. Accessed August 29, 2009.

4. Sufenta injection [prescribing information]. Decatur, IL: Taylor Pharmaceuticals; July 2007.

5. Schwartz AE, Matteo RS, Ornstein E, et al. Pharmacokinetics of sufentanil in obese patients. *Anesth Analg.* 1991;73:790-793.

6. Glenski JA, Friesen RH, Lane GA, et al. Low-dose sufentanil as a supplement to halothane/N2O anaesthesia in infants and children. *Can J Anaesth.* 1988;35:379-384.

7. Hickey PR, Hansen DD. Fentanyl- and sufentanil-oxygen-pancuronium anesthesia for cardiac surgery in infants. *Anesth Analgesia.* 1984;63:117-124.

8. Anand KJ, Phil D, Hickey PR. Halothane-morphine compared with high-dose sufentanil for anesthesia and post-operative analgesia in neonatal cardiac surgery. *N Eng J Med.* 1992;326:1-9.

9. Sufentanil. Lexi-Comp Online with AHFS (database). Hudson, OH: Lexi-Comp Inc; updated July 9, 2009.

10. Aronoff GR, Berns JS, Brier ME, et al. Drug prescribing in renal failure. 4th ed. Available at: http://www.kdp-baptist.louisville.edu/renalbook/. Accessed August 17, 2009.

11. Sufentanil. Lexi-Comp Online with AHFS (database). Bethesda, MD: American Society of Health-System Pharmacists; updated May 26, 2009.

12. Trissel LA, ed. *Handbook on Injectable Drugs.* 15th ed. Bethesda, MD: American Society of Health-System Pharmacists; 2009.

13. Moore RA, Yang SS, McNicholas KW, et al. Hemodynamic and anesthetic effects of sufentanil as the sole anesthetic for pediatric cardiovascular surgery. *Anesthesiology.* 1985;62:725-731.

14. Albanese J, Durbec O, Viviand X, et al. Sufentanil increases intracranial pressure in patients with head trauma. *Anesthesiology.* 1993;79:493-497.

15. Guay J, Gaudreault P, Tang A, et al. Pharmacokinetics of sufentanil in normal children. *Can J Anesth.* 1992;39:14-20.

Tacrolimus

1. Available at: http://www.usp.org/hqi/similarProducts/choosy.html. Accessed July 3, 2009.

2. Prograf [package insert]. Deerfield, IL: Astellas Pharma US Inc; May 2009.

3. McDiarmid SV, Busuttil RW, Ascher NL, et al. FK506 (Tacrolimus) compared with cyclosporine for primary immunosuppression after pediatric liver transplantation. *Transplantation.* 1995;59:530-536.

4. Yasuhara M, Hashida T, Toraguchi M, et al. Pharmacokinetics and pharmacodynamics of FK506 in pediatric patients receiving living-related donor liver transplantations. *Transplant Proc.* 1995;27:1108-1110.

5. McDiarmid SV, Colonna JO, Shaked A, et al. Differences in oral FK506 dose requirements between adult and pediatric liver transplant patients. *Transplantation.* 1993;56:1328-1332.

References

6. Tzakis AG, Reyes J, Todo S, et al. FK506 versus cyclosporine in pediatric liver transplantation. *Transplant Proc.* 1991;23:3010-3015.
7. Robinson BV, Boyle GJ, Miller SA, et al. Optimal dosing of intravenous tacrolimus following pediatric heart transplant. *J Heart Lung Transplant.* 1999;18:786-791.
8. Tzakis AG, Reyes J, Todo S, et al. Two-year experience with FK506 in pediatric patients. *Transplant Proc.* 1993;25:619-621.
9. Tzakis AG, Fung JJ, Todo S, et al. Use of FK506 in pediatric patients. *Transplant Proc.* 1991;23:924-92.
10. Busuttil RW, McDiarmid S, Klintmalm GM, et al. A comparison of tacrolimus (FK506) and cyclosporine for immunosuppression in liver transplantation. *N Engl J Med.* 1994;331:1110-1115.
11. Staatz CE, Taylor PJ, Lynch SV, et al. Population pharmacokinetics of tacrolimus in children who receive cut-down or full liver transplants. *Transplantation.* 2001;72:1056-1061.
12. Nash RA, Antin JH, Karanes C, et al. Phase 3 study comparing methotrexate and tacrolimus with methotrexate and cyclosporine for prophylaxis of acute graft-versus-host disease after marrow transplantation from unrelated donors. *Blood.* 2000;96:2062-2068.
13. Osunkwo I, Bessmertny O, Harrison L, et al. A pilot study of tacrolimus and mycophenolate mofetil graft-versus-host disease prophylaxis in childhood and adolescent allogeneic stem cell transplant recipients. *Biol Blood Marrow Transplant.* 2004;10:246-248.
14. Ohashi Y, Minegishi M, Fujie H, et al. Successful treatment of steroid-resistant severe acute GVHD with 24-h continuous infusion of FK506. *Bone Marrow Transplant.* 1997;19:625-627.
15. Taormina D, Abdallah HY, Venkataramanan R, et al. Stability and sorption of FK506 in 5% dextrose injection and 0.9% sodium chloride injection in glass, polyvinyl chloride, and polyolefin containers. *Am J Hosp Pharm.* 1992;49:119-122.
16. Firdaous I, Hassoun A, Otte JB, et al. Pediatric intravenous FK506—how much are we really infusing? *Transplantation.* 1994;57:1821-1823.
17. Trissel LA, ed. *Handbook on Injectable Drugs.* 15th ed. Bethesda, MD: American Society of Health-System Pharmacists; 2009.
18. Nakata Y, Yoshibayashi M, Yonemura T, et al. Tacrolimus and myocardial hypertrophy. *Transplantation.* 2000;69:1960-1962.
19. Brown NW, Gonde CE, Adams JE, et al. Low hematocrit and serum albumin concentrations underlie the overestimation of tacrolimus concentrations my microparticle enzyme immunoassay versus liquid chromatography—tandem mass spectrometry. *Clin Chem.* 2005;51:586-592.

Terbutaline Sulfate

1. Available at: http://ismp.org/Tools/confuseddrugnames.pdf. Updated April 1, 2005.
2. Available at: http://www.usp.org/hqi/similarProducts/choosy.html. Accessed July 3, 2009.
3. Terbutaline sulfate injection, USP [package insert]. Schaumburg, IL: AAP Pharmaceuticals LLC; March 2008.
4. National Asthma Education and Prevention Program. *Expert Panel Report 3 (EPR3): Guidelines for the Diagnosis and Management of Asthma.* Bethesda, MD: National Institutes of Health; August 2007.
5. Tipton WR, Nelson HS. Frequent parenteral terbutaline in the treatment of status asthmaticus in children. *Ann Allergy.* 1987;252-456.
6. Bremont F, Moisan V, Dutau G. Continuous subcutaneous infusion of Beta 2-agonists in infantile asthma. *Pediatr Pulmonol.* 1992;12:81-83.
7. Fuglsang G, Pedersen S, Borgstrom L. Dose-response relationships of intravenously administered terbutaline in children with asthma. *J Pediatr.* 1989;315-332.
8. Dietrich KA, Conrad SA, Romero MD. Creatine kinase (CK) isoenzymes in pediatric status asthmaticus treated with intravenous terbutaline. *Crit Care Med.* 1991;19:S39. Abstract.
9. DeNicola LK, Monem GF, Gayle MO, et al. Treatment of critical status asthmaticus in children. *Pediatr Clin North Am.* 1994;41:1293-1324.
10. Kambalapalli M, Nichani S, Upadhyayula S. Safety of intravenous terbutaline in acute severe asthma: a retrospective study. *Acta Paediatr.* 2005;94:1214-1217.
11. Stephanopoulos DE, Monge R, Schell KH, et al. Continuous intravenous terbutaline for pediatric status asthmaticus. *Crit Care Med.* 1998;26:1744-1748.
12. Payne DNR, Balfour-Lynn IM, Biggart EA. Subcutaneous terbutaline in children with chronic severe asthma. *Pediatric Pulmonol.* 2002;33:356-361.
13. Available at: http://kdpnet.louisville.edu/renalbook/pediatric/id/174/. Accessed October 2, 2009.
14. Trissel LA. *Handbook on Injectable Drugs.* 15th ed. Bethesda, MD: American Society of Health-System Pharmacists; 2009.
15. Hultquist C, Lindberg C, Nyberg L, et al. Pharmacokinetics of intravenous terbutaline in asthmatic children. *Dev Pharmacol Ther.* 1989;13:11-20.
16. Terbutaline. Lexi-Comp® Online with AHFS® (database). Hudson, OH: Lexi-Comp Inc; updated July 16, 2009.
17. Danziger Y, Garty M, Volwitz B, et al. Reduction of serum theophylline levels by terbutaline in children with asthma. *Clin Pharmacol Ther.* 1985;37:469-471.

Thiopental Sodium

1. Available at: http://ismp.org/Tools/highalertmedications.pdf. Accessed September 19, 2009.
2. Available at: http://www.usp.org/hqi/similarProducts/choosy.html. Accessed September 19, 2009.
3. Thiopental [package insert]. North Chicago, IL: Abbott Laboratories; February 1991.
4. American Academy of Pediatrics Committee on Drugs. Emergency drug doses for infants and children. *Pediatrics.* 1998;101:e1-e11.
5. Morton NS, Wee M, Christie G, et al. Propofol for induction of anaesthesia in children. *Anaesthesia.* 1988;43:350-355.
6. Mirakhur RK. Induction characteristics of propofol in children: comparison with thiopentone. *Anaesthesia.* 1988;43:593-598.
7. Badgwell JM, Cunliffe M, Lerman J. Thiopental attenuates dysrhythmias in children: comparison of induction regimens. *Tex Med.* 1990;86:36-38.
8. Viitanen H, Annila P, Rorarius M, et al. Recovery after halothane anaesthesia induced with thiopental, propofol-alfentanil or halothane for day-case adenoidectomy in small children. *Br J Anaesth.* 1998;81:960-962.
9. Wodey E, Chonow L, Beneux X, et al. Haemodynamic effects of propofol vs thiopental in infants: an echocardiographic study. *Br J Anaesth.* 1999;82:516-520.
10. Jonmarker C, Westrin P, Larsson S, et al. Thiopental requirements for induction of anesthesia in children. *Anesthesiology.* 1987;67:104-107.
11. Westrin P, Jonmarker C, Werner O. Thiopental requirements for induction of anesthesia in neonates and in infants one to six months of age. *Anesthesiology.* 1989;71:344-346.
12. Bhutada A, Sahni R, Rastogi S, et al. Randomised controlled trial of thiopental for intubation in neonates. *Arch Dis Child Fetal Neonatal Ed.* 2000;82:F34-F37.
13. Brett CM, Fisher DM. Thiopental dose-response relations in unpremedicated infants, children, and adults. *Anesth Analg.* 1987;66:1024-1027.
14. Demarquez JL, Galperine R, Billeaud C, et al. High-dose thiopental pharmacokinetics in brain injured children and neonates. *Dev Pharmacol Ther.* 1987;10:292-300.
15. Goldberg RN, Moscoso P, Bauer CR, et al. Use of barbiturate therapy in severe perinatal asphyxia: a randomized controlled trial. *J Pediatr.* 1986;109:851-856.
16. Eyre JA, Wilkerson AR. Thiopentone induced comas after severe birth asphyxia. *Arch Dis Child.* 1986;61:1084-1089.
17. Quandt CM, de los Reyes RA. Pharmacologic management of acute intracranial hypertension. *Drug Intell Clin Pharm.* 1984;18:105-112.
18. Sidi A, Cotev S, Hadani M, et al. Long-term barbiturate infusion to reduce intracranial pressure. *Crit Care Med.* 1983;11:478-481.
19. Quandt CM, de los Reyes RA, Diaz FG. Barbiturate-induced coma for the treatment of cerebral ischemia: review of outcome. *Clin Pharm.* 1982;1:549-551.

References

20. Russo H, Bressolle F, Duboin MP. Pharmacokinetics of high-dose thiopental in pediatric patients with increased intracranial pressure. *Ther Drug Monit.* 1997;19:63-70.
21. Krauss B, Green S. Procedural sedation and analgesia in children. *Lancet.* 2006;367:766-780.
22. Orlowski JP, Erenberg G, Lueders H, et al. Hypothermia and barbiturate coma for refractory status epilepticus. *Crit Care Med.* 1984;12:367-371.
23. Bonati M, Marraro G, Celardo A, et al. Thiopental efficacy in phenobarbital-resistant neonatal seizures. *Dev Pharmacol Ther.* 1990;15:16-20.
24. Amit R, Goitein KJ, Mathot I, et al. Prolonged electrocerebral silent barbiturate coma in intractable seizure disorders. *Epilepsia.* 1988;29:63-66.
25. Young GB, Blume WT, Bolton CF, et al. Anesthetic barbiturates in refractory status epilepticus. *Can J Neurol Sci.* 1980;7:291-292.
26. Aronoff GR, Berns JS, Brier ME, et al. Drug prescribing in renal failure. 4th ed. Available at: http://www.kdp-baptist.louisville.edu/renalbook/. Accessed August 28, 2009.
27. Russo H, Bressolle F. Pharmacodynamics and pharmacokinetics of thiopental. *Clin Pharmacokinet.* 1998;35:95-134.
28. Thiopental. Lexi-Comp® Online with AHFS® (database). Bethesda, MD: American Society of Health-System Pharmacists; updated August 13, 2009.
29. Trissel LA, ed. *Handbook on Injectable Drugs.* 15th ed. Bethesda, MD: American Society of Health-System Pharmacists; 2009.
30. Bohan KH, Mansuri TF, Wilson NM. Anticonvulsant hypersensitivity syndrome: implications for pharmaceutical care. *Pharmacotherapy.* 2007;27:1425-1439.
31. Bessmerty O, Pham T. Antiepileptic hypersensitivity syndrome: clinicians beware and be aware. *Curr Allergy Asthma Rep.* 2002;2:34-39.
32. Kaur S, Sarkar R, Thami GP, et al. Anticonvulsant hypersensitivity syndrome. *Pediatr Dermatol.* 2002;19:142-145.
33. Schalen W, Messeter K, Nordstrom H. Complications and side effects during thiopentone therapy in patients with severe head injuries. *Acta Anaesthesiol Scand.* 1992;36:369-377.
34. Sorbo S. The pharmacokinetics of thiopental in pediatric surgical patients. *Anesthesiology.* 1984;61:666-670.

Ticarcillin Disodium–Clavulanate Potassium

1. Available at: http://www.usp.org/hqi/similarProducts/choosy.html. Accessed November 2,2009.
2. Ticarcillin disodium-Clavulanate [package insert]. Research Triangle Park, NC: GlaxoSmithKline; July 2008.
3. Nelson JD, Bradley JS, eds. *Nelson's Pocket Book of Pediatric Antimicrobial Therapy.* 17th ed. Chicago, IL: American Academy of Pediatrics; 2009.
4. American Academy of Pediatrics. Pickering LK, Baker CJ, Kimberlin DW, et al., eds. *2009 Red Book: Report of the Committee on Infectious Diseases.* 28th ed. Elk Grove Village, IL: American Academy of Pediatrics; 2009.
5. Fricke G, Doerck M, Hafner D, et al. The pharmacokinetics of ticarcillin/clavulanate acid in neonates. *J Antimicrob Chemother.* 1989;24 Suppl B:111-120.
6. Fayed SB, Sutton AM, Turner TL, et al. The prophylactic use of ticarcillin/clavulanate in the neonate. *J Antimicrob Chemother.* 1987;19:113-118.
7. Miall-Allen VM, Whitelaw AG, Darrell JH. Ticarcillin plus clavulanic acid (Timentin) compared with standard antibiotic regimes in the treatment of early and late neonatal infections. *Br J Clin Pract.* 1988 ;42:273-279.
8. Burstein AH, Wyble LE, Gal P, et al. Ticarcillin-clavulanic acid pharmacokinetics in preterm neonates with presumed sepsis. *Antimicrob Agents Chemother.* 1994;38:2024-2028.
9. Dougherty SH, Sirinek KR, Schauer PR, et al. Ticarcillin/clavulanate compared with clindamycin/gentamicin (with or without ampicillin) for the treatment of intra-abdominal infections in pediatric and adult patients. *Am Surg.* 1995;61:297-230.
10. Jacobs RF, Elser JM. Timentin therapy for staphylococcus aureus infections in children: results of a multi-center trial. *Pediatr Infect Dis J.* 1989;8:441-444.
11. Meier H, Adam D, Heilmann HD. Penetration of ticarcillin/clavulanate into cartilage. *J Antimicrob Chemother.* 1989;24:101-105.
12. Pokorny WJ, Kaplan SL, Mason EO. A preliminary report of ticarcillin and clavulanate versus triple antibiotic therapy in children with ruptured appendicitis. *Surgery.* 1972;172:S54-S56.
13. Sirinek KR, Levine BA. A randomized trial of ticarcillin and clavulanate versus gentamicin and clindamycin in patients with complicated appendicitis. *Surgery.* 1972;172:30-35.
14. Blumer JL. Ticarcillin/clavulanate for the treatment of serious infections in hospitalized pediatric patients. *Pediatric Infect Dis J.* 1998;17:1211-1215.
15. Shenep JL, Hughes WT, Roberson PK, et al. Vancomycin, ticarcillin, and amikacin compared with ticarcillin–clavulanate and amikacin in the empirical treatment of febrile, neutropenic children with cancer. *N Engl J Med.* 1988;319:1053-1058.
16. Schaison G, Reinert P, Leverger G. Timentin (ticarcillin and clavulanic acid) in combination with aminoglycosides in the treatment of febrile episodes in neutropenic children. *J Antimicrob Chemother.* 1986;17C:177-181.
17. Bolton-Maggs PHB, Van Saene HKF, McDowell HP, et al. Clinical evaluation of ticarcillin with clavulanic acid, and gentamicin in the treatment of febrile episodes in neutropenic children. *J Antimicrob Chemother.* 1991;27:669-676.
18. Aronoff GR, Berns JS, Brier ME, et al. Drug prescribing in renal failure. 4th ed. Available at: http://www.kdp-baptist.louisville.edu/renalbook/. Accessed November 2, 2009.
19. Trissel LA, ed. *Handbook on Injectable Drugs.* 15th ed. Bethesda, MD: American Society of Health-System Pharmacists; 2009.
20. Robinson CA, Sawyer JE. Y-site compatibility of medications with parenteral nutrition. *J Pediatr Pharmacol Ther.* 2009;14:49-57.
21. Munckhof WJ, Carney J, Neilson G, et al. Continuous infusion of ticarcillin-clavulanate for home treatment of serious infections: clinical efficacy, safety, pharmacokinetics and pharmacodynamics. *Int J Antimicrob Agents.* 2005;25:514-522.
22. Kurtzman NA, Rogers PW, Harter HR. Neurotoxic reaction to penicillin and carbenicillin. *JAMA.* 1970;214:1320-1321.
23. Smith H, Lerner PI, Weinstein L. Neurotoxicity and massive intravenous therapy with penicillin. A study of possible predisposing factors. *Arch Intern Med.* 1967;120:47-53.
24. Barrons RW, Murray KM, Richey RM. Populations at risk for penicillin-induced seizures. *Ann Pharmacother.* 1992;26:26-29.
25. Manian FA, Stone WJ, Alford RH. Adverse antibiotic effects associated with renal insufficiency. *Rev Infect Dis.* 1990;12:236-249.
26. Kallay MC, Tabechian H, Riley GR, et al. Neurotoxicity due to ticarcillin in patient with renal failure. *Lancet.* 1979;1:608-609. Letter.
27. Fass RJ, Copelan EA, Brandt JT, et al. Platelet-mediated bleeding caused by broad-spectrum penicillins. *J Infect Dis.* 1987;155:1242-1248.
28. Sweet JM, Jones MP. Intrahepatic cholestasis due to ticarcillin-clavulanate. *Am J Gastroenterol.* 1995;90:675-676.

Tigecycline

1. Available at: http://www.usp.org/hqi/similarProducts/choosy.html. Accessed November 4, 2009.
2. Tigecycline [package insert]. Philadelphia, PA: Wyeth Pharmaceuticals Inc; March 2009.
3. Smith M, Ubkel JH, Fenton SJ, et al. The use of tetracyclines in pediatric patients. *J Pediatr Pharmacol Ther.* 2001;66-71.
4. Pankey GA, Steele RW. Tigecycline: a single antibiotic for polymicrobial infections. *Pediatr Infect Dis J.* 2007;26:77-78.
5. George DK, Crawford DH. Antibacterial-induced hepatotoxicity. Incidence, prevention and management. *Drug Saf.* 1996;15:79-85.
6. Hung WY, Kogelman L, Volpe G, et al. Tigecycline-induced acute pancreatitis: case report and literature review. *Int J Antimicrob Agents.* 2009;34:486-489.
7. Lipshitz J, Kruh J, Cheung P, et al. Tigecycline-induced Pancreatitis. *J Clin Gastroenterol.* 2008;43:93.

References

Tissue Plasminogen Activator (t-PA)-Alteplase

1. Available at: http://ismp.org/Tools/highalertmedications.pdf. ISMP 2008.
2. Available at: http://ismp.org/Tools/confuseddrugnames.pdf. Updated April 1, 2005.
3. Available at: http://www.usp.org/hqi/similarProducts/choosy.html. Accessed November 4, 2009.
4. Activase [prescribing information]. South San Francisco, CA: Genentech Inc; December 2005.
5. Alteplase. Lexi-Comp® Online with AHFS® (database). Hudson, OH: Lexi-Comp Inc; updated September 28, 2009.
6. Monagle P, Chalmers E, Chan A, et al. Antithrombotic therapy in neonates and children. *Chest.* 2008;133 (suppl)887S-968S. Available at: http://www.chestjournal.org/content/133/6_suppl/887S.full.html.
7. Dillon PW, Fox PS, Berg CJ, et al. Recombinant tissue plasminogen activator for neonatal and pediatric vascular thrombolytic therapy. *J Pediatr Surg.* 1993;28:1264-1269.
8. Farnoux C, Camard O, Pinquier D, et al. Recombinant tissue-type plasminogen activator therapy of thrombosis in 16 neonates. *J Pediatr.* 1998;133:137-140.
9. Levy M, Benson LN, Burrows PE, et al. Tissue plasminogen activator for the treatment of thromboembolism in infants and children. *J Pediatr.* 1991;118:467-472.
10. Van Overmeire B, Van Reempts PJ, Van Acker KJ. Intracardiac thrombosis formation with rapidly progressive heart failure in the neonate: treatment with tissue-type plasminogen activator. *Arch Dis Child.* 1992;67:443-445.
11. Glover ML, Camacho MT, Wolfsdorf J. The use of alteplase in a newborn receiving extracorporeal membrane oxygenation. *Ann Pharmacotherapy.* 1999;33:416-419.
12. Guerin V, Boisseau MR. Efficiency of alteplase in the treatment of venous arterial thrombosis in neonates. *Am J Hematol.* 1993;42:236-237.
13. Gupta AA, Leaker M, Andrew M, et al. Safety and outcomes of thrombolysis with tissue plasminogen activator for treatment of intravascular thrombosis in children. *J Pediatr.* 2001;139:682-688.
14. Kennedy LA, Drummond WH, Knight ME, et al. Successful treatment of neonatal aortic thrombosis with tissue plasminogen activator. *J Pediatr.* 1990;116:798-801.
15. Zenz W, Muntean W, Beitzke A, et al. Tissue plasminogen activator (alteplase) treatment for femoral artery thrombosis after cardiac catheterization in infants and children. *Br Heart J.* 1993;70:382-385.
16. Newall F, Browne M, Savoia H, et al. Assessing the outcome of systemic tissue plasminogen activator for the management of venous and arterial thrombosis in pediatrics. *J Pediatr Hematol Oncol.* 2007;29:269-273.
17. Nowak-Gottl U, Schwabe D, Schneider W, et al. Thrombolysis with recombinant tissue-type plasminogen activator in renal venous thrombosis in infancy. *Lancet.* 1992;430:1105. Letter.
18. Smets K, Vanhaesebrouck P, Voet D, et al. Use of tissue type plasminogen activator in neonates: case reports and review of the literature. *Am J Perinatol.* 1996;13:217-222.
19. Pyles LA, Pierpont ME, Steiner ME, et al. Fibrinolysis by tissue plasminogen activator in a child with pulmonary embolism. *J Pediatr.* 1990;116:801-804.
20. Gruber A, Nasel C, Lang W, et al. Intra-arterial thrombolysis for the treatment of perioperative childhood cardioembolic stroke. *Neurology.* 2000;54:1684-1686.
21. Fasano R, Kent P, Valentino L. Superior vena cava thrombus treated with low-dose, peripherally administered recombinant tissue plasminogen activator in a child. *J Pediatr Hematol Oncol.* 2005;27:692-695.
22. Tan H, Kizilkaya M, Alper F, et al. Thrombolytic therapy with tissue plasminogen activator for superior vena cava thrombosis in an infant with sepsis. *Acta Paediatrica.* 2005;94:239-253.
23. Coombs CJ, Richardson PW, Dowling GJ, et al. Brachial artery thrombosis in infants: an algorithm for limb salvage. *Plast Reconstr Surg.* 2006;117:1482-1488.
24. Wang M, Hays T, Balasa V, et al. Low-dose tissue plasminogen activator thrombolysis in children. *J Pediatr Hematol Oncol.* 2003;25:379-386.
25. Atkinson JB, Bagnall HA, Gomperts E. Investigational use of tissue plasminogen activator for occluded central venous catheters. *J Parenter Enter Nutr.* 1990;4:310-311.
26. Davis SN, Vermeulen L, Banton J, et al. Activity and dosage of alteplase dilution for clearing occlusions of venous-access devices. *Am J Health Syst Pharm.* 2000;57:1039-1045.
27. Jacobs BR, Haygood M, Hingl J. Recombinant tissue plasminogen activator in the treatment of central venous catheter occlusion in children. *J Pediatr.* 2001;139:593-596.
28. Shen V, Li X, Murdock M, et al. Recombinant tissue plasminogen activator (alteplase) for restoration of function to occluded central venous catheters in pediatric patients. *J Pediatr Hematol Oncol.* 2003;25:38-45.
29. Deitcher SR, Fesen MR, Kiproff PM, et al. Safety and efficacy of alteplase for restoring function in occluded central venous catheters: results of the cardiovascular thrombolytic to open occluded lines trial. *J Clin Oncol.* 2001;20:317-324.
30. Choi M, Massicotte MP, Marzinotto V, et al. The use of alteplase to restore patency of central venous lines in pediatric patients: a cohort study. *J Pediatr.* 2001;139:152-156.
31. Timoney JP, Malkin MG, Groeger JS, et al. Safe and cost effective use of alteplase for the clearance of occluded central venous access devices. *J Clin Oncol.* 2002;22:1918-1922.
32. Mehta JS, Adams GG. Recombinant tissue plasminogen activator following paediatric cataract surgery. *Br J Ophthalmol.* 2000;84:983-986.
33. Klais CM, Hattenbach LO, Steinkamp GW, et al. Intraocular recombinant tissue-plasminogen activator fibrinolysis of fibrin formation after cataract surgery in children. *J Cataract Refract Surg.* 1999;25:357-362.
34. Zalta AH, Sweeney CP, Zalta AK, et al. Intracameral tissue plasminogen activator use in a large series of eyes with valved glaucoma drainage implants. *Arch Ophthalmol.* 2002;120:1487-1493.
35. Krendel S, Pollack P, Hanly J. Tissue plasminogen activator in pediatric myocardial infarction. *Ann Emerg Med.* 2000;35:502-505.
36. Bishop NB, Pon S, Ushay HM, et al. Alteplase in the treatment of complicated parapneumonic effusion: a case report. *Pediatrics.* 2003;111:E188-E190. Available at: http://www.pediatrics.org/cgi/content/full/111/2/e188.
37. Diamond IR, Wales PW, Connolly B, et al. Tissue plasminogen activator for the treatment of intraabdominal abscesses in a neonate. *J Pediatr Surg.* 2003;38:1234-1236.
38. Levitas A, Zucker N, Zalzstein E, et al. Successful treatment of infective endocarditis with recombinant tissue plasminogen activator. *J Pediatr.* 2003;143:649-652.
39. Trissel LA. *Handbook on Injectable Drugs.* 15th ed. Bethesda, MD: American Society of Health-System Pharmacists; 2009.
40. Frazin BS. Maximal dilution of Activas. *Am J Hosp Pharm.* 1990;47:1016.
41. Zenz W, Muntean W, Gallist L, et al. Recombinant tissue plasminogen activator treatment in two infants with fulminant meningococcemia. *Pediatrics.* 1995;96:144-147.
42. Zenz W, Zoehrer B, Levin M, et al. Use of recombinant tissue plasminogen activator in children with meningococcal purpura fulminans: a retrospective study. *Crit Care Med.* 2004;32:1777-1780.

Tobramycin Sulfate

1. Available at: http://www.usp.org/hqi/similarProducts/choosy.html. Accessed November 14, 2009.
2. Tobramycin [package insert]. East Hanover, New Jersey: Novartis Pharmaceuticals; T2007-102.

References

3. Pannu N, Nadim MK. An overview of drug-induced acute kidney injury. *Crit Care Med*. 2008;36(4 Suppl):S216-S223.
4. Guthrie OW. Aminoglycoside induced ototoxicity. *Toxicology*. 2008;249:91-96.
5. Snavely SR, Hodges GR. The neurotoxicity of antibacterial agents. *Ann Intern Med*. 1984;101:92-104.
6. Paradelis AG. Aminoglycoside antibiotics and neuromuscular blockade. *J Antimicrob Chemother*. 1979;5:737-738.
7. Blouin RA, Mann HJ, Griffen WO, et al. Tobramycin pharmacokinetics in morbidly obese patients. *Clin Pharmacol Ther*. 1979;26:508-512.
8. Watterberg KL, Kelly W, Angelus P, et al. The need for a loading dose of gentamicin in neonates. *Ther Drug Monit*. 1989;11:16-20.
9. Gal P, Ransom JL, Weaver RL. Gentamicin in neonates: the need for loading doses. *Amer J Perinatol*. 1990;7:254-257.
10. American Academy of Pediatrics. Pickering LK, Baker CJ, Kimberlin DW, et al., eds. *2009 Red Book: Report of the Committee on Infectious Diseases*. 28th ed. Elk Grove Village, IL: American Academy of Pediatrics; 2009.
11. Prober CG, Stevenson DK, Benitz WE. The use of antibiotics in neonates weighing less than 1200 grams. *Pediatr Infect Dis J*. 1990;9:111-121.
12. Nelson JD, Bradley JS, eds. *Nelson's Pocket Book of Pediatric Antimicrobial Therapy*. 17th ed. Chicago, IL: American Academy of Pediatrics; 2009.
13. Nahata MC, Powell DA, Durrell DE, et al. Effect of gestational age and birth weight on tobramycin kinetics in newborn infants. *J Antimicrob Chemother*. 1984;14:59-65.
14. Nahata MC, Powell DA, Gregoire RP, et al. Tobramycin kinetics in newborn infants. *J Pediatr*. 1983;103:136-138.
15. Contopoulos-Ioannidis DG, Giotis ND, Baliatsa DV, et al. Extended-Interval aminoglycoside administration for children: A META-analysis. *Pediatrics*. 2004;114:e111-e118.
16. Langhendries JP, Battisti O, Bertrand JM, et al. Once-a-day administration of amikacin in neonates: Assessment of nephrotoxicity and ototoxicity. *Dev Pharmacol Ther*. 1993;20:220-230.
17. Marik PE, Lipman J, Kobilski S, et al. A prospective randomized study comparing once- versus twice-daily amikacin dosing in critically ill adult and paediatric patients. *J Antimicrob Chemother*. 1991;28:753-764.
18. Kafetzis DA, Sianidou L, Vlachos E, et al. Clinical and pharmacokinetic study of a single daily dose of amikacin in paediatric patients with severe gram-negative infections. *J Antimicrob Chemother*. 1991;27:105-112.
19. Trujillo H, Robledo J, Robledo C, et al. Single dose amikacin in paediatric patients with severe gram-negative infections. *J Antimicrob Chemother*. 1991;27:141-147.
20. Viscoli C, Dudley M, Ferrea G, et al. Serum concentration and safety of a single daily dose of amikacin in children undergoing bone marrow transplantation. *J Antimicrob Chemother*. 1991;27:113-120.
21. Sung L, Dupuis LL, Bliss B, et al. Randomized controlled trial of once- versus thrice-daily tobramycin in febrile neutropenic children undergoing stem cell transplantation. *J Natl Cancer Inst*. 2003;95:1869-1877.
22. Dupuis LL, Sung L, Taylor T, et al. Tobramycin pharmacokinetics in children with febrile neutropenia undergoing stem cell transplantation: once-daily versus thrice-daily administration. *Pharmacotherapy*. 2004;24:564-571.
23. Bouffet E, Fuhrmann C, Frappaz D, et al. Once daily antibiotic regimen in paediatric oncology. *Arch Dis Child*. 1994;70:484-487.
24. International Antimicrobial Therapy Cooperative Group of the European Organization for Research and Treatment of Cancer. Efficacy and toxicity of single daily doses of amikacin and ceftriaxone versus multiple daily doses of amikacin and ceftazidime for infection in patients with cancer and granulocytopenia. *Ann Intern Med*. 1993;119:584-593.
25. Krivoy N, Postovsky S, Elhasid R, et al. Pharmacokinetic analysis of amikacin twice and single daily dosage in immunocompromised pediatric patients. *Infection*. 1998;26:396-398.
26. Torfoss D, Hoiby EA, Tangen JM, et al. Tobramycin once versus three times daily, given with penicillin G, to febrile neutropenic cancer patients in Norway: a prospective, randomized, multicentre trial. *J Antimicrob Chemother*. 2007;59:711-717.
27. Chicella M. Once-daily aminoglycoside dosing in pediatrics. What is its role? *J Pediatr Pharm Pract*. 2000;5:98-103.
28. Wallace CS, Hall M, Kuhn RJ. Pharmacologic management of cystic fibrosis. *Clin Pharm*. 1993;12:657-674.
29. Smyth A, Tan KH, Hyman-Taylor P, et al. Once versus three-times daily regimens of tobramycin treatment for pulmonary exacerbations of cystic fibrosis—the TOPIC study: a randomized controlled trial. *Lancet*. 2005;365:573-578.
30. Beringer PM, Vinks AA, Jelliffe RW, et al. Pharmacokinetics of tobramycin in adults with cystic fibrosis: implications for once-daily administration. *Antimicrob Agents Chemother*. 2000;44:809-813.
31. Bates RD, Nahata MC, Jones JW, et al. Pharmacokinetics and safety of tobramycin after once-daily administration in patients with cystic fibrosis. *Chest*. 1997;112:1208-1213.
32. Aminimanizani A, Beringer PM, Kang J, et al. Distribution and elimination of tobramycin administered in single or multiple daily doses in adult patients with cystic fibrosis. *J Antimicrob Chemother*. 2002:50;553-559.
33. Bragonier R, Brown NM. The pharmacokinetics and toxicity of once-daily tobramycin therapy in children with cystic fibrosis. *J Antimicrob Chemother*. 1998:42:103-106.
34. Master V, Roberts GW, Coulthard KP, et al. Efficacy of once-daily tobramycin monotherapy for acute pulmonary exacerbations of cystic fibrosis: a preliminary study. *Pediatr Pulmonol*. 2001;3:367-376.
35. Henning S, Norris R, and Kirkpatrick CMJ. Target concentration intervention is needed for tobramycin dosing in paediatric patients with cystic fibrosis — a population pharmacokinetic study. *Br J Clin Pharmacol*. 2007;65:502-510.
36. Lam W, Tjon J, Seto W, et al. Pharmacokinetic modeling of a once-daily dosing regimen for intravenous tobramycin in paediatric cystic fibrosis patients. *J Antimicrob Chemother*. 2007:59:1135-1140.
37. Massie J, Cranswick N. Pharmacokinetic profile of once daily intravenous tobramycin in children with cystic fibrosis. *J Paediatri Child Health*. 2006;42:601-605.
38. Van Meter DJ, Corriveau M, Ahern JW, et al. A survey of once-daily dosage tobramycin therapy in patients with cystic fibrosis. *Pediatr Pulmonol*. 2009;44:325-329.
39. Aronoff GR, Berns JS, Brier ME, et al. Drug prescribing in renal failure. 4th ed. Available at: http://www.kdp-baptist.louisville.edu/renalbook/. Accessed August 28, 2009.
40. Loirat P, Rohan J, Baillet A, et al. Increased glomerular filtration rate in patients with major burns and its effect on the pharmacokinetics of tobramycin. *N Engl J Med*. 1978;299:915-919.
41. Buck ML. Pharmacokinetic changes during extracorporeal membrane oxygenation. *Clin Pharmacokinet*. 2003;42:403-417.
42. Armstrong DK, Hidalgo HA, Eldadah M. Vancomycin and tobramycin clearance in an infant during continuous hemo-filtration. *Ann Pharmacother*. 1993;27:224-227.
43. Trissel LA, ed. *Handbook on Injectable Drugs*. 15th ed. Bethesda, MD: American Society of Health-System Pharmacists; 2009.
44. Robinson CA, Sawyer JE. Y-site compatibility of medications with parenteral nutrition. *J Pediatr Pharmacol Ther*. 2009;14:49-57.
45. Mendelson J, Portnoy J, Dick V, et al. Safety of the bolus administration of gentamicin. *Antimicrob Agents Chemother*. 1976;9:633-638.
46. Dobbs SM, Mawer GE. Intravenous injection of gentamicin and tobramycin without impairment of hearing. *J Infect Dis*. 1976;134 (suppl):S114-S117.
47. Gillett AP, Falk RH, Andrews J, et al. Rapid intravenous injection of tobramycin: suggested dosage schedule and concentrations in serum. *J Infect Dis*. 1976;134:S110-S113.
48. Powell SH, Thompson WL, Luthe MA, et al. Once daily vs. continuous aminoglycoside dosing: efficacy and toxicity in animal and clinical studies of gentamicin, netilmicin and tobramycin. *J Infect Dis*. 1983;147:918-932.
49. Bodey GP, Chang HY, Rodriguez V, et al. Feasibility of administering aminoglycoside antibiotics by continuous intravenous infusion. *Antimicrob Agents Chemother*. 1975;8:328-333.
50. Giacoia GP, Schentag JJ. Pharmacokinetics and nephrotoxicity of continuous intravenous infusion of gentamicin in low birth weight infants. *J Pediatr*. 1986;109:715-719.
51. Beaubien AR, Desjardins S, Ormsby E, et al. Incidence of amikacin ototoxicity: a sigmoid function of total drug exposure independent of plasma levels. *Am J Otolaryngol*. 1989;10:234-243.

References

52. Beaubien AR, Ormsby E, Bayne A, et al. Evidence that amikacin ototoxicity is related to total perilymph area under the concentration-time curve regardless of concentration. *Antimicrob Agents Chemother.* 1991;35:1070-1074.
53. Brownsberger RJ, Morrelli HF. Neuromuscular blockade due to gentamicin sulfate.*West J Med.* 1988;148:215.
54. Warner WA, Sanders E. Neuromuscular blockade associated with gentamicin therapy. *JAMA.* 1971;215:1153-1154.
55. Massey KL, Hendeles L, Neims A. Identification of children for whom routine monitoring of aminoglycoside serum concentrations is not cost effective. *J Pediatr.* 1986;109:897-901.
56. Logsdon BA, Phelps SJ. Routine monitoring of gentamicin serum concentrations in pediatric patients with normal renal function is unnecessary. *Ann Pharmacother.* 1997;31:1514-1518.
57. Franson TR, Ritch PS, Quebbeman EJ. Aminoglycoside serum concentration sampling via central venous catheters: a potential source of clinical error. *JPEN J Parenter Enteral Nutr.* 1987;11:77-79.

Topotecan HCl

1. Available at: http://ismp.org/Tools/highalertmedications.pdf. ISMP 2008. Accessed August 29, 2009.
2. Available at: http://www.usp.org/hqi/similarProducts/choosy.html. Accessed August 29, 2009.
3. Hycamtin [package insert]. Research Triangle, NC: GlaxoSmithKline; November 2009.
4. Trissel LA, ed. *Handbook on Injectable Drugs.* 15th ed. Bethesda, MD: American Society of Health-System Pharmacists; 2009.
5. Walterhouse DO, Lyden ER, Breitfeld PP, et al. Efficacy of topotecan and cyclophosphamide given in a phase II window trial in children with newly diagnosed metastatic rhabdomyosarcoma: a Children's Oncology Group study. *J Clin Oncol.* 2004; 22(8):1360-1362.
6. Nitschke R, Parkhurst J, Sullivan J, et al. Topotecan in pediatric patients with recurrent and progressive solid tumors: a Pediatric Oncology Group phase II study. *J Pediatr Hematol Oncol.* 1998; 20(4):315-318.
7. Tubergen DG, Stewart CF, Pratt CB, et al. Phase I trial and pharmacokinetic (PK) and pharmacodynamics (PD) study of topotecan using a five-day course in children with refractory solid tumors: a pediatric oncology group study. *J Pediatr Hematol Oncol.* 1996;18(4):352-361.
8. Metzger ML, Stewart CF, Freeman BB, 3rd, et al. Topotecan is active against Wilms' tumor: results of a multi-institutional phase II study. *J Clin Oncol.* 2007;25:3130-136.
9. Wells RJ, Reid JM, Ames MM, et al. Phase I trial of cisplatin and topotecan in children with recurrent solid tumors: Children's Oncology Group Study 0942. *J Pediatr Hematol Oncol.* 2002;24(2):89-93.
10. Pratt CB, Stewart CF, Santana VM, et al. Phase I study of topotecan for pediatric patients with malignant solid tumors. *J Clin Oncol.*1994;12(3):539-543.
11. Santana VM, Zamboni WC, Kirstein MN, et al. A pilot study of protracted topotecan using a pharmacokinetically guided dosing approach in children with solid tumors. *Clin Cancer Res.* 2003;9(2):633-640.
12. Furman WL, Stewart CF, Kirstein M, et al. Protracted intermittent schedule of topotecan in children with refractory acute leukemia: a Pediatric Oncology Group Study. *J Clin Oncol.* 2002; 20(6):1617-1624.
13. Hijiya N, Stewart CF, Zhou Y, et al. Phase II study of topotecan in combination with dexamethasone, asparaginase, and vincristine in pediatric patients with acute lymphoblastic leukemia in first relapse. *Cancer.* 2008;112:1983-1991.
14. Topotecan. Lexi-Comp Online with AHFS (database). Hudson, OH: Lexi-Comp Inc; updated November 19, 2009.
15. Aronoff GR, Berns JS, Brier ME, et al. Drug prescribing in renal failure. 4th ed. Available at: http://www.kdp-baptist.louisville.edu/renalbook/. Accessed October 23, 2009.
16. National Comprehensive Cancer Network (NCCN) Antiemesis Panel Members. NCCN Clinical Practice Guidelines in Oncology. Antiemesis, v.1.2006. Available at www.nccn.org. Last accessed March 29, 2006.
17. Roila F, Feyer P, Maranzamo E, et al. Antiemetics in children receiving chemotherapy. *Supportive Care Cancer.* 2005;13:129-131.

Tromethamine

1. THAM solution [package insert]. Lake Forest, IL: Hospira; October 2005.
2. Tromethamine. Lexi-Comp® Online with AHFS® (database). Bethesda, MD: American Society of Health-System Pharmacists; updated September 2007.
3. Tromethamine. Lexi-Comp® Online with AHFS® (database). Hudson, OH: Lexi-Comp Inc; updated August 13, 2009.
4. Nahas GG, Sutin KM, Fermon C, et al. Guidelines for the treatment of acidaemia with THAM. *Drugs.* 1998;55(2):191-224.
5. Strauss J. Tris (hydroxymethyl) amino-methane (THAM): a pediatric evaluation. *Pediatrics.* 1968;41:667-689.
6. Tarail R, Bennett TE. Hypoglycemic activity of TRIS buffer in man and dog. *Proc Soc Exp Biol Med.* 1959;102:208-209.
7. Roberton NRC. Apnea after THAM administration in the newborn. *Arch Dis Child.* 1970;45:206-214.
8. Gupta JM, Dahlenburg GW, Davis JW. Changes in blood gas tensions following administration of amine buffer THAM to infants with respiratory distress syndrome. *Arch Dis Child.* 1967;42:416-427.
9. Baum JD, Robertson NRC. Immediate effects of alkaline infusion in infants with respiratory distress syndrome. *J Pediatr.* 1975;87:255.
10. Holmdahl MH, Wiklund L, Wetterberg T, et al. The place of THAM in the management of academia in clinical practice. *Acta Anaesthesiol Scand.* 2000;44:524-527.
11. Goldenberg VE, Wiegenstein L, Hopkins GB. Hepatic injury associated with tromethamine. *JAMA.* 1968;205:81-84.
12. Hooge MN, Verhoeven BH, Rutten WJ, et al. Irreversible ischemia of the hand after peripheral administration of tromethamol (THAM). *Intensive Care Med.* 2003;29:503.

Valproate Sodium

1. Valproate sodium injection [package insert]. North Chicago, IL: Abbott Laboratories.
2. American Academy of Pediatrics Committee on Drugs. Valproic acid: benefits and risks. *Pediatrics.* 1982;70:316-319.
3. Dreifuss FE, Santilli N, Langer DH, et al. Valproic acid hepatic fatalities: a retrospective review. *Neurology.* 1987;37:379-385.
4. Dreifuss FE, Langer DH, Moline KA, et al. Valproic acid hepatic fatalities. II. US experience since 1984. *Neurology.* 1989;39:201-207.
5. Bryant AE 3rd, Dreifuss FE. Valproic acid hepatic fatalities. III. U.S. experience since 1986. *Neurology.* 1996;46:465-469.
6. Rosenberg HK, Ortega W. Hemorrhagic pancreatitis in a young child following valproic acid therapy. Clinical and ultrasonic assessment. *Clin Pediatr.* 1987;26:98-101.
7. Cooper MA, Groll A. A case of chronic pancreatic insufficiency due to valproic acid in a child. *Can J Gastroenterol.* 2001;15:127-130.
8. Batalden PB, Van Dyne BJ, Cloyd J. Pancreatitis associated with valproic acid therapy. *Pediatrics.*1979;64:520-522.
9. Mathew NT, Kailasam J, Meadors L, et al. Intravenous valproate sodium (depacon) aborts migraine rapidly: a preliminary report. *Headache.* 2000;40:720-723.
10. Schwartz TH, Karpitskiy VV, Sohn RS. Intravenous valproate sodium in the treatment of daily headache. *Headache.* 2002;42:519-522.
11. Stillman MJ, Zajac D, Rybicki LA. Treatment of primary headache disorders with intravenous valproate: initial outpatient experience. *Headache.* 2004;44:65-69.
12. Reiter PD, Nickisch J, Merritt G. Efficacy and tolerability of intravenous valproic acid in acute adolescent migraine. *Headache.* 2005;45:899-903.

13. Taylor LM, Farzam F, Cook AM, et al. Clinical utility of a continuous intravenous infusion of valproic acid in pediatric patients. *Pharmacotherapy*. 2007;27:519-525.
14. Renbaugh JE, Sato S, et al. Sodium valproate: pharmacokinetics and effectiveness in treating intractable seizures. *Neurology*. 1980;30:1-6.
15. Sherard ES, Steiman GS, Couri D. Treatment of childhood epilepsy with valproic acid: results of the first 100 patients in a 6-month trial. *Neurology*. 1980;30:31-35.
16. Braathen G. Theorall K, Persson A, et al. Valproate in the treatment of absence epilepsy in children: a study of dose-response relationships. *Epilepsia*. 1988;29:548-552.
17. Herngren L, Lundberg B, Nergardh A. Pharmacokinetics of total and free valproate during monotherapy in infants. *J Neurol*. 1991;238:315-319.
18. Cloyd JC, Kriel RL, Fishcer JH. Valproic acid pharmacokinetics in children. II. Discontinuation of concomitant antiepileptic drug therapy. *Neurology*. 1985;35:1623-1627.
19. Cloyd JC, Fischer JH, Kriel RL, et al. Valproic acid pharmacokinetics in children. IV. Effects of age and antiepileptic drugs on protein binding and intrinsic clearance. *Clin Pharmacol Ther*. 1993;53:22-29.
20. Marlow N, Cooke RW. Intravenous sodium valproate in the neonatal intensive care unit. *J R Soc Med*. 1989;152:208-210.
21. Alfonso I, Alvarez LA, Gilman J, et al. Intravenous valproate dosing in neonates. *J Child Neurol*. 2000;15:827-829.
22. Hovinga CA, Chicella MF, Rose DF, et al. Use of intravenous valproate in three pediatric patients with convulsive or nonconvulsive status epilepticus. *Ann Pharmacother*. 1999;33:579-584.
23. Hodges BM, Mazur JE. Intravenous valproate in status epilepticus. *Ann Pharmacother*. 2001;35:1465-1470.
24. White JR, Santos CS. Intravenous valproate associated with significant hypotension in the treatment of status epilepticus. *J Child Neurol*. 1999;14:822-823.
25. Uberall MA, Trollmann R, Wunsiedler U, Wenzel D. Intravenous valproate in pediatric epilepsy patients with refractory status epilepticus. *Neurology*. 2000;54:2188-2189.
26. Venkataraman V, Wheless JW. Safety of rapid intravenous infusion of valproate loading doses in epilepsy patients. *Epilepsy Res*. 1999;147-153.
27. Chez MG, Hammer MS, Loeffel M, et al. Clinical experience of three pediatric and one adult case of spike-and-wave status epilepticus treated with injectable valproic acid. *J Child Neurol*. 1999;14:239-242.
28. Mehta V, Singhi P, Singhi S. Intravenous sodium valproate versus diazepam infusion for the control of refractory status epilepticus in children: a randomized controlled trial. *J Child Neurol*. 2007;22:1191-1197.
29. Temkin NR, Dikmen SS, Anderson GD, et al. Valproate therapy for prevention of posttraumatic seizures: a randomized trial. *J Neurosurg*. 1999;91:593-600.
30. Aronoff GR, Berns JS, Brier ME, et al. Drug prescribing in renal failure. 4th ed. Available at: http://www.kdp-baptist.louisville.edu/renalbook/. Accessed September 25, 2009.
31. Brewster D, Muir NC. Valproate plasma protein binding in the uremic condition. *Clin Pharmacol Ther*. 1980;27:76-82.
32. Peters CN, Pohlmann-Eden B. Intravenous valproate as an innovative therapy in seizure emergency situations including status epilepticus—experience in 102 adult patients. *Seizure*. 2005;14:164-169.
33. Kriel RL, Fischer JH, Cloyd JC, et al. Valproic acid pharmacokinetics in children: III. Very high dosage requirements. *Pediatr Neurol*. 1986;2:202-208.
34. Morton LD, O'Hara KA, Coots BP, et al. Safety of rapid intravenous valproate infusion in pediatric patients. *Pediatr Neurol*. 2007;36:81-83.
35. Limdi NA, Knowlton RK, Cofield SS, et al. Safety of rapid intravenous loading of valproate. *Epilepsia*. 2007;48:478-483.
36. Birnbaum AK, Kriel RL, Norberg SK, et al. Rapid infusion of sodium valproate in acutely ill children. *Pediatr Neurol*. 2003;28:300-303.
37. Wheless J, Venkataraman V. Safety of high intravenous valproate loading doses in epilepsy patients. *J Epilepsy*. 1998;11:319-324.
38. Ramsay RE, Cantrell D, Collins SD, et al. Safety and tolerance of rapidly infused Depacon. A randomized trial in subjects with epilepsy. *Epilepsy Res*. 2003;52:189-201.
39. Wheless J, Vazquez BR, Kanner AM, et al. Rapid insusion of valproate sodium is well tolerated in patients with epilepsy. *Neurology*. 2004;63:1507-1508.
40. Loiseau P. Sodium valproate, platelet dysfunction, and bleeding. *Epilepsia*. 1981;22:141-146
41. Acharya S, Bussel JB. Hematologic toxicity of sodium valproate. *J Pediatr Hematol Oncol*. 2000;22:62-65.
42. Cheung E, Wong V, Fung CW. Topiramate-valproate-induced hyperammonemic encephalopathy syndrome: case report. *J Child Neurol*. 2005;20:157-160.
43. Knudsen JF, Sokol GH, Flowers CM. Adjunctive topiramate enhances the risk of hypothermia associated with valproic acid therapy. *J Clin Pharm Ther*. 2008;33:513-519.
44. Longin E, Teich M, Koelfen W, et al. Topiramate enhances the risk of valproate-associated side effects in three children. *Epilepsia*. 2002;43:451-454.
45. Available at: http://www.fda.gov/Safety/MedWatch/SafetyInformation/SafetyAlertsforHumanMedicalProducts/ucm074939.htm. Accessed October 4, 2009.
46. Ueshima S, Aiba T, Makita T, et al. Characterization of non-linear relationship between total and unbound serum concentrations of valproic acid in epileptic children. *J Clin Pharm Ther*. 2008;33:31-38.
47. Anderson GD. A mechanistic approach to antiepileptic drug interactions. *Ann Pharmacother*. 1998;32:554-563.
48. Lheureux PE, Hantson P. Carnitine in the treatment of valproic acid-induced toxicity. *Clin Toxicol*. 2009;47:101-111.

Vancomycin HCl

1. Available at: http://www.usp.org/hqi/similarProducts/choosy.html. Accessed November 8, 2009.
2. Vancomycin [package insert]. Deerfield IL: Baxter Healthcare Corporation; February 2009.
3. Vancomycin. Lexi-Comp® Online with AHFS® (database). Hudson, OH: Lexi-Comp Inc; updated August 27, 2009.
4. Pai MP, Bearden DT. Antimicrobial dosing considerations in obese adult patients. *Pharmacotherapy*. 2007;27:1081-1091.
5. Bauer LA, Black DJ, Lill JS. Vancomycin dosing in morbidly obese patients. *Eur J Clin Pharmacol*. 1998;54:621-625.
6. Asbury WH, Darsey EH, Rose B, et al. Vancomycin pharmacokinetics in neonates and infants: a retrospective evaluation. *Ann Pharmacother*. 1993;27:490-494.
7. McDougal A, Ling EW, Levine M. Vancomycin pharmacokinetics and dosing in premature neonates. *Ther Drug Monitor*. 1995;17:319-326.
8. Grimsley C, Thomson AH. Pharmacokinetics and dose requirements of vancomycin in neonates. *Arch Dis Child*. 1999;81:F221-F227.
9. de Hoog M, Schoemaker RC, Mouton JW, et al. Vancomycin population pharmacokinetics in neonates. *Clin Pharmacol Ther*. 2000;67:360-367.
10. American Academy of Pediatrics. Pickering LK, Baker CJ, Kimberlin DW, et al., eds. *2009 Red Book: Report of the Committee on Infectious Diseases*. 28th ed. Elk Grove Village, IL: American Academy of Pediatrics; 2009.
11. Prober CG, Stevenson DK, Benitz WE. The use of antibiotics in neonates weighing less than 1200 grams. *Pediatr Infect Dis J*. 1990;9:111-121.
12. Reed MD, Kliegman RM, Weiner JS, et al. The clinical pharmacology of vancomycin in seriously ill preterm infants. *Pediatr Res*. 1987;22:360-363.
13. James A, Koren G, Milliken J, et al. Vancomycin pharmacokinetics and dose recommendations for preterm infants. *Antimicrob Agents Chemother*. 1987;31:52-54.
14. Gabriel MH, Kildoo CW, Gennrich JL, et al. Prospective evaluation of a vancomycin dosage guideline for neonates. *Clin Pharm*. 1991;10:129-132.
15. Schadd UB, McCracken GH, Nelson JD. Clinical pharmacology and efficacy of vancomycin in pediatric patients. *J Pediatr*. 1980;96:119-126.

References

16. Nelson JD, Bradley JS, eds. *Nelson's Pocket Book of Pediatric Antimicrobial Therapy*. 17th ed. Chicago, IL: American Academy of Pediatrics; 2009.
17. Tunkel AR, Hartman BJ, Kaplan SL, et al. Practice guidelines for the management of bacterial meningitis. *Clin Infect Dis.* 2004;39:1267-1284.
18. Rybak M, Lomaestro B, Rotschafer JC, et al. Therapeutic monitoring of vancomycin in adult patients: a consensus review of the American Society of Health-System Pharmacists, the Infectious Diseases Society of America, and the Society of Infectious Diseases Pharmacists. *Am J Health-Syst Pharm.* 2009;66:82-98.
19. Wilson W, Taubert K, Gewitz m, et al. Prevention of infective endocarditis. Guidelines from the American Heart Association Rheumatic Fever, Endocarditis, and Kawasaki Disease Committee, Council on Cardiovascular Disease in the Young, and the Councils on Clinical Cardiology, Council on Cardiovascular Surgery and Anesthesia and the Quality of Care and Outcomes Research Interdisciplinary Working Group. *Circulation.* 2007;115:1736-1754; correction *Circulation.* 2007;116:1736-1754.
20. Baddour LM, Wilson WR, Bayer AS, et al. Infective endocarditis: diagnosis, antimicrobial therapy, and management of complications: a statement for healthcare professionals from the Committee on Rheumatic Fever, Endocarditis, and Kawasaki Disease, Council on Cardiovascular Disease in the Young, and the Councils on Clinical Cardiology, Stroke, and Cardiovascular Surgery and Anesthesia, American Heart Association: endorsed by the Infectious Diseases Society of America. *Circulation.* 2005;111:e394-e434.
21. Inglesby TV, O'Toole T, Henderson DA, et al. Working Group on Civilian Biodefense. Anthrax as a biological weapon 2002: updated recommendations for management. *JAMA.* 2002;287:2236-2252.
22. Centers for Disease Control and Prevention. Update: investigation of bioterrorism-related anthrax and interim guidelines for exposure management and antimicrobial therapy, October 2001. *MMWR Morb Mortal Wkly Rep.* 2001;50:909-919.
23. Spafford PS, Sinkin RA, Cox X, et al. Prevention of central venous catheter-related coagulase-negative staphylococcal sepsis in neonates. *J Pediatr.* 1994;125:259-263.
24. Anon. Report from the hospital infection control practices advisory committee; comment period and public meeting. Preventing the spread of vancomycin resistance. *Federal Register.* 1994;59:2578-2563.
25. Baier RJ, Bocchini JA, Brown EG. Selective use of vancomycin to prevent coagulase-negative staphylococcal nosocomial bacteremia in high risk very low birth weight infants. *Pediatr Infect Dis J.* 1998;17:179-183.
26. Ocete E, Ruiz-Extremera A, Goicoechea A, et al. Low-dosage prophylactic vancomycin in central-venous catheters for neonates. *Early Human Dev.* 1998;53:S181-S186.
27. Henrickson KJ, Axtell RA, Hoover SM, et al. Prevention of central venous catheter-related infections and thrombotic events in immunocompromised children by the use of vancomycin/ciprofloxacin/heparin flush solution: a randomized, multicenter, double-blind trial. *J Clin Oncol.* 2000;18:1269-1278.
28. Swayne R, Rampling A, Newsom B. Intraventricular vancomycin for treatment of shunt-associated ventriculitis. *J Antimicrob Chemother.* 1987;19:249-253.
29. Pfausler B, Haring H, Wissel K. Cerebrospinal fluid pharmacokinetics of intraventricular vancomycin in patients with staphylococcal ventriculitis associated with CSF drainage. *Clin Infect Dis.* 1997;25:733-735.
30. Al-Jeraisy MA, Einhau S, Christensen ML, et al. Intraventricular vancomycin in pediatric patients with cerebrospinal fluid shunt infection. *J Pediatr Pharmacol Ther.* 2004;9:36-42.
31. Thompson JB, Einhaus S, Buckingham S, et al. Vancomycin for treating cerebrospinal fluid shunt infections in pediatric patients. *J Pediatr Pharmacol Ther.* 2005;10:14-25.
32. Aronoff GR, Berns JS, Brier ME, et al. Drug prescribing in renal failure. 4th ed. Available at: http://www.kdp-baptist.louisville.edu/renalbook/. Accessed November 13, 2009.
33. Amaker RD, Dipiro JT, Bhatia J. Pharmacokinetics of vancomycin in critically ill infants undergoing extracorporeal membrane oxygenation. *Antimicrob Agents Chemother.* 1996;40:1139-1142.
34. Chang D. Influence of malignancy on the pharmacokinetics of vancomycin in infants and children. *Pediatr Infect Dis J.* 1995;14:667-673.
35. Chang D, Liem L, Malogolowkin M. A prospective study of vancomycin pharmacokinetics and dosage requirements in pediatric cancer patients. *Pediatr Infect Dis J.* 1994;13:969-974.
36. Vancomycin. Lexi-Comp® Online with AHFS ® (database). Bethesda, MD: American Society of Health-System Pharmacists; updated August 27, 2009.
37. Trissel LA, ed. *Handbook on Injectable Drugs.* 15th ed. Bethesda, MD: American Society of Health-System Pharmacists; 2009.
38. Strauss AA. Di(2-ethylhexyl)phthalate (DEHP). *J Pediat Pharmacol Ther.* 2004;9:89-95.
39. Robinson CA, Sawyer JE. Y-site compatibility of medications with parenteral nutrition. *J Pediatr Pharmacol Ther.* 2009;14:49-57.
40. Koren G, James A. Vancomycin dosing in preterm infants: prospective verification of new recommendations. *J Pediatr.* 1987;110:797-798.
41. Alpert G, Campos JM, Harris MC, et al. Vancomycin dosage in pediatrics reconsidered. *Am J Dis Child.* 1984;138:20-22.
42. Albanèse J, Léone M, Bruguerolle B, et al. Cerebrospinal fluid penetration and pharmacokinetics of vancomycin administered by continuous infusion to mechanically ventilated patients in an intensive care unit. *Antimicrob Agents Chemother.* 2000;44:1356-1358.
43. James JK, Palmer SM, Levine DP, et al. Comparison of conventional dosing versus continuous-infusion vancomycin therapy for patients with suspected or documented gram-positive infections. *Antimicrob Agents Chemother.* 1996;40:696-700.
44. Wysocki M, Delatour F, Faurisson F, et al. Continuous versus intermittent infusion of vancomycin in severe Staphylococcal infections: prospective multicenter randomized study. *Antimicrob Agents Chemother.* 2001;45:2460-2467.
45. Byl B, Jacobs F, Wallemacq P, et al. Vancomycin penetration of uninfected pleural fluid exudate after continuous or intermittent infusion. *Antimicrob Agents Chemother.* 2003;47:2015-2017.
46. Ingram PR, Lye DC, Tambyah PA, et al. Risk factors for nephrotoxicity associated with continuous vancomycin infusion in outpatient parenteral antibiotic therapy. *J Antimicrob Chemother.* 2008;62:168-171.
47. Pawlotsky F, Thomas A, Kergueris MF, et al. Constant rate infusion of vancomycin in premature neonates: a new dosage schedule. *Br J Clin Pharmacol.* 1998;46:163-167.
48. Plan O, Cambonie G, Barbotte E, et al. Continuous-infusion vancomycin therapy for preterm neonates with suspected or documented Gram-positive infections: a new dosage schedule. *Arch Dis Child Fetal Neonatal Ed.* 2008;93:F418-F421.
49. Weathers L, Riggs D, Santeiro M, et al. Aerosolized vancomycin for treatment of airway colonization by methicillin-resistant Staphylococcus aureus. *Pediatr Infect Dis J.* 1990;9:220-221.
50. Maiz L, Canton R, Mir N, et al. Aerosolized vancomycin for the treatment of methicillin-resistant Staphylococcus aureus infection in cystic fibrosis. *Pediatr Pulmonol.* 1998;26:287-289.
51. Newfield P, Roizen MF. Hazard of rapid administration of vancomycin. *Ann Intern Med.* 1979;91:581.
52. Glicklich D, Figura I. Vancomycin and cardiac arrest. *Ann Intern Med.* 1984;101:880-881.
53. Healy DP, Sahai JV, Fuller SH, et al. Vancomycin-induced histamine release and "red man syndrome": comparison of 1- and 2-hour infusions. *Antimicrob Agents Chemother.* 1990;34:550-554.
54. Renz CL, Thurn JD, Finn HA, et al. Antihistamine prophylaxis permits rapid vancomycin infusion. *Crit Care Med.* 1999;27:1732-1737.
55. Bhatt-Mehta V, Schumacher RE, Faix RG, et al. Lack of vancomycin-associated nephrotoxicity in newborn infants: a case-control study. *Pediatrics.* 1999;103:e48.
56. Swinney VR, Rudd CC. Nephrotoxicity of vancomycin-gentamicin therapy in pediatric patients. *J Pediatr.* 1987;110:497-498.
57. Nahata MC. Lack of nephrotoxicity in pediatric patients receiving concurrent vancomycin and aminoglycoside therapy. *Chemotherapy.* 1987;33:302-304.
58. Timpe E. Nephrotoxicity with combination vancomycin-aminoglycoside therapy. *J Pediatr Pharmacol Ther.* 2005;10:174-182.
59. Chicella M, Adkins J, Mancao MY, et al. Impact of pediatric specific guidelines for vancomycin serum concentration monitoring on patient care. *J Pediatr Pharm Pract.* 1999;4:146-151.
60. Lee KR, Phelps SJ. Implementation of vancomycin monitoring criteria in a pediatric hospital. *J Pediatr Pharmacol Ther.* 2004;9:179-186.

61. Somerville AL, Wright DH, Rotschafer JC. Implications of vancomycin degradation products on therapeutic drug monitoring in patients with end-stage renal disease. *Pharmacotherapy.* 1999;9:702-707.
62. Kingery JR, Sowinski KM, Kraus MA, et al. Vancomycin assay performance in patients with end-stage renal disease receiving hemodialysis. *Pharmacotherapy.* 2000;20:653-656.

Vasopressin

1. Available at: http://www.usp.org/hqi/similarProducts/choosy.html. Accessed October 22, 2009.
2. Vasopressin injection, USP [package insert]. Schaumburg, IL: APP Pharmaceuticals LLC; April 2008.
3. Vasopressin. Lexi-Comp® Online with AHFS® (database). Hudson, OH: Lexi-Comp Inc; updated October 22, 2009.
4. Weigle CG, Tobin JR. Metabolic and endocrine disease in pediatric intensive care. In: Rogers MC, ed. *Textbook of Pediatric Intensive Care.* 2nd ed. Baltimore, MD: Williams & Wilkins; 1992:1252.
5. McDonald JA, Martha PM, Kerrigan J, et al. Treatment of the young child with postoperative central diabetes insipidus. *Am J Dis Child.* 1989; 143:201-204.
6. Rosenzweig EB, Stare TJ, Chen JM, et al. Intravenous arginine-vasopressin in children with vasodilatory shock after cardiac surgery. *Circulation.* 1999;100:II182-II186.
7. Vasudevan A, Lodha R, Kabra SK. Vasopressin infusion in children with catecholamine-resistant septic shock. *Acta Paediatr.* 2005;94:380-383.
8. Liedel JL, Meadow W, Nachman J, et al. Use of vasopressin in refractory hypotention in children with vasodilatory shock: five cases and a review of the literature. *Pediatr Crit Care Med.* 2002;3:15-18.
9. Holmes CL, Walley KR. Vasopressin in the ICU. *Curr Opin Crit Care.* 2004;10:442-448.
10. Dellinger RP, Carlet JM, Masur H, et al. Surviving sepsis campaign guidelines for management of severe sepsis and septic shock. *Crit Care Med.* 2004;32:858-873.
11. Durbin DR, Liacouras CA. Chapter 93: Gastrointestinal emergencies. In: Fleisher GR, Ludwig S, eds. *Textbook of Pediatric Emergency Medicine.* 4th ed. Philadelphia, PA: Lippincott Williams & Wilkins; 2000:1017-1041.
12. Hyams JS, Leichtner AM, Schwartz AN. Recent advance in diagnosis and treatment of gastrointestinal hemorrhage in infants and children. *J Pediatr.* 1985;106:1-9.
13. Tuggle DW, Bennett KG, Scott J, et al. Intravenous vasopressin and gastrointestinal hemorrhage in children. *J Pediatr Surg.* 1988;23:627-629.
14. Mann K, Berg RA, Nadkarni V. Beneficial effects of vasopressin in prolonged pediatric cardiac arrest: a case series. *Resuscitation.* 2002;52:149-156.
15. American Heart Association guidelines for cardiopulmonary resuscitation and emergency cardiovascular care. Part 12: pediatric advanced life support. *Circulation.* 2005;112 (suppl 1):167-187.
16. Aronoff GR, Berns JS, Brier ME, et al. Drug prescribing in renal failure. 4th ed. Available at: http://www.kdp-baptist.louisville.edu/renalbook/pediatric/. Accessed October 19, 2009.
17. Trissel LA. *Handbook on Injectable Drugs.* 15th ed. Bethesda, MD: American Society of Health-System Pharmacists; 2009.

Vecuronium Bromide

1. Available at: http://ismp.org/Tools/highalertmedications.pdf. ISMP 2008. Accessed August 29, 2009.
2. Available at: http://www.usp.org/hqi/similarProducts/choosy.html. Accessed August 29, 2009.
3. Available at: http://ismp.org/Tools/confuseddrugnames.pdf. Accessed August 29, 2009.
4. Vecuronium bromide [package insert]. Bedford, OH: Bedford Laboratories; June 2007.
5. Goudsouzian NG, Young ET, Moss J, et al. Histamine release during the administration of atracurium or vecuronium in children. *Br J Anaesth.* 1986;58:1229-1233.
6. Durrani Z, O'Hara J. Histaminoid reaction from vecuronium priming: a case report. *Anesthesiology.* 1987;67:130-132.
7. Rowlee SC. Monitoring neuromuscular blockade in the intensive care unit: the peripheral nerve stimulator. *Heart Lung.* 1999;28:352-362.
8. Martin LD, Bratton SL, O'Rourke PP. Clinical uses and controversies of neuromuscular blocking agents in infants and children. *Crit Care Med.* 1999;27:1358-1368.
9. Eldadah MK, Newth CJ. Vecuronium by continuous infusion for neuromuscular blockade in infants and children. *Crit Care Med.* 1989;17:989-992.
10. Woelfel SK, Dong ML, Brandom BW, et al. Vecuronium infusion requirements in children during halothane-narcotic-nitrous oxide, isoflurane-narcotic-nitrous oxide, and narcotic-nitrous oxide anesthesia. *Anesth Analg.* 1991;73:33-38.
11. Fitzpatrick KT, Black GW, Crean PM, et al. Continuous vecuronium infusion for prolonged muscle relaxation in children. *Can J Anaesth.* 1991;38:169-174.
12. Sloan MH, Lerman J, Bissonnette B. Pharmacodynamics of high dose vecuronium in children during balanced anesthesia. *Anesthesiology.* 1991;74:656-659.
13. Meretoja OA, Taivainen T, Ja'kanen L, et al. Synergism between atracurium and vecuronium in infants and children during nitrous oxide-oxygen-alfentanil anaesthesia. *Br J Anaesth.* 1994;73:605-607.
14. Trissel LA, ed. *Handbook on Injectable Drugs.* 15th ed. Bethesda, MD: American Society of Health-System Pharmacists; 2009
15. Vecuronium. Lexi-Comp Online with AHFS (database). Hudson, OH: Lexi-Comp Inc; updated September 25, 2009.
16. Margolis BD, Khachikian D, Friedman Y, et al. Prolonged reversible quadriparesis in mechanically ventilated patients who received long-term infusions of vecuronium. *Chest.* 1991;100:877-878.
17. Lagasse RS, Katz RI, Peterson M, et al. Prolonged neuromuscular blockade following vecuronium infusion. *J Clin Anesth.* 1990;2:269-271.
18. Segredo V, Caldwell JE, Matthay MA, et al. Persistent paralysis in critically ill patients after long-term administration of vecuronium. *N Engl J Med.* 1992;327:524-528.
19. Salviati L, Laverda AM, Zancan L, et al. Acute quadriplegic myopathy in a 17-month-old boy. *J Child Neurol.* 2000;15:63-66.
20. Yeaton P, Teba L. Sinus node exit block following administration of vecuronium. *Anesthesiology.* 1988;68:177-178.
21. Panacek EA, Sherman B. Hydrocortisone and pancuronium bromide: acute myopathy during status asthmaticus. *Crit Care Med.* 1988;16:732.
22. Watling SM, Dasta JF. Prolonged paralysis in intensive care unit patients after the use of neuromuscular blocking agents: a review of the literature. *Crit Care Med.* 1994;22:884-893.
23. Dupuic JY, Martin R, Tetrault JP. Atracurium and vecuronium interaction with gentamicin and tobramycin. *Can J Anaesth.* 1989;36:407-411.
24. Kronenfeld MA, Thomas SJ, Turndorf H. Recurrence of neuromuscular blockade after reversal of vecuronium in a patient receiving polymyxin/amikacin sternal irrigation. *Anesthesiology.* 1986;65:93-94.
25. Jeffrey JE, Tamburro RF, Schmidt GM, et al. Dilated nonreactive pupils secondary to neuromuscular blockade. *Anesthesiology.* 2000;92:1476-1487.

Verapamil HCl

1. Available at: http://ismp.org/Tools/highalertmedications.pdf. ISMP 2008.
2. Verapamil hydrochloride injection, USP [package insert]. Lake Forest, IL; Hospira; June 2005.

References

3. Strasburger JF. Cardiac arrhythmias in childhood. Diagnostic considerations and treatment. *Drugs*. 1991;42:974-983.
4. Rowland TW. Augmented ventricular rate following verapamil treatment for atrial fibrillation with Wolff-Parkinson-White syndrome. *Pediatrics*. 1983;72:245-246.
5. Verapamil. Lexi-Comp® Online with AHFS® (database). Hudson, OH: Lexi-Comp Inc; updated September 25, 2009.
6. Porter CJ, Gillette PC, Garson A, et al. Effects of verapamil on supraventricular tachycardia in children. *Am J Cardiol*. 1981;48:487-491.
7. Porter CJ, Garson A, Gillette PC. Verapamil: an effective calcium blocking agent for pediatric patients. *Pediatrics*. 1983;71:748-755.
8. 2005 American Heart Association Guidelines for Cardiopulmonary Resuscitation and Emergency Cardiovascular Care Part 12: Pediatric Advanced Life Support. *Circulation*. 2005;112(24 suppl):IV-167 to IV-187.
9. Radford D. Side effects of verapamil in infants. *Arch Dis Child*. 1983;58:465-466.
10. Epstein ML, Kiel EA, Victoria BE. Cardiac decompensation following verapamil therapy in infants with supraventricular tachycardia. *Pediatrics*. 1985;75:737-740.
11. Garson A Jr. Medicolegal problems in the management of cardiac arrhythmias in children. *Pediatrics*. 1987;79:84-88.
12. Kirk CR, Gibbs JL, Thomas R, et al. Cardiovascular collapse after verapamil in supraventricular tachycardia. *Arch Dis Child*. 1987;62:1265-1266.
13. Dick M II, Campbell RM. Advances in the management of cardiac arrhythmias in children. *Pediatr Clin North Am*. 1984;31:1175-1195.
14. Soler-Soler J, Sagrista-Sauleda J, Cabrera A, et al. Effect of verapamil in infants with paroxysmal supraventricular tachycardia. *Circulation*. 1979;59:876-879.
15. Sapire DW, O'Riordan AC, Black IF. Safety and efficacy of short and long-term verapamil therapy in children with tachycardia. *Am J Cardiol*. 1981;48:1091-1097.
16. Dhala A, Lewis DA, Garland J, et al. Verapamil sensitive incessant ventricular tachycardia in the newborn. *PACE*. 1996;19:1652-1654.
17. Shahar E, Barzilay Z, Frand M. Verapamil in the treatment of paroxysmal supraventricular tachycardia in infants and children. *J Pediatr*. 1981;98:323-326.
18. Somogyi A, Albrecht M, Kliems G, et al. Pharmacokinetics, bioavailability and ECG response of verapamil in patients with liver cirrhosis. *Br J Clin Pharmac*. 1981;12:51-60.
19. Liao WB, Bullard MJ, Kuo CT, et al. Anticholinergic overdose induced torsade de pointes successfully treated with verapamil. *Jpn Heart J*. 1996;37:925-931.
20. Trissel LA, ed. *Handbook on Injectable Drugs*. 15th ed. Bethesda, MD: American Society of Health-System Pharmacists; 2009.
21. Haug MT, DeRespino J, Zimmerman J, et al. Extended verapamil infusion for recurrent atrial tachyarrhythmias complicating acute myocardial infarction. *Clin Pharm*. 1984;3:540-544.
22. Chew CY, Hecht HS, Collett JT, et al. Influence of severity of ventricular dysfunction on hemodynamic responses to intravenously administered verapamil in ischemic heart disease. *Am J Cardiol*. 1981;47:917-922.
23. Reiter MJ, Shand DG, Aanonsen LM, et al. Pharmacokinetics of verapamil: experience with a sustained intravenous infusion regimen. *Am J Cardiol*. 1982;50:716-721.
24. Maiteh M, Daoud AS. Myoclonic seizure following intravenous verapamil injection: case report and review of the literature. *Ann Trop Paediatr*. 2001;21:271-272.
25. Ilan Y, Hillman M, Oren R. Intravenous verapamil for tachyarrhythmia in Duchenne's muscular dystrophy. *Pediatr Cardiol*. 1990;11:177-178.
26. Zalman F, Perloff JK, Durant NN, et al. Acute respiratory failure following intravenous verapamil in Duchenne's muscular dystrophy. *Am Heart J*. 1983;105:510-511.

VinBLAStine Sulfate

1. Available at: http://ismp.org/Tools/highalertmedications.pdf. ISMP 2008. Accessed August 29, 2009.
2. Available at: http://ismp.org/Tools/confuseddrugnames.pdf. Accessed August 29, 2009.
3. Available at: http://www.usp.org/hqi/similarProducts/choosy.html. Accessed August 29, 2009.
4. Vinblastine [package insert]. Bedford, OH: Bedford Laboratories; December 2001.
5. Trissel LA, ed. *Handbook on Injectable Drugs*. 15th ed. Bethesda, MD: American Society of Health-System Pharmacists; 2009.
6. Dorr RT, Alberts DS. Vinca alkaloid skin toxicity: antidote and drug disposition studies in the mouse. *J Natl Cancer Inst*. 1985;74:113-120.
7. Gadner H, Grois N, Arico M, et al. A randomized trial of treatment for multisystem Langerhans' cell histiocytosis. *J Pediatr*. 2001;138:728-734.
8. Nachman JB, Sposto R, Herzog P, et al. Randomized comparison of low-dose involved-field radiotherapy and no radiotherapy for children with Hodgkin's disease who achieve a complete response to chemotherapy. *J Clin Oncol*. 2002;20:3765-3771.
9. Schneider DT, Hilgenfeld E, Schwabe D, et al. Acute myelogenous leukemia after treatment for malignant germ cell tumors in children. *J Clin Oncol*. 1999;17:3226-3233.
10. Baranzelli MC, Kramar A, Bouffet E, et al. Prognostic factors in children with localized malignant nonseminomatous germ cell tumors. *J Clin Oncol*. 1999;17:1212-1218.
11. Vinblastine. Lexi-Comp® Online with AHFS® (database). Bethesda, MD: American Society of Health-System Pharmacists; updated January 2009.
12. Aronoff GR, Berns JS, Brier ME, et al. Drug prescribing in renal failure. 4th ed. Available at: http://www.kdpbaptist.louisville.edu/renalbook/. Accessed October 23, 2009.
13. Perry MC. Hepatoxicity of chemotherapeutic agents. *Semin Oncol*. 1982;9:65-74.
14. Weiss HD, Walker MD, Wiernik PH. Neurotoxicity of commonly used antineoplastic agents (second of two parts). *N Engl J Med*. 1974;291:127-133.
15. Kris MG, Pablo D, Gralla RJ, et al. Dyspnea following vinblastine or vindesine administration in patients receiving mitomycin plus vinca alkaloid combination therapy. *Cancer Treat Rep*. 1983;68:1029-1031.
16. Ballen KK, Weiss ST. Fatal acute respiratory failure following vinblastine and mitomycin administration for breast cancer. *Am J Med Sci*. 1988;295:558-560.
17. Hoelzer KL, Harrison BR, Luedke SW, et al. Vinblastine-associated pulmonary toxicity in patients receiving combination therapy with mitomycin and cisplatin. *Drug Intell Clin Pharm*. 1986;20:287-289.
18. Rao SX, Ramaswamy G, Leven M, et al. Fatal acute respiratory failure after vinblastine-mitomycin therapy in lung carcinoma. *Arch Inter Med*. 1985;145:1905-1907.
19. Ozols RF, Hogan WM, Ostchega Y, et al. MVP (mitomycin, vinblastine, and progesterone): a second-line regimen in ovarian cancer with a high incidence of pulmonary toxicity. *Cancer Treat Rep*. 1983;67:721-722.
20. Konits PH, Aisner J, Sutherland JC, et al. Possible pulmonary toxicity secondary to vinblastine. *Cancer*. 1982;50:2771-2774.
21. Israel RH, Olson JP. Pulmonary edema associated with intravenous vinblastine. *JAMA*. 1978;240:1585.
22. National Comprehensive Cancer Network (NCCN) Antiemesis Panel Members. NCCN Clinical Practice Guidelines in Oncology. Antiemesis, v.1.2006. Available at www.nccn.org. Accessed March 29, 2006.
23. Roila F, Feyer P, Maranzamo E, et al. Antiemetics in children receiving chemotherapy. *Support Care Cancer*. 2005;13:129-131.

VinCRIStine Sulfate

1. Available at: http://ismp.org/Tools/highalertmedications.pdf. ISMP 2008. Accessed August 29, 2009.
2. Available at: http://ismp.org/Tools/confuseddrugnames.pdf. Updated August 29, 2009.

3. Available at: http://www.usp.org/hqi/similarProducts/choosy.html. Accessed August 29, 2009.
4. Vincristine [package insert]. Lake Forest, IL: Hospira; December 2007.
5. Trissel LA, ed. *Handbook on Injectable Drugs.* 15th ed. Bethesda, MD: American Society of Health-System Pharmacists; 2009.
6. Cohen MR. Hazard warning: deaths due to accidental intrathecal injection of vincristine. *Hosp Pharm.* 1989;24:694.
7. Meggs WJ, Hoffman RS. Fatality resulting from intraventricular vincristine administration. *Clin Toxicol.* 1998;36(3):243-246.
8. Vincristine. Lexi-Comp® Online with AHFS® (database). Bethesda, MD: American Society of Health-System Pharmacists; updated January 2009.
9. MacCara ME. Extravasation: a hazard of intravenous therapy. *Drug Intell Clin Pharm.* 1983;17:713-717.
10. Arico M, Valsecchi MG, Conter V, et al. Improved outcome in high-risk childhood acute lymphoblastic leukemia defined by prednisone-poor response treated with double Berlin-Frankfurt-Muenster protocol II. *Blood.* 2002;100:420-426.
11. Nachman JB, Sposto R, Herzog P, et al. Randomized comparison of low-dose involved-field radiotherapy and no radiotherapy for children with Hodgkin's disease who achieve a complete response to chemotherapy. *J Clin Oncol.* 2002;20:3765-3771.
12. Dorr VJ, Morris D, Lorber M. Chemotherapy programs. In: Perry MC, ed. *The Chemotherapy Sourcebook.* 2nd ed. Baltimore, MD: Lippincott Williams & Wilkins; 1996:845-887.
13. Whitelaw DM, Cowan DH, Cassidy FR, et al. Clinical experience with vincristine. *Cancer Chemother Rep.* 1963;30:13-20.
14. Crom WR, Graff SS, Synold T, et al. Pharmacokinetics of vincristine in children and adolescents with acute lymphocytic leukemia. *J Pediatr.* 1994;125:642-649.
15. Perry MC. Hepatotoxicity of chemotherapeutic agents. *Semin Oncol.* 1982;9:65-74.
16. Aronoff GR, Berns JS, Brier ME, et al. Drug prescribing in renal failure. 4th ed. Available at: http://www.kdpbaptist.louisville.edu/renalbook/. Accessed October 23, 2009.
17. Legha SS. Vincristine neurotoxicity: pathophysiology and management. *Med Toxicol.* 1986;1:421-427.
18. Jeannine SM, Lindley C. Appropriateness of maximum-dose guidelines for vincristine. *Am J Health-Syst Pharm.* 1997;54:1755-1758.
19. Chan JD. Pharmacokinetic drug interactions of vinca alkaloids: summary of case reports. *Pharmacotherapy.* 1998;18:1304-1307.
20. National Comprehensive Cancer Network (NCCN) Antiemesis Panel Members. NCCN Clinical Practice Guidelines in Oncology. Antiemesis, v.1.2006. Available at www.nccn.org. Last accessed March 29, 2006.
21. Roila F, Feyer P, Maranzamo E, et al. Antiemetics in children receiving chemotherapy. *Support Care Cancer.* 2005;13:129-131.
22. Hansen MM, Ranek L, Walbom S, et al. Fatal hepatitis following irradiation and vincristine. *Acta Med Scand.* 1982;212:171-174.

Vitamin A

1. Available at: http://www.usp.org/hqi/similarProducts/choosy.html. Accessed August 27, 2009.
2. Aquasol [parenteral prescribing information]. Lake Forest, IL: Mayne Pharma (USA) Inc; April 2005.
3. Shenai JP, Kennedy KA, Chytil F, et al. Clinical trial of vitamin A supplementation in infants susceptible to bronchopulmonary dysplasia. *J Pediatr.* 1987;111:269-277.
4. Tyson JE, Wright LL, Oh W, et al. Vitamin A supplementation for extremely-low-birth-weight infants. *N Engl J Med.* 1999;340:1962-1968.
5. Ambalavanan N, Tyson JE, Kennedy KA, et al. Vitamin A supplementation for extremely low birth weight infants: outcome at 18 to 22 months. *Pediatr.* 2005;115:e249-e254.
6. Shenai JP. Vitamin A supplementation in very low birth weight neonates: rationale and evidence. *Pediatrics.* 1999;104:1369-1374.
7. Gleghorn EE, Eisenberg LD, Hack S, et al. Observations of vitamin A toxicity in three patients with renal failure receiving parenteral alimentation. *Am J Clin Nutr.* 1986;44:107-112.
8. Shenai JP, Mellen BG, Chytil F. Vitamin A status and postnatal dexamethasone treatment in bronchopulmonary dysplasia. *Pediatr.* 2000;106:547-553.

Vitamin K$_1$–Phytonadione

1. Available at: http://www.usp.org/hqi/similarProducts/choosy.html. Accessed July 2, 2009.
2. Phytonadione. Lexi-Comp® Online with AHFS® (database). Hudson, OH: Lexi-Comp Inc; updated August 13, 2009.
3. American Academy of Pediatrics, Committee on Fetus and Newborn Policy Statement. Controversies concerning vitamin K and the newborn. *Pediatrics.* 2003;112;191-192.
4. Lane PA, Hathaway WE. Vitamin K in infancy. *J Pediatr.* 1985;106:351-359.
5. American Academy of Pediatrics, Committee on Nutrition. Vitamin K compounds and water soluble analogues: use in therapy and prophylaxis in pediatrics. *Pediatrics.* 1961;28:501-507.
6. Hathaway WE. The bleeding newborn. *Clin Perinatol.* 1975;2:83-97.
7. Uses and hazards of vitamin K drugs. *Med Lett Drugs Ther.* 1963;5:97-98.
8. Montgomery RR, Hathaway WE. Acute bleeding emergencies. *Pediatr Clin North Am.* 1980;27:327-344.
9. Glader BE, Buchanan GR. The bleeding neonate. *Pediatrics.* 1976;58:548-555.
10. Nammacher MA, Willemin M, Hartmann JR, et al. Vitamin K deficiency in infants beyond the neonatal period. *J Pediatr.* 1970;76:549-554.
11. Walters TR, Koch HF. Hemorrhagic diathesis and cystic fibrosis in infancy. *Am J Dis Child.* 1972;124:641-642.
12. Phytonadione. Lexi-Comp® Online with AHFS® (database). Bethesda, MD: American Society of Health-System Pharmacists; updated.
13. Bolton-Maggs P, Brook L. The use of vitamin K for reversal of over-warfarinization in children. *Br J Haematol.* 2002;118:924-925. Letter.
14. Hanley JP. Warfarin reversal. *J Clin Pathol.* 2004:57;1132-1139.
15. Trissel LA. *Handbook on Injectable Drugs.* 15th ed. Bethesda, MD: American Society of Health-System Pharmacists; 2009.
16. Kumar D, Greer FR, Super DM, et al. Vitamin K status of premature infants: implications for current recommendations. *Pediatrics.* 2001;108:1117-1122.
17. Loughnan PM, McDougall PN, Balvin H, et al. Late onset haemorrhagic disease in premature infants who received intravenous vitamin K1. *J Paediatr Child Health.* 1996;32:268-269.

Voriconazole

1. Available at: http://www.usp.org/hqi/similarProducts/choosy.html. Accessed August 29, 2009.
2. Vfend [package insert]. New York, NY: Pfizer; May 2008.
3. Steinbach WJ, Benjamin DK. New antifungal agents under development in children and neonates. *Curr Opin Infect Dis.* 2005;18:484-489.
4. Fallon RM, Girotto JE. A review of clinical experience with newer antifungals in children. *J Pediatr Pharmacol Ther* .2008;13:124-140.
5. American Academy of Pediatrics. Antifungal drugs for systemic fungal infections. In: Pickering LK, Baker CJ, Kimberlin DW, et al., eds. *2009 Red Book: Report of the Committee on Infectious Diseases.* 28th ed. Elk Grove Village, IL: American Academy of Pediatrics; 2009:765-776.
6. Frankenbusch K, Eifinger F, Kribs A, et al. Severe primary cutaneous aspergillosis refractory to amphotericin B and the successful treatment with systemic voriconazole in two premature infants with extremely low birth weight. *J Perinatol.* 2006;26:511-514.
7. Muldrew KM, Maples HD, Stowe CD, et al. Intravenous voriconazole therapy in a preterm infant. *Pharmacotherapy.* 2005;25:893-898.
8. Maples HD, Stowe CD, Saccente SL, et al. Voriconazole serum concentrations in an infant treated for *Trichosporon beigelii* infection. *Pediatr Infect Dis J.* 2003;22:1022-1024.

References

9. Guzman-Cottrill JA, Zheng X, Chadwick EG. Fusarium solani endocarditis successfully treated with liposomal amphotericin B and voriconazole. *Pediatr Infect Dis J.* 2004;23:1059-1061.
10. Pannaraj PS, Walsh TJ, Baker CJ. Advances in antifungal therapy. *Pediatr Infect Dis J.* 2005;24:921-922.
11. Schwartz S, Ruhnke M, Ribaud P, et al. Improved outcome in central nervous system aspergillosis, using voriconazole treatment. *Blood.* 2005;106:2641-2645.
12. Chakraborty A, Workman MR, Bullock PR. Scedosporium apiospermum brain abscess treated with surgery and voriconazole. *J Neurosurg.* 2005;103:83-87.
13. Walsh TJ, Karlsson MO, et al. Pharmacokinetics and safety of intravenous voriconazole in children after single- or multiple-dose administration. *Antimicrob Agents Chemother.* 2004;48:2166-2172.
14. Walsh TJ, Lutsar I, Driscoll T, et al. Voriconazole in the treatment of aspergillosis, scedosporiosis and other invasive fungal infections in children. *Pediatr Infect Dis J.* 2002;21:240-248.
15. Aronoff GR, Berns JS, Brier ME, et al. Drug prescribing in renal failure. 4th ed. Available at: http://www.kdp-baptist.louisville.edu/renalbook/. Accessed November 9, 2009.
16. Peng LW, Lien YH. Pharmacokinetics of single, oral-dose voriconazole in peritoneal dialysis patients. *Am J Kidney Dis.* 2005;45:162-166.
17. Alffenaar JWC, Doedens RA, Kosterink JGW. High-dose voriconazole in a critically ill pediatric patient with neuroblastoma. *Pediatr Infect Dis J.* 2008;27:189-190.
18. Trissel LA, ed. *Handbook on Injectable Drugs.* 15th ed. Bethesda, MD: American Society of Health-System Pharmacists; 2009.
19. Voriconazole. Lexi-Comp Online with AHFS (database). Hudson, OH: Lexi-Comp Inc; updated October 23, 2009.
20. Bruggemann RJM, Antonius T, Van Heijst A, et al. Therapeutic drug monitoring of voriconazole in a child with invasive aspergillosis requiring extracorporeal membrane oxygenation. *Ther Drug Monit.* 2008;30:643-646.
21. Pasqualotto AC, Shah M, Wynn R, et al. Voriconazole plasma monitoring. *Arch Dis Child.* 2008;93:578-581.
22. Destino L, Sutton DA, Helon AL, et al. Severe osteomyelitis caused by Myceliophthora thermophila after a pitchfork injury. *Ann Clin Microbiol Antimicrob.* 2006;5:21.

Zidovudine

1. Available at: http://www.usp.org/hqi/similarProducts/choosy.html. Accessed August 29, 2009.
2. Available at: http://ismp.org/Tools/confuseddrugnames.pdf. Accessed August 29, 2009.
3. Retrovir [package insert]. Research Triangle Park, NC: GlaxoSmithKline; October 2006.
4. AIDSinfo. Recommendations for use of antiretroviral drugs in pregnant HIV-infected women for maternal health and interventions to reduce perinatal HIV transmission in the United States—April 29, 2009. Available at: http://aidsinfo.nih.gov/ContentFiles/PerinatalGL.pdf. Accessed October 18, 2009.
5. AIDSinfo. Guidelines for the use of antiretroviral agents in pediatric HIV infection—February 23, 2009. Available at: http://aidsinfo.nih.gov/contentfiles/PediatricGL_SupI.pdf. Accessed October 17, 2009.
6. American Academy of Pediatrics. Pickering LK, Baker CJ, Kimberlin DW, et al., eds. *2009 Red Book: Report of the Committee on Infectious Diseases.* 28th ed. Elk Grove Village, IL: American Academy of Pediatrics; 2009.
7. McKinney RE, Pizzo PA, Scott GB, et al. Safety and tolerance of intermittent intravenous and oral zidovudine therapy in human immunodeficiency virus-infected pediatric patients. *J Pediatr.* 1990;116:640-647.
8. Connor EM, Pizzo PA, Balis F, et al. Working Group on Antiretroviral Therapy: National Pediatric HIV Resource Center. Antiretroviral therapy and medical management of the human immunodeficiency virus-infected child. *Pediatr Infect Dis J.* 1993;12:513-522.
9. Mirochnick M, Capparelli E, Connor J. Pharmacokinetics of zidovudine in infants: a population analysis across studies. *Clin Pharmacol Ther.* 1999;66:16-24.
10. Blanche S, Caniglia M, Fischer A, et al. Zidovudine therapy in children with acquired immunodeficiency syndrome. *Am J Med.* 1988;85: 203-207.
11. Mueller BU, Jacobsen F, Butler KM, et al. Combination treatment with azidothymidine and granulocyte colony-stimulating factor in children with human immunodeficiency virus infection. *J Pediatr.* 1992;121:797-802.
12. Balis FM, Pizzo PA, Eddy J, et al. Pharmacokinetics of zidovudine administered intravenously and orally in children with human immunodeficiency virus infection. *J Pediatr.* 1989;114:880-884.
13. Pizzo PA, Eddy J, Falloon J, et al. Effect of continuous intravenous infusion of zidovudine (AZT) in children with symptomatic HIV infection. *N Engl J Med.* 1988;319:889-896.
14. Balis FM, Pizzo PA, Murphy RF, et al. The pharmacokinetics of zidovudine administered by continuous infusion in children. *Ann Intern Med.* 1989;110:279-285.
15. Aronoff GR, Berns JS, Brier ME, et al. Drug prescribing in renal failure. 4th ed. Available at: http://www.kdp-baptist.louisville.edu/renalbook/. Accessed August 17, 2009.
16. Trissel LA, ed. *Handbook on Injectable Drugs.* 15th ed. Bethesda, MD: American Society of Health-System Pharmacists; 2009.
17. Myers SA, Torrente S, Hinthorn D, et al. Life-threatening maternal and fetal macrocytic anemia from antiretroviral therapy. *Obstet Gynecol.* 2005;106:1189-1191.
18. Scalfaro P, Chesaux JJ, Buchwalder PA, et al. Severe transient neonatal lactic acidosis during prophylactic zidovudine treatment. *Intensive Care Med.* 1998;24:247-250.

Zoledronic Acid

1. Available at: http://www.usp.org/hqi/similarProducts/choosy.html. Accessed June 24, 2009.
2. Zometa [prescribing information]. East Hanover, NJ: Novartis Pharmaceuticals; March 2008.
3. Reclast [prescribing information]. East Hanover, NJ: Novartis Pharmaceuticals; May 2009.
4. Hogler W, Yap F, Little D, et al. Short-term safety assessment in the use of intravenous zoledronic acid in children. *J Pediatr.* 2004;145: 701-704.
5. Munns CF, Rajab MH, Hong J, et al. Acute phase response and mineral status following low dose intravenous zoledronic acid in children. *Bone.* 2007;41:366-370.
6. Brown JJ, Zacharin MR. Safety and efficacy of intravenous zolendronic acid in paediatric osteoporosis. *J Pediatr Endocrinol Metabol.* 2009;22:55-63.
7. Malmgren B, Astrom E, Soderhall S. No osteonecrosis in jaws of young patients with osteogenesis imperfecta treated with bisphosphonates. *J Oral Pathol Med.* 2008;37:196-200.

Index of Brand and Generic Drug Names

Index of Brand and Generic Drug Names